Essential Periodontics

T0342170

Dentistry Essentials series

The *Dentistry Essentials* are an international series of textbooks, designed to support lecture series or themes on core topics within dentistry.

Essential Physiology for Dental Students
by Kamran Ali, Elizabeth Prabhakar
February 2019

Essentials of Human Disease in Dentistry, 2nd Edition
by Mark Greenwood
April 2018

Essential Dental Therapeutics
by David Wray
September 2017

Essential Orthodontics
by Birgit Thilander, Krister Bjerklin, Lars Bondemark
July 2017

Essential Clinical Oral Biology
by Stephen Creanor
April 2016

Essential Periodontics

Edited by

Steph Smith, BChD, BChD (Hons), MDent, MChD
Department of Preventive Dental Sciences
Division of Periodontology
College of Dentistry, Imam Abdulrahman Bin Faisal University
Dammam, Kingdom of Saudi Arabia

Khalid Almas, BDS (Pak), MSc (Lond), FDSRCS (Edin),
FRACDS (Syd), MSc (Lond), DDPHRCS (Eng), FICD, FAAOM
Department of Preventive Dental Sciences
Division of Periodontology
College of Dentistry, Imam Abdulrahman Bin Faisal University
Dammam, Kingdom of Saudi Arabia

WILEY Blackwell

This edition first published 2022
© 2022 John Wiley & Sons Ltd

All rights reserved. No part of this publication may be reproduced, stored in a retrieval system, or transmitted, in any form or by any means, electronic, mechanical, photocopying, recording or otherwise, except as permitted by law. Advice on how to obtain permission to reuse material from this title is available at http://www.wiley.com/go/permissions.

The right of Steph Smith and Khalid Almas to be identified as the authors of the editorial material in this work has been asserted in accordance with law.

Registered Offices
John Wiley & Sons, Inc., 111 River Street, Hoboken, NJ 07030, USA
John Wiley & Sons Ltd, The Atrium, Southern Gate, Chichester, West Sussex, PO19 8SQ, UK

Editorial Office
9600 Garsington Road, Oxford, OX4 2DQ, UK

For details of our global editorial offices, customer services, and more information about Wiley products visit us at www.wiley.com.

Wiley also publishes its books in a variety of electronic formats and by print-on-demand. Some content that appears in standard print versions of this book may not be available in other formats.

Limit of Liability/Disclaimer of Warranty

The contents of this work are intended to further general scientific research, understanding, and discussion only and are not intended and should not be relied upon as recommending or promoting scientific method, diagnosis, or treatment by physicians for any particular patient. In view of ongoing research, equipment modifications, changes in governmental regulations, and the constant flow of information relating to the use of medicines, equipment, and devices, the reader is urged to review and evaluate the information provided in the package insert or instructions for each medicine, equipment, or device for, among other things, any changes in the instructions or indication of usage and for added warnings and precautions. While the publisher and authors have used their best efforts in preparing this work, they make no representations or warranties with respect to the accuracy or completeness of the contents of this work and specifically disclaim all warranties, including without limitation any implied warranties of merchantability or fitness for a particular purpose. No warranty may be created or extended by sales representatives, written sales materials or promotional statements for this work. The fact that an organization, website, or product is referred to in this work as a citation and/or potential source of further information does not mean that the publisher and authors endorse the information or services the organization, website, or product may provide or recommendations it may make. This work is sold with the understanding that the publisher is not engaged in rendering professional services. The advice and strategies contained herein may not be suitable for your situation. You should consult with a specialist where appropriate. Further, readers should be aware that websites listed in this work may have changed or disappeared between when this work was written and when it is read. Neither the publisher nor authors shall be liable for any loss of profit or any other commercial damages, including but not limited to special, incidental, consequential, or other damages.

Library of Congress Cataloging-in-Publication Data applied for:

ISBN 9781119619628 (paperback)

Cover Design: Wiley
Cover Image: © xsense/Shutterstock

Set in 10/12pt Adobe Garamond by Straive, Pondicherry, India
Printed and bound by CPI Group (UK) Ltd, Croydon, CR0 4YY

C100964_170322

Steph Smith

This book is dedicated to my wife, Sandra, and my children, Raymond and Lauren, for their love and inspiration, and their unconditional support that has made this book possible.

Khalid Almas

I dedicate this book to my parents, H. Mairaj Uddin Mughal and Hameeda Begum, for their immeasurable love, dedication, and perseverance to raise the family throughout the thick and thin of their lifetime and to inculcate the virtues of honesty, passion for knowledge, and steadfastness. I am thankful to my wife Pakeeza, daughters Arooba and Areej, and son Muhammad Nabeel for their unconditional support and profound love. Without their unwavering perseverance, this book would have not been possible.

Contents

About the editors

Steph Smith, BChD, BChD (Hons), MDent, MChD

Is Senior Lecturer of Periodontology at Imam Abdulrahman Bin Faisal University, College of Dentistry, Preventive Dental Sciences Department, Dammam, Saudi Arabia, and a volunteer/visiting Professor of Periodontology at Rawal Institute of Health Sciences, Rawal College of Dentistry, Islamabad, Pakistan. He has been Director of Clinical Affairs of the College of Dentistry at Imam Abdulrahman Bin Faisal University. He has taught Periodontics for many years and has been Course Director of undergraduate Periodontics on numerous occasions, including participating in postgraduate Periodontics courses.

Khalid Almas, BDS (Pak), MSc (Lond), FDSRCS (Edin), FRACDS (Syd), MSc (Lond), DDPHRCS (Eng), FICD, FAAOM

Is Professor of Periodontology and is a founder and former Program Director of Postgraduate Periodontics at Imam Abdulrahman Bin Faisal University, College of Dentistry, Preventive Dental Sciences Department, Dammam, Saudi Arabia. Formerly, Dr. Almas has served at University of Connecticut School of Dental Medicine as clinical Professor, Director of the predoctoral Periodontics program and Director International Fellowship in Advanced Periodontics. He has served as a faculty member at New York University, College of Dentistry, New York, USA, and King Saud University College of Dentistry, Riyadh, Saudi Arabia, and as Head of Department of Periodontology and Oral Medicine at de Montmorency College of Dentistry, Punjab Dental Hospital, University of Punjab, Lahore, Pakistan. He also maintains his volunteer/visiting Professor position at University of Connecticut, USA, and at the Rawal Institute of Health Sciences, Rawal College of Dentistry, Islamabad, Pakistan. He has also been named as one of the world's top 2% of Scientists in a global ranking list released by Stanford University, USA (2020 and 2021).

List of contributors

Tara Taiyeb Ali, FDSRCS (Edin), FAMM, MSc (Lond), BDS (UM)
Professor
Department of Periodontology
MAHSA University
Selangor, Malaysia

Khalid Almas, BDS (Pak), MSc (Lon), FRACDS (Syd), MSc (Tmu), FDSRCS (Edin), DDPHRCS (Eng), FAAOM (USA), FICD
Professor
Preventive Dental Sciences Department
Division of Periodontology
Imam Abdulrahman Bin Faisal University
College of Dentistry
Dammam, Saudi Arabia

Nehal Almehmadi, BDS
Research Assistant
College of Dentistry
Department of Oral Health Practice
Division of Periodontics
University of Kentucky
Lexington, KY, USA

Mohanad Al-Sabbagh, DDS, MS
Professor
College of Dentistry
Department of Oral Health Practice
Division of Periodontics
University of Kentucky
Lexington, KY, USA

Haider Al-Waeli, BDS, MSc, PhD
Resident
Faculty of Dentistry, University of Toronto &
Princess Margaret Cancer Centre
Department of Dental Oncology and Maxillofacial Prosthetics
Toronto, Ontario, Canada

Michel V. Furtado Araujo, DDS, MSc, MDS
Private Practice
Melbourne, FL, USA

Pierluigi Balice, DDS, MDSc
Clinical Assistant Professor
Department of Periodontics
UMKC School of Dentistry
Kansas City, MO, USA

Subraya Bhat, MDS, MFGDP (UK), FICOI (USA), Fellow of FAIMER
Associate Professor
Preventive Dental Sciences Department
Division of Periodontology
Imam Abdulrahman Bin Faisal University
College of Dentistry
Dammam, Saudi Arabia

Avinash S. Bidra, BDS, MS, FACP
Clinical Professor
Department of Reconstructive Sciences
University of Connecticut
School of Dental Medicine
UCONN Health
Farmington, CT, USA

Brittany Camenisch, DMD, MS
Adjunct Assistant Professor
College of Dentistry
Department of Oral Health Practice
Division of Periodontics
University of Kentucky
Lexington, KY, USA

Aditi Chopra, BDS, MDS
Assistant Professor
Department of Periodontology
Manipal College of Dental Sciences
Manipal, India

Ajay K. Dhingra, BDS, MDS, MSD
Assistant Professor
Department of Reconstructive Sciences
UConn School of Dental Medicine
Farmington, CT, USA

David G. Gillam, BA, BDS, MSc, DDS, FRSPH, MICR
Clinical Reader
Oral Bioengineering
Institute of Dentistry
Barts and the London School of Medicine and Dentistry
London, UK

Michael Glogauer, DDS, Dip Perio, PhD
Professor
Faculty of Dentistry, University of Toronto &
Princess Margaret Cancer Centre
Department of Dental Oncology and Maxillofacial Prosthetics
Toronto, Ontario, Canada

Anders Gustafsson, DDS, PhD
Professor and Vice President
Karolinska Institutet
Stockholm, Sweden

Nader Hamdan, BDS, MSc, MDent (Perio), FRCD(C), Diplomate ABP, FDS RCPS (Glasg)
Assistant Professor
Department of Dental Clinical Sciences
Faculty of Dentistry
Dalhousie University
Halifax, Nova Scotia, Canada

Fawad Javed, BDS, PhD
Assistant Professor
Department of Orthodontics and Dentofacial Orthopedics
Eastman Institute for Oral Health
University of Rochester, NY, USA

Feras Al Khatib, DMD, MS
Clinical Assistant Professor
Department of Growth, Development and Structure
Section of Orthodontics
Southern Illinois University School of Dental Medicine
Alton, IL, USA

Adriane Kilar, DMD
General Dentist
Massachusetts Institute of Technology
Cambridge, MA, USA

Ahmad Kutkut, DDS, MS, FICOI, DICOI
Associate Professor
College of Dentistry
Department of Oral Health Practice
Division of Prosthodontics & Restorative Dentistry
University of Kentucky
Lexington, KY, USA

Diana Macri, RDH, BSDH, MSEd
Associate Professor
Hostos Community College.
New York, NY, USA

Farheen Malek, BDS, MDS
Resident
Louisiana State University Health Sciences Center (LSUHSC)
School of Dentistry
New Orleans, LA, USA

Pratishtha Mishra, BDS, MDS, MS
Assistant Professor
College of Dentistry
Department of Oral Health Practice
Division of Periodontics and
Division of Oral Medicine, Oral Diagnosis, and Oral Radiology
University of Kentucky
Lexington, KY, USA

Ola Norderyd, LDS, Odont Dr
Professor and Senior Consultant in Periodontology
Centre for Oral Health
School of Health and Welfare
Jönköping University
Jönköping, Sweden

Karo Parsegian, DDS, PhD
Assistant Professor
School of Dentistry
Department of Periodontics and Dental Hygiene
University of Texas Health Science Center
Houston, TX, USA

Salim Rayman, RDH, BS, MPA
Professor
Hostos Community College
New York, NY, USA

Arif Salman, BDS, MDSc
Assistant Professor
West Virginia University School of Dentistry
Morgantown, WV, USA

Stuart L. Segelnick, DDS, MS, DICOI
Adjunct Associate Professor
University of Pennsylvania School of Dental Medicine
Adjunct Clinical Professor
New York University College of Dentistry, New York, NY, USA
Private Practice, Brooklyn, NY, USA

Zeeshan Sheikh, Dip Dh, BDS, MSc, PhD
Resident
Department of Dental Clinical Sciences
Faculty of Dentistry, Dalhousie University
Halifax, Nova Scotia, Canada

Yasir Dilshad Siddiqui, BDS, MSc, PhD
Postdoctoral Fellow
Department of Neural & Pain Sciences
School of Dentistry
University of Maryland
Baltimore, MD, USA

Mabi Singh, DMD MS
Associate Professor
Department of Diagnostic Sciences
Division Oral Medicine
Tufts School of Dental Medicine
Boston, MA, USA

Steph Smith, BChD, BChD (Hons), MDent, MChD
Senior Lecturer
Preventive Dental Sciences Department
Division of Periodontology
Imam Abdulrahman Bin Faisal University
College of Dentistry
Dammam, Saudi Arabia

Aditya Tadinada, BDS, MDSc
Associate Professor
Associate Dean for Graduate Research, Education and Training
University of Connecticut School of Dental Medicine
Farmington, CT, USA

Sejal R. Thacker, DDS, MDSc
Assistant Professor
School of Dental Medicine
Oral Health and Diagnostic Sciences, UConn Health
Division of Periodontology
University of Connecticut
Farmington, CT, USA

Murugan Thamaraiselvan, BDS, MDS
Associate Professor
Department of Periodontics
Saveetha Dental College and Hospital
Chennai, India

Achint Utreja, BDS, MS, PhD
Associate Professor
Department of Growth, Development and Structure
Southern Illinois University School of Dental Medicine
Alton, IL, USA

Mea A. Weinberg, DMD, MSD, RPh
Clinical Professor
Ashman Department of Periodontology and Implant Dentistry
New York University College of Dentistry
New York, NY, USA

Qiang Zhu, DDS, PhD
Professor
Division of Endodontology
University of Connecticut School of Dental Medicine
Farmington, CT, USA

Foreword

I am proud to write the Foreword to *Essential Periodontics*. Our knowledge about the periodontium and its diseases is continuously increasing. Advanced research in genomics, proteomics, and metabolomics is also being applied in the field of Periodontology, giving us a new understanding of the pathogenesis of periodontitis. High-throughput sequencing techniques have led to a new view on the oral microflora. The number of newly identified microbial species in the oral cavity is increasing on a yearly basis.

Periodontology is a very active research field. More than 2000 new articles in the field of Periodontology are added to PubMed each year. Over 15 000 articles have been published since the beginning of 2015. This new textbook incorporates as many new insights and future trends as possible and the new classification system, introduced in 2018, is used throughout the book.

Essential Periodontics is aimed at undergraduate students, general dentists as well as periodontists, but I am sure that this comprehensive book will provide valuable new knowledge to all categories of dental professionals, including dental hygienists and specialists in the fields of Prosthodontics and Orthodontics.

The authors have had very high ambitions for this book and in my view they have succeeded in creating a valuable new textbook that I can recommend to all dental colleagues.

Professor Dr. Anders Gustafsson
Vice President
Karolinska Institutet
Aula Medica
Stockholm, Sweden

Preface

The pursuit of knowledge paves the way for the acquisition of both intellectual and material wealth. Knowledge is considered one of the most valuable traits a person can acquire. Proper scientific method in the pursuit of scientific knowledge can include uncertainty even when correct, whereby such endeavours will lead to greater confluence of scientific truth. Over many centuries, the scientific study of the periodontium in health and disease has been pursued, and so knowledge has been attained of how to treat, manage, control, and prevent periodontal diseases. In addition, and imperative to this acquisition, is our patients' knowledge of their oral health, which includes their interpretation and perceptions of the information they have received, and this will inevitably lead to whether they seek care as a result of such knowledge.

In light of this, it has been the ambition of the authors to compile a curriculum-based periodontics textbook that is specifically aimed at the undergraduate dental student, but which can also be a valuable contribution to other dental specialties, including oral implantology, prosthodontics, restorative dentistry, orthodontics, as well as oral hygiene. General dental practitioners will also be able to obtain scientific and methodical solutions to their clinical cases in periodontics.

This textbook comprises evidence-based research and is also based on the 2018 Classification of Periodontal and Peri-Implant Diseases and Conditions. Specific chapters have been dedicated to this new classification. Also included are chapters on oral implantology, which include the restorative/prosthodontic aspects of implant treatment. These chapters provide a sound and scientific basis for students to familiarize themselves with the newest developments in this exciting field of periodontology.

It is envisaged that this textbook will be a source of inspiration for students in their acquisition of knowledge in the field of periodontics, to improve their clinical skills, as well as to be a valuable source of information regarding the education and care of their patients.

We are thankful to all chapter authors and contributors, who made this evidence-based book possible for the common good of the dental profession. A special thanks to Wiley-Blackwell staff in Asia, Europe, and the USA for their highly professional demeanour, continuous support, understanding, and patience. We also have a debt of gratitude for the facilities at Imam Abdulrahman Bin Faisal University: the superb, modern digital library and the extremely helpful staff, especially Mr. Muhammad Ajmal Khan, for his help in classic literature collection and updated articles. We also thank Dr. Muhammad Abbas Alhammali for his professional and dedicated contribution to the clinical pictures of periodontal instrumentation. Ms. Michelle Eve Bajon is thanked for her willingness to partake in the instrumentation pictures. The authors are also grateful to all those patients who offered their willingness to include their clinical pictures.

Last but not least, a special word of thanks to our past and present students, who made us think differently.

"Wherever the art of medicine is loved, there is also a love of humanity".

Steph Smith
Khalid Almas

CHAPTER 1

Introduction to periodontology/ periodontics

Khalid Almas and Steph Smith

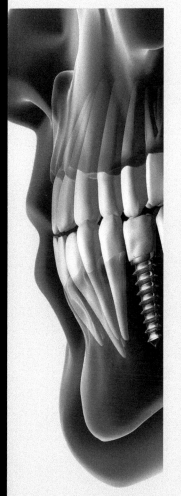

Periodontology has been defined as "the scientific study of the periodontium in health and disease." Periodontology or periodontics is the specialty of dentistry that studies the supporting structures of teeth, as well as diseases and conditions that affect them. The supporting tissues are known as the periodontium (*peri* = around, *odontos* = tooth), which includes the gingiva, alveolar bone, cementum, and the periodontal ligament.

Periodontal diseases, unlike caries, are not a byproduct of modern civilization. The diseases of the periodontium are as old as the recorded history of humankind. Studies in paleopathology indicate that destructive periodontal disease, including the awareness thereof, has accompanied early human beings in diverse cultures. A Sumerian text from 5000 BC describes that Sumerians were apparently suffering from periodontal disease. They practiced oral hygiene, including gingival massage in combination with various herbal medications. Hesy-Re (2686–2613 BC) was an Egyptian scribe who is often called the first "dentist," and is also credited as being the first man to recognize periodontal disease. Among the ancient Greeks, Hippocrates of Cos (460–377 BC), the father of modern medicine, discussed the function and eruption of the teeth and the etiology of periodontal disease. He believed that inflammation of the gums could be caused by accumulations of "pituita" or calculus, with gingival hemorrhage occurring in cases of persistent splenic maladies. Abu al-Qasim, also known as Albucasis (936–1013 AD), was a Spanish-Arabian physician. He had a clear understanding of the major etiological role of calculus deposits, and he described the techniques of scaling the teeth with the use of a set of instruments that he developed, splinting loose teeth with gold wire, and filing gross occlusal abnormalities. He invented and proposed the use of many elevators and scalers. Ambroise Paré (1509–1590), a Frenchman, was the outstanding surgeon of the Renaissance, and his contributions to dental surgery included gingivectomy for hyperplastic gingival tissues. Anton van Leeuwenhoek (1632–1723) of Delft, Holland, first described oral bacterial flora, and his drawings offered a reasonably good presentation of oral spirochetes and bacilli.

Modern dental practice essentially developed in eighteenth-century Europe, particularly in England and France. During the eighteenth century treatises were published, scientific lectures were given, the first surgeons were trained specifically in dentistry, nonsense remedies were rejected, and many inventions were patented. The nineteenth century is described as a time of advanced science and education, and by the dawn of the twentieth century, the realization that alveolar pyorrhea can be treated led to the recognition of periodontia as a dental specialty. The early twentieth century witnessed the dawn of modern periodontics, with major changes in the diagnosis, etiopathogenesis, classifications, and treatment modalities of periodontal diseases. Various periodontal surgical procedures and resective and regenerative approaches were born.

Essential Periodontics, First Edition. Edited by Steph Smith and Khalid Almas.
© 2022 John Wiley & Sons Ltd. Published 2022 by John Wiley & Sons Ltd.

However, the much-needed information exchange was impeded by inconsistent terminology. Over subsequent decades, periodontists on both sides of the Atlantic met repeatedly to develop countless classification systems that reflected scientific progress as well as clinical utility. As a result of this effort, new nomenclatures were published at arbitrary intervals by professional bodies such as the American Academy of Periodontology (AAP, established in 1914), the American Dental Association, the Arbeitsgemeinschaft für Paradentosen Forschung, and the World Dental Federation, among others. In addition individual authors also contributed various classifications.

Presently, apart from various regional and national periodontal societies, the AAP and the European Periodontal Federation are two major players representing the discipline of periodontics at an international level. Innovations, nomenclature, advances in the perio-systemic link, and periodontal medicine are progressing with evidence-based science. Also, in 2018 the new *Classification of Periodontal and Peri-Implant Diseases and Conditions* was published,

It is envisaged that one of the most ancient afflictions to humankind will be conquered one day to improve the quality of life of our patients.

FURTHER READING

American Academy of Periodontology (AAP). *Glossary of Periodontal Terms*, 4th edn. Chicago, IL: AAP; 2001.

Brkić Z, Pavlić V. Periodontology: the historical outline from ancient times until the 20th century. *Vojnosanit Pregl.* 2017; 74(2):193–199.

Dentino A, Lee S, Mailhot J, Hefti AF. Principles of periodontology. *Periodontol 2000.* 2013; 61(1):16–53.

El-Gammal SY. The role of Hippocrates in the development and progress of medical sciences. *Bull Indian Inst Hist Med Hyderabad.* 1993; 23(2):125–136.

Gold SI. Periodontics: the past. Part I. Early sources. *J Clin Periodontol.* 1985; 12:79–97.

Gurudath G, Vijayakumar KV, Arun R. Oral hygiene practices. Ancient historical review. *J Orofac Res.* 2012; 2(4):225–227.

Gurunluoglu R, Gurunluoglu A. Paul of Aegina: landmark in surgical progress. *World J Surg.* 2003; 27(1):18–25.

Herschfeld JJ. Dentistry in the writings of Albucasis during the golden age of Arabian medicine. *Bull Hist Dent.* 1987; 35(2):110–114.

Hujoel P, Zina LG, Cunha-Cruz J, Lopez R. Historical perspectives on theories of periodontal disease etiology. *Periodontol 2000.* 2012; 58(1):153–160.

Loukas M, Lanteri A, Ferrauiola J et al. Anatomy in ancient India: a focus on the Susruta Samhita. *J Anat.* 2010; 217(6):646–650.

Mitsis FJ, Taramidis G. Alveolar bone loss on neolithic man remains on 38 skulls of Khirokitia's (Cyprus) inhabitants. *J Clin Periodontol.* 1995; 22(10):788–793.

Shklar G. Stomatology and dentistry in the golden age of Arabian medicine. *Bull Hist Dent.* 1969; 17:17–24.

Yilmaz S, Efeoğlu E, Noyan U, Kuru B, Kiliç AR, Kuru L. The evolution of clinical periodontal therapy. *J Marmara Univ Dent Fac.* 1994; 2(1):414–423.

Ziskind B, Halioua B. Occupational medicine in ancient Egypt. *Med Hypotheses.* 2007; 69(4):942–945.

CHAPTER 2

Anatomy and histology of the periodontium

Aditi Chopra and Steph Smith

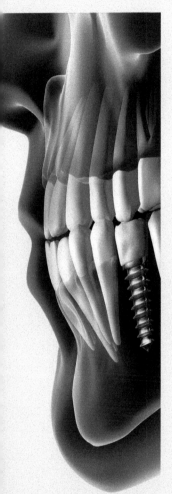

Contents

Learning objectives

- Macroscopic anatomy of the periodontium.
- Histology of the anatomic structures of the periodontium.
- Understanding of gingival and periodontal phenotypes.
- Dimensions and histology of the dento-gingival complex.
- Blood supply, lymphatic drainage, and nerve supply of the periodontium.

Essential Periodontics, First Edition. Edited by Steph Smith and Khalid Almas.
© 2022 John Wiley & Sons Ltd. Published 2022 by John Wiley & Sons Ltd.

Introduction

The oral cavity consists of two types of tissues: hard tissues, comprising 32 teeth and alveolar bone, and soft tissue, comprising the oral mucosa. The oral mucosa consists of three zones: *masticatory mucosa*, which includes the gingiva and the soft tissue covering of the hard palate; *specialized mucosa*, which covers the dorsum of the tongue; and the *oral mucous membrane*, lining the remainder of the oral cavity.

The root of each tooth is embedded into a socket of the alveolar process of the mandible and maxilla, called a gomphosis, also known as a dentoalveolar syndesmosis. It is a joint that binds the teeth to the sockets, and the fibrous connection between a tooth and its socket is a periodontal ligament. The tooth is furthermore supported in its position by the help of the tissues surrounding the tooth, i.e. the periodontium. The periodontium anchors the teeth in position and provides interdental linkage of the teeth within the dental arch. The periodontium, also called "the attachment apparatus" or "the supporting tissues of the teeth," undergoes certain changes with age and is also subjected to morphological changes related to functional alterations and alterations in the oral environment (Newman et al. 2019). The developmental, biological, and functional unit of the periodontium consists of four types of tissues: gingiva, root cementum, alveolar bone proper, and the periodontal ligament (Ainamo & Löe 1966; Cho & Garant 2000; Cleaton-Jones et al. 1978; Lindhe & Lang 2015; Listgarten 1964; Melcher & Bowen 1969; Newman et al. 2019; Ten Cate 1975, 1994) (Figure 2.1).

Gingiva

The gingiva is that part of the masticatory mucosa that covers the alveolar process of the jaw and surrounds the neck of the tooth (Ainamo & Löe 1966). Macroscopically, the gingiva is divided into three parts: interdental gingiva (Table 2.1), marginal (free) gingiva (Table 2.2), and attached gingiva (Table 2.3) (Ainamo & Löe 1966; Cho & Garant 2000; Cleaton-Jones et al. 1978; Lindhe & Lang 2015; Newman et al. 2019). The clinical characteristics of the gingiva are depicted in Table 2.4.

Gingival/periodontal phenotype

The gingival phenotype is determined by gingival thickness and the keratinized tissue width. The periodontal phenotype is determined by the gingival phenotype and the bone morphotype, i.e. the thickness of the buccal bone plate (Jepsen et al. 2018). Determination of the periodontal phenotype is necessitated for assessing therapy outcomes in periodontal and implant therapy, prosthodontics, and orthodontics. Three categories of periodontal phenotypes have been classified, i.e. thin scalloped, thick flat, and thick scalloped (Chambrone & Tatakis 2016; Cortellini & Bisada 2018; Kan et al. 2010; Zweers et al. 2014). For the diagnoses and factors determining the gingival/periodontal phenotypes, see Chapter 10.3.

Histology of the gingiva

Histologically, the gingiva is comprised of two parts: the gingival epithelium and the underlying connective tissue (Ainamo & Löe 1966; Cho & Garant 2000; Cleaton-Jones et al. 1978; Listgarten 1964).

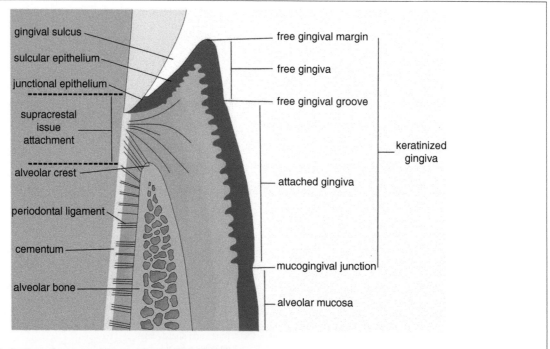

Figure 2.1 The periodontium. Courtsey of Dr. Abdulqader Alhammadi.

Table 2.1 The interdental gingiva.

- Also known as the papillary gingiva, it is a pyramidal-shaped tissue found between the two teeth, filling the space in the gingival embrasure below the contact point of adjacent teeth.
- In anterior regions of the dentition, the interdental papilla has a pyramidal form, while in molar regions, the papillae are flatter in the buccolingual direction (Newman et al. 2019).
- The shape of the interdental gingiva is determined by the contact relationships between the teeth; the width of the approximal tooth surfaces; the course of the cementoenamel junction; the distance between the contact point and the osseous crest; and the presence or absence of some degree of recession (Lindhe & Lang 2015).
- The facial and lingual surfaces are tapered toward the interproximal contact area, whereas the mesial and distal surfaces are slightly concave. The lateral borders and tips of the interdental papillae are formed by the marginal gingiva of the adjoining teeth. The intervening portion consists of attached gingiva.
- If a diastema is present, the gingiva is firmly bound over the interdental bone to form a smooth, rounded surface without interdental papillae (Lindhe & Lang 2015).
- The papillary gingiva between the buccal and lingual side is connected to form a valley of tissue, called the "col." In the premolar/molar regions of the dentition, the teeth have approximal contact surfaces rather than contact points. Thus, the interdental papillae in these areas often have one vestibular and one lingual/palatal portion separated by the col region.
- The col region is covered by a thin non-keratinized epithelium. This epithelium has many features in common with the junctional epithelium (Newman et al. 2019).

Table 2.2 The marginal gingiva.

- Also known as the free gingiva or unattached gingiva, as its inner surface is not attached to the tooth or periosteum of the alveolar bone (Ainamo & Löe 1966; Cleaton-Jones et al. 1978; Listgarten 1964; Melcher & Bowen 1969).
- In the coronal direction, the coral pink gingiva terminates in the free gingival margin, which has a scalloped outline (Newman et al. 2019).
- The gap between the marginal gingiva and tooth structure is known as the gingival sulcus. The depth of the sulcus can be examined using a periodontal probe, by estimating the distance the probe penetrates. The depth of the gingival sulcus corresponds to the free gingival groove on the outer surface of the gingival epithelium.
- The free gingival groove is positioned at a level corresponding to the level of the cementoenamel junction. The free gingival groove is not always clinically visible, and may only be present in about 30–40% of adults (Newman et al. 2019).
- The free gingival groove appears most frequently in the vestibular incisor and premolar regions of the mandible, and least frequently in the mandibular molar and maxillary premolar regions (Newman et al. 2019).
- Histologically, the free gingival groove represents a point between the free gingiva and the attached gingiva. Under ideal conditions, the depth of the gingival sulcus is 0 mm or close to 0 mm (Ainamo & Löe 1966). However, as determined in histological sections, the depth of the gingival sulcus in humans is approximately 1.8–3 mm (Cleaton-Jones et al. 1978; Listgarten 1964; Melcher & Bowen 1969; Ten Cate 1975, 1994).

Table 2.3 The attached gingiva.

- It is that portion of the masticatory mucosa that is firmly attached to the underlying alveolar bone (periosteum) and cementum by connective tissue fibers, thus being comparatively immobile in relation to the underlying tissue (Newman et al. 2019; Ten Cate 1994).
- It extends from the free gingival groove to the mucogingival junction. The mucogingival junction is an imaginary line that separates the alveolar mucosa and the attached gingiva, and can be visually identified by the distinct color change between the alveolar mucosa and attached gingiva.
- The alveolar mucosa is red, smooth, and shiny due to the presence of increased vascularity and a thinner non-keratinized epithelium, and contains no rete pegs.
- The color of the attached and marginal gingiva is generally described as "coral pink," being produced by the vascular supply, the thickness and degree of keratinization, and the presence of pigment-containing cells (Newman et al. 2019).
- The width of the attached gingiva on the buccal aspect can vary in size: the maximum in the anterior maxillary region being 3.5–4.5 mm; the mandibular anterior region 3.3–3.9 mm; the maxillary premolars 1.9 mm; and the mandibular premolars 1.8 mm (Ainamo 1978; Ainamo & Ainamo 1978; Bowers 1963). The width of the attached gingiva increases with age and in supra-erupted teeth (Ainamo 1978).
- On the lingual aspect of the mandible, the attached gingiva terminates at the junction of the lingual alveolar mucosa, which is continuous with the mucous membrane lining the floor of the mouth. The palatal surface of the attached gingiva in the maxilla blends with the firm and resilient palatal mucosa.
- The attached gingiva has numerous functions, including maintaining the integrity of and supporting the marginal gingiva; protecting the underlying anatomic and neurovascular structures; withstanding functional stress; resistance to tensional stresses; dissipating the pull on the marginal gingiva created by the movement of muscles of the adjacent alveolar mucosa; and helping to prevent soft tissue recession and attachment loss (Ten Cate 1994).

Table 2.4   Clinical characteristics of the gingiva.

Color	• The color of the gingiva is generally described as "coral pink" or pink with a varying degree of melanin pigmentation. The color of the gingiva is determined by its vascularity, thickness, and degree of keratinization of the epithelium, and the presence of pigment-containing cells.
	• Melanin is the most commonly found pigment in the gingival tissue. It is normally present in all individuals, but often not in sufficient quantities to be detected clinically.
	• The distribution of oral pigmentation can vary as follows: gingiva, 60%; hard palate, 61%; mucous membrane, 22%; and tongue, 15% (Ainamo & Löe 1966; Dummett & Barens 1971; Newman et al. 2019).
Contour	• The normal gingiva is scalloped with a knife edge. The contour of the gingiva depends upon the morphology of the underlying alveolar bone, oral hygiene practices, injury to the gingival tissues, and type of prosthesis.
	• Other factors that determine the contour of the gingiva include the shape of the teeth and their alignment in the arch; the location and size of the interproximal contact area; and the dimensions of the facial and lingual gingival embrasures.
	• The knife-edge papilla can become blunt or flat when there is loss of the interdental bone. The scalloping may become exaggerated when the gingival margins shift apically (gingival recession).
	• The marginal gingiva can appear as a straight line along teeth that have relatively flat surfaces.
	• On teeth with pronounced mesiodistal convexity (e.g. maxillary canines) or teeth in labial version, the normal arcuate contour is accentuated, and the gingiva is located farther apically.
	• On teeth in lingual version, the gingiva is horizontal and thickened. Additionally, a thickened shelf-like contour of the gingiva may be seen on a tooth in lingual version aggravated by local irritation caused by plaque accumulation (Ainamo & Löe 1966; Newman et al. 2019; Ten Cate 1994).
Size	• The bulk of cellular and intercellular elements of the gingival tissues along with the vascular supply determine the size of the gingiva.
	• The normal gingiva should adapt to the tooth without any bulge or enlargement. Any increase in the size of the gingiva may indicate the presence of a pathological condition (Newman et al. 2019).
Consistency	• The consistency of normal gingiva is related to the presence and/or absence of gingival fibers and ground substance. The normal gingiva is firm and resilient.
	• The onset of inflammation in the gingival tissues destroys the gingival fibers and extracellular matrix of the gingival tissues. The inflamed gingival tissue loses its resiliency and becomes soft and edematous (Newman et al. 2019).
Surface texture	• The gingival surface, when dried with gauze, can give the appearance of an "orange peel." The orange peel-like appearance is due to the presence of stippling (Dummett & Barens 1971; Newman et al. 2019).
	• Stippling is a form of adaptive specialization or reinforcement for function.
	• Stippling is a characteristic feature of the attached gingiva and central portion of the interdental papillae. The marginal gingiva and marginal borders of the interdental papilla are not stippled (Dummett & Barens 1971; Greene 1962; Rosenberg & Massler 1967).
	• Stippling varies with age. It is absent in infancy, appears in some children at about 5 years of age, increases until adulthood, and frequently begins to disappear in old age. Absence of stippling indicates the presence of gingival inflammation (Bimstein et al. 2003).
	• It is a feature of healthy gingiva, and reduction or loss of stippling is a common sign of gingival disease. When the gingiva is restored to health after treatment, the stippled appearance returns.
	• Microscopically, stippling is formed by the alternate rounded protuberances formed by the connective tissue projecting into the overlying epithelium, or the epithelium dips into the underlying connective tissue by forming rete pegs.
	• The subsurface of the epithelium is characterized by the presence of epithelial ridges that merge at various locations. The depressions seen on the outer surface of the epithelium correspond to these fusion sites between the epithelial ridges (Newman et al. 2019).
Position	• The position of the gingiva refers to the level at which the gingival margin is located in relation to the cementoenamel junction (CEJ).
	• This may be influenced by the position of the tooth; the phase of eruption; habits of the individual; and the nature of a prosthesis on the tooth.
	• With the CEJ taken as reference point, the position of the gingival margin can be either coronal to the CEJ, at the CEJ, or apical to the CEJ (in the case of gingival recession) (Newman et al. 2019).

Gingival epithelium

The gingival epithelium is divided into three parts: outer gingival epithelium, inner gingival epithelium (sulcular epithelium), and junctional epithelium. The outer epithelium starts at the gingival margin and extends to the mucogingival junction. The sulcular epithelium forms the inner lining of the gingival sulcus. The junctional epithelium is that part of the gingiva that is attached to the tooth surface and extends from the base of the gingival sulcus apically until the cementoenamel junction (CEJ) (Listgarten 1964). The gingival epithelium is separated from the underlying connective tissue by a basement membrane that is thrown into numerous folds, known as rete pegs (Ainamo & Löe 1966; Bartold & Narayanan 1998; Bartold et al. 2000; Cho & Garant 2000; Cleaton-Jones et al. 1978; Lindhe & Lang 2015; Listgarten 1964; Melcher & Bowen 1969; Newman et al. 2019; Schroeder 1997; Stern 1965; Ten Cate 1975, 1994). The connective tissue portions that project into the epithelium are called connective tissue papillae and are separated from each other by epithelial ridges: the so-called rete pegs. In normal, non-inflamed gingiva, rete pegs and connective tissue papillae are a characteristic morphological feature of the oral epithelium and the oral sulcular epithelium, but are however lacking in the junctional epithelium (Newman et al. 2019). The gingival epithelium provides a barrier against mechanical and chemical stimuli, as well as microbes and microbial products. It contains numerous receptors involved in signaling pathways of inflammation, including the immune response.

The *outer gingival epithelium* is a keratinized, stratified, squamous epithelium and is composed of four layers: stratum basale (basal layer), stratum spinosum (prickle cell layer), stratum granulosum (granular layer), and stratum corneum (cornified layer) (Ainamo & Löe 1966; Cleaton-Jones et al. 1978; Newman et al. 2019; Stern 1965). Each layer has a specific function characterized by the cells and type of filaments. The main cells of the gingival epithelium are the keratinocytes. The cells in the basal layer are either cylindric or cuboid, and are in contact with the basal lamina (basement membrane) that separates the epithelium and the connective tissue (Lindhe & Lang 2015).

The *basement membrane (basal lamina)* is a specialized extracellular matrix that is interposed between the underlying connective tissues and the oral epithelium. It has a physical barrier function; a selective permeability barrier function; as well as functions including cell polarization, migration, adhesion, and differentiation (Bosshardt & Lang 2005). The basal lamina consists of an electron-lucent zone called the lamina lucida (also known as the lamina rara), an electron-dense zone called the lamina densa, and a lamina fibroreticularis (also known as the sub-basal lamina). The lamina fibroreticularis forms a discontinuous layer consisting of reticular and anchoring fibrils and faces the connective tissue. Matrix constituents of the basement membrane are collagen types IV and VII, laminin, heparan sulfate proteoglycan, fibronectin, nidogen (entactin), and the proteoglycan perlecan (Bosshardt & Lang 2005).

The cell membrane of the basal epithelial cells facing the lamina lucida harbors hemidesmosomes, and cytoplasmic tonofilaments in the cell converge toward the hemidesmosomes. The hemidesmosomes of the basal epithelial cells abut the lamina lucida, which is mainly composed of the glycoprotein laminin (Lindhe & Lang 2015). From the lamina densa, anchoring fibers project in a fan-shaped fashion into the connective tissue and terminate freely in the connective tissue, and are connected to a reticular condensation of the underlying connective tissue fibrils (mainly collagen type IV), whereby the anchoring fibrils appear to form loops around the collagen fibers (Lindhe & Lang 2015). The basal lamina is permeable to fluids, but it acts as a barrier to particulate matter (Lindhe & Lang 2015). The cell layers of the gingival epithelium and characteristics thereof are depicted in Table 2.5; see also Figure 2.2.

The *differentiation of keratinocytes* involves the process of keratinization, entailing progressive biochemical and morphological events that occur in the cell as they migrate from the basal layer. Keratinization is considered a process of

---

Table 2.5 Cell layers and characteristics of the gingival epithelium.

Stratum basale
- The basal cells possess the ability to divide, and it is in the basal layer that the epithelium is renewed, so it is thereby considered the progenitor cell compartment of the epithelium (Newman et al. 2019).
- When two daughter cells are formed by cell division, an adjacent "older" basal cell is pushed into the spinous cell layer and starts, as a keratinocyte, to traverse the epithelium.
- Once the keratinocyte has left the basement membrane it can no longer divide, but maintains a capacity for production of protein (tonofilaments and keratohyalin granules). It takes approximately one month for a keratinocyte to reach the outer epithelial surface, where it is shed from the stratum corneum (Newman et al. 2019).
- The number of cells that divide in the basal layer equals the number of cells that are shed from the surface, thus the epithelium maintains a constant thickness.
- As the basal cell migrates through the epithelium, it becomes flattened, with its long axis parallel to the epithelial surface (Newman et al. 2019).

(Continued)

Table 2.5 (Continued)

Stratum spinosum

- This consists of 10–20 layers of relatively large, polyhedral cells, containing short cytoplasmic processes resembling spines. The cytoplasmic processes occur at regular intervals and give the cells a prickly appearance.
- Together with intercellular protein–carbohydrate complexes, a solid cohesion between the cells is provided by numerous desmosomes (pairs of hemidesmosomes) that are located between the cytoplasmic processes of adjacent cells (Newman et al. 2019).
- A desmosome is comprised of (i) the outer leaflets of the cell membranes of two adjoining cells, (ii) the thick inner leaflets of the cell membranes, and (iii) the attachment plaques, which represent granular and fibrillar material in the cytoplasm.

Stratum granulosum

- In this layer electron-dense keratohyalin bodies and clusters of glycogen containing granules start to appear.
- Such granules are related to the synthesis of keratin (Newman et al. 2019).

Stratum corneum

- The cytoplasm of the cells is filled with keratin, and the nucleus, the mitochondria, the endoplasmic reticulum, and the Golgi complex are absent (Newman et al. 2019).
- The lining mucosa has no stratum granulosum or corneum, and cells containing viable nuclei can be identified in all layers, from the basal layer to the surface of the epithelium (Lindhe & Lang 2015).

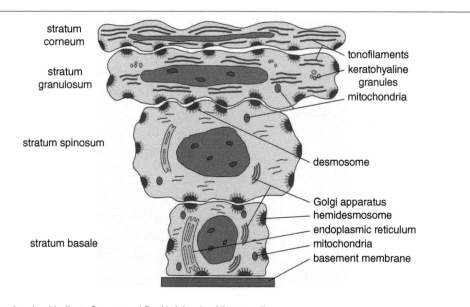

Figure 2.2 Cell layers of oral epithelium. Courtesy of Dr. Abdulqader Alhammadi.

differentiation rather than degeneration. It is a process of protein synthesis that requires energy and is dependent on functional cells, i.e. cells containing a nucleus and a normal set of organelles (Newman et al. 2019). The main morphological changes include (i) progressive flattening of the cell with an increasing prevalence of tonofilaments and desmosomes, (ii) intercellular junctions coupled to the production of keratohyalin granules, and (iii) decrease in the number of mitochondria, lamellae of rough endoplasmic reticulum, and Golgi complexes, and the disappearance of the nucleus. Thus, the entire apparatus for protein synthesis and energy production is lost (Bartold & Narayanan 1998; Bartold et al. 2000; Newman et al. 2019; Stern 1965). A complete keratinization process leads to the production of an orthokeratinized superficial horny layer, with no nuclei in the stratum corneum and a well-defined stratum granulosum (Lindhe & Lang 2015).

The oral epithelium is a keratinized, stratified, and squamous epithelium of which 75% is parakeratinized, 15% orthokeratinized, and 10% non-keratinized (Bral & Stahl 1977; Caffesse et al. 1977). In parakeratinized epithelia, the stratum corneum retains pyknotic nuclei, and the keratohyalin granules are dispersed, not giving rise to a stratum granulosum. The non-keratinized epithelium has neither granulosum or corneum strata, whereas superficial cells have viable nuclei. Apart from keratinocytes, the gingival epithelium contains numerous types of cells, proteins, non-keratinocytes, and inflammatory cells. Most of these cells do not contain desmosomes or tonofilaments. Table 2.6 depicts the various non-keratinocytes

Table 2.6 Non-keratinocytes of the gingival epithelium.

Cell type	Location in gingival epithelium	Function
Odland bodies (Keratinosomes)	Uppermost cells of the stratum spinosum	Act as modified lysosome. Contain acid phosphatase involved in destruction of organelles
Melanocytes	Basal and spinous layers of the gingival epithelium	Synthesize melanin in organelles called premelanosomes or melanosomes
Melanophages (Melanophores)	Stratum spinosum and stratum corneum	Phagocytose melanin granules
Langerhans cells	All suprabasal levels and in smaller amounts in sulcular epithelium; absent in the junctional epithelium	Antigen-presenting cells for lymphocytes
Merkel cells	Located in the deeper layers of the epithelium	Associated with nerve endings and act as tactile perceptors
Lymphocytes	Dispersed throughout layers	Innate and adaptive immunity

of the gingival epithelium (Bral & Stahl 1977; Caffesse et al. 1977).

The *sulcular epithelium* is non-keratinized and lacks granulosum and corneum strata. The cells are cuboidal in shape, and it normally does not contain Merkel cells (Newman et al. 2019). It extends from the coronal limit of the junctional epithelium to the crest of the gingival margin. It has the potential to keratinize if it is reflected and exposed to the oral cavity. Conversely, the outer epithelium loses its keratinization when it is placed in contact with the tooth (Bral & Stahl 1977). The sulcular epithelium may act as a semipermeable membrane through which injurious bacterial products pass into the gingiva and through which tissue fluid from the gingiva seeps into the sulcus. Unlike the junctional epithelium, the sulcular epithelium is not heavily infiltrated by polymorphonuclear neutrophil leukocytes, and it is found to be less permeable (Lindhe & Lang 2015).

The *junctional epithelium* (JE) is part of the marginal "free" gingiva, forming a collar peripheral to the cervical region of the tooth, and is thus not visible intra-orally. In the interproximal area, the JE adjacent to neighboring teeth fuse to form the epithelial lining of the interdental col. The coronal termination of the JE is a free surface and is located either at the bottom of the sulcus, at the gingival margin, or at the interdental col area. Under pristine conditions, the epithelial seal extends from the cementoenamel junction to the gingival margin, averaging about 2 mm in height. However, due to subclinical inflammation, the coronal termination of the JE corresponds usually to the bottom of the gingival sulcus. At its apical and lateral aspects, the JE is bordered by soft connective tissue and, at its coronal-most portion, by the sulcular epithelium. Toward the tooth surface, the JE cells form and maintain the epithelial attachment (Bosshardt & Lang 2005).

The JE consists of a collar-like band of stratified squamous non-keratinizing epithelium (Cabrini & Carranza 1966;

Listgarten 1964; Newman et al. 2019; Oksche & Hollrath 1986; Salonen & Pollanen 1997; Schroeder 1981; Yamasaki et al. 1979). The cells of the JE are arranged in two layers or strata: the basal layer facing the connective tissue and a suprabasal layer extending to the tooth surface. The basal cells and the adjacent 1–2 suprabasal cell layers are cuboidal to slightly spindle shaped. All remaining cells of the suprabasal layer are flat, oriented parallel to the tooth surface, and closely resemble each other. The innermost suprabasal cells (facing the tooth surface) are also called DAT cells (= directly attached to the tooth) (Bosshardt & Lang 2005). The DAT cells form and maintain the internal basal lamina that faces the tooth surface (Newman et al. 2019). (See Figure 2.3.) The JE is continuously renewed through cell division in the basal layer. The cells

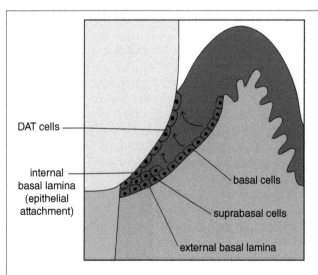

Figure 2.3 DAT cells of junctional epithelium. DAT, directly attached to the tooth. Courtesy of Dr. Abdulqader Alhammadi.

migrate to the base of the gingival sulcus, from where they are shed. The length of the JE ranges from 0.25 to 1.35 mm. It is 3–4 layers thick in early life, but the number of layers increases with age to 10–20 layers. The JE tapers from its coronal end, which may be 10–29 cells wide to 1–2 cells at its apical termination, located at the CEJ in healthy tissue. The JE has a free surface at the bottom of the gingival sulcus. The borderline between the JE and the underlying connective tissue does not have epithelial rete pegs, except when inflamed (Bosshardt & Lang 2005; Newman et al. 2019).

Within the basal epithelium cells, cytokeratin bundles are scarce, however, the Golgi fields are large, the rough endoplasmic reticulum is abundant, and polyribosomes are numerous (Bosshardt & Lang 2005). There are distinct differences between the oral sulcular epithelium, the oral epithelium, and the JE. The size of the JE cells is, relative to the tissue volume, larger than those of the oral epithelium; the intercellular spaces in the JE are, relative to the tissue volume, comparatively wider than in the oral epithelium; and the number of desmosomes is smaller in the JE than in the oral epithelium, including having occasional gap junctions (Bosshardt & Lang 2005; Newman et al. 2019). These features account for the JE's permeability (Bosshardt & Lang 2005).

The JE faces both the gingival connective tissue (i.e. the lamina propria of the gingiva) and the tooth surface. The external basal lamina is interposed between the basal cells of the JE and the gingival connective tissue. The external basal lamina of the JE resembles, in its structure and composition, other basement membranes that are interposed between an epithelium and a connective tissue (Bosshardt & Lang 2005). The internal basal lamina forms part of the interfacial matrix between the tooth-facing JE cells (DAT cells) and the tooth surface (Bosshardt & Lang 2005). The internal basal lamina (IBL) is distinctively different, structurally and molecularly. It has been suggested to be a specialized basal lamina, forming a strategic adhesive relationship with the tooth surface. It lacks most of the common basement membrane components such as collagen types IV and VII, most laminin isoforms, perlecan, and a lamina fibroreticularis, and is enriched in laminin-332 (Lm332) (Bosshardt & Lang 2005). The adhesive capacity of the IBL is further accomplished by JE cells secreting three unique epithelial proteins: amelotin (AMTN), odontogenic ameloblast-associated (ODAM), and secretory calcium-binding phosphoprotein proline-glutamine rich 1 (SCPPPQ1) (Fouillen et al. 2019). Thus, the IBL of the JE has its own characteristics and cannot be regarded as a basement membrane in the true sense (Bosshardt & Lang 2005). The IBL together with hemidesmosomes forms the interface between the tooth surface and the JE, and is known as the epithelial attachment (see Figure 2.4). The epithelial attachment normally is not static but dynamic. JE cells migrate in the coronal direction toward the free surface, where they desquamate. Thus, a remodeling of the epithelial attachment occurs (Bosshardt & Lang 2005). The hemidesmosomes consist of an attachment

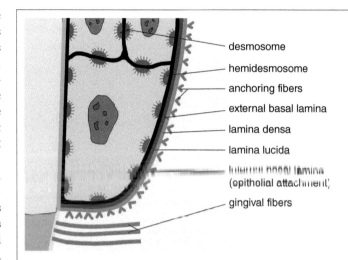

Figure 2.4 Junctional epithelial cell. Courtesy of Dr. Abdulqader Alhammadi.

plaque associated with cytokeratin filaments and the sub-basal dense plate, which is extracellularly located in the lamina lucida. The lamina densa directly faces the enamel, dentin, or cementum (fibrillar or afibrillar) (Bosshardt & Lang 2005). The elements of the epithelial attachment are produced and renewed by the adjacent DAT cells, thereby being part of the dynamics of the JE (Bosshardt & Lang 2005). The attachment of the JE to the tooth is reinforced by the gingival fibers, which brace the marginal gingiva against the tooth surface. The JE along with the gingival fibers form a functional unit, known as the dentogingival unit (Cho & Garant 2000; Listgarten 1964).

The JE exhibits several unique structural and functional characteristics that prevent pathogenic microbes from colonizing the subgingival tooth surface. This is achieved by, first, a firm attachment forming an "epithelial barrier" that prevents microbes and their products from entering the underlying tissues. Secondly, it allows access of gingival fluid, inflammatory cells, and components of the host defense to provide primary defense mechanisms. Thirdly, the rapid turnover rate of the JE helps to maintain the epithelial attachment to the tooth surface and promotes rapid repair of damaged tissue. The JE also secretes enzymes like defensins, which along with infiltrating neutrophils provide antimicrobial defense mechanisms at the dentogingival junction (Schroeder & Listgarten 1971, 1997; Ten Cate & Deporter 1975). Furthermore, large numbers of lysosomal bodies are found in JE cells. Enzymes contained within these lysosomes eradicate bacteria. Migrating polymorphonuclear neutrophil leukocytes are found routinely in the central region of the JE and near the tooth surface. In addition, lymphocytes and macrophages reside in and near the basal cell layer. Antigen-presenting cells and Langerhans and other dendritic cells are also present. The JE, particularly its basal cell layers, is well innervated by sensory nerve fibers (Bosshardt & Lang 2005).

Gingival connective tissue

The connective tissue of the gingiva is also known as the lamina propria. The lamina propria is divided into two parts: the reticular lamina and papillary lamina. The papillary lamina is that part of the lamina propria that is present between the rete pegs. The remaining connective tissue is called the reticular lamina. The gingival connective tissue is composed of collagen fibers (about 60% by volume), fibroblasts (5%), blood vessels, lymphatic vessels, nerves, and matrix (about 35%) (Listgarten 1964; Newman et al. 2019; Ten Cate 1994). The components of the gingival connective tissue are depicted in Table 2.7.

The dentogingival complex

The dentogingival complex comprises the relationship between the crest of the alveolar bone surrounding a tooth, the connective tissue attachment, the epithelial attachment, and the sulcus depth (Cook & Lim 2019; Gargiulo et al. 1961; Vacek et al. 1994). The dentogingival complex, also termed the "biological width" (Ingber et al. 1977) is a commonly used clinical term to describe the apico coronal variable dimensions of the supracrestal attached tissues. It is histologically composed of two components, the supracrestal connective tissue attachment and the junctional epithelial attachment, coronal to the alveolar bone crest (see Figure 2.1). The term "biological width" has also recently been proposed to be replaced by "supracrestal tissue attachment" (Jepsen et al. 2018). On average this dimension measures about 2 mm (Gargiulo et al. 1961; Ingber et al. 1977; Vacek et al. 1994). Table 2.8 depicts the relationship of the components of the dentogingival complex, as well as their clinical significance.

Table 2.7 Components of the gingival connective tissue.

Cells
- The most common cell of the gingival connective tissue is the fibroblast. Fibroblasts secrete collagen fibers and non-collagenous proteins that form the extracellular matrix of the gingival connective tissue.
- Fibroblasts play a major role in the development, maintenance, and repair of gingival connective tissue. They also degrade damaged collagen fibers by means of phagocytosis and secreting collagenase enzymes (Bartold & Narayanan 1998; Ten Cate & Deporter 1975).
- Other cells in the gingival connective tissue include mast cells, fixed macrophages, histiocytes, adipose cells, and eosinophils.

Ground substance
- This is the amorphous aqueous matrix that fills the space between fibers and cells.
- The ground substance is composed of proteoglycans, mainly hyaluronic acid and chondroitin sulfate, and glycoproteins, mainly fibronectin (Bartold & Narayanan 1998; Bartold et al. 2000).
- Fibronectin binds fibroblasts to the fibers and many other components of the intercellular matrix, thereby mediating cell adhesion and migration (Bartold & Narayanan 1998).

Fibers
- The three most common types of connective tissue fibers seen in the gingival connective tissue are collagen, reticular, and elastin.
- Collagen fibers, particularly collagen type I, form the bulk of the lamina propria and provide tensile strength to the gingival tissue.
- Type IV collagen branches between the collagen type I bundles and is continuous with fibers of the basement membrane and blood vessel walls.
- The elastic fiber system is composed of oxytalan, elaunin, and elastin fibers that are present between the collagen fibers (Bartold & Narayanan 1998; Bartold et al. 2000; Newman et al. 2019; Oksche & Hollrath 1986; Schroeder & Listgarten 1971, 1997; Stern 1965; Ten Cate & Deporter 1975).
- The collagen fibers in the gingiva are irregularly or randomly distributed, although they tend to be arranged in groups of bundles with a distinct orientation (Lindhe & Lang 2015; Newman et al. 2019). They can be divided into the following groups (see Figure 2.5):
- *Dentogingival fibers*: these project from the cementum of the supra-alveolar portion of the root, just beneath the JE, in a fan-like conformation, into the free gingival tissue of the facial, lingual, and interproximal surfaces, toward the crest and outer surface of the marginal gingiva, where they terminate short of the epithelium.
- *Dentoperiosteal fibers*: from the cementum of the supra-alveolar portion of the root they extend apically over the vestibular and lingual bone crest and terminate in the tissue of the attached gingiva, or blend with the periosteum of the bone. In the area of the free gingival groove, i.e. the border area between the free and attached gingiva, there is often a lack of support from the underlying oriented collagen fiber bundles.
- *Transseptal fibers*: these extend between the supra-alveolar cementum of approximating teeth and run straight across the interdental septum, to be embedded in the cementum of adjacent teeth.
- *Circular fibers*: these run their course in the free gingiva and encircle the tooth in a ring- or cuff-like fashion.

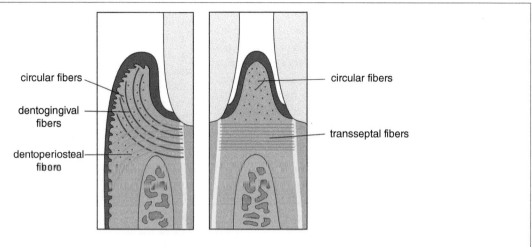

Figure 2.5 Gingival fiber groups. Courtesy of Dr. Abdulqader Alhammadi.

Table 2.8   Relationship of components of the dentogingival complex.

Dentogingival component	Location	Dimensions	Clinical significance
Histological sulcus	Gingival margin to the epithelial attachment	0.69–1.34 mm	May differ from the clinical sulcus depth
Epithelial attachment	Distance from coronal to apical portion of the attachment	0.97–1.14 mm	The most variable component
Connective tissue attachment	Distance from epithelial attachment to crest of alveolar bone	0.77–1.07 mm	The most consistent component

Source: Cook & Lim 2019/ With permission of Elsevier.

Zone of attached gingiva around healthy teeth/ implants and diseased teeth/implants with infrabony lesions

When the supracrestal tissue attachment (biological width) is attached to a healthy tooth or tissue-level implant, then the zone of attached gingiva (AG) is measured from the base of the sulcus to the mucogingival junction (MGJ). In clinical practice, though, clinicians cannot always observe the free gingival groove, and thus determine the zone of AG by measuring the full zone of keratinized tissue and then subtracting the sulcular depth (Ainamo & Löe 1966; Tarnow et al. 2021).

However, when the epithelial attachment and gingival fibers (biological width) are below the bone crest, such as with infrabony pockets on periodontally involved teeth, then the determination of the zone of AG may not always be valid, as the base of the pocket will be subcrestal and can thus not be used as a reference point (see Chapter 11). In this instance, the determination of the pocket depth will therefore have no clinical significance, and it cannot be deducted from the zone of keratinized tissue. The zone of AG should thus be measured from the bone crest, and not the base of the sulcus, to the MGJ (Tarnow et al. 2021). The same applies to periodontally involved tissue-level implants, and to periodontally involved bone-level implants placed at or below the bone crest, which have infrabony lesions (Tarnow et al. 2021). (See Chapter 33 for types of implant placement.)

Furthermore, the AG's apical aspect may be bound to bone or may be bound only to the tooth or implant, and not to the bone at all, thereby influencing the location of the MGJ in relation to the bone crest. The determination of the attachment of the zone of AG should therefore be based on the consideration of the MGJ in relation to the bone crest. In other words, the zone of AG should be measured from the bone crest to the MGJ (Tarnow et al. 2021).

It has thus been proposed that there is a need to modify how the definition of AG applies to healthy and diseased teeth and implants (Tarnow et al. 2021). This includes two scenarios: in type 1 scenarios, the MGJ is apical to the bone crest, and in type 2 scenarios, the MGJ is coronal to the bone crest. In many type 2 scenarios there will be an absence of AG, instead only having a zone of keratinized tissue (Tarnow et al. 2021).

Type 1 and type 2 scenarios have further implications regarding forced tooth eruption. In type 1 scenarios, forced tooth eruption will lead to an increase in the zone of keratinized

Table 2.9 Attached gingiva around healthy teeth/implants and diseased teeth/implants with infrabony lesions.

Healthy/diseased tooth/implant	Type 1/2 scenarios	Method of attachment of zone of attached gingiva (AG)
Healthy tooth	Type 1	The zone of AG is attached via the junctional epithelium, connective tissue fibers, and periosteum over bone
	Type 2	The zone of AG is attached via the junctional epithelium and connective tissue fibers, but is not attached to the bone
Healthy tissue-level implant	Type 1	The zone of AG is attached via the junctional epithelium, connective tissue fibers, and periosteum over bone
	Type 2	The zone of AG is attached via the junctional epithelium and the connective tissue fibers, but is not attached to the bone
Tooth with facial infrabony defect	Type 1	The zone of AG is attached only to the bone and not to the tooth
	Type 2	There is no AG, only a zone of keratinized tissue
Tissue-level implant with facial infrabony lesion	Type 1	The zone of AG is attached only to the bone and not to the tooth
	Type 2	There is no AG, only a zone of keratinized tissue
Healthy bone-level implant	Type 1	The zone of AG is attached only to the bone and not to the tooth
	Type 2	There is no AG, only a zone of keratinized tissue
Bone-level implant with facial infrabony lesion	Type 1	The zone of AG is attached only to the bone and not to the tooth
	Type 2	There is no AG, only a zone of keratinized tissue

Type 1 = mucogingival junction is apical to the bone crest. Type 2 = mucogingival junction is coronal to the bone crest.

tissue and AG. This is because the MGJ is bound to bone and remains at the same level as the tooth is erupted. In type 2 scenarios, forced tooth eruption may not increase the zone of AG; however, the zone of keratinized tissue will move coronally with the tooth, as the attachment is not bound to bone and is only attached to the tooth (Ainamo & Löe 1966; Hochman et al. 2014; Ingber 1976; Tarnow et al. 2021). (See also Chapter 27.2.)

Table 2.9 depicts the features of both types of scenarios determining the attachment of AG as they apply to healthy teeth and to infrabony pockets around diseased teeth and implants.

Cementum

Cementum is the calcified, avascular mesenchymal tissue that forms the outer covering of the anatomic root (Saygin et al. 2000). Cementum deposition is a continuous process that occurs at varying rates throughout life. The cementum often contains incremental lines, indicating alternating periods of formation and rest (Newman et al. 2019). Cementum is composed of inorganic and organic components. The inorganic content of cementum (hydroxyapatite) is 45–50%, which is less than that of bone (65%). The organic matrix of cementum is composed of type I (90%) and type III (about 5%) collagens along with non-collagenous proteins, such as proteoglycans, glycoproteins, and phosphoproteins (Yamamoto et al. 2016).

The cementum is formed when the mesenchymal cells of dental follicles transverse Hertwig's epithelial root sheath, attach to the root dentin, convert to cementoblasts, and start laying down cementum. Once the cementoblast deposits the cementum on the root surface, it continuously shifts away from the root surface. The formation of cementum and migration of cementoblasts are slow when the tooth is not erupting and is in its developing stage (Newman et al. 2019; Saygin et al. 2000; Tadokoro et al. 2002). Once the tooth erupts and moves coronally toward the occlusal plane, the formation of cementum is faster. During this stage, the cementoblast gets embedded into the deposited cementum and is referred to as a cementocyte. The cementum formed after the root erupts into the oral cavity is known as cellular (secondary) cementum. The cellular cementum contains large amounts of cementocytes. The early formed cementum without any cementocytes is called acellular cementum (Listgarten 1964; Yamamoto et al. 2000a). Since the deposition of cementum starts from the coronal end of the root near the enamel before the tooth erupts into the oral cavity, acellular cementum is found at or near the CEJ. The apical third or half of the root is covered with cellular cementum. Cellular cementum is more irregular and contains cells (cementocytes) in individual spaces (lacunae) that communicate with each other through a system of anastomosing canaliculi. Cellular cementum is less calcified than the acellular type. Sharpey's fibers occupy a smaller portion of cellular cementum and are separated by other fibers that are arranged

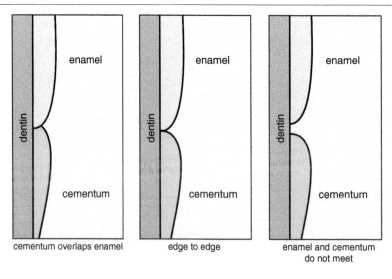

Figure 2.6 Types of cementoenamel junction. Courtesy of Dr. Abdulqader Alhammadi.

either parallel to the root surface or at random. Sharpey's fibers may be completely or partially calcified, or they may have a central, uncalcified core surrounded by a calcified border (Cleaton-Jones et al. 1978; Newman et al. 2019; Yamamoto et al. 2000a).

The deposition of cementum on the enamel forms the CEJ. As the cementum gets deposited on enamel, three types of CEJ have been observed: cementum overlaps the enamel (60–65%); an edge-to-edge butt joint exists (30%); and a gap junction, where cementum and enamel fail to meet (5–10%) (Listgarten 1968). The terminal apical area of the cementum where it joins the internal root canal dentin is known as the cementodentinal junction (2–3 μm wide) (Noyes et al. 1938). See Figure 2.6.

The functions of cementum include the following: attachment of periodontal ligament to the tooth; compensation for occlusal wear of tooth by apical deposition; as reparative tissue for root surfaces during functional adaptation of the tooth; maintaining and controlling the width of the periodontal ligament space; and protection of the underlying dentine.

Apart from the presence of cementocytes, cementum also contains two types of fibers: intrinsic (formed by cementoblast) and extrinsic fibers (formed by the fibroblast) (Yamamoto & Wakita 1992; Yamamoto et al. 2000b). Based on the presence and absence of fibers and cells and its location, cementum has been classified as in Table 2.10 (Yamamoto et al. 2000b).

Alveolar bone

The alveolar bone is a specialized part of maxillary and mandibular bone that forms and supports the tooth socket (alveoli). Alveolar bone is formed by intramembranous bone formation during the formation of the mandible and maxilla.

Table 2.10	Classification of cementum.
Acellular afibrillar cementum	Contains only the mineralized ground substance without any cells or fibers. It is the most coronal cementum with a thickness of 1–15 μm.
Acellular extrinsic fiber cementum	Is composed almost entirely of densely packed bundles of Sharpey's fibers, but lacks cells. Acellular extrinsic fiber cementum is formed predominantly by fibroblasts and less often by cementoblasts. It is found in the coronal and middle portions of the root, but may extend farther apically. It forms an important part of the attachment apparatus and connects the tooth with the bundle bone (alveolar bone proper). Its thickness is between 30 and 230 μm.
Cellular mixed stratified cementum	It is a co-product of fibroblasts and cementoblasts. In humans, it appears primarily in the apical third of the roots and apices and in furcation areas. It contains both extrinsic and intrinsic fibers as well as cementocytes. Its thickness ranges from 100 to 1000 μm.
Cellular intrinsic fiber cementum	Contains cementocytes and intrinsic fibers, but no extrinsic collagen fibers. It is found in the resorption lacunae.
Intermediate cementum	Is a poorly defined zone near the cementodentinal junction of certain teeth that appears to contain cellular remnants of Hertwig's sheath embedded in calcified ground substance.

Source: Based on Yamamoto et al. 2000b.

Composition of alveolar bone

The alveolar bone consists of 67% inorganic and 33% organic components. The inorganic matter is composed principally of calcium and phosphate, along with hydroxyl, carbonate, citrate, and trace amounts of other ions such as sodium, magnesium, and fluorine. The mineral salts are in the form of hydroxyapatite crystals of ultramicroscopic size and constitute approximately two-thirds of the bone structure (Schraer 1970). The organic matrix consists mainly of collagen type I (90%), with small amounts of non-collagenous proteins such as osteocalcin, osteonectin, bone morphogenetic protein, phosphoproteins, and proteoglycans. Osteopontin and bone sialoprotein are cell adhesion proteins that are important for the adhesion of both osteoclasts and osteoblasts (Ten Cate 1975).

The alveolar process that extends from the basal bone of the maxilla and mandible consists of (i) the supporting alveolar bone and (ii) the alveolar bone proper. The supporting alveolar bone is composed of both an outer layer of cortical bone and an inner region of cancellous bone (Newman et al. 2019; Saffar et al. 1997). (See Figure 2.7.)

The alveolar process is divisible into relative proportions of spongy bone and compact bone. Most of the facial and lingual portions of the sockets are formed by compact bone alone, with no or minimal cancellous bone. The interdental septum is composed primarily of cortical bone, with no cancellous bone. However, toward the apex of the tooth, increasing amounts of cancellous bone occupy the region between the cortical plates. The amount of cancellous bone is dependent on the location in the arch. The anterior region of the arch containing the incisors has very little cancellous bone. Cancellous bone is found predominantly in the interradicular and interdental spaces and in limited amounts facially or lingually, except in the palate. In the adult human, more cancellous bone exists in the maxilla than in the mandible (Melcher & Bowen 1969; Newman et al. 2019; Ten Cate 1975).

Supporting alveolar bone

See Figure 2.8.

Cortical plates form the outer (buccal) and inner (lingual) plates of the alveolar bone. The height and thickness of the facial and lingual bony plates are affected by the alignment of the teeth, the angulation of the root to the bone, and occlusal forces. The cortical bone of the alveolar process tends to be thinner in the maxilla than in the mandible. It is thickest in the mandible adjacent to the premolars and molars. On teeth in labial version, the labial bone margin is located farther apically compared to teeth that are in proper alignment. The bone margin has a thin knife edge, presenting with an accentuated arc in the apical direction. On teeth in lingual version, the facial bony plate is thicker than normal. The margin is blunt, rounded, and horizontal rather than arcuate (Newman et al. 2019).

In isolated areas where the root is denuded of bone and the root surface is covered only by periosteum and overlying gingiva, the defects are termed *fenestrations*. In these areas, the marginal bone is intact. When the denuded areas extend through the marginal bone, the defect is called a *dehiscence* (Newman et al. 2019). Such defects occur on approximately 20% of the teeth, appear more often facially than lingually, are more common on anterior teeth than posterior teeth, and are frequently bilateral. Predisposing factors may be prominent root contours, malposition, and labial protrusion of roots in combination with a thin bony plate (Newman et al. 2019). See Figure 2.9.

The tissue that covers the outer surface of the cortical plates is termed the periosteum, and that lining the internal bone cavities is called the endosteum. The periosteum consists of

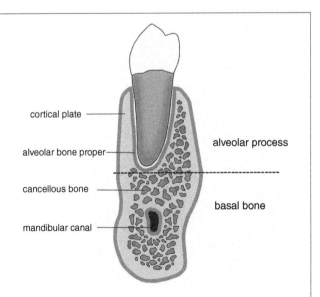

Figure 2.7 Alveolar and basal bone. Courtesy of Dr. Abdulqader Alhammadi.

cortical plate
alveolar bone proper
cancellous bone
mandibular canal
alveolar process
basal bone

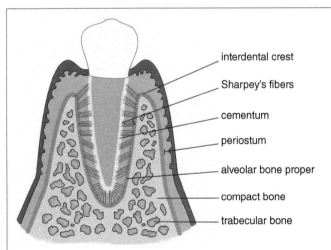

Figure 2.8 Alveolar bone. Courtesy of Dr. Abdulqader Alhammadi.

interdental crest
Sharpey's fibers
cementum
periostum
alveolar bone proper
compact bone
trabecular bone

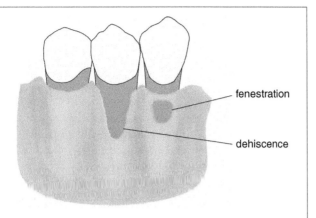

fenestration

dehiscence

Figure 2.9 Fenestration and dehiscence. Courtesy of Dr. Abdulqader Alhammadi.

two layers: an inner layer composed of osteoblasts surrounded by osteoprogenitor cells that can differentiate into osteoblasts, and an outer layer rich in blood vessels and nerves and composed of collagen fibers and fibroblasts. Bundles of periosteal collagen fibers penetrate the bone, thereby binding the periosteum to the bone (Newman et al. 2019).

Cancellous bone, also called bone spongiosa, fills the area between the cortical plates and the alveolar bone proper. It contains trabeculae of bone and marrow spaces. The trabeculae enclose irregularly shaped marrow spaces lined with a layer of thin, flattened endosteal cells. The trabecular pattern of cancellous bone can vary due to the effect of occlusal forces (Newman et al. 2019). Two types of spongy bone (spongiosa) can be observed: in type I, the trabeculae are regular and horizontal like a ladder (mandible); in type II, there are irregularly arranged, delicate, and numerous trabeculae (maxilla) (Yamamoto & Wakita 1992). The spongy bone is very thin or absent in the anterior regions of both the jaws.

Alveolar bone proper

The inner lining of the socket is formed by thin, compact bone called the alveolar bone proper. The alveolar bone proper is composed of lamellated bone systems and bundle bone. Bundle bone is the bone adjacent to the periodontal ligament (PDL) that provides the attachment site for Sharpey's fibers from the PDL (Yamamoto & Wakita 1992). The Sharpey's fibers are organized into bundles and calcified within the bone to provide a strong attachment between tooth and bone. Bundle bone is localized within the alveolar bone proper and merges with adjacent lamellar bone that comprises the alveolar process (Newman et al. 2019). Histologically, the inner lining of the alveolar bone (socket) has a series of openings (i.e. the cribriform plate), through which the neurovascular bundles link the PDL with the central component of the alveolar bone (Melcher & Bowen 1969; Ritchey & Orban 1953; Saffar et al. 1997; Sodek & McKee 2000; Ten Cate 1975). The lamellar part of alveolar bone proper merges with the cortical bone of the alveolar

process to form the alveolar crest. In a healthy individual, the alveolar crest is generally 1.5–2 mm below the CEJ of the tooth (Tadokoro et al. 2002). The alveolar bone proper is seen as the lamina dura in radiographs (Newman et al. 2019).

The *interdental septum* is the bone between adjacent sockets. It consists of cancellous bone that is bordered by the socket wall cribriform plates (i.e. lamina dura or alveolar bone proper) of approximating teeth and the facial and lingual cortical plates (Newman et al. 2019). The mesiodistal and faciolingual dimensions and shape of the interdental septum, including the alveolar crest, are governed by the size and convexity of the crowns of the two approximating teeth, the position of the CEJ between adjacent teeth, as well as by the position of the teeth in the jaw and their degree of eruption. If the interdental space is narrow, the septum may consist of only the cribriform plate. If the roots are too close together, an irregular "window" can appear in the bone between adjacent roots (Newman et al. 2019).

Alveolar crest position

A relationship between the CEJ and the crest of the alveolar bone has been suggested as follows (Cook et al. 2011; Kois 1996; Machado 2014):

- *Normal crest:* the midfacial alveolar crest is 3 mm and the proximal alveolar crest is 3–4.5 mm apical to the CEJ (in 85% of cases).
- *High crest:* the midfacial alveolar crest is less than 3 mm and the proximal alveolar crest is 3 mm apical to the CEJ (in 2% of cases).
- *Low crest:* the midfacial alveolar crest is greater than 3 mm and the proximal alveolar crest is greater than 4.5 mm apical to the CEJ (in 13% of cases).

The alveolar bone is constantly in a state of remodeling, with resorption and formation of bone occurring simultaneously to maintain the alveolar bone socket and tooth position. It is also the major pathway of bony changes in shape, resistance to forces, repair of wounds, and calcium and phosphate homeostasis in the body (Newman et al. 2019). The remodeling of the alveolar bone affects its height, contour, and density and is manifested in the following three areas: adjacent to the periodontal ligament, in relation to the periosteum of the facial and lingual plates, and along the endosteal surface of the marrow spaces (Newman et al. 2019).

In the adult, the marrow of the jaw is normally of the yellow type (fatty and inactive); however, foci of red bone marrow can be seen in the maxillary tuberosity, the maxillary and mandibular molar and premolar areas, and the mandibular symphysis and ramus angle, which may be visible radiographically as zones of radiolucency (Newman et al. 2019).

Periodontal ligament

The PDL is composed of a complex vascular and highly cellular connective tissue that surrounds the tooth root and connects it to the inner wall of the alveolar bone (Beertsen et al. 1997; Berkovitz 1990; Berkovitz et al. 1982; Ciancio et al. 1967). Coronally, it is continuous with the connective tissue of the gingiva; laterally, on the one side, it communicates with the alveolar bone marrow spaces through vascular channels in the bone, and on the other side, with the cementum on the root surface. The average width of the periodontal ligament space is around 0.2 mm. The PDL is comprised of fibers, cells, and ground substance (Beertsen et al. 1997). The components of the PDL are depicted in Table 2.11.

The PDL fibers are arranged in a systematic manner: see Table 2.12 and Figure 2.10. The functions of the PDL are depicted in Table 2.13.

Blood supply of the periodontium

There are numerous anastomoses present between different arteries and rather than individual groups of vessels, the entire system of blood vessels should be regarded as the unit supplying the soft and hard tissues of the maxilla and mandible (Newman et al. 2019) (see Figure 2.11).

The dental artery, which is a branch of the superior or inferior alveolar artery, dismisses the intraseptal artery before it enters the tooth socket. Before the dental artery enters the root canal, it puts out branches that supply the PDL. After entering the PDL, the blood vessels anastomose and form a polyhedral network that surrounds the root like a stocking. The majority

Table 2.11	Components of the periodontal ligament (PDL).
Ground substance	• The ground substance of the PDL fills the spaces between fibers and cells. • It consists of two main components: glycosaminoglycans, such as hyaluronic acid and proteoglycans, and glycoproteins, such as fibronectin and laminin (Berkovitz et al. 1982; Newman et al. 2019).
Cells	• Four types of cells have been identified in the PDL: connective tissue cells, epithelial rest cells of Malassez, immune system cells, and cells associated with neurovascular elements (Newman et al. 2019; Schroeder 1997). • Fibroblasts are the most common cells in the PDL. PDL fibroblasts appear as ovoid or elongated cells oriented along the principal fibers, exhibiting pseudopodia-like processes (Berkovitz et al. 1982). • These cells synthesize collagen and possess the capacity to degrade damaged collagen fibers by the process of intracellular degradation without involving collagenases (Ainamo & Löe 1966; Beertsen et al. 1997; Berkovitz 1990; Berkovitz et al. 1982; Cho & Garant 2000; Lindhe & Lang 2015; Newman et al. 2019). • Osteoblasts, cementoblasts, osteoclasts, and odontoclasts are also seen in the cemental and osseous surfaces of the PDL, where they help to regenerate and repair the lost cementum and alveolar bone. • The epithelial rests of Malassez form a latticework in the PDL and appear as isolated clusters of cells or interlacing strands. The epithelial rests are remnants of Hertwig's root sheath, which disintegrates during root development. • Epithelial rests are known to contain keratinocyte growth factors and can proliferate when stimulated to form periapical cysts and lateral root cysts (Fullmer et al. 1974). • Neutrophils, lymphocytes, macrophages, mast cells, and eosinophils have also been observed in the PDL (Berkovitz 1990).
Fibers	• The PDL comprises distinctly oriented collagen fibers that provide a hammock-like cushioning effect to occlusal forces and maintains the tooth in its position. • The principal fiber bundles consist of collagenous fibers that form a continuous anastomosing network between the tooth and alveolar bone to provide the framework and tone of the PDL (Cleaton-Jones et al. 1978; Machado 2014; Newman et al. 2019). • The fibers of the PDL are wavy in nature, with numerous folds that allow it to stretch and compress under occlusal loads (Cook et al. 2011; Kois 1996; Machado 2014). • The principal fibers are composed mainly of collagen type I, whereas reticular fibers are composed of collagen type III (Cook et al. 2011). • Apart from collagen fibers, oxytalan and eluanin fibers are also present in the PDL (Berkovitz et al. 1982; Ciancio et al. 1967). The oxytalan fibers run parallel to the root surface in a vertical direction and bend to attach to the cementum in the cervical third of the root. They help to regulate the vascular flow around the blood vessels of the PDL. Oxytalan fibers have been shown to develop de novo in the regenerated PDL (Ciancio et al. 1967). • The terminal portions of the PDL fibers are inserted into the cementum and alveolar bone. These terminal extensions are termed Sharpey's fibers. The Sharpey's fibers are more numerous toward the cementum than toward the alveolar bone. Once embedded in the wall of the alveolus or in the cementum, the Sharpey's fibers calcify to a significant extent.

Table 2.12   Periodontal ligament fibers.

Alveolar crest group	Alveolar crest fibers extend obliquely from the cementum just beneath the junctional epithelium to the alveolar crest. Fibers also run from the cementum over the alveolar crest and to the fibrous layer of the periosteum covering the alveolar bone. The alveolar crest fibers prevent the extrusion of the tooth and resist lateral tooth movements (Berkovitz et al. 1982).
Horizontal group	Horizontal fibers extend at right angles to the long axis of the tooth from the cementum to the alveolar bone.
Oblique group	Oblique fibers, the largest group in the periodontal ligament, extend from the cementum in a coronal direction obliquely to the bone. They bear the brunt of vertical masticatory stresses and transform them into tension on the alveolar bone.
Apical group	The apical fibers radiate in a rather irregular manner from the cementum to the bone at the apical region of the socket.
Interradicular group	The interradicular fibers fan out from the cementum to the alveolar bone in the furcation areas of multirooted teeth.

Source: Lindhe & Lang 2015; Newman et al. 2019.

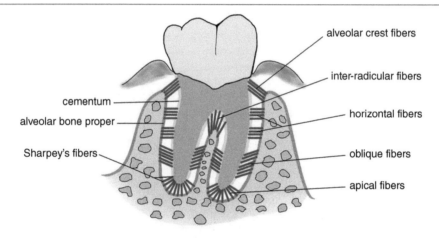

Figure 2.10 Periodontal ligament fibers. Courtesy of Dr. Abdulqader Alhammadi.

Table 2.13   Functions of the periodontal ligament (PDL).

Physical	Attachment of the teeth to the bone and maintenance of tooth position; effective transmission of occlusal forces to the alveolar bone by means of a "suspension bridge" or "hammock-like" arrangement of the principal fibers (Berkovitz et al. 1982); provides a soft tissue "casing" to protect the vessels and nerves from injury due to mechanical forces; and the maintenance of PDL width throughout its functional lifetime.
Formative and remodeling	The cells of the PDL have a formative and regenerative function that forms collagen fibers; residual mesenchymal cells develop into osteoblasts and cementoblasts; remodeling of the cementum and bone are necessary for physiological tooth movement; repair of injuries.
Nutritional and sensory	Blood vessels provide nutrients to the cementum, bone, and gingiva (Page et al. 1972); and an abundant supply of sensory nerve fibers transmit tactile, pressure, and pain sensations by the trigeminal pathways (Carranza et al. 1966). The neural bundles are divided into single myelinated fibers, which ultimately lose their myelin sheaths and end in one of four types of neural termination: (i) free endings, which have a tree-like configuration and carry pain sensation; (ii) Ruffini-like mechanoreceptors, located primarily in the apical area; (iii) coiled Meissner's corpuscles, also mechanoreceptors, found mainly in the mid-root region; and (iv) spindle-like pressure and vibration endings, which are surrounded by a fibrous capsule and located mainly in the apex (Carranza et al. 1966).

Source: Lindhe & Lang 2015; Newman et al. 2019.

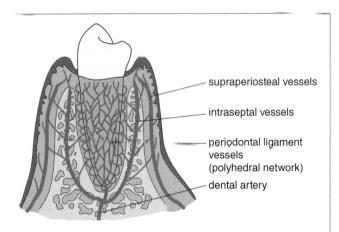

Figure 2.11 Blood supply of the periodontium. Courtesy of Dr. Abdulqader Alhammadi.

of the blood vessels in the PDL are found close to the alveolar bone. In the coronal portion of the PDL, the blood vessels run in a coronal direction, passing the alveolar bone crest, into the free gingiva. The intraseptal artery gives off branches that penetrate the alveolar bone proper in canals (Volkmann's canals) at all levels of the socket. They anastomose with blood vessels in the PDL space, and with other terminal branches from the intraseptal artery.

The supraperiosteal blood vessels are terminal branches of the sublingual artery, the mental artery, the buccal artery, the facial artery, the greater palatine artery, the infraorbital artery, and the posterior superior dental artery (Newman et al. 2019).

The main blood supply of the free gingiva is derived from the supraperiosteal blood vessels that, in the gingiva, anastomose with the intraseptal blood vessels and vessels of the PDL (Figure 2.12). During their course toward the free gingiva, the supraperiosteal blood vessels give off numerous branches to the subepithelial plexus, located immediately beneath the oral epithelium of the free and attached gingiva. This subepithelial plexus in turn yields thin capillary loops to each of the connective tissue papillae projecting into the oral epithelium. Beneath the sulcular epithelium, the subepithelial plexus forms capillary loops. Beneath the JE is a fine-meshed network of blood vessels termed the dentogingival plexus. The blood vessels in this plexus are mainly venules. In healthy gingiva, no capillary loops occur in the dentogingival plexus. The blood supply of the vestibular gingiva is mainly through supraperiosteal blood vessels (Newman et al. 2019).

The greater palatine artery, which is a terminal branch of the ascending palatine artery, runs through the greater palatine canal to the palate. As it runs in a frontal direction, it puts out branches that supply the gingiva and the masticatory mucosa of the palate (Newman et al. 2019).

Lymphatic system of the periodontium

Lymph capillaries form an extensive network in the connective tissue. Before entering the bloodstream, the lymph passes through lymph nodes in which the lymph is supplied with lymphocytes. The labial and lingual gingiva of the mandibular incisor region are drained to the submental lymph nodes. The palatal gingiva of the maxilla is drained to the deep cervical lymph nodes. The buccal gingiva of the maxilla and the buccal and lingual gingiva in the mandibular premolar and molar regions are drained to submandibular lymph nodes. The third molars are drained to the jugulodigastric lymph node (Newman et al. 2019).

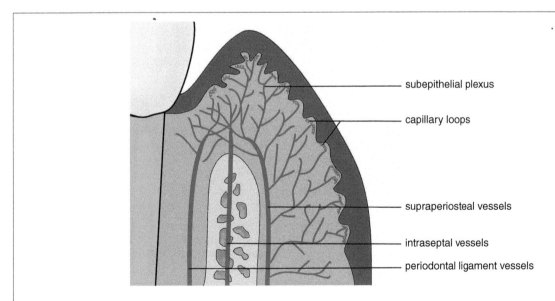

Figure 2.12 Blood supply of the gingiva. Courtesy of Dr. Abdulqader Alhammadi.

Nerve supply of the periodontium

The periodontium contains receptors that record pain, touch, and pressure (nociceptors and mechanoreceptors). Additionally, nerve components are found innervating the blood vessels of the periodontium. Nerves have their trophic center in the semilunar ganglion and are brought to the periodontium via the trigeminal nerve and its end branches (Newman et al. 2019). Receptors in the PDL, together with proprioceptors in muscles and tendons, play an important role in the regulation of chewing movements and chewing forces.

The mandibular teeth, including their PDL, are innervated by the inferior alveolar nerve, while the maxillary teeth are innervated by the superior alveolar plexus.

The gingiva on the labial aspect of maxillary incisors, canines, and premolars is innervated by superior labial branches from the infraorbital nerve. The buccal gingiva in the maxillary molar region is innervated by branches from the posterior superior dental nerve. The palatal gingiva is innervated by the greater palatal nerve, except for the area of the incisors, which is innervated by the long sphenopalatine nerve. The lingual gingiva in the mandibular incisors and canines is innervated by the mental nerve, and the gingiva at the buccal aspect of the molars by the buccal nerve. The innervation areas of these two nerves frequently overlap in the premolar region.

The small nerves of the periodontium follow the same course as the blood vessels. The nerves to the gingiva run superficially to the periosteum and give off branches to the oral epithelium on their way toward the free gingiva. The nerves enter the periodontal ligament through Volkmann's canals. In the periodontal ligament, the nerves join larger bundles that take a course parallel to the long axis of the tooth to supply certain parts of the PDL. Various types of neural terminations, such as free nerve endings and Ruffini's corpuscles, have been identified in the PDL (Newman et al. 2019).

REFERENCES

Ainamo A. Influence of age on the location of the maxillary mucogingival junction. *J Periodontal Res.* 1978; 13:189–193.

Ainamo A, Ainamo J. The width of attached gingiva on supra-erupted teeth. *J Periodontal Res.* 1978; 13:194–198.

Ainamo J, Löe H. Anatomical characteristics of gingiva: a clinical and microscopic study of the free and attached gingiva. *J Periodontol.* 1966; 37:5–13.

Bartold PM, Walsh LJ, Narayanan AS. Molecular and cell biology of the gingiva. *Periodontol 2000.* 2000; 24:28–55.

Bartold PM, Narayanan AS, eds. *Biology of the Periodontal Connective Tissues.* Chicago, IL: Quintessence; 1998.

Beertsen W, McCullough CAG, Sodek J. The periodontal ligament: a unique, multifunctional connective tissue. *Periodontol 2000.* 1997; 13:20–40.

Berkovitz BK. The structure of the periodontal ligament: an update. *Eur J Ortho.* 1990; 12(1):51–76.

Berkovitz BK, Moxham BJ, Newman HE, eds. *The Periodontal Ligament in Health and Disease.* London: Pergamon; 1982.

Bimstein E, Peretz B, Holan G. Prevalence of gingival stippling in children. *J Clin Pediatr Dent.* 2003; 27:163–165.

Bosshardt DD, Lang NP. The junctional epithelium: from health to disease. *J Dent Res.* 2005; 84(1):9–20.

Bowers GM. A study of the width of the attached gingiva. *J Periodontol.* 1963; 34(3):201–209.

Bral MM, Stahl SS. Keratinizing potential of human crevicular epithelium. *Periodontol.* 1977; 48:381–387.

Cabrini RL, Carranza FA Jr. Histochemistry of periodontal tissues: a review of the literature. *Int Dent J.* 1966; 16:466–479.

Caffesse RG, Karring T, Nasjleti CE. Keratinizing potential of sulcular epithelium. *Periodontol.* 1977; 48:140–146.

Carranza FA Jr, Itoiz ME, Cabrini RL et al. A study of periodontal vascularization in different laboratory animals. *J Periodontal Res.* 1966; 1(2):120–128.

Chambrone L, Tatakis DN. Long-term outcomes of untreated buccal gingival recessions: a systematic review and meta-analysis. *J Periodontol.* 2016; 87:796–808.

Cho MI, Garant PR. Development and general structure of the periodontium. *Periodontol 2000.* 2000; 24:9–27.

Ciancio SC, Neiders ME, Hazen SP. The principal fibers of the periodontal ligament. *Periodontics.* 1967; 5(2):76–81.

Cleaton-Jones P, Buskin SA, Kolchansky A. Surface ultrastructure of human gingiva. *J Periodontal Res.* 1978; 13(4):367–371.

Cook DR, Mealey BL, Verrett RG et al. Relationship between clinical periodontal biotype and labial plate thickness: an in vivo study. *Int J Periodontics Restorative Dent.* 2011; 31:344–354.

Cook R, Lim K. Update on perio-prosthodontics. *Dent Clin N Am.* 2019; 63:157–174.

Cortellini P, Bissada NF. Mucogingival conditions in the natural dentition: narrative review, case definitions, and diagnostic considerations. *J Clin Periodontol.* 2018; 45 (Suppl 20):S190–S198.

Dummett CO, Barens G. Oromucosal pigmentation: an updated literary review. *J Periodontol.* 1971; 42(11):726–736.

Fouillen A, Grenier D, Barbeau J et al. Selective bacterial degradation of the extracellular matrix attaching the gingiva to the tooth. *Eur J Oral Sci.* 2019; 127:313–322.

Fullmer HM, Sheetz JH, Narkates AJ. Oxytalan connective tissue fibers: a review. *J Oral Pathol.* 1974; 3:291–316.

Gargiulo AW, Wentz FM, Orban B. Dimensions and relations of the dentogingival junction in humans. *J Periodontol.* 1961; 32(3):261–267.

Greene AH. A study of the characteristics of stippling and its relation to gingival health. *J Periodontol.* 1962; 33:176–182.

Hochman MN, Chu SJ, Tarnow DP. Orthodontic extrusion for implant site development revisited: a new classification determined by anatomy and clinical outcomes. *Semin Orthod.* 2014; 20:208–227.

Ingber JS. Forced eruption: part II. A method of treating non-restorable teeth—periodontal and restorative consideration. *J Periodontol.* 1976; 47:203–216.

Ingber JS, Rose LF, Coslet JG. The "biologic width"—a concept in periodontics and restorative dentistry. *Alpha Omegan.* 1977; 70(3):62–65.

Jepsen S, Caton JG, Albandar JM et al. Periodontal manifestations of systemic diseases and developmental and acquired conditions: consensus report of workgroup 3 of the 2017 World Workshop on the Classification of Periodontal and Peri-Implant Diseases and Conditions. *J Clin Periodontol.* 2018; 45(Suppl 20):S219–S229.

Kan JY, Morimoto T, Rungcharassaeng K, Roe P, Smith DH. Gingival biotype assessment in the esthetic zone: visual versus direct measurement. *Int J Periodontics Restorative Dent.* 2010; 30:237–243.

Kois J. The restorative-periodontal interface: biological parameters. *Periodontol 2000.* 1996; 11:29–38.

Lindhe J, Lang NP, eds. *Clinical Periodontology and Implant Dentistry.* Chichester: Wiley; 2015.

Listgarten MA. The ultrastructure of human gingival epithelium. *Am J Anat.* 1964; 114:49.

Listgarten MA. A light and electron microscopic study of coronal cementogenesis. *Arch Oral Biol.* 1968; 13(1):93–114.

Machado AW. 10 commandments of smile esthetics. *Dental Press J Orthod.* 2014; 19:136–157.

Melcher AH, Bowen WH, eds. *Biology of the Periodontium.* New York: Academic Press; 1969.

Newman MG, Takei HH, Klokkevold PR et al. *Newman and Carranza's Clinical Periodontology.* St. Louis, MO: Elsevier Saunders; 2019.

Noyes FB, Schour I, Noyes HJ, eds. *A Textbook of Dental Histology and Embryology.* Philadelphia, PA: Lea & Febiger; 1938.

Oksche A, Hollrath L, eds. *The Periodontium Handbook of Microscopic Anatomy.* Berlin: Springer; 1986.

Page RC, Ammons WF, Schectman LR et al. Collagen fibre bundles of the normal marginal gingiva in the marmoset. *Arch Oral Biol.* 1972; 19(11):1039–1043.

Ritchey B, Orban B. The crests of the interdental alveolar septa. *J Periodontol.* 1953; 24(2):75–87.

Rosenberg HM, Massler M. Gingival stippling in young adult males. *J Periodontol.* 1967; 38:473–480.

Saffar JL, Lasfargues JJ, Cherruau M. Alveolar bone and the alveolar process: the socket that is never stable. *Periodontol 2000.* 1997; 13:76–90.

Salonen JI, Pollanen MT. Junctional epithelial cells directly attached to the tooth. *Acta Med Dent Helv.* 1997; 2:137–141.

Saygin NE, Giannobile W, Somerman MJ. Molecular and cell biology of cementum. *Periodontol 2000.* 2000; 24:73–98.

Schraer H, ed. *Biological Calcification.* New York: Appleton-Century-Crofts; 1970.

Schroeder HE. *Differentiation of Human Oral Stratified Epithelia.* New York: Karger; 1981.

Schroeder HE. Biological structure of the normal and diseased periodontium. *Periodontol 2000.* 1997; 13:1–148.

Schroeder HE, Listgarten MA, eds. *Monographs in Developmental Biology.* Basel: Karger; 1971.

Schroeder HE, Listgarten MA. The gingival tissues: the architecture of periodontal protection. *Periodontol 2000.* 1997; 13:91–120.

Sodek J, McKee MD. Molecular and cellular biology of alveolar bone. *Periodontol 2000.* 2000; 24:99–126.

Stern IB. Electron microscopic observations of oral epithelium. I. Basal cells and the basement membrane. *Periodontics.* 1965; 3:224–238.

Tadokoro O, Maeda T, Heyeraas KJ et al. Merkel-like cells in Malassez epithelium in the periodontal ligament of cats: an immunohistochemical, confocal-laser scanning and immuno electron-microscopic investigation. *J Periodontal Res.* 2002; 37(6):456–463.

Tarnow D, Hochman M, Chu S, Fletcher P. A new definition of attached gingiva around teeth and implants in healthy and diseased sites. *Int J Periodontics Restorative Dent.* 2021; 41(1):43–49.

Ten Cate AR. Formation of supporting bone in association with periodontal ligament organization in the mouse. *Arch Oral Biol.* 1975; 20:137–138.

Ten Cate AR. *Oral Histology: Development, Structure, and Function.* St Louis, MO: Mosby; 1994.

Ten Cate AR, Deporter DA. The degradative role of the fibroblast in the remodeling and turnover of collagen in soft connective tissue. *Anat Rec.* 1975; 182(1):1–13.

Vacek JS, Gher ME, Assad DA et al. The dimensions of the human dentogingival junction. *Int J Periodontics Restorative Dent.* 1994; 14:154–165.

Yamamoto T, Domon T, Takahashi S et al. The fibrillar structure of cement lines on resorbed root surfaces of human teeth. *J Periodontal Res.* 2000a; 35(4):208–213.

Yamamoto T, Domon T, Takahashi S et al. The fibrous structure of the cemento-dentinal junction in human molars shown by scanning electron microscopy combined with NaOH-maceration. *J Periodontal Res.* 2000b; 35(2):59–64.

Yamamoto T, Hasegawa T, Yamamoto T, Hongo H, Amizuka N. Histology of human cementum: its structure, function, and development. *Jpn Dent Sci Rev.* 2016; 52(3):63–74.

Yamamoto T, Wakita M. Bundle formation of principal fibers in rat molars. *J Periodontal Res.* 1992; 27(1):20–27.

Yamasaki A, Nikai H, Niitani K et al. Ultrastructure of the junctional epithelium of germ-free rat gingiva. *J Periodontol.* 1979; 50(12):641–648.

Zweers J, Thomas RZ, Slot DE, Weisgold AS, Van der Weijden GA. Characteristics of periodontal biotype, its dimensions, associations and prevalence: a systematic review. *J Clin Periodontol.* 2014; 41:958–971.

CHAPTER 3
Classification of periodontal and peri-implant diseases and conditions

Khalid Almas and Steph Smith

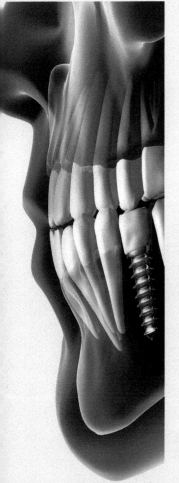

Contents

Learning objectives

- The chronological development of classifications for periodontal diseases.
- Description of the 1999 and 2018 AAP classification of periodontal diseases and conditions.
- Knowledge of key changes from the 1999 classification.
- Knowledge of new terminology used in the new classification.

Essential Periodontics, First Edition. Edited by Steph Smith and Khalid Almas.
© 2022 John Wiley & Sons Ltd. Published 2022 by John Wiley & Sons Ltd.

Introduction

Classification of periodontal diseases enables the development of frameworks to study the etiology, pathogenesis, and treatment of such diseases. It also provides the international healthcare community with a means of communicating in a common language. Classification systems furthermore provide practitioners with schemes to organize and execute treatment strategies for individual patients (Milward & Chapple 2003).

History of periodontal diseases classification systems

Over the last four decades, the American Academy of Periodontology (AAP) has presented multiple classifications of periodontal disease. However, many shortcomings in the 1977 classification were noticed, such as the lack of clear categorization of gingival disease, similarities of microbiological and host responses in some disease conditions, and the restriction of the age factor to certain diseases. During the period from 1977 to 1989, the classification transformed to include five categories of periodontal diseases in place of the traditional two categories in practice. The major changes from the 1977 to the 1989 classifications were the addition of the effect of systemic diseases on periodontal conditions and early-onset periodontitis (AAP 1989; Babay et al. 2019) (see Table 3.1).

The 1999 classification of periodontal disease dealt with these shortcomings and was based on different clinical entities, like necrotizing periodontitis, chronic periodontitis, aggressive periodontitis, and periodontitis as a secondary manifestation of systemic disease (1999 International Workshop 1999; Babay et al. 2019) (see Table 3.2).

Explanation of the 1999 classification

According to the 1999 International Workshop for a Classification of Periodontal Diseases and Conditions, in addition to increasing the number of disease classes from five to eight, the revision included several substantial deviations from preceding classifications. Briefly, gingival diseases were included as an independent entity (class I). Chronic periodontitis (class II) and aggressive periodontitis (class III) replaced adult periodontitis and early-onset periodontitis, respectively, thus eliminating the classifier "age." The refractory class was abandoned, periodontitis as a manifestation of systemic diseases (class IV) was modified and restricted to include only genetic and hematological diseases, and necrotizing periodontal diseases (class V) replaced necrotizing ulcerative periodontitis. Categories for abscesses of the periodontium (class VI), periodontitis associated with endodontic lesions (class VII), and developmental or acquired deformities and conditions (class VIII) completed the new classification system (1999 International Workshop 1999).

Although not perfect, this reflected the scientific understanding of the nature of periodontal diseases, as well as the practice of periodontics at that time.

Clinical and histological findings correlating with rapid loss of attachment and severe bone destruction, either localized or generalized (>30% of sites are involved), were considered as determinants for the diagnosis of aggressive periodontitis. Clinical cases not meeting these criteria were classified as chronic periodontitis. A substantial amount of new information from epidemiological and prospective studies evaluating the proposed systemic risk factors in chronic diseases has also been included since then (Babay et al. 2019).

The 2015 Task Force Report by the AAP added other parameters to the 1999 Classification of Periodontal Diseases and Conditions, such as radiographic bone loss in association with clinical attachment loss (CAL). Reduction of 1–2 mm CAL and up to 15% of root length or ≥2 mm and ≤3 mm bone loss was characterized as mild periodontitis, 3–4 mm CAL and 16–30% or >3 mm and ≤5 mm bone loss as moderate periodontitis, and CAL ≥5 mm and bone loss >30% as severe periodontitis. However, challenges in differentiating aggressive periodontitis from chronic periodontitis and the emergence of new scientific evidences such as peri-implant health and diseases

---

Table 3.1 Evolution of the AAP periodontal disease classification system.

1977	1986	1989

1. Juvenile periodontitis
2. Chronic marginal periodontitis
	I. Juvenile periodontitis
	  A. Prepubertal
	  B. Localized juvenile periodontitis
	  C. Generalized juvenile periodontitis
	II. Adult periodontitis
	III. Necrotizing ulcerative gingivo-periodontitis
	IV. Refractory periodontitis
		I. Early-onset periodontitis
		  A. Prepubertal periodontitis
		    1. Localized
		    2. Generalized
		  B. Juvenile periodontitis
		    1. Localized
		    2. Generalized
		  C. Rapidly progressive periodontitis
		II. Adult periodontitis
		III. Necrotizing ulcerative periodontitis
		IV. Refractory periodontitis
		V. Periodontitis associated with systemic disease

Source: Adapted from AAP 1989.

Table 3.2 1999 Classification of periodontal diseases and conditions (abbreviated version).

I. Gingival diseases
   A. Dental plaque-induced gingival diseases
   B. Non-plaque-induced gingival lesions

II. Chronic periodontitis (slight: 1–2 mm CAL; moderate: 3–4 mm CAL; severe: >5 mm CAL)
   A. Localized
   B. Generalized (>30% of sites are involved)

III. Aggressive periodontitis (slight: 1–2 mm CAL; moderate: 3–4 mm CAL; severe: >5 mm CAL)
   A. Localized
   B. Generalized (>30% of sites are involved)

IV. Periodontitis as a manifestation of systemic diseases
   A. Associated with hematological disorders
   B. Associated with genetic disorders
   C. Not otherwise specified

V. Necrotizing periodontal diseases
   A. Necrotizing ulcerative gingivitis
   B. Necrotizing ulcerative periodontitis

VI. Abscesses of the periodontium
   A. Gingival abscess
   B. Periodontal abscess
   C. Peri-coronal abscess

VII. Periodontitis associated with endodontic lesions
   A. Combined periodontic-endodontic lesions

VIII. Developmental or acquired deformities and conditions
   A. Localized tooth-related factors that modify or predispose to plaque-induced gingival diseases/periodontitis
   B. Mucogingival deformities and conditions around teeth
   C. Mucogingival deformities and conditions on edentulous ridges
   D. Occlusal trauma

Source: Based on CAL, clinical attachment loss.
1999 International Workshop 1999.

Table 3.3 Classification of periodontal and peri-implant diseases and conditions (2018).

- Periodontal health, gingival diseases and conditions (see Chapter 6)
  Periodontal health and gingival health
  Gingivitis: dental biofilm induced
  Gingival diseases: non-dental biofilm induced

- Periodontitis (see Chapter 7)
  Necrotizing periodontal diseases
  Periodontitis as manifestation of systemic diseases
  Periodontitis

- Periodontal manifestations of systemic diseases and developmental and acquired conditions (see Chapter 10)
  Systemic diseases or conditions affecting the periodontal supporting tissues
  Other periodontal conditions
    Periodontal abscesses
    Endodontic – periodontal lesions
  Mucogingival conditions and deformities
  Traumatic occlusal forces
  Prosthesis and tooth-related factors that modify or predispose to plaque-induced gingival diseases/periodontitis

- Peri-implant diseases and conditions (see Chapter 34)
  Peri-implant health
  Peri-implant mucositis
  Peri-implantitis
  Peri-implant soft and hard tissue deficiencies

Source: Modified from Caton et al. 2018.

workshop proceedings also included for the first time a new classification for peri-implant diseases and conditions (Caton et al. 2018) (see Table 3.3).

New terminology of 2018

Other salient features of the new classification are as follows (Babay et al. 2019):

- Introduction of the term "gingival pigmentation."
- Identifying smoking and diabetes as the major potential risk factors that can alter the grading of periodontal disease.
- Recognition of "periodontitis as a manifestation of systemic disease," such as Papillon Lefèvre syndrome.
- Systemic conditions affecting the periodontium when not related to dental plaque will be considered as "Systemic diseases or conditions affecting the periodontal supporting tissues."
- Management protocol of gingival recession based on the interproximal attachment loss.
- The term "periodontal biotype" was replaced with "periodontal phenotype," and "supracrestal tissue attachment" is the new term replacing "biological width."

were the main rationales for the new classification workshop in 2017 (Babay et al. 2019). Implant dentistry has become a major component of patient treatment planning and care since 1999. A classification scheme for periodontal and peri-implant diseases and conditions was thus considered necessary for clinicians to properly diagnose and treat patients, as well as for scientists to investigate the etiology, pathogenesis, natural history, and treatment of these diseases and conditions (Sheikh et al. 2020). This led to the development of a new classification, and a workshop was co-sponsored in 2017 by the AAP and the European Federation of Periodontology (EFP), which included expert participants from all over the world. In addition, the

It should be remembered that all classification systems have their faults, and this may always be the case for periodontal diseases, owing to their multifactorial and varied natural history. However, as nothing is guaranteed, the systems of the future are also likely to be controversial, stimulating debate and requiring further modification (Milward & Chapple 2003). It should be appreciated that the latest periodontal classification is based on evidence-based international knowledge agreed upon by world experts in the field.

REFERENCES

1999 International Workshop for a Classification of Periodontal Diseases and Conditions. *Ann Periodontol.* 1999; 4:1–112.

American Academy of Periodontology (AAP). *Proceedings of the World Workshop in Clinical Periodontics.* Chicago, IL: AAP; 1989: I/23–I/24.

Babay N, Alshehri F, Al Rowis R. Major highlights of the new 2017 classification of periodontal and peri-implant diseases and conditions. *Saudi Dent J.* 2019; 31(3):303–305.

Caton JG, Armitage G, Berglundh T et al. A new classification scheme for periodontal and peri-implant diseases and conditions – introduction and key changes from the 1999 classification. *J Periodontal.* 2018; 89(Suppl 1):S1–S8.

Milward MR, Chapple IL. Classification of periodontal diseases: where were we? Where are we now? Where are we going? *Dent Update.* 2003; 30(1):37–44.

Sheikh Z, Hamdan N, Glogauer, M. The new classification scheme for periodontal diseases and conditions. *J Ont Dent Assoc.* 2020; 97(5):24–28.

CHAPTER 4
Epidemiology and indices of periodontal disease

Ola Norderyd

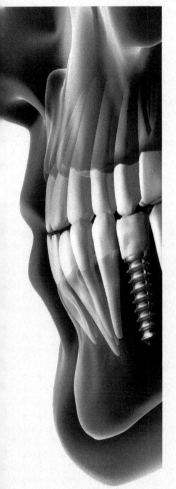

Contents

Learning objectives

- Presentation of trends in periodontitis epidemiology.
- Reasons for changes in periodontal health and disease over time in different populations.
- Consideration of the literature about the epidemiology of periodontitis.

Essential Periodontics, First Edition. Edited by Steph Smith and Khalid Almas.
© 2022 John Wiley & Sons Ltd. Published 2022 by John Wiley & Sons Ltd.

Introduction

Epidemiology entails the survey of the presence of specific diseases (prevalence), new cases/individuals with the disease (incidence), and the extent and severity of the disease in a population. Epidemiological investigations are important instruments for analyzing a population's treatment needs, the organization and planning of appropriate measures, and the evaluation of preventive actions and care.

Periodontitis is an inflammatory disease affecting the tooth-supporting tissues that leads to loss of periodontal attachment and surrounding bone. The two most important factors for the lifelong retainment of teeth in human beings is a healthy periodontium and being free from caries.

Indices

Periodontal diseases are common and their incidence varies in different populations. Prevalence estimates are influenced by different study design methods used, e.g. how periodontitis is defined at the individual level. Thus, comparisons between studies may be difficult.

The proposed standard today is to report prevalence and extent of teeth or tooth sites with gingival pocket depths (PD) ≥4 mm and ≥6 mm and with clinical attachment loss (CAL) ≥3 mm and ≥ 5mm (Holtfreter et al. 2015). This also makes it easier to see the distribution between different age groups in populations.

At the 2017 World Workshop on the Classification of Periodontal and Peri-implant Diseases and Conditions, a new classification of periodontitis was established (Caton et al. 2018; Papapanou et al. 2018) (see Chapter 3). The new classification system includes staging, current status, and grading as indicator of the rate of periodontitis progression. If CAL measurements are not available, radiographic bone loss (RBL) should be used instead. If this system is used in future epidemiological studies, it will make comparisons between studies more uniform. In brief, the new classification of periodontitis is divided into three parts: (i) extent, (ii) severity and complexity, and (iii) indicator of progression rate.

Extent of periodontitis

Localized (less than 30% of the teeth), generalized, or molar/incisor pattern.

Severity and complexity of periodontitis

- Stage I: CAL 1–2 mm or RBL <15%; maximum PD 4 mm.
- Stage II: CAL 3–4 mm or RBL 15–33%; maximum PD 5 mm.
- Stage III: CAL 5 mm or more or RBL extending to mid-third of root and beyond; PD 6 mm or more; up to four lost teeth due to periodontitis.
- Stage IV: stage III complexity and, in addition, need for complex rehabilitation due to periodontitis; tooth mobility degree 2 or more; five lost teeth or more due to periodontitis.

Indicator of progression rate of periodontitis

- Grade A: no bone loss over 5 years; % bone loss divided by age (in years) less than 0.25; non-smoker.
- Grade B: less than 2 mm bone loss over 5 years; % bone loss divided by age (in years) 0.25–1.0; smoking less than 10 cigarettes/day; diabetes with HbA1c less than 7.0%.
- Grade C: bone loss 2 mm or more over 5 years; % bone loss divided by age (in years) more than 1.0; smoking 10 cigarettes/day or more; diabetes with HbA1c 7.0% or more.

For a more detailed and in-depth description of the new classification system, see Papapanou et al. (2018). See also Chapter 7.3.

Figure 4.1 shows a panoramic radiograph of a 47-year-old male with generalized periodontitis, to offer an example of how to use the new classification.

- *Generalized periodontitis*: More than 30% of the teeth are involved.
- *Stage IV*: RBL extending to mid-third of root and beyond and PD 6 mm or more (clinical recordings are not shown). At the baseline examination, the patient had not yet lost any

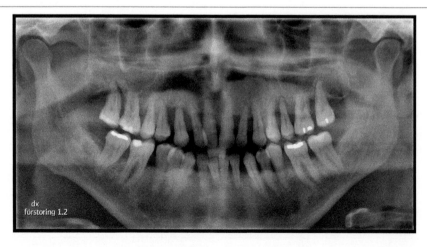

Figure 4.1 Generalized periodontitis. Courtesy of Dr. Ola Norderyd.

teeth because of periodontitis. However, several teeth had mobility of degree 2 or more. During the active periodontal treatment phase, six teeth were extracted and replaced by a tooth-supported cross-arch fixed partial denture.

■ *Grade C*: No previous clinical or radiographic data were available, but percentage bone loss divided by age on the most affected teeth was more than 1.0. The patient did not smoke and had no diagnosis of diabetes.

Epidemiological studies on periodontitis

Long-term (over decades) population studies on periodontal diseases are sparse. The best known are the Sri Lanka studies that followed a specific population of male tea workers over a period of 15 years (Löe et al. 1986). In this population, Harald Löe and co-workers identified three different patterns in the progression of periodontitis (CAL), two groups with no (11%) or moderate (81%) disease progression and a third group with rapid (8%) disease progression. In the group with rapid disease progression, the absence of periodontitis prevention and treatment together with insufficient oral hygiene led to complete edentulousness before the age of 50 years.

Other long-term studies include the Jönköping studies in Sweden, which started in 1973 with follow-up of a specified population every 10 years (Norderyd et al. 2015). The most recent examination was performed during 2013–2014. During the 40-year period, an increase in periodontally healthy individuals was seen, from 8% in 1973 to 45% in 2013 (Figure 4.2). The proportion of individuals with extensive periodontal problems had been fairly constant, except in 1973 when there was a high proportion of completely edentate persons. The average number of teeth, on the other hand, has increased continuously over the years, even for the group with pronounced periodontal disease experience (advanced and severe).

Country-wide epidemiological studies, termed the National Health and Nutrition Examination Survey (NHANES), have been conducted in the USA since the 1960s. The NHANES survey in 2009–2012 showed that nearly 50% of adult Americans 30 years and older had some form of periodontitis (mild, moderate, or severe) (Eke et al. 2015). The total proportion of individuals with severe periodontitis was 8.5%. In the NHANES investigation of 2009–2012, severe periodontitis was defined as a combination of PD >5 mm and CAL >6 mm. In this study, differences between ethnic groups and more periodontitis in individuals with lower socioeconomic status were seen.

From the Global Burden of Disease (GDB) 2010 study, a meta-analysis of 72 epidemiological studies on periodontal health and disease in different populations was performed (Kassebaum et al. 2014). Severe periodontitis was defined as PD ≥6 mm (this also corresponds to a Community Periodontal Index of Treatment Needs, CPITN, score of 4) or CAL of >6 mm. This global clinical review showed a prevalence and incidence peak of severe periodontitis of 11.2% and at the age of 38 years, respectively. Geographic differences were seen. Severe periodontitis was unusual before the age of 20 and there were no significant differences between males and females. In the GBD study from 2015, which analyzed 195 countries and territories, a severe periodontitis prevalence of 7.4% was presented (Kassebaum et al. 2015). In total, 538 million people were affected by severe periodontitis. In the most recent GDB study from 2017, oral disorders were among the most prevalent conditions (diseases) in the world, for both females and males (GBD 2017).

Risk for periodontitis

To define some terms:
■ Risk = the probability of a negative event.
■ Risk factor = trait or condition indicating increased risk of a person getting one or more diseases, e.g. occurrence of hereditary disease in the family or tobacco smoking.

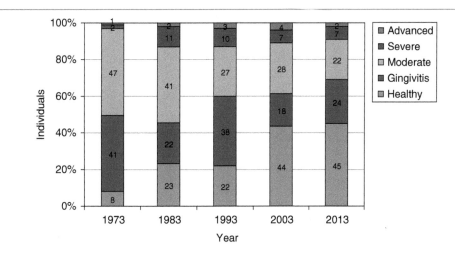

Figure 4.2 Distribution of periodontal health and periodontal disease experience for all individuals 20–70 years in Jönköping, Sweden, 1973–2013. Source: Norderyd et al. (2015). With permission of Swedish Dental Association.

- Risk marker = something that is associated with an increased risk of a certain disease, without any causal relationship being proven, e.g. a blood analysis result.

The most significant risk factors for periodontitis are heredity, tobacco smoking, and diabetes (Bergström & Preber 1994; Michalowicz et al. 2000; Thorstensson & Hugoson 1993). Risk factor analyses in periodontal epidemiology started with the Erie County studies performed in Buffalo, New York State (Grossi et al. 1994). In these studies, strong associations between severe periodontitis and certain subgingival bacteria, smoking, and diabetes were found. The presence of a microbial biofilm on the teeth is necessary to initiate periodontal disease (dysbiosis of the plaque), but it is difficult to detect as a risk factor in epidemiological studies. This is, above all, because of the high prevalence of proximal bacterial plaque in populations generally, regardless of the degree of periodontal disease

sensitivity. Bleeding on probing is a significantly better variable for predicting periodontal disease progression. The absence of bleeding over time is a reliable factor for maintaining (predicting) periodontal health (Lang et al. 1990).

More recent studies have focused on heredity, using the human genome, e.g. human genome-wide association studies (Shungin et al. 2019). Also, new methods have been developed using complex modeling to investigate relationships between population characteristics, oral health behaviors, and periodontitis (Holde et al. 2018).

In the future it will be of the utmost importance to continue to register changes and needs that will follow with an aging population with more teeth and with a global prevalence of severe periodontitis around 10% on average.

Also see Appendix 2 for the periodontal indices currently being used.

REFERENCES

Bergström J, Preber H. Tobacco use as a risk factor. *J Periodontol.* 1994; 65 Suppl 5S:545–550.

Caton JG, Armitage G, Berglundh T et al. A new classification scheme for periodontal and peri-implant diseases and conditions – introduction and key changes from the 1999 classification. *J Periodontol.* 2018; 89 Suppl 1:S1–S8.

Eke PI, Dye BA, Wei L et al. Update on prevalence of periodontitis in adults in the United States: NHANES 2009 to 2012. *J Periodontol.* 2015; 86(5):611–622.

GBD 2017 Disease and Injury Incidence and Prevalence Collaborators. Global, regional, and national incidence, prevalence, and years lived with disability for 354 diseases and injuries for 195 countries and territories, 1990–2017: a systematic analysis for the Global Burden of Disease Study 2017. *Lancet.* 2018; 392(10159):1789–1858.

Grossi SG, Zambon JJ, Ho AW et al. Assessment of risk for periodontal disease. I. Risk indicators for attachment loss. *J Periodontol.* 1994; 65(3):260–267.

Holde GE, Baker SR, Jönsson B. Periodontitis and quality of life: what is the role of socioeconomic status, sense of coherence, dental service use and oral health practices? An exploratory theory-guided analysis on a Norwegian population. *J Clin Periodontol.* 2018; 45(7):768–779.

Holtfreter B, Albandar JM, Dietrich T et al. Joint EU/USA Periodontal Epidemiology Working Group. Standards for reporting chronic periodontitis prevalence and severity in epidemiologic studies: proposed standards from the Joint EU/USA Periodontal Epidemiology Working Group. *J Clin Periodontol.* 2015; 42(5):407–412.

Kassebaum NJ, Bernabé E, Dahiya M et al. Global burden of severe periodontitis in 1990–2010: a systematic review and meta-regression. *J Dent Res.* 2014; 93(11):1045–1053.

Kassebaum NJ, Smith AGC, Bernabé E et al. GBD 2015 Oral Health Collaborators. Global, regional, and national prevalence, incidence, and disability-adjusted life years for oral conditions for 195 countries, 1990–2015: a systematic analysis for the global burden of diseases, injuries, and risk factors. *J Dent Res.* 2017; 96(4):380–387.

Lang NP, Adler R, Joss A, Nyman S. Absence of bleeding on probing. An indicator of periodontal stability. *J Clin Periodontol.* 1990; 17(10):714–721.

Löe H, Anerud A, Boysen H, Morrison E. Natural history of periodontal disease in man. Rapid, moderate and no loss of attachment in Sri Lankan laborers 14 to 46 years of age. *J Clin Periodontol.* 1986; 13(5):431–445.

Michalowicz BS, Diehl SR, Gunsolley JC et al. Evidence of a substantial genetic basis for risk of adult periodontitis. *J Periodontol.* 2000; 71(11):1699–1707.

Norderyd O, Koch G, Papias A et al. Oral health of individuals aged 3–80 years in Jönköping, Sweden during 40 years (1973–2013) II. Review of clinical and radiographic findings. *Swed Dent J.* 2015; 39(1):69–86.

Papapanou PN, Sanz M, Buduneli N et al. Periodontitis: consensus report of workgroup 2 of the 2017 World Workshop on the Classification of Periodontal and Peri-Implant Diseases and Conditions. *J Periodontol.* 2018; 89 Suppl 1:S173–S182.

Shungin D, Haworth S, Divaris K et al. Genome-wide analysis of dental caries and periodontitis combining clinical and self-reported data. *Nat Commun.* 2019; 10(1):2773. doi:10.1038/s41467-019-10630-1.

Thorstensson H, Hugoson A. Periodontal disease experience in adult long-duration insulin dependent diabetics. *J Clin Periodontol.* 1993; 20(5):352–358.

CHAPTER 5
Etiology and pathogenesis of periodontal diseases

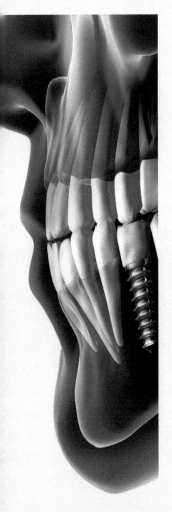

Contents

Essential Periodontics, First Edition. Edited by Steph Smith and Khalid Almas.
© 2022 John Wiley & Sons Ltd. Published 2022 by John Wiley & Sons Ltd.

5.1 THE DENTAL BIOFILM

Steph Smith

Contents

Learning objectives

- The stages of biofilm formation with the eventual formation of a climax community.
- The role of bacteriophages in the development and pathogenicity of the biofilm.
- Formation and functions of the biofilm matrix.
- Elements of biofilms that contribute to health of the host.
- Development and characteristics of a dysbiosis in gingivitis and periodontitis.
- Factors affecting the architecture and composition of the periodontal microbiome.
- Role of *Porphyromonas gingivalis* in the establishment of biofilms, as well as in periodontal disease.
- Characteristics of the subgingival microbiome in well-maintained patients with a history of periodontitis and its implications.
- Perspective on the role of biofilms in the development of disease and its implications in treating periodontitis.

Introduction

The mouth supports the growth of various microorganisms, including mycoplasma, bacteria, viruses, fungi, archaea, and protozoa. These microorganisms colonize mucosal and dental surfaces in the mouth to form highly diverse three-dimensional, structurally and functionally organized multispecies communities that are termed biofilms.

Unique processes that include various biochemical and biophysical principles contribute to the structure and function of dental plaque microbial communities. These processes may be studied at three spatial scales: the macro-, meso-, and microscale (Borisy & Valm 2021).

The *macroscale level* of dental plaque structure is described to be of the order of 1 mm to 1 cm or more, and includes the relevant microbially colonized human structures in the mouth, namely the epithelial mucosa of the cheek and gingiva, the papillary surface of the tongue dorsum, and the non-shedding, supragingival and subgingival hard surfaces of teeth (Dewhirst et al. 2010). At this macroscale, the different microbial communities are described in terms of the taxonomic composition, and the processes that contribute to the macroscale structure of dental plaque are mostly environmental characteristics, such as the surfaces available for attachment, oxygen availability, and exposure to host products delivered by saliva and gingival crevicular fluid (Human Microbiome Project Consortium 2012).

The *microscale level*, which is from 1 to 10 μm, is the scale of the individual cells themselves that comprise dental plaque. Relevant processes that dominate the assembly of dental plaque communities at this scale involve both physical and chemical intercellular interactions, among the microbes in the dental plaque community and between microbial cells and the host, as well as host contributions (i.e. diet and immune system interactions) (Borisy & Valm 2021; Lamont et al. 2018).

At the *mesoscale level*, which is from 10 to 1000 μm, the mesoscale architecture of the dental plaque biofilm is shaped by a combination of both environmental processes and intercellular interactions. This leads to the creation of ecological niches, metabolic cooperation, and persistence in its environment, and qualitatively resembles the spatial patterning governed by phenotypically different cells (Borisy & Valm 2021).

Biofilm formation is the primary mode of growth for bacteria in both natural and clinical environments. There is a highly interactive relationship (i.e. a reciprocal and dynamic balance) between the biofilm and the host, whereby these biofilm communities play an active and critical role in the normal development of the host and in the maintenance of oral health (Buduneli 2021; Kaplan 2010; Marsh & Zaura 2017). This relationship is characterized by active cross-talk between members of the resident oral microflora and the host's immune defenses, including both innate and adaptive immunity, without triggering an unwanted detrimental host response, while the host retains the ability to respond to a genuine microbial challenge (Cornejo Ulloa et al. 2019). Unless a major perturbation occurs in the environment of the biofilm, such as a major change in diet or an alteration to the immune status of the host, the microbial composition of the biofilm at a site usually remains stable over time (Marsh 2015).

Formation of the dental biofilm

There are distinct stages in dental biofilm formation (see Box 5.1.1).

The oral phageome

Metagenomic profiling of oral biofilms has led to an increased understanding of the potential role of phages in the development, regulation, and treatment of pathogenic microbiomes of the periodontium and other oral sites (Szafrański et al. 2021). A large population of viruses, mostly bacteriophages (phages), can infect specific bacterial species of the oral microbiome. They appear as free phage virions (phage particles) or as dormant prophages (i.e. within bacterial lysogens) (Szafrański et al. 2019, 2021).

Transmission of oral phages can take place between mother and children, family members, couples with intimate contact, and people in the same household. Person-to-person exchange of prophage-carrying oral bacteria may be a major route of phage transmission (Ly et al. 2016; Raya & H'bert 2009). Other potential routes of phage transmission can be indirect transfer by deposited oral material (e.g. food, utensils) or severe coughing (Kort et al. 2014).

Oral bacteria tend to be site specific, and oral phages follow a similar pattern (Koskella & Meaden 2013). Phage phylotypes may show a clear niche specificity, e.g. the buccal mucosa and tongue (Szafrański et al. 2019). Oral microbiomes and related phageomes may be affected by disease, aging, and different food intake. Most phage populations tend to be stable and highly personalized, and this stability of oral phage groups ensures a continuous phage effect on oral microorganisms (Abeles et al. 2014).

Phage infection

Tailed bacteriophages make up 96% of all phage isolates and are divided into families based on the tail morphology (Paez-Espino et al. 2019). The tailed phage particles attach to specific receptors, such as cell wall proteins, lipopolysaccharides, teichoic acids, capsular polysaccharides, pili, and flagella of permissive bacteria, and the phage nucleic acid is subsequently injected into the bacterial cell. Phages follow typical viral mechanisms of infection and multiply intracellularly by using the bacterial machinery for genomic replication. With a lytic infection, phage particles containing the phage genome are released by phage-mediated bacterial lysis. Phages can also persist in a chronic prophage stage (lysogenic state) by integrating into the bacterial genome or by forming an extrachromosomal, independently replicating plasmid-like episome (Howard-Varona

Box 5.1.1 Formation of the Dental Biofilm

Adsorption of conditioning biofilm

Within one minute after cleaning, tooth surfaces become coated with potentially more than 180 biologically active peptides, proteins, and glycoproteins, including keratins, mucins, proline-rich proteins, phosphoproteins (e.g. statherin), and histidine-rich proteins, which are derived mainly from saliva, as well as from gingival crevicular fluid (GCF) and bacteria (Hannig et al. 2005a; Siqueira & Oppenheim 2009; Siqueira et al. 2007). The pellicle is composed of two layers: a thin basal layer that is firmly attached, and a thicker globular layer (Hannig 1999; Hannig et al. 2005b). Many of these proteins retain enzymatic activity when they are incorporated into the pellicle, such as peroxidases, lysozyme, and α-amylase (Hannig et al. 2005c, 2008, 2009). Salivary biologically active molecules undergo conformational changes upon adsorption to surfaces, or undergo enzymatic cleavage of terminal residues, leading to the exposure of hidden molecular segments, which then serve as adhesion receptors for bacteria. For example, proteases may cleave peptide bonds, thus exposing arginine residues, making them available for binding (Gibbons et al. 1988; Jin & Yip 2002). This leads to the formation of a salivary pellicle, which is a biologically active substrate to which pioneer organisms can then attach (Rosan & Lamont 2000). Pellicle proteins with enzymatic activity furthermore affect the physiology and metabolism of adhering bacterial cells (Hannig et al. 2005c, 2008, 2009). The biological and chemical properties of the tooth surface thus become altered, whereby the exposed receptors confer specificity on the adhesive process, thus directly influencing the subsequent pattern of microbial colonization as microorganisms interact directly with this conditioning film (Gibbons et al. 1988; Hannig et al. 2005; Jin & Yip 2002).

Reversible adhesion followed by a more permanent attachment

Initially, reversible adhesion of a limited number of bacterial species to the tooth surface occurs. The initial colonizers of early dental plaque in the first few days are essentially composed of Gram-positive aerobic bacteria, mainly *Streptococcus spp.* as the dominant "pioneer" species, followed by increasing proportions of *Actinomyces naeslundii* (Lasserre et al. 2018). This is achieved by long-range physicochemical forces between the electrical charge of the molecules on the pellicle-coated surface and those on the bacterial cell surface (Bos et al. 1999). These include attractive van der Waals' forces and repulsive electrostatic interactions, and are influenced by the pH and ionic strength of the oral fluid. This is followed by stronger and more specific adhesin-receptor attachment mechanisms (Hojo et al. 2009), whereby early bacterial colonizers, e.g. *S. mitis* and *S. oralis*, by means of adhesins, stereochemically bind to complementary glycoprotein receptors in the acquired pellicle, thereby making the attachment more permanent. For example, salivary oligosaccharide-containing glycoproteins may serve as receptors for oral streptococci, and the salivary proline-rich protein 1 and statherin can serve as receptors for type I fimbriae of *A. viscosus* (Busscher et al. 2008; Nobbs et al. 2011).

Co-adhesion/co-aggregation

Once attached, the early colonizers start to multiply and their metabolism modifies the local environment. The consumption of oxygen and the production of reduced end products of metabolism by early colonizers make the environment more anaerobic. This is followed by microbial succession, whereby secondary colonizers, i.e. obligate anaerobes, bind to receptors on bacteria that are already attached (Teughels et al. 2019). This process is termed co-adhesion, i.e. the adherence of planktonic cells to already attached organisms on a surface. Co-aggregation entails the binding of bacteria that are in suspension (Kolenbrander 2011). This leads to the composition of the biofilm becoming more diverse (Kolenbrander et al. 2006), being composed supragingivally of a dense filament-containing plaque and subgingivally of flagellated bacteria, spirochaetes, and Gram-negative bacteria. Co-aggregation between different bacterial species is facilitated by (i) cation-dependent interactions requiring calcium ions; (ii) intergeneric specific cell-to-cell recognition via surface adhesins and receptors; (iii) the bridging of cells by multivalent molecules such as salivary mucins, agglutinin glycoproteins, and glucans, involving non-covalent, stereochemical interactions including a lectin-like protein on one partner cell recognizing a carbohydrate receptor on the other partner cell; (iv) extracellular vesicles; and (v) non-specific interactions involving cell-surface lipoproteins (Jin & Yip 2002; Lasserre et al. 2018; Rosan & Lamont 2000). *Fusobacterium nucleatum* co-adheres to most oral bacteria, thereby acting as a bridging organism between early and late colonizers. Thus, through co-aggregation, it allows the adhesion of late colonizers and periodontopathogens like *Porphyromonas gingivalis* (Curtis et al. 2020; Kolenbrander et al. 2006). Co-adhesion promotes microbial interactions by co-locating organisms next to physiologically relevant partner species, i.e. organisms with complementary metabolic functions, thereby facilitating nutritional cooperation and food chains, gene transfer, and cell–cell signaling (Marsh &

Zaura 2017). This has functional consequences, such as the protection of obligately anaerobic bacteria in aerobic environments by neighboring species that either consume oxygen or are oxygen tolerating (Marsh & Zaura 2017).

The oral cavity is a very complex ecosystem that can harbor more than 700 different identified microorganisms (Curtis et al. 2020; Lasserre et al. 2018). However, only a few numerically dominant bacterial species may be harbored in individual subgingival sites, with a large number of taxa being present in low abundance (Curtis et al. 2020) (see Table 5.1.1). Based on typical interspecies associations (depicted by the frequency with which different clusters of microorganisms are associated with each other) and sequential colonization, microbiota have been grouped in different colored complexes. The yellow complex comprises the oral streptococci, which together with *A. naeslundii* and *A. oris* (which are independent of defined complexes) are primary colonizers. *Rothia spp.* and *Corynebacterium spp.* have also been shown to serve as initiators of cell–cell co-aggregation interactions in early

biofilms (Curtis et al. 2020). Purple complex colonizers include *Veillonella parvula* and *A. odontolyticus*, and are also early colonizers. Green complex colonizers include *Eikenella corrodens, Aggregatibacter actinomycetemcomitans* serotype a, and different species of *Capnocytophaga*. The orange complex includes anaerobic bacteria, e.g. *Prevotella spp., Fusobacterium nucleatum, Eubacterium*, anaerobic streptococci, and motile *Campylobacter spp.* The red complex species include *P. gingivalis, Tannerella forsythia,* and *Treponema denticola* (Larsen & Fiehn 2017; Socransky et al. 1998). The microorganisms primarily considered to be late colonizers fall into the green, orange, and red complexes (Larsen & Fiehn 2017). The majority of the bacteria are anaerobic and have a proteolytic metabolism, which is favored by the local anaerobic conditions in the periodontal pocket, being rich in GCF. GCF is a tissue exudate resembling serum and is rich in proteins and blood products (Larsen & Fiehn 2017). This sequence is in accordance with the "ecological plaque hypothesis" of periodontal disease (Kolenbrander et al. 2006). The composition of the dental biofilm varies not only between different sites in the oral cavity, but also between individuals (Larsen & Fiehn 2017).

Theories have been suggested to explain the origins of disease-associated microbial species, including either an exogenous acquisition; translocation from reservoir sites such as the buccal mucosa, saliva, the depths of the tongue papillae, and crypts of the tonsils; or being present at healthy sites but in low numbers, thereby not being of clinical relevance, as well as being non-competitive with other members of the resident subgingival microbiota (Larsen & Fiehn 2017; Marsh & Devine 2011).

Plaque maturation
Some attached bacteria synthesize extracellular polymers to form a plaque matrix. The plaque matrix consolidates attachment of the biofilm, serving as a scaffold for the biofilm, facilitates the binding and retention of molecules, including enzymes, and also retards the penetration of charged molecules into the biofilm (Allison 2003; Vu et al. 2009). The plaque matrix also contributes to co-adherence of bacteria on the tooth surface and offers protection of biofilm bacteria (Larsen & Fiehn 2017). (See "The dental plaque biofilm matrix" later in this chapter.)

Bulk fluid is critical to the survival of species in a biofilm. This fluid provides nutrients, removes waste products, and acts as the vehicle for transport of bacterial cells from site to site in the oral cavity, as well as probably facilitating person-to-person transfer. The major bulk fluid in the oral cavity emanates from saliva and GCF, which emanates from the sulcus or periodontal pocket in dentate subjects (Socransky & Haffajee 2005). Bulk fluid is critical for the

---

Table 5.1.1 Examples of early and late colonizers in biofilm formation.

Early colonizers

Streptococcus gordonii, S. intermedius, S. mitis, S. oralis, S. sanguinis
  Rothia dentocariosa, R. aeria
  Actinomyces gerencseriae, A. israelii, A. naeslundii, A. oris, A. odontolyticus
  Aggregatibacter actinomycetemcomitans serotype a
  Capnocytophaga gingivalis, C. ochracea, C. sputigena
  Corynebacterium matruchotii, C. durum
  Eikenella corrodens
  Veillonella parvula, V. atypica

Late colonizers

Campylobacter gracilis, C. rectus, C. showae
  Eubacterium nodatum
  Aggregatibacter actinomycetemcomitans serotype b
  Fusobacterium nucleatum ss. nucleatum, F. nucleatum ss. vincentii, F. nucleatum ss. polymorphum, F. nucleatum ss. periodonticum, F. nucleatum ss. animalis
  Parvimonas micra
  Prevotella intermedia, P. loescheii, P. nigrescens
  Streptococcus constellatus
  Tannerella forsythia
  Porphyromonas gingivalis, P. endodontalis
  Treponema denticola

Source: Adapted from Curtis et al. 2020; Teughels et al. 2019.

sustained colonization of bacterial species. The inflammatory state of the gingival sulcus or periodontal pocket is important to the rate and nature of microbial colonization at or below the gingival margin. Gingivitis sites exhibit far more rapid plaque regrowth (Socransky & Haffajee 2005).

After the interplay of all the local habitat, host, and microbial determinants, a stable climax community is established, whereby the microorganisms achieve an equilibrium with each other and with the habitat provided by the host. This equilibrium is dynamic and minor perturbations may continuously occur, with adjustments being made by both the host and the colonizing species. Short-term changes in the host such as upper respiratory infection, a brief change in diet, and a lapse in oral hygiene procedures may modify the microbial community, but the community will return to its climax state once these factors are removed (Socransky & Haffajee 2005).

Subgingival microbiome characterizations utilizing rRNA gene sequencing have identified species whose proportions do not change from health to disease. These species are referred to as core species, constituting a core microbiome regardless of health status. The core microbiome is defined as a suite of species identified based on their high prevalence above a certain threshold of abundance (Diaz et al. 2016). The core microbiome is markedly larger within the oral cavity than in other body sites (Teles et al. 2021). Core species bacteria interact with health-associated and periodontitis-associated community members. Two of the most consistently detected species in this group are *Campylobacter gracilis* and *F. nucleatum ss. vincentii*, and they make up an important component of plaque structure due to their ability to co-aggregate with many other species, as well as upregulating the pathway of lysine fermentation to butyrate in disease (Curtis et al. 2020).

Plaque dispersal

Biofilm dispersal plays a critical role in the transmission of bacteria from environmental reservoirs to human hosts, in the transmission of bacteria between hosts, and in the exacerbation and spread of infection within a single host. Biological dispersal thus promotes colonization at other sites, leading to focal invasion and the spreading of infection (Kaplan 2010).

Following plaque maturation, biofilm dispersal occurs whereby detachment of bacteria from the biofilm makes them free to float in the surrounding body fluids, returning them to planktonic mode (Kaplan 2010). The regulation of biofilm dispersal is influenced by environmental conditions, such as nutrient levels, oxygen tension, pH, and temperature. However, biofilm dispersal is a selective advantage when environmental conditions become both unfavorable and favorable, as biological dispersal has fundamental importance for the expansion, reproduction, and survival of all species.

There are three known distinct modes of biofilm dispersal: erosion, sloughing, and seeding (Kaplan 2010). Erosion is the continuous release of single cells or small clusters of cells from a biofilm at low levels over the course of biofilm formation. Erosion involves cell detachment due to cell division, whereby one of the progeny cells at the outer surface of the biofilm colony may be located at a sufficient distance from the colony so that it is not subjected to the attractive forces of the biofilm matrix, and is thus liberated into the bulk fluid following cell separation. Sloughing is the sudden detachment of large portions of the biofilm, usually during the later stages of biofilm formation. Seeding dispersal, also known as central hollowing, is the rapid release of a large number of single cells or small clusters of cells from hollow cavities that form inside the biofilm colony. Erosion and sloughing can be either active or passive processes, whereas seeding dispersal is always an active process (Kaplan 2010).

Biofilm dispersal is accomplished by the production of extracellular enzymes that degrade adhesive components in the biofilm matrix. Enzymes implicated in active biofilm dispersal include glycosidases, proteases, and deoxyribonucleases. These enzymes mediate biofilm dispersal by enabling bacteria to degrade their own biofilm matrix polymers. One example is dispersin B, a glycoside hydrolase enzyme produced by *A. actinomycetemcomitans*. Dispersin B degrades a biofilm matrix polysaccharide that mediates attachment of *A. actinomycetemcomitans* cells to abiotic surfaces, intercellular adhesion, and resistance to killing by detergents and human phagocytic cells. *S. intermedius* produces hyaluronidase enzyme that degrades the glycosaminoglycan hyaluronan found in the extracellular matrix of connective tissue. By breaking down the connective tissue, hyaluronidase may provide nutrients for the bacteria or allow the spread of bacteria and toxins deeper into the tissue. In multispecies biofilms such as dental plaque, bacteria may produce interspecific matrix-degrading enzymes that degrade biofilm matrix polymers produced by other species, so as to provide bacteria with a source of nutrients, or as a defense mechanism that detaches and displaces competing species (Kaplan 2010).

et al. 2017, Silpe & Bassler 2019). Unfavorable host conditions such as suboptimal temperature or pH, ultraviolet radiation, presence of DNA-targeting antibiotics, reactive oxygen species, and foreign DNA can trigger latent phages (prophage stage) to enter the lytic cycle and propagate before the death of the bacterial host cell (Silpe & Bassler 2019; Stokar-Avihail et al. 2019). Prophages can also transfer genetic traits or cause genome excision of bacterial genes, thereby conferring novel properties on bacteria. Examples of prophage-encoded virulence factors are the life-threatening toxins of *Vibrio cholerae*, *Escherichia coli*, *Corynebacterium diphtheriae*, and *Clostridium botulinum* (Davies et al. 2016).

Phage interactions within microbiomes

An important feature of the interplay between phages and bacteria (oral/periodontal phageome) is the rapid adaptation of new phage-invading mechanisms and the ability of phages to kill bacteria, as well as bacterial inherent defenses against phage infection and bacterial countermeasures. Phages exhibit both virulence factors and defense mechanisms against counterattacks by the bacterial host (Hampton et al. 2020). Bacterial antiphage nucleases and bacteria-encoded restriction enzymes can cleave unmodified phage DNA (Barrangou et al. 2007). Mutation in bacterial receptors for phage recognition or changes in the expression of bacterial surface structures are additional mechanisms of resistance toward phage infection. However, phages can attach to another bacterial site or the phage receptor-binding proteins may mutate to fit the mutated bacterial receptor. Bacterial capsule or extracellular matrix may also inhibit access of phages to receptors on the bacterial surfaces, but some phages can drill through such barriers by means of polymer-degrading hydrolases (Pires et al. 2016; Vidakovic et al. 2018). Extracellular membrane vesicles released from bacteria can intercept phages or may block entrance of new phage DNA. Bacteria can also undergo abortive infection to limit phage replication; however, phages may also be able to overcome this (Doron et al. 2018; Toyofuku et al. 2019).

Most oral phages infect commensal bacteria, and only a few are linked to classical periodontopathogens: 4 to *T. forsythia*, 19 to *Prevotella intermedia/P. nigrescens*, and none to *P. gingivalis* (Al-Shayeb et al. 2020; Szafrański et al. 2021). Dormant *Aggregatibacter* prophages have been detected in both periodontal health and disease, but active *Aggregatibacter* phages have been observed to be associated with advanced periodontitis (Preus et al. 1987; Willi et al. 1997). It has been hypothesized that prophage activation and lysis of *A. actinomycetemcomitans* may expose the periodontium to bacterial virulence factors, such as leukotoxin, lipopolysaccharide, peptidoglycan, flagellin, and DNA (Preus et al. 1987; Stevens et al. 2013). In addition to systemic transmission of phage-infected oral bacteria, other atypical oral bacteria as well as enterococci, staphylococci, and pseudomonads may colonize the mouth and introduce novel phage populations (Zehnder & Guggenheim 2009).

Phage interactions with human cells

Although phages are not directly aggressive toward human cells, their immunomodulatory actions against specific bacteria might alter the oral microbiome (Sweere et al. 2019). Phages affect cell physiology and cell–cell signaling by inducing anti- and proinflammatory mediators, modulating innate and adaptive immunity, thereby exerting either beneficial effects or maladaptive pathogenic immune responses (Górski et al. 2012; Van Belleghem et al. 2019). Phage virions can attach to and be phagocytosed by neutrophils, monocytes, and dendritic cells. By means of occupying phagocyte receptors, they may compromise or act as phagocytosis-facilitating opsonins. Phage DNA attaches to toll-like receptor-9 and activates signaling transduction pathways, which launch immunoinflammatory responses aimed at eliminating invading phages, thus providing an overall beneficial effect, but they can also give rise to maladaptive immune responses (Gogokhia et al. 2019; Szafrański et al. 2021). Internalized phages may also modulate phagocytes. The filamentous single-stranded DNA phage Pf has been shown to induce toll-like receptor-3–dependent type I interferon in leukocytes, which suppresses tumor necrosis factor and phagocytosis and thus potentially extends the survivability of the host bacterium and the phage (Sweere et al. 2019). Oral phage virions may also transverse the periodontal epithelium and interact with immune cells within the tissues (Nguyen et al. 2017; Szafrański et al. 2021). By crossing the oral epithelial barrier (transcytosis), oral phages may also disseminate to extraoral sites, in the form of prophages of invasive lysogenic bacteria or as a cargo of phagocytic cells (Schmidt et al. 2019). [66] The prophage of *S. mitis* encodes a platelet-binding factor that can promote platelet activation and aggregation, with a subsequent risk of causing endocarditis (Bensing et al. 2001; Willner et al. 2011).

The dental plaque biofilm matrix

Origins and components of the biofilm matrix

The presence of a matrix is one of the defining features of microbial biofilms and is responsible for many of their emergent characteristics: those properties emerging when bacterial cells are together in a biofilm (Flemming & Wuertz 2019). The major classes of extracellular polymeric substances that form the matrix are common to most biofilms and comprise carbohydrates, proteins, nucleic acids, and cell wall polymers, such as peptidoglycans and lipids (Flemming & Wingender 2010). Many components of the dental plaque extracellular matrix are originally synthesized within microbial cells that are then actively secreted, such as polysaccharides, proteins, and DNA (Grohmann et al. 2018; Jakubovics et al. 2020). However, there may be extensive variation in the specific types and proportions of macromolecules between different types of biofilm (Jakubovics et al. 2020).

Extracellular vesicles from Gram-negative and Gram-positive bacteria are abundant in dental plaque. Gram-negative outer-membrane vesicles, including those of *P. gingivalis*, contain lipopolysaccharides and protect DNA within them. Gram-positive vesicles, such as those from *S. mutans*, are associated with extracellular DNA on the external surface (Ho et al. 2015; Liao et al. 2014). The fungus *C. albicans* also produces extracellular vesicles that play a role in biofilm matrix production by transporting proteins and polysaccharides (glucans and mannans) out of the cell (Zarnowski et al. 2018). Extracellular vesicles are also enriched in virulence factors, such as leukotoxin from *A. actinomycetemcomitans*, and arginine and lysine-specific gingipains from *P. gingivalis* (Kieselbach et al. 2015; Veith et al. 2014). Vesicles of *A. actinomycetemcomitans*, *P. gingivalis*, and *T. denticola* also contain a range of small ribonucleic acids that can be delivered directly to host cells and may play roles in immunomodulation (Choi et al. 2017).

Bacterial cell lysis also plays an important role in the accumulation of plaque matrix material. Lysis may occur as a natural consequence of cell senescence or may be induced by exogenous compounds that degrade the cell wall, such as antibiotics or bacteriocins, or by enzymes (autolysins) present within the bacterial cell. Cell lysis may be an important mechanism for delivery of extracellular DNA into the biofilm matrix, as well as peptidoglycan, phospholipids, and, in the case of Gram-negative bacteria, lipopolysaccharides (Jakubovics et al. 2020; Perry et al. 2009; Wenderska et al. 2012).

Bacteriophages and virus-like particles can be observed in association with microbial cells within dental plaque. These may provide a source of extracellular nucleic acids or proteins (Halhoul & Colvin 1975; Pride et al. 2012).

During the early phases of dental plaque growth, molecules from saliva (proteins and glycoproteins) adsorb onto tooth surfaces and promote microbial attachment and biofilm formation (Jakubovics & Kolenbrander 2010). Depending on the location of the dental plaque (above or below the gumline), these macromolecules from saliva and/or GCF may attach to dental plaque and integrate into the biofilm (Heller et al. 2017). Many of the proteins that adsorb to oral surfaces also interact with oral microorganisms, including glycoproteins, secretory immunoglobulin A, mucins, proline-rich proteins, amylase, and statherin (Carpenter 2020; Nobbs et al. 2011). Periodontal pockets containing various host inflammatory cells can provide additional sources of proteins, glycoproteins, nucleic acids, and lipids for dental plaque (Jakubovics et al. 2020).

Host cells are also found in dental plaque and contribute to the plaque matrix when they degrade. Epithelial cells from the tongue, oral mucosa, or gingiva can be found in dental plaque within one hour after introducing a clean tooth surface into the mouth (Tinanoff & Gross 1976). Periodontal disease and gingival bleeding can also lead to the accumulation of erythrocytes at or close to sites of dental plaque (Jakubovics et al. 2020).

Lysis of cellular contents of host immune cells (neutrophils and macrophages) during the process of generating extracellular "traps" for the purposes of catching invading microorganisms may generate the presence of nucleic acids, antimicrobial peptides, and proteins that are secreted from these cells, and be located within the plaque matrix (Hirschfeld et al. 2015).

Functions of the biofilm matrix

Adhesion/cohesion and mechanical resistance

The biofilm matrix facilitates interactions between macromolecules, which help to retain cells within the biofilm and to stabilize the overall structure. For example, matrix glucans promote adherence to glucan binding proteins of *S. mutans*, thereby shaping the overall architecture of the biofilm (Couvigny et al. 2018; Mieher et al. 2018).

Biofilms exhibit viscoelastic behavior when subjected to external stress factors. The biofilm will deform under a given stress (e.g. shear stress) and returns to a state that is similar to, but not necessarily identical to, the initial state after this given stress is removed (Peterson et al. 2015). This sturdiness against detachment forces is further influenced by the shear forces that the biofilm experiences during growth. Biofilms grown under higher shear stress exhibit stronger attachment and stronger cohesive forces than biofilms grown under lower shear (Cieplik et al. 2019; Paramonova et al. 2009). This may be accomplished by structural changes with regard to the physical arrangement and structure of extracellular polymers in the matrix; or due to a selection favouring bacterial subpopulations that produce biofilms with increased strength of their structural matrix under high-shear conditions (Cieplik et al. 2019).

Regulation of mass transfer and cell migration

The scaffold formed by the macromolecular biofilm matrix can impede the transfer of molecules and cells. A given molecule may be delayed in diffusion throughout a biofilm because its pathway is determined by interstitial voids in the biofilm structure; consequently, the route will be a three-dimensional one rather than the direct path found for free diffusion in bulk water (Thurnheer et al. 2003). In addition, the biofilm matrix can act as an ion-exchange resin that will reduce the rate of movement of charged molecules through the biofilm, as they may undergo electrostatic interactions with biofilm matrix components (Kurniawan et al. 2012). Mixed-species biofilms cultured in vitro with complex matrix components or tighter cell–cell interactions have been shown to retard the penetration of immunoglobulin G (IgG) and IgM antibodies, to the point where IgG does not reach the center of clusters a few hundred micrometers in diameter (Takenaka et al. 2009; Thurnheer et al. 2003). Proteases of periodontal pathogens can also cleave multiple complement proteins and antibodies, which will potentially protect biofilm bacteria from host immunity (Damgaard et al. 2015; Vincents et al. 2011).

Bacteria can potentially migrate within biofilms. Motility mediated by type IV pili and flagella is required for the formation of three-dimensional cap structures in *P. aeruginosa* biofilms (Barken et al. 2008). Flagella-driven motility is also important for *T. denticola* to form mixed-species biofilms with

P. gingivalis (Vesey & Kuramitsu 2004). Gliding motility driven by *Capnocytophaga gingivalis* has been shown to contribute to the organization of polymicrobial oral biofilms, and gliding *C. gingivalis* cells can transport non-motile bacteria to other areas of the biofilm (Shrivastava et al. 2018).

Signaling and host interactions

Cell–cell sensing and signaling are optimized by means of the biofilm matrix helping to position microbial cells in close proximity. This is further mediated by autoinducer-2, peptides, and extracellular proteases contained within the biofilm matrix (Shanker & Federle 2017; Wang & Kuramitsu 2005; Wright et al. 2013).

Many biofilm matrix molecules, including lipopolysaccharides, peptidoglycans, and extracellular DNA, are pathogen-associated molecular patterns (PAMPs) that are recognized by immune cells, such as neutrophils and macrophages. However, there is evidence that immune responses are attenuated by bacteria in biofilms (Jakubovics et al. 2020). *S. aureus* biofilms have been shown to dampen host immune responses and to induce macrophage dysfunction and cell death (Thurlow et al. 2011). *Prevotella intermedia* has been shown to resist phagocytosis by polymorphonuclear leukocytes (Yamanaka et al. 2009).

Extracellular pool of nutrients and genes

The matrix is an important source of extracellular nutrients for bacteria within the biofilm. Polysaccharides, proteins, and extracellular DNA may be broken down that can then be internalized by bacteria (Jakubovics et al. 2020). The extracellular DNA component of the matrix may also serve as a pool of genes, whereby extracellular DNA-mediated horizontal gene transfer within oral biofilms can occur, which facilitates antimicrobial resistance and the encoding of antibiotic-resistant forms of penicillin-binding proteins (Sukumar et al. 2016; Tribble et al. 2012).

Benefits of resident oral microbiota to the host

Natural microbial residents are essential for the normal development of the physiology, nutrition, and defenses of the host (Marsh 2000; Wilks 2007). Commensal microbiota play a protective role against exogenous pathogens, participate in food digestion and contribute to the synthesis of certain vitamins, and can educate our immune system. This host–microbe mutualism whereby the host and microbes live in harmony and in a co-dependent relationship is called symbiosis (Lasserre et al. 2018). A "commensal communism" paradigm has been proposed whereby oral microbiota and the mucosa form a unified "tissue" in which the host–microbe "cross-talk" is finely balanced to ensure microbial survival and to prevent the induction of damaging inflammation (Henderson & Wilson 1998). It has been suggested that a bidirectional balance exists between the microbiome and the host inflammatory response (homeostasis) (Curtis et al. 2020).

Resident subgingival bacteria help to maintain healthy tissue by regulating low levels of expression of intracellular adhesion molecule 1, E-selectin, and interleukin (IL)-8, which in turn regulate the establishment of a protective layer of neutrophils strategically positioned between the subgingival biofilm and the junctional epithelium (Dixon et al. 2004). Pathogenic and non-pathogenic bacteria may initiate different intracellular signaling pathways and innate immune responses in epithelial cells (Cosseau et al. 2008). Bacteria can down-regulate epithelial cell inflammatory responses by inhibiting the nuclear factor kappa B (NF-κB) pathway, but also actively stimulate beneficial pathways, including type I and II interferon responses, and exert significant effects on the cytoskeleton and adhesive properties of the host cell (Cosseau et al. 2008).

Resident microbiota at a site can prevent colonization by exogenous (and often pathogenic) microorganisms, this property being termed "colonization resistance." This may be accomplished by more effective (i) attachment to host receptors; (ii) competition for endogenous nutrients; (iii) creation of unfavorable growth conditions to discourage attachment and multiplication of invading organisms; and (iv) production of antagonistic substances (hydrogen peroxide, bacteriocins, etc.) (Scofield & Wu 2016; Van der Waaij et al. 1971). Colonization resistance can be impaired by factors that compromise the integrity of host defenses or perturb the stability of resident microbiota, such as the side effects of cytotoxic therapy or the long-term use of broad-spectrum antibiotics, thus permitting the overgrowth of oral yeasts (Johnston & Bodley 1972).

Resident anaerobic oral bacteria reduce nitrate secreted in saliva to nitrite. Nitrite affects the regulation of blood flow, blood pressure, gastric integrity, and tissue protection against ischemic injury. Nitrite is further converted to nitric oxide in the acidified stomach. Nitric oxide has antimicrobial properties against enteropathogens and plays a role in the regulation of gastric mucosal blood flow and mucus formation (Marsh 2015).

Perturbation of the biofilm ecosystem: microbial dysbiosis

Both synergistic and antagonistic interactions contribute to the ecological stability of the microbial community that characterizes oral health (Marsh & Zaura 2017). Changes in the oral environment will affect the ecology of the ecosystem. These changes can include temperature, atmosphere, pH, receptors for attachment, nutrients, host defenses, host genetics, health, and lifestyle (Marsh & Devine 2011). This will impact the outcome of the interactions among the biofilm microorganisms, thereby affecting the proportions of members of the community (Marsh & Zaura 2017).

The development of a periodontopathogen biofilm ecosystem entails the accumulation of a microbial biomass around the gingival margin, inducing an inflammatory response. The breakdown of inflammatory tissue generates nutrients for bacteria, such as degraded collagen fragments and heme-containing compounds, which are important sources of amino acids and iron. Inflammation results in an increased flow of GCF, delivering components of the host defenses, e.g. immunoglobulins, complement, neutrophils, and cytokines (Ebersole 2003), as well as host molecules that act as substrates for proteolytic bacteria. Host molecules also contain hemin, e.g. haptoglobin, hemopexin, and hemoglobin, which is an essential co-factor for the growth of potential periodontopathogens such as *P. gingivalis* (Olczak 2005). Moreover, the low redox potential found in inflamed subgingival sites favors the development of anaerobic species (Rosier et al. 2018).

Inflammation may be sensed directly by bacteria, leading to changes in their virulence phenotype. Inflammatory cytokines such as interleukin-1 beta and tumor necrosis factor have been shown to enhance the growth and virulence potential of certain bacteria that capture these cytokines through specific receptors (Luo et al. 1993; Porat et al. 1991). *Pseudomonas aeruginosa* has been shown to use its outer-membrane porin, OprF, to interact with interferon-gamma, leading to enhanced expression of quorum-sensing–dependent virulence determinants that impair epithelial cell function (Wu et al. 2005).

Distinct stages in glycoprotein breakdown involving bacteria with different metabolic capabilities may correlate with changes in the microbial composition of bacterial plaque (ter Steeg & van der Hoeven 1989). Isobutyric acid produced by *P. gingivalis* can stimulate the growth of *T. denticola*, while succinic acid generated by *T. denticola* can enhance the growth of *P. gingivalis* (Grenier 1992). *Prevotella intermedia* and *P. gingivalis* utilize gingipains to catabolize hemoglobin to increase hemin availability, whereby an increase in hemin availability can alter the phenotype of *P. gingivalis*, leading to increased virulence and protease activity and changes in the structure of its lipopolysaccharide (Larsen & Fiehn 2017). Increases in fermentable carbohydrates (and the resultant acidic conditions) and host proteins (including hemin-containing molecules) can thus bring about the development of numerous nutritional interdependencies and physical interactions among species, thereby disrupting the microbial interactions that control the balance of microbial communities in health (ter Steeg & van der Hoeven 1989). This includes the fostering of the outgrowth of proteolytic and asaccharolytic bacteria with iron-acquisition capacity, such as *P. gingivalis* (Lamont & Hajishengallis 2015; Maekawa et al. 2014).

Bacterial changes in the local environment can also alter gene expression and increase the competitiveness of species such as *P. gingivalis* within microbial communities (Marsh & Zaura 2017). Studies have shown elevated expression of proteolysis-related genes and genes for peptide transport and acquisition of iron, as well as the increased expression of genes involved in the synthesis of lipopolysaccharides that could thus enhance the proinflammatory potential of the microbial community (Duran-Pinedo et al. 2014; Marchesan et al. 2017).

The inflammatory response can influence the subgingival microbiota via the impact of the host defenses (Marsh & Zaura 2017). Innate immune defenses can inhibit susceptible species. Sensitive species will thus be eliminated, although some may survive due to cross-protection from neighboring organisms (Hajishengallis & Lamont 2014; Nyako et al. 2005). A subset of species that can tolerate the inflammatory response, termed inflammophilic pathobionts, can capitalize on the inflammatory spoils and will flourish (Hajishengallis 2014). Other periodontal pathogens, such as *P. gingivalis*, can subvert the host response by degrading complement, interfering with neutrophil function, and blocking phagocytosis (Myrak et al. 2014; Slaney & Curtis 2008).

Inflammatory responses will thus alter the competitiveness and outcome of multiple interactions among the microbes in the subgingival microbiota, leading to changes in the proportions of individual species in biofilms from inflamed sites (Diaz et al. 2016; Marsh & Zaura 2017). However, there are conflicting reports on whether the diversity of the resultant microbial communities is altered (Hong et al. 2015; Park et al. 2015). Qualitative changes in the microbial community profile may include an increase in the numbers of more harmful bacteria and/or a shift in the balance of the microbiota away from organisms that are potentially protective, i.e. the shift appears largely independent of the acquisition of new members of the microbiota (Curtis et al. 2020; Kumar et al. 2006). Rather, the microbial shift reflects changes in the abundance of individual organisms or consortia of organisms resident within the subgingival biofilm in health (Curtis et al. 2020). This microbial shift allows for the uncontrolled growth of the commensal microbial community, which includes a disease-associated community shift, or dysbiosis of the microbiota, leading to periodontitis through disruption of host tissue homeostasis. Dysbiosis is defined as a condition in which the balanced state of the ecosystem is disturbed, i.e. the selective expansion of periodontitis-associated microbial species at the expense of health-compatible species (Cho & Blaser 2012; Lamont et al. 2018; Rosier et al. 2018). Dysbiosis is thus driven by alterations to the local environmental conditions whereby the host inflammatory response is considered to be one likely driver of this altered ecology. It has thus been suggested that in periodontitis a bidirectional imbalance exists between the oral microbiome and the host inflammatory response, whereby uncontrolled inflammatory and immune responses are largely, if not entirely, responsible for periodontal tissue destruction. Periodontitis, therefore, is initiated by a dysbiotic polymicrobial community, with the subgingival microbiome and the host inflammatory response forming a feedback loop in which the dysbiotic community causes deleterious inflammatory responses and inflammation perpetuates dysbiosis (Abusleme et al. 2021). Dysbiosis is clearly associated with periodontitis; however, it remains unclear whether dysbiosis causes disease or results from disease (Curtis et al. 2020). Nevertheless, this cyclic process, or feed-forward loop, between dysbiosis and inflammation is probably the main driver of inflammatory diseases such as periodontitis (Teles et al. 2021).

Dysbiosis in gingivitis

Following abstention of oral hygiene, the development of gingivitis occurs concomitantly with an increase in bacterial biomass and a large shift in the composition of subgingival communities. This includes depletion of Gram-positive species such as *R. dentocariosa* and a shift in dominant Gram-negative morphotypes including rods, filaments, and spirochaetes, such as, among others, *Prevotella* spp. and *F. nucleatum ss. polymorphum* (Curtis et al. 2020)

Dysbiosis in periodontitis

The development of periodontitis is accompanied by the emergence of different Gram-negative species to those enriched during gingivitis. Among the enriched species is the red-complex triad consisting of *T. denticola*, *P. gingivalis*, and *Tanneralla forsythia* (Curtis et al. 2020). A distinctive feature of the microbiome alteration that accompanies periodontitis is an increased diversity in species. These diverse communities may indicate niches with a more diverse pool of available nutritional resources delivered through an increased inflammatory response, or alternatively niches in which the efficient utilization of complex nutritional substrata benefits a multispecies consortium, rather than a single microorganism. Hence, periodontitis communities may depend on a larger web of metabolic interactions than their healthy counterparts (Curtis et al. 2020).

Alternatively, the subgingival environment in periodontitis may represent a site of immune dysfunction that includes a lowered efficiency of both innate and adaptive responses, thereby allowing the proliferation of species normally controlled by the host defense (Curtis et al. 2020).

Although dysbiosis associated with periodontitis results from changes in dominant species, there is also a significant increase in the total load of health-associated species in periodontal disease compared with periodontal health. Furthermore, the properties of this group of bacteria have been shown to switch to a potentially more pathogenic behavior in disease compared with health, suggesting that they contribute to the overall microbial challenge to the host tissues. Microorganisms with the largest number of up-regulated putative virulence determinants have been shown to be health-associated streptococcal species. Thus, the overall virulence challenge in periodontitis may actually be a product of the entire microbial community (Curtis et al. 2020).

Subgingival communities associated with periodontal sites that exhibit loss of attachment over time have been shown to be different metabolically from communities of stable sites, suggesting that prior to detectable destruction of tissues, the environmental conditions of the site and the characteristics of the community are different to those in sites that remain stable (Curtis et al. 2020).

Factors affecting the composition of the periodontal microbiome

The periodontal microbiome is defined as a characteristic microbial community occupying a well-defined habitat that has distinct physio-chemical properties (Teles et al. 2020). The structure of the microbiome may be shaped by an individual's recent interaction with the environment, as well as by diet, medications, and overall health, with the least stable site being supragingival plaque (Ding & Schloss 2014).

Figure 5.1.1 depicts various factors affecting the composition of the periodontal microbiome. These factors are also inevitably involved in complex interactions in the etiopathogenesis of periodontal disease (Buduneli 2021).

Interspecies interactions

The composition of subgingival communities varies from individual to individual. Intersubject variability in the overall composition of the oral microbiome is governed at the individual

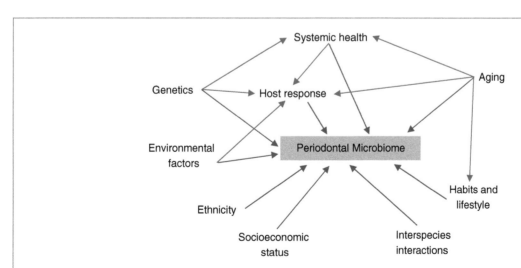

Figure 5.1.1 Factors affecting the composition of the periodontal microbiome. Source: Adapted from Buduneli 2021.

level by both the exposure and acquisition of oral microbial communities from the environment from birth to adulthood, as well as by the genetic landscape of the host (Curtis et al. 2020).

Biofilms have a diverse composition, are spatially and functionally organized, and include the close proximity of multiple species forming interactive microbial communities. Following attachment to a surface and the formation of a biofilm, microorganisms can exhibit a radically different phenotype (Marsh 2015). Interbacterial interactions influence behavior, virulence, and the relative proportions of various bacterial species (Kilian 2018; Shokeen et al. 2021). Furthermore, the combined properties of the biofilm bacteria are greater than the sum of the activities of the constituent species, which includes being engaged in a wide range of physical, metabolic, and molecular interactions (Marsh & Zaura 2017). These interactions, being both synergistic and antagonistic, contribute to the ecological stability of the microbial community that characterizes oral health. Also, the binding of bacteria to specific host receptors can induce significant changes in patterns of host cell gene expression (Marsh 2015). The oral microbiome is thus best described as a series of functions and interactions in both health and disease, rather than as a list of individual organisms. These functions also might not be provided by the same microbes in different people (Lloyd-Price et al. 2016; Takahashi 2015). Interspecies interactions thus determine biofilm architecture and composition, which includes interspecies adherence, metabolic interactions, interspecies signaling, competition for resources, as well as production of antimicrobial compounds for selective killing of other community members (Jakubovics 2015; Kolenbrander et al. 2010; Miller et al. 2019).

Interspecies adherence

F. nucleatum strains vary in the adherence properties that they possess. Individual strains may colonize distinct ecological niches and exert significant influence on the subsequent biofilm development within a specific ecological niche. In particular, an outer-membrane galactose-inhibitable protein adhesin is associated with adherence to Gram-negative oral bacteria that include key periodontal pathogens, and the presence of this adhesin on a *F. nucleatum* strain may correlate to the potential for periodontal disease in patients (Kaplan et al. 2009).

Numerous genes are also involved in synergistic pathogenic interactions involving adherence. For example, a specific interspecies contact between *P. gingivalis* with its partner species *S. gordonii* induces genes encoding the adhesins fimbrillin and minor fimbrium, both of which are directly involved in binding of *P. gingivalis* to *S. gordonii*, as well as in attachment to host cells, matrix material, and other host components (Hendrickson et al. 2017).

Metabolic interactions

The primary nutrients for oral microorganisms are host proteins and glycoproteins. These nutrients are obtained mainly from saliva for organisms in supragingival plaque and from GCF for those located in subgingival biofilms (Wei et al. 1999). Individual bacteria are dependent on the metabolic capability of other species for access to essential nutrients (Marsh & Zaura 2017). Thus, the metabolism of early colonizers alters the local environment, making conditions suitable for attachment and growth of later species (Marsh 2015). This may entail (i) the usage of an end product of metabolism of one organism being utilized as a primary nutrient by a secondary feeder; (ii) a consortium of microbes breaking down molecules that are normally recalcitrant to catabolism by an individual organism; or (iii) the catabolism of structurally complex host macromolecules enhancing metabolic cooperation among species. These nutritional interdependencies increase the metabolic efficiency of the microbial community (Larsen & Fiehn 2017; Periasamy & Kolenbrander 2010), thereby contributing to the temporal stability and resilience of oral microbial communities, and hence are able to co-exist and maintain a stable equilibrium, also termed microbial homeostasis (Marsh & Zaura 2017).

Interspecies signaling

Plaque bacteria communicate with one another in a cell density-dependent manner via small diffusible peptides, also called signaling molecules. The process of bacteria producing signaling molecules, transporting, sensing, and controlling a series of acts, is called a quorum-sensing system (Marsh & Zaura 2017). Quorum-sensing systems control bacterial surface adhesion, extracellular matrix production, synthesis of biosurfactants, the influencing of protein synthesis involved in biofilm formation, spore formation, the altering of gene transcription and expression among cells of a similar species, competence development, bacteriocin synthesis, stress resistance, and autolysis (Guo et al. 2014; Suntharalingam & Cvitkovitch 2005). Quorum sensing regulates the expression of biofilm-specific genes that involves the synthesis, secretion, and sensing of small chemical signals called autoinducers. As the cell density and autoinducer reach a threshold concentration of autoinducer, it triggers an increase in the transcription of biofilm-specific genes, whereby autoinducers have been shown to control several stages of biofilm formation, including surface attachment, matrix synthesis, the formation of fluid channels and pillar-like architecture, and dispersal (Kaplan 2010).

The close proximity of cells in biofilms increases the opportunity for horizontal gene transfer (HGT). HGT involves acquisition of DNA either from co-resident species or from exogenous sources. It allows oral bacteria to sample from an immense metagenome and in this way increase their adaptive potential to changes in the oral environment (Roberts & Kreth 2014). DNA can be transferred through transduction by bacterial viruses (bacteriophages), conjugation by bacterial pili, and transformation by DNA uptake involving naturally competent bacteria, and via membrane vesicles in Gram-negative bacteria (Olsen et al. 2013). Extracellular DNA is a component of the biofilm matrix and plays a role in adhesion and in possible nutrient storage, as well as being a potential source of phosphate and other ions (Jakubovics & Burgess 2015).

Diffusible peptides can facilitate the sharing of genes responsible for penicillin-binding proteins so as to induce penicillin resistance among commensal and pathogenic bacterial species (Hakenbeck et al. 1998). The reduced susceptibility of an organism to antimicrobial agents growing on a surface can be from 2- to 1000-fold greater than that of the same planktonic cells (Stewart & Costerton 2001). Resistance to antimicrobial agents can develop due to mutations affecting the drug target, the presence of efflux pumps, or the production of modifying enzymes, e.g. β-lactamase (Allison 2003). Another example is *S. mutans*, when exposed to low pH, releasing diffusible peptides to initiate a protective response among neighboring cells to regulate acid tolerance (Li et al. 2002). Neighboring cells of a different species can produce neutralizing enzymes such as β-lactamase, IgA protease, and catalase, which can protect inherently susceptible organisms from inhibitors (Brook 1989). Microbial communities can also give physical protection from phagocytosis to cells deep within a spatially organized consortium (Fux et al. 2005).

Antagonistic interactions

This implies that one of the interacting partners benefits at the expense of the other, whereby an organism obtains a competitive advantage during colonization and when competing with other microbes. Antagonistic compounds are for example bacteriocins, hydrogen peroxide, organic acids, different bacterial enzymes, and the release of lytic phages (Marsh & Zaura 2017). Bacteriocins and bacteriocin-like substances are antimicrobial and are produced by both Gram-positive and Gram-negative bacteria (Jakubovics & Burgess 2015). Varying concentrations of hydrogen peroxide produced by oral bacteria in different regions of the biofilm may influence the balance between symbiosis and dysbiosis, depending on the complex interplay between multiple antagonistic microbial interactions (Kreth et al. 2016). Phages are bacterial viruses that may lyse competing cells (Wang et al. 2016).

Tobacco products

Smoking affects the human microbiome directly, or indirectly via immunosuppressive mechanisms, oxygen deprivation, or biofilm formation (Buduneli 2021). Tobacco smoke contains thousands of chemicals that promote biofilm formation by increasing the adherence of bacteria to a stratum (Hutcherson et al. 2015).

- Exposure to tobacco smoke induces anaerobic environmental conditions that favour the growth of facultative anaerobic periodontopathogens. Smokers have pathogen-rich, commensal-poor biofilms in disease and the dysbiosis is established long before the onset of clinical signs of periodontitis (Mason et al. 2015; Shchipkova et al. 2010).
- In smokers, low taxonomic diversity has been related to higher disease severity (Bizarro et al. 2013).

- The microbial profile of periodontitis associated with smoking exhibits subgingival microbial communities that are less diverse than those of non-smokers, indicating significant differences in the prevalence and abundance of disease-associated and health-compatible bacteria (Shchipkova et al. 2010). The detection rates of *Tannerella forsythia, P. gingivalis*, and *Prevotella intermedia* have been found to be higher in groups of smokers than in groups of non-smokers in periodontitis patients (Mikhailova et al. 2017).
- Smoking favours the early acquisition and relatively unstable initial colonization of pathogens in both marginal and subgingival oral biofilms. This can result in sustained pathogen enrichment with periodontal pathogens (Kumar et al. 2011; Matthews et al. 2013). Smokers with periodontitis have been shown to have a robust core microbiome dominated by anaerobic bacteria (Ganesan et al. 2017). This can furthermore lead to a decrease in the ability of a subgingival microbiome to reset itself following episodes of disease, thereby lowering the resilience of the ecosystem and decreasing its resistance to future disease (Joshi et al. 2014).
- Essential metabolic functions of commensal bacteria are significantly influenced by exposure to smoke and the virulence of genes increases in pathogenic bacteria (Marsh 2015).
- Cigarette smoke extract has been suggested to augment *P. gingivalis* biofilm formation by increasing FimA avidity, which, in turn, supports initial interspecies interactions and subsequently promotes biofilm growth (Bagaitkar et al. 2009, 2011).
- Cigarette smoking has the potential to change the microbial diversity and composition of the buccal mucosa (Yu et al. 2017). Low concentrations of cigarette smoke condensate have also been shown to increase the invasion of human gingival epithelial cells by *P. gingivalis* (Imamura et al. 2015).
- Cigarette smoke extract exposure has been shown to regulate *P. gingivalis* genes, including detoxification and oxidative stress-related genes, DNA repair genes, and genes related to virulence, as well as the expression of outer-membrane proteins (Bagaitkar et al. 2009, 2011).
- Using 16S ribosomal RNA sequencing, a lower bacterial diversity has been reported in smokers when comparing the peri-implant microbiome between sites with healthy implants, peri-implantitis, and peri-implant mucositis (Tsigarida et al. 2015).
- Passive smoking, also known as environmental smoking or second-hand smoking, also has an effect on periodontal tissues. Parents who smoke harbor more potential pathogens and fewer interfering organisms, therefore acting as a source of pathogens that can colonize and/or infect their children (Brook 2011).
- Smokeless tobacco has been reported to induce metabolic alterations in oral bacteria, including oxidative stress (Sun et al. 2016).
- The risk of harm associated with electronic nicotine delivery systems (vaping) to the oral microbiome may be similar to or even greater than that associated with smoking tobacco: 1353 genes unique to individuals using electronic

cigarettes have been indicated to encode for antibiotic resistance, motility chemotaxis, stress response, HGT, iron acquisition, and cell wall and membrane transport. These functions were mostly found to be attributable to pathogenic species belonging to *Fusobacteria, Treponema, Prevotella*, and *Bacteroides* genera (Kumar et al. 2019).

■ Smokers have been shown to respond less favorably to periodontal treatment (scaling and root planing) than non-smokers (Queiroz et al. 2014). Moreover, supragingival periodontal treatment has been shown to affect only slightly the diversity of subgingival microbiota in smokers compared with non-smokers (Meulman et al. 2012).

■ Cessation of smoking has been indicated to alter the prevalence and levels of selected subgingival bacteria (Delima et al. 2010), thus being beneficial for promoting a health-compatible subgingival microbial community (Kanmaz et al. 2019).

Psychological stress

A systematic review has described a positive association between stress and periodontal diseases (Peruzzo et al. 2007). Psychological stress can directly affect periodontal health via biological mechanisms, and can have indirect effects through lifestyle changes such as ignoring oral hygiene measures, smoking more heavily, or consuming more fat and sugar (Leresche & Dworkin 2003). A bidirectional relationship between microorganisms and human neuroendocrine factors has been proposed (microbial endocrinology), whereby bacteria use host hormones to promote bacterial growth and infectious diseases (Genco et al. 1999; Lyte 1993).

Exposure to stress factors elevates the activity of the sympathetic nervous system, inducing chromaffin cells of the adrenal medulla to release increased levels of stress hormones, called catecholamines. The major catecholamines are epinephrine (adrenaline), norepinephrine (noradrenaline), and dopamine (Harbeck et al. 2015; Lymperopoulos et al. 2008). In response to psychological stress, cortisol, a glucocorticoid hormone, is secreted by stimulation of the hypothalamus–pituitary–adrenal axis. Cortisol has been shown to be positively associated with the severity of periodontal disease, systemic disease, age, sex, and lifestyle choices such as smoking and stress (Leresche & Dworkin 2003). These hormones affect various tissues in the human body, including the cardiovascular, metabolic, endocrine, neuronal, intestinal barrier, and immune systems (Lymperopoulos et al. 2008). Chronic stress induces a shift from T helper 1-linked cellular immunity toward T helper 2-linked humoral immunity and changes the course of infection (Verbrugghe et al. 2012).

Catecholamines have been shown to affect the growth of various bacterial species, thereby contributing to the clinical course of stress-associated periodontal diseases. The effects of catecholamines on bacteria cause changes in biofilm composition and behavior involving bacterial adherence and virulence, the infection dose, enzyme production, and the spread and severity of infections (Akcali et al. 2013; Boyanova 2017). Epinephrine and norepinephrine mainly affect bacterial gene expression, iron acquisition, and growth (Buduneli 2012). Noradrenaline reduces the growth of *P. gingivalis* and *A. actinomycetemcomitans*, but increases the growth of *Eikenella corrodens* (Semenoff-Segundo et al. 2012; Shapira & Frolow 2007). It also increases the expression of virulence factors like *P. gingivalis* gingipains, but simultaneously reduces expression of autoinducer, which is involved in the quorum-sensing process of *P. gingivalis* (Menezes et al. 2011; Shapira & Frolow 2007). Adrenaline and noradrenaline can induce changes in gene expression related to oxidative stress and virulence factors in *P. gingivalis* (Graziano et al. 2014). Other studies have described positive growth effects of norepinephrine on *Actinomyces naeslundii* and *Campylobacter gracilis*, together with inhibitory effects on *P. gingivalis* and *T. forsythia* (Roberts et al. 2002). Dopamine has been shown to enhance the growth of *Fusobacterium nucleatum*, whereas the growth of *P. gingivalis* may be unaffected (Jentsch et al. 2013).

Exposure to cortisol can significantly increase the growth of *P. gingivalis* over the first 24 hours, peaking after 12 hours (Akcali et al. 2014), although no growth effect has been observed with *T. forsythia, T. denticola*, and *A. actinomycetemcomitans* (Ardila & Guzman 2016).

Systemic health

Systemic diseases can increase the risk of, or even exacerbate, periodontitis by increasing the inflammatory burden, and/or by causing further alterations to the local microbiome, which includes the microbiome becoming more pathogenic. As already discussed, inflammation represents a strong ecological factor that drives dysbiosis, including the expansion of inflammophilic species. These species are better adapted to the inflammatory environment and furthermore are also more potent in inducing inflammation (Teles et al. 2021).

Diabetes

A disease-associated bacterial community framework is established in states of periodontal health in diabetic subjects, whereby periodontally healthy diabetic subjects exhibit significantly lower species richness than periodontally healthy controls, with lower levels of Gram-positive facultative species and higher levels of Gram-positive and Gram-negative anaerobic species (Ganesan et al. 2017). Increases in the pathogenic content of hyperglycemic microbiota, i.e., increases in the levels of species belonging to disease-associated genera, including *Porphyromonas, Prevotella, Campylobacter*, and *Fusobacterium*, make periodontally healthy individuals who are diabetic at risk of periodontitis (Long et al. 2017; Saeb et al. 2019).

Comparisons between normoglycemic and diabetic individuals with periodontitis show that bacterial samples from diabetic patients are distinct from those of normoglycemic individuals (Ganesan et al. 2017; Zhou et al. 2013). Diabetic individuals who have periodontitis exhibit significantly lower species richness, lower levels of anaerobic organisms, and higher levels of both Gram-positive and Gram-negative facultative organisms. Higher levels of species belonging to the genera *Lactobacillus*, *Corynebacterium*, and *Pseudomonas*, and lower levels belonging to the genera *Treponema*, *Porphyromonas*, *Prevotella*, and *Parvimonas*, have been observed in diabetic patients (Ganesan et al. 2017). This has been attributed to selective environmental pressure levels of glucose availability in GCF (Ganesan et al. 2017; Longo et al. 2018). The level of metabolic control furthermore shapes the periodontal microbiome, whereby microbial communities in periodontitis patients with high levels of glycated hemoglobin have been shown to be clearly distinct from those with well-controlled diabetes (Chopra & Kumar 2011). Glucose availability may favour the increase in levels of saccharolytic commensals, whereby a less traditionally pathogenic microbiome can mediate significant periodontal destruction in individuals with diabetes. The pathogenic capability of these bacteria, being generally considered as health compatible, has been suggested to be the result of the activation of virulence factors triggered in a proinflammatory milieu, in combination with immune resistance (Teles et al. 2021; Yost et al. 2015) (See also Chapter 23.1).

A multiplicative and not an additive effect on the periodontal microbiome has been suggested for diabetic smoker patients, including having a much higher relative risk of lower diversity, higher levels of Gram-negative facultative anaerobes, lower levels of Gram-negative anaerobes, and a smaller core microbiome (Ganesan et al. 2017).

Pregnancy

Broad microbial shifts occur during gestation and are affected by stage of pregnancy, delivery, and smoking, whereby significantly higher bacterial diversity has been noted in the third trimester. Pregnancy hormones have been suggested to act as a driver of compositional differences in pregnancy, particularly in the third trimester (Lin et al. 2018; Paropkari et al. 2016).

Overall, pregnancy is associated with lower levels of subgingival Gram-positive and Gram-negative anaerobes, and higher levels of Gram-negative facultatives, than controls. A greater abundance of species from the genera *Pseudomonas*, *Acidovorax*, *Enterobacter*, *Enterococcus*, *Diaphorobacterium*, and *Methylobacterium* is found in pregnancy, along with significant depletion of commensal organisms, including those from the genera *Neisseria*, *Veillonella*, and *Actinomyces* (Paropkari et al. 2016).

Rheumatoid arthritis

Patients with rheumatoid arthritis have been shown to have greater plaque biomass and an abundance of both Gram-positive and Gram-negative obligate anaerobes, with high levels of members of the genera *Cryptobacterium*, *Dialister*, *Fretibacterium*, *Prevotella*, *Treponema*, and *Selenomonas*, and less abundance and prevalence of health-associated species, such as *Rothia aeria*, *Kingella oralis*, and others belonging to the genera *Gemella*, *Granulicatella*, *Haemophilus*, *Neisseria*, *Streptococcus*, and *Actinomyces* (Corrêa et al. 2019; Lopez-Oliva et al. 2018).

It has been suggested that rheumatoid arthritis is a major modulator driving a healthy microbiome to one that is pathogenic prior to the establishment of periodontitis (Teles et al. 2021).

Bacteria produce large amounts of citrulline, and may play a role in the production of autoantigenic citrullinated peptides in rheumatoid arthritis. Subjects with rheumatoid arthritis, without periodontitis, show twofold increases in interleukin-2, interferon-gamma, tumor necrosis factor, and interleukin-33 compared with matched controls, which partly explains the chronic inflammatory selective pressure of rheumatoid arthritis on the microbiome (Corrêa et al. 2019).

Systemic lupus erythematosus

The altered immune response in systemic lupus erythematosus (a multisystem autoimmune disease) has been suggested to disrupt the balance between the host and the oral microbiota, favoring a unique dysbiotic condition that results in enhanced periodontal inflammation and tissue destruction (Teles et al. 2021).

These changes in the oral microbiome have been linked to increased local inflammation, as demonstrated by higher concentrations of salivary cytokines such as interleukin-6 and interleukin-17 in individuals with systemic lupus erythematosus and periodontitis compared with controls (Corrêa et al. 2017).

A distinct periodontitis-associated microbial shift has been reported with a decreased diversity and a higher bacterial load of *Prevotella*, *Selenomonas*, and *Treponema* (Corrêa et al. 2017).

Human immunodeficiency virus

Human immunodeficiency virus (HIV) itself and the antiretroviral treatment for HIV infection have the potential to alter the diversity and composition of the oral microbiome through inducing host–microbe dysbiosis, further linking to a variety of different complications of HIV, including more rapid progression of disease. Commensal bacteria can act as opportunistic pathogens in immunosuppressed individuals, with the oral cavity being a primary site for colonization (Patel et al. 2003; Saxena et al. 2012).

The oral bacteriome of both sub- and supragingival biofilms in HIV-1-infected participants, compared with non–HIV-1-infected individuals, has been shown to have increased richness and complexity, with higher relative abundance of potentially pathogenic species *Veillonella* and *Prevotella* in the subgingival biofilm (Gonçalves et al. 2019).

HIV-infected patients display decreased expression of histatin-5, a potent salivary antimicrobial peptide known to inhibit the growth of *Candida albicans*, which could be a potential mechanism of how HIV infection influences the mycobiome (Torres et al. 2009).

The role of *Porphyromonas gingivalis* in the pathogenesis of periodontitis

A pathogenic synergism exists within the microbial community that is characterized by the combined activity of an interacting consortium in which each member is only weakly virulent, but with a distinct role or function in order for the consortium to persist (van Steenbergen et al. 1984). Metatranscriptome analysis of biofilms in active periodontal disease sites shows evidence for the role of the entire community, not just a few pathogens, to be involved in biofilm dysbiosis (Yost et al. 2015). Thus, it should be noted that the presence of *P. gingivalis* does not necessarily prompt a pathological transition toward periodontal disease; rather, this bacterium signifies a risk factor for disease (Zenobia & Hajishengallis 2015). The presence of *P. gingivalis*, even at low abundance, alters the total commensal microbial load and composition. *P. gingivalis* thus contributes to destructive periodontitis in an indirect manner rather than having a direct effect on host tissue functions (Curtis 2015).

The host immune response to microbial communities changes the subgingival environment, causing low-abundant key opportunistic pathogens, for example among others *P. gingivalis*, to become the dominant bacteria in the biofilm, thus breaking the homeostasis between symbiotic microorganisms and the host (perturbation of the biofilm ecosystem) (Abdi et al. 2017). In other words, although *P. gingivalis* is often not prominent in number, its presence can shift biofilm communities from homeostasis with the host to a dysbiotic pathogenic state (Shokeen et al. 2021). The mechanisms through which *P. gingivalis* accomplishes these microbial changes are probably related to its virulent factors, which may inhibit the normal host-protective mechanisms in the periodontium (Yost et al. 2015). The virulence of *P. gingivalis* entails (i) colonization in the host; (ii) immune escape; (iii) immunosuppression; (iv) cellular entry and exit; (v) extraction of nutrients from the host; and (vi) release of virulence factors (How et al. 2016; Jia et al. 2019). These key virulence factors of *P. gingivalis* are regulated by local environmental conditions, involving host-related factors affecting virulence gene expression, and accessory pathogens that assist *P. gingivalis* in colonization and metabolic activities, and these conditions can differ among individuals (Kumar et al. 2006). Some individuals can resist the capacity of *P. gingivalis* to convert a symbiotic microbiota into a dysbiotic one by virtue of their intrinsic immune status (Kumar et al. 2006). In susceptible individuals, however, *P. gingivalis* can elevate the pathogenicity of the dysbiotic microbial community. By means of inducing differential immunoinflammatory responses, *P. gingivalis* can affect both the innate and adaptive immune responses by interacting with effector cells and complementary systems, thereby influencing inflammation and cytokine production (Abdi et al. 2017). The subversion of the host immune response can thus enhance the fitness of the community in a nutritionally favorable inflammatory environment (Kumar et al. 2006). In addition, *P. gingivalis* may also influence the composition of the polymicrobial biofilm through host-independent effects (Bao et al. 2014; Barth et al. 2013). Box 5.1.2 illustrates some important virulence factors of *P. gingivalis* (see also Figure 5.1.2).

The microbiome of well-maintained patients with a history of periodontitis

The question remains whether well-maintained patients with a history of periodontitis have the same subgingival microbiome as healthy subjects (Lu et al. 2020). Epidemiological studies have demonstrated that maintained patients still have a higher risk of recurrence compared with periodontally healthy individuals (Haffajee et al. 1998; Teles et al. 2008). A study using checkerboard DNA–DNA hybridization demonstrated that pathogenic bacteria in maintenance subjects remained significantly higher when compared with healthy subjects (Teles et al. 2008). Contrary to this, using the same method, another study did not find any significant difference between the same two groups of patients (Flemmig & Beikler 2011).

A study by Lu et al. (2020) was done on the subgingival microbiota in well-maintained periodontitis patients and healthy patients. When comparisons were made between the two groups, a significantly lower microbial richness and a significantly higher microbial diversity were found in the well-maintained group of patients compared with the healthy group. Furthermore, well-maintained individuals were shown to harbor a more pathogenic composition than healthy individuals. This included among others *Spirochaetes* and *Bacteroidetes* (at phylum level); significantly more abundant periodontitis-associated genera, such as *Treponema* and *Leptotrichia*, and less health-associated genera, such as *Streptococcus* and *Granulicatella* (at genus level); *Streptococcus 058*, *Neisseriamucosa*, *Neisseria flavescens*, *Granulicatella adiacens*, *Gemella morbillorum*, and *Neisseria oralis* were significantly lower (at species level); while *Leptotrichia hongkongensis*, *Capnocytophaga granulosa*, *Cardiobacterium hominis*, *Capnocytophaga 336*, *Capnocytophaga leadbetteri*, *Capnocytophaga sputigena*, *Selenomonas noxia*, *Capnocytophaga 326*, *Prevotella saccharolytica*, and *Treponema socranskii* were significantly higher (at species level) (Lu et al. 2020).

Network analysis was also performed with core genera to determine interactions among genera and microbial structure. The network of the well-maintained group of patients showed a much more complex pathogenic composition and more robust interactions than the health group. This included periodontitis-associated bacteria, such as the genus of *Porphyromonas*, *Tannerella*, *Prevotella*, and *Fusobacterium*, which formed an intertwined symbiotic network including multiple robust interactions with other microbiota. The healthy group showed a network that was sparse and balanced (Lu et al. 2020). It was suggested that increased microbial diversity together with robust interactions revealed a more

Box 5.1.2 Virulence factors of *Porphyromonas gingivalis*

Capsule

- Encapsulated *P. gingivalis* strains are more virulent than non-encapsulated strains, and the type of capsule influences the initial adhesion of *P. gingivalis* to periodontal pocket epithelial cells, as well as causing perturbation of epithelial cells (Dierickx et al. 2003; How et al. 2016).
- The level and mechanism of co-aggregation between *P. gingivalis* and *Fusobacterium nucleatum* have been shown to be capsular dependent (Rosen & Sela 2006).
- Encapsulated *P. gingivalis* can modulate the host response by reducing the synthesis of interleukin(IL)-1, IL-6, and IL-8 by fibroblasts (Singh et al. 2011).
- Increased encapsulation is also correlated with increased resistance to phagocytosis, thereby increasing bacterial survival within host cells (Singh et al. 2011).

Fimbriae

- *P. gingivalis* fimbriae/pili are filamentous structures located on the *P. gingivalis* surface that enhance adhesion to extracellular matrix proteins, oral epithelium cells, and other commensal bacteria, and take part in the formation of the biofilm (Nagano et al. 2013).
- Fimbriae also specifically interact with the $\alpha5\beta1$-integrin of epithelial cells, which mediates bacterial adherence to and entry into host cells, as well as endothelial cells (Enersen et al. 2013).
- Fimbriae can activate the $\beta2$ integrin CR3 in a TLR2-dependent manner, representing another cellular adhesion signaling pathway in neutrophils, natural killer (NK) cells, and macrophages, and simultaneously inhibit the production of IL-12, thereby enhancing the capacity of *P. gingivalis* to evade death (Hajishengallis et al. 2013).
- The bacterium is then captured by cellular pseudopodia, which enables invagination to occur through the endosomal pathway. The intracellular localization of *P. gingivalis* may be specific to the type of host cell, and includes various cellular compartments, such as the cytoplasm, endosomes, and autophagosomes (Amano et al. 2010). *P. gingivalis* inhibits apoptosis in gingival epithelial cells to promote its intracellular persistence (Yilmaz et al. 2004).
- *P. gingivalis* uses its fimbriae to interact with lectin in dendritic cells, followed by internalization and survival within the dendritic cell. This can contribute to the systemic dissemination of *P. gingivalis* as an atherogenic phenotype (Amano et al. 2010).
- Long fimbrial proteins can activate human gingival epithelial cells through TLR2 together with soluble CD14 receptor, thereby upregulating IL-8 expression and nuclear factor kappa B (NF-kB) activation, which are involved in bone resorption (Hajishengallis et al. 2013).

- Minor fimbriae can stimulate epithelial cells to produce IL-1β, tumor necrosis factor (TNF)-α, and IL-6, and thus enhance the differentiation of osteoclast precursor cells and bone resorption by osteoclasts (Hajishengallis et al. 2013).
- Minor fimbriae stimulate the expression of TNF-α, IL-1α, IL-1β, and IL-6 cytokines in macrophages via the TLR2/complement receptor 3 (CR3) pathway, thus regulating immunity and mediating tissue damage (Wang et al. 2010).

Outer-membrane vesicles

- *P. gingivalis* releases outer-membrane vesicles (OMVs) in an extracellular manner. These OMVs contain components of outer-membrane constituents, including lipopolysaccharide (LPS), muramic acid, capsule, fimbriae, and proteases termed gingipains (Furuta et al. 2009a).
- OMV proteins from *P. gingivalis* are important aggregation factors on the cell surface, and are associated with the formation and maintenance of periodontal biofilms (Enersen et al. 2013).
- *P. gingivalis* OMVs also enter into gingival epithelial cells via an endocytosis pathway entailing lipid rafts through the actin filament assembly, whereby they are routed to early endosomes and subsequently to lysosomes (Furuta et al. 2009a).
- OMVs degrade cellular transferrin receptors and focal adhesion complex proteins, which results in depletion of intracellular transferrin and the inhibition of cellular migration, leading to cellular impairment (Furuta et al. 2009b).

Gingipains

- Gingipains are cysteine proteases and exist in the outer membranes, vesicles, and extracellular structures of *P. gingivalis* (Yongking et al. 2011), and collectively account for 85% of the extracellular proteolytic activity of *P. gingivalis* at infection sites (de Diego et al. 2014).
- *P. gingivalis* gingipains participate in the adhesion to oral epithelial cells. They also affect the composition of multimicrobial biofilms quantitatively and qualitatively (Hocevar et al. 2018), by functioning as ligands in the co-aggregation of the bacterium with other oral bacteria, such as *T. denticola*, *T. forsythia*, and *A. actinomycetemcomitans*, thereby promoting the colonization of *P. gingivalis* in dental plaque (Bao et al. 2014; Ito et al. 2010; Sakanaka et al. 2016).
- Due to the proteolytic action of gingipains, *P. gingivalis* cleaves or degrades a variety of host proteins to escape immune defense mechanisms, including immunomodulatory proteins, signaling pathway

regulatory proteins, extracellular matrix proteins such as collagen, activation of the host matrix metalloproteinases, inactivation of plasma proteinase inhibitors, and cleavage of cell-surface receptors and adhesion molecules (Hocevar et al. 2018; Potempa et al. 2000).

- Gingipains degrade fibrinogen and host heme proteins, contributing to inhibition of blood coagulation and increased bleeding, thereby enhancing the availability of hemin for bacterial growth (Sroka et al. 2001).
- Gingipains degrade antibacterial peptides, such as neutrophil-derived α-defensins (Bao et al. 2014).
- Gingipains suppress IL-8 production, thereby disrupting neutrophil migration into gingival tissues (Kumar et al. 2006).
- *P. gingivalis* causes the production of high levels of IL-10 by CD4+ and CD8+ T cells, which in turn potently inhibits interferon (IFN)-γ production by Th1 cells, thus ameliorating protective cell-mediated immunity against periodontal bacteria (Gemmell et al. 2007).
- *P. gingivalis* gingipains hydrolyze IL-12, thereby reducing IL-12–induced IFN-γ production by CD4 cells, causing a shift to a Th2 response (Yun et al. 2001).
- Gingipains degrade T-cell receptors, such as CD4 and CD8, thereby manipulating the adaptive immune response by subverting T-cell function (Bao et al. 2014; Gaddis et al. 2012).
- Gingipains downregulate mCD14 expression, resulting in low responsiveness of macrophages to *P. gingivalis* infection, which includes inhibition of nitrogen oxide production by macrophages, leading to more severe chronic inflammation (Jia et al. 2019; Wilensky et al. 2015).
- *P. gingivalis* can withstand the bactericidal lytic activity in blood serum by combating the complement system, e.g. gingipains adsorb to C4b components, thereby inhibiting the classical and lectin pathways of the complement system (Hajishengallis et al. 2013; Hertz et al. 2018).

Lipopolysaccharides

- *P. gingivalis* LPS is a bacterial endotoxin that is released after the lysis of bacteria or as free vesicles outward from the outer membranes of living bacteria (Singhrao & Olsen 2018).
- After acute infection, acute-phase proteins such as LPS-binding protein (LBP) are produced by hepatocytes, lung, and gastrointestinal epithelial cells. High concentrations of LBP inhibit inflammation induced by LPS (Zweigner et al. 2001), while low-concentration LBP–LPS complexes are transported to membrane CD14 (mCD14) or soluble CD14 (sCD14) receptors, thereafter to be internalized by Toll-like receptors (TLRs) (Ding & Jin 2014; Tsukamoto et al. 2018).
- The ability of gingival epithelial cells to secrete chemokine IL-8 is diminished, thereby affecting the activation of neutrophils, eosinophils, and basophils, this phenomenon being described as chemokine paralysis. This results in resistance to oxidative burst-killing by polymorphonuclear neutrophils (Darveau et al. 1998).
- Depending on environmental factors, such as hemin levels and phosphate availability, *P. gingivalis* LPS can have heterogeneous forms and, acting as a pathogen-associated molecular pattern, can interact with both TLR2 and TLR4 receptors, leading to the initiation of differential immunoinflammatory responses (Darveau et al. 2004; Rangarajan et al. 2017).
- For example, *P. gingivalis*–derived LPS activates TLR2 receptors, inducing a strong Th2 response (Hirschfeld et al. 2001; Pulendran et al. 2001).
- *P. gingivalis* LPS inhibits osteoblastic differentiation and mineralization in periodontal ligament stem cells that participate in periodontal tissue regeneration (Kato et al. 2014).

disordered microbiome, and furthermore that the presence of periodontitis-associated bacteria in the well-maintained group of patients can indicate a more dysbiotic microbiome. This study therefore provided evidence that the subgingival microflora in well-maintained patients is more dysbiotic and pathogenic than in healthy individuals, thus indicating a high susceptibility of recurrence for well-maintained patients with a history of periodontitis (Lu et al. 2020).

The oral biofilm and implications for control of periodontitis

Periodontal treatment approaches are based on complete removal of subgingival biofilms and associated calculus deposits, but they may also comprise the adjunctive use of local and/or systemic antimicrobials (Flemmig & Beikler 2011).

Mechanical removal

This may be technically demanding and is further impeded by limited access and impaired visibility into deeper periodontal pockets (Petersilka et al. 2002). Plaque and calculus residues may still be detected in irregularities of instrumented root surfaces, such as fine grooves, ridges, or lacunae, and in areas where the operator may have changed from one curette to another (Rateitschak-Plüss et al. 1992). Removal of calculus and plaque in furcation sites of multirooted teeth may also be limited, even when subgingival debridement is aided by endoscopy (Fleischer et al. 1989; Michaud et al. 2007).

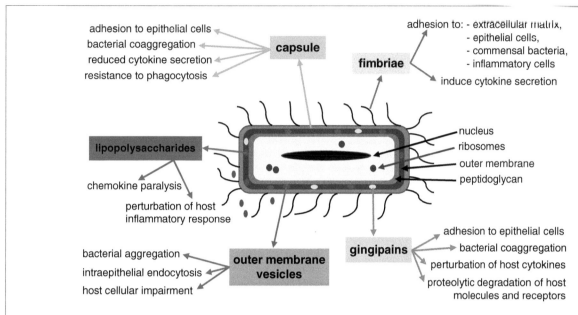

Figure 5.1.2 Virulence factors of *Porphyromonas gingivalis*. Courtesy of Dr. Steph Smith.

When forces are applied directly (e.g. by means of a curette), the viscoelastic nature of a biofilm may not be a crucial factor, but may be of importance when hydrodynamic forces are applied in a non-contact mode e.g. by means of sonic scalers during subgingival debridement or by brushing with powered toothbrushes. If enough energy is absorbed from the hydrodynamic forces and the viscoelastic deformation of the biofilm exceeds a given yield point, only then will biofilm removal occur (Busscher et al. 2010; Rmaile et al. 2014).

Antimicrobial therapy

Bacteria embedded in biofilms can be up to 1000 times more tolerant toward antimicrobials than their planktonic counterparts (Marsh 2004). The general consensus is that thorough subgingival debridement needs to be performed prior to adjunctive antimicrobial therapy in order to disrupt the subgingival biofilm structure (Jepsen & Jepsen 2016). The causes underlying the enhanced tolerance of biofilm-embedded bacteria toward antimicrobials are multifactorial (Mah & O'Toole 2001).

The degree of penetration of antimicrobials into the matrix depends on the thickness and the sorptive capacities of the biofilm, as well as on the respective antimicrobial-associated factors, such as its effective diffusivity within the biofilm, its reactivity with biofilm components, and its concentration and period of application (Stewart 2015). Some agents may exhibit retarded penetration, such as reactive oxidants, e.g. chlorine and hydrogen peroxide; and cationic molecules, including some antibiotics, chlorhexidine, or quaternary ammonium compounds (e.g. cetylpyridinium chloride). This may be ascribed to biofilm viscoelastic properties, reaction–diffusion

interactions, hydrophobic interactions, ionic interactions, and extracellular polymeric substances (De Beer et al. 1994; He et al. 2013; Sandt et al. 2007). It has also been demonstrated by confocal microscopy that positively charged chlorhexidine may only affect the outer layers of bacteria within biofilms formed in situ (Zaura-Arite et al. 2001).

Enhanced tolerance of biofilm bacteria toward antimicrobials may also be ascribed to the inactivation of antimicrobials by bacterial enzymes that originate either from lysed bacteria owing to antimicrobial exposure, or from active secretion by bacteria in the biofilm via membrane vesicles (Høiby et al. 2010; Mah & O'Toole 2001). Ampicillin has been shown to be unable to penetrate *Klebsiella pneumoniae* biofilms owing to the production of β-lactamase, an ampicillin-degrading enzyme (Anderl et al. 2000). Note should also be taken that some agents may be inactivated during their diffusion throughout the biofilm structure, and as a consequence this may lead to subinhibitory concentrations of antimicrobials in the deeper layers of biofilms, thus posing the risk of inducing drug resistances in bacteria (Block & Furman 2002; Cieplik et al. 2019; Roberts & Mullany 2010).

Summary

Microbial biofilm communities display properties that are more than the sum of the component species, and their characteristics cannot be inferred from studies of individual organisms (Diaz et al. 2014). In health, numerous interactions contribute to the stability and resilience of the ecosystem against environmental perturbations, presenting as a symbiotic homeostasis (Marsh 1989). When environmental pressures exceed thresholds that vary from patient to patient, then the competitiveness of certain bacteria is altered, which can then lead to a biofilm dysbiosis (Marsh & Zaura 2017). Shifts in the microbiome induced by inflammatory disease favor overgrowth of certain commensals, and this may also change the expression of virulence factors depending upon the repertoire of organisms that are present in a given niche. These virulence factors are furthermore up-regulated in presumed pathogens, as well as in health-associated commensals (Curtis et al. 2020). In susceptible patients, periodontal disease can develop due to a non-resolving innate and acquired immune response, which includes dysregulation in the production of proinflammatory mediators, leading to the production and release of host tissue–degrading enzymes (Page et al. 1997). The inflammatory response thus contributes to microbiome changes and to the expression of bacterial virulence factors (Curtis et al. 2020). Periodontal bacteria can then exploit mechanisms to evade host defenses, thereby enhancing their penetration into and colonization of host tissues, inducing direct tissue destruction through proteolytic and hydrolytic enzymes, as well as their toxic metabolites (Amano et al. 2014; Duran-Pinedo & Frias-Lopez 2015; Teles et al. 2013). Thus, to summarize in other words, the central component of the pathobiology in periodontitis is an aberrant (i.e. excessive) inflammatory immune response, which leads to the selective outgrowth of inflammatory pathobionts that can perpetuate periodontal inflammation, resulting in a vicious cycle for disease progression, whereby dysbiosis and inflammation reinforce each other (Loos & Van Dyke 2020). It is thus suggested that the inflammatory response and the microbiome are in bidirectional balance in oral health (homeostasis) and in bidirectional imbalance in periodontitis (Curtis et al. 2020).

Future considerations

There are still many unanswered questions regarding the role of the biofilm matrix in the complex interplay between bacteria and host. The biofilm matrix is a key factor regarding the enhancement of tolerance of biofilm-embedded bacteria toward mechanical removal, as well as toward antimicrobial approaches. Brushing and flossing remain the mainstay of oral hygiene, but these procedures may have limited efficacy in difficult-to-reach areas of the teeth, such as those present in periodontal pockets. New approaches designed to overcome these limitations include high-velocity water microdroplets, which can physically remove biofilms in interproximal spaces (Rmaile et al. 2014). Targeting the biofilm matrix, which includes disintegrating its bonds and shielding effects, can lead to the dispersal of biofilms and release of planktonic cells, as well as inducing changes in gene expression in bacteria, potentially making them more susceptible toward antimicrobials (McDougald et al. 2012). In this regard, matrix degrading or biofilm-dispersing enzymes have been considered as potential therapeutic agents (Kaplan 2009). Extracellular DNA is an important structural component within the biofilm matrix, and the dispersing effects of exogenously applied deoxyribonucleases on bacterial biofilms have been investigated in many in vitro studies (Okshevsky et al. 2015). However, many of these studies have been performed with monospecies biofilms, and extrapolating these results to complex biofilm communities such as dental plaque is difficult (Kaplan 2010). Other approaches targeting the biofilm matrix include bacteriophages, d-amino acids, modulation of cyclic dimeric guanosine monophosphate signaling pathways, or inhibitors of extracellular metabolic enzymes (Kaplan 2009; McDougald et al. 2012). Bacteriophages have been shown to incorporate polysaccharide depolymerase enzymes that can degrade the biofilm matrix of susceptible biofilms, leading to biofilm dispersal (Hughes et al. 1998). Engineered bacteriophages have been utilized to express glycoside hydrolase enzyme for simultaneously attacking bacterial cells and the biofilm matrix, and have shown a reduction of viable cell counts. However, bacteriophages are very difficult in clinical usage, as phages have to be customized according to the pathogens associated with biofilm formation (Lu & Collins 2007).

Identifying the microbiological profile of well-maintained periodontitis patients could establish essential baseline data for future applications in evaluating the effect of periodontal treatment. It is also important to assess the microbiological risk of maintained patients, as this can further lead to investigations as to why patients with a history of periodontitis may be more likely to suffer from peri-implant diseases (Lu et al. 2020).

REFERENCES

Abdi K, Chen T, Klein BA et al. Mechanisms by which *Porphyromonas gingivalis* evades innate immunity. *PLoS ONE*. 2017; 12:e0182164.

Abeles SR, Robles-Sikisaka R, Ly M et al. Human oral viruses are personal, persistent and gender-consistent. *ISME J*. 2014; 8(9):1753–1767.

Abusleme L, Hoare A, Hong B-Y, Diaz PI. Microbial signatures of health, gingivitis, and periodontitis. *Periodontol 2000*. 2021; 86(1):57–78. doi: 10.1111/prd.12362.

Akcali A, Huck O, Buduneli N, Davideau J-L, Tenenbaum H. Exposure of *Porphromonas gingivalis* to cortisol increases bacterial growth. *Arch Oral Biol*. 2014; 59(1):30–34.

Akcali A, Huck O, Tenenbaum H, Davideau JL, Buduneli N. Periodontal diseases and stress: a brief review. *J Oral Rehabil*. 2013; 40(1):60–68.

Al-Shayeb B, Sachdeva R, Chen L-X et al. Clades of huge phages from across Earth's ecosystems. *Nature*. 2020; 578(7795):425–431.

Allison DG. The biofilm matrix. *Biofouling.* 2003; 19:139–150.

Amano A, Chen C, Honma K et al. Genetic characteristics and pathogenic mechanisms of periodontal pathogens. *Adv Dent Res.* 2014; 26(1):15–22.

Amano A, Furuta N, Tsuda K. Host membrane trafficking for conveyance of intracellular oral pathogens. *Periodontol 2000.* 2010; 52:84–93.

Anderl JN, Franklin MJ, Stewart PS. Role of antibiotic penetration limitation in *Klebsiella pneumoniae* biofilm resistance to ampicillin and ciprofloxacin. *Antimicrob Agents Chemother.* 2000; 44:1818–1824.

Ardila CM, Guzman IC. Association of *Porphyromonas gingivalis* with high levels of stress-induced hormone cortisol in chronic periodontitis patients. *J Investig Clin Dent.* 2016; 7(4):361–367.

Bagaitkar J, Daep CA, Patel CK et al. Tobacco smoke augments *Porphyromonas gingivalis-Streptococcus gordonii* biofilm formation. *PLoS One.* 2011; 6(11):e27386.

Bagaitkar J, Williams LR, Renaud DE et al. Tobacco-induced alterations to *Porphyromonas gingivalis*-host interactions. *Environ Microbiol.* 2009; 11(5):1242–1253.

Bao K, Belibasakis GN, Thurnheer T et al. Role of *Porphyromonas gingivalis* gingipains in multi-species biofilm formation. *BMC Microbiol.* 2014; 14:258.

Barken KB, Pamp SJ, Yang L et al. Roles of type IV pili, flagellum-mediated motility and extracellular DNA in the formation of mature multicellular structures in *Pseudomonas aeruginosa* biofilms. *Environ Microbiol.* 2008; 10:2331–2343.

Barrangou R, Fremaux C, Deveau H et al. CRISPR provides acquired resistance against viruses in prokaryotes. *Science.* 2007; 315(5819):1709–1712.

Barth K, Remick DG, Genco CA. Disruption of immune regulation by microbial pathogens and resulting chronic inflammation. *J Cell Physiol.* 2013; 228:1413–1422.

Bensing BA, Siboo IR, Sullam PM. Proteins PblA and PblB of *Streptococcus mitis*, which promote binding to human platelets, are encoded within a lysogenic bacteriophage. *Infect Immun.* 2001; 69(10):6186–6192.

Bizarro S, Loos BG, Laine ML, Crielaard W, Zaura E. Subgingival microbiome in smokers and non-smokers in periodontitis: an exploratory study using traditional targeted techniques and a next-generation sequencing. *J Clin Periodontol.* 2013; 40(5):483–492.

Block C, Furman M. Association between intensity of chlorhexidine use and micro-organisms of reduced susceptibility in a hospital environment. *J Hosp Infect.* 2002; 51:201–206.

Borisy GG, Valm AM. Spatial scale in analysis of the dental plaque microbiome. *Periodontol 2000.* 2021; 86(1):97–112. doi: 10.1111/prd.12364.

Bos R, van der Mei HC, Busscher HJ. Physicochemistry of initial microbial adhesive interactions—its mechanisms and methods for study. *FEMS Microbiol Rev.* 1999; 23:179–230.

Boyanova L. Stress hormone epinephrine (adrenaline) and norepinephrine (noradrenaline) effects on anaerobic bacteria. *Anaerobe.* 2017; 44:13–19.

Brook I. Direct and indirect pathogenicity of beta-lactamase-producing bacteria in mixed infections in children. *Crit Rev Microbiol.* 1989; 16:161–180.

Brook I. The impact of smoking on oral and nasopharyngeal bacteria. *J Dent Res.* 2011; 90(6):704–710.

Buduneli N. Environmental factors and periodontal microbiome. *Periodontol 2000.* 2021; 85:112–123.

Busscher HJ, Jager D, Finger G, Schaefer N, van der Mei HC. Energy transfer, volumetric expansion, and removal of oral biofilms by non-contact brushing. *Scand J Dent Res.* 2010; 118:177–182.

Busscher HJ, Norde W, van der Mei HC. Specific molecular recognition and nonspecific contributions to bacterial interaction forces. *Appl Environ Microbiol.* 2008; 74:2559–2564.

Carpenter G. Salivary factors that maintain the normal oral commensal microflora. *J Dent Res.* 2020; 99:644–649.

Cho I, Blaser MJ. The human microbiome: at the interface of health and disease. *Nat Rev Genet.* 2012; 13(4):260–270.

Choi JW, Kim SC, Hong SH, Lee HJ. Secretable small RNAs via outer membrane vesicles in periodontal pathogens. *J Dent Res.* 2017; 96:458–466.

Chopra P, Kumar TS. Correlation of glucose level among venous, gingival and finger-prick blood samples in diabetic patients. *J Indian Soc Periodontol.* 2011; 15(3):288–291.

Cieplik F, Jakubovics NS, Buchalla W et al. Resistance toward chlorhexidine in oral bacteria—is there cause for concern? *Front Microbiol.* 2019; 10:587.

Cieplik F, Kara E, Muehler D et al. Antimicrobial efficacy of alternative compounds for use in oral care toward biofilms from caries-associated bacteria in vitro. *Microbiology Open.* 2019; 8:e00695.

Cornejo Ulloa PC, van der Veen MH, Krom BP. Review: modulation of the oral microbiome by the host to promote ecological balance. *Odontology.* 2019; 107(4):437–448.

Corrêa JD, Calderaro DC, Ferreira GA et al. Subgingival microbiota dysbiosis in systemic lupus erythematosus: association with periodontal status. *Microbiome.* 2017; 5(1):34.

Corrêa JD, Fernandes GR, Calderaro DC et al. Oral microbial dysbiosis linked to worsened periodontal condition in rheumatoid arthritis patients. *Sci Rep.* 2019; 9(1):8379.

Cosseau C, Devine DA, Dullaghan E et al. The commensal *Streptococcus salivarius* K12 downregulates the innate immune responses of human epithelial cells and promotes host–microbe homeostasis. *Infect Immun.* 2008; 76(9):4163–4175.

Couvigny B, Kulakauskas S, Pons N et al. Identification of new factors modulating adhesion abilities of the pioneer commensal bacterium *Streptococcus salivarius. Front Microbiol.* 2018; 9:273.

Curtis, M. Periodontal infections. In: *Clinical Periodontology and Implant Dentistry* (ed. NP Lang, J Lindhe). Chichester: Wiley; 2015: 169–182.

Curtis MA, Diaz PI, Van Dyke TE. The role of the microbiota in periodontal disease. *Periodontol 2000.* 2020; 83:14–25.

Damgaard C, Holmstrup P, Van Dyke TE, Nielsen CH. The complement system and its role in the pathogenesis of periodontitis: current concepts. *J Periodontal Res.* 2015; 50:283–293.

Darveau RP, Belton CM, Reife RA, Lamont RJ. Local chemokine paralysis, a novel pathogenic mechanism for *Porphyromonas gingivalis. Infect Immun.* 1998; 66:1660–1665.

Darveau RP, Pham T-TT, Lemley K et al. *Porphyromonas gingivalis* lipopolysaccharide contains multiple lipid A species that functionally interact with both toll-like receptors 2 and 4. *Infect Immun.* 2004; 72:5041–5051.

Davies EV, Winstanley C, Fothergill JL, James CE. The role of temperate bacteriophages in bacterial infection. *FEMS Microbiol Lett.* 2016; 363(5):fnw015.

De Beer D, Srinivasan R, Stewart PS. Direct measurement of chlorine penetration into biofilms during disinfection. *Appl Environ Microbiol.* 1994; 60:4339–4344.

de Diego I, Veillard F, Sztukowska MN et al. Structure and mechanism of cysteine peptidase Gingipain K(Kgp), a major virulence factor of *Porphyromonas gingivalis* in periodontitis. *J Biol Chem.* 2014; 289:32291–32302.

Delima SL, McBride RK, Preshaw PM, Haesman PA, Kumar PS. Response of subgingival bacteria to smoking cessation. *J Clin Microbiol.* 2010; 48(7):2344–2349.

Dewhirst FE, Chen T, Izard J et al. The human oral microbiome. *J Bacteriol.* 2010; 192(19):5002–5017.

Diaz PI, Hoare A, Hong BY. Subgingival microbiome shifts and community dynamics in periodontal diseases. *J Calif Dent Assoc.* 2016; 44(7):421–435.

Diaz PI, Strausbaugh LD, Dongari-Bagtzoglou A. Fungal-bacterial interactions and their relevance to oral health: linking the clinic and the bench. *Front Cell Infect Microbiol.* 2014; 4:101.

Dierickx K, Pauwels M, Laine ML et al. Adhesion of *Porphyromonas gingivalis* serotypes to pocket epithelium. *J Periodontol.* 2003; 74:844–848.

Ding PH, Jin L. The role of lipopolysaccharide-binding protein in innate immunity: a revisit and its relevance to oral/periodontal health. *J Periodont Res.* 2014; 49:1–9.

Ding T, Schloss PD. Dynamics and associations of microbial community types across the human body. *Nature.* 2014; 509(7500):357–360.

Dixon DR, Bainbridge BW, Darveau RP. Modulation of the innate immune response within the periodontium. *Periodontol 2000.* 2004; 35:53–74.

Doron S, Melamed S, Ofir G et al. Systematic discovery of antiphage defense systems in the microbial pangenome. *Science.* 2018; 359(6379):eaar4120.

Duran-Pinedo AE, Chen T, Teles R et al. Community-wide transcriptome of the oral microbiome in subjects with and without periodontitis. *ISME J.* 2014; 8(8):1659–1672.

Duran-Pinedo AE, Frias-Lopez J. Beyond microbial community composition: functional activities of the oral microbiome in health and disease. *Microbes Infect.* 2015; 17:505–516.

Ebersole JL. Humoral immune responses in gingival crevice fluid: local and systemic implications. *Periodontol 2000.* 2003; 31:135–166.

Enersen M, Nakano K, Amano A. *Porphyromonas gingivalis fimbriae. J Oral Microbiol.* 2013; 5:e20265.

Fleischer HC, Mellonig JT, Brayer WK, Gray JL, Barnett JD. Scaling and root planing efficacy in multirooted teeth. *J Periodontol.* 1989; 60:402–409.

Flemmig TF, Beikler T. Control of oral biofilms. *Periodontol 2000.* 2011; 55:9–15.

Flemming HC, Wingender J. The biofilm matrix. *Nat Rev Microbiol.* 2010; 8:623–633.

Flemming HC, Wuertz S. Bacteria and archaea on Earth and their abundance in biofilms. *Nat Rev Microbiol.* 2019; 17:247–260.

Furuta N, Takeuchi H, Amano A. Entry of *Porphyromonas gingivalis* outer membrane vesicles into epithelial cells causes cellular functional impairment. *Infect Immun.* 2009; 77:4761–4770.

Furuta N, Tsuda K, Omori H et al. *Porphyromonas gingivalis* outer membrane vesicles enter human epithelial cells via an endocytic pathway and are sorted to lysosomal compartments. *Infect Immun.* 2009; 77:4187–4196.

Fux CA, Costerton JW, Stewart PS, Stoodley P. Survival strategies of infectious biofilms. *Trends Microbiol.* 2005; 13:34–40.

Gaddis DE, Maynard CL, Weaver CT, Michalek SM, Katz J. Role of TLR2 dependent-IL-10 production in the inhibition of the initial IFN-g T cell response to *Porphyromonas gingivalis. J Leukoc Biol.* 2012; 93:21–31.

Ganesan SM, Joshi V, Fellows M et al. A tale of two risks: smoking, diabetes and the subgingival microbiome. *ISME J.* 2017; 11(9):2075–2089.

Gemmell E, Yamazaki K, Seymour GJ. The role of T-cells in periodontal disease: homeostasis and autoimmunity. *Periodontol 2000.* 2007; 43:14–40.

Genco RJ, Ho AW, Grossi SG, Dunford RG, Tedesco LA. Relationship of stress, distress and inadequate coping behaviors to periodontal disease. *J Periodontol.* 1999; 70(7):711–723.

Gibbons RJ, Hay DI, Cisar JO, Clark WB. Adsorbed salivary proline-rich protein 1 and statherin: receptors for type 1 fimbriae of *Actinomyces viscosus* T14V-11 on apatite surfaces. *Infect Immun.* 1988; 56:2990–2993.

Gogokhia L, Buhrke K, Bell R et al. Expansion of bacteriophages is linked to aggravated intestinal inflammation and colitis. *Cell Host Microbe.* 2019; 25(2):285–299.e8.

Gonçalves LS, Ferreira DDC, Heng NCK et al. Oral bacteriome of HIV-1-infected children from Rio de Janeiro, Brazil: next-generation DNA sequencing analysis. *J Clin Periodontol.* 2019; 46(12):1192–1204.

Górski A, Międzybrodzki R, Borysowski J et al. Phage as a modulator of immune responses: practical implications for phage therapy. *Adv Virus Res.* 2012; 83:41–71.

Graziano TS, Closs P, Poppi T et al. Catecholamines promote the expression of virulence and oxidative stress genes in

Porphyromonas gingivalis. J Periodontal Res. 2014; 49(5):660–669.

Grenier D. Nutritional interactions between two suspected periodontopathogens, *Treponema denticola* and *Porphyromonas gingivalis. Infect Immun.* 1992; 60:5298–5301.

Grohmann E, Christie PJ, Waksman G, Backert S. Type IV secretion in gram-negative and gram-positive bacteria. *Mol Microbiol.* 2018; 107:455–471.

Guo L, He X, Shi W. Intercellular communications in multispecies oral microbial communities. *Front Microbiol.* 2014; 5:328.

Haffajee AD, Cugini MA, Tanner A et al. Subgingival microbiota in healthy, well-maintained elder and periodontitis subjects. *J Clin Periodontol.* 1998; 25:346–353.

Hajishengallis G. The inflammophilic character of the periodontitis-associated microbiota. *Mol Oral Microbiol.* 2014; 29(6):248–257.

Hajishengallis G, Abe T, Maekawa T, Hajishengallis E, Lambris JD. Role of complement in host–microbe homeostasis of the periodontium. *Semin Immunol.* 2013; 25:65–72.

Hajishengallis G, Lamont RJ. Breaking bad: manipulation of the host response by *Porphyromonas gingivalis. Eur J Immunol.* 2014; 44:328–338.

Hajishengallis G, McIntosh ML, Nishiyama SI, Yoshimura F. Mechanism and implications of CXCR4-mediated integrin activation by *Porphyromonas gingivalis. Mol Oral Microbiol.* 2013; 28:239–249.

Hakenbeck R, Konog A, Kern I et al. Acquisition of five high-Mr penicillin-binding protein variants during transfer of high-level beta-lactam resistance from *Streptococcus mitis* to *Streptococcus pneumoniae. J Bacteriol.* 1998; 180:1831–1840.

Halhoul N, Colvin JR. Virus-like particles in association with a microorganism from human gingival plaque. *Arch Oral Biol.* 1975; 20:833–836.

Hampton HG, Watson BNJ, Fineran PC. The arms race between bacteria and their phage foes. *Nature.* 2020; 577(7790):327–336.

Hannig C, Hannig M, Attin T. Enzymes in the acquired enamel pellicle. *Eur J Oral Sci.* 2005; 113:2–13.

Hannig C, Hoch J, Becker K, Hannig M, Attin T. Lysozyme activity in the initially formed in situ pellicle. *Arch Oral Biol.* 2005; 50:821–828.

Hannig C, Spitzmuller B, Hannig M. Characterisation of lysozyme activity in the in situ pellicle using a fluorimetric assay. *Clin Oral Investig.* 2009; 13:15–21.

Hannig C, Spitzmuller B, Knausenberger S et al. Detection and activity of peroxidase in the in situ formed enamel pellicle. *Arch Oral Biol.* 2008; 53:849–858.

Hannig M. Ultrastructural investigation of pellicle morphogenesis at two different intraoral sites during a 24-h period. *Clin Oral Investig.* 1999; 3:88–95.

Hannig M, Khanafer AK, Hoth-Hannig W, Al-Marrawi F, Açil Y. Transmission electron microscopy comparison of methods for collecting in situ formed enamel pellicle. *Clin Oral Investig.* 2005; 9:30–37.

Harbeck B, Suefke S, Haas CS et al. No stress after 24-hour on-call shifts? *J Occup Health.* 2015; 57(5):438–447.

He Y, Peterson BW, Jongsma MA et al. Stress relaxation analysis facilitates a quantitative approach towards antimicrobial penetration into biofilms. *PLoS One.* 2013; 8:e63750.

Heller D, Helmerhorst EJ, Oppenheim FG. Saliva and serum protein exchange at the tooth enamel surface. *J Dent Res.* 2017; 96:437–443.

Henderson B, Wilson M. Commensal communism and the oral cavity. *J Dent Res.* 1998; 77:1674–1683.

Hendrickson EL, Beck DA, Miller DP et al. Insights into dynamic polymicrobial synergy revealed by time-coursed RNA-Seq. *Front Microbiol.* 2017; 8:261.

Hertz CE, Bayarri-Olmos R, Kirketerp-Møller N et al. Chimeric proteins containing MAP-1 and functional domains of C4b-binding protein reveal strong complement inhibitory capacities. *Front Immunol.* 2018; 9:1945.

Hirschfeld J, Dommisch H, Skora P et al. Neutrophil extracellular trap formation in supragingival biofilms. *Int J Med Microbiol.* 2015; 305:453–463.

Hirschfeld M, Weis JJ, Toshchakov V et al. Signaling by Toll-like receptor 2 and 4 agonists results in differential gene expression in murine macrophages. *Infect and Immun.* 2001; 69:1477–1482.

Ho MH, Chen CH, Goodwin JS, Wang BY, Xie H. Functional advantages of *Porphyromonas gingivalis* vesicles. *PLoS One.* 2015; 10:e0123448.

Hocevar K, Potempa J, Turk B. Host cell-surface proteins as substrates of gingipains, the main proteases of *Porphyromonas gingivalis. Biol Chem.* 2018; 399:1353–1361.

Høiby N, Bjarnsholt T, Givskov M, Molin S, Ciofu O. Antibiotic resistance of bacterial biofilms. *Int J Antimicrob Agents.* 2010; 35:322–332.

Hojo K, Nagaoka S, Ohshima T, Maeda N. Bacterial interactions in dental biofilm development. *J Dent Res.* 2009; 88:982–990.

Hong B-Y, Furtado Araujo MV et al. Microbiome profiles in periodontitis in relation to host and disease characteristics. *PLoS One.* 2015; 10:e0127077.

How, KY, Song, KP, Chan KG. *Porphyromonas gingivalis*: an overview of periodontopathic pathogen below the gum line. *Front Microbiol.* 2016; 7:53.

Howard-Varona C, Hargreaves KR, Abedon ST, Sullivan MB. Lysogeny in nature: mechanisms, impact and ecology of temperate phages. *ISME J.* 2017; 11(7):1511–1520.

Hughes KA, Sutherland IW, Jones MV. Biofilm susceptibility to bacteriophage attack: the role of phage-borne polysaccharide depolymerase. *Microbiology.* 1998; 144:3039–3047.

Human Microbiome Project Consortium. Structure, function and diversity of the healthy human microbiome. *Nature.* 2012; 486(7402):207–214.

Hutcherson JA, Scott DA, Bagaitkar J. Scratching the surface-tobacco-induced bacterial biofilms. *Tob Induced Dis.* 2015; 13(1):1.

Imamura K, Kokubu E, Kita D et al. Cigarette smoke condensate modulates migration of human gingival epithelial cells and their interactions with *Porphyromonas gingivalis. J Periodontal Res.* 2015; 50(3):411–421.

Ito R, Ishihara K, Shoji M, Nakayama K, Okuda K. Hemagglutinin/adhesin domains of *Porphyromonas gingivalis* play key roles in coaggregation with *Treponema denticola. FEMS Immunol Med Microbiol.* 2010; 60:251–260.

Jakubovics NS. Intermicrobial interactions as a driver for community composition and stratification of oral biofilms. *J Mol Biol.* 2015; 427:3662–3675.

Jakubovics NS, Burgess JG. Extracellular DNA in oral microbial biofilms. *Microbes Infect.* 2015; 17(7):531–537.

Jakubovics NS, Goodman SD, Mashburn-Warren L, Stafford GP, Cieplik F. The dental plaque biofilm matrix. *Periodontol 2000.* 2020; 86(1):32–56.

Jakubovics NS, Kolenbrander PE. The road to ruin: the formation of disease-associated oral biofilms. *Oral Dis.* 2010; 16:729–739.

Jentsch HFR, Marz D, Krüger M. The effects of stress hormones on growth of selected periodontitis related bacteria. *Anaerobe.* 2013; 24:49–54.

Jepsen K, Jepsen S. Antibiotics/antimicrobials: systemic and local administration in the therapy of mild to moderately advanced periodontitis. *Periodontol 2000.* 2016; 71:82–112.

Jia L, Han N, Du J et al. Pathogenesis of important virulence factors of *Porphyromonas gingivalis* via Toll-like receptors. *Front Cell Infect Microbiol.* 2019; 9:262.

Jin Y, Yip H-K. Supragingival calculus: formation and control. *Crit Rev Oral Biol Med.* 2002; 13(5): 426–441.

Johnston DA, Bodley GP. Oropharyngeal cultures of patients in protected environmental units: evaluation of semiquantitative technique during antibiotic prophylaxis. *Appl Microbiol.* 1972; 23(5):846–851.

Joshi V, Matthews C, Aspiras M et al. Smoking decreases structural and functional resilience in the subgingival ecosystem. *J Clin Periodontol.* 2014; 41(11):1037–1047.

Kanmaz B, Lamont G, Danacı G et al. Microbiological and biochemical findings in relation to clinical periodontal status in active smokers, non-smokers and passive smokers. *Tob Induc Dis.* 2019; 17:20.

Kaplan CW, Lux R, Haake SK, Wenyuan Shi. The *Fusobacterium nucleatum* outer membrane protein RadD is an arginine-inhibitable adhesin required for inter-species adherence and the structured architecture of multi-species biofilm. *Mol Microbiol.* 2009; 71(1):35–47.

Kaplan JB. Therapeutic potential of biofilm-dispersing enzymes. *Int J Artif Organs.* 2009; 32:545–554.

Kaplan JB. Biofilm dispersal. Mechanisms, clinical implications, and potential therapeutic uses. *J Dent Res.* 2010 Mar; 89(3):205–218.

Kato H, Taguchi Y, Tominaga K, Umeda M, Tanaka A. *Porphyromonas gingivalis* LPS inhibits osteoblastic differentiation and promotes pro-inflammatory cytokine production in human periodontal ligament stem cells. *Arch Oral Biol.* 2014; 59:167–175.

Kieselbach T, Zijnge V, Granström E, Oscarsson J. Proteomics of *Aggregatibacter actinomycetemcomitans* outer membrane vesicles. *PLoS One.* 2015; 10:e0138591.

Kilian M. The oral microbiome-friend or foe? *Eur J Oral Sci.* 2018; 126(Suppl. 1):5–12.

Kolenbrander PE. Multispecies communities: interspecies interactions influence growth on saliva as sole nutritional source. *Int J Oral Sci.* 2011; 3:49–54.

Kolenbrander PE, Palmer RJ Jr, Periasamy S, Jakubovics NS. Oral multispecies biofilm development and the key role of cell–cell distance. *Nat Rev Microbiol.* 2010; 8:471–480.

Kolenbrander PE, Palmer RJ Jr, Rickard AH et al. Bacterial interactions and successions during plaque development. *Periodontol 2000.* 2006; 42:47–79.

Kort R, Caspers M, van de Graaf A et al. Shaping the oral microbiota through intimate kissing. *Microbiome.* 2014; 2(1):41.

Koskella B, Meaden S. Understanding bacteriophage specificity in natural microbial communities. *Viruses.* 2013; 5(3):806–823.

Kreth J, Giacaman RA, Raghavan R, Merritt J. The road less traveled – defining molecular commensalism with *Streptococcus sanguinis. Mol Oral Microbiol.* 2016; 32(3):181–196.

Kumar PS, Clark P, Brinkman MC, Saxena D. Novel nicotine delivery systems. *Advance Dent Res.* 2019; 30(1):11–15.

Kumar PS, Leys EJ, Bryk JM et al. Changes in periodontal health status are associated with bacterial community shifts as assessed by quantitative 16S cloning and sequencing. *J Clin Microbiol.* 2006; 44:3665–3673.

Kumar PS, Matthews CR, Joshi V, de Jager M, Aspiras M. Tobacco smoking affects bacterial acquisition and colonization in oral biofilms. *Infect Immun.* 2011; 79(11):4730–4738.

Kurniawan A, Yamamoto T, Tsuchiya Y, Morisaki H. Analysis of the ion adsorption-desorption characteristics of biofilm matrices. *Microbes Environ.* 2012; 27:399–406.

Lamont RJ, Hajishengallis G. Polymicrobial synergy and dysbiosis in inflammatory disease. *Trends Mol Med.* 2015; 21(3):172–183.

Lamont RJ, Koo H, Hajishengallis G. The oral microbiota: dynamic communities and host interactions. *Nat Rev Microbiol.* 2018; 16(12):745–759.

Larsen T, Fiehn N-E. Dental biofilm infections – an update. *APMIS.* 2017; 125:376–384.

Lasserre JF, Brecx MC, Toma S. Oral microbes, biofilms and their role in periodontal and peri-implant diseases. *Materials.* 2018; 11:1802.

Leresche L, Dworkin SF. The role of stress in inflammatory disease, including periodontal disease: review of concepts and current findings. *Periodontol 2000.* 2003; 30:91–103.

Li Y-H, Tang N, Aspiras MB et al. A quorum-sensing signaling system essential for genetic competence in *Streptococcus mutans* is involved in biofilm formation. *J Bacteriol.* 2002; 84:2699–2708.

Liao S, Klein MI, Heim KP et al. Streptococcus mutans extracellular DNA is upregulated during growth in biofilms, actively released via membrane vesicles, and influenced by components of the protein secretion machinery. *J Bacteriol.* 2014; 196:2355–2366.

Lin W, Jiang W, Hu X et al. Ecological shifts of supragingival microbiota in association with pregnancy. *Front Cell Infect Microbiol.* 2018; 8:24.

Lloyd-Price J, Abu-Ali G, Huttenhower C. The healthy human microbiome. *Genome Medicine.* 2016; 8:51.

Long J, Cai Q, Steinwandel M et al. Association of oral microbiome with type 2 diabetes risk. *J Periodontal Res.* 2017; 52(3):636–643.

Longo PL, Dabdoub S, Kumar P et al. Glycaemic status affects the subgingival microbiome of diabetic patients. *J Clin Periodontol.* 2018; 45(8):932–940.

Loos BG, Van Dyke TE. The role of inflammation and genetics in periodontal disease. *Periodontol 2000.* 2020; 83:26–39.

Lopez-Oliva I, Paropkari AD, Saraswat S et al. Dysbiotic subgingival microbial communities in periodontally healthy patients with rheumatoid arthritis. *Arthritis Rheumatol.* 2018; 70(7):1008–1013.

Lu H, He L, Xu J et al. Well-maintained patients with a history of periodontitis still harbor a more dysbiotic microbiome than health. *J Periodontol.* 2020; 91:1584–1594.

Lu TK, Collins JJ. Dispersing biofilms with engineered enzymatic bacteriophage. *Proc Natl Acad Sci USA.* 2007; 104:11197–11202.

Luo G, Niesel DW, Shaban RA, Grimm EA, Klimpel GR. Tumor necrosis factor alpha binding to bacteria: evidence for a high-affinity receptor and alteration of bacterial virulence properties. *Infect Immun.* 1993; 61(3):830–835.

Ly M, Jones MB, Abeles SR et al. Transmission of viruses via our microbiomes. *Microbiome.* 2016; 4(1):64.

Lymperopoulos A, Rengo G, Zincarelli C, Soltys S, Koch WJ. Modulation of adrenal catecholamine secretion by in vivo gene transfer and manipulation of G protein–coupled receptor kinase-2 activity. *Mol Ther.* 2008; 16:302–307.

Lyte M. The role of microbial endocrinology in infectious disease. *J Endocrinol.* 1993; 137(3):343–345.

Maekawa T, Krauss J, Abe T et al. *Porphyromonas gingivalis* manipulates complement and TLR signaling to uncouple bacterial clearance from inflammation and promote dysbiosis. *Cell Host Microbe.* 2014; 15(6):768–778.

Mah TF, O'Toole GA. Mechanisms of biofilm resistance to antimicrobial agents. *Trends Microbiol.* 2001; 9:34–39.

Marchesan JT, Jiao Y, Moss K et al. Common polymorphisms in IFI16 and AIM2 genes are associated with periodontal disease. *J Periodontol.* 2017; 88(7):663–672.

Marsh PD. Host defenses and microbial homeostasis: role of microbial interactions. *J Dent Res.* 1989; 68:1567–1575.

Marsh PD. Role of the oral microflora in health. *Microb Ecol Health Dis.* 2000; 12:130–137.

Marsh PD. Dental plaque as a microbial biofilm. *Caries Res.* 2004; 38:204–211.

Marsh PD. Dental biofilms. In: *Clinical Periodontology and Implant Dentistry* (ed. NP Lang, J Lindhe). Chichester: Wiley; 2015: 169–182.

Marsh PD, Devine DA. How is the development of dental biofilms influenced by the host? *J Clin Periodontol.* 2011; 38(Suppl 11):28–35.

Marsh PD, Zaura E. Dental biofilm: ecological interactions in health and disease. *J Clin Periodontol.* 2017; 44(Suppl. 18):S12–S22.

Mason MR, Preshaw PM, Nagaraja HN et al. The subgingival microbiome of clinically healthy current and never smokers. *ISME J.* 2015; 9(1):268–272.

Matthews CR, Joshi V, de Jager M, Aspiras M, Kumar PS. Host-bacterial interactions during induction and resolution of experimental gingivitis in current smokers. *J Periodontol.* 2013; 84(1):32–40.

McDougald D, Rice SA, Barraud N, Steinberg PD, Kjelleberg S. Should we stay or should we go: mechanisms and ecological consequences for biofilm dispersal. *Nat Rev Microbiol.* 2012; 10:39–50.

Menezes AR, Liavie CJ, Milani RV, O'Keefe J, Lavie TJ. Psychological risk factors and cardiovascular disease: is it all in your head? *Postgrad Med.* 2011; 123(5):165–176.

Meulman T, Casarin RC, Peruzzo DC et al. Impact of supragingival therapy on subgingival microbial profile in smokers versus non-smokers with severe chronic periodontitis. *J Oral Microbiol.* 2012; 4(1):8640.

Michaud RM, Schoolfield J, Mellonig JT, Mealey BL. The efficacy of subgingival calculus removal with endoscopy-aided scaling and root planing: a study on multirooted teeth. *J Periodontol.* 2007; 78:2238–2245.

Mieher JL, Larson MR, Schormann N et al. Glucan binding protein C of *Streptococcus mutans* mediates both sucrose-independent and sucrose-dependent adherence. *Infect Immun.* 2018; e00146–18.

Mikhailova ES, Koroleva IV, Kolesnikova PA, Ermolaeva LA, Suvorov AN. The characteristics of microbiota of periodontal recesses in smoking patients with chronic generalised periodontitis. *Klin Lab Diagn.* 2017; 62(2):107–111.

Miller DP, Fitzsimonds ZR, Lamont RJ. Metabolic signaling and spatial Interactions in the oral polymicrobial community. *J Dent Res.* 2019; 98:1308–1314.

Mysak J, Podzimek S, Sommerova P et al. *Porphyromonas gingivalis*: major periodontopathic pathogen overview. *J Immunol Res.* 2014; 2014:476068.

Nagano K, Abiko Y, Yoshida Y, Yoshimura F. Genetic and antigenic analyses of *Porphyromonas gingivalis* FimA fimbriae. *Mol Oral Microbiol.* 2013; 28:392–403.

Nguyen S, Baker K, Padman BS et al. Bacteriophage transcytosis provides a mechanism to cross epithelial cell layers. *MBio.* 2017; 8(6):e01874–17.

Nobbs AH, Jenkinson HF, Jakubovics NS. Stick to your gums: mechanisms of oral microbial adherence. *J Dent Res.* 2011; 90:1271–1278.

Nyako EA, Watson CJ, Preston AJ. Determination of the pH of peri-implant crevicular fluid in successful and failing dental implant sites: a pilot study. *Arch Oral Biol.* 2005; 50:1055–1059.

Okshevsky M, Regina VR, Meyer RL. Extracellular DNA as a target for biofilm control. *Curr Opin Biotechnol.* 2015; 33:73–80.

Olczak T, Simpson W, Liu X, Genco CA. Iron and heme utilization in *Porphyromonas gingivalis. FEMS Microbiol Rev.* 2005; 29:119–144.

Olsen I, Tribble GD, Fiehn N-E, Wang B-Y. Bacterial sex in dental plaque. *J Oral Microbiol.* 2013; 2013:5.

Paez-Espino D, Zhou J, Roux S et al. Diversity, evolution, and classification of virophages uncovered through global metagenomics. *Microbiome.* 2019; 7(1):157.

Page RC, Offenbacher S, Schroeder HE, Seymour GJ, Kornman KS. Advances in the pathogenesis of periodontitis: summary of developments, clinical implications and future directions. *Periodontol 2000.* 1997; 14:216–248.

Paramonova E, Kalmykowa OJ, van der Mei HC, Busscher HJ, Sharma PK. Impact of hydrodynamics on oral biofilm strength. *J Dent Res.* 2009; 88:922–926.

Park O.-J, Yi H, Jeon JH et al. Pyrosequencing analysis of subgingival microbiota in distinct periodontal conditions. *J Dent Res.* 2015; 94:921–927.

Paropkari AD, Leblebicioglu B, Christian LM, Kumar PS. Smoking, pregnancy and the subgingival microbiome. *Sci Rep.* 2016; 6:30388.

Patel M, Coogan M, Galpin JS. Periodontal pathogens in subgingival plaque of HIV-positive subjects with chronic periodontitis. *Oral Microbiol Immunol.* 2003; 18(3):199–201.

Periasamy S, Kolenbrander PE. Central role of the early colonizer *Veillonella* sp. in establishing multispecies biofilm communities with initial, middle, and late colonizers of enamel. *J Bacteriol.* 2010; 192(12):2965–2972.

Perry JA, Cvitkovitch DG, Levesque CM. Cell death in *Streptococcus mutans* biofilms: a link between CSP and extracellular DNA. *FEMS Microbiol Lett.* 2009; 299:261–266.

Peruzzo DC, Benatti BB, Ambrosano GM et al. A systematic review of stress and psychological factors as possible risk factors for periodontal disease. *J Periodontol.* 2007; 78(8):1491–1504.

Petersilka GJ, Ehmke B, Flemmig TF. Antimicrobial effects of mechanical debridement. *Periodontol 2000.* 2002; 28:56–71.

Peterson BW, He Y, Ren Y et al. Viscoelasticity of biofilms and their recalcitrance to mechanical and chemical challenges. *FEMS Microbiol Rev.* 2015; 39:234–245.

Pires DP, Oliveira H, Melo LD, Sillankorva S, Azeredo J. Bacteriophage-encoded depolymerases: their diversity and biotechnological applications. *Appl Microbiol Biotechnol.* 2016; 100(5):2141–2151.

Porat R, Clark BD, Wolff SM, Dinarello CA. Enhancement of growth of virulent strains of *Escherichia coli* by interleukin-1. *Science.* 1991; 254(5030):430–432.

Potempa J, Banbula A, Travis J. Role of bacterial proteinases in matrix destruction and modulation of host responses. *Periodontol 2000.* 2000; 24:153–192.

Preus HR, Olsen I, Namork E. Association between bacteriophage-infected *Actinobacillus actinomycetemcomitans* and rapid periodontal destruction. *J Clin Periodontol.* 1987; 14(4):245–247.

Pride DT, Salzman J, Haynes M et al. Evidence of a robust resident bacteriophage population revealed through analysis of the human salivary virome. *ISME J.* 2012; 6:915–926.

Pulendran B, Kumar P, Cutler CW et al. Lipopolysaccharides from distinct pathogens induce different classes of immune responses in vivo. *J Immunol.* 2001; 167:5067–5076.

Queiroz AC, Suaid FA, de Andrade PF et al. Antimicrobial photodynamic therapy associated to nonsurgical periodontal treatment in smokers: microbiological results. *J Photochem Photobiol B.* 2014; 141:170–175.

Rangarajan M, Aduse-Opoku J, Paramonov N, Hashim A, Curtis M. Hemin binding by *Porphyromonas gingivalis* strains is dependent on the presence of A-LPS. *Mol Oral Microbiol.* 2017; 32:365–374.

Rateitschak-Plüss EM, Schwarz JP, Guggenheim R, Düggelin M, Rateitschak KH. Non-surgical periodontal treatment: where are the limits? *An SEM study. J Clin Periodontol.* 1992; 19:240–244.

Raya RR, H'Bert EM. Isolation of phage via induction of lysogens. *Methods Mol Biol.* 2009; 501:23–32.

Rmaile A, Carugo D, Capretto L et al. Removal of interproximal dental biofilms by high-velocity water microdrops. *J Dent Res.* 2014; 93:68–73.

Roberts A, Matthews JB, Socransky SS et al. Stress and the periodontal diseases: effects of catecholamines on the growth of periodontal bacteria in vitro. *Oral Microbiol Immunol.* 2002; 17(5):296–303.

Roberts AP, Kreth J. The impact of horizontal gene transfer on the adaptive ability of the human oral microbiome. *Front Cell Infect Microbiol.* 2014; 4:124.

Roberts AP, Mullany P. Oral biofilms: a reservoir of transferable, bacterial, antimicrobial resistance. *Expert Rev Anti Infect Ther.* 2010; 8:1441–1450.

Rosan B, Lamont RJ. Dental plaque formation. *Microbes Infect.* 2000; 2(13):1599–1607.

Rosen G, Sela MN. Coaggregation of *Porphyromonas gingivalis* and *Fusobacterium nucleatum* PK 1594 is mediated by capsular polysaccharide and lipopolysaccharide. *FEMS Microbiol Lett.* 2006; 256:304–310.

Rosier BT, Marsh PD, Mira A. Resilience of the oral microbiota in health: mechanisms that prevent dysbiosis. *J Dent Res.* 2018; 97(4):371–380.

Saeb ATM, Al-Rubeaan KA, Aldosary K et al. Relative reduction of biological and phylogenetic diversity of the oral microbiota of diabetes and pre-diabetes patients. *Microb Pathog.* 2019; 128:215–229.

Saktanala A, Takeuchi H, Kuboniwa M, Amano A. Dual lifestyle of *Porphyromonas gingivalis* in biofilm and gingival cells. *Microb Pathog.* 2016; 94:42–47.

Sandt C, Barbeau J, Gagnon M-A, Lafleur M. Role of the ammonium group in the diffusion of quaternary ammonium compounds in *Streptococcus mutans* biofilms. *J Antimicrob Chemother.* 2007; 60:1281–1287.

Saxena D, Li Y, Yang L et al. Human microbiome and HIV/AIDS. *Curr HIV/AIDS Rep.* 2012; 9(1):44–51.

Schmidt TS, Hayward MR, Coelho LP et al. Extensive transmission of microbes along the gastrointestinal tract. *eLife.* 2019; 8:e42693.

Scoffield JA, Wu H. Nitrite reductase is critical for *Pseudomonas aeruginosa* survival during co-infection with the oral commensal *Streptococcus parasanguinis. Microbiology.* 2016; 62(2):376–383.

Semenoff-Segundo A, Porto AN, Semenoff TA et al. Effects of two chronic stress models on ligature-induced periodontitis in Wistar rats. *Arch Oral Biol.* 2012; 57(1):66–72.

Shanker E, Federle MJ. Quorum sensing regulation of competence and bacteriocins in *Streptococcus pneumoniae* and *mutans. Genes.* 2017; 8:E15.

Shapira L, Frolow I. Experimental stress suppresses recruitment of macrophages but enhanced their *P. gingivalis* LPS-stimulated secretion of nitric oxide. *J Periodontol.* 2007; 71(3):476–481.

Shchipkova AY, Nagaraja HN, Kumar PS. Subgingival microbial profiles of smokers with periodontitis. *J Dent Res.* 2010; 89(11):1247–1253.

Shokeen B, Dinis MDB, Haghighi F, Tran NC, Lux R. Omics and interspecies interaction. *Periodontol 2000.* 2021; 85:101–111.

Shrivastava A, Patel VK, Tang Y et al. Cargo transport shapes the spatial organization of a microbial community. *Proc Natl Acad Sci USA.* 2018; 115:8633–8638.

Silpe JE, Bassler BL. A host-produced quorum-sensing autoinducer controls a phage lysis-lysogeny decision. *Cell.* 2019; 176(1–2):268–280.e13.

Singh A, Wyant T, Anaya-Bergman C et al. The capsule of *Porphyromonas gingivalis* leads to a reduction in the host inflammatory response, evasion of phagocytosis, and increase in virulence. *Infect Immun.* 2011; 79:4533–4542.

Singhrao SK, Olsen I. Are *Porphyromonas gingivalis* outer membrane vesicles microbullets for sporadic Alzheimer's disease manifestation? *J Alzheimers Dis Rep.* 2018; 2:219–228.

Siqueira WL, Oppenheim FG. Small molecular weight proteins/ peptides present in the in vivo formed human acquired enamel pellicle. *Arch Oral Biol.* 2009; 54:437–444.

Siqueira WL, Zhang W, Helmerhorst EJ, Gygi SP, Oppenheimer FG. Identification of protein components in in vivo human acquired enamel pellicle using LC-ESI-MS/MS. *J Proteome Res.* 2007; 6:2152–2160.

Slaney JM, Curtis MA. Mechanisms of evasion of complement by *Porphyromonas gingivalis. Front Biosci.* 2008; 13:188–196.

Socransky SS, Haffajee AD. Periodontal microbial ecology. *Periodontol 2000.* 2005; 38:135–187.

Socransky SS, Haffajee AD, Gugini MA, Smith C, Kent RL Jr. Microbial complexes in subgingival plaque. *J Clin Periodontol.* 1998; 25:134–144.

Sroka A, Sztukowska M, Potempa J, Travis J, Genco CA. Degradation of host heme proteins by lysine- and arginine-specific cysteine proteinases (gingipains) of *Porphyromonas gingivalis. J Bacteriol.* 2001; 183:5609–5616.

Stevens RH, Moura Martins Lobo dos Santos C, Zuanazzi D et al. Prophage induction in lysogenic *Aggregatibacter actinomycetemcomitans* cells co-cultured with human gingival fibroblasts, and its effect on leukotoxin release. *Microb Pathog.* 2013; 54:54–59.

Stewart PS. Antimicrobial tolerance in biofilms. *Microbiol Spectrum.* 2015; 3. doi: 10.1128/micro biols pec. MB-0010-2014.

Stewart PS, Costerton JW. Antibiotic resistance of bacteria in biofilms. *Lancet.* 2001; 358:135–138.

Stokar-Avihail A, Tal N, Erez Z, Lopatina A, Sorek R. Widespread utilization of peptide communication in phages infecting soil and pathogenic bacteria. *Cell Host Microbe.* 2019; 25(5):746–755.e5.

Sukumar S, Roberts AP, Martin FE, Adler CJ. Metagenomic insights into transferable antibiotic resistance in oral bacteria. *J Dent Res.* 2016; 95:969–976.

Sun J, Jin J, Beger RD et al. Metabolomics evaluation of the impact of smokeless tobacco exposure on the oral bacterium *Capnocytophaga sputigena. Toxicol in vitro.* 2016; 36:133–141.

Suntharalingam P, Cvitkovitch DG. Quorum sensing in streptococcal biofilm formation. *Trends Microbiol.* 2005; 13:3–6.

Sweere JM, Van Belleghem JD, Ishak H et al. Bacteriophage trigger antiviral immunity and prevent clearance of bacterial infection. *Science.* 2019; 363(6434):eaat9691.

Szafrański SP, Kilian M, Yang I et al. Diversity patterns of bacteriophages infecting *Aggregatibacter* and *Haemophilus* species across clades and niches. *ISME J.* 2019; 13(10):2500–2522.

Szafrański SP, Slots J, Stiesch M. The human oral phageome. *Periodontol 2000.* 2021; 86(1):79–96. doi: 10.1111/prd.12363.

Takahashi N. Oral microbiome metabolism: from "who are they?" to "what are they doing?" *J Dent Res.* 2015; 94:1628–1637.

Takenaka S, Pitts B, Trivedi HM, Stewart PS. Diffusion of macromolecules in model oral biofilms. *Appl Environ Microbiol.* 2009; 75:1750–1753.

Teles F, Wang Y, Hajishengallis G, Hasturk H, Marchesan JT. Impact of systemic factors in shaping the periodontal microbiome. *Periodontol 2000*. 2021; 85:124–160.

Teles R, Teles F, Frias-Lopez J, Paster B, Haffajee A. Lessons learned and unlearned in periodontal microbiology. *Periodontol 2000*. 2013; 62:95–162.

Teles RP, Patel M, Socransky SS, Haffajee AD. Disease progression in periodontally healthy and maintenance subjects. *J Periodontol*. 2008; 79:784–794.

ter Steeg PF, van der Hoeven JS. Development of periodontal microflora on human serum. *Microb Ecol Health Dis*. 1989, 2:1–10.

Teughels W, Laleman I, Quirynen M, Jakubovics N. Biofilm and periodontal microbiology. In: *Newman and Carranza's Clinical Periodontology* (ed. MG Newman, HH Takei, PR Klokkevold et al.). Philadelphia, PA: Elsevier; 2019: 528–691.

Thurlow LR, Hanke ML, Fritz T et al. *Staphylococcus aureus* biofilms prevent macrophage phagocytosis and attenuate inflammation in vivo. *J Immunol*. 2011; 186:6585–6596.

Thurnheer T, Gmür R, Shapiro S, Guggenheim B. Mass transport of macromolecules within an in vitro model of supragingival plaque. *Appl Environ Microbiol*. 2003; 69:1702–1709.

Tinanoff N, Gross A. Epithelial cells associated with the development of dental plaque. *J Dent Res*. 1976; 55: 580–583.

Torres SR, Garzino-Demo A, Meiller TF, Meeks V, Jabra-Rizk MA. Salivary histatin-5 and oral fungal colonisation in HIV+ individuals. *Mycoses*. 2009; 52(1):11–15.

Toyofuku M, Nomura N, Eberl L. Types and origins of bacterial membrane vesicles. *Nat Rev Microbiol*. 2019; 17(1):13–24.

Tribble GD, Rigney TW, Dao D-H et al. Natural competence is a major mechanism for horizontal DNA transfer in the oral pathogen *Porphyromonas gingivalis*. *MBio*. 2012; 3:e00231–11.

Tsigarida AA, Dabdoub SM, Nagaraja HN, Kumar PS. The influence of smoking on the peri-implant microbiome. *J Dent Res*. 2015; 94(9):1202–1217.

Tsukamoto H, Takeuchi S, Kubota K et al. Lipopolysaccharide (LPS)-binding protein stimulates CD14-dependent Toll-like receptor 4 internalization and LPS-induced TBK1-IKK-IRF3 axis activation. *J Biol Chem*. 2018; 293:10186–10201.

Van Belleghem JD, Dąbrowska K, Vaneechoutte M, Barr JJ, Bollyky PL. Interactions between bacteriophage, bacteria, and the mammalian immune system. *Viruses*. 2019; 11(1):10.

Van der Waaij D, Berghuis-de Vries JM, Lekker-Kerk van der Wees JEC. Colonisation resistance of the digestive tract in conventional and antibiotic-treated mice. *J Hyg*. 1971; 69:405–411.

van Steenbergen TJ, van Winkelhoff AJ, de Graaff J. Pathogenic synergy: mixed infections in the oral cavity. *Antonie van Leeuwenhoek*. 1984; 50:789–798.

Veith PD, Chen YY, Gorasia DG et al. *Porphyromonas gingivalis* outer membrane vesicles exclusively contain outer membrane and periplasmic proteins and carry a cargo enriched with virulence factors. *J Proteome Res*. 2014; 13:2420–2432.

Verbrugghe E, Boyen F, Gaastra W et al. The complex interplay between stress and bacterial infections in animals. *Vet Microbiol*. 2012; 155(2-4):115–127.

Vesey PM, Kuramitsu HK. Genetic analysis of *Treponema denticola* ATCC 35405 biofilm formation. *Microbiology*. 2004; 150:2401–2407.

Vidakovic L, Singh PK, Hartmann R, Nadell CD, Drescher K. Dynamic biofilm architecture confers individual and collective mechanisms of viral protection. *Nat Microbiol*. 2018; 3(1):26–31.

Vincents B, Guentsch A, Kostolowska D et al. Cleavage of IgG1 and IgG3 by gingipain K from *Porphyromonas gingivalis* may compromise host defense in progressive periodontitis. *FASEB J*. 2011; 25:3741–3750.

Vu B, Chen M, Crawford RJ, Ivanova EP. Bacterial extracellular polysaccharides involved in biofilm formation. *Molecules*. 2009; 14:2535–2554.

Wang BY, Kuramitsu HK. Interactions between oral bacteria: inhibition of *Streptococcus mutans* bacteriocin production by *Streptococcus gordonii*. *Appl Environ Microbiol*. 2005; 71:354–362.

Wang J, Gao Y, Zhao F. Phage-bacteria interaction network in human oral microbiome. *Environ Microbiol*. 2016; 18(7):2143–2158.

Wang M, Krauss JL, Domon H et al. Microbial hijacking of complement-toll-like receptor crosstalk. *Sci Signal*. 2010; 3:ra11

Wei GX, van der Hoeven JS, Smalley JW, Mikx FH, Fan MW. Proteolysis and utilization of albumin by enrichment cultures of subgingival microbiota. *Oral Microbiol Immunol*. 1999; 14:348–351.

Wenderska IB, Lukenda N, Cordova M et al. A novel function for the competence inducing peptide, XIP, as a cell death effector of *Streptococcus mutans*. *FEMS Microbiol Lett*. 2012; 336:104–112.

Wilensky A, Tzach-Nahman R, Potempa J, Shapira L, Nussbaum G. *Porphyromonas gingivalis* gingipains selectively reduce CD14 expression, leading to macrophage hypo-responsiveness to bacterial infection. *J Innate Immun*. 2015; 7:127–135.

Wilks M. Bacteria and early human development. *Early Hum Dev*. 2007; 83:165–170.

Willi K, Sandmeier H, Asikainen S, Saarela M, Meyer J. Occurrence of temperate bacteriophages in different *Actinobacillus actinomycetemcomitans* serotypes isolated from periodontally healthy individuals. *Oral Microbiol Immunol*. 1997; 12(1):40–46.

Willner D, Furlan M, Schmieder R et al. Metagenomic detection of phage-encoded platelet-binding factors in the human oral cavity. *Proc Natl Acad Sci USA*. 2011; 108(Suppl 1):4547–4553.

Wright CJ, Burns LH, Jack AA et al. Microbial interactions in building of communities. *Mol Oral Microbiol*. 2013; 28:83–101.

Wu L, Estrada O, Zaborina O et al. Recognition of host immune activation by *Pseudomonas aeruginosa*. *Science*. 2005; 309(5735):774–777.

Yamanaka T, Furukawa T, Matsumoto-Mashimo C et al. Gene expression profile and pathogenicity of biofilm-forming *Prevotella intermedia* strain 17. *BMC Microbiol*. 2009; 9:11.

Yilmaz O, Jungas T, Verbeke P, Ojcius DM. Activation of the phosphatidylinositol 3-kinase/Akt pathway contributes to survival of primary epithelial cells infected with the periodontal pathogen *Porphyromonas gingivalis*. *Infect Immun*. 2004; 72:3743–3751.

Yongqing T, Potempa J, Pike RN, Wijeyewickrema LC. The lysine-specific gingipain of *Porphyromonas gingivalis*: importance to pathogenicity and potential strategies for inhibition. *Adv Exp Med Biol*. 2011; 712:15–29.

Yost S, Duran-Pinedo AE, Teles R, Krishnan K, Frias-Lopez J. Functional signatures of oral dysbiosis during periodontitis progression revealed by microbial metatranscriptome analysis. *Genome Med*. 2015; 7(1):27.

Yu G, Phillips S, Gail MH et al. The effect of cigarette smoking on the oral and nasal microbiota. *Microbiome*. 2017; 5(1):3.

Yun PL, Decarlo AA, Collyer C, Hunter N. Hydrolysis of interleukin-12 by *Porphyromonas gingivalis* major cysteine proteinases may affect local gamma interferon accumulation and the Th1 or Th2 T-cell phenotype in periodontitis. *Infect Immun*. 2001; 69:5650–5660.

Zarnowski R, Sanchez H, Covelli AS et al. Candida albicans biofilm–induced vesicles confer drug resistance through matrix biogenesis. *PLoS Biol*. 2018; 16:e2006872.

Zaura-Arite E, Marle J, ten Cate JM. Confocal microscopy study of undisturbed and chlorhexidine-treated dental biofilm. *J Dent Res*. 2001; 80:1436–1440.

Zehnder M, Guggenheim B. The mysterious appearance of enterococci in filled root canals. *Int Endod J*. 2009; 42(4):277–287.

Zenobia C, Hajishengallis G. *Porphyromonas gingivalis* virulence factors involved in subversion of leukocytes and microbial dysbiosis. *Virulence*. 2015; 6(3):236–243.

Zhou MI, Rong R, Munro D et al. Investigation of the effect of type 2 diabetes mellitus on subgingival plaque microbiota by high-throughput 16S rDNA pyrosequencing. *PLoS One*. 2013; 8(4):e61516.

Zweigner J, Gramm HJ, Singer OC, Wegscheider K, Schumann RR. High concentrations of lipopolysaccharide-binding protein in serum of patients with severe sepsis or septic shock inhibit the lipopolysaccharide response in human monocytes. *Blood*. 2001; 98:3800–3808.

5.2   CALCULUS

Steph Smith and Khalid Almas

Contents

Learning objectives

- Composition of calculus, including organic and inorganic components.
- Differences in appearance, structure, location, colour, and formation between supragingival and subgingival calculus.
- Components involved in calculus formation and factors influencing formation of calculus.
- Attachment of calculus to tooth and implant surfaces.
- Methods of calculus detection.
- Methods to remove calculus and factors affecting removal efficacy.
- Agents used to prevent calculus formation.
- Clinical implications of calculus deposits on teeth.

Introduction

Dental calculus is calcified mineralized plaque containing a heterogeneous core, which is composed primarily of calcium phosphate mineral salts, covered by a soft, unmineralized, loose layer of bacteria. The calcified inorganic content is similar to that of bone, dentin, and cementum (Roberts-Harry & Clerehugh 2000). The surface of calculus is rough, and although it may not in itself induce inflammation in the adjacent periodontium, the surface may serve as a substrate for subgingival microbial colonization (Jepsen et al. 2011).

Composition of calculus

Calculus is composed of an organic matrix and an inorganic component (see Table 5.2.1).

Comparative features of supragingival and subgingival calculus

Table 5.2.2 depicts the comparative features of supragingival and subgingival calculus (Bosshardt & Lang 2015; Hinrichs & Thumbigere-Math 2019; Jepsen et al. 2011).

Calculus formation

- Usually starts between the 1st and 14th days of plaque formation, occurring within as little as 4 to 8 hours (Tibbetts & Kashiwa 1970). Calcifying plaques may become 50% mineralized in 2 days and 60–90% mineralized in 12 days (Muehlemann & Schroeder 1964; Sharawy et al. 1966). Calculus formation continues until it reaches a maximum, after which it may be reduced in amount. The time required to reach the maximal level has been reported to be between 10 weeks and 6 months (Conroy & Sturzenberger 1968; Volpe et al. 1969). The reduction in amount of calculus may be due to mechanical wear from food and from the cheeks, lips, and tongue movement (Hinrichs & Thumbigere-Math 2019).

- The development, amount, and composition of calculus vary from person to person, which includes heavy, moderate, and slight calculus formers and non-calculus formers, and also from site to site and over time (Corbett & Dawes 1998; Gürgan & Bilgin 2005; Turesky et al. 1962).

- The amount of calculus is influenced by numerous variables, such as age, sex, ethnic background, diet, location in the oral cavity, oral hygiene, bacterial composition, host response differences, access to professional cleaning, mental or physical handicaps, systemic diseases, and prescribed medications (White 1997). Moreover, there is a significant association between smoking and subgingival calculus deposition (Bergström 2005).

- Calculus deposition tends to occur where plaque is exposed to a salivary film of high velocity that promotes clearance of salivary sugar and acid from plaque, leading to a higher resting plaque pH. Furthermore, the abundant supply of urea from the major salivary gland secretions tends to increase the pH in plaque, thereby promoting calcium phosphate precipitation (Sissons et al. 1994).

Table 5.2.1 Composition of calculus.	
Organic component	The organic matrix is made up of protein–polysaccharide complexes, desquamated epithelial cells, leukocytes, and various types of microorganisms (Jin & Yip 2002). Between 1.9% and 9.1% of the organic component is carbohydrate, which is present in salivary glycoprotein (Hinrichs & Thumbigere-Math 2019). Salivary proteins account for 5.9–8.2% of the organic component of calculus and include most amino acids (Hinrichs & Thumbigere-Math 2019).
Inorganic component (constitutes 70–90% of the major bulk of calculus)	The *minor components* of the inorganic part consist of carbonate, sodium, copper, magnesium, silicon, iron, zinc, bromine, manganese, and fluorine (Hayashizaki et al. 2008). The *major components* of the inorganic part consist of:

Approximately 76% of calcium phosphate ($Ca_3[PO_4]_2$)		At least two-thirds of these calcium phosphate inorganic salts are in crystalline form (Bosshardt & Lang 2015): $Ca_5(PO_4)_3(OH)$ = hydroxyapatite (58%) $\beta\text{-}Ca_3(PO_4)_2$ = whitlockite (21%) $Ca_4H(PO_4)_3 \times 2H_2O$ = octacalcium phosphate (12%) $CaH(PO_4) \times 2H_2O$ = brushite (9%)
4% magnesium phosphate ($Mg_3[PO_4]_2$)		
3% calcium carbonate ($CaCO_3$)		
2% carbon dioxide (CO_2)		

Table 5.2.2 Comparison between supragingival and subgingival calculus.

Supragingival calculus	Subgingival calculus
Located coronal to the gingiva and is easily visible. When the gingival tissues recede, subgingival calculus becomes exposed and is therefore reclassified as supragingival, thus being composed of both initial supragingival calculus and previous subgingival calculus (see Figure 5.2.1)	Located apical to the gingival margin and is not visible; occasionally visible on dental radiographs
Firmly attached to enamel, including pits and irregularities of the tooth surface	Usually extends from the cementoenamel junction to close to the bottom of the pocket, but does not reach the junctional epithelium (calculus-free zone), and is adhered firmly to the tooth root. Related to pocket depth
Has claylike consistency or moderate hardness	Hard and dense
Is influenced by saliva, food pigments, and tobacco. Is creamy-whitish to dark yellow or brownish	Dark brown or greenish black in colour. Black pigmentation is derived from mineralized anaerobic microorganisms
Mainly observed on the buccal surfaces of the maxillary molars and the lingual surfaces of the mandibular anterior teeth; these are sites that are close to the orifices of salivary ducts	Usually randomly distributed, also mainly found on interproximal surfaces, the lingual surfaces of lower first molars, the buccal surfaces of mandibular anterior teeth, and maxillary molar teeth
Heterogeneously calcified, with islets of mineralized material within the covering plaque and non-mineralized areas within the calculus, accounting for the porous nature of calculus	Homogeneously calcified with the covering plaque containing no mineralized material and only mineralized material seen within the calculus itself
Supragingival plaque becomes mineralized due to the precipitation of mineral salts present in saliva	Is affected by mineral salts and hemorrhagic components in the inflammatory exudate from the gingival crevicular fluid, thus representing a secondary product of infection (plasma origin)
Sodium content is less. More brushite and octacalcium phosphate, less magnesium whitlockite	Sodium content increases with depth of pocket. Less brushite and octacalcium phosphate, more magnesium whitlockite. The ratio of calcium to phosphate is higher

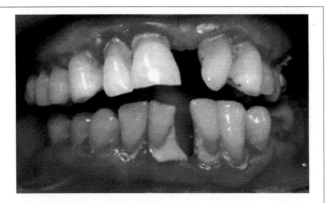

Figure 5.2.1 Supragingival calculus.

- The formation of calculus is always preceded by the development of a bacterial biofilm that undergoes mineralization due to the precipitation of mineral salts, although not all the plaque may become calcified (Jin & Yip 2002). The calcification of supragingival plaque and the attached component of subgingival plaque begins along the inner surface adjacent to the tooth structure (Hinrichs & Thumbigere-Math 2019). Studies have shown the presence of calcified masses with a spongy appearance and containing empty spaces and tubular holes. These holes appear to be areas of non-mineralized bacteria surrounded by a calcified matrix. There may also be areas where bacteria are calcified but surrounded by a non-mineralized space (Akcali & Lang 2018).

- Plaque mineralization occurs in numerous individual foci in the plaque intercellular matrix, and gradually some plaque microorganisms become calcified with increasing age of calculus (Donald 1997; Friskopp 1983). Also, calculus continually harbors viable bacterial plaque. *Aggregatibacter actinomycetemcomitans*, *Porphyromonas gingivalis*, and *Treponema denticola* have been found within the structural channels and lacunae of supragingival and subgingival calculus (Bosshardt & Lang 2015; Hinrichs & Thumbigere-Math 2019). Following the mineralization process, dental calculus loses its microbial virulence. However, subgingival dental calculus has been demonstrated to retain significant levels of endotoxin (White 1997).

- The initial mineralization of partially soluble calcium phosphate minerals and plaque bacteria is critical for the calcification of dental plaque (Jin & Yip 2002). However, this process is not simply a passive one, but is also active, supported by the supersaturation of saliva and plaque fluid with respect to calcium phosphate salts, bacterial enzymes, cell membrane-associated constituents, as well as the presence and degradation of nucleation inhibitors (Bosshardt & Lang 2015; Friskopp & Hammarström 1982). Osteopontin and bone sialoprotein are extracellular matrix proteins and are present in blood plasma, and osteopontin has been identified in gingival crevicular fluid (GCF) and calculus (Bosshardt & Lang 2015).

- Phosphatase liberated from dental plaque, desquamated epithelial cells, or bacteria precipitates calcium phosphate by hydrolyzing organic phosphates in saliva, thereby increasing the concentration of free phosphate ions (Hinrichs & Thumbigere-Math 2019).
- Esterase enzyme is present in cocci and filamentous organisms, leukocytes, macrophages, and desquamated epithelial cells of dental plaque. Esterase may initiate calcification by hydrolyzing fatty esters into free fatty acids, which then form soaps with calcium and magnesium. These soaps are later converted into less-soluble calcium phosphate salts (Hinrichs & Thumbigere-Math 2019).
- Bacterial plaque absorbs and concentrates partially soluble calcium and phosphate minerals derived from saliva, from the GCF, as well as from blood and pus entering the pocket from the surrounding soft tissues (Jepsen et al. 2011; Waerhaug 1955).
- Mineralization is characterized by binding of calcium ions to the carbohydrate–protein complexes (chelation) of the organic matrix. This has been referred to as the epitactic concept, also known as heterogeneous nucleation (Hinrichs & Thumbigere-Math 2019; Sharawy et al. 1966). This leads to the deposition of the precursor phases of calcium phosphate, such as octacalcium phosphate and dicalcium phosphate dihydrate (brushite) (Mandel 1960).
- This is followed by the precipitation of crystalline calcium phosphate salt crystals, which develop initially in the intercellular matrix and on the bacterial surfaces, and finally within the bacteria (Zander et al. 1960). Deposition of the less-soluble hydroxyapatite and whitlockite minerals follows during maturation (White 1997).
- Due to the diversity in bacterial proteolipids, not all microorganisms calcify. Plaque bacteria undergo extensive degradation, leaving only the cell walls for calculus formation (Jin & Yip 2002). Acidic phospholipids in the cell wall membranes are the key components involved in microbial calcification (Boyan & Boskey 1984).
- Calcium binds to phospholipid molecules in the bacterial cell wall, which facilitates the interaction of bound calcium with inorganic phosphate ions in solution, to form a calcium–phospholipid–phosphate complex (CPLX). Once CPLXs have formed, apatite deposition follows when sufficient calcium and phosphate ions are present and the concentration of inhibitors is low (Hauster et al. 1969).

- The pellicle beneath the bacterial plaque also undergoes calcification, thus facilitating the firm adherence of calculus to enamel, cementum, and/or dentin (Selvig 1970).
- The progression of mineralization occurs in incremental patterns from the inner zones of the bacterial plaque outward, thus producing concentric rings, called Liesegang rings, that reflect successive phases of mineralization (Bosshardt & Lang 2015).
- Calcification inhibitors include apatite nucleation inhibitors, such as magnesium (Mg), which blocks apatite crystallization and stabilizes calcium phosphate as amorphous mineral. Other inhibitors are crystal growth inhibitors, such as salivary statherin, proline-rich proteins (PRP), cystatins, histatins, and albumin, as well as pyrophosphate and zinc ions (Jin & Yip 2002).
- There are however enzymes that degrade calcification inhibitors. Salivary and plaque proteases can degrade calcification inhibitors such as statherin and PRP (Morita & Watanabe 1986). Acid and alkaline phosphatases are present in oral microorganisms, dental plaque and calculus, and saliva (Boyan & Boskey 1984). Acid and alkaline phosphatases may promote crystal growth by degrading pyrophosphate. They also hydrolyze phosphoproteins to produce inorganic phosphate ions, which are then transported for mineralization (Jin & Yip 2002).

Attachment of calculus to tooth and implant surfaces

Four modes of attachment to tooth surfaces have been described (Hinrichs & Thumbigere-Math 2019; Mandel 1960; Zander et al. 1960):

- Attachment by means of an organic pellicle on cementum and enamel.
- Mechanical locking into surface irregularities, such as caries lesions or resorption lacunae.
- Close adaptation of the undersurface of calculus to depressions or gently sloping mounds of the unaltered cementum surface.
- Penetration of bacterial calculus into cementum.

Attachment of calculus to pure titanium implant surfaces is less intimate than to root surface structures. Smooth machined implants have fewer microporosities for retention. Thus, calculus may be chipped off from implants without affecting them (Matarasso et al. 1996).

Detection of calculus

- *Visual examination*: Good lighting should be utilized to detect supra- and subgingival calculus just below the gingival margin. Light deposits of supragingival calculus that are wet with saliva are more difficult to visualize, and should thus be dried with compressed air (Aghanashini et al. 2016).

- *Tactile exploration*: This requires the skilled use of a fine-pointed explorer and probe. The explorer is held with a light but stable modified pen grasp, with light exploratory strokes being applied in a vertical direction. The pads of the thumb and middle finger should perceive the slight vibration conducted through the shank of the explorer (Aghanashini et al. 2016).

- *Radiographs*: Highly calcified interproximal calculus can be readily detected as radiopaque projections protruding into the interdental space. However, conventional oral radiography is considered to be a poor diagnostic method for the detection of calculus (Aghanashini et al. 2016). The sensitivity of conventional radiographs as a diagnostic test to detect subgingival calculus has been shown in a study to be only 43% (Buchanan et al. 1987) (see Figures 5.2.2 and 5.2.3). A study utilizing digital radiography that incorporates image enhancement found that when root surfaces were covered >30% in calculus with an increase in the horizontal size of calculus deposits, then the detection of calculus improved significantly. However, image enhancements with digital software did not significantly improve detection of dental calculus compared with the original image (Hyer et al. 2021).

- *Calculus detection systems* (Kamath & Nayak 2014):
  - *Perioscopy*: The perioscope is a miniature periodontal endoscope and is inserted into the periodontal pocket. It images the subgingival root surface, tooth surface, and calculus, and can be viewed on a monitor in real time, captured, and saved in computer files.
  - *Optical spectrometry*: An optical fiber in a device recognizes the characteristic spectral signals of calculus caused by the absorption, reflection, and diffraction of red light. Advantages of the device include its portability and emission of audible and luminous signals upon calculus detection.
  - *Autofluorescence-based technology:* Due to differences in composition of teeth and calculus, the fluorescence of calculus can be detected.

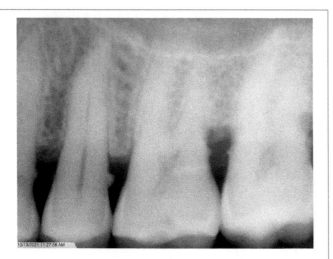

Figure 5.2.2 Subgingival calculus.

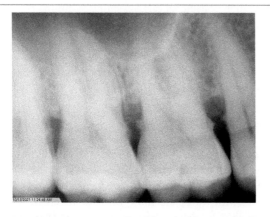

Figure 5.2.3 Subgingival calculus.

Removal of calculus

- *Hand instruments*: Scalers and curettes have the most access to supra- and subgingival calculus. Curettes can be used for root planing and effective debridement of subgingival calculus (Kamath & Nayak 2014).

- *Ultrasonic instruments:* These power-driven instruments oscillate at very high speeds, causing microvibrations that aid in calculus and subgingival plaque removal. Examples are magnetostrictive and piezoelectric devices (Kamath & Nayak 2014).

- *Laser ablation*: Experimental and clinical studies evaluating the efficacy and safety of emission wavelengths in the 3000 nm range have been indicated to be suitable for the effective removal of subgingival calculus, utilizing the pulsed Er:YAG laser, which includes a glass-fiber tip in contact mode under water irrigation (Aoki et al. 1994).

When comparing hand and ultrasonic instrumentation methods, no microscopic differences have been found regarding efficacy of calculus removal (Oosterwaal et al. 1987). Studies have found that the piezoelectric system is more efficient in calculus removal when compared to magnetostrictive and hand instrumentation, but that it left tooth surfaces rougher (Arabaci et al. 2007). Other studies have shown contradictory results, hence it is not clear whether hand or ultrasonic instrumentation is more efficient for removing plaque and calculus from the root surface (Kamath & Nayak 2014). Furthermore, studies have concluded that the effectiveness of these different treatment modalities in thorough calculus removal from root surfaces is impossible to determine (Aoki et al. 2000).

Regarding laser application, studies have concluded that the Er:YAG laser may provide a level of calculus removal similar to that provided by ultrasonic scaling (Eberhard et al. 2003). Studies comparing laser application to scaling and root planing showed that the in vivo efficiency of the Er:YAG laser was lower than that of hand instrumentation; however, laser application was associated with preservation of root cementum, whereas scaling and root planing can result in nearly complete removal of cementum (Oda et al. 2004; Schwarz et al. 2006).

Factors influencing the effectiveness of calculus removal

- *Pocket depth*: Studies correlating initial probing pocket depths with effectiveness of calculus removal utilizing hand instrumentation have shown that with probing depths of <5 mm, 90% of subgingival calculus can be removed, versus 77% in pockets with a probing depth of 5–6 mm, and 65% in pockets >6 mm (Rabbani et al. 1981). When initial probing depths were correlated with power-driven instruments, 14% of all surfaces showed residual calculus with probing depths <4 mm, versus 33% for probing depths of 4–5 mm and 59% for probing depths >5 mm (Gellin et al. 1986). Studies using a combination of hand instrumentation and power-driven instruments have shown similar results (Buchanan & Robertson 1987).
- *Tooth type*: Regarding the efficacy of hand instrumentation, single-rooted teeth may show 10% residual deposits, versus 30% for multirooted teeth (Gellin et al. 1986). Regarding ultrasonic instrumentation, 34% of surfaces of single-rooted teeth and 23.5% of surfaces of molar teeth can show residual calculus (Breininger et al. 1987).
- *Tooth surface*: Regarding hand instrumentation of molars, residual calculus may be found on 16% of approximal surfaces with initial probing pocket depths of 0–3 mm, versus 40% in pockets with an initial probing depth of 4–12 mm (Breininger et al. 1987). Studies utilizing phantom heads using hand instruments have shown 61.1% of treated surfaces to have residual deposits in maxillary molar furcations versus 39.5% in mandibular molar furcations, indicating more effective treatment of molars in the lower jaw (Oda & Ishikawa 1989). Similar observations have been reported for ultrasonic instruments, whereby 50.3% of surfaces in maxillary molars and 44.1% of surfaces in mandibular molars may be covered with residual calculus (Oda & Ishikawa 1989).
- *Repeated instrumentation*: A single episode of 10 min nonsurgical debridement using curettes has been shown to be as effective as two episodes of 10 min each within a 24 h interval (Anderson et al. 1996).
- *Access to tooth surfaces*: Studies have shown that after closed scaling of pockets >6 mm deep, 32% of the surfaces may be free of residual calculus, versus 48% after an open flap procedure and scaling (Caffesse et al. 1986). Open procedures with hand instruments have also been shown to be more effective compared to closed procedures for calculus removal in mandibular furcation areas (Parashis et al. 1993). Studies using a combination of curettes and ultrasonic scalers have shown an increased effectiveness of calculus removal in

pockets of 4–6 mm from 21% residual calculus using a closed approach, compared to 4% residual calculus when using open flap access. In pockets >6 mm deep, 19% residual calculus was found after instrumentation without a flap procedure versus 5% residual calculus after instrumentation in combination with a flap procedure (Brayer et al. 1989).
- *Operator experience*: Training of the operator can affect the efficacy of root debridement, especially when using hand instruments (Kamath & Nayak 2014). Studies on phantom heads have shown that approximately 15–24% of all surfaces may still have deposits after treatment by an inexperienced operator, compared with 13% residual deposits after root instrumentation by an experienced operator (Kocher et al. 1997).

Prevention of calculus formation

Calculus removal is labor- and time-consuming, which has led to the development of chemical approaches for calculus prevention and/or elimination. These measures include solubilizing calculus and the organic matrix, or the inhibition of plaque adhesion, formation, and mineralization (Jin & Yip 2002; Mandel 1995; White 1997). Inhibitors of calculus formation are however not capable of dissolving existing deposits, and their effects are mostly limited to the supragingival area. Anticalculus agents may be used alone or in dentifrices, at various concentrations with varied resultant outcomes. Pyrophosphate is the most common anticalculus agent used in dentifrices (Fairbrother & Heasman 2000; Kamath & Nayak 2014). Table 5.2.3 depicts the classification of various anticalculus agents.

Clinical implications

Dental calculus is not a primary cause of periodontal diseases. Calculus is always covered by an unmineralized layer of viable bacterial plaque, thereby having a secondary effect by providing a surface configuration conducive to further plaque accumulation and subsequent mineralization (Bosshardt & Lang 2015). Calculus may thus amplify the effects of bacterial plaque by keeping the bacterial deposits in close contact with the tissue surface, thereby influencing both bacterial ecology and tissue response (Friskopp & Hammarström 1980).

Calculus may be considered a secondary product of infection, rather than the cause of periodontal inflammation, as calcification of subgingival plaque requires a high flow of GCF. An increase in GCF flow is strongly induced by inflammation and provides the minerals that are required for plaque mineralization (Mandel & Gaffar 1986).

Calculus plays a secondary role in the development and progression of periodontitis, by providing an ideal porous vehicle for bacterial plaque retention and growth, thereby serving as a reservoir for toxic bacterial products and antigens. Calculus should thus be regarded a secondary etiological factor rather than a primary cause of periodontitis (Jepsen et al. 2011).

Table 5.2.3 Classification of anticalculus agents.

Dissolution agents	Acids, spring salts (containing salts of calcium, magnesium or sodium), alkaline springs (containing an alkali), sodium ricinoleate (sodium salt of ricinoleic fatty acid)
Plaque inhibition agents	Antiseptics (chloramine-T), Antibiotics (penicillin, cetylpyridinium chloride, niddamycin, triclosan)
Plaque attachment inhibitors	Silicones, ion exchange resins
Matrix disruption agents	Enzymes (mucinase), ascorbic acid, sodium percarbonate, copper sulfite, chelating agents, 30% urea
Inhibitors of crystal growth (mineralization)	Vitamin C, pyrophosphate, diphosphonate, bisphosphonates, sodium etidronate, zinc salts, calcium lactate, sodium fluoride, polymers and co-polymers, citroxain and sodium citrate, triclosan

Source: Fairbrother & Heasman 2000; Kamath & Nayak 2014; Mandel 1995; Reddy 2018.

It has been debated whether or not the rough surface of calculus may exert a detrimental effect on the soft tissues. However, it has clearly been established that surface roughness alone does not initiate gingivitis. Well-controlled clinical studies have shown that meticulous supragingival plaque control on a regular basis guarantees the depletion of the supragingival bacterial reservoir for subgingival recolonization, and furthermore that the removal of subgingival plaque on top of subgingival calculus results in healing of periodontal lesions and the maintenance of healthy gingival and periodontal tissues (Mobelli et al. 1995; Nyman et al. 1988). Animal studies have shown that if the calculus surface was disinfected using chlorhexidine, then a normal epithelial attachment with junctional epithelial cells forming hemidesmosomes and a basement membrane on calculus can be observed (Listgarten & Ellegaard 1973).

Calculus deposits may furthermore develop in areas that are difficult for oral hygiene access and, depending on their size, jeopardize proper oral hygiene practices. Factors such as anatomy, probing depth, instruments, and operator experience influence the efficacy of subgingival calculus removal. Although some agents have been proven to reduce calculus formation, their effects appear to be limited to supragingival calculus and complete prevention cannot be achieved with them (Jepsen et al. 2011).

REFERENCES

Aghanashini S, Puvvalla B, Mundinamane DB et al. A comprehensive review on dental calculus. *J Health Sci Res.* 2016; 7(2):42–50.

Akcali A, Lang NP. Dental calculus: the calcified biofilm and its role in disease development. *Periodontol 2000.* 2018; 76:109–115.

Anderson GB, Palmer JA, Bye FL, Smith BA, Caffesse RG. Effectiveness of subgingival scaling and root planing: single versus multiple episodes of instrumentation. *J Periodontol.* 1996; 67:367–373.

Aoki A, Ando Y, Watanabe H, Ishikawa I. in vitro studies on laser scaling of subgingival calculus with an erbium:YAG laser. *J Periodontol.* 1994; 65:1097–1106.

Aoki A, Miura M, Akiyama F et al. in vitro evaluation of Er:YAG laser scaling of subgingival calculus in comparison with ultrasonic scaling. *J Periodontal Res.* 2000; 35:266–277.

Arabaci T, Cicek Y, Canakci CF. Sonic and ultrasonic scalers in periodontal treatment: a review. *Int J Dent Hyg.* 2007; 5:2–12.

Bergström J. Tobacco smoking and subgingival dental calculus. *J Clin Periodontol.* 2005; 32:81–88.

Bosshardt DD, Lang NP. Dental calculus. In: *Clinical Periodontology and Implant Dentistry* (ed. NP Lang, J Lindhe). Chichester: Wiley; 2015: 183–190.

Boyan BD, Boskey AL. Co-isolation of proteolipids and calcium-phospholipid-phosphate complexes. *Calcif Tissue Int.* 1984; 36:214–218.

Brayer WK, Mellonig JT, Dunlap RM, Marinak KW, Carson RE. Scaling and root planing effectiveness: the effect of root surface access and operator experience. *J Periodontol.* 1989; 60:67–72.

Breininger DR, O'Leary TJ, Blumenshine RV. Comparative effectiveness of ultrasonic and hand scaling for the removal of subgingival plaque and calculus. *J Periodontol.* 1987; 58: 9–18.

Buchanan SA, Jenderseck RS, Granet MA et al. Radiographic detection of dental calculus. *J Periodontol.* 1987; 58:747–751.

Buchanan SA, Robertson PB. Calculus removal by scaling/root planing with and without surgical access. *J Periodontol.* 1987; 58:159–163.

Caffesse RG, Sweeney PL, Smith BA. Scaling and root planing with and without periodontal flap surgery. *J Clin Periodontol.* 1986; 13:205–210.

Conroy CW, Sturzenberger OP. The rate of calculus formation in adults. *J Periodontol.* 1968; 39(3):142–144.

Corbett TL, Dawes C. A comparison of the site-specificity of supragingival and subgingival calculus deposition. *J Periodontol.* 1998; 69:1–8.

Donald JW. Dental calculus: recent insight into occurrence, formation, prevention, removal and oral health effects of supragingival and subgingival deposits. *Eur J Oral Sci.* 1997; 105:508–522.

Eberhard J, Ehlers H, Falk W et al. Efficacy of subgingival calculus removal with Er:YAG laser compared to mechanical debridement: an in situ study. *J Clin Periodontol.* 2003; 30:511–518.

Fairbrother KJ, Heasman PA. Anticalculus agents. *J Clin Periodontol.* 2000; 27:285–301.

Friskopp J. Ultrastructure of non-decalcified supragingival and subgingival calculus. *J Periodontol.* 1983; 54:542–550.

Friskopp J, Hammarström, L. A comparative scanning electron microscopic study of supragingival and subgingival calculus. *J Periodontol.* 1980; 51:553–562.

Friskopp J, Hammarström L. An enzyme histochemical study of dental plaque and calculus. *Acta Odontol Scand.* 1982; 40:459–466.

Gellin RG, Miller MC, Javed T, Engler WO, Mishkin DJ. 6. *J Periodontol.* 1986; 57:672–680.

Gürgan CA, Bilgin E. Distribution of different morphologic types of subgingival calculus on proximal root surfaces. *Quintessence Int.* 2005; 36:202–208.

Hauster H, Chapman D, Dawson RM. Physical studies of phospholipids XI. Ca2+ binding to monolayers of phosphatidlserine and phosphatidyl inositol. *Biochim Biophys Acta.* 1969; 183:320–333.

Hayashizaki J, Ban S, Nakagaki H et al. Site specific mineral composition and microstructure of human supra-gingival dental calculus. *Arch Oral Biol.* 2008; 53(2):168–174.

Hinrichs JE, Thumbigere-Math V. The role of dental calculus and other local predisposing factors. In: *Newman and Carranza's Clinical Periodontology* (ed. MG Newman, HH Takei, PR Klokkevold et al.). Philadelphia, PA: Elsevier; 2019: 528–691.

Hyer JC, Deas DE, Palaiologou AA et al. Accuracy of dental calculus detection using digital radiography and image manipulation. *J Periodontol.* 2021; 92:419 427.

Jepsen S, Deschner J, Braun A, Schwarz F, Eberhard J. Calculus removal and the prevention of its formation. *Periodontol 2000.* 2011; 55:167–188.

Jin Y, Yip HK. Supragingival calculus: formation and control. *Crit Rev Oral Biol Med.* 2002; 13:426–441.

Kamath DG, Nayak SU. Detection, removal and prevention of calculus: literature review. *Saudi Dent J.* 2014; 26(1):7–13.

Kocher T, Rühling A, Momsen H, Plagmann HC. Effectiveness of subgingival instrumentation with power-driven instruments in the hands of experienced and inexperienced operators. A study on manikins. *J Clin Periodontol.* 1997; 24:498–504.

Listgarten MA, Ellegaard B. Electron microscopic evidence of a cellular attachment between junctional epithelium and dental calculus. *J Periodontal Res.* 1973; 8:143–150.

Mandel ID. Calculus formation: the role of bacteria and mucoprotein. *Dent Clin North Am.* 1960; 4:731–738.

Mandel ID. Calculus update: prevalence, pathogenicity and prevention. *J Am Dent Assoc.* 1995; 26:573–580.

Mandel ID, Gaffar A. Calculus revisited. *A review. J Clin Periodontol.* 1986; 13:249–257.

Matarasso S, Quaremb G, Corraggio F et al. Maintenance of implants. An in vitro study of titanium implant surface modifications subsequent to the application of different prophylaxis procedures. *Clin Oral Implants Res.* 1996; 7(1):64–72.

Mombelli A, Nyman S, Brägger N, Wennström J, Lang NP. Clinical and microbiological changes associated with an altered subgingival environment induced by periodontal pocket reduction. *J Clin Periodontol.* 1995; 22:780–787.

Morita M, Watanabe T. Relation between the presence of supragingival calculus and protease activity in dental plaque. *J Dent Res.* 1986; 65:703–705.

Muehlemann HR, Schroeder HE. Dynamics of supragingival calculus formation. *Adv Oral Biol.* 1964; 1:175–203.

Nyman S, Westfelt E, Sarhed G, Karring T. Role of "diseased" root cementum in healing following treatment of periodontal disease. *A clinical study. J Clin Periodontol.* 1988; 15:464–468.

Oda S, Ishikawa I. in vitro effectiveness of a newly designed ultrasonic scaler tip for furcation areas. *J Periodontol.* 1989; 60:634–639.

Oda S, Nitta H, Setoguchi T, Izumi Y, Ishikawa I. Current concepts and advances in manual and power-driven instruments. *Periodontol 2000.* 2004; 36:45–58.

Oosterwaal PJ, Matee MI, Mikx FH, van 't Hof MA, Renggli HH. The effect of subgingival debridement with hand and ultrasonic instruments on the subgingival microflora. *J Clin Periodontol.* 1987; 14:528–533.

Parashis AO, Anagnou-Vareltzides A, Demetriou N. Calculus removal from multirooted teeth with and without surgical access. (I). Efficacy on external and furcation surfaces in relation to probing depth. *J Clin Periodontol.* 1993; 20:63–68.

Rabbani GM, Ash MM Jr, Caffesse RG. The effectiveness of subgingival scaling and root planing in calculus removal. *J Periodontol.* 1981; 52:119–123.

Reddy S. *Essentials of Clinical Periodontology and Periodontics.* New Delhi: Jaypee Brothers Medical; 2018.

Roberts-Harry EA, Clerehugh V. Subgingival calculus: where are we now? *A comparative review. J Dent.* 2000; 28:93–102.

Schwarz F, Bieling K, Venghaus S et al. Influence of fluorescence-controlled Er:YAG laser radiation, the Vector system and hand instruments on periodontally diseased root surfaces in vivo. *J Clin Periodontol.* 2006; 33:200–208.

Selvig KA. Attachment of plaque and calculus to tooth surfaces. *J Periodontal Res.* 1970; 5:8–18.

Sharawy AM, Sabharwal K, Socransky SS, Robene RR. A quantitative study of plaque and calculus formation in normal and periodontally involved mouths. *J Periodontol.* 1966; 37(6):495–501.

Sissons CH, Wong L, Hancock EM, Cutress TW. The pH response to urea and the effect of liquid flow in "artificial mouth" microcosm plaques. *Arch Oral Biol.* 1994; 39:497–505.

Tibbetts L, Kashiwa H. A histochemical study of early plaque mineralization. *J Dent Res.* 1970; 19:202.

Turesky S, Renstrup G, Glickman I. Effects of changing the salivary environment on progress of calculus formation. *J Periodontol.* 1962; 33:45–50.

Volpe AR, Kupczak LJ, King WJ et al. in vivo calculus assessment. IV. Parameters of human clinical studies. *J Periodontol.* 1969; 40(2):76–86.

Waerhaug J. The source of mineral salts in subgingival calculus. *J Dent Res.* 1955; 34:563–568.

White DJ. Dental calculus: recent insights into occurrence, formation, prevention, removal and oral health effects of supragingival and subgingival deposits. *Eur J Oral Sci.* 1997; 105:508–522.

Zander H, Hazen S, Scott D. Mineralization of dental calculus. *Proc Soc Exp Biol Med.* 1960; 103:257–560.

5.3 GENETICS AND PERIODONTAL DISEASE

Steph Smith

Contents

Learning objectives

- The role of genetics and epigenetics in host susceptibility to periodontal diseases.
- The role of genetics in periodontal disease phenotype, subgingival bacterial colonization, periodontal disease pathogenicity, aggressive periodontitis, and periodontal wound healing.

Introduction

The pathogenesis of periodontal disease involves complex interactions among plaque bacteria, the host's genetic factors, and acquired environmental stressors (Zhang et al. 2020). Historical longitudinal studies on the rate of periodontal disease progression have described differences thereof in populations with a similar oral hygiene condition (Löe et al. 1978, 1986). Chronic inflammatory periodontal disease is characterized by clinical heterogeneity, depicting its nonlinearity, which includes large variations in the frequency and time periods of disease remission. This is related to stability or changes in the patients' immune fitness (Kuman 2018; Loos & Van Dyke 2020).

Genetics and epigenetics in periodontal disease susceptibility

Epidemiological studies have indicated that there is no positive correlation between the quantity of bacterial plaque and the severity of periodontitis (Löe et al. 1986): 20% of the risk for the development of periodontal disease is attributed to the deposition and accumulation of plaque, and 80% to environmental determinants and genetic variations within individuals (Bartold & Van Dyke 2019; Grossi et al. 1994; Kornman 2008). Therefore, plaque bacteria may initiate inflammation; however, it is intrinsic host factors and environmental stressors that modulate the magnitude, duration, and extent of the inflammatory response (Zhang et al. 2020). Most forms of periodontitis are polygenic, being caused by a combination of genetic and environmental factors (Chapple et al. 2017). Thus, apart from environmental stressors, the distinct differences in susceptibility to periodontal disease are clearly attributed to a genetic component (Zhang et al. 2020). Evidence suggests that up to one-third of the variability of periodontitis traits in humans is attributable to genetic variants, indicating that some individuals are highly susceptible to periodontal disease while others are resistant, with heritability being higher for severe, early-onset traits, and younger individuals (Shaddox et al. 2021; Zhang et al. 2011). Periodontitis may be associated with variations in as many as 20 genes, being considered as either a susceptibility (initiation of disease) or a disease-modifying (progression of disease) locus (Hart et al. 2000; Laine et al. 2012). Furthermore, genotype frequencies can vary across populations. This includes ethnic and racial differences in gene polymorphisms as well as gene–environment interactions associated with periodontitis (Zhang et al. 2011).

The causal factors that regulate the immune system are both intrinsic and acquired. Intrinsic causal factors are inherited risk factors, i.e. genetic susceptibility (Raghuraman et al. 2016). Epigenetic influences act through DNA remodeling of chromatin, induced by DNA methylation or histone modifications, which can selectively activate or deactivate genes, including those involved in DNA repair, cell proliferation, regulation, and inflammatory gene expression (Shaddox et al. 2021). Epigenetic changes thus contribute to gene expression and function, altered immune function, and the magnitude of the inflammatory response. Epigenetic modifications of DNA can be inherited, so can be intrinsic, and can also be partly acquired during life (Raghuraman et al. 2016). Acquired epigenetic changes can be induced by aging, microbial exposure, dietary factors, systemic conditions (e.g. obesity, diabetes, osteoporosis, and depression), environmental factors (e.g. pollution), as well as modifiable risk and lifestyle factors, such as smoking, stress, and alcohol consumption (Raghuraman et al. 2016).

Periodontal transcriptome studies regarding the role of genetics in various aspects of periodontal disease, including periodontal wound healing, are depicted in Table 5.3.1.

Future considerations

Studies are emerging that incorporate global profiling data, which have enabled comprehensive assessments of biofilm bacteria–host interactions in periodontal disease, whereby novel single-nucleotide polymorphisms, genes, pathways, metabolites, and bacterial species are being studied that have not been previously associated with periodontal disease. However, replication in other studies utilizing similar designs should also be performed in different populations, and should furthermore be validated biologically, in vitro and in vivo (Zhang et al. 2020). The exploration of epigenetics can lead to the development of improved epigenetic regulation techniques to modulate wound healing. This, together with a clearer understanding of specific cellular pathways that are involved in development, proliferation, stem cell renewal, and differentiation, can provide new and more efficient therapies in wound healing (Zhu et al. 2010).

Table 5.3.1 Role of genetics in various aspects of periodontal disease.

Periodontal disease phenotype
- It has been hypothesized that relatively common in the population are disease-associating genetic variants or single-nucleotide polymorphisms which are present in the coding, regulatory, or intergenic sequences of genes (Zhang et al. 2020).
- The disease phenotype is determined by the totality of these variants, each of which contributes to the clinical disease in varying degrees (Gibson 2012; Kinane & Hart 2003).
- Important, however, is the fact that the carriage rate of genetic polymorphisms may vary among ethnic populations. Therefore, possible positive associations between a genetic polymorphism and disease within one population cannot always be extrapolated to other populations (Laine et al. 2012).
- Furthermore, disease susceptibility, clinical heterogeneity, disease progression, and response to treatment are substantiated by epigenetics. Epigenetics entails the mechanisms of how the environment interacts with the genome of individuals, this being accomplished via cell signaling cascades, which then produce persistent and heritable changes in gene expression, without any concomitant changes in the DNA sequence (Laine et al. 2012; Zhang et al. 2010).
- Epigenetic processes occur during different stages of normal development, as well as in disease states, and play an important role in damaged tissues (Cutroneo & Chiu 2000; Wang et al. 2009).
- In periodontal disease, epigenetics will comprise the interface between genetic and environmental factors, thereby giving rise to certain periodontal disease phenotypes, which are due to epigenetic changes influencing host responses to bacteria as well as the host inflammatory processes in periodontal tissues (Barros & Offenbacher 2014; Benakanakere et al. 2015; Loo et al. 2010; Stefani et al. 2013).
- It is therefore the genetic makeup and the epigenetic program modulated by environmental stimuli that will determine the periodontal inflammatory response, and thus the disease phenotype, when challenged by plaque pathogens (Zhang et al. 2020). Thus, due to gene–environment interactions, genetic effects may differ across populations in the presence of environmental variability (Zhang et al. 2011).
- One mechanism of gene–environment interaction is the interaction between environmental genotoxic agents and individual polymorphic genetic assets, which can result in DNA damage, thereby triggering cell loss and tissue degeneration (De Flora et al. 1996).
- Another mechanism in gene–environment interactions is the genetic control of an individual's susceptibility to environmental factors, which include modulation of the effects of multiple risk factors (Ordovas & Shen 2008). Examples are (i) the interaction between the risk factor smoking and interleukin (IL) polymorphism increasing the risk for periodontal disease in IL-1 genotype-positive smokers, thus increasing the levels of expression of inflammatory mediators (Laine et al. 2001; Schenkein 2002); or (ii) dietary factors may produce epigenetic alterations in DNA, resulting in long-lasting changes in the expression of selected genes, such as a calorie-restriction diet that can dampen the inflammatory response and reduce active periodontal breakdown associated with an acute microbial challenge (Branch-Mays et al. 2008; Zhang et al. 2011).

Subgingival bacterial colonization
- Homeostasis at the mucosal surface is co-determined by colonizing bacteria and the host immune response, which is underpinned by the host's genetics. Resident microbes foster normal immune-system development and mediate both innate and adaptive immune responses to achieve a symbiosis at the mucosal surface (Zhang et al. 2020).
- T-regulatory (Treg) cells have been recognized for immune tolerance and biofilm control, whereby a reciprocal and functional metabolite-driven loop including short-chain fatty acids from microbes controls the numbers of Treg cells. Local Treg cells alter the bacterial composition and determine which bacteria are tolerated, and are thus important for the maintenance of mucosal or oral tolerance so as to avoid damaging immune reactions to commensal microorganisms (Alvarez et al. 2018).
- The host inflammatory or immune defense state thus impacts subgingival microbial colonization, and genetic variants can influence this colonization by causing a shift in the composition of the microbial community from periodontal health to periodontitis (Stefani et al. 2013; Zhang et al. 2020).
- Therefore, the subversion of host defenses from health to disease permits colonization with larger numbers of bacterial species, especially those non-pathogenic commensals that will favour pathogen growth, i.e. host genetic variants can affect the microbial colonization in a given ecological niche by specific microbes (Loo et al. 2010; Shaddox et al. 2021).
- Evidence suggests that in human biofilms, host genetic variants (most often single-nucleotide polymorphisms) could thus impact the threshold for dysbiosis, and based on the above, the term "genetic dysbiosis" defines the disruption of the homeostasis at the mucosal surface, i.e. an imbalance between the integrity of epithelial barrier function and colonizing microorganisms (Shaddox et al. 2021).
- Two mechanisms of host defense subversion (genetic dysbiosis) have been proposed:
  - Single-nucleotide polymorphism variants can compromise genes that are associated with pathways of bacterial sensing and recognition (Griffen et al. 2012). Variants in the promoter or coding sequence of pattern recognition receptor genes, or genes encoding binding partners of pattern recognition receptors in the downstream signaling events, can thus affect the colonizing capacities of certain bacteria in the plaque biofilm (Griffen et al. 2012).

(Continued)

Table 5.3.1 (Continued)

- ○ Variant-affected genes lead to an excessively inflammatory environment in the subgingival niche, favouring the growth of specific biofilm bacteria. Association studies have indicated specific single-nucleotide polymorphisms in IL-1, IL-6, and Fc-gamma receptor genes to be potentially predisposing to subgingival colonization with periodontopathogenic bacteria, such as *Aggregatibacter actinomycetemcomitans* (Cavalla et al. 2018; Divaris et al. 2012; Socransky et al. 2000). Furthermore, the hyperinflammatory response causes an increased production of gingival crevicular fluid, thereby providing nutrients for plaque bacteria. Thus, inflammation-associated metabolic changes of bacteria can influence the mass and structure of the subgingival biofilm. Additionally, the excessive inflammatory response can cause tissue breakdown, which then also feeds pathogenic bacteria, thereby affecting biofilm formation (Nibali et al. 2014).
- In summary, host genetic variants could impact the threshold for dysbiosis and the individual ability to resolve the self-perpetuating cycle of dysbiosis and inflammation generated by an acute stimulus (Kollam & Weiss 2006; Nibali et al. 2014). However, other studies have shown no differences in supra- and subgingival species, suggesting that any host genetic effects may not affect mature bacterial communities (Nibali et al. 2016; Papapostolou et al. 2011).

Periodontal disease pathogenicity

- Periodontitis may be associated with alterations to both structural components of the periodontal tissues and inflammatory mediators. Studies have described 310 single-nucleotide polymorphisms for 75 genes encoding structural components of the periodontal tissues and 50 genes encoding endogenous inflammatory mediators (Suzuki et al. 2004).
- Epithelial barrier activity is critical in the pathogenicity of both gingivitis and periodontitis (Zhang et al. 2020). Cytokeratin family proteins that are expressed in the upper spinous layer of the epithelium are important in the establishment of the epithelial barrier (Moutsopoulos et al. 2014).
- The down-regulation of epithelial homeostasis-associated genes (such as keratin 1, keratin 2, and keratin 3) can lead to a compromised gingival or mucosal epithelial barrier, enabling easier penetration of plaque pathogens and their metabolites into the connective tissue compartment, thereby directly inducing inflammation in the subepithelial region and accelerating alveolar bone loss (Collin et al. 1992).
- Specific ethnic and racial differences in disease-susceptibility gene polymorphisms have also been reported to be strongly associated with susceptibility to periodontal disease. This includes gene nucleotide polymorphisms for IL-1, IL-6, IL-10, FcγR, tumor necrosis factor (TNF)-α, vitamin D receptor (VDR), CD14, Toll-like receptors (TLR2 and TLR4), and MMP-1 (Laine et al. 2012; Zhang et al. 2011).
- These genetic polymorphisms may cause a change in the encoded protein, or its expression, resulting in alterations of pathways involved in cytokine and chemokine activities, B-cell receptor signaling, as well as defense and immunity proteins in both innate and adaptive immune responses, and may be the most up-regulated in periodontitis gingival tissues (Collin et al. 1992; Laine et al. 2012).
- For example, the transcription of genes associated with chemotaxis and transendothelial migration of leukocytes is significantly increased during the induction of gingival inflammation (Kim et al. 2016).
- TLR-4 is the primary receptor for bacterial lipopolysaccharide (LPS) produced by *A. actinomycetemcomitans*, *Porphyromonas gingivalis*, and *Veillonella parvula* (Shaddox et al. 2021). Variations in the TLR-4 gene can generate structural changes within the TLR-4 protein that affect the ability of the receptor to associate with ligand and/or its co-receptors (Rallabhandi et al. 2006). This can lead to an increased risk of infectious disease, including an association with chronic periodontitis susceptibility (Chrzęszczyk et al. 2015).
- Single-nucleotide polymorphism of the IL-1A −889 C/T) gene has been shown to be associated with a greater risk of chronic periodontitis (da Silva et al. 2017). A composite genotype composed of the alleles IL-1A −889 and IL-1B +3953 has been reported to have a positive association with chronic periodontitis in Caucasians (Nikolopoulos et al. 2008).
- Vitamin D plays a role in metabolic pathways involving antibacterial and anti-inflammatory properties (Krishnan & Feldman 2011; Svensson et al. 2016). Both chronic and aggressive periodontitis have been associated with vitamin D deficiency and with single-nucleotide polymorphism in the vitamin D receptor gene (Chen et al. 2012; Deng et al. 2011).
- Matrix metalloproteinases (MMPs) constitute a family of endopeptidases that regulate cell-matrix composition, which includes cleavage of components of the extracellular matrix and basement membrane, allowing cell migration and triggering the activity of signaling molecules (Shaddox et al. 2021). MMP-1 promoter single-nucleotide polymorphism has been shown to be associated with a greater risk of chronic periodontitis (Song et al. 2013).
- The homeostasis of IL-17, which is secreted by T-helper 17 lymphocytes, is imperative for balancing mucosal defense and inflammatory responses. IL-17 signaling in epithelial cells plays a protective role against pathogen invasion by recruiting adequate neutrophils to mucosal surfaces (Collin et al. 1992; Offenbacher et al. 2009). The excessive secretion of IL-17 can lead to a range of inflammatory mucocutaneous diseases, and the absence of IL-17 activity may severely compromise antimicrobial defense mechanisms. For example, genetic mutations disrupting IL-17 signaling can make patients prone to fungal infection (Demmer et al. 2008).

Table 5.3.1 (Continued)

Aggressive periodontal disease

- Aggressive periodontitis has a strong genetic component and it is more prevalent within families, with a familial aggregation among young patients (Boisson et al. 2013).
- A limited number of studies have indicated different single-nucleotide polymorphisms of a specific gene to be risk factors associated with different forms of periodontitis (Stabholz et al. 2010). These include gene–gene and gene–environment interactions (Moore 2003; Van der Velden 2017).
- Genetic variants that are linked to the immune response can influence the activation of several cellular signaling pathways (Renz et al. 2011). These pathways may affect the expression of IL-1, IL-4, IL-6, IL-10, TNF, E-selectins, FcγR, CD14, TLRs, caspase recruitment domain 15, and vitamin D receptor (Kulkarni & Kinane 2014; Laine et al. 2012; Loos et al. 2005).
- Hyperinflammatory genotypes (as in IL-1 or IL-6 hyper-producers) have been theorized to possibly predispose subgingival environments to being more conducive to the growth of *A. actinomycetemcomitans*, including recolonization with this bacterium following periodontal treatment (Nibali et al. 2011; Nikolopoulos et al. 2008).
- Genetic polymorphisms that affect neutrophil functions in aggressive periodontitis have also been studied, indicating an oxidative burst in response to challenge with *A. actinomycetemcomitans* (Nibali et al. 2013).
- It is also hypothesized that individuals with increased expression levels of FcγRI receptor on phagocytes, and elevated levels of immunoglobulin (Ig)A reactive to periodontal pathogens may be at higher risk for aggressive periodontitis, this being attributed to antibody-dependent cell-mediated cytotoxicity, superoxide generation, and the release of inflammatory mediators (Nibali et al. 2013).
- Disease phenotypes are also affected by their environment, for example smoking may potentiate the associations of certain genotypes with aggressive periodontitis (Vieira & Albandar 2014).

Periodontal wound healing

- During the healing process, different programs of variant gene expression are required by various cells necessary for cell proliferation, differentiation, and migration (Zhu et al. 2010).
- This acquisition is brought about by epigenetic modifications, which include histone post-translational modifications (PTMs), DNA methylation, higher-order chromatin remodeling, and non-coding regulatory RNA editing (Dongdong et al. 2014).
- Trauma, the environment, and stress trigger epigenetic processes that can include covalent chemical modifications of chromatin, affecting all DNA-associated processes, including the transcription of genes in the genome (Mehler 2008).
- This then includes either activation or suppression of specific genes, which then further modulate intracellular signaling pathways. These intracellular signaling pathways trigger cell migration and proliferation, which are needed during wound healing (Bannister & Kouzarides 2011; Srivastava et al. 2010; Zhang et al. 2020).
- Dysregulated epigenetic conditions may contribute to a delayed inflammatory process through changed gene expression patterns, such as in diabetic patients, and may thus exacerbate a chronic state of inflammation (Breton et al. 2009; den Dekker et al. 2019).

REFERENCES

Alvarez C, Rojas C, Rojas L et al. Regulatory T lymphocytes in periodontitis: a translational view. *Mediators Inflamm.* 2018; 2018:7806912.

Bannister AJ, Kouzarides T. Regulation of chromatin by histone modifications. *Cell Res.* 2011; 21:381–395.

Barros SP, Offenbacher S. Modifiable risk factors in periodontal disease: epigenetic regulation of gene expression in the inflammatory response. *Periodontol 2000.* 2014; 64:95–110.

Bartold PM, Van Dyke TE. An appraisal of the role of specific bacteria in the initial pathogenesis of periodontitis. *J Clin Periodontol.* 2019; 46:6–11.

Benakanakere M, Abdolhosseini M, Hosur K, Finoti LS, Kinane DF. TLR2 promoter hypermethylation creates innate immune dysbiosis. *J Dent Res.* 2015; 94:183–191.

Boisson B, Wang C, Pedergnana V et al. An ACT1 mutation selectively abolishes interleukin-17 responses in humans with chronic mucocutaneous candidiasis. *Immunity.* 2013; 39(4):676–686.

Branch-Mays GL, Dawson DR, Gunsolley JC et al. The effects of a calorie-reduced diet on periodontal inflammation and disease in a non-human primate model. *J Periodontol.* 2008; 79:1184–1191.

Breton CV, Byun HM, Wenten M et al. Prenatal tobacco smoke exposure affects global and gene-specific DNA methylation. *Am J Respir Crit Care Med.* 2009; 180:462–467.

Cavalla F, Biguetti C, Lima Melchiades J et al. Genetic association with subgingival bacterial colonization in chronic periodontitis. *Genes (Basel).* 2018; 9(6):271.

Chapple ILC, Bouchard P, Cagetti MG et al. Interaction of lifestyle, behaviour or systemic diseases with dental caries and periodontal diseases: consensus report of group 2 of the joint EFP/ORCA workshop on the boundaries between caries and periodontal diseases. *J Clin Periodontol.* 2017; 44(Suppl 18):S39–S51.

Chen L-L, Li H, Zhang P-P, Wang S-M. Association between vitamin D receptor polymorphisms and periodontitis: a meta-analysis. *J Periodontol.* 2012; 83(9):1095–1103.

Chrzęszczyk D, Konopka T, Ziętek M. Polymorphisms of toll-like receptor 4 as a risk factor for periodontitis: meta-analysis. *Adv Clin Exp Med.* 2015; 24(6):1059–1070.

Collin C, Moll R, Kubicka S, Ouhayoun JP, Franke WW. Characterization of human cytokeratin 2, an epidermal cytoskeletal protein synthesized late during differentiation *Exp Cell Res.* 1992; 202(1):132–141.

Cutroneo KR, Chiu JF. Comparison and evaluation of gene therapy and epigenetic approaches for wound healing. *Wound Repair Regen.* 2000; 8:494–502.

da Silva FR, Guimaraes-Vasconcelos AC, de-Carvalho-Franca LF et al. Relationship between -889 C/T polymorphism in interleukin-1A gene and risk of chronic periodontitis: evidence from a meta-analysis with new published findings. *Med Oral Patol Oral Cir Bucal.* 2017; 22(1):e7–e14.

De Flora S, Izzotti A, Randerath K et al. DNA adducts and chronic degenerative diseases. Pathogenetic relevance and implications in preventive medicine. *Mutat Res.* 1996; 366:197–238.

Demmer RT, Behle JH, Wolf DL et al. Transcriptomes in healthy and diseased gingival tissues. *J Periodontol.* 2008; 79(11):2112–2124.

den Dekker A, Davis FM, Kunkel SL, Gallagher KA. Targeting epigenetic mechanisms in diabetic wound healing. *Transl Res.* 2019; 204:39–50.

Deng H, Liu F, Pan YH et al. BsmI, TaqI, ApaI, and FokI polymorphisms in the vitamin D receptor gene and periodontitis: a meta-analysis of 15 studies including 1338 cases and 1302 controls. *J Clin Periodontol.* 2011; 38(3):199–207.

Divaris K, Monda KL, North KE et al. Genome-wide association study of periodontal pathogen colonization. *J Dent Res.* 2012; 91(7 Suppl):21S–28S.

Dongdong T, Meirong L, Xiaobing F, Weidong H. Causes and consequences of epigenetic regulation in wound healing. *Wound Rep Reg.* 2014; 22:305–312.

Gibson G. Rare and common variants: twenty arguments. *Nat Rev Genet.* 2012; 13(2):135–145.

Griffen AL, Beall CJ, Campbell JH et al. Distinct and complex bacterial profiles in human periodontitis and health revealed by 16S pyrosequencing. *ISME J.* 2012; 6(6):1176–1185.

Grossi SG, Zambon JJ, Ho AW et al. Assessment of risk for periodontal disease. I. Risk indicators for attachment loss. *J Periodontol.* 1994; 65:260–267.

Hart TC, Marazita ML, Wright JT. The impact of molecular genetics on oral health paradigms. *Crit Rev Oral Biol Med.* 2000; 11(1):26–56.

Kellam P, Weiss RA. Infectogenomics: insights from the host genome into infectious diseases. *Cell.* 2006; 124(4):695–697.

Kim YG, Kim M, Kang JH et al. Transcriptome sequencing of gingival biopsies from chronic periodontitis patients reveals novel gene expression and splicing patterns. *Hum Genomics.* 2016; 10(1):28.

Kinane DF, Hart TC. Genes and gene polymorphisms associated with periodontal disease. *Crit Rev Oral Biol Med.* 2003; 14(6):430–449.

Kornman KS. Mapping the pathogenesis of periodontitis: a new look. *J Periodontol.* 2008; 79:1560–1568.

Krishnan AV, Feldman D. Mechanisms of the anti-cancer and anti inflammatory actions of vitamin D. *Annu Rev Pharmacol Toxicol.* 2011; 51(1):311–336.

Kulkarni C, Kinane DF. Host response in aggressive periodontitis. *Periodontol 2000.* 2014; 65:79–91.

Kuman M. The chronic diseases require nonlinear mathematical description. *Adv Complement Alt Med.* 2018; 1(3):1–4. ACAM.000514.

Laine ML, Crielaard W, Loos BG. Genetic susceptibility to periodontitis. *Periodontol 2000.* 2012; 58(1):37–68.

Laine ML, Farre MA, Gonzalez G et al. Polymorphisms of the interleukin-1 gene family, oral microbial pathogens, and smoking in adult periodontitis. *J Dent Res.* 2001; 80:1695–1699.

Löe H, Anerud A, Boysen H, Morrison E. Natural history of periodontal disease in man: rapid, moderate and no loss of attachment in Sri Lankan laborers 14 to 46 years of age. *J Clin Periodontol.* 1986; 13(5):431–445.

Löe H, Anerud A, Boysen H, Smith M. The natural history of periodontal disease in man: the rate of periodontal destruction before 40 years of age. *J Periodontol.* 1978; 49(12):607–620.

Loo WT, Jin L, Cheung MN, Wang M, Chow LW. Epigenetic change in E-cadherin and COX-2 to predict chronic periodontitis. *J Transl Med.* 2010; 8:110.

Loos BG, John RP, Laine ML. Identification of genetic risk factors for periodontitis and possible mechanisms of action. *J Clin Periodontol.* 2005; 32(Suppl. 6):159–179.

Loos BG, Van Dyke TE. The role of inflammation and genetics in periodontal disease. *Periodontol 2000.* 2020; 83:26–39.

Mehler MF. Epigenetic principles and mechanisms underlying nervous system functions in health and disease. *Prog Neurobiol.* 2008; 86:305–341.

Moore JH. The ubiquitous nature of epistasis in determining susceptibility to common human diseases. *Hum Hered.* 2003; 56:73–82.

Moutsopoulos NM, Konkel J, Sarmadi M et al. Defective neutrophil recruitment in leukocyte adhesion deficiency type I disease causes local IL-17-driven inflammatory bone loss. *Sci Transl Med.* 2014; 6(229):229ra40.

Nibali L, Di Iorio A, Onabolu O, Lin GH. Periodontal infectogenomics: systematic review of associations between host genetic variants and subgingival microbial detection. *J Clin Periodontol.* 2016; 43(11):889–900.

Nibali L, Henderson B, Sadiq ST, Donos N. Genetic dysbiosis: the role of microbial insults in chronic inflammatory diseases. *J Oral Microbiol.* 2014; 6(1):22962.

Nibali L, Madden I, Franch CF et al. IL6 -174 genotype associated with *Aggregatibacter actinomycetemcomitans* in Indians. *Oral Dis.* 2011; 17(2):232–237.

Nibali L, Pelekos G, D'Aiuto F et al. Influence of IL-6 haplotypes on clinical and inflammatory response in aggressive periodontitis. *Clin Oral Investig.* 2013; 17(4):1235–1242.

Nikolopoulos GK, Dimou NL, Hamodrakas SJ, Bagos PG. Cytokine gene polymorphisms in periodontal disease: a meta-analysis of 53 studies including 4178 cases and 4590 controls. *J Clin Periodontol.* 2008; 35(9):754–767.

Offenbacher S, Barros SP, Paquette DW et al. Gingival transcriptome patterns during induction and resolution of experimental gingivitis in humans. *J Periodontol.* 2009; 80(12):1963–1982.

Ordovas JM, Shen J. Gene–environment interactions and susceptibility to metabolic syndrome and other chronic diseases. *J Periodontol.* 2008; 79:1508–1513.

Papapostolou A, Kroffke B, Tatakis DN, Nagaraja HN, Kumar PS. Contribution of host genotype to the composition of health-associated supragingival and subgingival microbiomes. *J Clin Periodontol.* 2011; 38(6):517–524.

Raghuraman S, Donkin I, Versteyhe S, Barres R, Simar D. The emerging role of epigenetics in inflammation and immunometabolism. *Trends Endocrinol Metab.* 2016; 27:782–795.

Rallabhandi P, Bell J, Boukhvalova MS et al. Analysis of TLR4 polymorphic variants: new insights into TLR4/MD-2/CD14 stoichiometry, structure, and signaling. *J Immunol.* 2006; 177(1):322–332.

Renz H, von Mutius E, Brandtzaeg P et al. Gene–environment interactions in chronic inflammatory disease. *Nat Immunol* 2011; 12:273–277.

Schenkein HA. Finding genetic risk factors for periodontal diseases: is the climb worth the view? *Periodontol 2000.* 2002; 30:79–90.

Shaddox LM, Morford LA, Nibali L. Periodontal health and disease: the contribution of genetics. *Periodontol 2000.* 2021; 85:161–181.

Socransky SS, Haffajee AD, Smith C, Duff GW. Microbiological parameters associated with IL-1 gene polymorphisms in periodontitis patients. *J Clin Periodontol.* 2000; 27(11):810–818.

Song GG, Kim JH, Lee YH. Toll-like receptor (TLR) and matrix metalloproteinase (MMP) polymorphisms and periodontitis susceptibility: a meta-analysis. *Mol Biol Rep.* 2013; 40(8):5129–5141.

Srivastava S, Mishra RK, Dhawan J. Regulation of cellular chromatin state: insights from quiescence and differentiation. *Organogenesis.* 2010; 6:37–47.

Stabholz A, Soskolne WA, Shapira L. Genetic and environmental risk factors for chronic periodontitis and aggressive periodontitis. *Periodontol 2000.* 2010; 53:138–153.

Stefani FA, Viana MB, Dupim AC et al. Expression, polymorphism and methylation pattern of interleukin-6 in periodontal tissues. *Immunobiology.* 2013; 218:1012–1017.

Suzuki A, Ji G, Numabe Y et al. Single nucleotide polymorphisms associated with aggressive periodontitis and severe chronic periodontitis in Japanese. *Biochem Biophys Res Commun.* 2004; 317:887–892.

Svensson D, Nebel D, Nilsson BO. Vitamin D3 modulates the innate immune response through regulation of the hCAP-18/LL-37 gene expression and cytokine production. *Inflamm Res.* 2016; 65(1):25–32.

Van der Velden U. What exactly distinguishes aggressive from chronic periodontitis: is it mainly a difference in the degree of bacterial invasiveness? *Periodontol 2000.* 2017; 75:24–44.

Vieira AR, Albandar JM. Role of genetic factors in the pathogenesis of aggressive periodontitis. *Periodontol 2000.* 2014; 65:92–106.

Wang KC, Helms JA, Chang HY. Regeneration, repair and remembering identity: the three Rs of Hox gene expression. *Trends Cell Biol.* 2009; 19:268–275.

Zhang J, Sun X, Xiao L et al. Gene polymorphisms and periodontitis. *Periodontol 2000.* 2011; 56:102–124.

Zhang S, Yu N, Arce RM. Periodontal inflammation: Integrating genes and dysbiosis. *Periodontol 2000.* 2020; 82:129–142.

Zhang TY, Meaney MJ. Epigenetics and the environmental regulation of the genome and its function. *Annu Rev Psychol.* 2010; 61:439–466, C1–C3.

Zhu XL, Meng HX, Xu L et al. Combined association of CCR2-V64I and MCP-1-2518A/G polymorphisms with generalized aggressive periodontitis in Chinese. *Chin J Dent Res.* 2010; 13:109–114.

5.4 IMMUNOPATHOGENESIS OF PERIODONTAL DISEASE

Steph Smith

Contents

Learning objectives

- Interaction between periodontal pathogens and host susceptibility during the initiation of periodontal disease.
- Basic immunological mechanisms involved in the pathogenesis of periodontal disease.
- Mechanisms of connective tissue destruction.
- Basic immunological mechanisms of alveolar bone destruction.
- Mechanisms of resolution of inflammation.

Introduction

Periodontal disease (PD) is a complex inflammatory disease that includes a tissue-degrading, non-linear inflammatory response to colonizing plaque bacteria (Kantarci et al. 2015). The diagnosis and treatment planning of PD are based on an understanding of etiology (plaque) and patient susceptibility. Susceptibility to disease (pathogenesis) involves interaction between the host, bacteria, environmental factors, as well as differential gene expression (Ohlrich et al. 2009). Susceptibility, clinical heterogeneity, disease progression, and response to treatment are furthermore substantiated by epigenetics. Epigenetics comprises the interface between genetic and environmental factors, giving rise to certain phenotypes (Barros & Offenbacher 2014), whereby epigenetic changes can influence host responses to bacteria and host inflammatory processes in periodontal tissues (Benekanakere et al. 2015; Loo et al. 2010; Stefani et al. 2013). Extensive knowledge has been gained using in vitro and animal model studies; however, the utilization of reductionist models of disease based on artificial oral infection leaves significant challenges in discerning the complexity of the in situ biology of the pathogenesis of periodontitis (Kantarci et al. 2015).

Periodontal pathogens

Periodontal health is associated with a symbiotic oral microbiome (Dongari-Bagtzoglou 2008), including putative pathogens, however, not being pathogenic (Kolenbrander et al. 2010). Presently, the development of PD is considered as the result of an ecological succession of subgingival plaque bacteria, including an increase in bacterial load, with the emergence of keystone pathogens (Oliveira et al. 2016). Various hypotheses have been proposed regarding the development of PD, including the ecological plaque hypothesis (Marsh 1994), the keystone pathogen hypothesis (Hajishengallis et al. 2012), and the polymicrobial synergy and dysbiosis model (Hajishengallis & Lamont 2012; Lamont & Hajishengallis 2015). Unlike many infectious diseases, PD appears to be an infection mediated by the overgrowth of commensal organisms, with the identification of a "true pathogen" being elusive (Cekici et al. 2014). Evidence does exist that specific microbes are associated with progressive forms of PD; however, a landmark study has shown that many people who carry specific periodontal pathogens do not develop PD (Cullinan et al. 2003). The mere presence of these bacteria in the absence of disease progression suggests that PD is the net effect of the immune response (Cekici et al. 2014). in vitro studies and a limited number of in vivo studies, specifically utilizing biopsy specimens from advanced periodontitis lesions, have described bacterial invasion of epithelial cells (Baek et al. 2018; Bartold & Van Dyke 2019). However, such studies are largely lacking in healthy periodontal tissues, gingivitis, or early periodontitis lesions (Bartold & Van Dyke 2019). Furthermore, there is no in vivo evidence of keystone pathogenic bacteria migrating across intact basement membranes from within gingival epithelial cells into the underlying connective tissues (Bartold & Van Dyke 2019). Also, in vivo evidence is non-existent regarding any interactions between invading bacteria and fibroblasts, osteoblasts, or osteoclasts (Bartold & Van Dyke 2019). Histopathological studies do not support in vitro investigations of direct interactions of bacteria with neutrophils, fibroblasts, lymphocytes, or bone cells (Bartold & Van Dyke 2019). It has thus been suggested that without in vivo confirmation of such in vitro findings, the validity of such investigations should be questioned (Bartold & Van Dyke 2019).

Patient susceptibility

PD is recognized as a continuum of inflammation in response to bacteria in the dental biofilm (Cekici et al. 2014). This is however modified by multiple host response genes in combination with environmental factors and systemic diseases (Bartold & Van Dyke 2013, 2019). Of the risk for the development of PD, 20% is attributed to the deposition and accumulation of plaque (Grossi et al. 1994) and 80% to environmental determinants and genetic variations within individuals (see also Chapter 5.3), which in turn perpetuate a dysregulated immune-inflammatory response (Bartold & Van Dyke 2019; Grossi et al. 1994; Kornman 2007). Plaque control methods for the management of PD are only partially effective and fail in high-risk individuals (Bartold & Van Dyke 2019). The ultimate outcome of disease is determined by the presence of specific periodontal pathogens together with, importantly, a patient's innate susceptibility (Hirschfeld & Wasserman 1978). Superimposed on this are environmental factors that impact disease expression and progression, by means of affecting the manner of the host response to periodontopathic bacterial complexes (Cekici et al. 2014; Hirschfeld & Wasserman 1978; Ohlrich et al. 2009). Although not proven in human studies, animal studies have shown systemic inflammation to exacerbate periodontal inflammation and destruction (Zeng et al. 2017). Evidence from studies regarding gut dysbiosis, which is directly related to inflammation, shows that controlling gut inflammation limits the proliferation of disease-associated bacteria (Dongari-Bagtzoglou 2008). Periodontal pathogens are part of the normal oral microbiome, and their emergence and overgrowth always occur after the initial onset of periodontal inflammation (Bartold & Van Dyke 2019; Lindhe et al. 1980; Listgarten 1988; Tanner et al. 2007). The inference cannot thus be made that they cause PD, as inflammation-mediated environmental changes could just as probably have selected for them (Bartold & Van Dyke 2019; Kamada et al. 2013). It is therefore suggested that it is inflammation that drives periodontal dysbiosis, and that an overemphasis has been placed on keystone pathogens being responsible for the initiation of periodontitis, at the expense of considering the host response and genetic and environmental factors (Bartold & Van Dyke 2019).

Emerging evidence suggests that the inflammatory response within the individual is responsible for the changes in the periodontal microbiome, and therefore determines the risk for PD (Bartold & Van Dyke 2019; Socransky & Haffajee 2005). Early colonizing plaque bacteria induce gingival inflammation, and the innate immune response causes changes in the subgingival environment, allowing for increases in certain endogenous commensal bacteria (Socransky & Haffajee 2002, 2005). It is thus only after the initial resultant immunoinflammatory changes within the gingiva that an overgrowth of the bacterial load occurs, which includes the selection of specific pathogenic bacteria based on their growth requirements (mimicking a bacterial dysbiosis) (Bartold & Van Dyke 2019). Therefore, PD is not a conventional bacterial infectious disease, but is rather considered an inflammatory disease that is triggered by an inappropriate inflammatory reaction to the normal microbiota in the bacterial biofilm, which is subsequently exacerbated by the overgrowth of disease-associated bacterial species (Bartold & Van Dyke 2017, 2019). In light of this, an inverted paradigm hypothesis for the pathogenesis of PD has been proposed, whereby infection is driven and exacerbated by inflammation (Bartold & Van Dyke 2019) (see Figure 5.4.1). The concept is thus suggested that to enable the management of PD, inflammation should be controlled, thereby controlling infection (Bartold & Van Dyke 2017, 2019).

Immunoinflammatory mechanisms in the periodontium

Plaque biofilms contain complexes of periodontal pathogens; however, many people carry the organisms without manifesting disease progression (Cullinan et al. 2003). In this context, most people are in balance with their biofilm and it is the function of the immune response to maintain this homeostasis in the presence of the plaque biofilm. When this balance is disturbed, disease may result. There is presently general acceptance that tissue destruction is mediated via the effects of the immune response and is not a direct consequence of the bacteria per se (Seymour et al. 2015).

The development of gingivitis is considered a well-controlled immunological response, which includes proper innate immune responses ensuring effective adaptive immunity, which in turn potentiate the innate defense against periodontopathogens (Silva et al. 2015). The purpose is thus to eliminate infectious agents and to maintain local homeostasis and tissue integrity. The T-cell response is considered to be the

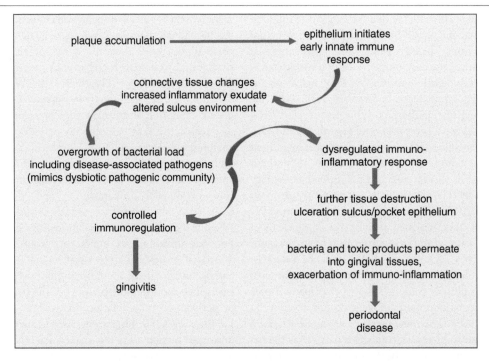

Figure 5.4.1 Inverted model for the pathogenesis of periodontal disease. An innate immune response is initiated by plaque bacteria. With unresolved continuous inflammation, the inflammatory exudate increases, accompanied by alteration of the sulcus environment. Increasing inflammation allows for the overgrowth of the bacterial load, including the selection of specific pathogenic bacteria based on their growth requirements. Gingivitis develops whereby there is an association between a controlled immune response and the subgingival microbiome. With a dysregulated immune response, however, uncontrolled gingival inflammation develops with a breach in the sulcular epithelium. A new environment develops followed by the permeation of pathogenic bacteria and their toxins into the tissues, consequently exacerbating inflammation, eventually leading to periodontal disease. Source: Adapted from Bartold & Van Dyke 2019.

default response responsible for this balance. PD progression will however be determined by the nature of the immune-inflammatory response (Teng 2006b). This response differs among individuals, depending on antimicrobial and pro- and anti-inflammatory cytokine responses, environmental factors, and the subjects' genetic makeup (Bartold & Van Dyke 2019; Tawfig 2016). Although many in vitro studies have elucidated the various and complex host–immune bacterial interactions,

effective modeling systems are still required to mimic or reflect the exact molecular mechanisms that may occur in vivo (Bartold & Van Dyke 2019; Teng 2006a). The overlapping intersections of innate and adaptive immunity are blurred and the underlying biological mechanisms are increasing in complexity (Paul 2011) (see Figure 5.4.2). Box 5.4.1 describes the basic proposed immunological mechanisms of inflammation during the development of PD.

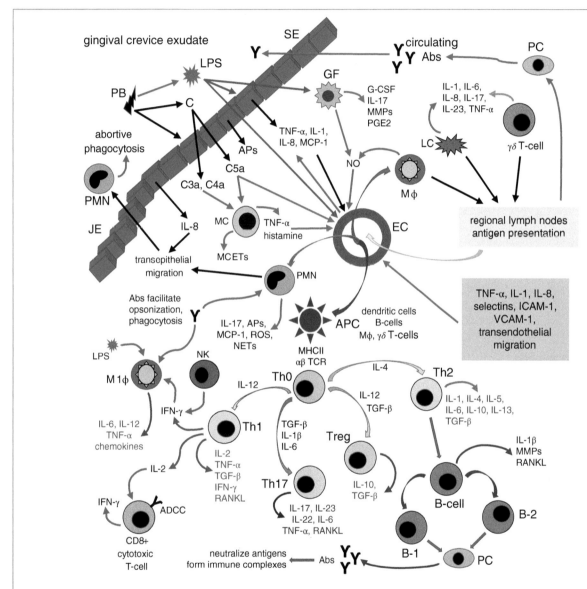

Figure 5.4.2 Immunoinflammatory mechanisms in the periodontium. αβ TCR, alpha beta T-cell receptor on Th0 cell; ADCC, antibody-dependent cellular cytotoxicity; APC, antigen-presenting cell (dendritic cells, B cells, Mφ and ΥδT cells); Aps, antimicrobial peptides; C, complement activation; CD8+, T-cytotoxic cell; EC, endothelial cells; G-CSF, granulocyte colony-stimulating factor; GF, gingival fibroblast; ICAM-1, intercellular adhesion molecule-1; IFN-γ, interferon gamma; IL, interleukin; JE, junctional epithelium; LC, Langerhans cells; LPS, lipopolysaccharide; Mφ, macrophages; MC, mast cells; MCETs, mast cell extracellular traps; MCP-1, monocyte chemoattractant protein-1; MHC11, MHC class 11 receptor on APC; MMPs, matrix metalloproteinases; NETs, neutrophil extracellular traps; NK, natural killer cell; NO, nitric oxide; PB, periodontal bacteria; PC, plasma cell; PMN, neutrophils; RANKL, receptor activator of nuclear factor-kappa B (NFκB) ligandl; ROS, reactive oxygen species; SE, sulcular epithelium; TGF-β, transforming growth factor-beta; Th, T-helper cells; TNF-α, tumor necrosis factor-alpha; Treg, T-regulatory cells; VCAM-1, vascular cell adhesion molecule-1; Υ = Abs, antibodies; ΥδT-cell, gamma delta T cell. Courtesy of Dr. Steph Smith.

Box 5.4.1 Immunoinflammatory mechanisms in the periodontium (see also Figure 5.4.2)

Innate immunity

Initial inflammation in periodontal tissues is considered a physiological defense mechanism rather than pathology (Cekici et al. 2014). Innate immune mechanisms include the barrier function of oral epithelium, together with vascular and cellular aspects of inflammation. The innate (non-specific) component of the immune response is not aimed specifically at any antigen (Kinane et al. 2008). Host pathogen recognition receptors (PRRs), such as CD14 and Toll-like receptors (TLRs), are expressed on epithelial cells, endothelial cells, mast cells, dendritic cells, lymphocytes, macrophages, polymorphonuclear neutrophils (PMNs), osteoblasts, and osteoclast precursors. PRRs recognize pathogen-associated molecular patterns (PAMPs), such as lipopolysaccharide (LPS), bacterial lipoproteins and lipoteichoic acids, peptidoglycans, flagellin, and DNA of bacteria and viruses. (Cekici et al. 2014; Meyle et al. 2017). For example, LPS binds to LPS-binding protein (CD14) and selects TLRs on epithelial cells, PMNs, monocytes, macrophages, and mast cells, thereby activating these cells (Sanz et al. 2017). In humans, however, the role of and response to biofilm-specific antigens have yet to be established, as dental plaque is a complex biofilm. Different people may have individually specific pathogenic complexes that may not be pathogenic in all people. Nevertheless, co-infection with multiple organisms can possibly modulate the immune response (Seymour et al. 2015).

PRR–PAMP interaction leads to production of cytokines and chemokines. Cytokines play a central role in the modulation of inflammation. Proinflammatory cytokines are for example tumor necrosis factor (TNF)-α, interleukin (IL)-1, IL-6, IL-8, IL-12, and anti-inflammatory cytokines are IL-1 receptor antagonist (IL-1RA), IL-4, IL-10, and transforming growth factor-beta (TGF-β) (Nicu & Loos 2016). TNF-α and IL-1 are secreted by monocytes/macrophages, PMNs, fibroblasts, epithelial cells, endothelial cells, and osteoblasts (Yucel-Lindberg & Båge 2013). Chemokines, IL-8, and monocyte chemoattractant protein-1 (MCP-1) are secreted by monocytes, lymphocytes, epithelial cells, endothelial cells, and fibroblasts, in response to IL-1, TNF-α, and LPS, and attract phagocytes to the site of infection (Cekici et al. 2014).

PAMPs of commensal bacteria and putative pathogens engage TLRs on epithelial cells. TLR signaling increases the innate antimicrobial resistance of epithelial cells to release IL-1α, and via an autocrine loop secrete IL-1α to up-regulate expression of antimicrobial peptides, including defensins, calprotectin, and cathelicidin (Sanz et al. 2017).

PMNs are also storehouses of antimicrobial proteins. Antimicrobial peptides serve as danger-associated molecular patterns (DAMPs), activating inflammasomes of epithelial cells and PMNs. The resultant production of inflammasome superoxides is toxic to both microbes and host tissues, causing local tissue damage and micro-abscess formation (Sanz et al. 2017). Antimicrobial peptides secreted by epithelial cells and PMNs activate the complement cascade, mast cells, and macrophages, and are chemotactic for Langerhans cells, CD4+, and CD8+ cells. They also up-regulate IL-8 production by epithelial cells, enhancing PMN recruitment (Marshall 2004).

Complement proteins in gingival crevicular fluid enter the gingival sulcus by percolation through the junctional epithelium and are rapidly activated by oral microbes, eliciting an inflammatory response (Sanz et al. 2017). Even in the presence of pathogen-specific antibodies (Abs), activation of the complement cascade is mostly via the alternative pathway, which is done by bacterial polysaccharides, LPS, or aggregated IgA, through factor P (properdin) that cleaves C3 (Cekici et al. 2014). C3b acts as an opsonin, facilitating phagocytosis and intracellular killing of bacteria by PMNs. Activated complement generating anaphylatoxins C3a, C4a, and C5a attracts monocytes, lymphocytes, and PMNs. Complement proteins also directly kill bacteria and stimulate mast cells (Yucel-Lindberg & Båge 2013).

Mast cells (MCs) possess complement receptor 3 (CR3) and FcγR, thereby recognizing pathogens that have been opsonized by either complement or immunoglobulin (Ig)G respectively. In the absence of opsonins, antigen recognition is mediated by cell-surface receptors such as TLRs or the mannose receptor (Marshall 2004; Okayama et al. 2000).

Activated MCs mediate a variety of antimicrobial activities. Opsonin-mediated binding leads to endocytosis and internalization of bacteria via the endosome–lysosome pathway, whereby bacteria are killed through a combination of oxidative and non-oxidative killing systems (Féger et al. 2002). Antimicrobial peptides such as cathelicidin LL-37, ß-defensins, and piscidins are present in MC granules and are secreted, indicating a possible extracellular phagocytosis-independent bactericidal mechanism (von Köckritz-Blickwede et al. 2008). However, degranulation of MCs can lead to an excessive release of proteolytic enzymes with tryptase-, chymase-, or carboxypeptidase-like activities, metalloproteases, cytokines, chemokines, or arachidonic acid metabolites, thereby exacerbating the inflammatory response and tissue damage (Martin & Leibovich 2005). Another form of extracellular killing of bacteria is by means of dying MCs forming mast cell extracellular traps (MCETs), which are strongly dependent on the production of reactive oxygen species (ROS). MCETs are composed of DNA, histones, MC-specific protease tryptase, and antimicrobial peptides. In addition to killing microbes, MCETs contribute to minimizing tissue damage by sequestering harmful compounds at infection sites, thereby preventing diffusion into surrounding non-infected tissue (von Köckritz-Blickwede et al. 2008).

The initial reaction of antigen contact with host cells includes a release of vasodilating agents causing an increase of vascular permeability (Nedzi-Góra et al. 2017). Activated MCs release preformed and newly synthesized inflammatory mediators, cytokines, and chemokines that recruit neutrophils to infection sites. MCs are the only cell type known to prestore TNF-α in their secretory granules, which is immediately released upon pathogen stimulation to initiate the early phase of the inflammatory response (von Köckritz-Blickwede et al. 2008). MCs secrete histamine in response to IL-1, IL-6, C3a, and C5a (Nedzi-Góra et al. 2017). Macrophages infiltrating inflamed tissues (Brennan et al. 2003) and gingival fibroblasts (Daghigh et al. 2002) secrete nitric oxide, causing vascular relaxation. The release of vasoactive amines and TNF-α increases vascular permeability and stimulates expression of vascular adhesion molecules such as intercellular adhesion molecule-1 (ICAM-1), vascular cell adhesion molecule -1 (VCAM-1), and P- and E-selectin on endothelial cell surfaces. Thus, tissue-derived cytokines and chemokines, such as IL-8 and MCP-1, together with adhesion ligands on endothelial cells, will then induce transendothelial migration and recruitment of inflammatory cells into the tissues (Cortés-Vieyra et al. 2016; Tawfig 2016).

PMNs are the first line of defense and produce cytokines and chemokines, which influence the immune response (Cortés-Vieyra et al. 2016; Mocsai 2013). PMN recruitment controls bacterial infections; however, PMN homeostasis is also imperative, so as to prevent collateral damage to the host (Hajishengallis & Hajishengallis 2014). PMN recruitment to the periodontium is also independent of commensal bacteria, this serving an immune surveillance function in periodontal health (Zenobia et al. 2013).

Regarding neutrophil homeostasis, granulopoiesis and neutrophil release from bone marrow is regulated by granulocyte colony-stimulating factor (G-CSF). During acute inflammation, G-CSF is released from fibroblasts, macrophages, and dendritic cells (Hajishengallis et al. 2015; Nicu & Loos 2016; von Vietinghoff & Ley 2008). Tissue-associated PMNs then release chemokines, i.e. monocyte chemoattractant protein-1 (MCP-1) and CCL20, which are ligands for CCR2 and CCR6 chemokine

receptors on TH17 cells. Th17 cells as well as PMNs and fibroblasts then secrete IL-17, which in turn up-regulates the production of G-CSF, promoting the release of PMNs from bone marrow (Cortés-Vieyra et al. 2016; Hajishengallis et al. 2015; Pelletier et al. 2010). This creates a positive loop for neutrophil recruitment (Zenobia & Hajishengallis 2015). Thereafter, PMNs undergo apoptosis and are cleared by resident macrophages and dendritic cells. Phagocytosis by macrophages of apoptotic PMNs triggers an anti-inflammatory reduction in IL-23 secretion by macrophages, causing reduced levels of IL-17 (Stark et al. 2005). This leads to less G-CSF production, and consequently less PMN production. Thus, a negative feedback loop, i.e. a neutrostat regulatory circuit (neutrostat IL-23–IL-17-G-CSF axis), is thus established that maintains steady-state PMN levels (Cortés-Vieyra et al. 2016; Hajishengallis et al. 2015; Zenobia & Hajishengallis 2015). The clearance of transmigrated apoptotic neutrophils is thus crucial for the regulation of neutrophil production in the bone marrow (Hajishengallis et al. 2015).

PMNs are present in large numbers in inflamed periodontal tissues, their presence correlating with the severity of PD, whereby tissue destruction results from collateral damage from activated PMNs (Cortés-Vieyra et al. 2016). Activation of PMNs involves priming and activation. Priming occurs with the initial exposure of PMNs to inflammatory cytokines and PAMPs (e.g. LPS). Primed PMNs respond more readily to activating agents, survive longer, and show delayed apoptosis. Maximal PMN degranulation and ROS release occur only in cells that have been primed before activation (Nicu & Loos 2016). Peripheral PMNs from periodontitis patients exhibit hyper-reactivity following stimulation by complement and bacteria, and hyperactivity in terms of excess ROS release in the absence of exogenous stimulation. The majority of PMNs then undergo transmigration by exiting through the vascular basement membrane using endothelial cell–cell junctions (paracellular route). However, about 10% will migrate transcellularly, i.e. directly through the center of an endothelial cell (Mocsai 2013; Nicu & Loos 2016; Woodfin et al. 2011).

Endogenous and exogenous chemoattractants, including PAMPs, LPS, IL-8, and C5a, bind to chemoattractant receptors on PMNs. Endogenous chemokines are produced by macrophages, fibroblasts, endothelial cells, platelets, T cells, and epithelial cells (Sanz et al. 2017). This determines the direction of migration for PMNs (Nicu & Loos 2016; Roberts et al. 2015). Phagocytic activation of PMNs is facilitated by receptors, i.e. opsonic C3b fragments and opsonic IgG Abs, as well as PAMP binding to PMN TLR ligands

(Herrmann & Meyle 2015). Phagocytosis in the absence of opsonization is mediated by CD14 receptors for LPS (Nicu & Loos 2016). Peripheral blood PMNs from PD patients can be of both hyperactive and hyper-reactive phenotypes. Intrinsic hyper-responsiveness of PMNs in PD has been hypothesized, whereby genetic polymorphism of PMN receptors may be responsible in certain percentages of the population (Nicu et al. 2007). However, even normal PMNs persisting in periodontal tissues can induce tissue damage, by undergoing necrosis in the absence of normal apoptosis. LPS inhibit apoptosis whereby PMNs die predominantly via necrosis, leading to the uncontrolled release of toxic PMN products into the tissues (Turina et al. 2005). PMNs in PD patients may also be dysfunctional, exhibiting reduced neutrophil chemotactic accuracy and velocity (Roberts et al. 2015). This may allow for a longer presence and greater potency of bacteria in periodontal tissues. IL-8, interferon-alpha (IFN-α) (due to viral infection), and G-CSF secretion may induce especially hyper-responsive PMNs to release extracellular ROS (Cooper et al. 2013; Matthews et al. 2007). PMNs in PD showing defective chemotactic accuracy will potentially undergo increased tissue transit times and, furthermore, if apoptosis of PMNs is disturbed with extracellular degranulation of excess ROS production, together with neutrophil elastase and matrix metalloproteinase secretion, this can lead to exacerbated collateral host tissue destruction (Cooper et al. 2013; Fuchs et al. 2007; Roberts et al. 2015). Oxidative stress manifested with increased cytokine secretion in close proximity to alveolar bone can also trigger receptor activator of nuclear factor-kappa B (NF-κB) ligand (RANKL)-mediated bone resorption (Cooper et al. 2013).

ROS, IL-8 (produced by macrophages and epithelial and endothelial cells), bacteria, LPS, and other bacterial toxins induce the release of PMNs' nuclear DNA, histone-rich proteins, and cathelicidin antimicrobial peptides as a biological 'spider's web' into the surrounding tissues, comprising the formation of neutrophil extracellular traps (NETs) (Cooper et al. 2013; Nicu & Loos 2016). This process is considered a new form of programmed cell death, namely NETosis, which is distinct from necrosis and apoptosis (Brinkmann et al. 2004). NETs allow PMNs to immobilize and kill bacteria and deactivate microbial virulence factors independently of phagocytosis (Fuchs et al. 2007; Martinelli et al. 2004). NETs may serve as adjuvants to phagocytosis by other PMNs (Brinkmann et al. 2004); initiate activation of the classical pathway of the complement cascade (Leffler et al. 2012); and prime and increase proliferation of CD4+ and CD8+ cells, together with IFN-ɣ release (Tillack et al. 2012). PD may however be associated with excessive production of

NETs, which are a rich source of autoantigens and concentrated degradative enzymes, leading to localized chronic inflammation, with an autoimmune component (Cooper et al. 2013; Matthews et al. 2007).

Bacterially derived chemotactic substances and C5a induce migration of PMNs into the gingival sulcus. However, PMNs in the sulcus are unable to phagocytose bacteria located in the tooth-associated biofilm. In this situation, PMNs disgorge their lysosomal contents into the gingival sulcus, a process termed "abortive phagocytosis." These lysosomal enzymes can return into the tissues, causing local destruction of connective tissues (Seymour et al. 2015). Within the gingival sulcus, PMNs also release IL-1, IL-1RA, and high levels of IL-17. IL-17 in turn induces the production of IL-8 by sulcus epithelial cells. IL-8, a chemoattractant for PMNs, is also a strong stimulus for NET formation, thus establishing a positive feedback loop to contain developing bacterial infection. IL-17 in PD may thus have a protective role in maintaining the PMN barrier in the gingival sulcus (Seymour et al. 2015). The release of TNF-α and IL-17 from MCs and PMNs undergoing NETosis leads to increased cell adhesion molecule expression, such as endothelial cell leukocyte adhesion molecule-1 (ELAM-1) and ICAM-1, which, together with increased IL-8 production by epithelial cells, establishes a fast flow of PMNs through the junctional epithelium and into the gingival sulcus (Seymour et al. 2015).

Inflammation can become deregulated when PMN homeostasis is altered, whereby PMNs recruit Th17 cells and these in turn can recruit more PMNs (Pelettier et al. 2010; Zenobia & Hajishengallis 2015). Both PMNs and Th17 cells secrete IL-17, which stimulates osteoblastic expression of RANKL, thus inducing osteoclastogenesis (Yago et al. 2009). Furthermore, LPS–TLR activation of PMNs has been indicated to induce membrane-bound RANKL expression by PMNs, thereby also inducing osteoclastogenesis (Chakravarti et al. 2009). In chronic inflammatory diseases, up-regulated expression of membrane-bound RANKL (mRANKL) by circulating neutrophils can induce osteoclastogenesis by direct cell contact with osteoclasts (Hu et al. 2017).

Natural killer (NK) cells get activated by major histocompatibility complex class I-like molecules (MHC1), and are a major source of IFN-ɣ (Gonzales 2015). NK cells kill target cells, without prior sensitization, by direct contact, and indirectly by IFN-ɣ (Meyle & Chapple 2015). NK cells kill herpesvirus-infected cells either by means of antibody-independent mechanisms, or via virus-specific antibody-dependent cell-mediated cytotoxicity (ADCC) (Slots 2010).

Monocytes/macrophages play a major role in initial inflammatory reactions and immunomodulation (Ebersole et al. 2017). Phenotype plasticity and polarization of macrophages determine the innate and adaptive immune-response outcomes of antigen recognition (Benoit et al. 2008; Locati et al. 2013; Mantovani et al. 2013). Polarized M1 macrophages can switch to M2 macrophages when stimulated by IL-4 (Tacke & Zimmermann 2014). M1 macrophages are prevalent in gingival tissues in periodontitis lesions, while M2 macrophages are prominent in gingival tissues in gingivitis lesions (Zhou et al. 2019). M2 macrophages are highly phagocytic and are responsible for tissue remodeling (Zhang et al. 2010). Gram-negative bacteria, NK-derived and Th1-derived IFN-Υ (secreted as autocrine or paracrine molecule), TNF-α, *Porphyromonas gingivalis* LPS, lipoproteins, and *Aggregatibacter actinomycetemcomitans* (Huang et al. 2016; Zhang et al. 2010) induce the activation and polarization of resting macrophages into M1 inflammatory macrophages. M1 macrophages then secrete inflammatory cytokines, i.e. TNF-α, IL-1β, IL-6, IL-12, and chemokines (Zhou et al. 2019). M1 macrophages phagocytose bacteria and initiate as well as augment inflammatory responses, leading to cytotoxicity, the undermining of epithelium integrity, degradation of connective tissue matrix, loss of fibroblast function/viability, fibrosis, and enhanced osteoclastogenesis with alveolar bone resorption (Hajishengallis 2014; Labonte et al. 2017; Locati et al. 2013; Zhou et al. 2019).

Th2-related cytokines IL-4 and IL-13 and oral commensal bacteria (Huang et al. 2016) trigger the polarization and activation of anti-inflammatory (wound healing) M2a macrophages, which then secrete chemokines, anti-inflammatory cytokines, i.e. IL-4, IL-10, IL-1RA, and TGF-β (Hajishengallis 2014; Liu et al. 2014; Zhou et al. 2019). These are wound-healing cell types that control the inflammatory response and aid in tissue repair and cellular regeneration (Mantovani et al. 2013). These cells clear apoptotic phagocytes and damaged matrix from inflammatory tissues (Zhou et al. 2019). Stimulation of M0 macrophages with immune complexes, IL-1RA, and LPS leads to polarization of M2b immunoregulatory macrophages that express major histocompatibility complex (MHC)-II, IL-6, IL-10, TNF-α, and chemokines (Labonte et al. 2017; Tugal et al. 2013). Host-derived IL-10, TGF-β, and glucocorticoids trigger the polarization and activation of M2c macrophage immunosuppressive phenotypes, which secrete IL-10, TGF-β, IL-1RA, CD14, and chemokines (Liu et al. 2014; Mantovani et al. 2013; Tugal et al. 2013; Zhang et al. 2010).

Adaptive immunity

Innate immunity activates adaptive immune responses (Cekici et al. 2014). The innate immune response determines the nature of the subsequent adaptive response, and simultaneously the adaptive response controls the effectiveness of the innate response (Ocymour ot al. 2010).

$\Upsilon\delta$ T cells are intraepithelial lymphocytes localized exclusively within crevicular and oral epithelium, both in normal as well as in diseased gingiva (Lundqvist & Hammarstrom 1993; Sanz et al. 2017). In humans, Vγ9Vδ2 T cells represent the major subtype of $\Upsilon\delta$ T cells in blood, but make up only 1–5% of all circulating peripheral T- cells. However, the number of Vγ9Vδ2 T cells increase during early responses to infection by intracellular pathogens (Skyberg et al. 2011). Vγ9Vδ2 T cells bridge innate and adaptive immune responses, (Sanz et al. 2017), their various functions including production of cytokines and chemokines, recruitment and activation of PMNs, differentiation of monocytes into proinflammatory cells, and the phenotypic maturation of dendritic cells (Sabbione et al. 2014). They are capable of phagocytosis (Wu et al. 2009) and behave like professional antigen-presenting cells (APC), relocating to draining lymph nodes in a manner similar to dendritic cells (Born et al. 2006). Vγ9Vδ2 T cells show antigen cross-presentation activity, by capturing bacterial antigens and presenting them to naïve CD8+ and CD4+ $\alpha\beta$ T cells (Sanz et al. 2017), thereby routing antigens to the MHC I and MHC II pathways, respectively (Moser & Eberl 2011). This leads to the induction and differentiation of CD8+ cytotoxic T cells, and Th1 and Th2 responses, respectively, including the promotion of B-cell activation and cytotoxic responses against infected and transformed cells (Born et al. 2006; Moser & Eberl 2011; Sabbione et al. 2014; Sanz et al. 2017). Stimulation of Langerhans dendritic cells and $\gamma\delta$ T cells in PD increases production of IL-1, IL-6, IL-8, IL-17, IL-23, and TNF-α proinflammatory cytokines, thereby replacing the antimicrobial function of PMNs in gingivitis. The production of IL-17 is also mechanistically associated with bone loss in PD (Sanz et al. 2017). A bi-directional cross-talk between $\gamma\delta$ T cells and PMNs has also been suggested, whereby $\gamma\delta$ T cells promote recruitment, activation, and phagocytic activity of PMNs against invading pathogens, and in turn PMNs suppress the activation of $\gamma\delta$ T cells by means of ROS production, and in doing so contribute to the resolution of inflammation (Sabbione et al. 2014).

The nature of APCs, such as dendritic cells, B cells, and macrophages, can modulate the Th1/Th2 profile. In gingivitis, the predominant APC is a Langerhans dendritic cell, whereas in periodontitis it is primarily a B cell (Seymour et al. 2015). APCs reach regional lymph nodes and present antigens to naïve CD4+ T lymphocytes (Th0 cells) (Cutler & Jotwani 2004; Kinane et al. 2008;

Labonte et al. 2017; Liu et al. 2014). MHC II receptors on APCs, together with antigens, interact with alpha beta T-cell receptors (αβ TCRs) on activated Th0 cells (Labonte et al. 2017; Tubo et al. 2014; Tugal et al. 2013). APCs including pre-plasma cells (B cells) and activated Th0 cells then enter the bloodstream and travel back to the gingiva, whereafter cell-mediated and humoral immunity is further initiated (Kinane et al. 2008). MHC II-αβ TCR interaction leads to maturation and development of phenotypically differentiated T cells, i.e. CD4+ Th1 and Th2 cells, effector Th17, and suppressor T-regulatory (Treg) cells, as well as CD8+ cell clones (Tawfig 2016; Wassenaar et al. 1995). Naïve T cells when incubated with TGF-β and IL-2 undergo up-regulation of transcription factor Foxp3 and develop into Treg cells, which play an important function in suppressing autoimmune responses. Naïve T cells incubated with TGF-β and IL-6 express the transcription factor RORγt, and become Th17 cells (Seymour et al. 2015).

These cells subsequently express subsets of cytokines, and it is the balance of cytokines that will define the immune response, and in doing so will determine whether PD remains stable or leads to progression and tissue destruction (Appay et al. 2008; Cullinan et al. 2003; Seymour et al. 2015; Weaver & Hatton 2009) (see Figure 5.4.2). Th1 and Th2 cells are associated with cellular and humoral acquired immunity, respectively (Murphy & Reiner 2002), and can simultaneously be present in infected periodontal tissues (Silva et al. 2015). A strong innate immune response results in high levels of IL-12 secreted by both PMNs and macrophages, leading to a Th1 response, cell-mediated immunity, and a stable periodontal lesion. Evidence that T cells are involved in recruitment and activation of PMNs at infection sites suggests that in the stable lesion, activation of PMNs is crucial in keeping infection under control (Campbell 1990). Also, NK cells in gingival tissues producing IFN-γ enhance the phagocytic activity of both PMNs and macrophages, thereby strengthening Th1 responses and hence containment of infection (Seymour et al. 2015). Poor innate immune responses with polyclonal B-cell activation lead to a Th2 response, resulting in low levels of IL-12, non-protective Ab, and a progressive periodontal lesion (Seymour et al. 2015). Also, plaque bacteria having a suppressive effect on Th1 responses may be fundamental in the conversion of a stable lesion to a progressive one (Evans et al. 1989).

TLRs on dendritic cells, PMNs, and macrophages recognize PAMPs. Stimulation of TLRs by PAMPs induces different immune responses, as determined by the resulting cytokine profiles (Seymour et al. 2015). TLR4 stimulation promotes expression of IL-12 and INF-γ–

inducible protein-10 (IP-10), indicating a Th1 response. TLR2 stimulation promotes inhibitory IL-12p40 (a subunit of IL-12), characterizing a Th2 response (Re & Strominger 2001). For example, *Escherichia coli*–derived LPS activates TLR4 receptors, inducing a strong Th1 response, while *Porphyromonas gingivalis*–derived LPS activates TLR2 receptors, inducing a strong Th2 response (Hirschfeld et al. 2001; Pulendran et al. 2001). *P. gingivalis* cysteine proteases (gingipains) hydrolyze IL-12, thereby reducing IL-12–induced IFN-γ production by CD4 cells, causing a shift to a Th2 response (Yun et al. 2001). Also, stress-induced stimulation of the sympathetic nervous system as well as hypothalamic–pituitary–adrenal (HPA) axis activation may lead to selective suppression of Th1 responses, with a shift toward Th2 dominance, thus leading to increased PD (Breivik et al. 2000; Seymour et al. 2015). It is generally accepted that PD is associated with a shift toward a Th2 phenotype response, producing high levels of IL-4 and low levels of IFN-γ (Berglundh & Donati 2005; Kinane & Bartold 2007; Seymour et al. 2015).

Two subsets of CD8+ cell clones have been described. CD8+ cytotoxic T cells produce high levels of IFN-γ, but no IL-4 or IL-5, mediating cytolytic activity and suppressing B cells. CD8+ suppressor T cells produce high levels of IL-4 and IL-5, mediating suppression of the proliferative response of cytotoxic CD8+ T cells, thereby suppressing cell-mediated immunity and providing help to B cells (Seymour et al. 2015; Wassenaar et al. 1995).

Th2-activated B-1 and B-2 cells transform into plasma cells, which produce Abs as part of adaptive humoral immunity. Plasma cells can produce Abs both in lymph nodes and locally within periodontal tissues. B cells can be activated either by specific Abs or by polyclonal activators. Polyclonal activation of B cells is likely to produce Abs of low affinity without the induction of the memory component (Tew et al. 1989). Periodontal pathogens, including *P. gingivalis, A. actinomycetemcomitans*, and *Fusobacterium nucleatum*, are known to be strong polyclonal B-cell activators (Ito et al. 1988). Polyclonal B-cell activation with associated production of non-specific and/or low-avidity Abs may not be capable of controlling PD. Furthermore, B cells are major sources of IL-1, and continued B-cell activation may contribute to subsequent tissue destruction (Gemmell & Seymour 1998; Seymour et al. 2015).

Matrix metalloproteinases (MMP)-1, -2, -3, and -9 have been correlated with B cells, suggesting a possible B-cell contribution to tissue destruction in PD (Korostoff et al. 2000). Also, a possible link between B cells and alveolar bone destruction in PD has been described. Both IL-1 and TNF-α regulate the balance of RANKL and osteoprotegerin (OPG) (Hofbauer et al. 1999), and B cells are known to secrete increased levels of IL-1β (Seymour et al. 2015). Activated T cells and B cells produce both soluble (sRANKL) and membrane-bound (mRANKL) RANKL (Horowitz et al. 2010), whereby the coupling of osteoblast-produced RANKL with osteoclast-expressed RANK results in bone loss in PD (Seymour et al. 2015).

B-1 cells are mostly involved in T-cell-independent Ab responses, generating polyspecific and low-affinity Abs (Gonzales 2015). Expansion of polyclonal B cells also includes the secretion of large amounts of IL-1 and, together with generation of non-specific Abs, continuous tissue breakdown occurs (Boch et al. 2001; Gonzales 2015). B-1 cells may also interact with T cells, undergo class switching, and produce IgG autoantibodies with high affinity, which may be directed against host tissue components (Kinane et al. 2008). Specifically, B-1a cells produce autoantibodies and large proportions thereof are found in subjects with autoimmune diseases and PD (Afar et al. 1992; Berglundh et al. 2002). Collagen type I-specific T-cell clones and anticollagen type I and III Abs have been described in gingival tissues (Hirsch et al. 1988). Cross-reactivity of human heat shock protein 60 (HSP60), expressed by stressed endothelial cells, and *P. gingivalis* GroEL, a bacterial homolog, has been observed in PD (Tabeta et al. 2000).

B-2 cells are responsible for T-cell-dependent Ab responses to specific microbial antigens (Brinkmann et al. 2004). B-2 cells develop into memory cells and long-lived plasma cells, producing Abs with high affinity (Seymour et al. 2015). Abs with high avidity have been suggested to confer resistance to continued or repeated infection (Kinane et al. 2008). B-2 cell-associated Abs neutralize antigens, form immune complexes, and, in conjunction with innate immunity, opsonize antigens for phagocytosis by neutrophils and macrophages (Kinane et al. 2008, Teng 2006b). Circulating Abs produced by plasma cells in lymph nodes leave the bloodstream and enter the gingival crevice in the transudate, thus inhibiting and controlling initial bacterial colonization in the gingival sulcus (Kinane et al. 2008). Abs trigger cytotoxic effector cells, such as CD8+ cells, in ADCC reactions against intracellular antigens (Teng 2006b).

The return to tissue homeostasis includes the gradual decrease of proinflammatory molecules due to reduction in levels of inflammatory stimuli. However, the process of returning to tissue homeostasis also involves the active resolution of inflammation. This requires endogenous and exogenous derived proresolving molecules such as lipoxins, resolvins, and protectins, which are released during inflammation. Lipoxins reduce PMN infiltration, chemotaxis, adhesion, and the production of proinflammatory mediators, and stimulate the uptake of apoptotic PMNs by macrophages (Nicu & Loos 2016; Serhan 2008).

The dysregulation of chronic inflammation drives the further destruction of connective tissue and alveolar bone during the development of PD (Bartold & Van Dyke 2019; Ohlrich et al. 2009). A switch from chronic gingivitis to a periodontal lesion is controlled and mediated by a balance between Th1/Th2 cells, with chronic periodontitis being mediated by Th2 cells (Ohlrich et al. 2009), involving predominantly larger proportions of B cells and plasma cells (Berthelot & Le Goff 2010; Lappin et al. 2001; Ohlrich et al. 2009).

Connective tissue destruction of the periodontium

The integrity and composition of connective tissue in the periodontium are physiologically regulated by the control of proteolytic activity, during both health and disease. This includes both synthesis and degradation of matrix constituents. The synthesis of collagens is influenced by growth factors, hormones, cytokines, and lymphokines (Potempa et al. 2000). This occurs during development, inflammation, and wound repair. Degradation involves a balance between the amount and activity of matrix-degrading proteolytic enzymes (matrix metalloproteinases, MMPs) and their associated tissue inhibitors (Séguier et al. 2001). During inflammation, however, degradation can become excessive (Potempa et al. 2000). Connective tissue degradation can occur by means of cytokines and inflammatory mediators affecting MMP enzyme release; bacterial products and host enzymes; the phagocytosis of matrix components; and the release of reactive oxygen species

(Bartold & Narayanan 1998). Table 5.4.1 depicts the basic mechanisms of connective tissue degradation of the periodontium.

Immunopathogenesis of periodontal bone loss

Skeletal homeostasis involves a dynamic balance between osteoblastic and osteoclastic activity (Teng 2006b). This balance is controlled by the endocrine system, and is influenced by the immune system, including an osteoimmunological regulation (osteoimmunology) that depends on lymphocyte- and macrophage-derived cytokines (Hienz et al. 2015; Walsh et al. 2006). Osteoimmunology comprises both the innate and adaptive immune mechanisms controlling normal and pathological skeletal turnover (Henderson & Kaiser 2018). Many cytokines are involved in bone homeostasis, and their imbalance leads to enhanced osteoclastic activity without an increase in bone formation, thus driving alveolar bone loss

Table 5.4.1 Connective tissue degradation of the periodontium.

Cytokines and inflammatory mediators

- Certain patients with a genetic predisposition to create a "dysregulated" hyper-reactive polymorphonuclear (PMN) phenotype show release of increased amounts of interleukin (IL)-1β, IL-6, IL-8, and tumor necrosis factor (TNF)-α (Nicu et al. 2007).
- As a result of the inflammatory process in periodontal disease (PD), growth factors and cytokines are secreted by platelets, keratinocytes, macrophages, and fibroblasts. These cytokines in turn induce matrix metalloproteinase (MMP) synthesis by resident gingival cells and macrophages, thereby initiating degradation of connective tissue (Reynolds et al. 1994).
- IL-1, IL-6, TNF-α, and prostaglandin (PGE)2 stimulate MMP production by fibroblasts and keratinocytes (Seymour et al. 2015; Tewari et al. 1994).
- Lipopolysaccharide (LPS) and TNF-α stimulate keratinocytes to secrete MMPs; LPS stimulates fibroblasts to secrete PGE2 and stimulates macrophages to secrete MMPs (Bartold & Narayanan 1998).
- PGE2 suppresses cell proliferation and inhibits collagen synthesis. PGE2 and IL-6 stimulate bone resorption (Schwartz et al. 1997).

Matrix metalloproteinases released from the host

- MMPs are secreted by PMNs, macrophages, plasma cells, fibroblasts, endothelial cells, keratinocytes, bone cells, and CD8+ and CD4+ T cells and B cells (Birkedal-Hansen 1995; Korostoff et al. 2000; Séguier et al. 2001).
- MMPs are present in periodontal tissues as pro-forms, active forms, complexed species, fragmented species, and cell bound (Birkedal-Hansen 1995; Séguier et al. 2001).
- MMPs are collagenases, gelatinases, and stromelysins. MMP activity is tightly regulated through gene expression, proenzyme activation, and enzyme inhibition by endogenous tissue inhibitors (Bartold & Narayanan 1998).
- Activation of MMPs is induced by independent or cooperative cascades involving pathogen proteases and host MMPs, as well as by reactive oxygen species (ROS) through direct enzyme oxidation (Cavalla et al. 2017). MMPs are activated by plasmin (a proteinase). The inactive precursor of plasmin is plasminogen, which is activated by urokinase-type plasminogen activator (u-PA) and tissue-type plasminogen activator (t-PA), secreted by fibroblasts and epithelial and endothelial cells. Plasmin and its activating proteinases are regulated by extracellular proteinase inhibitors, such as α_2-macroglobulin, α_1-proteinase inhibitor, α_2-antiplasmin, plasminogen activator inhibitor-1 (PA-1), and plasminogen activator inhibitor-2 (PA-2) (Bartold & Narayanan 1998).
- Inhibitors of MMPs are α_2-macroglobulin, tissue inhibitor of metalloproteinases (TIMP-1 and TIMP-2), interferon (IFN)-γ, IL-4, IL-10, glucocorticoids, and retinoid hormones (Bartold & Narayanan 1998). Inhibitors are expressed by fibroblasts, keratinocytes, monocytes/macrophages, endothelial cells, and osteoblasts (Kinane 2000). TIMPs control MMP activity tightly, both at the level of activation and at subsequent substrate degradation (Bartold & Narayanan 1998).
- MMP-1 (collagenase-1) hydrolyzes type I, II, III, VI, VIII, and X collagens and gelatin; MMP-8 (collagenase-2) hydrolyzes type I and III collagen; MMP-2 (gelatinase-A) and MMP-9 (gelatinase-B) hydrolyze gelatin, elastin, and collagen types IV, VII, X, and XI; and MMP-7 (matrilysin) is secreted by suprabasal junctional epithelial cells and degrades extracellular matrix (Bartold & Narayanan 1998; Cavalla et al. 2017).
- MMPs regulate periodontal inflammation. They release cytokines/chemokines from the extracellular matrix, increasing their bioavailability and modifying their bioactivity. Conversely, MMPs cleave cytokines/chemokines, generating truncated products, thereby acting as competitive antagonists (Bartold & Narayanan 1998; Kinane 2000). MMPs also regulate complement activity (Butler & Overall 2013).
- MMPs modulate bone resorption. MMP-13 is required for differentiation of preosteoclasts, osteoclast activation, and direct bone collagen matrix degradation (Cavalla et al. 2017).
- Cysteine proteinases, cathepsin B and L, are secreted from gingival fibroblasts as proenzymes. Cathepsin B could also contribute to collagen degradation indirectly through activation of MMP-1 (Cox et al. 2006).

Bacterial products

- Bacterial proteinases have a putative physiological role regarding bacterial growth (Potempa et al. 2000). Direct degradation of connective tissue by periodontal bacteria is accomplished by utilizing both exopeptidases and endopeptidases to degrade peptides into free amino acids, thereby obtaining their carbon and energy sources (Grenier 1992; Potempa et al. 2000).
- Indirect degradation by bacterial proteinases may be via stimulation of synthesis of MMPs by host cells, including the subsequent proteolytic activation of their zymogens. *Porphyromonas gingivalis* can boost the collagen-degrading ability of gingival fibroblasts, by increasing MMP activation and lowering TIMP-1 levels (Zhou & Windsor 2006). Furthermore, inactivation of α1-proteinase inhibitor can cause loss of control of host cysteine proteinases and neutrophil elastase, leading to excessive endogenous proteolytic activity (Nelson et al. 1999; Sorsa et al. 1992).
- Bacterial enzymes can also function as antigens, thereby stimulating cytokine production by host cells (Bartold & Narayanan 1998).
- By means of uncontrolled activation of the kallikrein/kinin pathway and coagulation cascade, bacterial gingipains contribute to the local generation of bradykinin and thrombin. This leads to PGE2 synthesis by osteoblasts, endothelium, and periodontal ligament (PDL) cells, thereby indirectly stimulating bone resorption (Potempa et al. 2000).

Table 5.4.1 (Continued)

Phagocytosis

- Physiological turnover of connective tissues by fibroblasts and macrophages entails initial proteolytic digestion of collagens by means of enzymes associated with the cell surface, or adjacent to the cell within the matrix. Internalization and further breakdown of collagen peptides are accomplished by the formation of phagolysosomes, wherein lysosomal enzymes, such as cathepsin L, are located (Bartold & Narayanan 1998). Collagen molecules that become denatured in the extracellular environment are phagocytosed by surrounding fibroblasts (Seymour et al. 2015).

The release of reactive oxygen species

- The production of ROS is associated with enhanced expression of proinflammatory cytokines that are both directly and indirectly responsible for connective tissue destruction and bone resorption.
- Connective tissue damage resulting from host–microbial interactions can directly be caused by excess ROS activity together with a compromised plasma antioxidant capacity, or indirectly as a result of the activation of redox-sensitive transcription factors and the creation of a proinflammatory state (Chapple & Matthews 2007).
- LPS, TNF-α, granulocyte colony-stimulating factor, IL-8, IL-1, IL-6, and platelet-activating factor have a priming effect on the PMN oxidative burst and, together with fibroblasts, generate and secrete ROS (Chapple & Matthews 2007). *P. gingivalis* LPS as well as hypoxia induce a NOX4-dependent increase in H_2O_2 release in PDL fibroblasts and, together with a reduction of catalase, increase ROS production (Gölz et al. 2014).
- ROS can lead to altered metabolic activity of connective tissues, by enhancing or deactivating proteolytic activity and by altering cellular activity (Waddington et al. 2000).
- ROS may cause direct degradation of connective tissue components and cause modifications to structures of connective tissue components, causing loss of function of periodontal tissues, including attachment loss in PD. Fibroblasts affected by ROS produce reduced levels of collagen, as well as excessive levels of MMPs, thereby promoting degradation of connective tissue and bone matrix (Sczepanik et al. 2020; Waddington et al. 2000).
- ROS may further indirectly potentiate extracellular matrix degradation by MMPs, via the activation of latent enzymes, such as collagenases and gelatinases, and via inactivation of enzyme inhibitors, such as TIMP (Waddington et al. 2000).

(Walsh et al. 2006). In PD, both microbial and host-derived factors are involved in bone resorption and remodeling (Schwartz et al. 1997). Host innate immunity recognizes PAMPs through PRRs, such as Toll-like receptors (TLR) and CD14 receptors, resulting in resident cells and eventually lymphocytes secreting various networks of cytokines (Cekici et al. 2014; Meyle et al. 2017; Teng 2006b). Alveolar bone resorption in PD can thus be directly or indirectly induced by the cellular inflammatory infiltrate (Schwartz et al. 1997; Taubman et al. 2005). Osteoclasts differentiate under the control of the RANK/RANKL/OPG system; however, the dysregulation of secreted cytokines, produced in pathological conditions, will modulate osteoclastogenesis, causing the progression of PD (Benedetto et al. 2013) (see Figure 5.4.3). Box 5.4.2 describes the basic proposed immunological mechanisms involved in periodontal bone loss during the development of PD.

Resolution of inflammation

Periodontitis results from the loss of homeostasis between resident commensal microbiota and the host-creating oral microbiome dysbiosis, chronic infection, and unresolved inflammation, which leads to a host-mediated destruction of the soft and hard periodontal tissues, including the alveolar bone (Bashutski et al. 2011). Early bacterial colonization on the tooth surface stimulates an inflammatory response, which

is usually self-limiting, and is resolved by cleaning of the teeth (Van Dyke & Sima 2020). After the acute phase, neutrophils begin to undergo programmed cell death (apoptosis), followed by an influx of mononuclear phagocytes and macrophages that phagocytize remaining bacteria and apoptotic neutrophils. The natural termination sequence of the acute phase of inflammation (resolution of inflammation pathways) is initiated by the generation of specialized proresolving lipid mediators (SPMs). As inflammation resolves, macrophages are cleared from the lesion through the lymphatics by a process called efferocytosis (Van Dyke 2020).

In susceptible individuals, however, the resultant and robust inflammatory response alters the growth environment, thereby altering the composition of the microbiome. The changing microbiome amplifies the inflammatory response, thereby inducing a cycle of increasing inflammation with consequent changes in the microbiome. Neutrophils are not cleared, macrophages assume a proinflammatory phenotype, and acquired immunity becomes activated with the accumulation of various lymphocytes (Van Dyke 2020). These events are thus characterized by excess inflammation and the loss of the ability to control the pathogenicity of the subgingival biofilm (Van Dyke & Sima 2020). Acute inflammation is therefore not resolved and it is this chronic immuno-inflammatory lesion that characterizes periodontitis (Van Dyke 2020). Thus, in susceptible individuals the cycle of uncontrolled and increasing inflammation, which includes microbiome changes and the

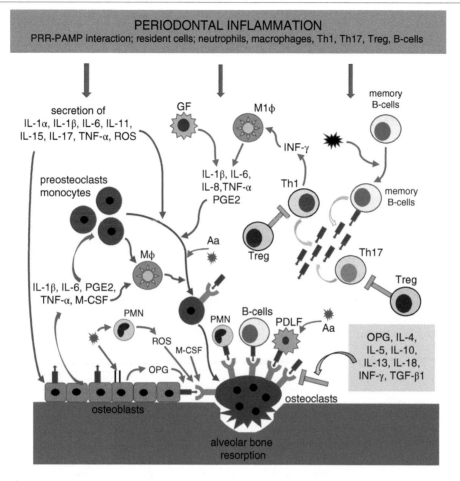

Figure 5.4.3 Immunopathogenesis of periodontal bone loss. Aa, cytolethal toxin and capsular polysaccharide from Aggregatibacter actinomycetemcomitans; GF, gingival fibroblasts; Mφ, tissue macrophages; M1φ, M1 macrophage; M-CSF, macrophage colony-stimulating factor; OPG, osteoprotegerin; PDLF, periodontal ligament fibroblasts; ROS, reactive oxygen species; II, Toll-like receptor (TLR); ■→, soluble/membrane-bound RANKL; ✳, *Porphyromonas gingivalis* lipopolysaccharide; |——, inhibition; ✳, periodontal bacteria; ■▷, RANKL–RANK interaction. Courtesy of Dr. Steph Smith.

Box 5.4.2   Immunopathogenesis of periodontal bone loss (see Figure 5.4.3)

In periodontal disease (PD), an increased inflammatory infiltrate of T cells, B cells, macrophages, and neutrophils, with a concurrent increase in inflammatory cytokine secretion, interacts with resident cells (Baek et al. 2018). Epithelial cells (ECs), dendritic cells (DCs), gingival fibroblasts (GFs), periodontal ligament fibroblasts (PDLFs), and osteoblasts respond via pathogen recognition receptors (PRRs) to pathogen-associated molecular patterns (PAMPs) and secrete proinflammatory cytokines and chemokines (Hans & Hans 2011). ECs secrete interleukin(IL)-8, causing polymorphonuclear neutrophil (PMN) recruitment and migration, and increases monocyte adhesion in blood vessels (Han et al. 2000; Trevani et al. 2003). PMNs secrete IL-1, IL-6, and tumor necrosis

factor (TNF)-α (Kinane 2000). Reactive oxygen species (ROS) generated from PMNs with increased cytokine secretion in close proximity to alveolar bone can also trigger receptor activator of nuclear factor-κB ligand (RANKL)-mediated bone resorption (Cooper et al. 2013; Sczepanik et al. 2020).

M1 macrophages are a major source of TNF-α and IL-1β, and, under dysregulation, play a critical role in an autocrine/paracrine manner in the regulation of bone resorption (Benedetto et al. 2013; Sima & Glogauer 2013; Tugal et al. 2013). DCs (such as Langerhans cells) have been suggested to have an immune-dampening function (Sima & Glogauer 2013) and secrete IL-12 and IL-18, causing interferon (IFN)-γ secretion by T cells

(Tew et al. 2012). GFs secrete TNF-α, IL-6, IL-8, and prostaglandin E2 (PGE2), and PDLFs secrete IL-1β, IL-6, TNF-α, and membrane-bound RANKL (mRANKL) (Scheres et al. 2010; Yucel-Lindberg & Båge 2013). TNF-α also contributes to periodontal damage by its direct effect on osteoclastogenesis, independent of RANKL (Yarilina et al. 2011).

Osteoblasts are induced by inflammatory cytokines, hormones, and PGE2 to express mRANKL (Yarilina et al. 2011). Macrophage colony-stimulating factor (M-CSF) is expressed by osteoblasts, and induces proliferation and differentiation of preosteoclasts into osteoclasts (Bartold et al. 2010; Koide et al. 2010). In the presence of M-CSF, osteoclast precursors differentiate into osteoclasts by means of cell-to-cell interactions with mRANKL on osteoblasts (Koide et al. 2010). Osteoblasts also produce osteoprotegerin (OPG), a soluble decoy receptor for RANKL, which inhibits osteoclastogenesis by blocking RANKL–RANK interaction (Benedetto et al. 2013; Hienz et al. 2015; Koide et al. 2010). Osteoblasts thus tightly regulate osteoclastic bone resorption as well as bone formation (Koide et al. 2010).

Osteoblasts express Toll-like receptors (TLRs), i.e. TLR2 and TLR4 (Henderson & Kaiser 2018), whereby interaction with lipopolysaccharide (LPS) increases osteoblastic expression of RANKL, IL-1, PGE2, and TNF-α, thereby inducing osteoclastic activity, viability, and differentiation (Bartold & Van Dyke 2013; Dumitrescu et al. 2004; Matsumoto et al. 2012; Ohlrich et al. 2009). LPS–TLR4 interaction with osteoblasts also suppresses OPG expression in osteoblasts (Lerner 2006). LPS also induces the formation of multinucleate osteoclasts, including bone-resorbing activity in osteoclasts (Park et al. 2012). Cytolethal toxin from *Aggregatibacter actinomycetemcomitans* (Aa) and *Porphyromonas gingivalis* LPS induce PDLF expression of RANKL (Hienz et al. 2015, Walsh et al. 2006). LPS from various bacteria, DNA, and Aa capsular polysaccharide induce osteoclast differentiation from bone marrow cells (Hienz et al. 2015; Udagawa et al. 2007). *Prevotella intermedia* LPS inhibits differentiation of osteoblasts and mineralization of bone (Hienz et al. 2015).

Antigen-presenting cells initiate adaptive immunity including the activation of T and B cells. Although T and B cells produce RANKL, they might not be involved in physiological bone resorption. However, in inflammatory PD, activated T cells can cause bone resorption through excessive production of soluble RANKL (sRANKL) (Hienz et al. 2015; Kawai et al. 2006; Taubman et al. 2005). The larger proportion of lymphocytes consists of B cells (Han et al. 2019), the majority thereof expressing RANKL, TNF-α, and IL-6 in response to periodontal pathogen stimulation (Benedetto et al. 2013; Han et al. 2007, 2019).

More specifically, memory B cells, a functional subset of B cells, express both sRANKL and mRANKL (Park et al. 2012). Th1 and Th17 cells also secrete IL-1α, IL-1β, IL-6, IL-11, IL-15, IL-17, INF-γ, and TNF-α. These cytokines stimulate osteoblasts and Th17 cells to express RANKL (Teng 2006b). INF-γ, which is produced by Th1 cells, induces proinflammatory IL-1β, TNF-α, and PGE2 production by macrophages; however, INF-γ inhibits osteoclastogenesis by interfering with the RANKL–RANK signaling pathway (Takayanagi et al. 2000).

Certain subsets of periodontitis patients have a genetic predisposition to create higher levels of a dysregulated hyperactive PMN phenotype, which is characterized by the overproduction of ROS and proteases (Sczepanik et al. 2020). The increased production of ROS is associated with the enhanced expression of proinflammatory cytokines, i.e., IL-1, IL-6, and TNF-α, leading to the expression of increased levels of RANKL mRNA, relating to the differentiation of macrophage/monocyte precursor cells into osteoclasts. Furthermore, an ROS-mediated increase in the RANKL/osteoprotegerin ratio causes the homeostatic relationship between bone formation and bone resorption to be uncoupled, including the stimulation of osteoclast activity as well as osteoblast death, resulting in bone loss (Sczepanik et al. 2020).

The main sources of RANKL are osteoblasts, Th1, Th17 cells, and B cells (Bartold et al. 2010; Benedetto et al. 2013; Sima & Glogauer 2013). Osteocytes have also been indicated to be a major source of RANKL; however, the role of osteocyte-derived RANKL may be limited to bone remodeling (Chen et al. 2014). Also, LPS–TLR activation of PMNs has been indicated to induce mRANKL expression by PMNs, thereby also inducing osteoclastogenesis (Leffler et al. 2012). In chronic inflammatory diseases the up-regulated expression of mRANKL by circulating neutrophils can induce osteoclastogenesis by direct cell contact with osteoclasts, influencing bone mineral density (Hu et al. 2017; Sczepanik et al. 2020; Tillack et al. 2012).

In response to M-CSF, sRANKL, inflammatory interleukins, TNF-α, ROS, and contact with osteocalcin, hematopoietic precursors undergo differentiation into monocyte- and macrophage-derived colony-forming cells, peripheral blood monocytes, and tissue macrophages, which then fuse into mature multicellular osteoclasts, leading to alveolar bone loss (Hienz et al. 2015; Sczepanik et al. 2020; Teng 2006b). RANKL exerts its biological effects directly through binding to RANK on osteoclast and preosteoclast cell surfaces (Teng 2006b). Regulatory T cells attenuate RANKL expression by other activated T cells (Chen et al. 2014).

OPG is produced by resident epithelial cells, periodontal fibroblasts, osteoblasts, endothelial cells, and marrow stromal cells (Bartold et al. 2010; Benedetto et al. 2013; Schwartz et al. 1997). GFs are heterogenic; although augmenting chronic inflammation by IL-6 and IFN secretion, they may also produce OPG in response to LPS and IL-1, thereby suppressing osteoclast formation (Hienz et al. 2015). OPG binds RANKL, thereby inhibiting RANKL/RANK interactions, thus preventing osteoclast formation

(Benedetto et al. 2013; Hienz et al. 2015). OPG as well as IL-4, IL-5, IL-10, IL-13, IL-18, INF-γ, and transforming growth factor (TGF)-β1 inhibit bone resorption (Teng 2006b). Cementoblasts stimulated by LPS express decreased levels of RANKL and increased levels of OPG and osteopontin, thereby possibly protecting against bone and root resorption (Dumitrescu et al. 2004; Ebersole et al. 2013).

eventual chronic inflammatory destruction of the periodontal tissues, is directly related to a failure of resolution of inflammation pathways. Excess inflammation actually inhibits bacterial clearance and sets up maintenance of the chronic inflammatory lesion and infection (Van Dyke & Sima 2020). In other words, tissue destruction in periodontitis is due to a sustained microbial challenge and microbiome dysbiosis, caused by a failure of endogenous resolution pathways (Tanner et al. 2007; Van Dyke 2011).

The inflammatory response is a protective biological process designed to eliminate harmful stimuli and promote return of the affected tissue to its preinflammatory state and function (homeostasis) (Loos & Van Dyke 2020). At the peak of an acute inflammatory response, proinflammatory mediators induce the generation of SPMs that stimulate their receptor targets, this process therefore being considered as the beginning of resolution (Recchiuti & Serhan 2012). Resolution of inflammation is an active, specific-receptor-mediated, biochemical and metabolic process, and is not merely a passive termination of inflammation. SPMs include lipoxins, resolvins, protectins, and maresins (Serhan & Chiang 2013). These

SPMs originate from the enzymatic conversion of omega-3 polyunsaturated fatty acids in the human diet (Loos & Van Dyke 2020) (see Figure 5.4.4). Lipoxins are derived from arachidonic acid (AA), resolvins from eicosapentaenoic acid (EPA), and protectins and maresins from docosahexaenoic acid (DHA) (Recchiuti & Serhan 2012). They are responsible for the mediation of the active resolution of inflammation; they do not inhibit inflammation (Ebersole et al. 2013; Serhan & Chiang 2013; Serhan et al. 2008). They function as agonists, and not as antagonists (Perretti et al. 2015; Serhan 2017). They bind to receptors that are only active in inflammation and proactively signal termination of inflammation, e.g. inflammasomes are disassembled and the production of IL-1β is stopped, prostaglandin (PGE) production is terminated, along with cessation of the expression of genes encoding inflammatory mediators, such as the cytokines TNF-α and IL-12 (Van Dyke 2020). There is thus a feed-forward signal versus non-specific inhibition (Ebersole et al. 2013).

Lipoxins are involved in the initiating steps that permit the diapedesis of leukocytes. SPMs, i.e. resolvins, protectins, and maresins, stop neutrophil migration and initiate neutrophil

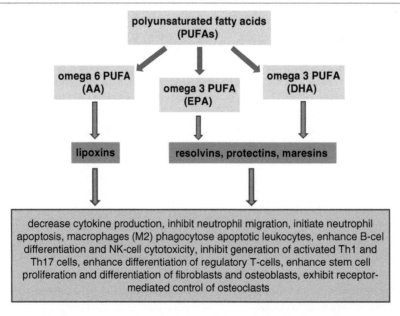

Figure 5.4.4 Various actions of pro-resolving lipid mediators in the resolution of inflammation. AA, arachidonic acid; DHA, docosahexaenoic acid; EPA, eicosapentaenoic acid; NK, natural killer cell. Courtesy of Dr. Steph Smith.

apoptosis. They are also chemotactic for activated mononuclear phagocytes whereby SPMs change the phenotype of these phagocytes from proinflammatory to anti-inflammatory, which entails the differentiation of proresolution macrophages by favouring pro-healing (M2-like) macrophage over proinflammatory (M1-like) macrophage activation (Damgaard et al. 2017; Van Dyke 2020). These actions lead to phagocytosis of remaining microbes and apoptotic neutrophils, and the counter-regulation of chemokines and cytokines (Recchiuti & Serhan 2012; Serhan 2017). SPMs are thus powerful regulators of inflammation-stimulatory molecules, promote infection clearance, prevent recurrence of infection, and are also involved in stem cell proliferation and differentiation (Serhan et al. 2018; Van Dyke 2017). They activate wound healing with tissue regeneration, instead of fibrosis and scarring, and directly improve bone healing and regeneration, thus preventing tissue damage in inflammation (Hasturk et al. 2007; Ortega-Gomez et al. 2013). Besides having actions beyond the control of white blood cell function, SPMs exhibit receptor-mediated control of osteoclasts, as well as stem cells that differentiate into fibroblasts and osteoblasts (Cianci et al. 2016; Gao et al. 2013; Kizil et al. 2015).

In summary, the cellular events regulated by SPMs efficiently control the bacterial biofilm and its environment, including suppression or elimination of pathogens, resulting in significant regeneration of bone and connective tissues for the reestablishment of a healthy periodontium (Van Dyke 2011).

Summary

Tissue homeostasis in the periodontium entails a balanced interaction between the host and the subgingival tooth-associated biofilm. A clinically healthy periodontium contains a minimal number of B cells and plasma cells, and a predominantly T-cell-rich infiltrate. Also, neutrophils constantly and proactively patrol the periodontium, in numbers lower than those present in gingivitis or periodontitis. Small populations of innate lymphoid cells that include a network of antigen-presenting cells, such as macrophages, dendritic cells, and gamma delta T cells, are also present in healthy gingiva. These cells are thought to contribute to protective immunity and maintenance of tissue homeostasis (Dutzan et al. 2016; Moutsopoulos & Konkel 2018).

Resistance or susceptibility to periodontitis is determined by multiple factors, including genetic, epigenetic, and environmental, such as smoking, stress, and a high-fat diet. Other factors include aging, immune deficiencies, and systemic diseases. These factors can act individually or in combination, and may modify the host response in either a protective or a destructive direction (Hajishengallis et al. 2020).

Periodontitis-associated microbiota is considerably diverse and complex, and the bacteria involved in disease act through polymicrobial synergy and dysbiosis (Lamont & Hajishengallis 2015; Lamont et al. 2018). Periodontitis is not caused by a single or a select few bacterial species, and therefore does not qualify as an infection per se, but is rather associated with a dysbiosis, whereby infection is driven and exacerbated by inflammation (Bartold & Van Dyke 2019). A dysbiosis is defined as an alteration in the abundance or influence of individual species within the polymicrobial community, relative to their abundance or influence in health (Hajishengallis et al. 2020).

Gingivitis can remain stable in individuals and may not necessarily progress to periodontitis. However, in the absence of adequate oral hygiene, selection for the further growth of potential pathobiotic bacteria (dysbiosis) can occur in a nutritionally favorable inflammatory environment. This conversion of the original bacterial homeostatic community into a dysbiotic one can thus increase the community's proinflammatory potential (Herrero et al. 2018). Although bacteria are required for disease pathogenesis, it is predominantly the host inflammatory response to this dysbiotic microbial challenge that ultimately determines whether damage is inflicted upon the periodontal tissues (Hasturk et al. 2012). In individuals with susceptibility to periodontitis, the initial inflammatory response to the subgingival biofilm can thus further develop into exacerbated inflammation, whereby a positive feedback loop of dysbiosis and inflammation in the susceptible individual can ultimately cause the host response to be ineffective, becoming dysregulated and destructive, thereby causing overt and chronic periodontitis (Hajishengallis 2015; Hajishengallis et al. 2020).

Future considerations

Although extensive research has been done, detailed mechanisms regarding the pathogenesis of PD have not been fully elucidated (Nicu & Loos 2016). Clinical studies utilizing sophisticated experimental designs are needed for the translation of basic biological processes that occur early in the transition from health to disease. Studies are also needed on the microenvironmental changes that select for a more pathogenic microbial ecology (Kawai et al. 2006). The identification of genetic and biological markers indicating increased susceptibility to PD by means of whole-genome microarrays and RNA sequencing is recommended (Meyle et al. 2017).

With a paradigm shift possibly moving away from using inhibitors of inflammation to using mediators of inflammation resolution as treatment (Van Dyke 2020), large-scale in vivo and ex vivo studies evaluating the effects of treatment with specialized proresolving mediators in individuals with periodontitis may shed more light on the complex molecular mechanisms involved in the resolution of periodontal inflammation (Loos & Van Dyke 2020). The potential of safe, effective, easy to-deliver treatments that may resolve inflammation in the mouth can also potentially reset systemic inflammatory responses. Lipoxin analogs could revolutionize treatment of many diseases that have chronic inflammation as a core component (Van Dyke 2020). Furthermore, profiling the resolution capacity through "-omics" of oral samples, including saliva and gingival crevicular fluid, will increase the sensitivity and specificity of diagnostic tools for periodontitis (Van Dyke & Sima 2020). Such research can lead to individualized targeted therapy for patients suffering from PD (Cekici et al. 2014).

Current research on therapies that increase the level of antioxidants and/or antioxidant activity is also ongoing, and these may prove to be viable additions to current approaches related to both the prevention and the treatment of periodontitis (Sczepanik et al. 2020). Antioxidants and detoxification enzymes have been shown to enhance cytoprotective effects by decreasing inflammation downstream of oxidative tissue damage (Scannapieco & Gershovich 2020).

Probiotics have also been indicated to prevent PD (Myneni et al. 2020; Sima et al. 2016). Probiotic bacteria may reverse inflammatory damage to epithelia, by means of stimulating the up-regulation of structural proteins. These bacteria may also colonize and proliferate sufficiently to deprive pathogenic bacteria of nutrients and thus inhibit their growth. Probiotic bacteria can produce antimicrobial products, such as acetic acid and lactic acid, that inhibit Gram-negative bacteria. Probiotics may also influence the host to down-regulate pathways that might damage host tissues, while simultaneously up-regulating other pathways that inhibit the growth or virulence of pathogens (Scannapieco & Gershovich 2020; Sima et al. 2016).

Another proposed preventive modality for PD is the development of periodontal vaccines, which includes targeting antigens of specific oral Gram-negative anaerobic pathogens that have been implicated in the pathogenesis of PD (Myneni et al. 2020; Scannapieco & Gershovich 2020). A vaccine-induced host response should ideally maximize protective immunity while minimizing its potentially destructive aspects. However, complex pathogenic mechanisms in periodontitis, together with the involvement of polymicrobial dysbiotic communities rather than specific pathogens, complicate the development of a periodontitis vaccine (Hajishengallis et al. 2020). To date, no periodontal vaccine trials in humans have been proven to prevent the formation of polymicrobial biofilms known to cause PD or to suppress alveolar bone loss. Further research is needed to evaluate long-term outcomes, as well as to evaluate multispecies vaccines in human models (Myneni et al. 2020).

REFERENCES

Afar B, Engel D, Clark EA. Activated lymphocyte subsets in adult periodontitis. *J Periodontal Res.* 1992; 27:126–133.

Appay V, van Lier RAW, Sallusto F, Roederer M. Phenotype and function of human T lymphocyte subsets: consensus and issues. *Cytometry A.* 2008; 73(11):975–983.

Baek K, Ji S, Choi Y. Complex intratissue microbiota forms biofilms in periodontal lesions. *J Dent Res.* 2018; 97:192–200.

Barros SP, Offenbacher S. Modifiable risk factors in periodontal disease: epigenetic regulation of gene expression in the inflammatory response. *Periodontol 2000.* 2014; 64:95–110.

Bartold PM, Cantley MD, Haynes DR. Mechanisms and control of pathologic bone loss in periodontitis. *Periodontol 2000.* 2010; 53:55–69.

Bartold PM, Narayanan AS. *Biology of the Periodontal Connective Tissues.* Batavia, IL: Quintessence; 1998.

Bartold PM, Van Dyke TE. Periodontitis: A host-mediated disruption of microbial homeostasis. Unlearning learned concepts. *Periodontol 2000.* 2013; 62(1):203–217.

Bartold PM, Van Dyke TE. Host modulation: controlling the inflammation to control the infection. *Periodontol 2000.* 2017; 75:317–329.

Bartold PM, Van Dyke TE. An appraisal of the role of specific bacteria in the initial pathogenesis of periodontitis. *J Clin Periodontol.* 2019; 46:6–11.

Bashutski JD, Eber RM, Kinney JS et al. The impact of vitamin D status on periodontal surgery outcomes. *J Dent Res.* 2011; 90(8):1007–1012.

Benakanakere M, Abdolhosseini M, Hosur K, Finoti LS, Kinane DF. TLR2 promoter hypermethylation creates innate immune dysbiosis. *J Dent Res.* 2015; 94:183–191.

Benedetto AD, Gigante I, Colucci S, Grano M. Periodontal disease: linking the primary inflammation to bone loss. *Clin Dev Immunol.* 2013; 2013:503754. doi: 10.1155/2013/503754.

Benoit M, Desnues B, Mege JL. Macrophage polarization in bacterial infections. *J Immunol.* 2008; 181:3733–3739.

Berglundh T, Donati M. Aspects of adaptive host response in periodontitis. *J Clin Periodontol.* 2005; 32(Suppl 6):87–107.

Berglundh T, Liljenberg B, Tarkowski A, Lindhe J. The presence of local and circulating autoreactive B cells in patients with advanced periodontitis. *J Clin Periodontol.* 2002; 29:281–286.

Berthelot JM, Le Goff B. Rheumatoid arthritis and periodontal disease. *Joint Bone Spine.* 2010; 77(6):537–541.

Birkedal-Hansen H. Role of matrix metalloproteinases in human periodontal diseases. *J Periodontol.* 1995; 64:474–484.

Boch JA, Wara-aswapati N, Auron PE. Interleukin 1 signal transduction – current concepts and relevance to periodontitis. *J Dent Res.* 2001; 80:400–407.

Born WK, Reardon CL, O'Brien RL. The function of γδ T cells in innate immunity. *Curr Opin Immunol.* 2006; 18(1):31–38.

Breivik T, Thrane PS, Gjermo P, Opstad PK. Glucocorticoid receptor antagonist RU 486 treatment reduces periodontitis in Fischer 344 rats. *J Periodontal Res.* 2000; 35:385–390.

Brennan PA, Thomas GJ, Langdon JD. The role of nitric oxide in oral diseases. *Arch Oral Biol.* 2003; 48:93–100.

Brinkmann V, Reichard U, Goosmann C et al. Neutrophil extracellular traps kill bacteria. *Science.* 2004; 303:1532–1535.

Butler GS, Overall CM. Matrix metalloproteinase processing of signaling molecules to regulate inflammation. *Periodontol 2000.* 2013; 63:123–148.

Campbell PA. Editorial review. The neutrophil, a professional killer of bacteria may be controlled by T cells. *Clin Exp Immunol.* 1990; 79:141–143.

Cavalla F, Hernández-Rios P, Sorsa T, Biguetti C, Hernández MH. Matrix metalloproteinases as regulators of periodontal inflammation. *Int J Mol Sci.* 2017; 18:440. doi: 10.3390/ijms18020440.

Cekici A, Kantarci A, Hasturk H, Van Dyke TE. Inflammatory and immune pathways in the pathogenesis of periodontal disease. *Periodontol 2000.* 2014; 64(1):57–80.

Chakravarti A, Raquil M-A, Tessier P, Poubelle PE. Surface RANKL of Toll-like receptor 4-stimulated human neutrophils activates osteoclastic bone resorption. *Blood.* 2009; 114(8):1633–1644.

Chapple ILC, Matthews JB. The role of reactive oxygen and antioxidant species in periodontal tissue destruction. *Periodontol 2000.* 2007; 43:160–232.

Chen B, Wu W, Sun W et al. RANKL expression in periodontal disease: where does RANKL come from? *BioMed Res Int.* 2014; 2014:731039. doi: 10.1155/2014/731039.

Cianci E, Recchiuti A, Trubiani O et al. Human periodontal stem cells release specialized proresolving mediators and carry immunomodulatory and pro-healing properties regulated by lipoxins. *Stem Cells Transl Med.* 2016; 5(1):20–32.

Cooper PR, Palmer LJ, Chapple ILC. Neutrophil extracellular traps as a new paradigm in innate immunity: friend or foe? *Periodontol 2000.* 2013; 63:165–197.

Cortés-Vieyra R, Rosales C, Uribe-Querol E. Neutrophil functions in periodontal homeostasis. *J Immunol Res.* 2016; 2016:Article ID 1396106. doi: 10.1155/2016/1396106.

Cox SW, Eley BM, Kiili M et al. Collagen degradation by interleukin-1b-stimulated gingival fibroblasts is accompanied by release and activation of multiple matrix metalloproteinases and cysteine proteinases. *Oral Dis.* 2006; 12:34–40.

Cullinan MP, Hamlet SM, Westerman B et al. Acquisition and loss of *Porphyromonas gingivalis*, *Actinobacillus actinomycetemcomitans* and *Prevotella intermedia* over a 5-year period: effect of a triclosan/copolymer dentifrice. *J Clin Periodontol.* 2003; 30:532–541.

Cutler CW, Jotwani R. Antigen-presentation and the role of dendritic cells in periodontitis. *Periodontol 2000.* 2004; 35:135–157.

Daghigh F, Borghaei RC, Thornton RD et al. Human gingival fibroblasts produce nitric oxide in response to proinflammatory cytokines. *J Periodontol.* 2002; 73:392–400.

Damgaard C, Kantarci A, Holmstrup P et al. *Porphyromonas gingivalis*-induced production of reactive oxygen species, tumor necrosis factor-☒, interleukin-6, CXCL8 and CCL2 by neutrophils from localized aggressive periodontitis and healthy donors: modulating actions of red blood cells and resolvin E1. *J Periodontal Res.* 2017; 52(2):246–254.

Dongari-Bagtzoglou A. Pathogenesis of mucosal biofilm infections: challenges and progress. *Expert Rev Anti Infect Ther.* 2008; 6:201–208.

Dumitrescu AL, El-Aleem SA, Morales-Aza B, Donaldson LF. A model of periodontitis in the rat: effect of lipopolysaccharide on bone resorption, osteoclast activity, and local peptidergic innervation. *J Clin Periodontol.* 2004; 31(8):596–603.

Dutzan N, Konkel JE, Greenwell-Wild T, Moutsopoulos NM. Characterization of the human immune cell network at the gingival barrier. *Mucosal Immunol.* 2016; 9(5):1163–1172.

Ebersole JL, Dawson D III, Emecen-Huja P et al. The periodontal war: microbes and immunity. *Periodontol 2000.* 2017; 75(1):52–115.

Ebersole JL, Dawson DR, Morford LA et al. Periodontal disease immunology: "double indemnity" in protecting the host. *Periodontol 2000.* 2013; 62(1):163–202.

Evans RI, Mikulecky M, Seymour GJ. Effect of initial treatment of chronic inflammatory periodontal disease in adults on spontaneous peripheral blood lymphocyte proliferation. *J Clin Periodontol.* 1989; 16:271–277.

Féger F, Varadaradjalou S, Gao Z, Abraham SN, Arock M. The role of mast cells in host defense and their subversion by bacterial pathogens. *Trends Immunol.* 2002; 23:151–157.

Fuchs TA, Abed U, Goosmann C et al. Novel cell death program leads to neutrophil extracellular traps. *J Cell Biol.* 2007; 176:231–241.

Gao L, Faibish D, Fredman G et al. Resolvin E1 and chemokine-like receptor 1 mediate bone preservation. *J Immunol.* 2013; 190(2):689–694.

Gemmell E, Seymour GJ. Cytokine profiles of cells extracted from human periodontal diseases. *J Dent Res.* 1998; 77:16–26.

Gölz L, Memmert S, Rath-Deschner B et al. LPS from *P. gingivalis* and hypoxia increases oxidative stress in periodontal ligament fibroblasts and contributes to periodontitis. *Mediators Inflamm.* 2014; 2014:986264. doi: 10.1155/2014/986264.

Gonzales JR. T- and B-cell subsets in periodontitis. *Periodontol 2000.* 2015; 69:181–200.

Grenier D. Effect of protease inhibitors on in vitro growth of *Porphyromonas gingivalis*. *Microb Ecol Health Dis.* 1992; 5:133–138.

Grossi SG, Zambon JJ, Ho AW et al. Assessment of risk for periodontal disease. I. Risk indicators for attachment loss. *J Periodontol.* 1994; 65:260–267.

Hajishengallis E, Hajishengallis G. Neutrophil homeostasis and periodontal health in children and adults. *J Dent Res.* 2014; 93(3):231–237.

Hajishengallis G. The inflammophilic character of the periodontitis-associated microbiota. *Mol Oral Microbiol.* 2014; 29:248–257.

Hajishengallis G. Periodontitis: from microbial immune subversion to systemic inflammation. *Nat Rev Immunol.* 2015; 15(1):30–44.

Hajishengallis G, Chavakis T, Hajishengallis E, Lambris JD. Neutrophil homeostasis and inflammation: novel paradigms from studying periodontitis. *J Leukoc Biol.* 2015; 98(4):539–548.

Hajishengallis G, Chavakis T, Lambris JD. Current understanding of periodontal disease pathogenesis and targets for host-modulation therapy. *Periodontol 2000.* 2020; 84:14–34.

Hajishengallis G, Darveau RP, Curtis MA. The keystone-pathogen hypothesis. *Nat Rev Microbiol.* 2012; 10:717–725.

Hajishengallis G, Lamont RJ. Beyond the red complex and into more complexity: the polymicrobial synergy and dysbiosis (PSD) model of periodontal disease etiology. *Mol Oral Microbiol.* 2012; 27:409–419.

Han X, Kawai T, Taubman MA. Interference with immune cell-mediated bone resorption in periodontal disease. *Periodontol 2000.* 2007; 45:76–94.

Han X, Lin X, Seliger AR et al. Expression of receptor activator of nuclear factor-κB ligand by B cells in response to oral bacteria. *Oral Microbiol Immunol.* 2009; 24(3):190–196.

Han Y, Jin Y, Miao Y, Shi T, Lin X. Improved RANKL expression and osteoclastogenesis induction of CD27+CD38- memory B cells: a link between B cells and alveolar bone damage in periodontitis. *J Periodontal Res.* 2019; 54:73–80.

Han YW, Shi W, Huang GTJ et al. Interactions between periodontal bacteria and human oral epithelial cells: fusobacterium nucleatum adheres to and invades epithelial cells. *Infect Immun.* 2000; 68(6):3140–3146.

Hans M, Hans VM. Toll-like receptors and their dual role in periodontitis: a review. *J Oral Sci.* 2011; 53(3):263–271.

Hasturk H, Kantarci A, Goguet-Surmenian E et al. Resolvin E1 regulates inflammation at the cellular and tissue level and restores tissue homeostasis in vivo. *J Immunol.* 2007; 179(10):7021–7029.

Hasturk H, Kantarci A, Van Dyke TE. Paradigm shift in the pharmacological management of periodontal diseases. *Front Oral Biol.* 2012; 15:160–176.

Henderson B, Kaiser F. Bacterial modulators of bone remodeling in the periodontal pocket. *Periodontol 2000.* 2018; 76:97–108.

Herrero ER, Fernandes S, Verspecht T et al. Dysbiotic biofilms deregulate the periodontal inflammatory response. *J Dent Res.* 2018; 2018:22034517752675.

Herrmann JM, Meyle J. Neutrophil activation and periodontal tissue injury. *Periodontol 2000.* 2015; 69:111–127.

Hienz SA, Paliwal S, Ivanovski S. Mechanisms of bone resorption in periodontitis. *J Immunol Res.* 2015; 2015:615486. doi: 10.1155/2015/615486.

Hirsch HZ, Tarkowski A, Miller EJ et al. Autoimmunity to collagen in adult periodontal disease. *J Oral Pathol.* 1988; 17:456–459.

Hirschfeld L, Wasserman B. A long-term survey of tooth loss in 600 treated periodontal patients. *J Periodontol.* 1978; 49:225–237.

Hirschfeld M, Weis JJ, Toshchakov V et al. Signaling by Toll-like receptor 2 and 4 agonists results in differential gene expression in murine macrophages. *Infect and Immun.* 2001; 69:1477–1482.

Hofbauer LC, Lacey DL, Dunstan CR et al. Interleukin-1beta and tumor necrosis factor-alpha, but not interleukin-6, stimulate osteoprotegerin ligand gene expression in human osteoblastic cells. *Bone.* 1999; 25:255–259.

Horowitz MC, Fretz JA, Lorenzo JA. How B cells influence bone biology in health and disease. *Bone.* 2010; 47:472–479.

Hu X, Sun Y, Xu W, Lin T, Zeng H. Expression of RANKL by peripheral neutrophils and its association with bone mineral density in COPD. *Respirology.* 2017; 22:126–132.

Huang CB, Alimova Y, Ebersole JL. Macrophage polarization in response to oral commensals and pathogens. *Pathog Dis.* 2016; 74(3):ftw011. doi: 10.1093/femspd/ftw011.

Ito H, Harada Y, Matsuo T, Ebisu S, Okada H. Possible role of T cells in the establishment of IgG plasma cell-rich periodontal lesion augmentation of IgG synthesis in the polyclonal B cell activation response by autoreactive T cells. *J Periodontal Res.* 1988; 23:39–45.

Kamada N, Seo SU, Chen GY, Nunez G. Role of the gut microbiota in immunity and inflammatory disease. *Nat Rev Immunol.* 2013; 13:321–335.

Kantarci A, Hasturk H, Van Dyke TE. Animal models for periodontal regeneration and peri-implant responses. *Periodontol 2000.* 2015; (68):66–82.

Kawai T, Matsuyama T, Hosokawa Y et al. B and T lymphocytes are the primary sources of RANKL in the bone resorptive lesion of periodontal disease. *Am J Pathol.* 2006; 169(3):987–998.

Kinane DF. Regulators of tissue destruction and homeostasis as diagnostic aids in periodontology. *Periodontol 2000.* 2000; 24:215–225.

Kinane DF, Bartold PM. Clinical relevance of the host responses of periodontitis. *Periodontol 2000.* 2007; 43:278–293.

Kinane DF, Berglundh T, Lindhe J. Pathogenesis of Periodontitis. In: J Lindhe, NP Lang, T Karring, eds. *Clinical Periodontology and Implant Dentistry*, 5th edn. Oxford: Blackwell; 2008: 285–306.

Kizil C, Kyritsis N, Brand M. Effects of inflammation on stem cells: together they strive? *EMBO Rep.* 2015; 16(4):416–426.

Koide M, Kinugawa S, Takahashi N, Udagawa N. Osteoclastic bone resorption induced by innate immune responses. *Periodontol 2000.* 2010; 54:235–246.

Kolenbrander PE, Palmer RJ Jr, Periasamy S, Jakubovics NS. Oral multispecies biofilm development and the key role of cell–cell distance. *Nat Rev Microbiol.* 2010; 8:471–448.

Kornman KS. Mapping the pathogenesis of periodontitis: a new look. *J Periodontol.* 2008; 79:1560–1568.

Korostoff JM, Wang JF, Sarment DP et al. Analysis of in situ protease activity in chronic adult periodontitis patients: expression of activated MMP-2 and a 40 kDa serine protease. *J Periodontol.* 2000; 71:353–360.

Labonte AC, Sung SJ, Jennelle LT, Dandekar AP, Hahn YS. Expression of scavenger receptor-AI promotes alternative activation of murine macrophages to limit hepatic inflammation and fibrosis. *Hepatology.* 2017; 65:32–43.

Lamont RJ, Hajishengallis G. Polymicrobial synergy and dysbiosis in inflammatory disease. *Trends Mol Med.* 2015; 21:172–183.

Lamont RJ, Koo H, Hajishengallis G. The oral microbiota: dynamic communities and host interactions. *Nat Rev Microbiol.* 2018; 16:745–759.

Lappin DF, MacLeod CP, Kerr A, Mitchell T, Kinane DF. Anti-inflammatory cytokine IL-10 and T cell cytokine profile in periodontitis granulation tissue. *Clin Exp Immunol.* 2001; 123:294–300.

Leffler J, Martin M, Gullstrand B et al. Neutrophil extracellular traps that are not degraded in systemic lupus erythematosus activate complement exacerbating the disease. *J Immunol.* 2012; 188:3522–3531.

Lerner UH. Inflammation-induced bone remodeling in periodontal disease and the influence of post-menopausal osteoporosis. *J Dent Res.* 2006; 85(7):596–607.

Lindhe J, Liljenberg B, Listgarten M. Some microbiological and histopathological features of periodontal disease in man. *J Periodontol.* 1980; 51:264–269.

Listgarten MA. The role of dental plaque in gingivitis and periodontitis. *J Clin Periodontol.* 1988; 15:485–487.

Liu YC, Zou XB, Chai YF, Yao YM. Macrophage polarization in inflammatory diseases. *Int J Biol Sci.* 2014; 10:520–529.

Locati M, Mantovani A, Sica A. Macrophage activation and polarization as an adaptive component of innate immunity. *Adv Immunol.* 2013; 120:163–184.

Loo WT, Jin L, Cheung MN, Wang M, Chow LW. Epigenetic change in E-cadherin and COX-2 to predict chronic periodontitis. *J Transl Med.* 2010; 8:110.

Loos BG, Van Dyke TE. The role of inflammation and genetics in periodontal disease. *Periodontol 2000.* 2020; 83:26–39.

Lundqvist C, Hammarstrom M-L. T-cell receptor $\Upsilon\delta$-expressing intraepithelial lymphocytes are present in normal and chronically inflamed human gingiva. *Immunology.* 1993; 79:38–45.

Mantovani A, Biswas SK, Galdiero MR, Sica A, Locati M. Macrophage plasticity and polarization in tissue repair and remodeling. *J Pathol.* 2013; 229:176–185.

Marsh PD. Microbial ecology of dental plaque and its significance in health and disease. *Adv Dent Res.* 1994; 8:263–271.

Marshall JS. *Mast-cell response to pathogens. Nature Rev.* 2004; 4:787–799.

Marshall RI. Gingival defensins: linking the innate and adaptive immune responses to dental plaque. *Periodontol 2000.* 2004; 35:14–20.

Martin P, Leibovich SJ. Inflammatory cells during wound repair: the good, the bad and the ugly. *Trends Cell Biol.* 2005; 15:599–607.

Martinelli S, Urosevic M, Daryadel A et al. Induction of genes mediating interferon-dependent extracellular trap formation during neutrophil differentiation. *J Biol Chem.* 2004; 279:44123–44132.

Matsumoto C, Oda T, Yokoyama S et al. Toll-like receptor 2 heterodimers, TLR2/6 and TLR2/1 induce prostaglandin E production by osteoblasts, osteoclast formation and inflammatory periodontitis. *Biochem Biophys Res Commun.* 2012; 428(1):110–115.

Matthews JB, Wright HJ, Roberts A, Cooper PR, Chapple IL. Hyperactivity and reactivity of peripheral blood neutrophils in chronic periodontitis. *Clin Exp Immunol.* 2007; 147:255–264.

Meyle J, Chapple I. Molecular aspects of the pathogenesis of periodontitis. *Periodontol 2000.* 2015; 69:7–17.

Meyle J, Dommisch H, Groeger S et al. The innate host response in caries and periodontitis. *J Clin Periodontol.* 2017; 44:1215–1225.

Mocsai A. Diverse novel functions of neutrophils in immunity, inflammation, and beyond. *J Exp Med.* 2013; 210(7):1283–1299.

Moser B, Eberl M. Gammadelta T-APCs: a novel tool for immunotherapy? *Cell Mol Life Sci.* 2011; 68(14):2443–2452.

Moutsopoulos NM, Konkel JE. Tissue-specific immunity at the oral mucosal barrier. *Trends Immunol.* 2018; 39(4):276–287.

Murphy KM, Reiner SL. The lineage decisions of helper T-cells. *Nat Rev Immunol.* 2002; 2(12):933–944.

Myneni SRV, Wang HH, Brocavich K. Biological strategies for the prevention of periodontal disease: probiotics and vaccines. *Periodontol 2000.* 2020; 84(1):161–175.

Nedzi-Góra M, Kowalski J, Górska R. The immune response in periodontal tissues. *Arch Immunol Ther Exp.* 2017; 65:421–429.

Nelson D, Potempa J, Kordula T, Travis J. Purification and characterization of a novel cysteine proteinase (periodontain) from *Porphyromonas gingivalis*. Evidence for a role in the inactivation of human a1-proteinase inhibitor. *J Biol Chem.* 1999; 274:12245–12251.

Nicu EA, Loos BG. Polymorphonuclear neutrophils in periodontitis and their possible modulation as a therapeutic approach. *Periodontol 2000.* 2016; 71:140–163.

Nicu EA, Van der Velden U, Everts V et al. Hyper-reactive PMNs in FcgammaRIIa 131 H/H genotype periodontitis patients. *J Clin Periodontol.* 2007; 34:938–945.

Ohlrich EJ, Cullinan MP, Seymour GJ. The immunopathogenesis of periodontal disease. *Aust Dent J.* 2009; 54:(1 Suppl): S2–S10.

Okayama Y, Kirshenbaum AS, Metcalfe DD. Expression of a functional high-affinity IgG receptor, FcΥRI, on human mast cells: up-regulation of IFN-Υ. *J Immunol.* 2000; 164:4332–4339.

Oliveira RR, Fermiano D, Feres M et al. Levels of candidate periodontal pathogens in subgingival biofilm. *J Dent Res.* 2016; 95:711–718.

Ortega-Gomez A, Perretti M, Soehnlein O. Resolution of inflammation: an integrated view. *EMBO Mol Med.* 2013; 5(5):661–674.

Park YD, Kim YS, Jung YM et al. *Porphyromonas gingivalis* lipopolysaccharide regulates interleukin (IL)-17 and IL-23 expression via SIRT1 modulation in human periodontal ligament cells. *Cytokine.* 2012; 60(1):284–293.

Paul WE. Bridging innate and adaptive immunity. *Cell.* 2011; 147:1212–1215.

Pelletier M, Maggi L, Micheletti A et al. Evidence for a crosstalk between human neutrophils and Th17 cells. *Blood.* 2010; 115(2):335–343.

Perretti M, Leroy X, Bland EJ, Montero-Melendez T. Resolution pharmacology: opportunities for therapeutic innovation in inflammation. *Trends Pharmacol Sci.* 2015; 36(11):737–755.

Potempa J, Banbula A, Travis J. Role of bacterial proteinases in matrix destruction and modulation of host responses. *Periodontol 2000.* 2000; 24:153–192.

Pulendran B, Kumar P, Cutler CW et al. Lipopolysaccharides from distinct pathogens induce different classes of immune responses in vivo. *J Immunol.* 2001; 167:5067–5076.

Re F, Strominger JL. Toll-like receptor 2 (TLR2) and TLR4 differentially activate human dendritic cells. *J Biol Chem.* 2001; 276:37692–37699.

Recchiuti A, Serhan CN. Pro-resolving lipid mediators (SPMs) and their actions in regulating mirna in novel resolution circuits in inflammation. *Front Immunol.* 2012; 3:298.

Reynolds JJ, Hembry RM, Meikle MC. Connective tissue degradation in health and periodontal disease and the roles of matrix metalloproteinases and their natural inhibitors. *Adv Dent Res.* 1994; 8(2):312–319.

Roberts HM, Ling MR, Insall R et al. Impaired neutrophil directional chemotactic accuracy in chronic periodontitis patients. *J Clin Periodontol.* 2015; 42:1–11.

Sabbione F, Gabelloni ML, Ernst G et al. Neutrophils suppress γδ T-cell function. *Eur J Immunol.* 2014; 44:819–830.

Sanz M, Beighton D, Curtis MA et al. Role of microbial biofilms in the maintenance of oral health and in the development of dental caries and periodontal diseases. Consensus report of group 1 of the Joint EFP/ORCA workshop on the boundaries between caries and periodontal disease. *J Clin Periodontol.* 2017; 44 (Suppl. 18):S5–S11. doi: 10.1111/jcpe.12682.

Scannapieco FA, Gershovich E. The prevention of periodontal disease—an overview. *Periodontol 2000.* 2020; 84:9–13.

Scheres N, Laine ML, de Vries TJ, Everts V, van Winkelhoff AJ. Gingival and periodontal ligament fibroblasts differ in their inflammatory response to viable *Porphyromonas gingivalis*. *J Periodontal Res.* 2010; 45(2):262–270.

Schwartz Z, Goultschin J, Dean DD, Boyan BD. Mechanisms of alveolar bone destruction in periodontitis. *Periodontol 2000.* 1997; 14(1):158–172.

Sczepanik FSC, Grossi ML, Casati M et al. Periodontitis is an inflammatory disease of oxidative stress: we should treat it that way. *Periodontol 2000.* 2020; 84:45–68.

Séguier S, Gogly B, Bodineau A, Godeau G, Brousse N. Is collagen breakdown during periodontitis linked to inflammatory cells and expression of matrix metalloproteinases and tissue inhibitors of metalloproteinases in human gingival tissue? *J Periodontol.* 2001; 72(10):1398–1406.

Serhan CN. Controlling the resolution of acute inflammation: a new genus of dual anti-inflammatory and pro-resolving mediators. *J Periodontol.* 2008; 79:1520–1526.

Serhan CN. Treating inflammation and infection in the 21st century: new hints from decoding resolution mediators and mechanisms. *FASEB J.* 2017; 31(4):1273–1288.

Serhan CN, Chiang N. Resolution phase lipid mediators of inflammation: agonists of resolution. *Curr Opin Pharmacol.* 2013; 13(4):632–640.

Serhan CN, Chiang N, Dalli J. New pro-resolving n-3 mediators bridge resolution of infectious inflammation to tissue regeneration. *Mol Aspects Med.* 2018; 64:1–17.

Serhan CN, Chiang N, Van Dyke TE. Resolving inflammation: dual anti-inflammatory and pro-resolution lipid mediators. *Nat Rev Immunol.* 2008; 8(5):349–361.

Seymour GJ, Trombelli L, Berglundh T. (2015). Pathogenesis of gingivitis. In: NP Lang, J Lindhe, eds. *Clinical Periodontology and Implant Dentistry*. Chichester: Wiley; 2015: 241–269.

Silva N, Abusleme L, Bravo D et al. Host response mechanisms in periodontal diseases. *J Appl Oral Sci.* 2015; 23(3):329–355.

Sima C, Aboodi GM, Lakschevitz FS et al. Nuclear factor erythroid 2-related factor 2 down-regulation in oral neutrophils is associated with periodontal oxidative damage and severe chronic periodontitis. *Am J Pathol.* 2016; 186(6):1417–1426.

Sima C, Glogauer M. Macrophage subsets and osteoimmunology: tuning of the immunological recognition and effector systems that maintain alveolar bone. *Periodontol 2000.* 2013; 63:80–101.

Skyberg JA, Thornburg T, Rollins M et al. Murine and bovine γδ T-cells enhance innate immunity against *Brucella abortus* infections. *PLoS ONE.* 2011; 6(7):e21978.

Slots J. Herpesviral–bacterial interactions in periodontal diseases. *Periodontol 2000.* 2010; 52:117–140.

Socransky SS, Haffajee AD. Dental biofilms: difficult therapeutic targets. *Periodontol 2000.* 2002; 28(1):12–55.

Socransky SS, Haffajee AD. Periodontal microbial ecology. *Periodontol 2000.* 2005; 8(1):135–187.

Sorsa T, Ingman T, Suomalainen K et al. Identification of proteases from periodontopathogenic bacteria as activators of latent human neutrophil and fibroblast-type interstitial collagenases. *Infect Immun.* 1992; 60:4491–5492.

Stark MA, Huo Y, Burcin TL et al. Phagocytosis of apoptotic neutrophils regulates granulopoiesis via IL-23 and IL-17. *Immunity.* 2005; 22(3):285–294.

Stefani FA, Viana MB, Dupim AC et al. Expression, polymorphism and methylation pattern of interleukin-6 in periodontal tissues. *Immunobiology.* 2013; 218:1012–1017.

Tabeta K, Yamazaki K, Hotokezaka H, Yoshie H, Hara K. Elevated humoral immune response to heat shock protein 60 family in periodontitis patients. *Clin Exp Immunol.* 2000; 120:285–293.

Tacke F, Zimmermann HW. Macrophage heterogeneity in liver injury and fibrosis. *J Hepatol.* 2014; 60:1090–1096.

Takayanagi H, Ogasawara K, Hida S et al. T-cell-mediated regulation of osteoclastogenesis by signaling cross-talk between RANKL and INF-γ. *Nature.* 2000; 408:600–605.

Tanner AC, Kent R Jr, Kanasi E et al. Clinical characteristics and microbiota of progressing slight chronic periodontitis in adults. *J Clin Periodontol.* 2007; 34:917–930.

Taubman MA, Valverde P, Han X, Kawai T. Immune response: the key to bone resorption in periodontal disease. *J Periodontol.* 2005; 76(11):2033–2041.

Tawfig N. Proinflammatory cytokines and periodontal disease. *J Dent Probl Solut.* 2016; 3(1):12–17.

Teng Y-TA. Protective and destructive immunity in the periodontium: part 1—innate and humoral immunity and the periodontium. *J Dent Res.* 2006a; 85(3):198–208.

Teng Y-TA. Protective and destructive immunity in the periodontium. part 2 T cell-mediated immunity in the periodontium. *J Dent Res.* 2006; 85(3):209–219.

Tew J, Engel D, Mangan D. Polyclonal B-cell activation in periodontitis. *J Periodontal Res.* 1989; 24:225–241.

Tew JG, ElShikh ME, ElSayed RM, Schenkein HA. Dendritic cells, antibodies reactive with oxLDL, and inflammation. *J Dent Res.* 2012; 91(1):8–16.

Tewari DS, Bian Y, Tewari M et al. Mechanistic features associated with induction of metalloproteinases in human gingival fibroblasts by interleukin-1. *Arch Oral Biol.* 1994; 39:657–664.

Tillack K, Breiden P, Martin R, Sospedra M. T-lymphocyte priming by neutrophil extracellular traps links innate and adaptive immune responses. *J Immunol.* 2012; 188:3150–3159.

Trevani AS, Chorny A, Salamone G et al. Bacterial DNA activates human neutrophils by a CpG-independent pathway. *Eur J Immunol.* 2003; 33(11):3164–3174.

Tubo NJ, Jenkins MK. TCR signal quantity and quality in CD4+ T cell differentiation. *Trends Immunol.* 2014; 35(12):591–596.

Tugal D, Liao X, Jain MK. Transcriptional control of macrophage polarization. *Arterioscler Thromb Vasc Biol.* 2013; 33:1135–1144.

Turina M, Miller FN, McHugh PP, Cheadle WG, Polk HC Jr. Endotoxin inhibits apoptosis but induces primary necrosis in neutrophils. *Inflammation.* 2005; 29:55–63.

Udagawa N, Sato N, Yang S et al. Signal transduction of lipopolysaccharide-induced osteoclast differentiation. *Periodontol 2000.* 2007; 43(1):56–64.

Van Dyke TE. Pro-resolving lipid mediators: potential for prevention and treatment of periodontitis. *J Clin Periodontol.* 2011; 38(Suppl 11):119–125.

Van Dyke TE. Pro-resolving mediators in the regulation of periodontal disease. *Mol Aspects Med.* 2017; 58:21–36.

Van Dyke TE. Shifting the paradigm from inhibitors of inflammation to resolvers of inflammation in periodontitis. *J Periodontol.* 2020; 91(Suppl. 1):S19–S25.

Van Dyke TE, Sima C. Understanding resolution of inflammation in periodontal diseases: is chronic inflammatory periodontitis a failure to resolve? *Periodontol 2000.* 2020; 82:205–213.

von Köckritz-Blickwede M, Goldmann O, Thulin P et al. Phagocytosis-independent antimicrobial activity of mast cells by means of extracellular trap formation. *Blood.* 2008; 111(6):3070–3080.

von Vietinghoff S, Ley K. Homeostatic regulation of blood neutrophil counts. *J Immunol.* 2008; 181(8):5183–5188.

Waddington RJ, Moseley R, Embery G. Reactive oxygen species: a potential role in the pathogenesis of periodontal diseases. *Oral Dis.* 2000; 6:138–151.

Walsh MC, Kim N, Kadono Y et al. Osteoimmunology: interplay between the immune system and bone metabolism. *Annu Rev Immunol.* 2006; 24:33–63.

Wassenaar A, Reinhardus C, Thepen T, Abraham Inpijn L, Kievits F. Cloning, characterization, and antigen specificity of T-lymphocyte subsets extracted from gingival tissue of chronic adult periodontitis patients. *Infect Immun.* 1995; 63:2147–2153.

Weaver CT, Hatton RD. Interplay between the Th17 and TReg cell lineages: a (co-)evolutionary perspective. *Nat Rev Immunol.* 2009; 9(12):883–889.

Woodfin A, Voisin MB, Beyrau M et al. The junctional adhesion molecule JAM-C regulates polarized transendothelial migration of neutrophils in vivo. *Nat Immunol.* 2011; 12:761–769.

Wu Y, Wu W, Wong WM et al. Human gamma delta T cells: a lymphoid lineage cell capable of professional phagocytosis. *J Immunol.* 2009; 183(9):5622–5629.

Yago T, Nanke Y, Ichikawa N et al. IL-17 induces osteoclastogenesis from human monocytes alone in the absence of osteoblasts, which is potently inhibited by anti-TNF-α antibody: a novel mechanism of osteoclastogenesis by IL-17. *J Cell Biochem.* 2009; 108(4):947–955.

Yarilina A, Xu K, Chen J, Ivashkiv LB. TNF activates calcium-nuclear factor of activated T cells (NFAT)c1 signaling pathways in human macrophages. *Proc Nat Acad Sci USA.* 2011; 108(4):1573–1578.

Yucel-Lindberg T, Båge T. Inflammatory mediators in the pathogenesis of periodontitis. *Expert Rev Mol Med.* 2013; 15(e7). doi: 10.1017/erm.2013.8.

Yun PL, Decarlo AA, Collyer C, Hunter N. Hydrolysis of interleukin-12 by *Porphyromonas gingivalis* major cysteine proteinases may affect local gamma interferon accumulation and the Th1 or Th2 T-cell phenotype in periodontitis. *Infect Immun.* 2001; 69:5650–5660.

Zeng MY, Inohara N, Nunez G. Mechanisms of inflammation-driven bacterial dysbiosis in the gut. *Mucosal Immunol.* 2017; 10:18–26.

Zenobia C, Hajishengallis G. Basic biology and role of interleukin-17 in immunity and inflammation. *Periodontol 2000.* 2015; 69(1):142–159.

Zenobia C, Luo XL, Hashim A et al. Commensal bacteria dependent select expression of CXCL2 contributes to periodontal tissue homeostasis. *Cell Microbiol.* 2013; 15(8):1419–1426.

Zhang S, Barros SP, Niculescu MD et al. Alteration of PTGS2 promoter methylation in chronic periodontitis. *J Dent Res.* 2010; 89:133–137.

Zhou J, Windsor LJ. *Porphyromonas gingivalis* affects host collagen degradation by affecting expression, activation, and inhibition of matrix metalloproteinases. *J Periodontal Res.* 2006; 41:47–54.

Zhou L-N, Bi C-S, Gao L-N et al. Macrophage polarization in human gingival tissue in response to periodontal disease. *Oral Dis.* 2019; 25:265–273.

5.5 HISTOPATHOGENESIS OF PERIODONTAL DISEASE

Steph Smith

Contents

Learning objectives

- Histopathological features occurring in the periodontal tissues during the development of gingivitis and periodontitis.
- Structural and functional characteristics that determine the integrity of the junctional epithelium.
- Histopathological mechanisms causing loss of attachment of junctional epithelium and the destruction of connective tissues, leading to the formation of the periodontal lesion and a periodontal pocket.
- Disease activity and site specificity of periodontitis.

Histopathogenesis of periodontal disease

The initial and early lesions of gingivitis are considered to be well-controlled immunological responses to the oral microbiome (Bartold & Van Dyke 2019, Ohlrich et al. 2009). However, with the persistence of the plaque biofilm, the immunological response does not resolve. Subsequently, prolonged chronic inflammation leads to the development of the established lesion of gingivitis, whereby a full transition from the innate immune response to the acquired immune response has occurred (Kurgan & Kantarci 2018; Ohlrich et al. 2009). This is histologically characterized by neutrophils, lymphocytes, and macrophages, with a predominance of B cells and plasma cells, including immunoglobulin (Ig)G1 and IgG3 subclasses of B lymphocytes. However, following this, in some people as a result of their own innate susceptibility and/or environmental factors, a dysregulation of immune-inflammatory mechanisms causes the development of the advanced lesion of gingivitis. This includes a loss of epithelial attachment, the breakdown of connective tissue, and bone resorption (Bartold & Van Dyke 2019; Hirschfeld & Wasserman 1978).

During the early stages of inflammation, the sulcular epithelium shows formation of rete pegs. The basal cell layer of the junctional epithelium (JE) starts to proliferate in an attempt to maintain epithelial integrity and to increase the physical barrier between the biofilm and the connective tissue, as evidenced by the epithelium proliferating to form deeper rete pegs (Kurgan & Kantarci 2018). The periodontal sulcus also starts deepening, although there is no loss of dentogingival attachment. In the established lesion, the JE is replaced with loosely adherent pocket epithelium that allows the bacterial biofilm to migrate deep into the periodontal sulcus. The pocket epithelium is heavily infiltrated with leukocytes, predominantly neutrophils, and shows increased permeability, allowing the passage of substances in and out of the connective tissue. The pocket epithelium shows ingrowth of rete pegs into the surrounding connective tissue (Birkedal-Hansen 1995; Kurgan & Kantarci 2018). Progressive degeneration and necrosis of the epithelium lead to ulceration of the lateral wall of the periodontal pocket, resulting in exposure of the underlying inflamed connective tissue. Breakdown of the basement membrane with subsequent ulceration of the pocket epithelium leads to increased permeability (Newman et al. 2019). This allows for the continued ingress of bacteria and microbial products, leading to a perpetual and exacerbated inflammatory process, including suppuration (Bartold & Van Dyke 2019). Acute inflammation can also be superimposed on the underlying chronic changes (Newman et al. 2019).

During this inflammatory process, fibroblast functions become altered, whereby cell proliferation and collagen production are impaired and components of the extracellular matrix are degraded. Connective tissue destruction results from the synergistic action of both bacteria and host-derived proteinases, namely matrix metalloproteinases (MMPs), leading to an imbalance of these proteinases over their inhibitors, namely tissue inhibitors of metalloproteinases (TIMPs) (Birkedal-Hansen 1995). The loss of collagen is due to extracellular collagenases (MMPs) and other enzymes secreted by various cells in healthy and inflamed tissue, such as fibroblasts, polymorphonuclear neutrophils (PMNs), and macrophages, as well as fibroblasts phagocytizing collagen fibers. Just apical to the JE, collagen fibers are destroyed. Also, the inserted collagen fibrils at the ligament–cementum interface become degraded and destroyed, including the fibrils of the cementum matrix (Newman et al. 2019).

As a consequence of the loss of collagen just apical to the JE and at the ligament–cementum interface, the apical cells of the JE proliferate along the root surface and extend finger-like projections that are two or three cells in thickness (Newman et al. 2019). In addition, MMPs degrade components of both the external and internal basal lamina of the JE, causing the JE to lose cohesiveness, thus becoming detached from the tooth surface. Furthermore, as a result of inflammation, PMNs invade the coronal end of the JE in increasing numbers. The PMNs are not joined to one another or to the epithelial cells by desmosomes. When the relative volume of PMNs reaches approximately 60% or more of the JE, the tissue loses cohesiveness and detaches from the tooth surface (Newman et al. 2019). Thus, the coronal portion of the JE detaches from the root as the apical portion migrates, resulting in its apical shift (Kurgan & Kantarci 2018). This occurs in conjunction with the breakdown and loss of attachment of connective tissue to the tooth surface, together with bone loss, thus leading to pocket formation characterizing the advanced lesion of gingivitis (periodontitis) (Birkedal-Hansen 1995; Paul 2011).

With continued inflammation, the gingiva increases in bulk, and the crest of the gingival margin extends coronally. The apical cells of the JE continue to migrate along the root, and its coronal cells continue to separate from it. The epithelium of the lateral wall of the pocket proliferates to form bulbous, cordlike extensions into the inflamed connective tissue. Leukocytes and edema from the inflamed connective tissue infiltrate the epithelium that lines the pocket, resulting in various degrees of degeneration and necrosis (Newman et al. 2019).

Periodontal pocket formation is a pathological process, whereby the host response causes tissue destruction; however, it is also the host response that is responsible for restricting the spreading of infection into deeper areas (Paul 2011; Pöllänen et al. 2012). This is reflected in the dual changes occurring in the connective tissue, namely simultaneous collagen fiber breakdown and fiber bundle thickening, involving alterations in type I, type III, and type VI collagens (Lorencini et al. 2009). Normally, the distance between the apical end of the JE and the alveolar bone is relatively constant. The distance from attached plaque to bone is never less than 0.5 mm and never more than 2.7 mm. The distance between the apical extent of calculus and the alveolar crest in human periodontal pockets is most constant, having a mean length of 1.97 mm (Newman et al. 2019).

The histopathological development of gingivitis and periodontitis is loosely divided into initial, early, established, and advanced lesions, as described by Page and Schroeder (1976) (see Figure 5.5.1).

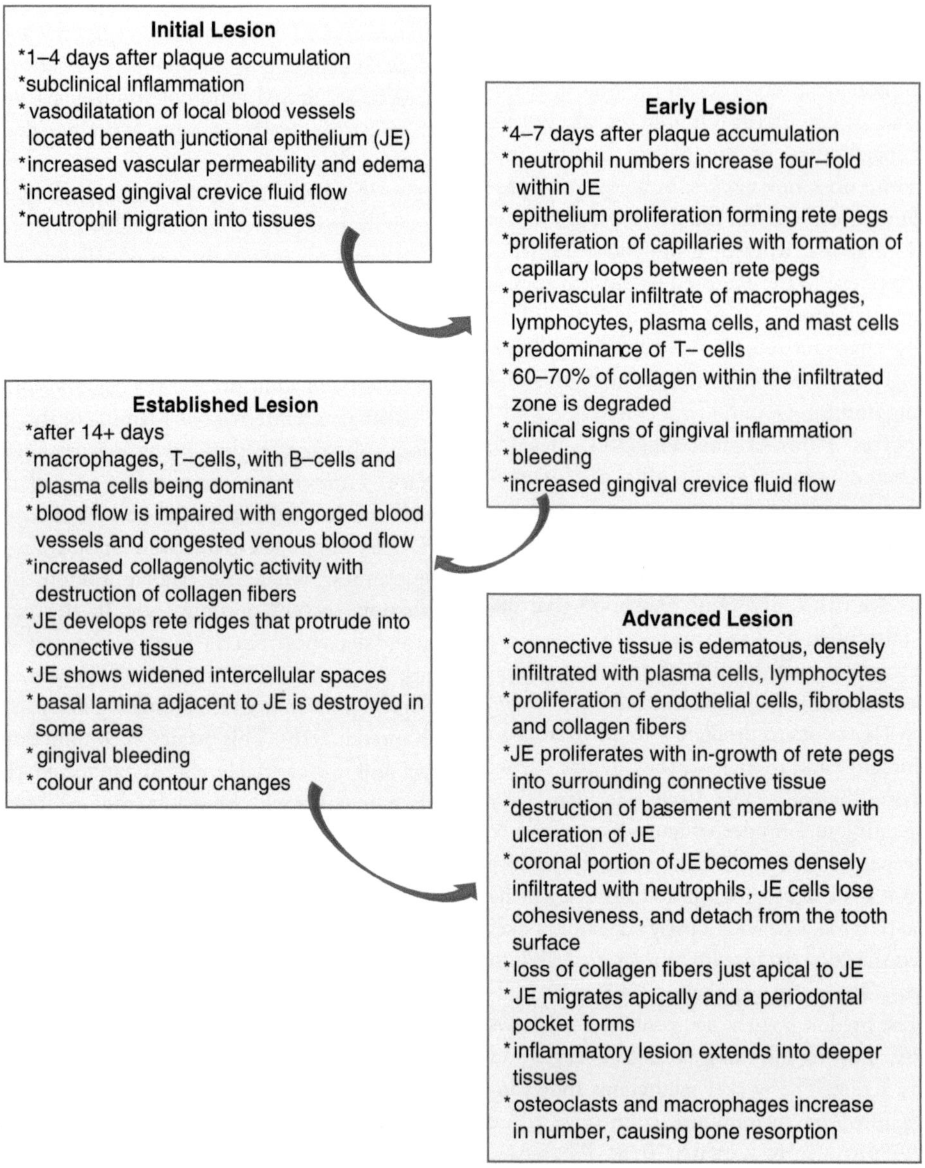

Initial Lesion
*1–4 days after plaque accumulation
*subclinical inflammation
* vasodilatation of local blood vessels
  located beneath junctional epithelium (JE)
*increased vascular permeability and edema
*increased gingival crevice fluid flow
*neutrophil migration into tissues

Early Lesion
*4–7 days after plaque accumulation
* neutrophil numbers increase four–fold
  within JE
* epithelium proliferation forming rete pegs
*proliferation of capillaries with formation of
  capillary loops between rete pegs
* perivascular infiltrate of macrophages,
  lymphocytes, plasma cells, and mast cells
* predominance of T– cells
* 60–70% of collagen within the infiltrated
  zone is degraded
* clinical signs of gingival inflammation
* bleeding
*increased gingival crevice fluid flow

Established Lesion
*after 14+ days
*macrophages, T–cells, with B–cells and
  plasma cells being dominant
* blood flow is impaired with engorged blood
  vessels and congested venous blood flow
*increased collagenolytic activity with
  destruction of collagen fibers
*JE develops rete ridges that protrude into
  connective tissue
*JE shows widened intercellular spaces
* basal lamina adjacent to JE is destroyed in
  some areas
* gingival bleeding
* colour and contour changes

Advanced Lesion
* connective tissue is edematous, densely
  infiltrated with plasma cells, lymphocytes
* proliferation of endothelial cells, fibroblasts
  and collagen fibers
*JE proliferates with in-growth of rete pegs
  into surrounding connective tissue
*destruction of basement membrane with
  ulceration of JE
* coronal portion of JE becomes densely
  infiltrated with neutrophils, JE cells lose
  cohesiveness, and detach from the tooth
  surface
*loss of collagen fibers just apical to JE
* JE migrates apically and a periodontal
  pocket forms
*inflammatory lesion extends into deeper
  tissues
* osteoclasts and macrophages increase
  in number, causing bone resorption

Figure 5.5.1 Histopathogenesis of periodontal disease. Courtesy of Dr. Steph Smith.

Junctional epithelium and loss of attachment

A hallmark in the progression of gingivitis to periodontitis is the conversion of the JE to pocket epithelium (Bosshardt & Lang 2005). It has thus been suggested that the initiation of pocket formation is either attributed to the detachment of DAT (directly attached) cells from the tooth surface or to the development of an intraepithelial split (Takata & Donath 1988). Studies have indicated that the initiation of pocket development is due to cleavage within the second or third cell layer of DAT cells in the most coronal portion of the JE-facing biofilms, and that it is not due to the detachment of DAT cells from the tooth (Fujita et al. 2018). However, it

remains unclear whether detachment of JE cells from the tooth surface or destruction of cell junctional complexes is more responsible for pocket development (Bosshardt 2018). Box 5.5.1 describes the process of loss of attachment affecting the JE.

In summary, the defense mechanisms in a healthy periodontium are generally sufficient to control the constant microbiological challenge through a normally functioning JE and a concentrated mass of inflammatory and immune cells and macromolecules transmigrating through the JE. The destruction of the structural integrity of the JE, which includes disruption of cell-to-cell contacts and detachment from the tooth surface, causes a disequilibrium of this delicate defense system. The thinning of the epithelium and its ulceration increase the

Box 5.5.1 Junctional epithelium and loss of attachment

Healthy junctional epithelium attachment

- The free surface of the junctional epithelium (JE) facing the gingival sulcus is characterized by an open system, which lacks a physical barrier in the form of a keratinized cell layer (Bosshardt 2018).
- However, the JE attachment is a dynamic structure, including unique functional and structural (cellular and extracellular) characteristics, providing a potent antimicrobial defense system. Rather than simply providing an attachment to the tooth surface, the JE actively hinders bacterial advancement into periodontal tissues by means of its structural framework.
- This is accomplished by cell attachment to the tooth surface via hemidesmosomes and an internal basal lamina (IBL), an attachment to the surrounding gingival connective tissue via an external basement lamina (EBL), and cell-to-cell attachment within the JE (Bosshardt 2018; Pöllänen et al. 2012).
- JE in clinically healthy periodontal tissue is only interconnected by desmosomes and occasionally by gap junctions, and not by tight junctions, and has wide intercellular spaces (Fujita et al. 2018).
- Multiprotein cell junction complexes are symmetrical structures found between cells and are crucial for the maintenance of the physical and functional integrity of tissues. Epithelial cadherin (E-cadherin) plays a crucial role in maintaining the structural integrity and function of desmosomal epithelial intercellular junctions, as well as in preventing bacterial invasion (Wheelock & Jensen 1992).
- Gap junctions are clusters of transmembranous hydrophilic channels that allow direct exchange of molecules, including ions, sugars, and small peptides, between adjacent cells. Gap junctional intercellular communication plays a critical role in cellular coordination in tissue homeostasis. Connexins are structural proteins of these gap junctions (Fujita et al. 2018).
- Rapid renewal and constant shedding of the JE cells toward the sulcus together with gingival crevicular fluid (GCF) flow efficiently inhibit bacterial colonization.
- The epithelial attachment mechanism is considered to be of high strength, which includes continuous remodeling of the epithelial attachment occurring via basal cells undergoing mitosis, as well as DAT cells migrating toward the sulcus bottom, where they desquamate (Bosshardt & Lang 2005).
- The EBL and IBL function as barriers to bacterial advancement, yet allow the passage of leukocytes and their antimicrobial agents as well as antibodies into the gingival crevice. The EBL functions merely as a

protective barrier, whereas the IBL is dedicated to maintaining the attachment to the tooth (Bosshardt & Lang 2005).
- The IBL has been suggested to be a specialized basal lamina, comprising an extracellular matrix, forming a strategic adhesive relationship with the tooth surface. This extracellular matrix contains no type IV and VII collagens, and is enriched in laminin-332 (Lm332) (Fouillen et al. 2019).
- The adhesive capacity of the IBL is further accomplished by JE cells secreting three unique epithelial proteins: amelotin (AMTN), odontogenic ameloblast-associated (ODAM), and secretory calcium-binding phosphoprotein proline-glutamine rich 1 (SCPPPQ1) (Wheelock & Jensen 1992). The IBL thus cannot be regarded as a basement membrane in the true sense (Bosshardt & Lang 2005).

Junctional epithelium and innate immune defense

- JE plays an active role in innate host defense by producing natural antimicrobial peptides, proteins, and cytokines/chemokines. Calprotectin, an antimicrobial peptide, expressed in neutrophils, monocytes, and gingival keratinocytes, protects gingival keratinocytes against binding and invasion by *Porphyromonas gingivalis* (Pöllänen et al. 2012).
- Antimicrobial peptides such as human β-defensin-1 (hBD-1) and human β-defensin-2 (hBD-2) are expressed by JE cells. Cathelicidin LL-37 is produced by JE cells and polymorphonuclear neutrophils (PMNs) that is both antimicrobial and chemotactic. α-Defensins are produced by PMNs in the JE (Page & Schroeder 1976), and are bound to junctional and pocket epithelium. JE cells lateral to DAT cells produce matrilysin (MMP-7), which activates the precursor peptide of α-defensin (Pöllänen et al. 2012).
- Cytokines such as interleukin (IL)-8, produced by basal JE cells, are chemotactic for PMNs. IL-1α, IL-1β, and tumor necrosis factor (TNF)-α, produced by JE cells and macrophages in the coronal portion of the JE, are proinflammatory cytokines contributing to innate defense. Large numbers of lysosomal bodies in JE cells contain enzymes that participate in the eradication of bacteria (Bosshardt & Lang 2005).
- Cell-to-cell adherence and communication between JE cells are mediated only by a few desmosomes and occasional gap junctions. The low number of desmosomes and wide intercellular spaces enable sulcular fluid as well as PMNs to transmigrate through the JE.
- Cell-to-cell attachment is accomplished by integrins (on membranes of JE cells), which are responsible for

mediating cell–matrix and cell–cell interactions; and E-cadherin and carcino-embryonic Ag-related cell adhesion molecule 1(CEACAM1), which are responsible for intercellular adhesion (Heymann et al. 2001).

- CEACAM1 is also expressed on the surface of PMNs, thus playing a role in the guidance of PMNs through the JE (Heymann et al. 2001).
- CEACAM1 also participates in the regulation of cell proliferation, stimulation, and co-regulation of activated T cells, and is a cell receptor for certain bacteria (Bosshardt & Lang 2005; Singer et al. 2000).
- Other adhesion molecules on JE cell membranes, such as intercellular adhesion molecule–1 (ICAM-1), also known as CD54, which functions as a ligand for β2 integrins present on leukocytes, as well as lymphocyte function antigen-3 (LFA-3), mediate cell–cell interactions in inflammatory lesions, thereby guiding PMN and leucocyte migration to inflammatory sites at the sulcus bottom (Bosshardt & Lang 2005).
- By means of the above, PMNs are located in the central region of the JE, and lymphocytes and macrophages are found in and near the basal cell layer. Langerhans and other dendritic cells (antigen presenting cells) are present as well (Bosshardt & Lang 2005).
- Thus, the presence of inflammatory cells in the subepithelial portion of the lamina propria and in the JE itself is regarded as part of normal homeostasis, and as an essential element of defense (Bosshardt & Lang 2005).

Failure of epithelial barrier function

- During inflammation, the host response itself is a major source contributing to the disintegration of the JE (Bosshardt 2018).
- Periodontopathogens increase the expression of IL-8 by epithelial cells, which is chemotactic for PMNs; however, IL-8 may also reduce gap junctional intercellular communication (Fujita et al. 2006).
- PMNs are essential in the first line of innate defense against plaque bacteria, and contact with bacteria causes PMN release of granular contents, as well as adherence to and phagocytosis of bacteria.
- Impaired PMN functions are generally considered to be related to periodontal tissue destruction; however, innate PMN hyperreactivity may also play a role in periodontitis (Gustafsson et al. 2006).
- Tissue damage can thus occur due to excess release of enzymes, reactive oxygen species, and MMPs from hyperreactive PMNs. Proteases such as elastase, cathepsin G, MMP-8, and MMP-9 released from PMNs can degrade host cellular and extracellular components. PMN proteinases are capable of degrading basal lamina components, such as Lm332 (Pöllänen et al. 2003).

- If PMN-dependent defense becomes insufficient, inflammation may become prolonged, with a domination of lymphocytes, macrophages, and plasma cells in the inflammatory infiltrate (Pöllänen et al. 2003).
- In susceptible patients, periodontopathogenic bacteria may trigger a Th1 cytokine response, resulting in the release of proinflammatory cytokines, e.g. IL-1, IL-6, IL-8, TNF-α, and PGE2, eventually leading to destruction of the dento-epithelial junction, resulting in the failure of the epithelial barrier function (Pöllänen et al. 2012).

Effects of bacteria on junctional epithelium

- Under these impaired defense conditions, bacteria and their products may enter the JE (Schroeder & Attström 1980).
- Subgingival spreading of bacteria may then occur, whereby bacterial virulence factors may overwhelm the defense mechanisms of the JE, which include the proteolytic disruption of the epithelial structural and functional integrity (Schroeder & Attström 1980).
- *Aggregatibacter actinomycetemcomitans* and *P. gingivalis* have been shown to adhere to, invade, and replicate in epithelial cells (Quirynen et al. 2001).
- Bacterial fimbriae and flagellae promote colonization, adherence, and invasion into host cells. Lipoteichoic acids (LTAs) arrest growth and decrease mitosis in epithelial cells. Lipopolysaccharides (LPS) increase epithelial cell permeability and penetrate gingival epithelium (Bosshardt & Lang 2005).
- *P. gingivalis* may exploit pattern recognition receptors (PRRs) of the host to undermine bacterial killing, or use them to enable protected entry routes to host defense cells (Hajishengallis & Lambris 2011). Some periodontopathogens may escape PMN phagocytosis and even cause PMN death when ingested (Pöllänen et al. 2012).
- *P. gingivalis* releases enzymes (Arg-gingipain and Lys-gingipain) through outer membrane vesicles (OMVs) or as soluble proteins (Fouillen et al. 2019). *P. gingivalis* gingipains degrade components of epithelial cell-to-cell junctional complexes, including proteolysis of focal contact components, adherens junction proteins, and adhesion signaling molecules (Hintermann et al. 2002).
- *P. gingivalis* and *A. actinomycetemcomitans* have been shown to decrease the expression of E-cadherin in cultured gingival epithelial cells (Katz et al. 2000; Noguchi et al. 2003).
- *A. actinomycetemcomitans* outer membrane proteins and IL-1β in cultured human gingival epithelium cells have been shown to reduce connexin levels, thereby reducing gap junctional intercellular communication (Fujita et al. 2008).

- This furthermore can lead to reduced adhesion to extracellular matrices, changes in morphology, impaired motility, and apoptosis of epithelial cells (Fujita et al. 2018).
- Periodontopathogens secreting short chain fatty acids impair the rapid renewal of coronal JE/DAT cells. Bacterial metabolites, LPS, and other toxins are able to cause epithelial cell death at high concentrations.
- *A. actinomycetemcomitans* induces apoptosis in gingival epithelial cells by activating the transforming growth factor (TGF)-β receptor I-smad2-caspase-3 signaling pathway. Apoptosis in epithelial cells triggers the destruction of epithelial barrier function (Abuhussein et al. 2014; Yoshimoto et al. 2014).
- Degeneration and detachment of DAT cells, loss of cellular continuity, and cell death in the coronal part of the JE can lead to the development of an intraepithelial split (Bosshardt & Lang 2005; Pöllänen et al. 2012).
- Gingipains may also disturb the ICAM-1-dependent adhesion of PMNs to oral epithelial cells, thereby causing perturbation of innate immunity of the JE (Tada et al. 2003).
- Bacterial interactions with CEACAM1 may result in altered structural organization of the JE (Heymann et al. 2001).
- Bacterial products and cytokines are able to increase production of MMP-13 by epithelial cells, causing degradation of the underlying basement membrane, thereby facilitating epithelial growth into the connective tissue (Uitto et al. 1998).
- Thus, bacterial products penetrating the JE at the bottom of the sulcus may directly perturb the structural and functional integrity of the JE (Fujita et al. 2018) (see Figure 5.5.2).

Disintegration of the functional and structural integrity of junctional epithelium
- With increasing degrees of gingival inflammation, which includes an increased rate of GCF passing through the intercellular spaces of the JE, together with an increased number of migrating T and B lymphocytes, monocytes/macrophages, and PMNs, a distension of the intercellular spaces occurs, leading to disruption of the functional and structural integrity of the JE, resulting in a focal disintegration of the JE (Schroeder & Listgarten 1997).
- Therefore, under impaired defense conditions, these virulence factors are responsible for the specific

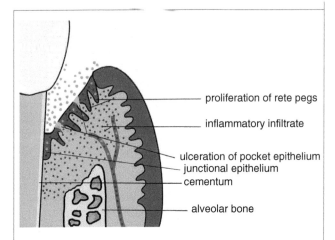

proliferation of rete pegs

inflammatory infiltrate

ulceration of pocket epithelium
junctional epithelium
cementum

alveolar bone

Figure 5.5.2 Histopathogenesis of loss of attachment. Courtesy of Dr. Abdulqader Alhammadi.

degradation of cell junctional complexes and the disturbance of the ICAM-1-dependent adhesion of PMNs to epithelial cells, thereby leading to the breakdown of the JE (Bosshardt 2018).
- The proteolytic disruption of JE integrity may then initiate pocket formation, which includes residual JE proliferating further apically, so as to maintain an epithelial attachment.
- Thus, perturbation of the structural and functional integrity of the JE leads to the creation of a space referred to as a periodontal pocket (Bosshardt 2018).
- The epithelium that lines the pocket wall is therefore an unattached epithelium, extending from the sulcular epithelium to the JE. It is characterized by thinning and ulceration of the epithelium, thereby increasing the possibility for invasion of bacteria and their products into the underlying soft connective tissues (Bosshardt & Lang 2005; Fouillen et al. 2019; Tada et al. 2003).
- Pocket epithelium is furthermore characterized by increased permeability, as well as high infiltration of T cells, B cells, plasma cells, and increased migration of PMNs.
- In the periodontal pocket there is now a larger surface for bacteria to directly deliver their toxins, thereby preventing reattachment and aggravating cellular dysfunction of the JE (Fouillen et al. 2019).
- This leads to a self-perpetuating cycle whereby, with increasing size of the pocket, a larger surface area is made available for bacterial colonization and for attack of the specialized IBL by proteases, thus reducing JE cell cohesion (Fouillen et al. 2019).

chance of the apical as well as the horizontal expansion of the biofilm, thus allowing for invasion of microorganisms and their products into the soft connective tissue, thereby aggravating the situation, leading to pocket formation and bone loss. Depending on the severity and duration of disease, a vicious circle of inflammatory destruction may thus develop, which includes deepening of the pocket with further bone destruction (Bosshardt 2018).

Periodontal disease activity

Periodontal pockets go through periods of exacerbation and quiescence as a result of episodic bursts of activity followed by periods of remission. Bone loss has been shown to occur in an episodic manner (Newman et al. 2019).

- *Periods of exacerbation (periods of activity)*: Characterized by a buildup of unattached plaque comprising Gram-negative, motile, and anaerobic bacteria. Bone and connective tissue attachment is lost and the pocket deepens. This period may last for days, weeks, or months, and it is eventually followed by a period of remission or quiescence. Active periods show bleeding, either spontaneously or with probing, and greater amounts of gingival exudate. Histologically, the pocket epithelium appears thin and ulcerated, and an inflammatory infiltrate composed predominantly of plasma cells and PMNs can be seen (Newman et al. 2019).
- *Periods of quiescence (periods of inactivity)*: Characterized by proliferation of Gram-positive bacteria. There is a reduced inflammatory response with little or no loss of bone and connective tissue attachment, and a more stable condition is established.

Site specificity of periodontal disease

Inflammation of gingival tissue is a prerequisite for the development of periodontitis; however, gingivitis may not ultimately result in progression to periodontitis. In some sites or individuals gingivitis never progresses to periodontitis, and other sites in the same individual can progress to periodontitis (Kurgan & Kantarci 2018).

Periodontal destruction does not occur in all parts of the mouth at the same time; rather, it occurs on a few teeth at a time or even only on some aspects of some teeth at any given time. Sites of periodontal destruction are often found next to sites with little or no destruction. Therefore, the severity of periodontitis increases with the development of new disease sites and/or with the increased breakdown of existing sites (Newman et al. 2019).

REFERENCES

Abuhussein H, Bashutski JD, Dabiri D et al. The role of factors associated with apoptosis in assessing periodontal disease status. *J Periodontol.* 2014; 85(8):1086–1095.

Bartold PM, Van Dyke TE. An appraisal of the role of specific bacteria in the initial pathogenesis of periodontitis. *J Clin Periodontol.* 2019; 46:6–11.

Birkedal-Hansen H. Role of matrix metalloproteinases in human periodontal diseases. *J Periodontol.* 1995; 64:474–484.

Bosshardt DD. The periodontal pocket: pathogenesis, histopathology and consequences. *Periodontol 2000.* 2018; 76:43–50.

Bosshardt DD, Lang NP. The junctional epithelium: from health to disease. *J Dent Res.* 2005;84(1):9–20.

Fouillen A, Grenier D, Barbeau J et al. Selective bacterial degradation of the extracellular matrix attaching the gingiva to the tooth. *Eur J Oral Sci.* 2019; 127:313–322.

Fujita T, Ashikaga A, Shiba H et al. Regulation of IL-8 by Irsogladine maleate is involved in abolishment of *Actinobacillus actinomycetemcomitans*-induced reduction of gap-junctional intercellular communication. *Cytokine.* 2006; 34:271–277.

Fujita T, Ashikaga A, Shiba H et al. Irsogladine maleate counters the interleukin-1beta-induced suppression in gap intercellular communication but does not affect the interleukin-1

beta-induced zonula occludens protein-1 levels in human gingival epithelial cells. *J Periodontal Res.* 2008; 43(1):96–102.

Fujita T, Yoshimoto T, Kajiya M et al. Regulation of defensive function on gingival epithelial cells can prevent periodontal disease. *Jpn Dent Sci Rev.* 2018; 54:66–75.

Gustafsson A, Ito H, Åsman B, Bergström K. Hyperreactive mononuclear cells and neutrophils in chronic periodontitis. *J Clin Periodontol.* 2006; 33(2):126–129.

Hajishengallis G, Lambris JD. Microbial manipulation of receptor crosstalk in innate immunity. *Nat Rev Immunol.* 2011; 11(3):187–200.

Heymann R, Wroblewski J, Terling C, Midtvedt T, Öbrink B. The characteristic cellular organization and CEACAM1 expression in the junctional epithelium of rats and mice are genetically programmed and not influenced by the bacterial microflora. *J Periodontol.* 2001; 72:454–460.

Hintermann E, Haake SK, Christen U, Sharabi A, Quaranta V. Discrete proteolysis of focal contact and adherens junction components in *Porphyromonas gingivalis*-infected oral keratinocytes: a strategy for cell adhesion and migration disabling. *Infect Immun.* 2002; 70:5846–5856.

Hirschfeld L, Wasserman B. A long-term survey of tooth loss in 600 treated periodontal patients. *J Periodontol.* 1978; 49:225–237.

Katz J, Sambandam V, Wu JH, Michalek SM, Balkovetz DF. Characterization of *Porphyromonas gingivalis*-induced degradation of epithelial cell junctional complexes. *Infect Immun*. 2000; 68(3):1441–1449.

Kurgan S, Kantarci A. Molecular basis for immunohistochemical and inflammatory changes during progression of gingivitis to periodontitis. *Periodontol 2000*. 2018; 76:51–67.

Lorencini M, Silva JAF, Almeida CA et al. A new paradigm in the periodontal disease progression: gingival connective tissue remodeling with simultaneous collagen degradation and fibers thickening. *Tissue Cell*. 2009; 41(1):43–50.

Newman MG, Takei HH, Klokkevold PR et al. *Newman and Carranza's Clinical Periodontology*. St. Louis, MO: Elsevier Saunders; 2019.

Noguchi T, Shiba H, Komatsuzawa H et al. Syntheses of prostaglandin E2 and E-cadherin and gene expression of beta-defensin-2 by human gingival epithelial cells in response to *Actinobacillus actinomycetemcomitans*. *Inflammation*. 2003; 27(6):341–349.

Ohlrich EJ, Cullinan MP, Seymour GJ. The immunopathogenesis of periodontal disease. *Aust Dent J*. 2009; 54:(1 Suppl): S2–S10.

Page RC, Schroeder HE. Pathogenesis of inflammatory periodontal disease. A summary of current work. *Lab Invest*. 1976; 34:235–249.

Paul WE. Bridging innate and adaptive immunity. *Cell*. 2011; 147:1212–1215.

Pöllänen MT, Laine MA, Ihalin R, Uitto V-J. Host-bacteria crosstalk at the dentogingival junction. *Int J Dent*. 2012; 2012: Article ID 821383. doi:10.1155/2012/821383.

Pöllänen MT, Salonen JI, Uitto VJ. Structure and function of the tooth-epithelial interface in health and disease. *Periodontol 2000*. 2003; 31:12–31.

Quirynen M, Papaioannou W, van Steenbergen TJ et al. Adhesion of *Porphyromonas gingivalis* strains to cultured epithelial cells from patients with a history of chronic adult periodontitis or from patients less susceptible to periodontitis. *J Periodontol*. 2001; 72:626–633.

Schroeder HE, Attström R. Pocket formation: a hypothesis. In: *The Borderland between Caries and Periodontal Disease II* (ed. T Lehner G Cimasoni). New York: Academic Press; 1980, 99–123.

Schroeder HE, Listgarten MA. The gingival tissues: the architecture of periodontal protection. *Periodontol 2000*. 1997; 13:91–120.

Singer BB, Scheffrahn I, Öbrink B. The tumor growth-inhibiting cell adhesion molecule CEACAM1 (C-CAM) is differently expressed in proliferating and quiescent epithelial cells and regulates cell proliferation. *Cancer Res*. 2000; 60:1236–1244.

Tada H, Sugawara S, Nemoto E et al. Proteolysis of ICAM-1 on human oral epithelial cells by gingipains. *J Dent Res*. 2003; 82:796–801.

Takata T, Donath K. The mechanism of pocket formation. A light microscopic study on undecalcified human material. *J Periodontol*. 1988; 59:215–221.

Uitto VJ, Airola K, Vaalamo M et al. Collagenase-3 (matrix metalloproteinase-13) expression is induced in oral mucosal epithelium during chronic inflammation. *Am J Pathol*. 1998; 152(6):1489–1499.

Wheelock MJ, Jensen PJ. Regulation of keratinocyte intercellular junction organization and epidermal morphogenesis by E-cadherin. *J Cell Biol*. 1992; 117(2):415–425.

Yoshimoto T, Fujita T, Ouhara K et al. Smad2 is involved in *Aggregatibacter actinomycetemcomitans*-induced apoptosis. *J Dent Res*. 2014; 93(11):1148–1154.

CHAPTER 6
Periodontal health, gingival diseases and conditions

Steph Smith

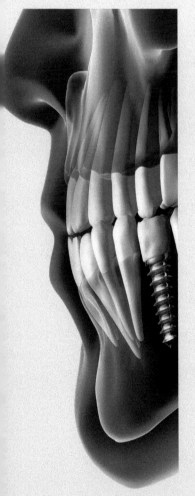

Contents

Learning objectives

- Holistic definition of periodontal health within a histological context.
- Determinants, indicators, and proposed outcomes of periodontal health.
- Biological changes, signs, symptoms, and severity of plaque-induced gingivitis.
- Case definition of plaque-induced gingivitis.
- Role of bleeding on probing in determining a gingivitis case.
- Classification of non-dental biofilm-induced gingival diseases and conditions.

Essential Periodontics, First Edition. Edited by Steph Smith and Khalid Almas.
© 2022 John Wiley & Sons Ltd. Published 2022 by John Wiley & Sons Ltd.

Periodontal health and gingival health

Periodontal diseases are complex and multifactorial, involving an interplay between subgingival microbiota, host immune and inflammatory responses, as well as environmental modifying factors (Bartold & Van Dyke 2013). By definition, periodontal health is a state free from inflammatory disease, meaning the absence of clinical inflammation associated with gingivitis or periodontitis (Lang & Bartold 2018). Periodontal health should furthermore be considered within the context of a holistic evaluation of all factors responsible for the emergence of disease, as well as the restoration and maintenance of health (Zaura & ten Cate 2015). Periodontal health can exist before disease commences, and can be restored to an anatomically reduced periodontium (Lang & Bartold 2018). However, gingivitis affects up to 95% of the population worldwide, and chronic periodontitis affects up to 65% of the North American population 65 years and older (Eke et al. 2012; Li et al. 2010). Periodontal health should therefore be considered in the context of returning to clinical health from disease (Lang & Bartold 2018).

Histological determinants of periodontal health

During the development of periodontitis, environmental changes within the sulcus caused by gingival inflammation cause a shift in the composition of the subgingival biofilm, resulting in a state of dysbiosis, with an ensuing exacerbation of periodontal inflammation, leading to heightened host-driven tissue damage (Darveau et al. 2012). For periodontal health to be attained, or maintained, a redirection of the subgingival biofilm composition needs to be achieved that will be compatible with gingival health (Teles et al. 2012) Histologically, with increasing inflammation there is an increase in lymphocyte infiltration, with a concomitant decrease in the numerical density of fibroblasts. With long-standing optimal oral hygiene however, lymphocyte infiltration has been shown to significantly decrease, together with a significant increase in the numerical density of fibroblasts (Brecx et al. 1987b). Nevertheless, the numerical density of polymorphonuclear lymphocytes subjacent to the junctional epithelium remains relatively stable in both inflammatory and healthy gingival tissues, even during prolonged time periods (Brecx et al. 1987a). Therefore, during the status of clinically healthy gingiva, there is histologically the presence of a small inflammatory cell infiltrate. This signifies an important physiological process of polymorphonuclear surveillance in maintaining homeostasis within the periodontium (Brecx et al. 1987a; Lang & Bartold 2018).

Determinants of clinical periodontal health

There are three main categories that determine clinical periodontal health, namely microbiological, host, and environmental (see Table 6.1) (Lang & Bartold 2018). Within these categories, the controllable and uncontrollable predisposing

Table 6.1 Determinants of clinical periodontal health.

Microbiological	Supragingival plaque composition Subgingival biofilm composition
Host	Local predisposing factors Periodontal pockets Dental restorations Root anatomy Tooth position and crowding Systemic modifying factors Host immune function Systemic health Genetics
Environmental	Smoking Medications Stress Nutrition

and modifying factors should be assessed for each patient, so as to attain and maintain clinical periodontal health (Lang & Bartold 2018). Predisposing factors are agents or conditions that contribute to the accumulation of dental plaque. Modifying factors are agents or conditions that alter the way in which patients respond to subgingival plaque accumulation (Lang & Bartold 2018). Although oral hygiene remains an imperative factor in attaining and maintaining periodontal health, it only accounts for 20% of the direct risk for developing periodontitis. The remaining 80% of direct and indirect risk, as well as modifying factors, may be responsible for the development of periodontal diseases (Grossi et al. 1994).

Indicators of clinical periodontal health

The term "clinically healthy periodontium" has been suggested for patients who have experienced periodontal disease (gingivitis or periodontitis), undergone treatment, then returned to a state of clinical health on either a full periodontium (in the case of gingivitis) or a reduced periodontium (in the case of periodontitis) (Lang & Bartold 2018). Table 6.2 outlines the clinical indicators of clinical periodontal health (Lang & Bartold 2018).

Proposed outcomes of periodontal health

Different levels of periodontal health have been proposed; these levels depend upon whether the periodontium has normal attachment and bone levels or reduced support, as well as the ability to control modifying factors and the consideration of relative treatment outcomes. When evaluating periodontal treatment outcomes, specific measurable biological and clinical outcomes should be determined, so as to ascertain whether a positive response to treatment is consistent with progression toward periodontal health and stability (Lang & Bartold 2018).

Table 6.2 Clinical indicators of periodontal health.

Periodontal probing depth (PPD)	• PPD or probing attachment levels should not be used alone, but in conjunction with bleeding on probing (BOP), as well as modifying and predisposing factors (Lang & Bartold 2018). • PPD, attachment levels, and bone height are not adequate predictors for sites that may become reinfected and undergo recurrent disease (Lindhe & Nyman 1984). • Historical evidence of disease (increased PPD, recession and loss of attachment, bone loss) may be of less relevance in the context of periodontal health on a reduced periodontium (Matuliene et al. 2008). • Deep pockets may exist as healthy pockets if they remain stable and uninflamed with careful supportive periodontal care over very long periods of time (Knowles et al. 1979; Lindhe & Nyman 1984).
Bleeding on probing (BOP)	• Bleeding is an earlier sign of gingivitis than the visual signs of inflammation (redness and swelling) (Lindhe & Nyman 1984). • Sites that bleed following probing with light pressure (0.25N) are associated with a significantly increased percentage of cell-rich and collagen-reduced connective tissue, but no increase in vascularity or vessel lumen size that would justify the bleeding tendency (Greenstein 1984). • BOP is a limited but useful prognostic indicator in monitoring periodontal tissue after active therapy (Lang et al. 1986). • The absence of BOP at repeated examinations represents periodontal health and is a very reliable indicator for disease progression or periodontal stability (Joss et al. 1994; Lang et al. 1990). • BOP is most reliable for monitoring patients in daily practice over time. Non-bleeding sites may be considered as clinically healthy and periodontally stable (Joss et al. 1994; Lang et al. 1990).
Radiographic features	• The distance from the cementoenamel junction to the alveolar crest in healthy individuals can vary between 1.0 and 3.0 mm (Wikner et al. 1990). • The periodontal ligament space can vary and is not considered a useful indicator of health (Lang & Bartold 2018).
Tooth mobility	• In teeth with non-inflamed periodontal tissue, tooth mobility is determined by the height of the periodontal tissue support and the width of the periodontal ligament (Lang & Bartold 2018). • A magnitude of movement up to 0.2 mm is regarded as physiological (Nyman & Lang 1994). • In a clinically healthy situation, increased tooth mobility associated with widening of the periodontal ligament usually represents a tooth in occlusal trauma (Lang & Bartold 2018). • For a tooth with a reduced, but healthy, periodontium, increased tooth mobility cannot be used as a sign of disease (Lang & Bartold 2018). • Hypermobility of a periodontally healthy tooth with reduced support but normal width of periodontal ligament should be considered physiological tooth mobility (Lang & Bartold 2018). • Increased tooth mobility in periodontally healthy teeth due to widening in the periodontal ligament is the result of uni- or multidirectional forces inducing resorption of the alveolar bone walls in pressure zones, but without loss of connective tissue attachment, irrespective of the height of the supportive bone, thus representing a physiological adaptation to altered function, rather than a sign of pathology (Lindhe & Ericsson 1976; Nyman & Lang 1994; Svanberg 1974). • Hence, it is not recommended to use tooth mobility as a sign of either health or disease status (Lang & Bartold 2018).

This will include accounting for modifiable clinical indicators of periodontitis such as attachment and bone loss and periodontal probing depth (PPD), modifiable inflammatory markers, and modifiable systemic risk factors. Thus, periodontal treatment will move from a solely biofilm-based protocol to a more holistic, inflammation-based model, whereby emphasis is placed on controlling the inflammation to control the infection and the ongoing destruction of the periodontium (Lang & Bartold 2018). Thus, the assessment of periodontal health is based largely on the inflammatory response; however, this does not diminish the importance of the periodontal microbiome (Lang & Bartold 2018). Furthermore, gingivitis is generally not a painful or functionally destructive state resulting in loss of function. Gingival inflammation may be a sufficient cause for destruction of the periodontium, but insufficient on its own to cause destructive forms of periodontal disease in all people (Chapple et al. 2017; Lang et al. 2009). It has been suggested that when making a distinction between pristine periodontal health (defined as a total absence of clinical inflammation) and clinical periodontal health (characterized by an absence or minimal levels of clinical inflammation), the implication can be made that a certain amount (extent/severity) of gingival inflammation of the dentition is compatible with a patient being defined as periodontally healthy

Table 6.3   Proposed outcomes of periodontal health.

	Levels of periodontal health	Bleeding on probing	Normal gingival sulcus depth	Normal bone heights	Modifying factors	Predisposing factors
	Pristine periodontal health Total absence of clinical inflammation Physiological immune surveillance Normal periodontium with no attachment or bone loss Not likely to be observed clinically	No	Yes	Yes	Controlled	Controlled
	Gingivitis	Yes	Yes	Yes	May be present	May be present
Intact periodontium	Clinical periodontal health Absence or minimal levels of clinical inflammation Periodontium with normal support	No/minimal	Yes	Yes	Controlled	Controlled
	Periodontal disease stability Successful treatment through control of local, systemic and modifying factors	No/minimal	No	No	Controlled	Controlled
Reduced periodontium	Periodontal disease remission/ control Treatment resulted in reduction (although not total resolution) of inflammation Some improvement in periodontal probing depth and attachment levels, but not optimal control of local or systemic contributing factors	Significantly reduced	No	No	Not fully controlled	Not fully controlled

(Lang & Bartold 2018). Thus, gingival inflammation may not be a disease but a variant of health (Murakami et al. 2018). Table 6.3 depicts the proposed levels of therapeutic outcomes of periodontal health, depending upon whether the periodontium has normal attachment and bone level or reduced support, and the ability to control modifying and predisposing factors (Lang & Bartold 2018).

Gingivitis: dental biofilm induced

Plaque-induced gingivitis is a site-specific inflammatory response of the gingival tissues resulting from bacterial plaque accumulation located at and below the gingival margin (Trombelli et al. 2018). It is the most common form of periodontal disease, prevalent at all ages in dentate populations (Murakami et al. 2018; White et al. 2012). Plaque accumulates more rapidly at inflamed gingival sites than non-inflamed sites, creating a complex dynamic between the dental plaque biofilm

and the host's immune-inflammatory response (Hillam & Hull 1977). Although gingivitis is considered as a precursor of periodontitis, not all inflammatory sites are destined to progress to periodontitis (Murakami et al. 2018; Trombelli et al. 2018).

Biological changes, signs, symptoms, and severity of plaque-induced gingivitis

The biological changes occurring during plaque-induced gingival inflammation, entailing the transcription of genes from non-inflamed to inflamed gingival units, are host–bacterial interactions, including microbial pattern recognition molecules; host cell chemotaxis; phagocytosis and degranulation; novel cellular/molecular pathway signaling, including cytokine signaling and cell adhesion; T-lymphocyte responses; angiogenesis; and epithelial immune responses (Offenbacher et al. 2009).

Common clinical signs of plaque-induced gingivitis include erythema, edema, bleeding, tenderness, and enlargement (Tonetti et al. 2015). These may manifest clinically as swelling, seen as loss of the knife-edged gingival margin and blunting of papillae; bleeding on gentle probing; redness; and discomfort on gentle probing (Chapple et al. 2018).

Symptoms a patient may report include bleeding gums (metallic/altered taste), pain (soreness), halitosis, difficulty eating, appearance (swollen red gums), and reduced oral health-related quality of life (Chapple et al. 2018).

Presently there are no objective clinical criteria for defining severity, as no robust evidence exists to clearly differentiate mild, moderate, and severe gingivitis. Definitions therefore remain a matter of professional opinion (Chapple et al. 2018). The severity can be influenced by tooth and root anatomy, restorative and endodontic considerations, and other tooth-related factors (Murakami et al. 2018).

Classification of plaque-induced gingivitis and modifying factors

Table 6.4 depicts the classification of plaque-induced gingivitis and modifying factors.

Plaque-induced gingivitis case definition

Although clinical gingival inflammation is a well-defined site-specific condition, the discrimination between a plaque-induced gingivitis case (a patient affected by gingivitis), with a certain extent/severity of inflamed gingival sites, and a periodontally healthy patient will facilitate surveillance studies to monitor the prevalence and distribution of gingivitis consistently within a cohort, as well as among different populations (Hugoson & Norderyd 2008). The concept of a gingivitis case is thus intended to be the means to define the disease on a

dentition-wide basis, at the patient level (Trombelli et al. 2018). It will furthermore help in setting priorities for therapeutic actions/programs, as well as enable oral health professionals to assess the effectiveness of their preventive measures and treatment regimens. This may then also be applicable to patients who have experienced attachment loss in the past and who have been successfully treated (Hugoson & Norderyd 2008; Trombelli et al. 2018).

The definition of a gingivitis case should be based on the full-mouth evaluation of all sites available for examination (Trombelli et al. 2018). It has thus been suggested that the extent, or the number of gingival sites exhibiting inflammation, can be described as either being localized, whereby <30% of sites are affected, or being generalized, whereby ≥30% of sites are affected (Murakami et al. 2018).

Bleeding on probing to define and grade a gingivitis case

A gingivitis case can be simply, objectively, and accurately defined and graded using a bleeding on probing score (BOP%) (Ainamo & Bay 1975). This is accomplished by assessing the proportion of bleeding sites (dichotomous yes/no evaluation) with stimulation by a standardized (dimensions and shape) manual probe with a controlled (~25 g) force to the bottom of the sulcus/pocket at six sites (mesio-buccal, buccal, disto-buccal, mesio-lingual, lingual, disto-lingual) on all present teeth (Trombelli et al. 2018).

Use of a BOP score is an objective, universally accepted, reliable, and accurate clinical sign that is easily assessed and recorded as part of a comprehensive periodontal examination (Lenox & Kopczyk 1973). BOP may thus be used for discriminating between a healthy and gingivitis patient, and for classifying a gingivitis case as being either localized or generalized (Murakami et al. 2018). With suitable training, general dental practitioners can achieve and maintain high levels of intra-examiner consistency in assessing bleeding (Eaton et al. 1997). The BOP score can also effectively be used to inform and motivate patients, as well as to monitor the efficacy of preventive and treatment strategies aimed at controlling periodontal diseases (Lang et al. 1986, 1990).

It should be kept in mind however, that a BOP score is a measure of the extent of gingival inflammation, rather than of the severity of the inflammatory condition. Severity of gingival inflammation may be well defined on a site-specific basis (Lang & Bartold 2018); however, the incorporation of gingival volume and color changes being merged with BOP% at a patient level would result in a subjective, time-consuming, and impractical procedure for establishing a universally acceptable gingivitis case definition (Trombelli et al. 2018).

A significant factor in determining the BOP response is the probing force having a direct and linear effect on BOP prevalence. Forces greater than 0.25 N (25 g) increase the risk of false-positive readings, while usage of a constant force will result in greater reproducibility of bleeding scores (Karayiannis

---

Table 6.4 Classification of plaque-induced gingivitis and modifying factors.

A. Associated with bacterial dental biofilm only
B. Potential modifying factors of plaque-induced gingivitis
  1. Systemic conditions
    a. Sex steroid hormones
      1. Puberty
      2. Menstrual cycle
      3. Pregnancy
      4. Oral contraceptives
    b. Hyperglycemia
    c. Leukemia
    d. Smoking
    e. Malnutrition
  2. Oral factors enhancing plaque accumulation
    a. Prominent subgingival restoration margins
    b. Hyposalivation
C. Drug-influenced gingival enlargements

Source: Murakami et al. 2018, with permission of John Wiley & Sons.

et al. 1992; Van der Velden 1980). Different clinicians may apply probing forces that can vary significantly and often exceed the 25 g threshold. Greater probing forces may exceed the pain threshold from a patient perspective in healthy sites (Freed et al. 1983, Heins et al. 1998), and even more so in inflamed sites (Heft et al. 1991). Other factors to consider are technique-related factors, such as angulation/placement of the probe (Trombelli et al. 2018), and instrument characteristics, such as different probe tip diameters exhibiting varying abilities to penetrate gingival tissues. It has been suggested that a probe tip diameter of 0.6 mm provides the best discrimination between diseased and healthy sites (Garnick & Silverstein 2000).

Besides the underlying tissue inflammation affecting the gingival response to mechanical stimulation by a probe, patient-related factors may also play a role. These factors can include genetic background, smoking, anticoagulant therapy, and periodontal tissue phenotype (Trombelli et al. 2018).

Table 6.5 depicts a diagnostic look-up table for a gingivitis case definition on a patient level, which includes patients with gingival health; or dental plaque-induced gingivitis including the extent thereof, this being on an intact periodontium; or a reduced periodontium but without a history of periodontitis; or with a reduced periodontium who have been successfully treated for periodontitis, provided that no BOP-positive sites show a probing depth ≥4 mm (Chapple et al. 2018; Trombelli et al. 2018).

Gingival diseases: non-dental biofilm induced

Non-plaque-induced pathological lesions that are limited to the gingival tissues may be manifestations of a systemic condition or a medical disorder. However, their clinical course may be impacted by plaque accumulation and subsequent gingival inflammation (Holmstrup et al. 2018). Dental healthcare providers should be familiar with these lesions, thus enabling them to diagnose, treat, or refer for treatment.

Classification of non-plaque-induced gingival diseases and conditions

Table 6.6 depicts a classification of the most relevant non-plaque-induced gingival diseases and conditions (Holmstrup et al. 2018). For a more detailed appraisal of these lesions, including their features, the reader is referred to Holmstrup et al. (2018).

Table 6.5 Diagnostic table for gingivitis case definition on a patient level.

		Health	Gingivitis	Localized gingivitis	Generalized gingivitis
Intact periodontium	Probing attachment loss	No	No	No	No
	Probing pocket depths (assuming no pseudo-pockets)	≤3 mm	≤3 mm		
	Bleeding on probing	<10%	Yes (≥10%)	≥10%, ≤30%	>30%
	Radiological bone loss	No	No	No	No
Reduced periodontium non-periodontitis patient	Probing attachment loss	Yes	Yes	Yes	Yes
	Probing pocket depths (all sites and assuming no pseudo-pockets)	≤3 mm	≤3 mm	≤3 mm	≤3 mm
	Bleeding on probing	<10%	Yes (≥10%)	≥10%, ≤30%	>30%
	Radiological bone loss	Possible	Possible	Possible	Possible
Successfully treated stable periodontitis patient	Probing attachment loss	Yes	Yes	Yes	Yes
	Probing pocket depths (all sites and assuming no pseudo-pockets)	≤4 mm (no site ≥4 mm with bleeding on probing)	≤3 mm	≤3 mm	≤3 mm
	Bleeding on probing	<10%	Yes (≥10%)	≥10%, ≤30%	>30%
	Radiological bone loss	Yes	Yes	Possible	Possible

Table 6.6   Classification of non-plaque-induced gingival diseases and conditions.

1. Genetic/developmental abnormalities	Hereditary gingival fibromatosis (HGF). Is a rare disease, may occur isolated, or as part of a syndrome
2. Specific infections	
2.1 Bacterial origin	Necrotizing periodontal disease (NPD). NPD encompasses necrotizing gingivitis (NG), necrotizing periodontitis (NP), and necrotizing stomatitis (NS), representing various stages of the same disease
2.1.1 Other bacterial infections	Are uncommon, may be due to loss of homeostasis between non-plaque-related pathogens and innate host resistance. Examples are acute streptococcal gingivitis, *Neisseria gonorrhoeae, Treponema pallidum*, and orofacial tuberculosis
2.2 Viral origin	Coxsackie virus (hand-foot-and-mouth disease), Herpes simplex 1/2 (primary or recurrent), Varicella zoster virus (chicken pox or shingles affecting V nerve), *Molluscum contagiosum* virus, human papilloma virus (squamous cell papilloma, condyloma acuminatum, verrucca vulgaris, and focal epithelial hyperplasia)
2.3 Fungal	Candidosis, other mycoses (e.g. histoplasmosis, aspergillosis)
3. Inflammatory and immune conditions and lesions	
3.1 Hypersensitivity reactions	Contact allergy, plasma cell gingivitis, erythema multiforme
3.2 Autoimmune diseases of skin and mucous membranes	Pemphigus vulgaris, pemphigoid, lichen planus, lupus erythematosus
3.3 Granulomatous inflammatory conditions	Crohn's disease, sarcoidosis
4. Reactive processes	
4.1 Epulides	Fibrous epulis, calcifying fibroblastic granuloma, pyogenic granuloma (vascular epulis), peripheral giant cell granuloma (or central)
5. Neoplasms	
5.1 Premalignant	Leukoplakia, erythroplakia
5.2 Malignant	Squamous cell carcinoma, leukemia, lymphoma
6. Endocrine, nutritional, and metabolic diseases	
6.1 Vitamin deficiencies	Vitamin C deficiency (scurvy)
7. Traumatic lesions	
7.1 Physical/mechanical insults	Frictional keratosis, toothbrushing-induced gingival ulceration, factitious injury (self-harm)
7.2 Chemical (toxic) insults	Etching, chlorhexidine acetylsalicylic acid, cocaine, hydrogen peroxide, dentifrice detergents, paraformaldehyde or calcium hydroxide
7.3 Thermal insults	Burns of mucosa
8. Gingival pigmentation	Gingival pigmentation/melanoplakia, smoker's melanosis, drug-induced pigmentation (antimalarials; minocycline), amalgam tattoo

Source: Adapted from Holmstrup et al. 2018.

REFERENCES

Ainamo J, Bay I. Problems and proposals for recording gingivitis and plaque. *Int Dent J.* 1975; 25:229–235.

Bartold PM, Van Dyke TE. Periodontitis: a host-mediated disruption of microbial homeostasis. Unlearning learned concepts. *Periodontol 2000.* 2013; 62:203–217.

Brecx MC, Gautschi M, Gehr P, Lang NP. Variability of histologic criteria in clinically healthy human gingiva. *J Periodontal Res.* 1987a; 22:468–472.

Brecx MC, Schlegel K, Gehr P, Lang NP. Comparison between histological and clinical parameters during human experimental gingivitis. *J Periodontal Res.* 1987b; 22:50–57.

Chapple IL, Bouchard P, Cagetti MG et al. Interaction of lifestyle, behaviour or systemic diseases with dental caries and periodontal diseases: consensus report of group 2 of the joint EFP/ORCA workshop on the boundaries between caries and periodontal diseases. *J Clin Periodontol.* 2017; 44(Suppl.18):S39–S51.

Chapple ILC, Mealey BL, Van Dyke TE et al. Periodontal health and gingival diseases and conditions on an intact and a reduced periodontium: consensus report of workgroup 1 of the 2017 World Workshop on the Classification of Periodontal and Peri-Implant Diseases and Conditions. *J Clin Periodontol.* 2018; 45(Suppl 20):S68–S77.

Darveau RP, Hajishengallis G, Curtis MA. *Porphyromonas gingivalis* as a potential community activist for disease. *J Dent Res.* 2012; 91:816–820.

Eaton KA, Rimini FM, Zak E, Brookman DJ, Newman HN. The achievement and maintenance of inter-examiner consistency in the assessment of plaque and gingivitis during a multicenter study based in general dental practices. *J Clin Periodontol.* 1997; 24:183–188.

Eke PI, Dye BA, Wei L, Thornton-Evans GO, Genco RJ. Prevalence of periodontitis in adults in the United States. *J Dent Res.* 2012; 91:914–920.

Freed HK, Gapper RL, Kalkwarf KL. Evaluation of periodontal probing forces. *J Periodontol.* 1983; 54:488–492.

Garnick JJ, Silverstein L. Periodontal probing: probe tip diameter. *J Periodontol.* 2000; 71:96–103.

Greenstein G. The role of bleeding upon probing in the diagnosis of periodontal disease. A literature review. *J Periodontol.* 1984; 55:684–688.

Grossi SG, Zambon JJ, Ho AW et al. Assessment of risk for periodontal disease. I. Risk indicators for attachment loss. *J Periodontol.* 1994; 65:260–267.

Heft MW, Perelmuter SH, Cooper BY, Magnusson I, Clark WB. Relationship between gingival inflammation and painfulness of periodontal probing. *J Clin Periodontol.* 1991; 18:213–215.

Heins PJ, Karpinia KA, Maruniak JW, Moorhead JE, Gibbs CH. Pain threshold values during periodontal probing: assessment of maxillary incisor and molar sites. *J Periodontol.* 1998; 69:812–828.

Hillam DG, Hull PS. The influence of experimental gingivitis on plaque formation. *J Clin Periodontol.* 1977; 4:56–61.

Holmstrup P, Plemons J, Meyle J. Non–plaque-induced gingival diseases. *J Clin Periodontol.* 2018; 45(Suppl 20):S28–S43.

Hugoson A, Norderyd O. Has the prevalence of periodontitis changed during the last 30 years? *J Clin Periodontol.* 2008; 35:338–345.

Joss A, Adler R, Lang NP. Bleeding on probing. A parameter for monitoring periodontal conditions in clinical practice. *J Clin Periodontol.* 1994; 21:402–408.

Karayiannis A, Lang NP, Joss A, Nyman S. Bleeding on probing as it relates to probing pressure and gingival health in patients with a reduced but healthy periodontium. A clinical study. *J Clin Periodontol.* 1992; 19:471–475.

Knowles JW, Burgett FG, Nissle RR et al. Results of periodontal treatment related to pocket depth and attachment level. Eight years. *J Periodontol.* 1979; 50:225–233.

Lang NP, Adler R, Joss A, Nyman S. Absence of bleeding on probing. An indicator of periodontal stability. *J Clin Periodontol.* 1990; 17:714–721.

Lang NP, Bartold PM. Periodontal health. *J Clin Periodontol.* 2018; 45(Suppl 20):S9–S16.

Lang NP, Joss A, Orsanic T, Gusberti FA, Siegrist BE. Bleeding on probing. A predictor for the progression of periodontal disease. *J Clin Periodontol.* 1986; 13:590–596.

Lang NP, Schätzle MA, Löe H. Gingivitis as a risk factor in periodontal disease. *J Clin Periodontol.* 2009; 36(Suppl.10):3–8.

Lenox JA, Kopczyk RA. A clinical system for scoring a patient's oral hygiene performance. *J Am Dent Assoc.* 1973; 86:849–852.

Li Y, Lee S, Hujoel P et al. Prevalence and severity of gingivitis in American adults. *Am J Dent.* 2010; 23:9–13.

Lindhe J, Ericsson I. The influence of trauma from occlusion on reduced but healthy periodontal tissues in dogs. *J Clin Periodontol.* 1976; 3:110–122.

Lindhe J, Nyman S. Long-term maintenance of patients treated for advanced periodontal disease. *J Clin Periodontol.* 1984; 11:504–514.

Matuliene G, Pjetursson BE, Salvi GE et al. Influence of residual pockets on progression of periodontitis and tooth loss: results after 11 years of maintenance. *J Clin Periodontol.* 2008; 35:685–695.

Murakami S, Mealey BL, Mariotti A, Chapple ILC. Dental plaque–induced gingival conditions. *J Clin Periodontol.* 2018; 45(Suppl 20): S17–S27.

Nyman SR, Lang NP. Tooth mobility and the biological rationale for splinting teeth. *Periodontol 2000.* 1994; 4:15–22.

Offenbacher S, Barros SP, Paquette DW et al. Gingival transcriptome patterns during induction and resolution of experimental gingivitis in humans. *J Periodontol.* 2009; 80:1963–1982.

Svanberg G. Influence of trauma from occlusion on the periodontium of dogs with normal and inflamed gingivae. *Odontol Revy.* 1974; 25:165–178.

Teles FR, Teles RP, Uzel NG et al. Early microbial succession in redeveloping dental biofilms in periodontal health and disease. *J Periodontal Res.* 2012; 47:95–104.

Tonetti MS, Chapple ILC, Jepsen S, Sanz M. Primary and secondary prevention of periodontal and peri-implant diseases. *J Clin Periodontol.* 2015; 42(Suppl. 16):S1–S4.

Trombelli L, Farina R, Silva CO, Tatakis DN. Plaque-induced gingivitis: case definition and diagnostic considerations. *J Clin Periodontol.* 2018; 45(Suppl 20):S44–S67.

Van der Velden U. Influence of probing force on the reproducibility of bleeding tendency measurements. *J Clin Periodontol.* 1980; 7:421–427.

White DA, Tsakos G, Pitts NB et al. Adult Dental Health Survey 2009: common oral health conditions and their impact on the population. *Br Dent J.* 2012; 213:567–572.

Wikner S, Söder PO, Frithiof L, Wouters F. The approximal bone height and intrabony defects in young adults, related to the salivary buffering capacity and counts of *Streptococcus mutans* and lactobacilli. *Arch Oral Biol.* 1990; 35(Suppl.):213S–215S.

Zaura E, ten Cate JM. Towards understanding oral health. *Caries Res.* 2015;49(Suppl 1):55–61.

CHAPTER 7
Periodontitis

Steph Smith and Khalid Almas

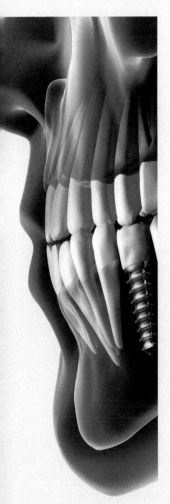

Contents

Learning objectives

- Aspects related to the definition and making of a clinical diagnosis of periodontitis.
- Classification and case definitions of various forms of periodontitis.
- Diagnosing a case definition of periodontitis by means of staging and grading.
- The diagnostic tools used for diagnosing gingivitis and periodontitis.
- Steps to staging and grading a periodontitis case.

Essential Periodontics, First Edition. Edited by Steph Smith and Khalid Almas.
© 2022 John Wiley & Sons Ltd. Published 2022 by John Wiley & Sons Ltd.

Clinical definition of periodontitis

Periodontitis is characterized by microbial-associated host-mediated inflammation that results in loss of periodontal attachment. This is detected as clinical attachment loss (CAL) by circumferential assessment of the erupted dentition with a standardized periodontal probe with reference to the cementoenamel junction (CEJ) (Tonetti et al. 2018a).

Definition of a periodontitis case

In defining a patient as a periodontitis case, a periodontitis case definition system should include three components:
- Identification of a patient as a periodontitis case.
- Identification of the specific type of periodontitis.
- Description of the clinical presentation and other elements that affect clinical management, prognosis, and potentially broader influences on both oral and systemic health (Papapanou et al. 2018).

Within a clinical context, it is imperative that the clinician is able to specifically detect and identify areas of attachment loss, either during periodontal probing or by direct visual detection of the interdental CEJ. Note should also be taken that some clinical conditions other than periodontitis may present with CAL (Tonetti et al. 2018a). Box 7.1 depicts the various clinical parameters that should be taken into account when identifying a periodontitis case.

Classification of forms of periodontitis

Once a diagnosis of a periodontitis case has been made, the clinician must then identify the different forms of periodontitis based on pathophysiology (Tonetti et al. 2018a), namely:
- Necrotizing periodontal disease.
- Periodontitis as manifestation of systemic diseases.
- Periodontitis.

Box 7.1 Clinical parameters for identifying a periodontitis case

A patient is a periodontitis case if:
- Interdental clinical attachment loss (CAL) is detectable at ≥ 2 non-adjacent teeth; or
- Buccal or oral CAL ≥ 3 mm with pocketing >3 mm is detectable at ≥ 2 teeth
  and
- The observed CAL cannot be ascribed to non-periodontal causes such as:
  - Gingival recession of traumatic origin.
  - Dental caries extending in the cervical area of the tooth.
  - The presence of CAL on the distal aspect of a second molar and associated with malposition or extraction of a third molar.
  - An endodontic lesion draining through the marginal periodontium.
  - The occurrence of a vertical root fracture.

The differential diagnosis is based on history and the specific signs and symptoms of necrotizing periodontal disease (NPD) and the presence or absence of an uncommon systemic disease that definitively alters the host immune response. The majority of clinical cases of periodontitis present with a range of phenotypes that require different approaches to clinical management (Tonetti et al. 2018a).

Necrotizing periodontal disease

NPD is a group of conditions that share a characteristic phenotype of three prominent and typical clinical features – namely necrosis of the gingival papilla or periodontal tissues, bleeding, and pain – and are associated with host immune response impairments (Papapanou et al. 2018; Tonetti et al. 2018a). NPD patients are frequently susceptible to future recurrence of disease, including the possibility of NPD also becoming a "chronic condition," with a slower rate of destruction (Herrera et al. 2018). A differential diagnosis with other conditions must be established, such as vesicular-bullous diseases, primary or recurrent herpetic gingivostomatitis, oral manifestations mimicking NPD lesions, and toothbrush abrasion (Tonetti et al. 2018a).

The case definitions for NPD are *necrotizing gingivitis* (NG), *necrotizing periodontitis* (NP), and *necrotizing stomatitis* (NS) (Papapanou et al. 2018). Studies have suggested that NG and NP may represent different stages of the same disease, which may then progress to more severe forms, namely NS and noma (Novak 1999; Rowland 1999). Table 7.1 depicts the case definitions of NG, NP, and NS, and the pathophysiology of NPD.

Classification of necrotizing periodontal diseases

Table 7.2 depicts a proposed classification of necrotizing periodontal diseases (Herrera et al. 2018; Papapanou et al. 2018; Tonetti et al. 2018a).

Periodontitis as a manifestation of systemic diseases

Periodontitis as a direct manifestation of systemic disease should follow the classification of the primary disease according to the respective International Statistical Classification of Diseases and Related Health Problems (ICD) codes (Albandar et al. 2018) (see Chapter 10.1).

Periodontitis

Descriptive definition of periodontitis

Periodontitis is defined as an inflammatory disease of the supporting tissues around teeth, which can cause irreversible loss of periodontal ligament and alveolar bone, leading to tooth mobility, and if left untreated can lead to tooth exfoliation (Fine et al. 2018).

In susceptible individuals, a non-progressive gingivitis lesion may convert from a symbiotic microbial and immune state to a dysbiotic microbiome concomitantly with an aberrant and exaggerated host inflammatory response. The destruction of the

Table 7.1   Case definitions and pathophysiology of necrotizing periodontal disease.

Case definitions for necrotizing periodontal disease (NPD)

Necrotizing gingivitis (NG)	An acute inflammatory process of the gingival tissues characterized by the presence of necrosis/ulcer of the interdental papillae, gingival bleeding, and pain. Other signs/symptoms may include halitosis, pseudo-membranes, regional lymphadenopathy, fever, and sialorrhea (in children) (Papapanou et al. 2018).
Necrotizing periodontitis (NP)	An inflammatory process of the periodontium characterized by the presence of necrosis/ulcer of the interdental papillae, gingival bleeding, halitosis, pain, and rapid bone loss. Other signs/symptoms may include pseudo-membrane formation, lymphadenopathy, and fever (Papapanou et al. 2018).
Necrotizing stomatitis (NS)	A severe inflammatory condition of the periodontium and the oral cavity in which soft tissue necrosis extends beyond the gingiva and bone denudation may occur through the alveolar mucosa, with larger areas of osteitis and formation of bone sequestrum. It typically occurs in severely systemically compromised patients. Atypical cases have also been reported, in which NS may develop without the prior appearance of NG/NP lesions (Papapanou et al. 2018).

Pathophysiology of necrotizing periodontal diseases
NG is characterized by the presence of ulcers within the stratified squamous epithelium and the superficial layer of the gingival connective tissue, surrounded by a non-specific acute inflammatory infiltrate. Four zones are included: a superficial bacterial zone, a neutrophil-rich zone, a necrotic zone, and a spirochetal/bacterial infiltration zone (Papapanou et al. 2018).

Host immune response	NPDs are strongly associated with impairment of the host immune system, which includes chronically, severely compromised patients (e.g. AIDS patients, children suffering from severe malnourishment, extreme living conditions, or severe infections) and may constitute a severe or even life-threating condition. Host immune impairment may also be associated with temporarily and/or moderately compromised patients (e.g. in smokers or psycho-socially stressed adult patients) (Herrera et al. 2018; Papapanou et al. 2018). Severe viral infections may include measles, herpes viruses, and chicken pox (Herrera et al. 2018).
Microbiology	*Prevotella intermedia* and *Treponema, Selenomonas*, and *Fusobacterium* species have been considered as "constant flora" in NPD lesions (Loesche et al. 1982; Riviere et al. 1991).
Risk factors	Various risk factors have been described, namely malnutrition, HIV, psychological stress and insufficient sleep, inadequate oral hygiene, pre-existing gingivitis, previous history of NPD, tobacco and alcohol consumption, young age (15–34 years old), and seasonal variations (Herrera et al. 2018).

Table 7.2   Classification of necrotizing periodontal diseases.

Category	Patients	Predisposing factors	Clinical condition
NPD in chronically, severely compromised patients	In adults	HIV±AIDS with CD4+ counts <200 and detectable viral load Other severe systemic conditions (immunosuppression)	NG, NP, NS, noma Possible progression
	In children	Severe malnourishment	
		Extreme living conditions	
		Severe viral infections	
NPD in temporarily and/or moderately compromised patients	In gingivitis patients	Uncontrolled factors: stress, nutrition, smoking, habits	Generalized NG Possible progression to NP
		Previous NPD: residual craters	
		Local factors: root proximity, tooth malposition	Localized NG Possible progression to NP
		Common predisposing factors for NPD	NG Infrequent progression
	In periodontitis patients		NP Infrequent progression

NG, necrotizing gingivitis; NP, necrotizing periodontitis; NPD, necrotizing periodontal disease; NS, necrotizing stomatitis.
Source: Adapted from Herrera et al. 2018; Papapanou et al. 2018.

periodontal tissues can be episodic, non-linear, and disproportionate to various risk factors (Goodson et al. 1982).

Diagnosing a case definition of periodontitis: staging and grading

Clinical cases of periodontitis that do not present with the local characteristics of NPD, or the systemic characteristics of an immune disorder with a secondary manifestation of periodontitis, should be diagnosed as "periodontitis" and be further defined using the two dimensions of the matrix definition system, namely staging and grading. This case definition system should describe the clinical presentation as well as other elements that will affect clinical management, prognosis, and the potentially broader influences on both oral and systemic health (Papapanou et al. 2018). A case definition system is also needed to be a dynamic process that will require revisions over time (Tonetti et al. 2018a). It should be emphasized that these case definitions are guidelines that should be applied using sound clinical judgment to arrive at the most appropriate clinical diagnosis (Tonetti et al. 2018a).

Staging

The purpose of staging a periodontitis patient is:
- To classify the measurable severity and extent of the currently destroyed and damaged tissue attributable to periodontitis.
- To assess the specific factors that may determine the complexity of controlling the current disease, as well as those in the management of the long-term function and esthetics of the dentition (Papapanou et al. 2018; Tonetti et al. 2018a).

Staging involves four categories (stages I through IV) and is determined after considering several variables. Table 7.3 depicts the staging of a periodontitis case (Caton et al. 2018).

Severity score in staging
The severity score is primarily based on interdental CAL in recognition of low specificity of both pocketing and marginal bone loss, although marginal bone loss is also included as an additional descriptor. The score is assigned based on the worst-affected tooth in the dentition. Only attachment loss attributable to periodontitis is used for the score (Caton et al. 2018).

Complexity score in staging
The complexity score is based on the local treatment complexity, assuming the wish/need to eliminate local factors, and takes into account factors like the presence of vertical defects, furcation involvement, tooth hypermobility, drifting and/or flaring of teeth, tooth loss, ridge deficiency, and loss of masticatory function. Besides the local complexity, it is recognized that individual case management may be complicated by medical factors or co-morbidities (Caton et al. 2018).

Extent and distribution
This provides information about how many teeth are affected by periodontitis. For each stage, the extent and distribution can be described as being localized (<30% of teeth involved), generalized, or having a molar/incisor pattern (Papapanou et al. 2018; Tonetti et al. 2018a). It does not give information about the percentage of teeth with slight, moderate, or severe destruction. Distribution refers to affected teeth, such as first molars and/or incisors (e.g. Stage III periodontitis with a generalized molar distribution).

Narrative descriptions of the stages are as follows:
- *Stage I (mild disease)*: CAL 1–2 mm, probing depth ≤4 mm, radiographic evidence of horizontal bone loss ≤15%, and will require non-surgical treatment. No post-treatment tooth loss is expected, indicating the case has a good prognosis going into maintenance care.
- *Stage II (moderate disease)*: CAL 3–4 mm, probing depth ≤5 mm, radiographic evidence of horizontal bone loss between 15 and 33%, and will require non-surgical and surgical treatment. No post-treatment tooth loss is expected, indicating the case has a good prognosis going into maintenance care.
- *Stage III (severe disease)*: CAL ≥5 mm, probing depth ≥6 mm, radiographic evidence of horizontal and/or vertical bone loss beyond 33%, and may have furcation involvement of class II or III. This will require surgical and possibly regenerative treatments. There is the potential for loss of up to 4 teeth. The complexity of implant and/or restorative treatment is increased. The patient may require multispecialty treatment. The overall case has a fair prognosis going into maintenance care.
- *Stage IV (very severe disease)*: Includes all of stage III features. Fewer than 20 teeth may be present and there is the potential for loss of 5 or more teeth. Advanced surgical treatment and/or regenerative therapy may be required, including augmentation treatment to facilitate implant therapy. Very complex implant and/or restorative treatment may be needed. The patient will often require multispecialty treatment. The overall case has a questionable prognosis going into maintenance care.

Staging of post-treatment patients
Successfully treated patients should also be periodically staged during the monitoring phase of treatment. For post-treatment patients, CAL and radiographic bone loss (RBL) remain the primary stage determinants. However, in most patients certain baseline complexity factors may have been resolved through treatment (Tonetti et al. 2018a). In such instances requiring the removal of a stage-shifting complexity factor, the stage should not retrogress to a lower stage, as the original stage complexity factor should always be considered in the maintenance phase of management. An exception to this may be successful periodontal regeneration involving improvement of tooth support, which includes improved CAL and RBL of the specific tooth (Tonetti et al. 2018a).

Grading

Individuals presenting with different severity/extent and resulting complexity of management may present different rates of

Table 7.3 Periodontitis stage.

Periodontitis stage		Stage I	Stage II	Stage III	Stage IV
Severity	Interdental clinical attachment loss at site of greatest loss	1–2 mm	3–4 mm	≥5 mm	≥5 mm
	Radiographic bone loss	Coronal third (<15%)	Coronal third (15–33%)	Extending to middle or apical third of the root	Extending to middle or apical third of the root
	Tooth loss	No tooth loss due to periodontitis		Tooth loss due to periodontitis of ≤4 teeth	Tooth loss due to periodontitis of ≥5 teeth
Complexity	Local	Maximum probing depth ≤4 teeth Mostly horizontal bone loss	Maximum probing depth ≤5 teeth Mostly horizontal bone loss	In addition to stage II complexity: Probing depth ≥6 mm Vertical bone loss ≥3 mm Furcation involvement Class II or III Moderate ridge defect	In addition to stage III complexity: Need for complex rehabilitation due to: Masticatory dysfunction Secondary occlusal trauma (tooth mobility degree ≥2) Severe ridge defect Bite collapse, drifting, flaring Less than 20 remaining teeth (10 opposing pairs)
Extent and distribution	Add to stage as descriptor	For each stage, describe extent as localized (<30% of teeth involved), generalized, or molar/incisor pattern			

Source: Adapted from Caton et al. 2018.

progression of the disease and/or risk factors. Grade is therefore used as an indicator of the rate of periodontitis progression (Caton et al. 2018). The purpose of grading a periodontitis patient is thus:

- To obtain supplemental information about the biological features of the disease, including a history-based analysis of the accumulated knowledge of direct or indirect evidence of the rate of periodontitis progression (Tonetti & Sanz 2019).
- To assess the future risk for further progression and to analyze possible poor outcomes of treatment, thereby guiding the intensity of therapy and monitoring. This is accomplished by considering the general health status and other exposures such as smoking or the level of metabolic control in diabetes, which is crucial in comprehensive patient management (Tonetti & Sanz 2019).

Diabetes-associated periodontitis should not be regarded as a distinct diagnosis, but rather as an important modifying factor to be included in the clinical diagnosis of periodontitis as a descriptor (Jepsen et al. 2018). Tobacco smoking is now regarded as a chronic relapsing medical disorder with major adverse effects on the periodontium, and also as a modifying factor to be included in the clinical diagnosis of periodontitis as a descriptor (Jepsen et al. 2018).

A further purpose of grading is to assess whether risk of the disease or its treatment may negatively affect the systemic health of the patient, thereby guiding systemic monitoring and co-therapy with medical colleagues (Tonetti et al. 2018a). It is envisaged in the future that the consideration of the increased risk of periodontitis to be an inflammatory co-morbidity for a specific patient can be achieved by utilizing biomarkers, especially in the early detection of periodontitis. Examples of such biomarkers are C-reactive protein values and indicators of bone loss/CAL (Papapanou et al. 2018; Tonetti & Sanz 2019; Tonetti et al. 2018a).

Grading includes three levels (grade A – low risk, grade B – moderate risk, grade C – high risk for progression) (Caton et al. 2018). Clinicians should initially assume grade B disease and seek specific evidence to shift toward grade A or C, if available. Once the grade is established based on evidence of progression, it can be modified based on the presence of risk factors (Caton et al. 2018). Table 7.4 depicts the grading of a periodontitis case (Caton et al. 2018).

Table 7.4 Periodontitis grade.

Periodontitis grade			Grade A: Slow rate of progression	Grade B: Moderate rate of progression	Grade C: Rapid rate of progression
Primary criteria	Direct evidence of progression	Longitudinal data (radiographic bone loss or CAL)	Evidence of no loss over 5 years	<2 mm over 5 years	≥2 mm over 5 years
	Indirect evidence of progression	% bone loss/age	<0.25	0.25–1.0	>1.0
		Case phenotype	Heavy biofilm deposits with low levels of destruction	Destruction commensurate with biofilm deposits	Destruction exceeds expectation given biofilm deposits; specific clinical patterns suggestive of periods of rapid progression and/or early-onset disease (e.g. molar/incisor pattern, lack of expected response to standard bacterial control therapies)
Grade modifiers	Risk factors	Smoking	Non-smoker	Smoker < 10 cigarettes/day	Smoker ≥ 10 cigarettes/day
		Diabetes	Normoglycemic/no diagnosis of diabetes	HbA1c <7.0% in patients with diabetes	HbA1c ≥7.0% in patients with diabetes
Risk of systemic impact of periodontitis	Inflammatory burden	High sensitivity CRP (hsCRP)	<1 mg/L	1–3 mg/L	>3 mg/L
Biomarkers	Indicators of CAL/bone loss	Saliva, gingival crevicular fluid, serum	?	?	?

CAL, clinical attachment loss; CRP, C-reactive protein.
Source: Adapted from Caton et al. 2018.

Narrative descriptions of the grades are as follows:

- *Grade A (slow progression)*: No bone loss or CAL over five years, no smoking, no diabetes, heavy biofilm, but no tissue destruction.
- *Grade B (moderate progression)*: Less than 2 mm bone loss or CAL over five years, half pack or less per day smoking, HbA1c less than 7%, biofilm commensurate with destruction.
- *Grade C (rapid progression)*: Greater than 2 mm of bone loss or CAL over five years, half pack or more per day smoking, HbA1c 7% or higher, tissue destruction exceeds amount of biofilm.

Clinicians should approach grading by assuming a moderate rate of progression (grade B) and look for direct and indirect measures of actual progression in the past as a means of improving the establishment of prognosis for the individual patient. If the patient has risk factors that have been associated with more disease progression or less responsiveness to bacterial reduction therapies, the risk factor information can be used to modify the estimate of the patient's future course of disease. A risk factor should therefore shift the grade score to a higher value independently of the primary criterion represented by the rate of progression. For example, a stage and grade case definition could be characterized by moderate attachment loss (stage II), the assumption of moderate rate of progression (grade B) modified by the presence of poorly controlled Type II diabetes (a risk factor that is able to shift the grade definition to rapid progression or grade C).

Diagnosing gingivitis and periodontitis

Implementation of the new classification of periodontal diseases as introduced by Caton et al. (2018) enables clinicians and educators to identify well-defined clinical cases, and thereby identify subjects meeting the criteria for a specific diagnosis. The need to explore the reasons for tooth loss is also an important consideration in the staging classification, since the lack of implication of this parameter, namely that tooth loss was due to periodontitis, can lead to the paradox that periodontitis severity has improved after the loss of the most compromised teeth (Tonetti & Sanz 2019). Utilizing specific and defined criteria, a diagnosis can then be linked with treatment and prevention (Tonetti & Sanz 2019). These defined criteria are used for the following diagnoses:

- Periodontal health (Lang & Bartold 2018).
- Gingivitis (Trombelli et al. 2018).
- Reduced but healthy periodontium (successfully treated periodontitis).
- Gingival inflammation in a periodontitis patient (treated periodontitis with persistent inflammation) (Chapple et al. 2018; see Chapter 6).
- Necrotizing periodontal disease (Herrera et al. 2018).
- Periodontitis as a manifestation of systemic diseases (Albandar et al. 2018; Jepsen et al. 2018).
- Periodontitis (Papapanou et al. 2018; Tonetti et al. 2018a).

Diagnostic tools

- *Bleeding on probing* (BOP) has been indicated to be the most reliable and validated diagnostic tool for the assessment of gingival inflammation (Murakami et al. 2018). The new classification (Caton et al. 2018) requires the identification of 10% BOP sites to distinguish between periodontal health and gingivitis, thereby requiring a full-mouth assessment and recording (see Chapter 6).

Furthermore, besides the need for diagnosing, the recording of BOP together with plaque represents a key approach in assessing patient oral hygiene, as well as in the planning of individualized preventive programs (Tonetti & Sanz 2019).

- *Clinical attachment loss* is considered as the primary definition of periodontitis (Tonetti & Sanz 2019). An adequate proxy measure of CAL is marginal alveolar bone loss that is apparent on diagnostic-quality radiographs. Probing pocket depths do not allow for the discrimination of periodontal health, gingivitis, periodontitis, reduced but healthy periodontium, and gingival health in a periodontitis patient (Tonetti & Sanz 2019). The signs of CAL must also be discriminated from other conditions associated with CAL, namely gingival recession, vertical root fractures, endo-periodontal lesions, loss on the distal aspect of lower second molars associated with impacted wisdom teeth, or attachment loss secondary to cervical decay or restorations. Interdental attachment loss can be discerned either visually, or by means of the periodontal probe tip reaching the root surface in the interdental space (Tonetti & Sanz 2019).

Steps to staging and grading a periodontitis case

Once a diagnosis of a periodontitis case has been made, it can then be characterized by the process of staging and grading (Papapanou et al. 2018; Tonetti et al. 2018a). The American Academy of Periodontology released a document titled "Three Steps to Staging and Grading a Patient" (Tonetti et al. 2018b) (Table 7.5).

Table 7.5 Steps to staging and grading a patient.	
Step 1: Initial case overview to assess disease	Screen: • Full-mouth probing depths • Full-mouth radiographs • Missing teeth Mild to moderate periodontitis will typically be either stage I or II Severe to very severe periodontitis will typically be either stage III or IV
Step 2: Establish stage	For mild to moderate periodontitis (typically stage I or II): • Confirm clinical attachment loss (CAL) • Rule out non-periodontitis causes of CAL (e.g. cervical restorations or caries, root fractures, CAL due to traumatic causes) • Determine maximum CAL or radiographic bone loss (RBL) • Confirm RBL patterns For moderate to severe periodontitis (typically stage III or IV): • Determine maximum CAL or RBL • Confirm RBL patterns • Assess tooth loss due to periodontitis • Evaluate case complexity factors (e.g. severe CAL frequency, surgical challenges)
Step 3: Establish grade	• Calculate RBL (% of root length x 100) divided by age • Assess risk factors (e.g. smoking, diabetes) • Measure response to scaling, root planing, and plaque control • Assess expected rate of bone loss • Conduct detailed risk assessment • Account for medical and systemic inflammatory considerations

Source: Adapted from Tonetti et al. 2018b.

SUMMARY

This chapter describes the specific criteria to classify forms of periodontitis, the classification and case definitions of necrotizing periodontal diseases, as well as the clinical parameters for identifying a periodontitis case. Diagnostic tools, i.e. bleeding upon probing and clinical attachment loss, are used to diagnose, among others, periodontal health, gingivitis and periodontitis. The steps to be implemented by clinicians in staging and grading a periodontitis case enables them to characterize a periodontitis case.

REFERENCES

Albandar JM, Susin C, Hughes FJ. Manifestations of systemic diseases and conditions that affect the periodontal attachment apparatus: case definitions and diagnostic considerations. *J Clin Periodontol.* 2018; 45(Suppl 20):S171–S189.

Caton J, Armitage G, Berglundh T et al. A new classification scheme for periodontal and periimplant diseases and conditions – introduction and key changes from the 1999 classification. *J Clin Periodontol.* 2018; 45(Suppl 20):S1–S8.

Chapple ILC, Mealey BL, van Dyke TE et al. Periodontal health and gingival diseases and conditions on an intact and a reduced periodontium: consensus report of workgroup 1 of the 2017 World Workshop on the Classification of Periodontal and Peri-Implant Diseases and Conditions. *J Clin Periodontol.* 2018; 45(Suppl 20):S68–S77.

Fine DH, Patil AG, LoosBG. Classification and diagnosis of aggressive periodontitis. *J Clin Periodontol.* 2018; 45(Suppl 20):S95–S111.

Goodson JM, Tanner AC, Haffajee AD, Sornberger GC, Socransky SS. Patterns of progression and regression of advanced destructive periodontal disease. *J Clin Periodontol.* 1982; 9:472–481.

Herrera D, Retamal-Valdes B, Alonso B, Feres M. Acute periodontal lesions (periodontal abscesses and necrotizing periodontal diseases) and endo-periodontal lesions. *J Clin Periodontol.* 2018; 45(Suppl 20):S78–S94.

Jepsen S, Caton JG, Albandar JM et al. Periodontal manifestations of systemic diseases and developmental and acquired conditions: consensus report of workgroup 3 of the 2017 World Workshop on the Classification of Periodontal and Peri-Implant Diseases and Conditions. *J Clin Periodontol.* 2018; 45(Suppl 20):S219–S229.

Lang NP, Bartold PM. Periodontal health. *J Clin Periodontol.* 2018; 45(Suppl 20):S9–S16.

Loesche WJ, Syed SA, Laughon BE, Stoll J. The bacteriology of acute necrotizing ulcerative gingivitis. *J Periodontol.* 1982; 53:223–230.

Murakami S, Mealey BL, Mariotti A, Chapple ILC. Dental plaque-induced gingival conditions. *J Clin Periodontol.* 2018; 45(Suppl 20):S17–S27.

Novak MJ. Necrotizing ulcerative periodontitis. *Ann Periodontol.* 1999; 4:74–78.

Papapanou PN, Sanz M, Buduneli N et al. Periodontitis: consensus report of Workgroup 2 of the 2017 World Workshop on the Classification of Periodontal and Peri-Implant Diseases and Conditions. *J Clin Periodontol.* 2018; 45(Suppl 20):S162–S170.

Riviere GR, Wagoner MA, Baker-Zander SA et al. Identification of spirochetes related to *Treponema pallidum* in necrotizing ulcerative gingivitis and chronic periodontitis. *N Engl J Med.* 1991; 325:539–543.

Rowland RW. Necrotizing ulcerative gingivitis. *Ann Periodontol.* 1999; 4:65–73.

Tonetti MS, Greenwell H, Kornman KS. Staging and grading of periodontitis: framework and proposal of a new classification and case definition. *J Clin Periodontol.* 2018a; 45(Suppl 20):S149–S161.

Tonetti MS, Greenwell H, Kornman KS. Staging and grading of periodontitis: framework and proposal of a new classification and case definition. *J Periodontol.* 2018b; 89(Supp 1):S159–S172. Retrieved from http://perio.org/sites/default/files/files/Staging%20and%20Grading%20Periodontitis.pdf.

Tonetti MS, Sanz M. Implementation of the new classification of periodontal diseases: Decision making algorithms for clinical practice and education. *J Clin Periodontol.* 2019; 46:398–405.

Trombelli L, Farina R, Silva CO, Tatakis DN. Plaque-induced gingivitis: case definition and diagnostic considerations. *J Clin Periodontol.* 2018; 45(Suppl 20):S44–S67.

CHAPTER 8
Aggressive periodontitis

Steph Smith

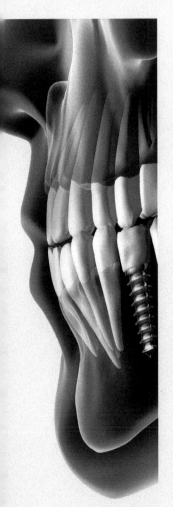

Contents

Learning objectives

- Understanding the reasons why aggressive periodontitis can be considered as a unique entity.
- The case definition for aggressive periodontitis.
- Features unique to aggressive periodontitis as pertaining to epidemiology, microbiology, the host response, the radiographic pattern of bone loss, and the genetic aspects of the disease.
- Classification and clinical features of both localized and aggressive forms of the disease.
- Various treatment modalities.

Essential Periodontics, First Edition. Edited by Steph Smith and Khalid Almas.
© 2022 John Wiley & Sons Ltd. Published 2022 by John Wiley & Sons Ltd.

Introduction

The 1999 Classification Workshop supported the distinction between chronic periodontitis (CP) and aggressive periodontitis (AgP) as being two different diseases (Armitage 1999). The literature has however reported conflicting findings on AgP, due to the fact that the classification is too broad and the disease has not been studied from its inception. Also, there exists a paucity of longitudinal studies, which include multiple time points and different populations (Papapanou et al. 2018a). In order to support the contention that CP and AgP are indeed different diseases, specific differences in etiology and pathophysiology are required to indicate the possible presence of distinct periodontitis entities. Although localized early-onset periodontitis has a distinct and well-recognized clinical presentation, it has been stated that variations in clinical presentation regarding extent and severity do not support the concept of different diseases. Also, specific etiological or pathophysiological elements that may account for this distinct presentation are insufficiently defined. Likewise, mechanisms accounting for the development of generalized periodontitis in young individuals are poorly understood (Papapanou et al. 2018a).

In 2018, the American Academy of Periodontology and the European Federation of Periodontology published the official proceedings from the 2017 World Workshop on the Classification of Periodontal Diseases (Caton et al. 2018). According to this new classification scheme, the diseases previously recognized as CP or aggressive AgP were grouped under a single category named periodontitis, thereby introducing the notion that AgP and CP are not different diseases, but variations of a single condition (Papapanou et al. 2018b; Tonetti et al. 2018). The main rationale for this decision was the lack of specific microbial profiles associated with CP or AgP, and a lack of specific patterns of the immuno-inflammatory response (Montenegro et al. 2020).

A systematic review assessing specific periodontal pathogens suggested that the presence or absence of these microorganisms could not distinguish between patients with CP and those with AgP (Mombelli et al. 2002). Another systematic review study that compiled data on 6376 patients and 23 920 subgingival biofilm samples suggested an association of *Aggregatibacter actinomycetemcomitans* with AgP, but neither this species nor other species studied were unique to, or could differentiate between, CP and AgP (Montenegro et al. 2020). This same review study indicated that the number of studies not showing statistically significant differences in bacterial species between CP and AgP was found to be always higher than that of studies showing differences (Montenegro et al. 2020). As pertaining to the host response, a systematic review reported insufficient evidence to support the existence of distinct cytokine profiles for patients with AgP and CP (Duarte et al. 2015). It has furthermore been suggested that due to the lack of specific differences between the subgingival microbiota of AgP and CP, the treatment of these clinical conditions also may not differ substantially (Montenegro et al. 2020).

According to the new periodontal disease classification, the previously termed aggressive periodontitis is now classified as periodontitis grade C, and localized aggressive periodontitis (previously termed juvenile periodontitis) is now classified as localized periodontitis grade C, incisor-molar pattern (Shaddox et al. 2021).

From a pathophysiological point of view, both localized aggressive periodontitis (LAgP) and CP are entities resulting from inflammatory responses to a bacterial biofilm, which result in bone loss (Graves et al. 2011). However, LAgP demonstrates a unique phenotype presenting with a substantial variation in clinical presentation with respect to extent and severity throughout the age spectrum (Graves et al. 2011). More specifically, there is evidence supporting the consideration of LAgP as a distinct entity, pertaining to disease localization, a high rate of progression, age of onset, a higher prevalence rate in individuals of African descent, and because of its pattern of familial aggregation (Armitage & Cullinan 2000; Brown et al. 1996; Diehl et al. 2005; Fine et al. 2007). This suggests that there are population subsets with distinct disease trajectories due to differences in exposure and/or susceptibility (Papapanou et al. 2018a).

Case definition for aggressive periodontitis

A new case definition for patients presenting with AgP has been recommended that includes the following distinctive criteria (Albander 2014):

- An early age of onset, usually before 25 years of age, this being a possible predictor of the disease's severity. Patients are clinically healthy except for the presence of periodontitis.
- Loss of periodontal tissue occurs at multiple permanent teeth.
- Periodontal destruction is detectable clinically and radiographically. Radiographically, lesions are depicted as vertical bone loss at the proximal surfaces of posterior teeth, usually similar bilaterally. In advanced cases the bone loss may be depicted as being horizontal.
- There is a relatively high progression rate of periodontal tissue loss.
- The primary teeth may also be affected.

Various studies have described distinctive features of AgP (Table 8.1).

Classification and clinical features

Localized aggressive periodontitis (localized periodontitis grade C, incisor-molar pattern)

- LAgP in the primary dentition of the African-American population has been described in children aged between 5 and 8 years, including the first and second primary molars mostly affected, with a possible initiation in the first primary molar, and an unusual pattern of external root resorption around these teeth (Miller et al. 2018).

Table 8.1   Features unique to aggressive periodontitis

Epidemiology
- Epidemiological studies indicate differences in the prevalence of localized aggressive periodontitis (LAgP) in various ethnic and racial populations, which can vary considerably between continents (Susin et al. 2014).
- The prevalence of LAgP is less than 1% and that of generalized aggressive periodontitis (GAgP) is 0.13%. Black people are at higher risk than white people, and males are at higher risk of GAgP than females (Joshipura et al. 2015).
- A higher prevalence of LAgP is seen in individuals of African and Middle Eastern descent, and a relatively low prevalence has been found in individuals of Caucasian descent (Elamin et al. 2010; Eres et al. 2009; Kissa et al. 2016; Lopez et al. 2009).
- Disease prevalence has been found to be 1–5% in the African population and in groups of African descent, 2.6% in African-Americans, 0.5–1.0% in Hispanics in North America, 0.3–2.0% in South America, and 0.2–1.0% in Asia. Among Caucasians, the disease prevalence is 0.1% in northern and central Europe, 0.5% in southern Europe, and 0.1–0.2% in North America. In Asia the prevalence rate is 1.2% for LAgP and 0.6% for GAgP in Baghdad and in the Iranian population, and 0.47% in the Japanese population (Joshipura et al. 2015).
- Genetic risk factors have also been described to be associated with GAgP in South India (Joshipura et al. 2015).

Microbiology
- Specific subpopulations of bacteria may be prevalent in specific populations, and a particularly thin biofilm composed of Gram-negative bacteria has been reported on root surfaces of LAgP subjects (Takeuchi et al. 2003).
- Studies have implicated *Aggregatibacter actinomycetemcomitans* (A.a) to be a risk marker in younger individuals, whereas this was not the case in older subjects (Aberg et al. 2009; Faveri et al. 2009; Gajardo et al. 2005).
- Studies show that in a subset of African and Middle Eastern subjects, A.a may occur in the early stages of disease.
- Specific A.a virulence factors can suppress the host response, allowing for the overgrowth of a toxic combination of other bacteria in the local environment, thereby hypothetically implicating toxic lipopolysaccharides, leukotoxin, and cytolethal distending toxin to be involved in disease activity (Fine et al. 2018).
- Other studies have indicated *Porphyromonas gingivalis, Tannerella forsythia*, and *Selenomonads* to be markers of risk (Chahboun et al. 2015; Feng et al. 2014; Li et al. 2015).
- Different combinations of bacteria that may occur in different ethnic populations can show similar clinical patterns of destruction, as similar metabolic end-products will challenge the host (Loos et al. 2015; Mombelli et al. 2002).

Host response
- Platelets, neutrophils, and monocytes in whole blood of LAgP patients display increased integrin and selectin surface expression, demonstrating a heightened proinflammatory phenotype, which includes increased platelet-leucocyte aggregates in the circulation together with a compromised capacity to generate proresolving lipid mediators (Fredman et al. 2011).
- Hyperactive neutrophil phenotypes produce an excess of proinflammatory mediator leukotriene B4, and show reduced production of proresolving mediator lipoxin A4, demonstrating that LAgP subjects exhibit a failure of resolution of inflammation (Van Dyke & Sima 2020).
- Polymorphonuclear neutrophils (PMNs) exhibit a number of functional abnormalities, including impaired chemotaxis, phagocytic abnormalities, and increased reactive oxygen species (ROS) generation (Fredman et al. 2011).
- Macrophages exhibit impaired phagocytosis (Fredman et al. 2011).
- Macrophage inflammatory protein (MIP) 1a, interleukin (IL)-1b, and tumor necrosis factor alpha (TNF-α) may be elevated prior to disease (Fine et al. 2014; Shaddox et al. 2011).
- These cytokines could act as potential risk markers at the site level. The relevance of these cytokines to clinical classification and disease initiation and progression, however, still needs to be determined (Aberg et al. 2009; Fine et al. 2014; Shaddox et al. 2011).
- Antibody responsiveness can be elevated at either a peripheral or a local level (Ebersole et al. 2000).

Radiographic pattern of bone loss (see Figure 8.1)
- Untreated AgP has a much faster rate of progression than chronic periodontitis (CP) (Onabolu et al. 2015), and the rate of bone loss in AgP can be three to four times higher than that of CP (Baer 1971).
- However, not all periodontal sites show continuous, quantifiable disease progression, as the rate of disease progression varies between subjects, and between different sites within the same subject (Brown et al. 1996; Mros & Berglundh 2010).
- At the early stage, periodontal lesions show a vertical pattern of alveolar bone loss at the proximal surfaces of the permanent first molars (Gjermo et al. 1984; Hørmand et al. 1979).
- These bone defects are usually arc shaped, and may extend from the distal surface of the second premolar to the mesial surface of the second molar (Albandar 2014; Baer 1971; Nibali et al. 2018).
- Also, the incisors are often affected, although the bone loss here is usually horizontal, because the alveolar bone is thinner than at the proximal surfaces of molars (Albandar 2014).

(Continued)

Table 8.1 (Continued)

- In advanced cases of AgP, the bone loss may be generalized and show a horizontal pattern (Albandar 2014).
- However, there are variances of the above. Some subjects may show significant bone loss around the incisors, and only moderate bone loss around the molars; whereas other subjects may show involvement of only the molars, with little or no involvement of incisors (Albandar 2014).

Genetic factors
- The role of genetics is considered more important in younger patients with AgP than in older subjects with CP (Van der Velden 2017).
- The familial pattern of the disease is an important feature that suggests a genetic predisposition, although this is a generic factor that is too broad to be used in a case definition (Albandar 2014).
- Genetic predisposition is a hallmark of this disease; however, in susceptible individuals the presence and intensity of other etiological factors, such as subgingival periodontal pathogens, smoking, and poor oral hygiene, may determine the clinical features and their severity, thereby contributing to the onset of the disease at an early age, and also lead to a more severe and /or generalized form of the disease (Albandar 2014).
- Other individuals who are genetically predisposed but harbor only low levels of virulent pathogens, and in addition lack other risk factors, may develop LAgP and the onset of the periodontal tissue loss may occur at an older age (Albandar 2014).
- For other studies regarding genetics and AgP, see Chapter 5.4.

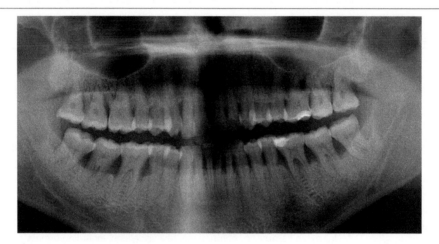

Figure 8.1 Radiographic pattern of bone loss in aggressive periodontitis.

- LAgP starts at circumpubertal age, involving interproximal attachment loss of first molars and/or incisors (Novak & Novak 1996).
- There is a lack of inflammation, with the presence of deep periodontal pockets and advanced bone loss (Novak & Novak 1996).
- The amount of plaque is minimal, being inconsistent with the amount of destruction, and rarely mineralizes to form calculus, but the plaque is highly pathogenic due to elevated levels of bacteria like *Aggregatibacter actinomycetemcomitans* and *Porphyromonas gingivalis* (Novak & Novak 1996).
- Secondary clinical features include disto-labial migration of incisors with diastema formation, mobility of the involved teeth, sensitivity of the denuded root, deep dull radiating pain to the jaw, periodontal abscess, and lymph node enlargement (Novak & Novak 1996).

Generalized aggressive periodontitis (periodontitis grade C)

- Generalized aggressive periodontitis (GAgP) has generalized interproximal attachment loss affecting at least three permanent teeth other than incisors and the first molar (Albandar 2014).
- Individuals are under the age of 30 years, with destruction occurring episodically.
- The rate of disease progression in GAgP may be higher than in LAgP (Albandar 2014).
- A higher proportion of sites with bilateral symmetrical periodontal destruction compared with severe CP (Brito et al. 2018).
- The presence of minimal plaque, which is inconsistent with destruction (Novak & Novak 1996).

- Gingival response appears as severely acute inflamed tissue that is ulcerated and red in color, with spontaneous bleeding indicating a destructive stage (Novak & Novak 1996).
- Or gingival response can appear as pink gingiva free of inflammation, with some degree of stippling and deep periodontal pockets, representing a quiescent stage (Novak & Novak 1996).
- It is generally recognized that CP may be superimposed on both localized and generalized forms of AgP (Armitage & Cullinan 2010).

Treatment

Patients with GAgP respond well to scaling and root planing in the short term (six months); however, after six months relapse may occur with disease progression, despite frequent recall visits and oral hygiene reinforcement (Teughels et al. 2014).

Systemic antibiotics like tetracycline, metronidazole, the combination of metronidazole and amoxicillin, clindamycin, and azithromycin have been used as adjuncts in the treatment of AgP. Meta-analysis studies have indicated that systemic antibiotics (metronidazole and amoxicillin combination) combined with non-surgical periodontal therapy resulted in a significant additional effect for the treatment of AgP (Keestra et al. 2015; Rebeis et al. 2019).

Local antimicrobial agents like 1% chlorhexidine gel, 40% tetracycline gel, tetracycline fibers, and chlorhexidine chip have been used in the treatment of LAgP and GAgP. Studies have concluded that the adjunct effect of local antimicrobials is not clear and does not seem to improve on the adjunct effect of systemic antibiotics. This type of treatment modality should thus rather be utilized on an individual basis (Keestra et al. 2015).

Access surgery (modified Widman flap) in combination with systemic antibiotics has been shown to be effective when compared to access surgery alone (Keestra et al. 2015).

Implant treatment in patients with GAgP has been suggested not to be contraindicated, provided that adequate infection control and an individualized maintenance program are assured (Kim & Sung 2012). However, in a prospective long-term cohort study, it was shown that patients with treated GAgP are more susceptible to mucositis and peri-implantitis, with lower implant survival and success rates (Swierkot et al. 2012).

Future recommendations

In light of the above, a more restrictive definition of LAgP should be created to enable the identification of the disease in its earliest stages, thereby enhancing knowledge on the diagnosis, pathogenesis, prevention, and management of this form of periodontitis (Fine et al. 2018). The new proposed definition should not only be based on clinical observations, such as the usual medical and dental history, clinical charting, and radiographic examinations, but should also focus on obvious phenotypic indictors in defined populations, namely (i) the age of the subject, (ii) location of lesions, and (iii) extent of disease (stages) (Fine et al. 2018). The age would include (i) childhood (prepubertal), (ii) adolescence (puberty), and (iii) early adulthood (post adolescence). Staging would include stage 1, a disease limited to one tooth; stage 2, limited to two teeth; stage 3, limited to three teeth (molars and incisors); and stage 4, the classic Löe and Brown (1991) definition of disease (Fine et al. 2018). Future advancement in the understanding of the genetic predisposition to AgP can also lead to the inclusion of specific genetic profiles in future case definitions. Future diagnostic methods of AgP should also possibly enable early diagnosis of the disease, so as to detect and prevent cases of AgP before the development of significant tissue loss (Albandar 2014).

REFERENCES

Aberg CH, Sjodin B, Lakio L et al. Presence of *Aggregatibacter actinomycetemcomitans* in young individuals: a 16-year clinical and microbiological follow-up study. *J Clin Periodontol.* 2009; 36:815–822.

Albandar JM. Aggressive periodontitis: case definition and diagnostic criteria. *Periodontol 2000.* 2014; 65:13–26.

Armitage GC. Development of a classification system for periodontal diseases and conditions. *Ann Periodontol.* 1999; 4:1–6.

Armitage GC, Cullinan MP. Comparison of the clinical features of chronic and aggressive periodontitis. *Periodontol 2000.* 2010; 53:12–27.

Baer PN. The case for periodontosis as a clinical entity. *J Periodontol.* 1971; 42:516–520.

Brito LF, Taboza ZA, Silveira VR et al. Aggressive periodontitis presents a higher degree of bilateral symmetry in comparison with chronic periodontitis. *J Oral Sci.* 2018; 60(1):97–104.

Brown LJ, Albandar JM, Brunelle JA, Löe H. Early-onset periodontitis: progression of attachment loss during 6 years. *J Periodontol.* 1996; 67:968–975.

Caton JG, Armitage G, Berglundh T et al. A new classification scheme for periodontal and peri-implant diseases and conditions—introduction and key changes from the 1999 classification. *J Periodontol.* 2018; 89(Suppl 1):S1–S8.

Chahboun H, Arnau MM, Herrera D, Sanz M, Ennibi OK. Bacterial profile of aggressive periodontitis in Morocco: a cross-sectional study. *BMC Oral Health.* 2015; 15:25.

Diehl SR, Wu T, Michalowicz BS et al. Quantitative measures of aggressive periodontitis show substantial heritability and consistency with traditional diagnoses. *J Periodontol.* 2005; 76:279–288.

Duarte PM, Bastos MF, Fermiano D et al. Do subjects with aggressive and chronic periodontitis exhibit a different cytokine/chemokine profile in the gingival crevicular fluid? A systematic review. *J Periodontal Res.* 2015; 50:18–27.

Ebersole JL, Cappelli D, Steffen MJ. Antigenic specificity of gingival crevicular fluid antibody to *Actinobacillus actinomycetemcomitans. J Dent Res.* 2000; 79:1362–1370.

Elamin AM, Skaug N, Ali RW, Bakken V, Albandar JM. Ethnic disparities in the prevalence of periodontitis among high school students in Sudan. *J Periodontol.* 2010; 81:891–896.

Eres G, Saribay A, Akkaya M. Periodontal treatment needs and prevalence of localized aggressive periodontitis in a young Turkish population. *J Periodontol.* 2009; 80:940–944.

Faveri M, Figueiredo LC, Duarte PM et al. Microbiological profile of untreated subjects with localized aggressive periodontitis. *J Clin Periodontol.* 2009; 36:739–749.

Feng X, Zhang L, Xu L et al. Detection of eight periodontal microorganisms and distribution of *Porphyromonas gingivalis* fimA genotypes in Chinese patients with aggressive periodontitis. *J Periodontol.* 2014; 85:150–159.

Fine DH, Markowitz K, Fairlie K et al. Macrophage inflammatory protein-1alpha shows predictive value as a risk marker for subjects and sites vulnerable to bone loss in a longitudinal model of aggressive periodontitis. *PLoS One.* 2014; 9:e98541.

Fine DH, Markowitz K, Furgang D et al. *Aggregatibacter actinomycetemcomitans* and its relationship to initiation of localized aggressive periodontitis: longitudinal cohort study of initially healthy adolescents. *J Clin Microbiol.* 2007; 45:3859–3869.

Fine DH, Patil AG, Loos BG. Classification and diagnosis of aggressive periodontitis. *J Periodontol.* 2018; 89(Suppl 1):S103–S119.

Fredman G, Oh SF, Ayilavarapu S et al. (2011) Impaired phagocytosis in localized aggressive periodontitis: rescue by resolvin E1. *PLoS One.* 2011; 6(9): e24422.

Gajardo M, Silva H, Gomez L et al. Prevalence of periodontopathic bacteria in aggressive periodontitis patients in a Chilean population. *J Periodontol.* 2005; 76:289–294.

Gjermo P, Bellini HT, Pereira Santos V, Martins JG, Ferracyoli JR. Prevalence of bone loss in a group of Brazilian teenagers assessed on bite-wing radiographs. *J Clin Periodontol.* 1984; 11:104–113.

Graves DT, Oates T, Garlet GP. Review of osteoimmunology and the host response in endodontic and periodontal lesions. *J Oral Microbiol.* 2011; 3:5304. doi: 10.3402/jom.v3i0.5304.

Hørmand J, Frandsen A. Juvenile periodontitis. Localization of bone loss in relation to age, sex, and teeth. *J Clin Periodontol.* 1979; 6:407–416.

Joshipura V, Yadalam U, Brahmavar B. Aggressive periodontitis: a review. *J Int Clin Dent Res Organ.* 2015; 7:11–17.

Keestra JAJ, Grosjean I, Coucke W, Quirynen M, Teughels W. Non-surgical periodontal therapy with systemic antibiotics in untreated aggressive periodontitis patients: a systematic review and meta-analysis. *J Periodont Res.* 2015; 50:689–706.

Kim KK, Sung HM. Outcomes of dental implant treatment in patients with GAP: a systematic review. *J Adv Prosthodont.* 2012; 4:210–217.

Kissa J, Chemlali S, El Houari B et al. Aggressive and chronic periodontitis in a population of Moroccan school students. *J Clin Periodontol.* 2016; 43:934–939.

Li Y, Feng X, Xu L et al. Oral microbiome in Chinese patients with aggressive periodontitis and their family members. *J Clin Periodontol.* 2015; 42:1015–1023.

Löe H, Brown LJ. Early onset periodontitis in the United States of America. *J Periodontol.* 1991; 62:608–616.

Loos BG, Papantonopoulos G, Jepsen S, Laine ML. What is the contribution of genetics to periodontal risk? *Dent Clin North Am.* 2015; 59:761–780.

Lopez R, Frydenberg M, Baelum V. Clinical features of early periodontitis. *J Periodontol.* 2009; 80:749–758.

Miller K, Treloar T, Guelmann M, Rody WJ Jr, Shaddox LM. Clinical characteristics of localized aggressive periodontitis in primary dentition. *J Clin Pediatr Dent.* 2018; 42:95–102.

Mombelli A, Casagni F, Madianos PN. Can presence or absence of periodontal pathogens distinguish between subjects with chronic and aggressive periodontitis? A systematic review. *J Clin Periodontol.* 2002; 29(suppl 3):10–21. Discussion 37–38.

Montenegro SCL, Retamal-Valdes B, Bueno-Silva B et al. Do patients with aggressive and chronic periodontitis exhibit specific differences in the subgingival microbial composition? A systematic review. *J Periodontol.* 2020; 91:1503–1520.

Mros ST, Berglundh T. Aggressive periodontitis in children: a 14–19-year follow-up. *J Clin Periodontol.* 2010; 37:283–287.

Nibali L, Tomlins P, Akcalı A. Radiographic morphology of intrabony defects in the first molars of patients with localized aggressive periodontitis: Comparison with health and chronic periodontitis. *J Periodont Res.* 2018; 53:582–588.

Novak KF, Novak MJ. Early-onset periodontitis. *Curr Opin Periodontol.* 1996; 3:45–58.

Onabolu O, Donos N, Tu Y-K, Darbar U, Nibali L. Periodontal progression based on radiographic records: an observational study in chronic and aggressive periodontitis. *J Dent.* 2015; 43:673–682.

Papapanou PN, Sanz M, Buduneli N et al. Periodontitis: consensus report of Workgroup 2 of the 2017 World Workshop on the Classification of Periodontal and Peri-Implant Diseases and Conditions. *J Clin Periodontol.* 2018a; 45(Suppl 20):S162–S170.

Papapanou PN, Sanz M, Buduneli N et al. Periodontitis: consensus report of workgroup 2 of the 2017 World Workshop on the Classification of Periodontal and Peri-Implant Diseases and Conditions. *J Periodontol.* 2018b; 89(Suppl 1):S173–S182.

Rebeis ES, Albuquerque-Souza E, Paulino da Silva M et al. Effect of periodontal treatment on *Aggregatibacter actinomycetemcomitans* colonization and serum IgG levels against A. *actinomycetemcomitans* serotypes and Omp29 of aggressive periodontitis patients. *Oral Dis.* 2019; 25:569–579.

Shaddox LM, Morford LA, Nibali L. Periodontal health and disease: the contribution of genetics. *Periodontol 2000.* 2021; 85:161–181.

Shaddox LM, Wiedey J, Calderon NL et al. Local inflammatory markers and systemic endotoxin in aggressive periodontitis. *J Dent Res.* 2011; 90:1140–1144.

Susin C, Haas AN, Albandar JM. Epidemiology and demographics of aggressive periodontitis. *Periodontol 2000.* 2014; 65:27–45.

Swierkot K, Lottholz P, Flores-de-Jacoby L, Mengel R. Mucositis, peri-implantitis, implant success, and survival of implants in patients with treated generalized aggressive periodontitis: 3- to 16-year results of a prospective long-term cohort study. *J Periodontol.* 2012; 83:1213–1225.

Takeuchi Y, Umeda M, Ishizuka M, Huang Y, Ishikawa I. Prevalence of periodontopathic bacteria in aggressive periodontitis patients in a Japanese population. *J Periodontol.* 2003; 74:1460–1469.

Teughels W, Dhondt R, Dekeyser C, Quirynen M. Treatment of aggressive periodontitis. *Periodontol 2000.* 2014; 65:107–133.

Tonetti MS, Greenwell H, Kornman KS. Staging and grading of periodontitis: framework and proposal of a new classification and case definition. *J Clin Periodontol.* 2018; 45(Suppl 20):S149–S161.

Van der Velden U. What exactly distinguishes aggressive from chronic periodontitis: is it mainly a difference in the degree of bacterial invasiveness? *Periodontol 2000.* 2017; 75:24–44.

Van Dyke TE, Sima C. Understanding resolution of inflammation in periodontal diseases: is chronic inflammatory periodontitis a failure to resolve? *Periodontol 2000.* 2020; 82:205–213.

CHAPTER 9
Periodontal conditions and the female patient

Mea A. Weinberg and Stuart L. Segelnick

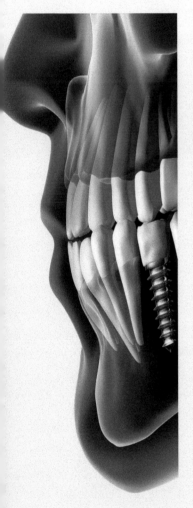

Contents

Learning objectives

- Effects of estrogen and progesterone on the periodontium.
- Role of female sex hormones affecting the periodontium at different ages.
- Oral contraceptive formulations and their impact on gingival tissues.
- Effect of sex hormones on the periodontium during pregnancy.

Essential Periodontics, First Edition. Edited by Steph Smith and Khalid Almas.
© 2022 John Wiley & Sons Ltd. Published 2022 by John Wiley & Sons Ltd.

Introduction

Female sex steroid hormones are important for sexual function and skeletal growth, and also play a role in the physiological changes in the periodontium. From puberty to the start of menses to pregnancy, perimenopause, and menopause, periodontal conditions in the female are altered as there are fluctuations in the blood levels of the sex hormones. Additionally, different formulations of oral contraceptives may also be responsible for gingival tissue changes.

Female sex hormones

Female sex hormones are secreted from the ovaries, adrenal cortex, and during pregnancy from the placenta. The main female sex hormones include estrogen and progesterone. Sex hormones are believed to have an influence on the entire body, including the oral cavity (Bhardwaj & Bhardwaj 2012).

Estrogen, mainly estradiol in perimenopause and estrone post menopause, is responsible for distinctive changes in the uterus and vagina that regulate the development of female characteristics and are at the highest levels during ovulation (Mariotti 1994). Additionally, estrogen is involved in skeletal growth and bone homeostasis (Weitzmann 2006). Estradiol, the most numerous and potent estrogen in premenopausal women, has a direct effect on the periodontal tissues by binding to estrogen receptors that are located on the cells in the periodontium, e.g. gingival fibroblasts of the lamina propria that regulate collagen production and secretion, periosteal fibroblasts, periodontal ligament (PDL) fibroblasts, and osteoblast-like cells (Bhardwaj & Bhardwaj 2012; Mariotti 1994; Mascarenhas et al. 2003; Novella et al. 2012). The function of progesterone in females includes preparation for and maintenance of pregnancy, which involves changes in the mucous membrane lining of the uterus. Receptors for progesterone are also found on the cells in the gingival tissues, namely on periosteal fibroblasts, fibroblasts in the lamina propria and PDL, and osteoblasts (Singh et al. 2013; Vittek et al. 1982). Table 9.1 depicts the effects of both estrogen and progesterone on the periodontium during gingival health, gingivitis, and periodontitis.

Estrogen acts on the immune system in two ways: in low doses it is proinflammatory by stimulating cytokine production and in high doses it decreases cytokine production (Ioannidou 2017). Normally, estrogen prevents bone loss by inhibiting the production of proinflammatory cytokines, including interleukin (IL)-1, IL-6, IL-10, and tumor necrosis factor (TNF)-α in bone marrow and bone cells (Galien & Garcia 1997; Johnson et al. 2002; Luo et al. 2014). IL-6 is both proinflammatory by stimulating osteoclast bone resorption and anti-inflammatory (Hienz et al. 2015). However, when estrogen levels are reduced in perimenopause

Table 9.1 Effects of estrogen and progesterone on the periodontium.

Estrogen	Progesterone
Proliferation of gingival fibroblasts resulting in production and maturation of gingival connective tissue, but with no net effect on gingival collagen production (Mariotti 1994; Ramamurthy 2015)	Inhibits proliferation of gingival fibroblasts and collagen synthesis, which delays gingival tissue repair (Mascarenhas et al. 2003; Novella et al. 2012)
Increased vascular cell permeability, proliferation, vasodilation, and vascular protection (Novella et al. 2012; Ramamurthy 2015)	Increases proliferation, dilation, and permeability of gingival blood vessels (Güncü et al. 2005; Singh et al. 2013)
Inhibits cyclooxygenase-derived vasoconstrictor substances, including thromboxane A2 (Meyer et al. 2015; Novella et al. 2012)	Stimulates production of prostaglandin (PGE2) in gingival crevicular fluid (proinflammatory; bone destruction) (Bhardwaj & Bhardwaj 2012; Ferris 1993; Markou et al. 2009)
Inhibits polymorphonuclear neutrophil (PMN) chemotaxis (Ito et al. 1995; Mariotti 1994; Ozveri et al. 2001; Reinhardt et al. 1994)	
Increases gingival inflammation due to an exaggerated response to bacteria (Gapski et al. 2003; Güncü et al. 2005; Reinhardt et al. 1994)	
Reduces T-cell-mediated inflammation (Josefsson et al. 1992)	
Stimulates PMN phagocytosis (Khan & Ahmed 2016)	
Inhibits production of interleukin-6 (proinflammatory) during gingival inflammation (Gordon et al. 2001)	
Regulates cytodifferentiation of stratified squamous epithelium. Reduces effectiveness of the epithelial barrier; decreases keratinization (Jafri et al. 2015; Mariotti 1994; Sarita et al. 2018)	

and menopause, there are higher levels of IL-6 that stimulate osteoclasts, inducing alveolar bone resorption (Lapp et al. 1995). Progesterone, however, reduces IL-6 production by gingival fibroblasts (Lapp et al. 1995).

Periodontal changes in the female

The status of the periodontal tissues at any given time results from the cumulative and synergistic effects of the levels of estrogen and progesterone (Ramamurthy 2015). Alteration in the proportionate concentration levels of these hormones affects the overall regulatory mechanisms within the periodontal tissues, such as that occurring during puberty, the menstrual cycle, pregnancy, and menopause (Ramamurthy 2015).

Puberty

During puberty both estradiol and progesterone are produced. Estradiol and progesterone begin to affect the gingival tissues during the onset of puberty, whereby a peak prevalence of gingivitis has been determined at 12 years, 10 months in females (Ashutosh et al. 2018). The levels of estrogen and progesterone reach a point during puberty that stays constant during the reproductive phases thereafter. Increased levels in these hormones during puberty have been related to an alteration of subgingival bacteria, and an increased prevalence of gingival inflammation without a corresponding change in mean plaque levels (Güncü et al. 2005; Markou et al. 2009; Tevatia 2017; Tiainen et al. 1992). It has been documented that *Prevotella intermedia*, part of the orange complex cluster of periodontopathic bacteria, uses estradiol and progesterone in place of vitamin K as a "growth factor," allowing it to feed off the hormones and multiply (Markou et al. 2009; Nagakawa et al. 1994). Besides increased levels of *P. intermedia*, *Capnocytophaga* spp. are also increased during puberty, which has been linked to increased bleeding (Markou et al. 2009).

Menses

An edematous and erythematous gingiva, including increased gingival bleeding due to increased permeability of gingival blood vessels, has been reported during menstruation or at the onset of puberty. This has been ascribed to a most likely exaggerated response to increased levels of progesterone that peak around 10 days and then decrease just before menstruation (Ashutosh et al. 2018; Singh et al. 2013). Other factors involved in the inflammation include stimulating prostaglandin production and increasing polymorphonuclear neutrophil (PMN) chemotaxis (Miyagi et al. 1992). However, the majority of women who have "healthy" gingival tissues most likely will not show any signs of inflammation related to menstruation (Amar & Chung 1994; Güncü et al. 2005). Essentially, most periodontal changes during menstruation, with fluctuations of estrogen and progesterone levels, have been found to

be inflammatory and temporary, specifically regarding the production of gingival crevicular fluid (GCF) proinflammatory IL-6 (Aydinyurt et al. 2018). Some studies, however, have not found a change in IL-6 levels during the menstrual cycle (Becerik et al. 2010). TNF-α levels have been described to be highest during the premenstrual day and lowest during the menstruation day (Aydinyurt et al. 2018; Khosravisamani et al. 2014).

Oral contraceptives

Since their introduction in 1960, the formulation of oral contraceptives (OCs) has changed dramatically. In past years, the concentration of estrogen was 50–150 µg and progestin 10 mg. Currently, the concentrations of the majority of OCs are 20–30 µg estrogen (e.g. ethinyl estradiol) and 1.5 mg or less progestin (e.g. norethindrone, desogestrel) (Institute of Medicine 1991; Smadi & Zakaryia 2018). The progesterone component in current OCs has a more distinct progestogen effect compared to older-generation OCs, where the progesterone component had more of an androgenic effect, which resulted in many undesirable adverse side effects (Jones 1995; Smadi & Zakaryia 2018). Recent studies have concluded that the combined newer-generation OCs, even with lower doses of estrogen, can still affect the periodontal tissues (increased gingival inflammation) independent of plaque accumulation (Domingues et al. 2012).

Pregnancy

Peak estrogen and progesterone levels occur in the third trimester of pregnancy, are higher than during menstruation, and may affect gingival tissues and the subgingival bacteria (Al-Qahtani et al. 2019; Patel et al. 2012; Steinberg et al. 2008). Gingivitis gradually increases from the first to the third trimesters (González-Jaranay et al. 2017). The mechanism of the effect of sex hormones on gingival inflammation in pregnancy is relatively controversial (Wu et al. 2016). Some studies report that the inflammation is not related to an increase in GCF IL-1β and TNF-α levels, even though these may be elevated (de Souza Massoni et al. 2019).

Women with gingivitis during the first trimester of pregnancy have been documented to have elevated levels of *Porphyromonas gingivalis* (Pg), which may be due to the presence of *Tannerella forsythia* and progesterone levels (Figuero et al. 2010). High levels of Pg and *Aggregatibacter actinomycetemcomitans* (A.a) have been reported during the third trimester (Figuero et al. 2010). Periodontal changes that occur during pregnancy most likely improve during the postpartum period (González-Jaranay et al. 2017).

It has been concluded that periodontal disease in pregnant women is a risk factor for preterm low-birth-weight babies (Walia & Saini 2015). There are many possible mechanisms proposed, with the underlying cause being endotoxins that stimulate the production of proinflammatory cytokines and prostaglandins from Gram-negative bacterial infections seen in periodontal disease. These proinflammatory mediators have the potential to cross the placenta and cause fetal toxicity, resulting in low-birth-weight babies (Saini et al. 2010).

Due to hormonal changes (primarily estrogen, which increases vascular endothelial growth factor [VEGF] production in macrophages), a pyogenic granuloma or pregnancy tumor may be seen in about 5% of pregnant women in the second or third trimester. It is a benign, vascular lesion, usually occurring on the gingival papillae (Gondivkar et al. 2010).

Menopause

Menopausal and postmenopausal estradiol levels decrease to a low level, which may increase the incidence of women developing periodontitis (Haas et al. 2009). With low estrogen levels there is an increase in macrophage, monocyte, and osteoclast activity, which may influence the increased production of GCF IL-16 and TNF-α. This may reduce bone density and cause cancellous and cortical bone loss; however, the exact mechanisms of bone loss are unclear (Nazir 2017; Reinhardt et al. 1994; Singh et al. 2018).

REFERENCES

Al-Qahtani A, Al-Twaijri S, Tulbah H, Al-Fouszan A, Abu-Shaheen A. Gynecologists' knowledge of the association between periodontal health and female sex hormones. *Cureus.* 2019; 11(4):e4513.

Amar S, Chung KM. Influence of hormonal variation in the periodontium on women. *Periodontol 2000.* 1994; 6:79–87.

Ashutosh N, Priyanka B, Jaspreet K. Ascendancy of sex hormones on the periodontium during reproductive life cycle of women. *J Int Clin Dent Res Organ.* 2018; 10(1):3–11.

Aydinyurt HS, Yuncu YZ, Tekin Y, Ertugrul AS. IL-6, TNF-α levels and periodontal status changes during the menstrual cycle. *Oral Dis.* 2018; 24:1599–1605.

Becerik S, Ozcaka Z, Nalbantsoy A et al. Effects of menstrual cycle on periodontal health and gingival crevicular fluid markers. *J Periodontol.* 2010; 81(5):673–681.

Bhardwaj A, Bhardwaj SV. Effect of androgens, estrogens and progesterone on periodontal tissues. *J Orofac Res.* 2012; 2(3):165–170.

de Souza Massoni RS, Fabio Aranha AM, Matos FZ et al. Correlation of periodontal and microbiological evaluations, with serum levels of estradiol and progesterone, during different trimesters of gestation. *Sci Rep.* 2019; 9:11762.

Domingues RS, Ferraz BF, Greghi SL et al. Influence of combined oral contraceptives on the periodontal condition. *J Appl Oral Sci.* 2012; 20(2):253–259.

Ferris GM. Alteration in female sex hormones: their effect on oral tissues and dental treatment. *Compendium.* 1993; 14(12):1558–1570.

Figuero E, Carrillo-De-Albornoz A, Herrera D, Bascones-Martínez, A. Gingival changes during pregnancy: II. Influence of hormonal variations on the subgingival biofilm. *J Clin Periodontol.* 2010; 37(3):230–240.

Galien R, Garcia T. Estrogen receptor impairs interleukin-6 expression by preventing protein binding on the NF-kappaB site. *Nucleic Acids Res.* 1997; 25(12):2424–2429.

Gapski MP, KAS, Wang H-L. Influence of sex hormones on the periodontium. *J Clin Periodontol.* 2003; 30:671–681.

Gondivkar SM, Gadbail A, Chole R. Oral pregnancy tumor. *Contemp Clin Dent.* 2010; 1(3):190–192.

González-Jaranay M, Téllez L, Roa-López A, Gómez-Moreno G, Moreu G. Periodontal status during pregnancy and postpartum. *PLoS One.* 2017; 12(5):e0178234.

Gordon CM, LeBoff MS, Glowacki J. Adrenal and gonadal steroids inhibit IL-6 secretion by human marrow cells. *Cytokine.* 2001; 16(5):178–186.

Güncü GN, Tözüm TF, Çaglayan F. Effects of endogenous sex hormones on the periodontium – review of literature. *Aust Dent J.* 2005; 50(3):138–145.

Haas AN, Rösing CK, Oppermann RV, Albandar JM, Susin C. Association among menopause, hormone replacement therapy, and periodontal attachment loss in southern Brazilian women. *J Periodontol.* 2009; 80(9):1380–1387.

Hienz SA, Paliwal S, Ivanovski S. Mechanisms of bone resorption in periodontitis. *J Immunol Res.* 2015; 2015:615486.

Institute of Medicine (US). Committee on the Relationship Between Oral Contraceptives and Breast Cancer. *Oral Contraceptives & Breast Cancer.* Washington, DC: National Academies Press; 1991: 143–151.

Ioannidou E. The sex and gender intersection in chronic periodontitis. *Front Public Health.* 2017; 5:189.

Ito I, Hayashi T, Yamada K et al. Physiological concentration of estradiol inhibits polymorphonuclear leukocyte chemotaxis via a receptor mediated system. *Life Sciences.* 1995; 56(25):2247–2253.

Jafri Z, Bhardwaj A, Sawai M, Sultan N. Influence of female sex hormones on periodontium: a case series. *J Nat Sci Biol Med.* 2015; Suppl 1:S146–S149.

Johnson RB, Gilbert JA, Cooper RC et al. Effect of estrogen deficiency on skeletal and alveolar bone density in sheep. *J Periodontol.* 2002; 73(4):383–391.

Jones EE. Androgenic effects of oral contraceptives: implications for patient compliance. *Am J Med.* 1995; 98(1A):116S–119S.

Josefsson E, Tarkowski A, Carlsten H. Anti-inflammatory properties of estrogen. I. in vivo suppression of leukocyte production in bone marrow and redistribution of peripheral blood neutrophils. *Cell Immunol.* 1992; 142(1):67–78.

Khan D, Ahmed SA. The immune system is natural target for estrogen action: opposing effects of estrogen in two prototypical autoimmune diseases. *Front Immunol.* 2016; 6:635.

Khosravisamani M, Malij G, Seyfi S et al. Effect of the menstrual cycle on inflammatory cytokines in the periodontium. *J Periodontal Res.* 2014; 49(6):770–776.

Lapp CA, Thomas ME, Lewis JB. Modulation by progesterone of interleukin-6 production by gingival fibroblasts. *J Periodontol.* 1995; 66:279–284.

Luo K, Ma S, Guo J, Huang Y, Yan F, Xiao Y. Association between postmenopausal osteoporosis and experimental periodontitis. *Biomed Res Int.* 2014; 2014:316134.

Mariotti A. Sex steroid hormones and cell dynamics in the periodontium. *Crit Rev Oral Biol Med.* 1994; 5(1):27–53.

Markou E, Eleana B, Lazaros T, Antonios K. The influence of sex steroid hormones on gingiva of women. *Open Dent J.* 2009; 3:114–119.

Mascarenhas P, Gapski R, Al-Shammari K, Wang HL. Influence of sex hormones on the periodontium. *J Clin Periodontol.* 2003; 30:671–681.

Meyer MR, Fredette NC, Barton M, Prossnitz ER. G protein-coupled estrogen receptor inhibits vascular prostanoid production and activity. *J Endocrinol.* 2015; 227(1):61–69.

Miyagi M, Aoyama H, Morishita M, Iwamoto Y. Effects of sex hormones on chemotaxis of human peripheral polymorphonuclear leukocytes and monocytes. *J Periodontol.* 1992; 63:8–32.

Nakagawa S, Fugii H, Machida Y, Okud K. A longitudinal study from prepuberty to puberty of gingivitis. Correlation between the occurrence of *Prevotella intermedia* and sex hormones. *J Clin Periodontol.* 1994; 21:658–665.

Nazir MA. Prevalence of periodontal disease, its association with systemic diseases and prevention. *Int J Health Sci.* 2017; 11(2):72–80.

Novella S, Dantas AP, Segarra G, Medina P, Hermenegildo C. Vascular aging in women: is estrogen the fountain of youth? *Front Physio.* 2012; 3:165.

Ozveri ES, Bozkurt A, Haklar G et al. Prevention and repair of multiorgan failure by human umbilical cord blood stem cells and premarin in experimental heatstroke. *Inflamm Res.* 2001; 50(12):585–891.

Patel SN, Kalburgi NB, Koregol AC et al. Female sex hormones and periodontal health-awareness among gynecologists – a questionnaire survey. *Saudi Dent J.* 2012; 24:99–104.

Ramamurthy J. Role of estrogen and progesterone in the periodontium. *Res J Pharm Biol Chem Sci.* 2015; 6(4):1540–1547.

Reinhardt RA, Masada MP, Payne JB, Allison AC, DuBois LM. Gingival fluid IL-1 beta and IL-6 levels in menopause, *J Clin Periodontol.* 1994; 21(1):22–25.

Saini R, Saini S, Saini SR. Periodontitis: a risk for delivery of premature labor and low-birth-weight babies. *J Nat Sci Biol Med.* 2010; 1(1):40–42.

Sarita SS, Narayan J, Yadalam U et al. Influence of female sex hormones on periodontium – a review. *Int J Curr Res.* 2018; 10(02):64990–64994.

Singh M, Radhika S, Negi R et al. Periodontal status in pre- and post-menopausal women: a review. *Asian Pac J Health Sci.* 2018; 5(2):136–141.

Singh P, Dev YP, Kaushal S. Progesterone supplementation – beware of changes in the oral cavity. *J Hum Reprod Sci.* 2013; 6(2):165.

Smadi L, Zakaryia A. The association between the use of new oral contraceptive pills and periodontal health. *J Int Oral Health.* 2018; 10:127–131.

Steinberg BJ, Minsk L, Gluch JI et al. Women's oral health issues. In: A Clouse, K Sherif, ed., *Women's Health in Clinical Practice.* Totawa, NJ: Humana Press; 2008: 273–293.

Tevatia S. Puberty induced gingival enlargement. *Biomed J Sci & Tech Res.* 2017; 1(1). doi: 10.26717/bjstr.2017.01.000126.

Tiainen L, Aslkainen S, Saxén L. Puberty-associated gingivitis. *Commun Dent Oral Epidemiol.* 1992; 20:87–89.

Vittek J, Munnangi PR, Gordon GG, Rappaport SC, Southren AL. Progesterone receptors in human gingiva. *IRSC Med Sci.* 1982; 10:381–384.

Walia M, Saini N. Relationship between periodontal diseases and preterm birth: recent epidemiological and biological data. *Int J Appl Basic Res.* 2015; 5(1):2–6.

Weitzmann MN, Pacifici R. Estrogen deficiency and bone loss: an inflammatory tale. *J Clin Inves.* 2006; 116:1186–1194.

Wu M, Chen SW, Su WL et al. Sex hormones enhance gingival inflammation without affecting Il-1β and TNF-α in periodontally healthy women during pregnancy. *Mediators Inflamm.* 2016; 2016:4897890.

CHAPTER 10

Periodontal manifestations of systemic diseases and developmental and acquired conditions

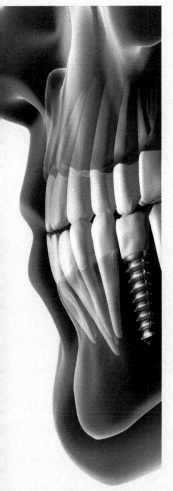

Contents

Essential Periodontics, First Edition. Edited by Steph Smith and Khalid Almas.
© 2022 John Wiley & Sons Ltd. Published 2022 by John Wiley & Sons Ltd.

10.1 SYSTEMIC DISEASES OR CONDITIONS AFFECTING THE PERIODONTAL SUPPORTING TISSUES

Anders Gustafsson

Contents

Learning objectives

- Systemic disorders impacting the loss of periodontal tissue by influencing periodontal inflammation as well as systemic conditions influencing the pathogenesis of periodontal diseases.
- Systemic disorders resulting in loss of periodontal tissue independent of dental plaque biofilm-induced inflammation.
- Knowledge of specific systemic conditions affecting the periodontium, e.g. Down's syndrome, hematological diseases, neoplasms, and HIV.

Introduction

The pathogenesis of periodontitis includes an individual with a varied host response to periodontal pathogens. An altered, deficient, or exaggerated host immune response may lead to more severe forms of the disease, explaining the many differences in disease severity among different individuals (Caton et al. 2018). However, systemic diseases, disorders, and conditions can also alter host tissues and physiology, leading to impairment of the host's barrier function and immune defence against periodontal pathogens. Such systemic diseases and disorders have been implicated as risk indicators or risk factors in periodontal disease, thereby creating the opportunity for the progression of destructive periodontal disease (Albandar et al. 2018; Jepsen et al. 2018). These disorders are due to innate mechanisms or may be acquired via environmental factors or lifestyle, causing alterations in the host immune response to periodontal infection. They may also instigate metabolic changes in the periodontal tissues, or cause defects in the gingiva or periodontal tissues (Albandar et al. 2018). Certain classes of systemic medications are associated with an increased loss of periodontal tissue, for example medications used in the treatment of malignancies (Albandar et al. 2018). The classification of these systemic conditions includes mainly rare systemic conditions (such as Papillon–Lefèvre syndrome, leucocyte adhesion deficiency, and others) with a major effect on the course of periodontitis, and more common conditions (such as diabetes mellitus) with variable effects, as well as conditions affecting the periodontium independently of dental plaque biofilm-induced inflammation (such as neoplastic diseases) (Jepsen et al. 2018). It is important, however, to recognize that these conditions themselves do not cause periodontitis; rather, they may predispose to the disease, or accelerate or increase its progression (Caton et al. 2018). Table 10.1.1 depicts the classification of systemic diseases or conditions affecting the periodontal supporting tissues. For more detailed case definitions and diagnostic considerations, see Albandar et al. (2018).

Down's syndrome

Down's syndrome (DS) is a genetic disorder that results from a trisomy on chromosome 21 (Carrada et al. 2016). It is present in approximately 1 in 600 to 1 in 1000 live births (Frydman et al. 2012). Patients with DS have been shown to have an increased susceptibility to periodontal disease (PD) (Brown 1978), ranging from 36% to 100% (Frydman et al. 2012). DS patients have been described as developing extensive gingivitis at an early age, which becomes more generalized and rapidly progressive PD in young adulthood (Scalioni et al. 2018). By the end of the fourth decade of life, these patients are then often experiencing severe tooth mobility and tooth loss (Sterling 1992). An increased susceptibility to PD is usually manifested clinically by significantly more missing teeth, greater bleeding on probing, as well as higher gingival and plaque indices (Khocht et al. 2010), although with dental caries being found to be less prevalent (Siosen et al. 2000). It is thus important for clinicians to know that DS patients need a thorough prophylaxis already from an early age.

The clinical and radiographic appearance of PD in patients with DS often resembles the pattern of bone loss observed in aggressive PD, with most lesions detected in the mandibular incisors. Other affected teeth can also include the maxillary and mandibular first molars, with the canines being the least affected (Modeer et al. 1990). However, it has been stated that poor oral hygiene *per se* may not explain the severity of the generalized PD observed in DS patients (Carrada et al. 2016).

Other mechanisms such as impairment of the immune system, including reduced T- and B-cell counts, the absence of a normal lymphocyte expansion observed in infancy, the lack of antibody responses to immunizations, a decreased immunoglobulin-A secretion in saliva, as well as high levels of tumor necrosis factor (TNF)-α and interferon (IFN)-γ cytokine secretion, together with an altered expression of immune-related genes in children with DS (Rostami et al. 2012), are thus also possibilities accentuating other pathophysiological molecular mechanisms involved in children with DS (Ferreira et al. 2016). Other studies have also described a diminished chemotaxis of neutrophils, a decreased phagocytic ability, as well as a shortened half-life of neutrophils (Yavuzyilmaz et al. 1993).

Advanced tissue destruction has also been ascribed to the induction of both endogenous and exogenous collagenase activity, whereby increased amounts and activity of neutrophil-derived matrix metalloproteinase-2 (MMP), as well as MMP-8 and MMP-9, have been described, due to activation by *Aggregatibacter actinomycetemcomitans* and *Porphyromonas gingivalis,* respectively (Halinen et al. 1996; Tiranathanagul et al. 2004). *P. gingivalis* has been reported to increase collagen degradation by human gingival fibroblasts, coinciding with increased activation of MMPs and lowered tissue inhibitor of metalloproteinase protein levels (Santos et al. 1996; Zhou & Windsor 2006). Comparisons made between patients who have mental challenges and those with DS have shown a preponderance in DS patients for higher amounts of periodontal pathogens, including among others *P. gingivalis, Tannerella forsythia*, and *A. actinomycetemcomitans* (Amano et al. 2000; Sakellari et al. 2001). Studies have also shown certain periodontopathic bacteria to be specifically associated with particular other species in the gingival sulcus microbiome, and in this manner thus contributing to the increased prevalence and severity of PD in DS patients (Carrada et al. 2016; Nuernberg et al. 2019). Other studies have not found these same results, however (Amano et al. 2000). Furthermore, a potential etiology of a co-infection by bacteria and viruses, namely Epstein–Barr virus type 1 and human cytomegalovirus, has been proposed (Hanookai et al. 2000). Tissue tropism associated with viruses may thus also explain the destruction seen in specific areas of the dentition in DS patients (Ting et al. 2000).

Table 10.1.1   Systemic diseases or conditions associated with degradation of periodontal tissues.

Systemic disorders impacting the loss of periodontal tissue by influencing periodontal inflammation	Genetic disorders	**Diseases associated with immunological disorders:** Down's syndrome, leukocyte adhesion deficiency syndromes, Papillon–Lefèvre syndrome, Haim–Munk syndrome, Chédiak–Higashi syndrome, severe neutropenia (congenital neutropenia, cyclic neutropenia), primary immunodeficiency diseases (chronic granulomatous disease, hyperimmunoglobulin E syndromes), Cohen syndrome
		Diseases affecting the oral mucosa and gingival tissue: Epidermolysis bullosa (dystrophic epidermolysis bullosa, Kindler syndrome), plasminogen deficiency
		Diseases affecting connective tissues: Ehlers–Danlos syndrome (types I, IV, VIII), angioedema (C1-inhibitor deficiency), systemic lupus erythematosus
		Metabolic and endocrine disorders: Glycogen storage disease, Gaucher disease, hypophosphatasia, hypophosphatemic rickets, Hajdu–Cheney syndrome, diabetes mellitus, obesity, osteoporosis
	Acquired immunodeficiency diseases	Acquired neutropenia HIV infection
	Inflammatory diseases	Epidermolysis bullosa acquisita, inflammatory bowel disease, arthritis (rheumatoid arthritis, osteoarthritis)
Other systemic disorders that influence the pathogenesis of periodontal diseases	Emotional stress and depression	
	Smoking (nicotine dependence)	
	Medications	
Systemic disorders that can result in loss of periodontal tissue independent of periodontitis	Neoplasms	Primary neoplastic diseases of periodontal tissue (oral squamous cell carcinoma, odontogenic tumors, other primary neoplasms of periodontal tissue), secondary metastatic neoplasms of periodontal tissue
	Other disorders that may affect periodontal tissue	Granulomatosis with polyangiitis, Langerhans cell histiocytosis, giant cell granulomas, hyperparathyroidism, systemic sclerosis (scleroderma), vanishing bone disease (Gorham–Stout syndrome)

Source: Adapted from Albandar et al. 2018.

Hematological diseases

Hematological diseases affect a large number of people globally. These diseases are disorders affecting the blood and blood-forming organs. Hematological diseases include rare genetic disorders, anemia, sickle cell disease, and hematological malignancies. Many of these diseases are very serious conditions where periodontitis is but one of many symptoms. Patients with leukemia often have gingival swelling, leading to periodontal pockets, and sometimes spontaneous gingival bleeding. Severe neutropenia and agranulocytosis frequently lead to severe periodontitis with rapidly progressing bone loss and subsequent tooth loss.

Patients with severe hematological diseases require specialist treatment in close collaboration with medical specialists. Generally, these patients need extensive prophylaxis, before and after treatment of their hematological disease (Ruchlemer et al. 2018).

Rare genetic disorders

There are numerous very rare genetic disorders that lead to severe periodontitis. Papillon–Lefèvre syndrome affects one to four individuals per million and leads to very rapid bone and tooth loss. Leucocyte adhesion deficiency (LAD) is another very rare disease that leads to severe periodontitis, with a prevalence of fewer than 10 cases per million. These disorders must be treated in close collaboration between dental and medical practitioner.

Neoplasms of the periodontium

Various forms of cancers can occur in all tissues of the body, as well as the periodontium. The most common is oral squamous cell carcinoma, which is a big health problem in some parts of the world. Oral cancers are among the top 15 most common cancers globally, with 500 550 new cases reported in 2018. The number of deaths due to oral cancer in 2018 was 177 384 (67% in males), giving an age-standardized rate of 2.8 per 100 000 males and 1.2 per 100 000 females. In 2018 the incidence of oral cancer was the highest among all cancers in Melanesia and South Asia among males, and it is the leading cause of cancer-related mortality among males in India and Sri Lanka (Bray et al. 2018).

The most important risk factors for oral squamous cell cancer are the usage of tobacco, smoking or chewing of tobacco products, human papilloma virus, and betel nuts.

Other oral cancers are, however, much less prevalent than squamous cell carcinoma, odontogenic tumors, and tumors of the salivary glands. Most salivary gland tumors are benign, with only 20% being malignant, but they can cause severe clinical problems, since they can obstruct salivary flow (Ogle 2020).

All cancers should be treated in close collaboration with a medical specialist.

HIV and periodontitis

Epidemiology of HIV infection

According to the World Health Organization, HIV is still a major global threat to human health. The disease killed more than 32 million people by the end of 2018. In 2018 alone, 770 000 people died from HIV-related causes. In the same year, 37.9 million people were living with HIV, and 1.7 million people were infected. Africa is the most affected continent, with 25.7 million people living with HIV and accounting for almost two-thirds of all new HIV infections.

Increased testing for HIV together with effective preventive measures, and the development and introduction of antiretroviral therapy (ART), have had a tremendous effect on the spread and mortality of HIV. Lifelong ART was being given to 62% of all adults and 52% of all children living with HIV in 2018. The incidence of HIV infections fell by 37% between 2000 and 2018, and HIV-related deaths fell by 45%, with 13.6 million lives saved by ART during the same period.

Diagnosis and treatment of HIV

Presently, HIV infection is diagnosed through rapid diagnostic tests (RDTs), which detect the presence or absence of antibodies toward the virus. Most often these tests provide same-day results, which are essential for same-day diagnosis and early treatment and care. There is no cure for HIV infection. However, effective ART drugs can control the virus and help prevent transmission, so that people with HIV can live a long and normal life. It is estimated that currently 79% of people with HIV know their status. In 2018, 23.3 million people living with HIV were receiving ART globally.

Oral and periodontal signs and symptoms of HIV infection

Oral candidiasis, Kaposi's sarcoma, lymphoma, and hairy leukoplakia used to be associated with HIV infection, but have decreased after the introduction of ART. HIV/AIDS-associated periodontal lesions such as linear gingival erythema, necrotizing ulcerative periodontitis (NUP), and necrotizing ulcerative gingivitis (NUG) have also decreased after the introduction of ART. However, chronic periodontitis is still a problem in patients with HIV infection. Most clinical/epidemiological studies in recent years show that periodontitis is more prevalent and more severe, although many studies are hampered by not having a socioeconomically comparable control group. Two recent studies using comparable control groups showed no differences in the prevalence or severity of periodontitis, suggesting that lifestyle is an important confounder (Spolsky et al. 2018; Williams-Wiles & Vieira 2019).

Treatment modalities or protocols

Normal non-surgical periodontal treatment has been shown to be equally effective in HIV-infected patients compared to the same treatment in non-infected patients. The increased prevalence and severity of periodontitis make stringent prophylaxis and frequent follow-up visits important.

Future trends in management

ART has already made HIV a more or less chronic disease. Future progress in antiviral treatment and the possibility of an effective vaccine will most probably decrease oral problems related to HIV infection.

REFERENCES

Albandar JM, Susin C, Hughes FJ. Manifestations of systemic diseases and conditions that affect the periodontal attachment apparatus: case definitions and diagnostic considerations. *J Clin Periodontol.* 2018; 45(Suppl 20):S171–S189.

Amano A, Kishima T, Kimura S et al. Periodontopathic bacteria in children with Down syndrome. *J Periodonol.* 2000; 71:249–255.

Bray F, Ferlay J, Soerjomataram I et al. Global cancer statistics 2018: GLOBOCAN estimates of incidence and mortality worldwide for 36 cancers in 185 countries. *CA Cancer J Clin.* 2018; 68:394–424.

Brown RH. A longitudinal study of periodontal disease in Down's syndrome. *NZ Dent J.* 1978; 74:137–144.

Carrada CF, Scalioni FAR, Cesar DE et al. Salivary periodontopathic bacteria in children and adolescents with Down Syndrome. *PLoS One.* 2016; 11. doi: 10.1371/journal.pone.0162988.

Caton JG, Armitage G, Berglundh T et al. A new classification scheme for periodontal and peri-implant diseases and conditions – introduction and key changes from the 1999 classification. *J Clin Periodontol.* 2018; 45(Suppl 20):S1–S8.

Ferreira R, Michel RC, Greghi SLA et al. Prevention and periodontal treatment in Down syndrome patients: a systematic review. *PLoS One.* 2016; 11(6):e0158339.

Frydman A, Nowzari H. Down syndrome-associated periodontitis: a critical review of the literature. *Compendium.* 2012; 33:356–361.

Halinen S, Sorsa T, Ding Y et al. Characterization of matrix metalloproteinase (MMP-8 and -9) activities in the saliva and in gingival crevicular fluid of children with Down's syndrome. *J Periodontol.* 1996; 67:748–754.

Hanookai D, Nowzari H, Contreras A et al. Herpesvirus and periodontopathic bacteria in trisomy 21 periodontitis. *J Periodontol.* 2000; 71:376–384.

Jepsen S, Caton JG, Albandar JM et al. Periodontal manifestations of systemic diseases and developmental and acquired conditions: consensus report of workgroup 3 of the 2017 World Workshop on the classification of periodontal and peri-implant diseases and conditions. *J Clin Periodontol.* 2018; 45(Suppl 20):S219–S229.

Khocht A, Janal M, Turner B. Periodontal health in Down syndrome: contributions of mental disability, personal, and professional dental care. *Spec Care Dentist.* 2010; 30: 118–123.

Modeer T, Barr M, Dahllof G. Periodontal disease in children with Down's syndrome. *Scand J Dent Res.* 1990; 98:228–234.

Nuernberg MAA, Ivanaga CA, Haas AN et al. Periodontal status of individuals with Down's syndrome: sociodemographic, behavioural and family perception influence. *J Intellect Disabil Res.* 2019; 63(10):1181–1192.

Ogle OE. Salivary gland diseases. *Dent Clin North Am.* 2020; 64(1):87–104.

Rostami MN, Douraghi M, Mohammadi AM, Nikmanesh B. Altered serum pro-inflammatory cytokines in children with Down's syndrome. *Eur Cytokine Netw.* 2012; 23:64–67.

Ruchlemer R, Amit-Kohn M, Tvito A et al. Bone loss and hematological malignancies in adults: a pilot study. *Support Care Cancer.* 2018; 26(9):3013–3020.

Sakellari D, Belibasakis G, Chadjipadelis T et al. Supragingival and subgingival microbiota of adult patients with Down's syndrome. Changes after periodontal treatment. *Oral Microbiol Immunol.* 2001; 16:376–382.

Santos R, Shanfeld J, Casamassimo P. Serum antibody response to *Actinobacillus Actinomycetemcomitans* in Down's syndrome. *Spec Care Dentist.* 1996; 16:80–83.

Scalioni FAR, Carrada CF, Martins CC, Ribeiro RA, Paiva SM. Periodontal disease in patients with Down syndrome: a systematic review. *J Am Dent Assoc.* 2018; 149(7):628–639.e11.

Siosen PB, Furgang D, Steinberg LM, Fine DH. Proximal caries in juvenile periodontitis patients. *J Periodontol.* 2000; 71:710–716.

Spolsky VW, Clague J, Shetty V. Cohort study of HIV-positive and -negative methamphetamine users. *J Am Dent Assoc.* 2018; 149(7):599–607.

Sterling ES. Oral and dental considerations in Down syndrome. In: I Lott, E McCoy, ed. *Down Syndrome Advances in Medical Care.* New York: Wiley-Liss; 1992: 135–145.

Ting M, Contreras A, Slots J. Herpesvirus in localized juvenile periodontitis. *J Periodontal Res.* 2000; 35:17–25.

Tiranathanagul S, Yongchaitrakul T, Pattamapun K, Pavasant P. *Actinobacillus actinomycetemcomitans* lipopolysaccharide activates matrix metalloporteinase-2 and increases receptor activator of nuclear factor-kappaB ligand expression in human periodontal ligament cells. *J Periodontol.* 2004; 75:1647–1654.

Williams-Wiles L, Vieira AR. HIV status does not worsen oral health outcomes. *J Clin Periodontol.* 2019; 46(6):640–641.

Yavuzyilmaz E, Ersoy F, Sanal O, et al. Neutrophil chemotaxis and periodontal status in Down's syndrome patients. *J Nihon Univ Sch Dent.* 1993; 35:91–95.

Zhou J, Windsor LJ. *Porphyromonas gingivalis* affects host collagen degradation by affecting expression, activation, and inhibition of matrix metalloproteinases. *J Periodontal Res.* 2006; 41:47–54.

10.2.1 PERIODONTAL ABSCESS

Steph Smith

Contents

Learning objectives

- Case definition of a periodontal abscess.
- Prevalence, clinical features, diagnosis, and differential diagnosis.
- Classification of periodontal abscesses based on etiology.
- Microbiology, pathophysiology, and histopathology.
- Treatment and principles of antibiotic therapy.

Introduction

Periodontal abscesses represent common dental emergencies requiring immediate management that may result in rapid destruction of the periodontium, thus having a negative impact on the prognosis of the affected tooth. Periodontal abscesses have been suggested as the main cause for tooth extraction during the phase of supportive periodontal therapy (Chace & Low 1993). Furthermore, in certain circumstances, periodontal abscesses may have severe systemic consequences (Herrera et al. 2000c, 2014).

Case definition of a periodontal abscess

A periodontal abscess is a localized accumulation of pus located within the gingival wall of the periodontal pocket/sulcus, resulting in significant tissue breakdown, this occurring during a limited period of time, and with easily detectable clinical symptoms (Herrera et al. 2000c; Papapanou et al. 2018).

Prevalence

Periodontal abscesses represent approximately 7.7–14.0% of all dental emergencies, being ranked the third most prevalent infection demanding emergency treatment, after dentoalveolar abscesses and pericoronitis (Herrera et al. 2018). Abscesses occur more often in molar sites, which represent >50% of all sites affected by abscess formation; however, the lower anterior incisors may also be predominantly affected (Jaramillo et al. 2005). A higher number of abscesses have been reported in interproximal areas (Smith & Davies 1986), whereas other studies have observed more frequent abscess formation at buccal sites (Chan & Tien 2010; Herrera et al. 2000a).

Clinical features, diagnosis, and differential diagnosis

Periodontal abscesses are differentiated from periodontitis lesions by the following: (i) they have a rapid onset; (ii) there is rapid destruction of periodontal tissues, thereby necessitating the importance of prompt treatment; and (iii) pain or discomfort, leading patients to seek urgent care (Papapanou et al. 2018). In periodontitis patients, signs and symptoms may indicate a history of periodontal disease or previous periodontal therapy, together with the presence of deep periodontal pockets and usually tooth vitality (Herrera et al. 2015).

The primary detectable signs/symptoms are an ovoid elevation in the gingiva along the lateral part of the root and bleeding on probing, together with a deep periodontal pocket (Papapanou et al. 2018). Other signs/symptoms include pain, tenderness of the gingiva, swelling, and sensitivity to percussion of the affected tooth, as well as suppuration on probing, either through a fistula or, most commonly, through the pocket opening. Suppuration may be spontaneous or occur when pressure is applied to the outer surface of the lesion. Other related symptoms are tooth elevation and increased tooth mobility (Herrera et al. 2000c, 2018).

Radiographically, there may either be a normal appearance of the interdental bone or evident bone loss, including just a widening of the periodontal ligament space, or pronounced bone loss involving most of the affected root, including furcation lesions (Herrera et al. 2015, 2018).

Extraoral findings are not common, but may include facial swelling (3.6%), elevated body temperature, malaise, regional lymphadenopathy (7–40%), or increased blood leukocytes (Herrera et al. 2018).

Severe systemic consequences may also be associated with systemic dissemination of a localized infection, either through dissemination occurring during therapy or related to an untreated abscess (Herrera et al. 2018).

The differential diagnosis is of the utmost importance, and may include the following, among others: self-inflicted gingival injuries, sickle cell anemia, dento-alveolar abscesses, pericoronitis, endo-periodontal abscess, lateral periapical cyst, pyogenic granuloma, osteomyelitis, non-Hodgkin's lymphoma, squamous cell carcinoma, or metastatic carcinoma (Herrera et al. 2018).

Classification of periodontal abscesses

The classification is based on etiology, depending on the origin of the acute infectious process (Herrera et al. 2018). Two types of abscesses may occur (see Table 10.2.1.1).

Periodontitis-related abscess

As an acute exacerbation of a chronic lesion

May occur in an untreated periodontitis patient or as a recurrent infection during supportive periodontal therapy (Silva et al. 2008). The abscess is the result of an acute exacerbation of a chronic infection residing in the periodontal tissues (Herrera et al. 2015). The acute infection originates from bacteria present at the subgingival biofilm in a deepened periodontal pocket, whereby marginal closure of the pocket leads to an extension of the infection into the surrounding periodontal tissues (DeWitt et al. 1985; Herrera et al. 2018). Deep pockets and concavities associated with furcation lesions favour the development of these acute conditions (Herrera et al. 2015). Additionally, the composition of the subgingival microbiota can change and, together with increased bacterial virulence or a decreased host defense, inefficient drainage may lead to increased suppuration (Herrera et al. 2018).

Post-therapy periodontal abscesses

The lesions occur immediately after professional prophylaxis, usually related to small fragments of remaining calculus that are obstructing the pocket entrance or have been forced into previously non-inflamed periodontal tissues (Dello Russo 1985). Other instances may include the incomplete surgical removal of subgingival calculus or the post-surgical presence of foreign bodies in the periodontal tissues, such as sutures, regenerative

Table 10.2.1.1 Proposed classification of periodontal abscesses, based on etiological factors.

Periodontal abscess in periodontitis patient	Acute exacerbation Untreated periodontitis Non-responsive to periodontal therapy Supportive periodontal therapy After treatment Post scaling Post surgery Post medication Systemic antimicrobials Nifedipine and other drugs
Periodontal abscess in non-periodontitis patients	Impaction Dental floss, orthodontic elastic, toothpick, rubber dam, popcorn hulls Harmful habits Wire or nail biting, clenching Orthodontic factors Orthodontic forces, cross-bite Gingival overgrowth Alteration of root surface Severe anatomic alterations Invaginated tooth, dens evaginatus, odontodysplasia Minor anatomic alterations Cemental tears, enamel pearls, developmental grooves Iatrogenic conditions Perforations Severe root damage Fissure or fracture, cracked tooth syndrome External root resorption

Source: Adapted from Herrera et al. 2018.

devices, or pieces of periodontal pack (Garrett et al. 1997). Treatment with systemic antibiotics without appropriate subgingival debridement may lead to the subgingival biofilm being partially protected from the action of the antibiotic, resulting in an acute infection (Helovuo et al. 1993).

Non-periodontitis-related abscess

In this instance external local factors are responsible, which may include the impaction of foreign bodies, harmful habits, orthodontic appliances, and gingival overgrowth (Herrera et al. 2015, 2018). Other external factors include anatomic factors affecting root morphology, such as invaginated roots, presence of fissures, developmental grooves, external root resorption, root tears, or iatrogenic endodontic perforations (Herrera et al. 2015, 2018).

Microbiology

Periodontal abscesses have a microbial composition similar to that observed in periodontitis (Herrera et al. 2018). The most prevalent bacterial species identified are *Porphyromonas gingivalis* (50–100%), *Prevotella intermedia*, *Prevotella melaninogenica*, *Fusobacterium nucleatum*, *Tannerella forsythia*, *Treponema* species, *Campylobacter* species, *Capnocytophaga* species, and *Aggregatibacter actinomycetemcomitans* (Eguchi et al. 2008; Herrera et al. 2018; Jaramillo et al. 2005).

Pathophysiology

Occlusion of the periodontal pocket lumen, due to trauma or tissue tightening, has been hypothesized to prevent proper drainage, resulting in extension of the infection from the pocket into the soft tissues of the pocket wall (Herrera et al. 2015). The invasion of bacteria into the soft tissue pocket wall initiates the induction of an inflammatory process. Chemotactic factors released by bacteria attract polymorphonuclear leucocytes (PMN) and other inflammatory cells. This triggers the release of catabolic cytokines, leading to destruction of the connective tissues, encapsulation of the bacterial infection, and the production of pus. Once the abscess is formed, the rate of destruction within the abscess will depend on the growth of bacteria inside the foci, their virulence, and an acidic environment that favors the activity of lysosomal enzymes (DeWitt et al. 1985).

Histopathology

When observing the lesion from the outside to the inside, the following have been observed: a normal oral epithelium and lamina propria; an acute inflammatory infiltrate; an intense focus of inflammation, with the presence of PMNs and lymphocytes in an area of destroyed and necrotic connective tissue; and a destroyed and ulcerated pocket epithelium (DeWitt et al. 1985).

Treatment

Treatment is usually performed in two stages (Herrera et al. 2015).

Management of the acute lesion

- *Mechanical therapy*, which includes incision and surgical drainage through the pocket, and scaling and planing of the root surface with/without periodontal surgery.
- *Locally or systemically administered antibiotics*. For abscesses with marked swelling, tension, and pain, the initial treatment recommended is the administration of systemic antibiotics alone, and once the acute condition has receded,

mechanical debridement, including root planing, should be performed. In principle, high dosages of antibiotic delivered over short time periods (5 days) are recommended (Herrera et al. 2015). Antibiotic therapy may not always be able to resolve the infection (Herrera et al. 2015), as the presence of resistant strains of periodontal pathogens has been described (Herrera et al. 2000b; Jaramillo et al. 2005). Therefore, essential for definitive treatment, antibiotic usage should always be in combination with the first treatment option, which includes incision, drainage, and mechanical debridement, with or without surgical flaps (Herrera et al. 2015). Proposed antibiotic regimes that have been used are:

- Systemic metronidazole (200 mg three times a day for 5 days) (Smith & Davies 1986).
- Systemic tetracycline therapy for 2 weeks (Hafström et al. 1994).
- Amoxicillin/clavulanate, 500 mg + 125 mg three times a day for 8 days (Herrera et al. 2000b).
- Azithromycin, 500 mg once a day for 3 days (Herrera et al. 2000b).

Management of the original and/or residual lesion

This includes appropriate treatment once the emergency situation has been controlled (Herrera et al. 2015).

REFERENCES

Chace RJ, Low SB. Survival characteristics of periodontally-involved teeth: a 40-year study. *J Periodontol.* 1993; 64:701–705.

Chan YK, Tien WS. Clinical parameters of periodontal abscess: a case series of 14 abscesses. *Malays Dent J.* 2010; 31:6–7.

Dello Russo MM. The post-prophylaxis periodontal abscess: etiology and treatment. *Int J Periodontics Restorative Dent.* 1985; 1:29–37.

DeWitt GV, Cobb CM, Killoy WJ. The acute periodontal abscess: microbial penetration of the soft tissue wall. *Int J Periodontics Restorative Dent.* 1985; 5:38–51.

Eguchi T, Koshy G, Umeda M et al. Microbial changes in patients with acute periodontal abscess after treatment detected by PadoTest. *Oral Dis.* 2008; 14(2):180–184.

Garrett S, Polson AM, Stoller NH et al. Comparison of a bioabsorbable GTR barrier to a non-absorbable barrier in treating human class II furcation defects. A multi-center parallel design randomized single-blind study. *J Periodontol.* 1997; 68:667–675.

Hafström CA, Wikström MB, Renvert SN, Dahlén GG. Effect of treatment on some periodontopathogens and their antibody levels in periodontal abscesses. *J Periodontol.* 1994; 65:1022–1028.

Helovuo H, Hakkarainen K, Paunio K. Changes in the prevalence of subgingival enteric rods, staphylococci and yeasts after treatment with penicillin and erythromycin. *Oral Microbiol Immunol.* 1993; 8:75–79.

Herrera D, Alonso B, de Arriba L et al. Acute periodontal lesions. *Periodontol 2000.* 2014; 65:149–177.

Herrera D, Retamal-Valdes B, Alonso B, Feres M. Acute periodontal lesions (periodontal abscesses and necrotizing periodontal diseases) and endo-periodontal lesions. *J Clin Periodontol.* 2018; 45(Suppl 20):S78–S94.

Herrera D, Roldan S, Gonzalez I, Sanz M. The periodontal abscess (I). Clinical and microbiological findings. *J Clin Periodontol.* 2000a; 27:387–394.

Herrera D, Roldán S, O´Connor A, Sanz M. The periodontal abscess: II. Short-term clinical and microbiological efficacy of two systemic antibiotics regimes. *J Clin Periodontol.* 2000b; 27:395–404.

Herrera D, Roldan S, Sanz M. The periodontal abscess: a review. *J Clin Periodontol.* 2000c; 27:377–386.

Herrera D, van Winkelhoff AJ, Sanz M. Abscesses in the periodontium. In: J Lindhe, NP Lang, ed. *Clinical Periodontology and Implant Dentistry.* Oxford: Wiley-Blackwell; 2015: 463–471.

Jaramillo A, Arce RM, Herrera D et al. Clinical and microbiological characterization of periodontal abscesses. *J Clin Periodontol.* 2005; 32:1213–1218.

Papapanou PN, Sanz M, Nurcan Buduneli N et al. Periodontitis: consensus report of Workgroup 2 of the 2017 World Workshop on the Classification of Periodontal and Peri-Implant Diseases and Conditions. *J Clin Periodontol.* 2018; 45(Suppl 20):S162–S170.

Silva GL, Soares RV, Zenóbio EG. Periodontal abscess during supportive periodontal therapy: a review of the literature. *J Contemp Dent Pract.* 2008; 9:82–91.

Smith RG, Davies RM. Acute lateral periodontal abscesses. *Br Dent J.* 1986; 161:176–178.

10.2.2 ENDODONTIC-PERIODONTAL LESIONS

Steph Smith and Qiang Zhu

Contents

Learning objectives

- Case definition, the signs and symptoms of endodontic-periodontal lesions (EPLs).
- Etiology, pathophysiology, and microbiological aspects of EPLs.
- Risk factors involved for the occurrence of EPLs.
- How to diagnose and classify EPLs.
- The differential diagnosis of periodontal and periapical abscesses.
- Treatment of EPLs.

Case definition of an endodontic-periodontal lesion

An endodontic-periodontal lesion (EPL) is a pathologic communication between the pulpal and periodontal tissues at a given tooth that may occur in an acute or a chronic form (Papapanou et al. 2018).

- When EPLs are associated with a recent traumatic or iatrogenic event (e.g. root fracture or perforation), the most common manifestation is an abscess accompanied by pain.
- When EPLs are associated with periodontal disease, they normally present with slow and chronic progression without evident symptoms (Herrera et al. 2018).

Signs and symptoms (Herrera et al. 2018)

- Deep periodontal pockets – reaching to or close to apex.
- Altered or negative responses to pulp vitality tests.
- Bone resorption in apical or furcation region.
- Spontaneous pain or pain with palpation and percussion.
- Purulent exudate.
- Tooth mobility.
- Sinus tract.
- Gingival color alterations.

Etiology

An established EPL is always associated with varying degrees of microbial contamination of the dental pulp and the supporting periodontal tissues, and can be:

- *Associated with endodontic and periodontal infections*, which are triggered:
  - By a carious lesion that affects the pulp and, secondarily, affects the periodontium.
  - By periodontal destruction that secondarily affects the root canal.
  - Or by both events concomitantly ("true-combined" lesion). The periodontal condition has an important impact on the prognosis of the EPL (Herrera et al. 2018).
- *Associated with trauma and iatrogenic factors*, due to:
  - Root/pulp chamber/furcation perforation (e.g. because of root canal instrumentation or tooth preparation for post-retained restorations).
  - Root fracture or cracking (e.g. because of trauma or tooth preparation for post-retained restorations).
  - External root resorption (e.g. because of trauma).
  - Pulp necrosis (e.g. because of trauma) draining through the periodontium.

These conditions usually have a *poor prognosis* as they affect the tooth structure (Herrera et al. 2018).

Pathophysiology

Communication pathways exist between the dental pulp and the periodontium, which includes the apical foramina, accessory/lateral canals (which are more prevalent in the apical third and furcation area), and dentinal tubules. Pathological communication between these, including the migration of microorganisms and inflammatory mediators between the root canal and the periodontium, can thus lead to EPLs (Herrera et al. 2018).

Microbiology

No major differences have been found between microorganisms located in endodontic and periodontal lesions, including the presence of any specific bacterial profile associated with EPLs. The latter are attributed to both sites of infection (root canal and periodontal pockets) being anaerobic environments exposed to similar nutrients (Herrera et al. 2018). The bacterial species that have most often been identified are *Porphyromonas gingivalis*, *Tannerella forsythia*, *Parvimonas micra*, *Fusobacterium*, *Prevotella*, and *Treponema* (Pereira et al. 2011; Rupf et al. 2000; Xia & Qi 2013). These species and genera have also recently been shown to be associated with chronic or aggressive periodontitis (Oliveira et al. 2016; Perez-Chaparro et al. 2014).

Risk factors for the occurrence of endodontic-periodontal lesions (Herrera et al. 2018)

- Advanced periodontitis.
- Trauma.
- Iatrogenic events.
- Palatal grooves.
- Furcation involvements.
- Porcelain fused to metal (PFM) crowns.
- Active carious lesions.

Diagnosis of endodontic-periodontal lesions

The diagnosis and classification should be based on the *present disease status* and the *prognosis* of the tooth involved, which would determine the first step of the treatment planning, i.e. whether to *maintain* or *extract* the tooth (Herrera et al. 2018). Determining the primary source of infection as a basis for a classification is not relevant for the treatment of EPL, as both the root canal and the periodontal tissues would require treatment (Al-Fouzan 2014; Chapple & Lumley 1999; Meng 1999).

The three main prognostic groups for a tooth with an EPL are (Herrera et al. 2018) (i) hopeless, (ii) poor, and (iii) favorable:

- A hopeless prognosis is associated with EPL caused by trauma or iatrogenic factors (Figure 10.2.2.1).
- A prognosis ranging from favorable to hopeless for an EPL associated with endodontic and periodontal infections will depend on:
  - The extension of the periodontal destruction around the affected tooth.
  - The presence and severity of the periodontal disease affecting the patient's oral health.

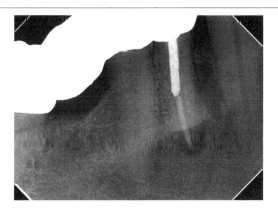

Figure 10.2.2.1 Tooth #28 shows irregular radiolucency in the mesial side of the root. Narrow isolated deep probing in the mesial buccal side confirms root fracture. Tooth #28 was extracted.

Diagnosis includes the following (Herrera et al. 2018):

- Assessment of the patient's history, clinical and radiographic examination.
- If there is a patient history of trauma, endodontic instrumentation, or post preparation: detailed clinical and radiographic examinations to seek the presence of perforations, fractures, cracking, or external root resorption, and root anatomy, this being done to assess the integrity of the root and to help with making a differential diagnosis.
- If this is not identified, then a full-mouth periodontal assessment should be performed (to assess presence, absence, and extent of periodontal disease), including probing depth, attachment level, bleeding on probing, suppuration, and mobility, as well as tooth vitality and percussion tests. The presence of a periodontal pocket reaching or close to the apex, combined with the absence of pulp vitality, would indicate the presence of an EPL.

Differential diagnosis of periodontal and periapical abscesses

Table 10.2.2.1 provides some general guidelines for the differential diagnosis.

Classification of endodontic-periodontal lesions

An EPL should be classified according to signs and symptoms feasible to assess at the time that the lesion is detected and that have a direct impact on its treatment, such as the presence or the absence of fractures and perforations, the presence or absence of periodontitis, and the extent of the periodontal destruction around the affected teeth (Herrera et al. 2018). Table 10.2.2.2 depicts the proposed classification of EPLs.

Table 10.2.2.1 Differential diagnosis of periodontal and periapical abscesses.

	Periapical abscess	Periodontal abscess
History	Previous pulpal and apical symptoms Trauma	Periodontal signs and symptoms
Location	In apical area below attached gingiva	Gingiva and/or attached gingiva
Pulp test	No response	Pulp response normal (if no endodontic treatment before)
Periodontal breakdown	No periodontal breakdown Generally no connection with pocket unless drainage through the sulcus Or narrow localized pocket to the lesion	Periodontal pocket and alveolar bone resorption
Radiograph evaluation	Lesion around apical area Gutta percha in the sinus tract goes to apex Or unusual periodontal bone resorption	No apical lesion Gutta-perch point in the sinus tract stops before going to the apex

Treatment

The primary endodontic lesion with a secondary periodontal involvement is always first started with the initialization of root canal treatment. Periodontal healing normally occurs after endodontic therapy (Figure 10.2.2.2).

Saving teeth associated with traumatic or iatrogenic events may be attempted by repairing the perforation, by halting the process of resorption with calcium hydroxide, or by removing the diseased root in multirooted teeth (Figure 10.2.2.3).

If the EPL is clearly due to periodontal disease without endodontic involvement, then there is no need for endodontic consideration. Generally, symptomatic retrograde pulpitis does not occur until the apical foramen is involved due to deep periodontal pockets reaching the apex.

In cases where there are concomitant pulpal-periodontal lesions whereby the disease processes exist independently in both tissues, then both endodontic and periodontal treatment is needed.

Table 10.2.2.2 Classification of endodontic-periodontal lesions.

Endo-periodontal lesion with root damage	Root fracture or cracking	
	Root canal or pulp chamber perforation	
	External root resorption	
Endo-periodontal lesion without root damage	Endo-periodontal lesion in periodontitis patients	Grade 1 – narrow deep periodontal pocket in 1 tooth surface
		Grade 2 – wide deep periodontal pocket in 1 tooth surface
		Grade 3 – deep periodontal pockets in more than 1 tooth surface
	Endo-periodontal lesion in non-periodontitis patients	Grade 1 – narrow deep periodontal pocket in 1 tooth surface
		Grade 2 – wide deep periodontal pocket in 1 tooth surface
		Grade 3 – deep periodontal pockets in more than 1 tooth surface

Source: Herrera et al. 2018, with permission of John Wiley & Sons.

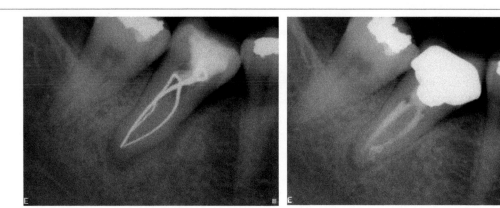

Figure 10.2.2.2 Tooth #31 shows an apical lesion and radiolucency extend along the mesial side of the root to the marginal ridge. One year after root canal retreatment, a radiograph revealed the complete resolution of radiolucency along the mesial side of the root. The apical radiolucency had significantly reduced.

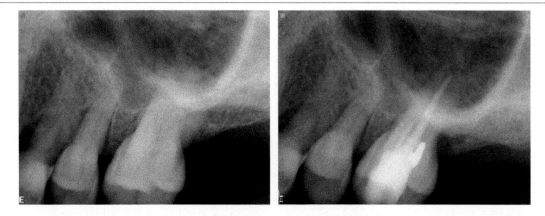

Figure 10.2.2.3 Tooth #14 had a vertical fracture on the distal buccal root and was treated by root canal therapy followed by distal buccal root amputation.

REFERENCES

Al-Fouzan KS. A new classification of endodontic periodontal lesions. *Int J Dent.* 2014; 2014:919173.

Chapple IL, Lumley PJ. The periodontal-endodontic interface. *Dent Update.* 1999; 26(8):331–336.

Herrera D, Retamal-Valdes B, Alonso B, Feres M. Acute periodontal lesions (periodontal abscesses and necrotizing periodontal diseases) and endo-periodontal lesions. *J Periodontol.* 2018; 89(Suppl 1):S85–S102.

Meng HX. Periodontic-endodontic lesions. *Ann Periodontol.* 1999; 4:84–90.

Oliveira RR, Fermiano D, Feres M et al. Levels of candidate periodontal pathogens in subgingival biofilm. *J Dent Res.* 2016; 95:711–718.

Papapanou PN, Sanz M, Buduneli N et al. Periodontitis: consensus report of Workgroup 2 of the 2017 World Workshop on the Classification of Periodontal and Peri-Implant Diseases and Conditions. *J Clin Periodontol.* 2018; 45(S20):S162–S170.

Pereira CV, Stipp RN, Fonseca DC, Pereira LJ, Höfling JF. Detection and clonal analysis of anaerobic bacteria associated to endodontic-periodontal lesions. *J Periodontol.* 2011; 82:1767–1775.

Perez Chaparro PJ, Gonçalves C, Figueiredo LC et al. Newly identified pathogens associated with periodontitis: a systematic review. *J Dent Res.* 2014; 93:846–858.

Rupf S, Kannengiesser S, Merte K et al. Comparison of profiles of key periodontal pathogens in periodontium and endodontium. *Endod Dent Traumatol.* 2000; 16:269–275.

Xia M, Qi Q. Bacterial analysis of combined periodontal-endodontic lesions by polymerase chain reaction-denaturing gradient gel electrophoresis. *J Oral Sci.* 2013; 55:287–291.

10.3 MUCOGINGIVAL CONDITIONS AND DEFORMITIES

Steph Smith

Contents

Learning objectives

- The concept of mucogingival conditions not being necessarily associated with the development of a pathosis.
- Classifications of periodontal phenotypes and gingival recessions.
- Predisposing factors for development of gingival recessions and the different clinical conditions associated with them.

Introduction

A normal mucogingival condition is defined as the absence of pathosis, this being within an individual's variability of anatomy and morphology, and is thus associated with periodontal health, for example an individual's periodontal phenotype. Other mucogingival conditions and deformities that are not necessarily associated with the development of pathosis are, for example a lack of keratinized tissues, decreased vestibular depth, an aberrant frenum/muscle position, gingival excess, and an abnormal color (Cortellini & Bissada 2018).

Classification of mucogingival conditions and deformities (Cortellini & Bissada 2018)

- Gingival/periodontal phenotype.
- Gingival recession.
- Lack of keratinized gingiva.
- Decreased vestibular depth.
- Aberrant muscle/frenum position.
- Gingival excess.
- Abnormal color.

Gingival/periodontal phenotype

A phenotype can be site specific and indicates a dimension that may change over time, and describes the appearance of an organ based on a multifactorial combination of genetic traits, environmental factors, and clinical intervention. The gingival phenotype is determined by gingival thickness and the keratinized tissue width. The periodontal phenotype is determined by the gingival phenotype and the bone morphotype, i.e. the thickness of the buccal bone plate (Jepsen et al. 2018).

Determination of the periodontal phenotype is necessary for assessing therapy outcomes in periodontal and implant therapy, prosthodontics, and orthodontics (Cortellini & Bissada 2018). The term has been extended to include peri-implant dimensions to describe the peri-implant phenotype (Kao et al. 2020).

Classification of periodontal phenotype

Three categories of periodontal phenotypes have been classified (Zweers et al. 2014):
- *Thin scalloped phenotype* is associated with slender triangular crowns; a subtle cervical convexity; interproximal contacts being close to incisal edges and a narrow zone of keratinized tissue (KT); clear, thin, delicate gingiva; and relatively thin alveolar bone.
- *Thick flat phenotype* is associated with square-shaped tooth crowns; pronounced cervical convexity; large interproximal contacts located more apically; a broad zone of KT; thick, fibrotic gingiva, and comparatively thick alveolar bone.
- *Thick scalloped phenotype* is associated with thick fibrotic gingiva; slender teeth; a narrow zone of KT; and pronounced gingival scalloping.

To diagnose the periodontal phenotype, a periodontal probe can be used to determine the visual detection thereof through the gingival sulcus. Visual detection of the probe is associated with a thin periodontal phenotype, and the inability to visualize the probe is associated with a thick/average periodontal phenotype (Kan et al. 2010).

Individual cases should not be referred to as being a thick phenotype versus a thin phenotype, but should rather be assessed based on genetic and environmental factors. Variations in gingival phenotype exist among individuals, in patterns of bilateral symmetry as well as regarding tooth location within individuals (Kao et al. 2020).

Determinants of periodontal phenotype

Discernment of the different phenotypes is based upon the anatomic characteristics of the components of the masticatory complex (Cortellini & Bissada 2018; Kao et al. 2020):
- *Gingival thickness* varies among different individuals as well as in different areas of the mouth within the same individual (Kao et al. 2020); maxillary central incisors present with the greatest mean thickness, followed by lateral incisors and canines (Kao et al. 2020); a positive correlation has been shown between keratinized tissue width and gingival thickness in maxillary anterior teeth (Kao et al. 2020); and is usually thinner in thin periodontal phenotypes, especially around the cuspids (Cortellini & Bissada 2018). Individuals with thin tissue and narrow gingival width tend to have a higher incidence of gingival recession (Kao et al. 2020). Pocket depth may also be greater in subjects with a thick gingival phenotype (Kao et al. 2020).
- *Keratinized tissue width* can range in a thin phenotype from 2.75 mm to 5.44 mm and in a thick phenotype from 5.09 mm to 6.65 mm. Maxillary lateral incisors have the greatest keratinized tissue width, followed by central incisors and canines (Kao et al. 2020).
- *Bone morphotype*: a mean buccal bone thickness of 0.343 mm for a thin phenotype and 0.754 mm for a thick/average phenotype has been described (Cortellini & Bissada 2018).
- *Tooth position*: a buccal position of the tooth in the alveolar process is frequently associated with a thin gingiva and a thin labial bone plate (Cook et al. 2011; Muller & Kononen 2005).

When assessing periodontal phenotypes based on gingival thickness, a thick phenotype is more frequently observed (51.9%) than a thin phenotype (42.3%). When assessment is based on the gingival morphotype, then there is usually a more equal distribution, i.e. thick 38.4%, thin 30.3%, and normal 45.7%. In general, thin phenotypes have an increased risk for pathosis, including recession, inflammation, or periodontitis/peri-implantitis, compared to thick ones (Kao et al. 2020; Kim & Neiva 2015; Scheyer et al. 2015). This may thus influence the integrity of the periodontium throughout the patient's life, and constitute a risk when applying orthodontic, implant, and restorative treatments (Ahmad 2005; Johal et al. 2010; Kois 2001).

Gingival recession

Gingival recession is defined as the apical shift of the gingival margin with respect to the cementoenamel junction (CEJ). It is associated with attachment loss and with exposure of the root surface to the oral environment (Cortellini & Bissada 2018; Pini Prato 1999).

Table 10.3.1 depicts the predisposing factors responsible for the development of gingival recession (Cortellini & Bissada 2018).

Classification of gingival recession

From a clinical diagnostic point of view, it has been shown that recessions associated with the integrity of the interdental attachment have the potential for complete root coverage. Full root coverage has also been reported in sites with limited clinical attachment loss (CAL), whereas loss of interdental attachment reduces the potential for complete root coverage, and very severe CAL impairs that possibility (Tatakis et al. 2015; Tonetti & Jepsen 2014). The development of modern advanced surgical techniques has also led to the improvement of forecasting potential root coverage, this being in contrast to previous classification systems (Pini-Prato 2011). A new treatment-oriented recession classification based on the interdental CAL measurement has thus been proposed (Cairo et al. 2011). Table 10.3.2 outlines the proposed classification of recession, together with predicted potential treatment outcomes (Cairo et al. 2011; Pini-Prato 2011; Tonetti & Jepsen 2014).

Clinical conditions associated with gingival recession

Table 10.3.3 depicts various clinical conditions that may be encountered with gingival recession, including the findings of clinical studies.

For information regarding prevention of the occurrence of gingival recession or to treat single or multiple recessions, the reader is referred to reviews and reports from the 2014 European Federation of Periodontology and 2015 American Academy of Periodontology workshops (Cairo et al. 2014; Graziani et al. 2014). See also Chapter 17.

Table 10.3.1 Predisposing factors for the development of gingival recession.

Periodontal phenotype and attached gingiva	• A thin periodontal phenotype, absence of attached gingiva, and reduced thickness of the alveolar bone due to abnormal tooth position in the arch can lead to the development of gingival recession (Kao et al. 2020; Kassab & Cohen 2003; Kim & Neiva 2015; Zweers et al. 2014).
	• 2 mm of keratinized tissue and 1 mm of attached gingiva are desirable around teeth to maintain periodontal health, even though a minimum amount of keratinized tissue is not needed to prevent attachment loss when optimal plaque control is present (Kim & Neiva 2015).
	• Periodontal health can be maintained in sites exhibiting a thin gingival phenotype, provided good oral hygiene is performed and iatrogenic factors are absent (Kao et al. 2020).
Impact of toothbrushing	• Systematic reviews have concluded that data are inconclusive to support or refute the association between toothbrushing and gingival recession (Heasman et al. 2017; Rajapakse et al. 2007).
	• However, improper toothbrushing method has been proposed as the most important mechanical factor contributing to the development of gingival recession (Kassab & Cohen 2003; Khocht et al. 1993; Sarfati et al. 2010).
	• Other potential risk factors are duration of toothbrushing, brushing force, frequency of changing the toothbrush, brush (bristle) hardness, toothbrushing technique, and toothbrushing frequency (Cortellini & Bissada 2018).
Impact of cervical restorative margins	• Sites with minimal or no gingiva associated with intrasulcular restorative margins are more prone to gingival recession and inflammation (Kim & Neiva 2015).
Impact of orthodontics	• Gingival recession may develop during or after orthodontic therapy, depending on the direction of the orthodontic movement (Joss-Vassalli et al. 2010; Renkema et al. 2013, 2015).
	• If a facially positioned tooth is moved in a lingual direction within the alveolar process, the apico-coronal tissue dimension on its facial aspect will increase in width (Karring et al. 1982).
	• The bucco-lingual thickness of the gingiva plays an important role in soft tissue alteration during orthodontic treatment (Kim & Neiva 2015).
	• There is a higher probability of recession during tooth movement in areas with <2 mm of gingiva, thus gingival augmentation may be indicated before initiation of orthodontic treatment in these areas (Cortellini & Bissada 2018; Kim & Neiva 2015).
Other conditions	• The following could contribute to the development of gingival recession: persistent gingival inflammation (e.g. bleeding on probing, swelling, edema, redness, and/or tenderness), shallow vestibular depth, frenum position, and clefts or fissures that restrict access for effective oral hygiene (Merijohn 2016).

Table 10.3.2 Classification of gingival recession based on interdental clinical attachment loss.

Recession type 1 (RT1)	Gingival recession with no loss of interproximal attachment. Interproximal cementoenamel junction (CEJ) is clinically not detectable at both mesial and distal aspects of the tooth. 100% root coverage can be predicted.
Recession type 2 (RT2)	Gingival recession associated with loss of interproximal attachment. The amount of interproximal clinical attachment loss (CAL) is less than or equal to the buccal attachment loss (measured from the buccal CEJ to the apical end of the buccal sulcus/pocket). By applying different root coverage procedures with limited interdental CAL, 100% root coverage is predictable.
Recession type 3 (RT3)	Gingival recession associated with loss of interproximal attachment. The amount of interproximal CAL is greater than the buccal attachment loss (measured from the buccal CEJ to the apical end of the buccal sulcus/pocket). In this instance, full root coverage is not achievable.

Source: Adapted from Cairo et al. 2011.

Table 10.3.3 Clinical conditions associated with gingival recession.

Long-term outcomes of untreated facial gingival recession defects	Untreated facial gingival recession in subjects with good oral hygiene will probably result in an increase in recession depth during long-term follow-up. However, the presence of keratinized tissue and/or greater gingival thickness may decrease the likelihood of a recession depth increase, or of the development of new gingival recession (Chambrone & Tatakis 2016).
Tooth loss	Limited evidence suggests that existing or progressing gingival recession does not lead to tooth loss (Agudio et al. 2016; Chambrone & Tatakis 2016).
Gingival augmentation in recession sites with thin gingival phenotype	Thin gingival phenotypes in recession sites augmented by grafting procedures remain more stable over time compared to non-augmented sites, which may show a limited increase in recession over time. However, in highly motivated patients, the development and/or progression of gingival recession and inflammation can be prevented (Agudio et al. 2016; Chambrone & Tatakis 2016).
Esthetics	A survey among dentists has shown that esthetics account for 90.7% of the justification for root coverage procedures (Zaher et al. 2005). However, esthetic ratings among patients are based on subjective assessment, and their perception of gingival recessions and the desire for treatment should be evaluated carefully before proceeding to treatment. The Smile Esthetic Index (SEI) has been proposed to assess the esthetic component of the smile, to be utilized by the dentist in the diagnostic phase and for setting appropriate treatment plans (Rotundo et al. 2015).
Dentin hypersensitivity	Dentin hypersensitivity (DH) is a common and transient oral condition, affecting quality of life. It is characterized by short and sharp pain, resulting immediately on stimulation of exposed dentin, and resolving on stimulus removal (Boiko et al. 2010; Holland et al. 1997). Risk factors include gingival recession, an erosive diet, and lifestyle (West et al. 2013). Treatment modalities include the use of different agents applied to the root surfaces or the application of root coverage procedures (De Oliveira et al. 2013; West et al. 2013). However, evidence is lacking that surgical root coverage procedures predictably reduce cervical DH (Cortellini & Bissada 2018).
Tooth conditions	Different conditions of the tooth, including root caries (Nuttall et al. 1998) and non-carious cervical lesions (NCCL) (Bartlett & Shah 2006; Pecie et al. 2011) may be associated with gingival recession, the prevalence being found to be high, and the severity of NCCL appearing to increase with age (Pecie et al. 2011; Pini-Prato et al. 2010). Historically, NCCL have been classified according to their appearance: wedge-shaped, disc-shaped, flattened, and irregular areas (Bartlett & Shah 2006; Pecie et al. 2011). However, these dental lesions cause modifications of the root/tooth surface, potentially causing disappearance of the original cementoenamel junction (CEJ) and/or the formation of concavities (steps) of different depths, with extension on the root surface (Pini-Prato et al. 2010). A classification has thus been proposed that includes four different scenarios of tooth-related conditions associated with gingival recession (Pini-Prato et al. 2010): Class A = detectable CEJ; Class B = undetectable CEJ; Class + = presence of a cervical step >0.5 mm; Class − = absence of a cervical step. The presence of NCCL is associated with a reduced probability of complete root coverage (Pini-Prato et al. 2015; Santamaria et al. 2010).

Source: Adapted from Cortellini & Bissada 2018.

REFERENCES

Agudio G, Cortellini P, Buti J, Pini Prato GP. Periodontal conditions of sites treated with gingival-augmentation surgery compared to untreated contralateral homologous sites: a 18- to 35-year long-term study. *J Periodontol.* 2016; 87:1371–1378.

Ahmad I. Anterior dental aesthetics: gingival perspective. *Br Dent J.* 2005; 199:195–202.

Bartlett DW, Shah P. A critical review of non-carious cervical (wear) lesions and the role of abfraction, erosion, and abrasion. *J Dent Res.* 2006; 85:306–312.

Boiko OV, Baker SR, Gibson BJ et al. Construction and validation of the quality of life measure for dentin hypersensitivity (DHEQ). *J Clin Periodontol.* 2010; 37:973–980.

Cairo F, Nieri M, Cincinelli S, Mervelt J, Pagliaro U. The interproximal clinical attachment level to classify gingival recessions and predict root coverage outcomes: an explorative and reliability study. *J Clin Periodontol.* 2011; 38:661–666.

Cairo F, Nieri M, Pagliaro U. Efficacy of periodontal plastic surgery procedures in the treatment of localized facial gingival recessions. *A systematic review. J Clin Periodontol.* 2014; 41(Suppl. 15):S44–S62.

Chambrone L, Tatakis DN. Long-term outcomes of untreated buccal gingival recessions. A systematic review and meta-analysis. *J Periodontol.* 2016; 87:796–808.

Cook DR, Mealey BL, Verrett RG et al. Relationship between clinical periodontal biotype and labial plate thickness: an in vivo study. *Int J Periodontics Restorative Dent.* 2011; 31:345–354.

Cortellini P, Bissada NF. Mucogingival conditions in the natural dentition: narrative review, case definitions, and diagnostic considerations. *J Clin Periodontol.* 2018; 45(Suppl 20):S190–S198.

De Oliveira DWD, Oliveira-Ferreira F, Flecha OD, Goncxalves PF. Is surgical root coverage effective for the treatment of cervical dentin hypersensitivity? *A systematic review. J Periodontol.* 2013; 84:295–306.

Graziani F, Gennai S, Rolda NS et al. Efficacy of periodontal plastic procedures in the treatment of multiple gingival recessions. *J Clin Periodontol.* 2014;41(Suppl. 15):S63–S76.

Heasman PA, Ritchie M, Asuni A et al. Gingival recession and root caries in the ageing population: a critical evaluation of treatments. *J Clin Periodontol.* 2017; 44(Suppl 18):S178–S193.

Holland GR, Nearhi MN, Addy M, Ganga-rosa L, Orchardson R. Guidelines for the design and conduct of clinical trials on dentin hypersensitivity. *J Clin Periodontol.* 1997; 24:808–813.

Jepsen S, Caton JG, Albandar JM et al. Periodontal manifestations of systemic diseases and developmental and acquired conditions: consensus report of Workgroup 3 of the 2017 World Workshop on the Classification of Periodontal and Peri-Implant Diseases and Conditions. *J Clin Periodontol.* 2018; 45(Suppl 20):S219–S229.

Johal A, Katsaros C, Kiliaridis S et al. Orthodontic therapy and gingival recession: a systematic review. *Orthod Craniofac Res.* 2010; 13:127–141.

Joss-Vassalli I, Grebenstein C, Topouzelis N, Sculean A, Katsaros C. Orthodontic therapy and gingival recession: a systematic review. *Orthod Craniofac Res.* 2010; 13:127–141.

Kan JY, Morimoto T, Rungcharassaeng K, Roe P, Smith DH. Gingival biotype assessment in the esthetic zone: visual versus direct measurement. *Int J Periodontics Restorative Dent.* 2010; 30:237–243.

Kao RT, Curtis DA, Kim DM et al. American Academy of Periodontology best evidence consensus statement on modifying periodontal phenotype in preparation for orthodontic and restorative treatment. *J Periodontol.* 2020; 91:289–298.

Karring T, Nyman S, Thilander B, Magnusson I. Bone regeneration in orthodontically produced alveolar bone dehiscences. *J Periodontal Res.* 1982; 17:309–315.

Kassab MM, Cohen RE. The etiology and prevalence of gingival recession. *J Am Dent Assoc.* 2003; 134:220–225.

Khocht A, Simon G, Person P, Denepitiya JL. Gingival recession in relation to history of hard toothbrush use. *J Periodontol.* 1993; 64:900–905.

Kim DM, Neiva R. Periodontal soft tissue non-root coverage procedures: a systematic review from the AAP regeneration workshop. *J Periodontol.* 2015; 86(S2): S56–S72.

Kois JC. Predictable single tooth peri-implant esthetics: five diagnostic keys. *Compend Contin Educ Dent.* 2001; 22:199–206.

Merijohn GK. Management and prevention of gingival recession. *Periodontol 2000.* 2016; 71:228–242.

Muller HP, Kononen E. Variance components of gingival thickness. *J Periodontal Res.* 2005; 40:239–244.

Nuttall N, Steele JG, Nunn J et al. *A Guide to the UK Adult Dental Health Survey 1998.* London: British Dental Association; 2001: 1–6.

Pecie R, Krejci I, Garcia-Godoy F, Bortolotto T. Noncarious cervical lesions – a clinical concept based on the literature review. Part 1: prevention. *Am J Dent.* 2011; 24:49–56.

Pini Prato GP. Mucogingival deformities. *Ann Periodontol.* 1999; 4:1–6.

Pini-Prato G. The Miller classification of gingival recession: limits and drawbacks. *J Clin Periodontol.* 2011; 38:243–245.

Pini-Prato G, Franceschi D, Cairo F, Nieri M, Rotundo R. Classification of dental surface defects in areas of gingival recession. *J Periodontol.* 2010; 81:885–890.

Pini-Prato G, Magnani C, Zaheer F, Rotundo R, Buti J. Influence of inter-dental tissues and root surface condition on complete root coverage following treatment of gingival recessions: a 1-year retrospective study. *J Clin Periodontol.* 2015; 42:567–574.

Rajapakse PS, McCracken GI, Gwynnett E et al. Does tooth brushing influence the development and progression of non-inflammatory gingival recession? *A systematic review. J Clin Periodontol.* 2007; 34:1046–1061.

Renkema AM, Fudalej PS, Renkema AAP et al. Gingival labial recessions in orthodontically treated and untreated individuals – a pilot case–control study. *J Clin Periodontol.* 2013; 40:631–637.

Renkema AM, Navratilova Z, Mazurova K, Katsaros C, Fudalej PS. Gingival labial recessions and the post-treatment proclination of mandibular incisors. *Eur J Orthod.* 2015; 37:508–513.

Rotundo R, Nieri M, Bonaccini D et al. The Smile Esthetic Index (SEI): a method to measure the esthetics of the smile. An intrarater and interrater agreement study. Eur *J Oral Implantol.* 2015; 8:397–403.

Santamaria MP, Bovi Ambrosano GM, Zaffalon Casati M et al. The influence of local anatomy on the outcome of treatment of gingival recession associated with non-carious cervical lesions. *J Periodontol.* 2010; 81:1027–1034.

Sarfati A, Bourgeois D, Katsahian S, Mora F, Bouchard P. Risk assessment for buccal gingival recession defects in an adult population. *J Periodontol.* 2010; 81:1419–1425.

Scheyer ET, Sanz M, Dibart S et al. Periodontal soft tissue non–root coverage procedures: a consensus report from the AAP regeneration workshop. *J Periodontol.* 2015; 86: S73–S76.

Tatakis DN, Chambrone L, Allen EP et al. Periodontal soft tissue root coverage procedures: a consensus report from the AAP regeneration workshop. *J Periodontol.* 2015; 86(S2):S52–S55.

Tonetti MS, Jepsen S. Clinical efficacy of periodontal plastic surgery procedures: consensus Report of Group 2 of the 10th European Workshop on Periodontology *J Clin Periodontol.* 2014;41(S15): S36–S43.

West NX, Sanz M, Lussi A et al. Prevalence of dentin hypersensitivity and study of associated factors: a European population-based cross-sectional study. *J Dent.* 2013; 41:841–851.

Zaher CA, Hachem J, Puhan MA, Mombelli A. Interest in periodontology and preferences for treatment of localized gingival recessions. *J Clin Periodontol.* 2005; 32:375–382.

Zweers J, Thomas RZ, Slot DE, Weisgold AS, Van der Weijden GA. Characteristics of periodontal biotype, its dimensions, associations and prevalence: a systematic review. *J Clin Periodontol.* 2014; 41:958–971.

10.4 TRAUMATIC OCCLUSAL FORCES

Steph Smith

Contents

Learning objectives

- Various case definitions related to occlusal trauma.
- How to diagnose trauma from occlusion, including the clinical and radiographic indicators associated with occlusal trauma.
- The effects of occlusal trauma on the initiation and progression of periodontal disease, including the effects of occlusal discrepancies.
- The effects of occlusal trauma on gingival recession and the effects of orthodontic forces on the periodontium.

Case definitions

- *Excessive occlusal force* is defined as an occlusal force that exceeds the reparative capacity of the periodontal attachment apparatus, which results in occlusal trauma and/or causes excessive tooth wear (loss) (Fan & Caton 2018).
- *Occlusal trauma* describes injury resulting in tissue changes within the attachment apparatus, including periodontal ligament (PDL), supporting alveolar bone, and cementum, as a result of occlusal force(s) (AAP 2001). Occlusal trauma may occur in an intact periodontium or in a reduced periodontium caused by periodontal disease (Fan & Caton 2018).
- *Primary occlusal trauma* is injury resulting in tissue changes from excessive occlusal forces applied to a tooth or teeth with a normal periodontium. It occurs in the presence of normal clinical attachment levels, normal bone levels, and excessive occlusal force(s) (AAP 2001).
- *Secondary occlusal trauma* is injury resulting in tissue changes from normal or excessive occlusal forces applied to a tooth or teeth with reduced periodontal support. It occurs in the presence of attachment loss, bone loss, and normal/excessive occlusal force(s) (AAP 2001).
- *Fremitus* is a palpable or visible movement of a tooth when subjected to occlusal forces (AAP 2001).
- *Bruxism or tooth grinding* is a habit of grinding, clenching, or clamping the teeth. The force generated may damage both tooth and attachment apparatus (AAP 2001).

Diagnosis of trauma from occlusion

The diagnosis is usually based on histological changes in the periodontium. Therefore, clinical and radiographic surrogate indicators are used in making a presumptive diagnosis of occlusal trauma (Fan & Caton 2018). A differential diagnosis should also be considered when, for example, severity of mobility is affected by loss of clinical attachment, or whether wear facets are caused by functional contacts or by parafunctional habits, such as bruxism. Supplementary diagnostic procedures, such as pulp vitality tests and the evaluation of parafunctional habits, should be utilized in the making of a differential diagnosis (Fan & Caton 2018).

Proposed clinical and radiographic indicators of occlusal trauma are the following (Jin & Cao 1992; Pihlstrom et al. 1986):
- Fremitus
- Mobility
- Occlusal discrepancies
- Wear facets
- Tooth migration
- Fractured tooth
- Thermal sensitivity
- Discomfort/pain on chewing
- Widened PDL space
- Root resorption
- Cemental tear

Abfraction

Excessive occlusal forces have long been proposed to be a causative factor in the development of abfraction (Grippo 1991; Lee & Eakle 1984, 1996). The lesion of abfraction has been described as a wedge-shaped defect occurring at the cementoenamel junction of affected teeth, this being caused by flexure and eventual fatigue of enamel and dentin (Lee & Eakle 1984, 1996). Abfraction has been proposed to be an etiological factor in non-carious cervical lesions (NCCLs); other known etiologies for NCCLs include abrasion, erosion, corrosion, or combinations thereof (Grippo 1991, 1992; Piotrowski et al. 2001). Abfraction is however not currently supported by appropriate clinical evidence, and is still regarded as a biomechanically based theoretical concept, thus a definitive diagnosis is not possible (Fan & Caton 2018). Therefore, in cases of NCCLs, toothbrushing habits, diet, eating disorders, as well as occlusal relationships and parafunctional habits should be thoroughly evaluated (Fan & Caton 2018).

Effects of occlusal trauma on the initiation and progression of periodontitis

Histological changes within the periodontium reflect an adaptive response to occlusal trauma (Glickman & Smulow 1969). The location and severity of the lesions may vary, based on the magnitude and direction of the applied forces (Fan & Caton 2018). This includes distinct zones of tension and pressure within the adjacent periodontium.

On the pressure side, these changes may include increased vascularization and permeability, hyalinization/necrosis of the PDL, hemorrhage, thrombosis, bone resorption, and, in some instances, root resorption and cemental tears.

On the side of tension, these changes may include elongation of the PDL fibers and apposition of alveolar bone and cementum (Glickman & Smulow 1969; Macapanpan & Weinmann 1954).

With sustained occlusal trauma, the density of the alveolar bone decreases and the width of the PDL space increases, which leads to increased tooth mobility, as well as a radiographic widening of the PDL space. This widening of the PDL is either limited to the alveolar crest or may include the entire width of the alveolar bone (Macapanpan & Weinmann 1954; Stahl 1968). In addition, fremitus or palpable functional tooth mobility may also be a significant clinical sign of occlusal trauma (Fan & Caton 2018).

In the presence of plaque-induced periodontitis and occlusal trauma, a greater loss of bone volume and increased mobility have been found, but loss of connective tissue attachment is reported to be the same as on teeth not being subjected to occlusal trauma, but subjected to periodontitis alone (Polson 1974). In some studies, when occlusal trauma is superimposed on periodontitis, an accelerated loss of connective tissue attachment can occur (Lindhe & Svanberg 1974). However, in the absence of plaque-induced inflammation, occlusal trauma does not cause irreversible bone loss or loss of connective tissue attachment. Therefore, occlusal trauma is not a causative agent of periodontitis. Results from animal studies suggest that occlusal trauma does not cause periodontitis, but it may be a co-factor that can accelerate the periodontal breakdown in the presence of periodontitis (Fan & Caton 2018).

Regarding the association between occlusal discrepancies and the progression of periodontitis, multiple types of occlusal contacts, including premature contacts in centric relation, posterior protrusive contact, non-working contacts, combined working and non-working contacts, and the length of slide between centric relation and centric occlusion have been shown to be associated with significantly deeper probing depths, more clinical attachment loss, more mobility, and an increasing assignment to a less favorable prognosis (Harrel & Nunn 2009; Nunn & Harrel 2001). Clinical studies have demonstrated the added benefit of occlusal therapy in the management of periodontal disease, but they do not provide strong evidence to support routine occlusal therapy. Occlusal therapy is not a substitute for conventional periodontal treatment for resolving plaque-induced inflammation. Overall, in the presence of occlusal trauma, occlusal therapy may slow the progression of periodontitis and improve the prognosis (Fan & Caton 2018).

Effects of excessive occlusal forces on gingival recession

Studies have failed to establish a relationship between the presence of occlusal discrepancies, tooth mobility, recession, and the initial width of gingival tissues, or between occlusal treatment and changes in the width of the gingiva (Bernimoulin & Curilović 1977; Geiger & Wasserman 1976; Harrel & Nunn 2004). Hence, existing data do not provide any solid evidence to substantiate the effects of occlusal forces on NCCLs and gingival recession (Fan & Caton 2018).

Effects of orthodontic forces on the periodontium

Existing evidence suggests that orthodontic treatment has minimal detrimental effects on the periodontium (Fan & Caton 2018). Orthodontic therapy has been shown to be associated with 0.03 mm of gingival recession, 0.13 mm of alveolar bone loss, and 0.23 mm increase in pocket depth when compared with no treatment (Bollen et al. 2008). Furthermore, in patients with good plaque control, teeth with a reduced but healthy periodontium have been shown to undergo successful tooth movement without compromising the periodontal support (Boyd et al. 1989; Eliasson et al. 1982). However, non-controlled orthodontic forces have been shown to negatively affect the periodontium and can result in root resorption, pulpal disorders, and alveolar bone resorption (see also Chapter 27.2).

REFERENCES

American Academy of Periodontology (AAP). Glossary of periodontal terms. 2001. Retrieved from www.perio.org.

Bernimoulin J, Curilović Z. Gingival recession and tooth mobility. *J Clin Periodontol.* 1977; 4:107–114.

Bollen AM, Cunha-Cruz J, Bakko DW, Huang GJ, Hujoel PP. The effects of orthodontic therapy on periodontal health: a systematic review of controlled evidence. *J Am Dent Assoc.* 2008; 139:413–422.

Boyd RL, Leggott PJ, Quinn RS, Eakle WS, Chambers D. Periodontal implications of orthodontic treatment in adults with reduced or normal periodontal tissues versus those of adolescents. *Am J Orthod Dentofacial Orthop.* 1989; 96:191–198.

Eliasson LA, Hugoson A, Kurol J, Siwe H. The effects of orthodontic treatment on periodontal tissues in patients with reduced periodontal support. *Eur J Orthod.* 1982; 4:1–9.

Fan J, Caton JG. Occlusal trauma and excessive occlusal forces: narrative review, case definitions, and diagnostic considerations. *J Clin Periodontol.* 2018; 45(Suppl 20):S199–S206.

Geiger AM, Wasserman BH. Relationship of occlusion and periodontal disease: part IX – incisor inclination and periodontal status. *Angle Orthod.* 1976; 46:99–110.

Glickman I, Smulow JB. The combined effects of inflammation and trauma from occlusion in periodontitis. *Int Dent J.* 1969; 19:393–407.

Grippo JO. Abfractions: a new classification of hard tissue lesions of teeth. *J Esthet Dent.* 1991; 3:14–19.

Grippo JO. Non-carious cervical lesions: the decision to ignore or restore. *J Esthet Dent.* 1992: 55–64.

Harrel SK, Nunn ME. The effect of occlusal discrepancies on gingival width. *J Periodontol.* 2004; 75:98–105.

Harrel SK, Nunn ME. The association of occlusal contacts with the presence of increased periodontal probing depth. *J Clin Periodontol.* 2009; 36:1035–1042.

Jin LJ, Cao CF. Clinical diagnosis of trauma from occlusion and its relation with severity of periodontitis. *J Clin Periodontol.* 1992; 19:92–97.

Lee WC, Eakle WS. Possible role of tensile stress in the etiology of cervical erosive lesions of teeth. *J Prosthet Dent.* 1984; 52:374–380.

Lee WC, Eakle WS. Stress-induced cervical lesions: review of advances in the past 10 years. *J Prosthet Dent.* 1996; 75:487–494.

Lindhe J, Svanberg G. Influence of trauma from occlusion on progression of experimental periodontitis in the beagle dog. *J Clin Periodontol.* 1974; 1:3–14.

Macapanpan LC, Weinmann JP. The influence of injury to the periodontal membrane on the spread of gingival inflammation. *J Dent Res.* 1954; 33:263–272.

Nunn ME, Harrel SK. The effect of occlusal discrepancies on periodontitis. I. Relationship of initial occlusal discrepancies to initial clinical parameters. *J Periodontol.* 2001; 72:485–494.

Pihlstrom BL, Anderson KA, Aeppli D, Schaffer EM. Association between signs of trauma from occlusion and periodontitis. *J Periodontol.* 1986; 57.1–6.

Piotrowski BT, Gillette WB, Hancock EB. Examining the prevalence and characteristics of abfraction-like cervical lesions in a population of U.S. veterans. *J Am Dent Assoc.* 2001; 132:1694–1701.

Polson AM. Trauma and progression of marginal periodontitis in squirrel monkeys. II. Co-destructive factors of periodontitis and mechanically produced injury. *J Periodontal Res.* 1974; 9:108–113.

Stahl SS. The responses of the periodontium to combined gingival inflammation and occluso-functional stresses in four human surgical specimens. *Periodontics.* 1968; 6:14–22.

10.5 PROSTHESIS AND TOOTH-RELATED FACTORS THAT MODIFY OR PREDISPOSE TO PLAQUE-INDUCED GINGIVAL DISEASES/PERIODONTITIS

Steph Smith

Contents

Learning objectives

- Prostheses and tooth-related factors affecting the integrity of the supracrestal tissue attachment.
- Prosthesis and tooth-related factors that modify or predispose the periodontium to plaque-induced gingival diseases/periodontitis.

Introduction

Factors related to the presence, design, fabrication, delivery, and materials of tooth-supported prostheses have been suggested to influence the periodontium. The anatomy, position, and relationships of teeth within the dental arches are also factors that have been associated with plaque retention, gingivitis, and periodontitis. Table 10.5.1 is a summary of some relevant findings regarding the above-mentioned factors (Ercoli & Caton 2018).

Table 10.5.1 Prosthesis and tooth-related factors that modify or predispose to plaque-induced gingival diseases/periodontitis.

Biological width (supracrestal tissue attachment)	• Defined as the cumulative apical–coronal dimensions of the junctional epithelium (JE) and supracrestal connective tissue attachment (SCTA) (AAP 2001). • To clearly define a "fixed" biological width dimension is difficult, as the dimensions of the JE and SCTA can vary considerably (Gargiulo et al. 1995; Schmidt et al. 2013). • In areas where crowns are placed with their interproximal margins situated <1 mm between the crown margin and alveolar crest, with clear encroachment of the crown margins within the SCTA, greater papillary bleeding indexes may be observed, and are associated with increased probing depths (Gunay et al. 2000). • In humans it is not possible to determine if the negative effects on the periodontium associated with restoration margins located within the SCTA are caused by bacterial plaque, trauma, or a combination of these factors (Ercoli & Caton 2018).
Fixed dental restorations and prostheses	• Direct restorations with overhangs greater than 0.2 mm are associated with crestal bone loss, increases in bleeding on probing, and probing depths that exceed these values found at sites with well-fitting restorations and unrestored teeth (Bjorn et al. 1969; Pack et al. 1990; Rodriguez-Ferrer et al. 1980). • For indirect restorations, overhangs between 0.5 and 1 mm are associated with an increase in gingival inflammation, more apical crestal bone levels, and increases in probing depth, while overhangs of less than 0.2 mm are not (Bjorn et al. 1970; Boeckler et al. 2010; Hey et al. 2014). • The above-mentioned changes are likely caused by the overhang acting as a plaque-retentive factor and causing a qualitative shift toward a microflora more characteristic of periodontitis (Ercoli & Caton 2018). • Permanent changes to the periodontium, such as gingival recession, appear to be mostly related to trauma to the periodontium exerted by the procedures, instruments, and materials required to place and record the margins in a subgingival location (Ercoli & Caton 2018). • Plaque control and compliance with periodontal maintenance are important to maintain the health of the periodontium when subgingival margins are adopted in the prosthetic design (Ercoli & Caton 2018).
Dental materials	• Different dental materials act similarly to enamel as plaque-retentive factors to initiate gingivitis (Ercoli & Caton 2018; Konradsson et al. 2007). • Dental materials' surface characteristics, such as surface-free energy and roughness, as well as their location in relation to the gingiva, have been associated with variable periodontal responses (Ababnaeh et al. 2011; Quirynen et al. 1990). • Metal ions and particles, especially nickel and palladium, have been associated with hypersensitivity reactions, appearing as localized gingivitis in areas of gingival contact with the dental material, do not respond to plaque-control measures, and may lead to contact stomatitis having a lichenoid-type appearance (Muris et al. 2014). • Limited evidence suggests that the replacement of such prostheses with zirconia-based protheses will be associated with resolution of the allergic reaction (Gokcen-Rohlig et al. 2010).

(Continued)

Table 10.5.1 (Continued)	
Removable dental prostheses	• No differences have been reported in probing depths, bleeding upon probing, gingival recession, microbial count and species between teeth that support removable dental prostheses (RDPs) and teeth that do not (Costa et al. 2017). • In studies with no available information on the level of self-performed plaque control, periodontal maintenance, or baseline periodontal conditions, RDPs have been associated with increased prevalence of caries, gingivitis, and periodontitis (Kern & Wagner 2001). • However, if plaque control is established, the prostheses are correctly designed and regularly checked, and indicated maintenance procedures are performed, then RDPs do not cause greater plaque accumulation, periodontal loss of attachment, or increased mobility (Bergman 1987; Dhingra 2012; Maeda et al. 2008). • If these factors are lacking, then RDPs, including overdentures, could act as plaque-retentive factors and indirectly cause gingivitis and periodontitis (Budtz-Jorgensen 1994; Ettinger & Jakobsen 1996). • Distal extension RDPs, when not properly maintained and relined, have the potential to apply greater forces and torque to abutment teeth, causing a traumatic increase in mobility (Akaltan & Kaynak 2005).
Tooth shape and position	• The anatomy (shape) of teeth and their approximation have been shown to affect the height of the interproximal papilla (Kim et al. 2014). • Cross-bite, misalignment/rotation of teeth, and crowding of the maxillary and mandibular anterior teeth have been shown to be associated with increased plaque retention, gingivitis, greater probing depths, bone loss, and clinical attachment loss (al-Jasser & Hashim 1995; Behlfelt et al. 1981; El-Mangoury et al. 1987; Helm & Petersen 1989). • Other studies assessing effects of crowding on the periodontium have not found associations with plaque retention and gingivitis (Geiger et al. 1974; Ingervall et al. 1977). • Traumatic toothbrushing, tooth malposition within the alveolar process, together with a thin periodontal biotype may pose a greater risk for gingival recession (Khocht et al. 1993; Richman 2011).
Open contacts	• Adequate proximal tooth contacts are considered important to prevent food impaction between teeth. A statistically greater occurrence of food impaction at sites with open contacts has been shown to be associated with increased probing depths in these areas (Hancock et al. 1980; Jernberg et al. 1983).
Cervical enamel projections (CEP) and enamel pearls (EP)	• Tooth anatomic factors, such as CEP and EP, have been associated with furcation invasion, increased probing depths, and loss of clinical attachment (Lim et al. 2016; Matthews & Tabesh 2004). • The extent of CEP extension toward the furcation area is classified into three classes: grade I = a distinct change in cementoenamel junction (CEJ) attitude with enamel projecting toward the furcation; grade II = the CEP approaching the furcation, but not actually making contact with it; grade III = the CEP extends into the furcation proper (Masters & Hoskins 1964). • A low prevalence of grade III CEP (4.3–6.3%) is however considered to be more detrimental to the furcation tissues compared to grade I and II CEP (Blanchard et al. 2012). • EPs are spheroidal in shape, occurring in 1–5.7% in furcation areas of all molar teeth, their dimension ranging from 0.3 to 2 mm, and are most often isolated. EPs can act as a plaque-retentive factor, becoming part of the subgingival microbial ecosystem during the development of periodontitis (Goldstein 1979; Moskow & Canut 1990).
Developmental grooves	• The palatal groove, the most frequent developmental groove, is most often located in the maxillary lateral incisor (Withers et al. 1981). • 43% of grooves do not extend more than 5 mm apical to the CEJ and only 10% are present 10 mm or more apical to the CEJ (Kogon 1986). • Grooves are also present on other teeth and mostly in the interproximal areas, with few of these grooves extending to the tooth apex (Albaricci et al. 2008; Dabebneh & Rodan 2013). • Developmental grooves are indirectly involved in the initiation of periodontal disease via plaque retention that causes localized gingivitis and periodontitis (Andreana 1998; Gound & Maze 1998; Leines et al. 1994).

Table 10.5.1 (Continued)	
Tooth fractures	• Tooth fractures occurring coronal to the gingival margin and not extending into the surrounding periodontal tissues will not initiate gingivitis or periodontitis, unless the surface characteristics of the fracture area predispose to greater plaque retention (Ercoli & Caton 2018).
Root proximity	• In the maxilla, root proximity (RP) is most prevalent between the first and second molars and between the central and lateral incisors; in the mandible, RP is seen between the central and lateral incisors (Vermylen et al. 2005a, b). • A classification has been proposed that defines the location of the measured site of RP – i.e. cervical, middle, or apical third of the root – and divides the severity of the RP into type 1 >0.5 to ≤0.8 mm; type 2 >0.3 to ≤0.5 mm; and type 3 ≤0.3 mm (Vermylen et al. 2005a). • Sites with interproximal root distance <0.6 mm have been shown to be 28% and 56% more likely to lose >0.5 mm and >1.0 mm of bone, respectively, over a period of 10 years; however, the biological mechanisms underlying this increased bone loss are unclear (Kim et al. 2008).
Root resorption	• Root resorption can be classified into surface, inflammatory, and replacement resorption (Andreason 1985; Carrotte 2004) and, depending on its location, as internal or external, cervical or apical (Bartok et al. 2012; Darcey & Qualtrough 2013). • Root resorption located within the cervical third of the root can easily communicate with the subgingival microbial ecosystem. Plaque retention at such sites can cause gingivitis and periodontitis (Bartok et al. 2012; Darcey & Qualtrough 2013). • Cemental tears can potentially lead to localized periodontal breakdown, although the biological mechanism involved has not been elucidated (Haney et al. 1992; Ishikawa et al. 1996).
Root fractures	• Root fractures can be classified based on the trajectory of the fracture (vertical, transverse, or oblique), its extent (complete or incomplete), location (apical, midroot, or cervical regions), and on the healing/repair mode (Andreasen et al. 2012a). • Fractures located within the midroot and apical regions have been shown to have a very favorable prognosis (78% and 89% tooth survival, respectively); fractures located within the cervical one-third of the root usually have a significantly worse prognosis for tooth retention (33%) (Andreasen et al. 2012a, b; Cvek et al. 2002). • Fractures located within the cervical third of a root are more likely to be colonized by subgingival plaque, acting as a plaque-retentive factor, thus indirectly causing gingivitis and periodontitis. They can also directly traumatize the surrounding periodontium due to mobility of the fractured tooth surfaces. Fractures located within the anatomic crown or slightly into the cervical third of the root can be successfully repaired with adhesive techniques (Eichelsbacher et al. 2009; Giachetti et al. 2010). • Vertical root fractures are defined as longitudinal fractures that can begin on the internal canal wall and extend outward to the external root surface. They occur most often on endodontically treated teeth, but may also be present on non-endodontically treated teeth, especially molars and premolars, as a result of apical extensions of coronal tooth fractures (Chan et al. 1999). • A localized pocket, with loss of attachment and bone, is usually associated with the fractured tooth, and extends to variable lengths along the fracture line (Lommel et al. 1978; Luebke 1984). • Narrow, deep, V- or U-shaped osseous defects are generally associated with the fractured area, with bone resorption and inflammation related to bacterial infection from the gingival margin and root canal system (Lustig et al. 2000; Meister et al. 1980).

Source: Adapted from Ercoli & Caton 2018.

REFERENCES

Ababnaeh KT, Al-Omari M, Alawneh TN. The effect of dental restoration type and material on periodontal health. *Oral Health Prev Dent.* 2011; 9:395–403.

Akaltan F, Kaynak D. An evaluation of the effects of two distal extension removable partial denture designs on tooth stabilization and periodontal health. *J Oral Rehabil.* 2005; 32:823–829.

al-Jasser N, Hashim H. Periodontal findings in cases of incisor cross-bite. *Clin Pediatr Dent.* 1995; 19:285–287.

Albaricci MF, de Toledo BE, Zuza EP, Gomes DA, Rosetti EP. Prevalence and features of palato-radicular grooves: an in-vitro study. *J Int Acad Periodontol.* 2008; 10:2–5.

American Academy of Peridontology (AAP). Glossary of periodontal terms. 2001. Retrieved from www.perio.org.

Andreana S. A combined approach for treatment of developmental groove associated periodontal defect. *A case report. J Periodontol.* 1998; 69:601–607.

Andreasen JO. External root resorptions: its implication in dental traumatology, pedodontics, periodontics, orthodontics, and endodontics. *Int Endodont J.* 1985; 18:109–118.

Andreasen JO, Ahrensburg SS, Tsilingaridis G. Root fractures: the influence of type of healing and location of fracture on tooth survival rates – an analysis of 492 cases. *Dent Traumatol.* 2012a; 28:404–409.

Andreasen JO, Ahrensburg SS, Tsilingaridis G. Tooth mobility changes subsequent to root fractures: a longitudinal clinical study of 44 permanent teeth. *Dent Traumatol.* 2012b; 28:410–414.

Bartok RI, Vaideanu T, Dimitriu B et al. External radicular resorption: selected cases and review of the literature. *J Med Life.* 2012; 5:145–148.

Behlfelt K, Eriksson L, Jacobson L, Linder-Aronson S. The occurrence of plaque and gingivitis and its relationship to tooth alignment within the dental arches. *J Clin Periodontol.* 1981; 8:329–337.

Bergman B. Periodontal reactions related to removable partial dentures: a literature review. *J Prosthet Dent.* 1987; 58:454–458.

Bjorn AL, Bjorn H, Grkovic B. Marginal fit of restorations and its relation to periodontal bone level. I. *Metal fillings. Odontol Revy.* 1969; 20:311–321.

Bjorn AL, Bjorn H, Grkovic B. Marginal fit of restorations and its relation to periodontal bone level. II. Crowns. *Odontol Revy.* 1970; 21:337–346.

Blanchard SB, Derderian GM, Averitt TR, John V, Newell DH. Cervical enamel projections and associated pouch-like opening in mandibular furcations. *J Periodontol.* 2012; 83:198–203.

Boeckler AF, Lee H, Psoch A, Setz JM. Prospective observation of CAD/CAM titanium-ceramic-fixed partial dentures: 3-year followup. *J Prosthodont.* 2010; 19:592–597.

Budtz-Jorgensen E. Effects of denture-wearing habits on periodontal health of abutment teeth in patients with overdentures. *J Clin Periodontol.* 1994; 21:265–269.

Carrotte P. Endodontics: part 9. Calcium hydroxide, root resorption, endo-perio lesions. *Br Dent J.* 2004; 197:735–743.

Chan CP, Lin CP, Tseng SC, Jeng JH. Vertical root fracture in endodontically versus nonendodontically treated teeth. A survey of 315 cases in Chinese patients. *Oral Surg Oral Med Oral Pathol Oral Radiol Endod.* 1999; 87:504–507.

Costa L, do Nascimento C, de Souza VO, Pedrazzi V. Microbiological and clinical assessment of the abutment and non-abutment teeth of partial removable denture wearers. *Arch Oral Biol.* 2017; 75:74–80.

Cvek M, Mejare I, Andreasen JO. Healing and prognosis of teeth with intra-alveolar fractures involving the cervical part of the root. *Dent Traumatol.* 2002; 18:57–65.

Dababneh R, Rodan R. Anatomical landmarks of maxillary bifurcated first premolars and their influence on periodontal diagnosis and treatment. *J Int Acad Periodontol.* 2013; 15:8–15.

Darcey J, Qualtrough A. Resorption: part 1. Pathology, classification and aetiology. *Br Dent J.* 2013; 214:439–451.

Dhingra K. Oral rehabilitation considerations for partially edentulous periodontal patients. *J Prosthodont.* 2012; 21:494–513.

Eichelsbacher F, Denner W, Klaiber B, Schlagenhauf U. Periodontal status of teeth with crown-root fractures: results two years after adhesive fragment reattachment. *J Clin Periodontol.* 2009; 36:905–911.

El-Mangoury NH, Gaafar S, Mostafa YA. Mandibular anterior crowding and periodontal disease. *Angle Orthod.* 1987; 57:33–38.

Ercoli C, Caton JG. Dental prostheses and tooth-related factors. *J Clin Periodontol.* 2018; 45(Suppl 20):S207–S218.

Ettinger RL, Jakobsen J. Periodontal considerations in an overdenture population. *Int J Prosthodont.* 1996; 9:230–238.

Gargiulo A, Krajewski J, Gargiulo M. Defining biologic width in crown lengthening. *CDS Rev.* 1995; 88:20–23.

Geiger AM, Wasserman BH, Turgeon LR. Relationship of occlusion and periodontal disease part VIII – relationship of crowding and spacing to periodontal destruction and gingival inflammation. *J Periodontol.* 1974; 45:43–49.

Giachetti L, Bertini F, Rotundo R. Crown-root reattachment of a severe subgingival tooth fracture: a 15-month periodontal evaluation. *Int J Periodontics Restorative Dent.* 2010; 30:393–399.

Gokcen-Rohlig B, Saruhanoglu A, Cifter ED, Evlioglu G. Applicability of zirconia dental prostheses for metal allergy patients. *Int J Prosthodont.* 2010; 23:562–565.

Goldstein AR. Enamel pearls as a contributing factor in periodontal breakdown. *J Am Dent Assoc.* 1979; 99:210–211.

Gound TG, Maze GI. Treatment options for the radicular lingual groove: a review and discussion. *Pract Periodontics Aesthet Dent.* 1998; 10:369–375.

Gunay H, Seeger A, Tschernitschek H, Geurtsen W. Placement of the preparation line and periodontal health—a prospective 2-year clinical study. *Int J Periodontics Restorative Dent.* 2000; 20:171–181.

Hancock EB, Mayo CV, Schwab RR, Wirthlin MR. Influence of interdental contacts on periodontal status. *J Periodontol.* 1980; 51:445–449.

Haney JM, Leknes KN, Lie T, Selvig KA, Wikesjo UM. Cemental tear related to rapid periodontal breakdown — a case report. *J Periodontol.* 1992; 63:220–224.

Helm S, Petersen PE. Causal relation between malocclusion and periodontal health. *Acta Odontol Scand.* 1989; 47:223–228.

Hey J, Beuer F, Bensel T, Boeckler AF. Single crowns with CAD/CAM-fabricated copings from titanium: 6-year clinical results. *J Prosthet Dent.* 2014; 112:150–154.

Ingervall B, Jacobson U, Nyman S. A clinical study of the relationship between crowding of teeth, plaque and gingival condition. *J Clin Periodontol.* 1977; 4:214–222.

Ishikawa I, Oda S, Hayashi J, Arakawa S. Cervical cemental tears in older patients with adult periodontitis. *Case reports. J Periodontol.* 1996; 67:15–20.

Jernberg GR, Bakdash MB, Keenan KM. Relationship between proximal tooth open contacts and periodontal disease. *J Periodontol.* 1983; 54:529–533.

Kern M, Wagner B. Periodontal findings in patients 10 years after insertion of removable partial dentures. *J Oral Rehabil.* 2001; 28:991–997.

Khocht A, Simon G, Person P, Denepitiya JL. Gingival recession in relation to history of hard toothbrush use. *J Periodontol.* 1993; 64:900–905.

Kim T, Miyamoto T, Nunn ME, Garcia RI, Dietrich T. Root proximity as a risk factor for progression of alveolar bone loss: the Veterans Affairs dental longitudinal study. *J Periodontol.* 2008; 79:654–659.

Kim YK, Kwon EY, Cho YJ et al. Changes in the vertical position of interdental papillae and interseptal bone following the approximation of anterior teeth. *Int J Periodontics Restorative Dent.* 2014; 34:219–224.

Kogon SL. The prevalence, location and conformation of palato-radicular grooves in maxillary incisors. *J Periodontol.* 1986; 57:231–234.

Konradsson K, Claesson R, van Dijken JW. Dental biofilm, gingivitis and interleukin-1 adjacent to approximal sites of a bonded ceramic. *J Clin Periodontol.* 2007; 34:1062–1067.

Lejnes KN, Lie T, Selvig KA. Root grooves – a risk factor in periodontal attachment loss. *J Periodontol.* 1994; 65:859–863.

Lim HC, Jeon SK, Cha JK et al. Prevalence of cervical enamel projection and its impact on furcation involvement in mandibular molars: a cone-beam computed tomography study in Koreans. *Anat Rec.* 2016; 299:379–384.

Lommel TJ, Meister F, Gerstein H, Davies EE, Tilk MA. Alveolar bone loss associated with vertical root fractures.

Report of six cases. *Oral Surg Oral Med Oral Pathol.* 1978; 45:909–919.

Luebke RG. Vertical crown-root fractures in posterior teeth. *Dent Clin North Am.* 1984; 28:883–894.

Lustig JP, Tamse A, Fuss Z. Pattern of bone resorption in vertically fractured, endodontically treated teeth. *Oral Surg Oral Med Oral Pathol Oral Radiol Endod.* 2000; 90:224–227.

Maeda Y, Kinoshita Y, Gacho H, Yang TC. Influence of bonded composite resin ringed on root caries on abutment tooth periodontal tissues: a longitudinal prospective study. *Int J Prosthodont.* 2008; 21:37–39.

Masters DH, Hoskins SW. Projection of cervical enamel into molar furcations. *J Periodontol.* 1964; 35:49–53.

Matthews DC, Tabesh M. Detection of localized tooth-related factors that predispose to periodontal infections. *Periodontol 2000.* 2004; 34:136–150.

Meister F Jr, Lommel TJ, Gerstein H. Diagnosis and possible causes of vertical root fractures. *Oral Surg Oral Med Oral Pathol.* 1980; 49:243–253.

Moskow BS, Canut PM. Studies on root enamel (2). Enamel pearls. A review of their morphology, localization nomenclature, occurrence, classification, histogenesis and incidence. *J Clin Periodontol.* 1990; 17:275–281.

Muris J, Scheper RJ, Kleverlaan CJ et al. Palladium-based dental alloys are associated with oral disease and palladium-induced immune responses. *Contact Dermatitis.* 2014; 71:82–91.

Pack AR, Coxhead LJ, McDonald BW. The prevalence of overhanging margins in posterior amalgam restorations and periodontal consequences. *J Clin Periodontol.* 1990; 17:145–152.

Quirynen M, Marechal M, Busscher HJ et al. The influence of surface free energy and surface roughness on early plaque formation. *J Clin Periodontol.* 1990; 17:138–144.

Richman C. Is gingival recession a consequence of an orthodontic tooth size and/or tooth position discrepancy? A paradigm shift. *Compend Contin Educ Dent.* 2011; 32:62–69.

Rodriguez-Ferrer HJ, Strahan JD, Newman HN. Effect of gingival health of removing overhanging margins of interproximal subgingival amalgam restorations. *J Clin Periodontol.* 1980; 7:457–462.

Schmidt JC, Sahrmann P, Weiger R, Schmidlin PR, Walter C. Biologic width dimensions – a systematic review. *J Clin Periodontol.* 2013; 40:493–504.

Vermylen K, De Quincey GN, van 't Hof MA, Wolffe GN, Renggli HH. Classification, reproducibility and prevalence of root proximity in periodontal patients. *J Clin Periodontol.* 2005a; 32:254–259.

Vermylen K, De Quincey GN, Wolffe GN, van 't Hof MA, Renggli HH. Root proximity as a risk marker for periodontal disease: a case-control study. *J Clin Periodontol.* 2005b; 32:260–265.

Withers JA, Brunsvold MA, Killoy WJ, Rahe AJ. The relationship of palato-gingival grooves to localized periodontal disease. *J Periodontol.* 1981; 52:41–44.

CHAPTER 11
Periodontal soft and hard tissue pathology

Steph Smith

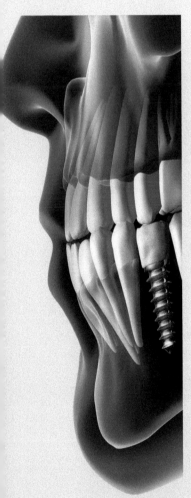

Contents

Learning objectives

- Definition of a periodontal pocket.
- Classification of pockets.
- Pocket depths in relation to variations in attachment and bone loss.
- Histopathogenesis of alveolar bone loss.
- Pathways of inflammation affecting the development of bony lesions.
- Factors that will determine the morphology of bony lesions.
- Classification of various bony lesions.
- Etiology of furcation lesions.
- Diagnosis and classification of furcation lesions.
- Factors to consider when determining a prognosis for furcation lesions.
- Available treatment approaches for furcation lesions.

Essential Periodontics, First Edition. Edited by Steph Smith and Khalid Almas.
© 2022 John Wiley & Sons Ltd. Published 2022 by John Wiley & Sons Ltd.

The periodontal pocket

The periodontal pocket is defined as a pathologically deepened gingival sulcus. Deepening of the gingival sulcus may occur as a result of coronal movement of the gingival margin, apical displacement of the gingival attachment, or a combination of the two processes (Newman et al. 2019).

Classification of pockets

- *A gingival pocket* (also called a "pseudo-pocket") is formed by gingival enlargement without destruction of the underlying periodontal tissues. The sulcus is deepened because of the increased bulk of the gingiva (Newman et al. 2019) (Figure 11.1A).
- *A periodontal pocket* is formed due to the destruction of the supporting periodontal tissues. Based on the location of the base of the pocket in relation to the underlying bone, periodontal pockets can be classified as follows:
  - A *suprabony pocket* (supracrestal or supra-alveolar) occurs when the bottom of the pocket and the pocket wall are coronal to the underlying alveolar bone. The pattern of destruction of the underlying bone is horizontal (Newman et al. 2019) (Figure 11.1.B).
  - An *intrabony pocket* (infrabony, subcrestal, or intra-alveolar) occurs when the bottom of the pocket is apical to the level of the adjacent alveolar bone. The lateral pocket wall lies between the tooth surface and the alveolar bone. The pattern of bone destruction is vertical (angular) (Newman et al. 2019) (Figure 11.1.C).
- *Simple pockets, compound pockets, complex pockets.* Pockets can be classified according to involved tooth surfaces, including one, two, or more tooth surfaces (simple pocket). They can be of different depths and types on different surfaces of the same tooth and on approximal surfaces of the same interdental space (compound pocket). Pockets can also be spiral (i.e. originating on one tooth surface and twisting around the tooth to involve one or more additional surfaces; complex pocket). These types of pockets are most common in furcation areas (Krayer & Rees 1993; Newman et al. 2019).

Relationship of attachment loss and bone loss to pocket depth

The severity of bone loss is generally but not always correlated with pocket depth. Extensive attachment and bone loss may be associated with shallow pockets if the attachment loss is accompanied by recession of the gingival margin, and slight bone loss can occur with deep pockets (Newman et al. 2019).

- Pockets of the *same depth* may be associated with different degrees of attachment loss (see Figure 11.2).
- Pockets of *different depths* may be associated with the same amount of attachment loss (see Figure 11.3). The distance between the junctional epithelium and the cementoenamel junction remains the same despite different pocket depths.

Bone loss and patterns of bone destruction

One of the characteristic signs of destructive periodontal disease is loss of alveolar bone support. The extent and severity of alveolar bone loss are usually assessed by a combination of radiographic and clinical means, which serve as adjuncts to the clinician (Papapanou & Tonetti 2000). The understanding of the anatomy, histology, and pattern of bone loss for the diagnosis of and prognosis for periodontal disease is of major importance in determining the therapy that must be rendered

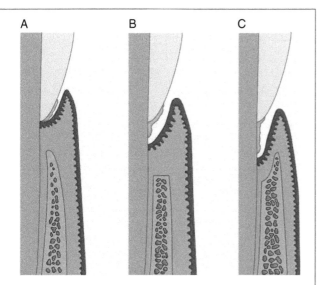

Figure 11.1 Classification of periodontal pockets. Courtesy of Dr. Abdulqader Alhammadi.

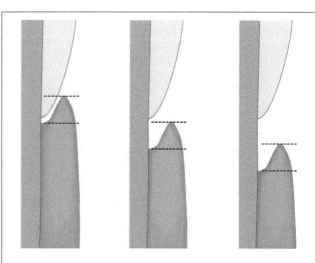

Figure 11.2 Pockets of the same depth may be associated with different degrees of attachment loss. Courtesy of Dr. Abdulader Alhammadi.

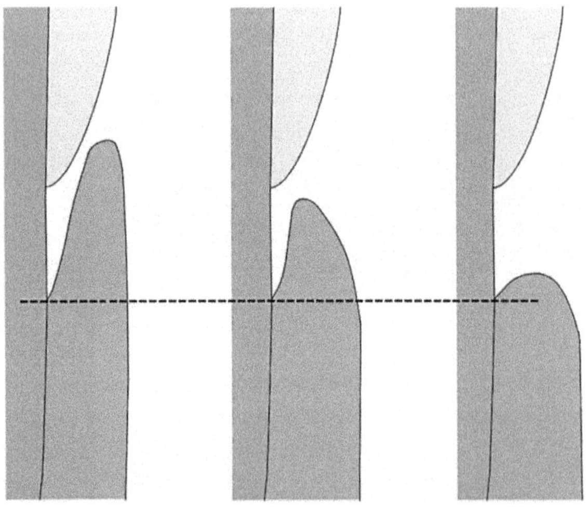

Figure 11.3 Different pocket depths associated with the same amount of clinical attachment loss. Courtesy of Dr. Abdulqader Alhammadi.

(Newman et al. 2019). The formation of an osseous periodontal lesion is considered to be the result of an apical downgrowth of subgingival plaque with a concomitant resorption of bone within a 2 mm radius from the root surface. The loss of bone is the ultimate and last event of the inflammatory process. The existing bone level is thus the result of past episodes of bone loss from the effects of periodontitis. It is the loss of bone that will determine the retention, maintenance, or loss of the dentition in periodontal disease (Papapanou & Tonetti 2000).

The more remotely located bone structures and the root surface retain their integrity and form the anatomical boundaries of the osseous lesion (Heins et al. 1988; Waerhaug 1979). Each individual defect affecting a specific tooth in the dentition of a certain patient thus presents a unique anatomy (see "Factors affecting the morphology of defects"). The degree of bone loss also does not necessarily correlate with the depth of the periodontal pocket, the severity of ulceration of the pocket wall, or the presence or absence of an exudate (Papapanou & Tonetti 2000).

Histopathogenesis of alveolar bone loss

The inflammatory infiltrate often reaches the bone and elicits a response before there may be evidence of crestal resorption or loss of attachment (Moskow & Polson 1991). Gingival inflammation extends along the collagen fiber bundles and follows the course of the blood vessels through the loosely arranged tissues around them into the alveolar bone (Weinmann 1941). Along its course from the gingiva to the bone, the inflammation destroys the gingival and transseptal fibers, reducing them to disorganized granular fragments interspersed among the inflammatory cells and edema (Ooya & Yamamoto 1978). However, the transseptal fibers are continuously recreated across the crest of the interdental septum as the bone

destruction progresses, forming a firm covering over the bone that is encountered during periodontal flap surgery after the superficial granulation tissue is removed (Newman et al. 2019).

After inflammation reaches the bone (see "Inflammatory pathways from the gingiva into the supporting periodontal tissues"), it spreads into the marrow spaces and replaces the marrow with a leukocytic and fluid exudate, new blood vessels, and proliferating fibroblasts, as well as an increased number of mononuclear phagocytes and multinuclear osteoclasts. In the marrow spaces, resorption proceeds from within and causes a thinning of the surrounding bony trabeculae and an enlargement of the marrow spaces; this is followed by the destruction of the bone and a reduction in bone height. Bone destruction in periodontal disease involves the activity of living cells along viable bone, and is not a process of bone necrosis (Newman et al. 2019).

For bone loss to occur, the range of effectiveness in which bacterial biofilm can induce horizontal bone loss is about 1.5–2.5 mm. Interproximal angular defects can appear only in spaces that are wider than 2.5 mm (Tal 1984). If periodontal disease is allowed to progress untreated, the rate of bone loss may vary, with averages of about 0.2 mm per year for facial surfaces and about 0.3 mm per year for proximal surfaces (Löe et al. 1978).

Areas of bone formation are also found immediately adjacent to sites of active bone resorption and along trabecular surfaces at a distance from the inflammation in an apparent effort to reinforce the remaining bone, i.e. buttressing bone formation may thus be observed (Glickman & Smulow 1965; Newman et al. 2019).

Inflammatory pathways from the gingiva into the supporting periodontal tissues

- *Facially and lingually* (Figure 11.4A): from the gingiva into the periodontal ligament (1), from the periosteum into the bone by penetrating into the marrow spaces through vessel channels in the outer cortex (2), and from the gingiva along the outer periosteal surface (3).
- *Interproximally* (Figure 11.4B): from the gingiva into the bone (1), less frequently from the gingiva into the periodontal ligament, from there into the interdental septum (2), and from the bone into the periodontal ligament (3).

Factors affecting the morphology of bone destruction

The osseous contours produced by periodontal disease are affected by the existing normal variations within the morphological features of alveolar bone. Such anatomic features are the following:
- Thickness, width, and crestal angulation of the interdental septa.
- Thickness of the facial and lingual alveolar plates.
- Presence of fenestrations and dehiscences.
- Alignment of the teeth.

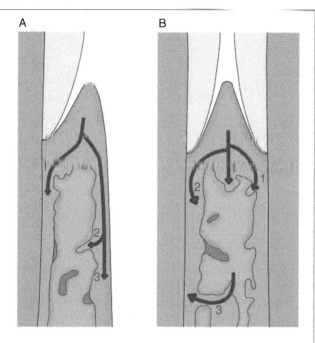

Figure 11.4 Inflammatory pathways from the gingiva into the supporting periodontal tissues. Courtesy of Dr. Abdulqader Alhammadi.

- Root and root trunk anatomy.
- Root position within the alveolar process.
- Proximity with another tooth surface.

Classification of bony lesions

Classifications of bony lesions are generally based upon specific morphological criteria, their purpose being to guide clinicians with their diagnosis, treatment, and prognosis (Papapanou & Tonetti 2000).

Horizontal bone loss

Horizontal bone loss is the most common pattern of bone loss in periodontal disease. The bone is reduced in height, but the bone margin remains approximately perpendicular to the tooth surface. The interdental septa and the facial and lingual plates are affected, but not necessarily to an equal degree around the same tooth (Newman et al. 2019).

Vertical or angular defects

Vertical or angular defects occur in an oblique direction, leaving a hollowed-out trough in the bone alongside the root; the base of the defect is located apical to the surrounding bone. In most instances, angular defects have accompanying infrabony periodontal pockets; and on the other hand, infrabony pockets must always have an underlying angular defect. Goldman and Cohen (1958) classified angular defects on the basis of the number of osseous walls. Angular defects are depicted in Figure 11.5, and may be three-walled (Figure 11.5A), two-walled (Figure 11.5B), or one-walled (Figure 11.5C).

Vertical defects that occur interdentally can generally be seen on the radiograph, although thick, bony plates can obscure them. Angular defects may also appear on facial and lingual or palatal surfaces, although these defects may be more difficult to visualize on radiographs. Radiographically detected vertical defects have been reported to appear most often on the distal and mesial surfaces (Nielsen et al. 1980; Papapanou & Tonetti 2000). However, three-wall defects are more frequently found on the mesial surfaces of the upper and lower molars (Larato 1970). Surgical exposure is usually the only sure way to determine the presence and configuration of vertical osseous defects (Newman et al. 2019).

Circumferential defects

These are continuous defects that involve more than one surface of a tooth, in a shape that is similar to a trough.

Combined osseous defects

These occur when the number of walls in the apical portion of the defect is greater than that in its occlusal portion. For example (see Figure 11.6), a facial wall is half the height of the distal (1) and lingual (2) walls, therefore the osseous defect has three walls in its apical half and two walls in its occlusal half.

Osseous craters

Osseous craters are a specific type of two-wall defect: they present as concavities in the crest of the interdental bone that is confined within the facial and lingual walls. It is described as a cup- or bowl-shaped defect in the interdental alveolar

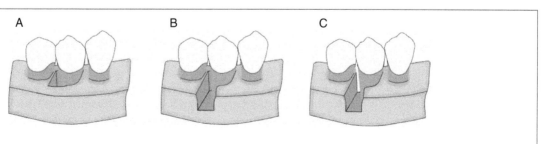

Figure 11.5 Angular defects. Courtesy of Dr. Abdulqader Alhammadi.

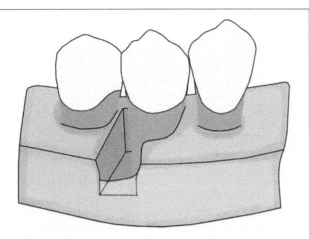

Figure 11.6 Combined lesion. The osseous defect has three walls in its apical half and two walls in its occlusal half. Courtesy of Dr. Abdulqader Alhammadi.

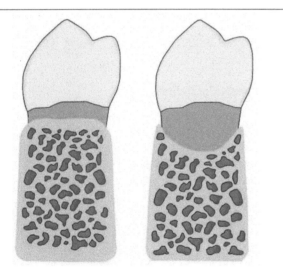

Figure 11.7 Osseous crater. Courtesy of Dr. Abdulqader Alhammadi.

bone, with bone loss nearly equal on the roots of two contiguous teeth, and with the buccal and lingual alveolar crest having a more coronal position, although the facial and lingual/palatal walls may be of unequal height (Glickman & Smulow 1965; Papapanou & Tonetti 2000). This defect can be considered as the result of the apical spread of periodontitis along two adjacent roots in a relatively narrow (mesiodistally) interproximal area (Figure 11.7). Craters have been found to make up about one-third of all defects and about two-thirds of all mandibular defects, occurring twice as often in posterior segments as in anterior segments (Manson 1976; Manson & Nicholson 1974). The high frequency of interdental craters can be due to the following reasons: (i) the

interdental area collects biofilm and is difficult to clean; (ii) the normal flat or even slightly concave buccolingual shape of the interdental septum in the lower molars may favor crater formation; or (iii) vascular patterns from the gingiva to the center of the crest may provide a pathway for inflammation (Manson 1976; Manson & Nicholson 1974; Saari et al. 1968).

Bulbous bone contours

Bulbous bone contours are bony enlargements that are caused by exostoses, adaptation to function, or buttressing bone formation. They are found more frequently in the maxilla than in the mandible.

Reversed architecture

Reversed (or negative) alveolar bone architecture is the result of a loss of interdental bone, without a concomitant loss of radicular (buccal or lingual/palatal) bone, thereby reversing the normal (or positive) architecture. Negative architecture is more common in the maxilla of patients with periodontitis (Nielsen et al. 1980).

Ledges

Ledges are plateau-like bone margins that are caused by the resorption of thickened bony plates (Newman et al. 2019).

Furcation involvement

See the next section.

Furcation lesions

Furcation involvement is defined as bone resorption and attachment loss in the bifurcation and trifurcation of multirooted teeth that result from plaque-associated periodontal disease (Cattabriga et al. 2000; Newman et al. 2019).

The complex and irregular anatomy of furcations lends itself to a greater radicular surface for the exposure to bacterial toxins and the potential buildup of calculus. The distal location in the dental arch and difficult access may conceivably impair both self-performed and professional plaque-control procedures in the furcation area, limiting their effectiveness. Furcation defects therefore represent a formidable problem regarding the prognosis and treatment of periodontal disease (Cattabriga et al. 2000). Higher mortality and compromised prognoses for molars with furcal involvement have been reported in various retrospective studies of tooth loss. Furthermore, lack of proper access for instrumentation resulting in reduced efficacy of periodontal therapy has been consistently found in multirooted teeth with furcal involvement, regardless of the treatment modality employed. Consequently, there may be a persistence of pathogenic microbial flora (Al-Shammari et al. 2001; Cobb 1996).

Histopathology

Microscopically, furcation involvement presents no unique pathological features. It is simply the apical extension of the periodontal pocket along a multirooted tooth. During its early stages, widening of the periodontal space occurs with cellular and fluid inflammatory exudation, and this is followed by epithelial proliferation into the furcation area from an adjoining periodontal pocket. Extension of the inflammation into the bone leads to resorption and a reduction in bone height. The bone-destructive pattern may produce horizontal loss, but angular osseous defects associated with intrabony pockets may also exist. Biofilm, calculus, and bacterial debris occupy the denuded furcation space (Newman et al. 2019).

Etiological factors associated with the development of furcation defects

Plaque-associated inflammation

Extension of inflammatory periodontal disease processes into the furcation area leads to interradicular bone resorption and formation of furcation defects, the lesions thus being an extension of existing periodontal pockets (Al-Shammari et al. 2001).

Pulpal pathology

The high incidence of molar teeth with accessory canals supports an association of pulpal pathology in the etiology of furcation involvement (Al-Shammari et al. 2001).

Trauma from occlusion

Although some controversy still exists, it has been reported that furcations are some of the more susceptible areas of the periodontium to excessive occlusal forces. The periodontal fiber orientation in furcation areas facilitates a more rapid spread of inflammation and may account for the increased susceptibility to occlusal forces (Al-Shammari et al. 2001).

Vertical root fractures

Vertical root fractures are associated with rapid, localized alveolar bone loss. Furcation defects can result if the fracture extends into the furcation area (Al-Shammari et al. 2001).

Iatrogenic factors

Molars with a crown or a proximal restoration have been shown to have a significantly higher percentage of furcation involvement than non-restored teeth (Wang et al. 1993).

Contributing anatomic factors (Al-Shammari et al. 2001):

- Furcation entrance width.
- Root trunk length.
- Presence of root concavities.
- Cervical enamel projections.
- Bifurcation ridges.
- Enamel pearls.

Diagnosis of furcation lesions

Clinical assessment

- *Probing*: The buccal furcation entrance of the maxillary molars and the buccal and lingual furcation entrances of the mandibular molars are normally accessible for examination using the Nabers probe. The examination of approximal furcations is more difficult. Large contact areas between teeth further impair access to approximal furcation entrances. In maxillary molars, the mesial furcation should be probed from the palatal aspect of the tooth, and the distal furcation should be probed from the palatal aspect of the tooth (Newman et al. 2019; Parihar & Katoch 2015).
- *Bone sounding or transgingival probing with local anesthesia*: This method may aid in the diagnosis of furcation defects by more accurately determining the underlying bony contours. The probe should be "walked" along the tissue–tooth interface so that the operator can feel the topography. The probe may also be passed horizontally through the tissue to provide more three-dimensional information regarding bony contours, i.e. the thickness, height, and shape of the underlying base (Al-Shammari et al. 2001; Glickman 1953; Greenberg et al. 1976).

Radiographic assessment

Radiographs may aid in the diagnosis of furcation defects, but are of limited value if used as the sole diagnostic tool, especially in early and moderate defects. Thus, radiographs must always be obtained to confirm findings made during probing of a furcation-involved tooth. Correlating the radiographic findings with clinical evidence is essential to properly diagnose the degree of involvement (Al-Shammari et al. 2001). The radiographic examination includes intraoral periapical radiographs and vertical bitewing radiographs (Cattabriga et al. 2000; Lindhe & Lang 2015) (see also Chapter 12.2).

Classification of furcation lesions

Glickman (1953)

- *Grade I*: Pocket formation into the flute, but intact interradicular bone (incipient). The pocket is suprabony, involving the soft tissue; there is slight bone loss in the furcation area. Radiographic change is not usual, as bone loss is minimal.
- *Grade II*: Loss of interradicular bone and pocket formation, but not extending through to the opposite side. Alveolar bone is destroyed on one or more aspects of the furcation, but a portion of the alveolar bone and periodontal ligament remains intact, permitting only partial penetration of the probe into the furcation. The lesion is essentially a cul-de-sac. The depth of the horizontal component of the

pocket will determine whether the furcation involvement is early or advanced. The radiograph may or may not reveal the grade II furcation involvement.

- *Grade III*: Through-and-through lesion. The interradicular bone is completely absent, but the facial and/or lingual orifices of the furcation are occluded by gingival tissue. Therefore, the furcation opening cannot be seen clinically, but is essentially a through-and-through tunnel. There may be a crater-like lesion in the interradicular area, creating an apical or vertical component along with the horizontal loss of bone. Radiographs of the mandibular molars can depict a radiolucent area between the roots. Maxillary molars may present a radiographic diagnostic difficulty due to roots overlapping each other.
- *Grade IV*: Through-and-through lesion with gingival recession, leading to a clearly visible furcation area. The interradicular bone is completely destroyed. The gingival tissue is also recessed apically so that the furcation opening is clinically visible, these involvements thus exhibiting tunnels without the orifices being occluded. The radiographic picture is essentially the same as that of grade III lesions.

Hamp et al. (1975)

- *Degree I*: Horizontal loss of periodontal tissue support less than 3 mm.
- Degree II: Horizontal loss of support >3 mm, but not encompassing the total width of the furcation.
- *Degree III*: Horizontal through-and-through destruction of the periodontal tissue in the furcation.

Ramfjord and Ash (1979)

- *Class I*: Beginning involvement. Tissue destruction <2 mm (less than one-third of tooth width) into the furcation.
- *Class II*: Cul-de-sac. Tissue destruction >2 mm (more than one-third of tooth width), but not through and through.
- *Class III*: Through-and-through involvement

Tarnow and Fletcher (1984)

Sub-classification based on the degree of vertical involvement:
- *Subclass A*: 0–3 mm.
- Subclass B: 4–6 mm.
- Subclass C: >7 mm.

Factors to consider in the determination of prognosis (Al-Shammari et al. 2000)

- Degree of involvement.
- Crown/root ratio; length of roots.
- Root anatomy/morphology.
- Degree of root separation.
- Strategic value of the tooth.
- Residual tooth mobility.
- Need for endodontic treatment.
- Prosthetic requirements.
- Periodontal condition of adjacent teeth.
- Ability to maintain oral hygiene.
- Long-term prognosis.
- Quality of bone/ability to place implants.
- Operator's skill and experience.
- Financial considerations.

Treatment approaches according to Glickman classification of furcation lesions (Al-Shammari et al. 2001; Glickman 1953)

Grade I

- Scaling and root planing.
- Odontoplasty.

Grade II

- Scaling and root planing.
- Odontoplasty.
- Open debridement/pocket elimination.
- Regenerative procedures (guided tissue regeneration (GTR), bone grafts, bone morphogenetic proteins (BMPs).
- Root resection (amputation, hemisection).
- Bicuspidization (root separation).
- Tunnel preparation.
- Extraction/implant placement.

Grades III and IV

- Open debridement/pocket elimination.
- Regenerative procedures (GTR, bone grafts, BMPs).
- Root resection (amputation, hemisection).
- Bicuspidization (root separation)/
- Tunnel preparation/
- Extraction/implant placement.

REFERENCES

Al-Shammari KF, Kazor CE, Wang H-L. Molar root anatomy and management of furcation defects. *J Clin Periodontol.* 2001; 28(8):730–740.

Cattabriga M, Pedrazzoli V, Wilson TG Jr. The conservative approach in the treatment of furcation lesions. *Periodontol 2000.* 2000; 22:133–153.

Cobb CM. Non-surgical pocket therapy. *Mechanical. Ann Periodontol.* 1996; 1(1):443–490.

Glickman I. *Clinical Periodontology.* Philadelphia, PA: WB Saunders; 1953.

Glickman I, Smulow J. Buttressing bone formation in the periodontium. *J Periodontol.* 1965; 36(5):365–370.

Goldman HM, Cohen DW. The intrabony pocket: classification and treatment. *J Periodontol.* 1958; 29(4):272–291.

Greenberg J, Laster L, Listgarten MA. Transgingival probing as a potential estimator of alveolar bone level. *J Periodontol.* 1976, 47(9):514–517.

Hamp SE, Nyman S, Lindhe J. Periodontal treatment of multirooted teeth. Results after 5 years. *J Clin Periodontol.* 1975; 2(3):126–135.

Heins PJ, Thomas RG, Newton JW. The relationship of interradicular width and alveolar bone loss. A radiometric study of a periodontitis population. *J Periodontol.* 1988; 59(2):73–79.

Krayer JW, Rees TD. Histologic observations on the topography of a human periodontal pocket viewed in transverse step-serial sections. *J Periodontol.* 1993; 64(7):585–588.

Larato DC. Intrabony defects in the dry human skull. *J Periodontol.* 1970; 41(9):496–498.

Lindhe J, Lang NP, eds. *Clinical Periodontology and Implant Dentistry.* Oxford: Wiley-Blackwell; 2015.

Löe H, Anerud A, Boysen H, Smith M. The natural history of periodontal disease in man: the rate of periodontal destruction before forty years of age. *J Periodontol.* 1978; 49(12):607–620.

Manson JD. Bone morphology and bone loss in periodontal disease. *J Clin Periodontol.* 1976; 3(1):14–22.

Manson JD, Nicholson K. The distribution of bone defects in chronic periodontitis. *J Periodontol.* 1974; 45(2):88–92.

Moskow BS, Polson AM. Histologic studies on the extension of the inflammatory infiltrate in human periodontitis. *J Clin Periodontol.* 1991; 18(7):534–542.

Newman MG, Takei HH, Klokkevold PR, et al. *Newman and Carranza's Clinical Periodontology.* St. Louis, MO: Elsevier Saunders; 2019.

Nielsen JI, Glavind L, Karring T. Interproximal periodontal intrabony defects: prevalence, localization and etiological factors. *J Clin Periodontol.* 1980; 7(3):187–198.

Ooya K, Yamamoto H. A scanning electron microscopic study of the destruction of human alveolar crest in periodontal disease. *J Periodontal Res.* 1978; 13(6):498–503.

Papapanou PN, Tonetti MS. Diagnosis and epidemiology of periodontal osseous lesions. *Periodontol 2000.* 2000; 22:8–21.

Parihar AS, Katoch V. Furcation involvement & its treatment: a review. *J Adv Med Dent Sci Res.* 2015; 3(1):81–87.

Ramfjord SP, Ash MM Jr. *Periodontology and Periodontics.* Philadelphia, PA: WB Saunders; 1979.

Saari JT, Hurt WC, Briggs NL. Periodontal bony defects on the dry skull. *J Periodontol.* 1968; 39(5):278–283.

Tal H. Relationship between interproximal distance of roots and the prevalence of intrabony pockets. *J Periodontol.* 1984; 55(10):604–607.

Tarnow D, Fletcher P. Classification of the vertical component of furcation involvement. *J Periodontol.* 1984; 55(5):283–284.

Waerhaug J. The angular bone defect and its relationship to trauma from occlusion and downgrowth of subgingival plaque. *J Clin Periodontol.* 1979; 6(2):61–82.

Wang H-L, Burgett FG, Shyr Y. The relationship between restoration and furcation involvement on molar teeth. *J Periodontol.* 1993; 64(4):302–305.

Weinmann JP. Progress of gingival inflammation into the supporting structures of the teeth. *J Periodontol.* 1941; 12(2):71–82.

CHAPTER 12
The periodontal examination

Steph Smith and Aditya Tadinada

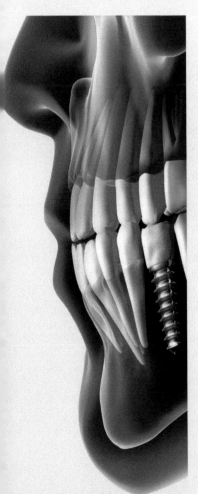

Contents

Learning Objectives

- Components of a comprehensive periodontal examination.
- Medical and dental history of the periodontal patient.
- Purposes of photographic documentation.
- Elements of clinical examination and periodontal charting.
- Relevance of radiographs in diagnosing periodontal diseases.
- Normal radiographic anatomy of the periodontium.
- Types and usage of different radiographs as diagnostic aids.
- Expectations and limitations of intraoral and extraoral radiographic techniques.
- Radiographic features of periodontal lesions.
- Usage and applicability of cone beam computed tomography in diagnosis and therapy of periodontal disease.

Essential Periodontics, First Edition. Edited by Steph Smith and Khalid Almas.
© 2022 John Wiley & Sons Ltd. Published 2022 by John Wiley & Sons Ltd.

Clinical examination and charting

A periodontal examination is an important data-collection activity that is necessary to arrive at a diagnosis and develop a treatment plan (Armitage 2004). Proper diagnosis is essential to intelligent treatment. A diagnosis furthermore determines whether a disease is present, including its severity and extent. Some patients may be unaware of any problems; however, others may report bleeding gums, loose teeth, spreading of the teeth with the appearance of spaces where none existed before, a foul taste in the mouth, or an itchy feeling in the gums. There may be pain of varied types and duration, including constant, dull, gnawing pain; dull pain after eating; deep radiating pain in the jaws; acute throbbing pain; sensitivity when chewing; sensitivity to hot and cold; burning sensation in the gums; or extreme sensitivity to inhaled air (Armitage 2004; Newman et al. 2019).

Diagnostic procedures must thus be systematic and organized for specific purposes so that they provide a meaningful explanation of the patient's periodontal problem. Therefore, the periodontal examination should entail a sequence of procedures for the diagnosis of periodontal diseases (Newman et al. 2019).

Overall appraisal of the patient

From the first meeting, the clinician should attempt an overall appraisal of the patient. This includes consideration of the patient's mental and emotional status, temperament, attitude, and physiological age (Newman et al. 2019).

Health history

Most of the health history is obtained at the first visit, and should be supplemented by pertinent questioning at subsequent visits. The health history can be obtained verbally by questioning the patient and recording the responses in the patient chart, or by means of a questionnaire that the patient completes prior to the appointment. The reasons for a health history are the following:

- Certain systemic diseases, conditions, behavioral factors, and medications can have an impact on periodontal disease, its treatment, and treatment outcomes.
- Certain conditions may require special precautions or modifications of the periodontal treatment procedure.
- Oral infections can have an influence on the occurrence and severity of a variety of systemic diseases and conditions (Newman et al. 2019).

A health history should include the following pertinent aspects (Newman et al. 2019):

- Date of the last physical exam and the frequency of physical exams and physician visits. If the patient is under the care of a physician, the nature and duration of the problem and its therapy should be noted.
- Hospitalizations and types of operations, including anesthetic, hemorrhagic, or infectious complications.

- All medical problems, e.g. cardiovascular, hematological, endocrine, including infectious diseases, sexually transmitted diseases, high-risk behavior for HIV infection, and possible occupational disease.
- Abnormal bleeding tendencies, such as nosebleeds, prolonged bleeding from minor cuts, spontaneous ecchymosis, and a tendency toward excessive bruising. These symptoms should be correlated with the medications that the patient is taking.
- Information is needed for females regarding the onset of puberty, menopause, menstrual disorders, excessive menstrual bleeding, hysterectomy, pregnancies, and miscarriages.
- List of all medications being taken, either prescribed or obtained over the counter. All possible effects of these medications should be analyzed to determine their effect, if any, on the oral tissues and also to avoid administering medications that would cause adverse interactions. Special inquiry should be made about anticoagulants, corticosteroids, and bisphosphonates.
- The patient's allergy history, including hay fever, asthma, sensitivity to foods, sensitivity to drugs (e.g. aspirin, codeine, barbiturates, sulfonamides, antibiotics, procaine, laxatives), and sensitivity to dental materials (e.g. latex, eugenol, acrylic resins).
- A family history of bleeding disorders, cardiovascular disease, diabetes, or periodontal diseases.
- Information on current usage and history of alcohol, recreational drugs, and tobacco use.

Dental history

The dental history should include the following (Newman et al. 2019):

- Visits to the dentist: frequency thereof, date of the most recent visit, nature of the treatment, history of frequency of dental prophylaxis, scaling and root planing, and periodontal maintenance.
- Patient's oral hygiene regimen, including toothbrushing frequency, time of day, method, type of toothbrush and dentifrice, and interval when brushes are replaced. Usage of mouthwashes, interdental brushes, other devices, water irrigation, and dental floss.
- Any orthodontic treatment, including its duration and the approximate date of termination.
- Experience of pain in the teeth or in the gingiva, the manner in which the pain is provoked, its nature and duration, and the manner in which it is relieved.
- Presence of gingival bleeding; when it first occurred; whether it occurs spontaneously, on brushing or eating, at night, or with regular periodicity; whether it is associated with the menstrual period or other specific factors; its duration and the manner by which it is stopped.
- A bad taste in the mouth and areas of food impaction.
- Assess whether the patient's teeth feel "loose," if patient has difficulty chewing, and whether there is tooth mobility.

- General dental habits, such as grinding or clenching of the teeth during the day or at night, tobacco smoking or chewing, nail biting, or biting on foreign objects.
- Previous periodontal problems, the nature of the condition, if it was previously treated, the type of treatment received (surgical or non-surgical), and whether the problem was resolved.
- The wearing of a removable prosthesis. Is it detrimental to the existing dentition or the surrounding soft tissues?
- Implant therapy to replace any missing teeth.

Study models

Alginate impressions should be taken of the patient's dentition for the manufacture of study models. The study models may then be kept for record purposes, studying the patient's occlusion, patient education, as well as before and after treatment comparisons.

Photographic documentation

At the beginning of the clinical examination, intraoral photos should be taken before the tissue is probed and manipulated so as to obtain a baseline of the patient's mouth with gingiva and biofilm intact. Photographic documentation is important for record-keeping, education of both the clinician and the patient, communication with referrals and colleagues, and planning and treatment of especially high aesthetic demand cases (Newman et al. 2019).

Clinical examination (Newman et al. 2019)

Examination of extraoral structures

- Temporomandibular joints.
- Muscles of mastication.
- Lymph nodes of the head and neck.

Examination of the oral cavity

- Cleanliness of the oral cavity – accumulated food debris, biofilm, calculus, tooth surface stains, biofilm coating of tongue dorsum, oral malodor.
- Abnormalities and pathologies of the lips, floor of the mouth, tongue, palate, vestibule, and oropharyngeal region.

Examination of the periodontium

- Visual periodontal assessment of the gingival margin to assess biofilm and calculus accumulation.
- Changes in the soft tissue – color, consistency, surface texture, pigmentation, marginal bleeding, suppuration.
- Visual examination of attached gingiva, mucogingival junction, frenum attachments.
- Examination of the teeth – erosion, abrasion, attrition, faceting, stains, hypersensitivity, proximal contact relations, tooth mobility (see Table 12.1), pathological migration of teeth, sensitivity to percussion, overbite, openbite, crossbite, functional occlusion.

Table 12.1 Grading of tooth mobility.

Physiological	Most often occurs in a horizontal direction, although some axial mobility occurs to a lesser degree
Abnormal/ Pathological	Most often occurs facio-lingually
Score (Miller index)	
0	No detectable movement apart from physiological tooth movement
1	Mobility greater than normal (physiological)
2	Mobility up to 1 mm in bucco-lingual direction
3	Mobility >1 mm in bucco-lingual direction in combination with vertical deformability

Source: Adapted from Newman et al. 2019.

- Periodontal probing of the gingival crevice, pain on probing, probing of subgingival tooth surface to assess probing depths, gingival recession, clinical attachment loss, bleeding on probing, tooth surface aberrations, concavities, subgingival calculus and furcations, periodontal defects, interdental craters. See also Chapter 16.1.2.

Tooth mobility

The most commonly used index system to record tooth mobility is that devised by Miller (1950). Mobility is graded clinically by holding the tooth firmly between the handles of two metallic instruments or with one metallic instrument and one finger (Newman et al. 2019).

Causes of increased tooth mobility (Newman et al. 2019)

- Bone loss:
  - The severity and distribution of bone loss.
  - However, the severity of tooth mobility does not necessarily correspond to the amount of bone loss.
  - The severity and distribution of bone loss at individual root surfaces, the length and shape of the roots, and the root size compared with that of the crown should also be taken into consideration.
- Trauma from occlusion:
  - Occurs when the composite of all occlusal forces on a specific tooth exceeds the tolerance or adaptability of its periodontium.
  - The tissue injury to the periodontium can result in excessive tooth mobility, a widened periodontal ligament (PDL) space, vertical or angular bone destruction, infrabony pockets, and pathological migration, especially of the anterior teeth.

- Sensitivity to percussion is a feature of acute inflammation of the periodontal ligament.
- Premature tooth contacts in the posterior region that deflect the mandible anteriorly contribute to the destruction of the periodontium of the maxillary anterior teeth and to pathological migration.
- Loss of posterior teeth can lead to the mandibular anterior dentition placing increased trauma against the palatal surface of the maxillary anterior dentition, causing facial "flaring" of those teeth.
- Examination of the dentition with the jaws closed can reveal:
- *An excessive overbite*: may cause impingement of the teeth on the gingiva and food impaction in the anterior region, followed by gingival inflammation, gingival enlargement, and pocket formation.
- *An openbite relationship*: especially in the anterior region, whereby reduced mechanical cleansing by the passage of food may lead to accumulation of plaque and debris, calculus formation, and extrusion of teeth.
- *A crossbite*: may be bilateral or unilateral, or may affect only a pair of antagonists. A crossbite can cause trauma from occlusion, food impaction, spreading of the mandibular teeth, and associated gingival and periodontal disturbances.
- *Abnormalities of functional occlusal relationships*: this involves abnormalities in cusp–fossa or cusp–marginal ridge relationships (occlusal discrepancies) on working and non-working sides of the dentition during, for example, centric relation, disclusion, lateral excursion, and protrusion, whereby there may be a loss of resistance to vertical loading on posterior teeth.
- Extension of inflammation from the gingiva or the periapical area into the PDL.
- Periodontal surgery may temporarily increase tooth mobility immediately after the intervention and for a short period.
- Pregnancy, the menstrual cycle, or the use of hormonal contraceptives, due to physicochemical changes in the periodontal tissues.
- Pathological processes of the jaws that destroy the alveolar bone or the roots of the teeth, such as osteomyelitis and tumors of the jaws.

Periodontal charting

The periodontal chart is a permanent record that assists the clinician in arriving at a diagnosis and prognosis, developing a treatment plan, and longitudinally evaluating the response to therapy. Various types and styles of periodontal charts are available (see www.periodontalchart-online.com and Appendix 1). Acceptable charting systems should be simple, easy to fill out and read, and contain relevant information required for making a diagnosis. Relevant information to be included in the periodontal chart can include:
- Probing depths.
- Gingival marginal bleeding and bleeding with probing.

- Clinical attachment loss.
- Gingival margin and attached gingiva.
- Recession.
- Furcation lesions.
- Mobility.
- Open contacts/food impaction.
- Caries.
- Existing restorations/defective restorations/overhangs.
- Extracted teeth/missing teeth/teeth to be extracted.
- Unerupted/impacted teeth.

In addition to clinical information in the periodontal chart, other information relevant to the subsequent development and execution of the treatment plan is usually entered in the progress notes of the patient's chart (Armitage 2004; Newman et al. 2019).

For the purposes of further detailed examination and diagnosis, see the following chapters:
- Calculus – Chapter 5.2.
- Periodontal pocket – Chapter 11.
- Bone loss and patterns of bone destruction – Chapter 11.
- Furcation lesions – Chapter 11.

According to the 2017 Classification of Periodontal Diseases:
- Gingival health, gingivitis, and other gingival diseases – Chapter 6.
- Periodontal health – Chapter 6
- Mucogingival conditions and deformities – Chapter 10.3.
- Necrotizing periodontal diseases – Chapter 7.
- Periodontitis – Chapter 7.
- Aggressive periodontitis – Chapter 8.
- Periodontal abscesses – Chapter 10.2.1.
- Endodontic-periodontal lesions – Chapter 10.2.2.
- Trauma from occlusion – Chapter 10.4.
- Prosthesis- and tooth-related factors – Chapter 10.5.
- Peri-implant health, peri-implant mucositis, peri-implantitis – Chapter 34.
- Systemic conditions affecting the periodontium – Chapter 10.1.

Systems for the numbering and naming of teeth

- *Universal Notation System*. The universal system of notation for the permanent dentition uses "numbers" for each of the teeth. The maxillary teeth are numbered from 1 through 16, beginning with the right third molar. Beginning with the mandibular left third molar, the teeth are numbered 17 through 32.
- *Palmer Notation System*. The Palmer notation consists of a symbol (⌋ ⌊ ⌐ ⌐) designating in which quadrant the tooth is found and a number indicating the position from the midline (Figure 12.1). Adult teeth are numbered 1 through 8. For example, _4| will be the Palmer notation for an upper right first premolar tooth.
- *FDI World Dental Federation Notation System*. This uses a two-number system for the location and naming of each tooth (Figure 12.2). The jaw is divided into four quadrants

	Upper Right								**Upper Left**							
	8⌋	7⌋	6⌋	5⌋	4⌋	3⌋	2⌋	1⌋	⌊1	⌊2	⌊3	⌊4	⌊5	⌊6	⌊7	⌊8
	8⌐	7⌐	6⌐	5⌐	4⌐	3⌐	2⌐	1⌐	⌐1	⌐2	⌐3	⌐4	⌐5	⌐6	⌐7	⌐8
	Lower Right								**Lower Left**							

Figure 12.1 The Palmer Notation System.

Right upper quadrant = **1**	Left upper quadrant = **2**
18 17 16 15 14 13 12 11	**21 22 23 24 25 26 27 28**
48 47 46 45 44 43 42 41	**31 32 33 34 35 36 37 38**
Lower right quadrant = **4**	Lower left quadrant = **3**

Figure 12.2 The FDI World Dental Federation Notation System.

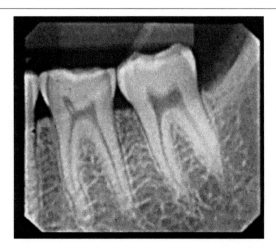

Figure 12.3 Radiographic anatomy of alveolar bone.

between the central incisors and the upper and lower dental arches. The first number refers to the quadrant of a tooth. Adult teeth are numbered 1 through 8. The notation "21" would therefore refer to the permanent left upper central incisor.

Radiographic examination of the periodontium

Radiographs are valuable for the diagnosis of periodontal disease, estimation of severity, determination of prognosis, and evaluation of treatment outcome. However, radiographs are an adjunct to the clinical examination, not a substitute for it. Radiographic information must be considered as one of the key elements of the diagnostic workup in conjunction with clinical findings and patient history. Radiographs demonstrate changes in the calcified tissue; they do not reveal current cellular activity, but rather reflect the effects of past cellular experience on the bone and roots (Newman et al. 2019).

Each of the periodontal structures has a different biochemical composition and, as a result, each of these components has a different density and differential absorption of X-rays. Current radiographic techniques make it extremely challenging to image the soft tissue components, the gingiva, and the PDL. Most radiographic techniques focus on imaging the hard tissues, comprising the cementum overlaying on the root of the tooth and the surrounding alveolar bone. The PDL is assessed on the basis of the PDL space it occupies (Prakash et al. 2015). Enlargement of the PDL space is often considered a response to inflammation (van der Waal 1991; White & Pharoah 2014).

Radiographic anatomy of the periodontium

Evaluation of bone changes in periodontal disease is based mainly on the appearance of the interdental bone, because the relatively dense root structure obscures the facial and lingual bony plates (Figure 12.3).

The interdental bone is normally outlined by a thin, radiopaque line adjacent to the PDL and at the alveolar crest, referred to as the lamina dura. Because the lamina dura represents the cortical bone lining the tooth socket, the shape and position of the root and changes in the angulation of the X-ray beam produce considerable variations in its appearance (Newman et al. 2019). The mesial and distal PDL spaces are usually thin and of even width (Whaites & Drage 2021).

The interdental crestal bone is continuous with the lamina dura of the adjacent teeth, and the junction of the two forms a sharp angle (Whaites & Drage 2021). In the posterior regions, the corticated margins of the interdental crestal bone are evenly thin and smooth (Figure 12.2). In the anterior regions, the interdental crestal bone has thin, even, pointed margins. However, cortication at the top of the crest is not always evident, owing mainly to the small amount of bone between the anterior teeth (Whaites & Drage 2021) (Figure 12.4).

The relationship between the crestal bone margin and the cementoenamel junction (CEJ) is normally depicted by a distance of 2–3 mm (Whaites & Drage 2021). The width and shape of the interdental bone and the angle of the crest normally vary according to the convexity of the proximal tooth surfaces and the level of the CEJ of the approximating teeth. The angulation of the crest of the interdental septum is

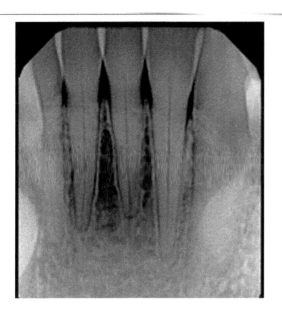

Figure 12.4 Radiographic anatomy of alveolar bone.

generally parallel to a line between the CEJs of the approximating teeth. When there is a difference in the level of the CEJs, the crest of the interdental bone appears angulated rather than horizontal (Newman et al. 2019).

Although these features may not always be evident, their absence from radiographs does not necessarily mean that periodontal disease is present (Whaites & Drage 2021). Absence of these features may be due to technique errors, overexposure, and normal anatomic variations in alveolar bone shape and density. Furthermore, radiographs show evidence of earlier bone loss when there was active disease, therefore bone loss observed in radiographs is not an indicator of the presence of inflammation (Whaites & Drage 2021).

Methods of radiographic imaging

The clinician has two primary methods of imaging the periodontal structures: intraoral and extraoral radiographic techniques (Corbet et al. 2009).

Intraoral radiography

Periapical radiographs

Intraoral periapical radiographs (IOPA) acquired with the parallelling technique using position indicator devices (PIPs) depict the teeth and the periapical structures with the least possible distortion. In this technique, the image receptor is placed parallel to the long axis of the tooth (White & Pharoah 2014). From a practical standpoint, while using this technique the operator must strive to align the X-ray beam, the tooth, and the image receptor in a parallel orientation (Shah et al. 2014) (Figure 12.5).

However, when this method is not achievable because of patient limitations or unavailability of PIPs, an older method called the bisecting angle technique can be used (Figure 12.6). The bisecting angle technique is achieved by placing the image receptor on the lingual/palatal side of the tooth and the central ray (CR) is directed perpendicular to the long axes of both the tooth and the image receptor (Bilhan et al. 2015; White & Pharoah 2014). If the direction of the X-ray beam is not at right angles to the long axis of the tooth, this technique results in image distortion. The area of interest is depicted either too long (elongated) or too short (foreshortening). Elongation can make the bone margin appear closer to the crown; the level of the facial bone may be more distorted than that of the lingual. Inappropriate horizontal angulation results in tooth overlap, changes in the shape of the interdental bone image, alterations of the radiographic width of the PDL space and the appearance of the lamina dura, and may distort the extent of furcation involvement (Newman et al. 2019). This method is more technique sensitive than the parallelling technique and depends on the clinical situation, operator's skill, and patient's cooperation (Bilhan et al. 2015).

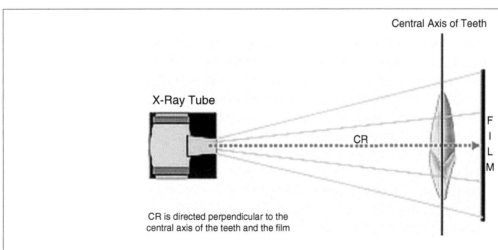

Figure 12.5 Paralleling technique. CR, central ray.

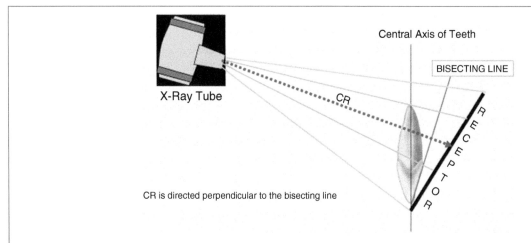

Central Axis of Teeth

X-Ray Tube

BISECTING LINE

CR

RECEPTOR

CR is directed perpendicular to the bisecting line

Figure 12.6 Bisecting angle technique. CR, central ray.

Horizontal and vertical bitewing radiographs

Some cases presenting with a shallow palate or floor of the mouth may not allow ideal placement of the periapical film. In these instances, periapical radiographs frequently do not reveal the correct relationship between the alveolar bone and the CEJ. Bitewing radiographs offer an alternative method that better images periodontal bone levels and the crowns of the teeth. The projection geometry of the bitewing films allows evaluation of the relationship between the interproximal alveolar crest and the CEJ without distortion (Newman et al. 2019). Bitewings are typically used to detect interproximal caries, but are also useful in evaluating the normal crestal bone architecture and any changes in the bone levels because of periodontal pathology (White & Pharoah 2014). The hallmark of periodontitis is alveolar bone loss and it can be well visualized on bitewing radiographs (Zaki et al. 2015). Often there is calculus associated with periodontal pathology and this can also be visualized on bitewing radiographs (White & Pharoah 2014; Zaki et al. 2015). When clinicians refer to bitewing radiographs, they refer to horizontal bitewings for detection of interproximal caries and crestal bone levels (Figure 12.7), but when the

clinical examination requires evaluation of severe bone loss, vertical bitewings (Figure 12.8) can also be acquired by using a specific holding device for vertical bitewings and orienting the image receptor vertically (White & Pharoah 2014). Bitewing radiography is also the preferred imaging technique to depict periodontal bone levels in the posterior dentition (Newman et al. 2019).

Radiographic imaging follows the principles of shadow casting and when the receptor is placed on the lingual aspect of the teeth, the structures nearest to the receptor are best depicted on the radiographic image (White & Pharoah 2014). The resolution of intraoral imaging is better than extraoral imaging

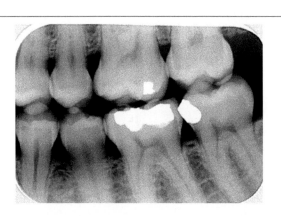

Figure 12.7 Horizontal bitewing.

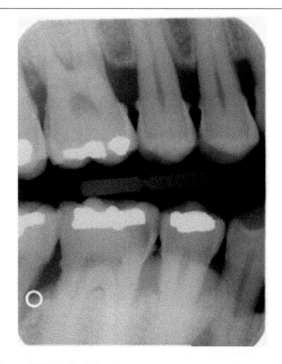

Figure 12.8 Vertical bitewing.

modalities and so the PDL space, which is a key pointer for evaluating pathology, is better depicted on intraoral imaging (Bagis et al. 2015). Widening of the PDL space is often indicative of an inflammatory response and is an important feature in evaluating periodontal and pulpal pathology (van der Waal 1991, White & Pharoah 2014).

Since periapical and bitewing radiographs are two-dimensional (2D) in nature, there are several inherent limitations. These limitations can include the following (Bagis et al. 2015, White & Pharoah 2014):

- Bone loss is detectable only when sufficient calcified tissue has been resorbed to alter the attenuation of the X-ray beam.
- Information is provided only on the hard tissues of the periodontium.
- The most obvious is the inability to depict circumferential bone levels. All 2D images show the mesial and distal bone levels and it is difficult to assess the buccal and lingual/palatal bone plates.
- Only part of a complex bony defect is shown, and one wall of a bone defect may obscure the rest of the defect.
- Exposure factors can have a marked effect on the apparent crestal bone height, whereby overexposure can cause "burn-out" when using film-based imaging.
- Dense tooth or restoration shadows may obscure buccal or lingual bone defects, and buccal or lingual calculus deposits.
- Bone resorption in the furcation area may be obscured by an overlying root or bone shadow.

Extraoral radiography

A variety of extraoral radiographs like lateral cephalometric radiographs or antero-posterior (AP) and postero-anterior (PA) skull views show the periodontal structures in varying clarity, but the imaging modality that is most used by dentists is the orthopantomogram (OPG) or panoramic radiograph (White & Pharoah 2014).

Panoramic radiographs

Panoramic radiography is also called rotational panoramic radiography or pantomography. In this technique, the film and the X-ray source rotate around the patient, who remains stationary, to produce a series of individual images in a single film (Pramod 2011). Panoramic radiographs provide an overview of the maxillary and mandibular arches in one film (Figure 12.9).

Indications for the usage of panoramic radiographs (Pramod 2011):

- Radiographic examination of patients with limited mouth opening.
- For patient education.
- Detection of any pathology involving the jaws, including the extent of a large lesion.
- Generalized assessment of bone levels.
- Evaluation of impacted teeth.
- Evaluation of traumatic injuries.
- Evaluation of multiple unerupted supernumerary teeth.
- Identification of diseases of the temporomandibular joint.

Disadvantages of panoramic radiographs (Pramod 2011):

- Images are not as sharp as in an intraoral film or the resolution is very low.
- Structures in the anterior region may not be well defined.
- Images may show superimposition, especially in the premolar region.
- Images do not have the resolution to reliably demonstrate changes in the PDL space (Bagis et al. 2015).
- Soft tissue and air shadows can overlie the required hard tissue structures (Whaites & Drage 2021).
- Ghost or artifactual shadows can overlie the structures in the focal trough (Whaites & Drage 2021).
- The tomographic movement together with the distance between the focal trough and image receptor produce distortion and magnification of the final image (approximately × 1.3) (Whaites & Drage 2021).

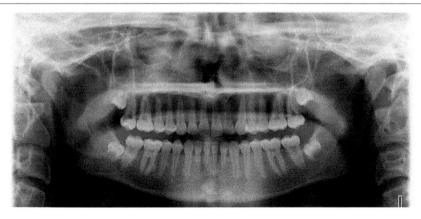

Figure 12.9 Panoramic radiograph.

Radiographic appearance of periodontal disease

See Figures 12.10–12.15. In periodontal disease the interdental bone undergoes changes that affect the lamina dura, crestal radiodensity, size and shape of the medullary spaces, and height and contour of the bone. Early destructive changes of bone that do not remove sufficient mineralized tissue cannot be captured on radiographs. Even slight radiographic changes of the periodontal tissues suggest that the disease has progressed beyond its earliest stages. Furthermore, even when radiographic changes are clearly evident, radiographic examination may underestimate the extent of bone loss. Thus, the earliest signs of periodontal disease and the assessment of periodontal bone levels should be based on combined clinical–radiographic evaluation (Armitage 2004).

Radiographs are an indirect method for determining the amount of bone loss in periodontal disease; they show the amount of remaining bone rather than the amount lost. X-ray angulation may account for the underestimation of the severity of bone loss. The difference between the alveolar crest height and the radiographic appearance can range from 0 to 1.6 mm (Armitage 2004).

Differentiation between treated versus active periodontal disease can only be achieved clinically. Radiographs can only assess the amount of periodontal bone that is present and deduce the extent of bone loss. Therefore, radiographically detectable changes in the normal cortical outline of the interdental bone merely serve as corroborating evidence of destructive periodontal disease (Armitage 2004).

The earliest radiographic change in periodontitis resulting from bone resorption activated by extension of gingival inflammation into the periodontal bone can present as fuzziness and disruption of lamina dura crestal cortication continuity. In the posterior region this may be seen as a blunting of the sharp angle formed by the lamina dura and the alveolar crest (Zaki et al. 2015). However, no correlation has been found between crestal lamina dura in radiographs and the presence or absence of clinical inflammation, bleeding on probing, periodontal pockets, or loss of attachment. Therefore, the presence of an intact crestal lamina dura may be an indicator of periodontal health, whereas its absence lacks diagnostic relevance (Armitage 2004; Pramod 2011).

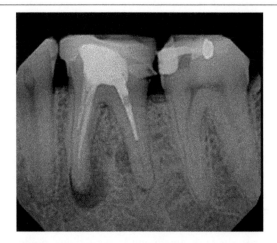

Figure 12.10 Widened periodontal ligament with apical pathology.

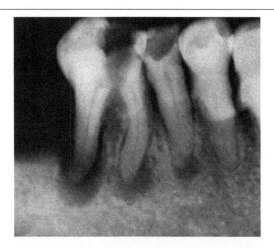

Figure 12.11 Occlusal caries with widened periodontal ligament space and apical pathology.

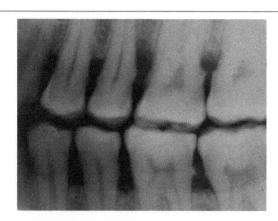

Figure 12.12 Crestal bone loss with radiographic calculus.

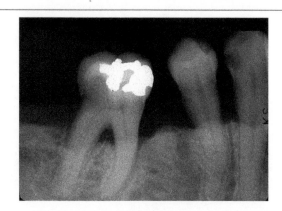

Figure 12.13 Furcation involvement.

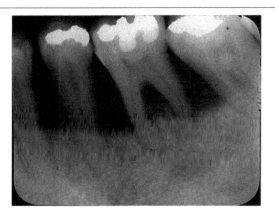

Figure 12.14 Aggressive periodontitis with furcation involvement.

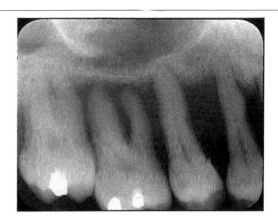

Figure 12.15 Periodontitis with severe bone loss.

Radiographs do not reveal the extent of involvement on the facial and lingual surfaces, as bone destruction of these surfaces is masked by the dense root structure. Frequently a radiopaque horizontal line can be observed across the roots of a tooth. This opaque line demarcates the portion of the root where the labial or lingual bony plate has been partially or completely destroyed from the remaining bone-supported portion. Bone destruction on the mesial and distal root surfaces may be partially hidden by superimposed anatomy, such as a dense mylohyoid ridge. In most cases, it can be assumed that bone loss seen interdentally continues in either the facial or lingual aspect, creating a trough-like lesion. These lesions may terminate on the radicular surface or may communicate with the adjacent interdental area to form one continuous lesion (Armitage 2004).

The height of interdental bone may be reduced, with the crest perpendicular to the long axis of the adjacent teeth, demarcated as horizontal bone loss, or angular or arcuate defects, demarcated as angular or vertical bone loss. With horizontal bone loss, the bone loss is parallel with the CEJ, usually involving multiple teeth. With angular defects the continued periodontal bone loss and widening of the PDL space can be depicted as being uneven and oblique, resulting in a wedge-shaped radiolucency at the mesial or distal aspect of the crest, with the apex of the area pointing in the direction of the root. Angular defects (focal bone loss) are usually centered upon one tooth more than the adjacent tooth (Armitage 2004; Rams et al. 1995). Severe vertical bone loss, extending from the alveolar crest and involving the tooth apex, in which necrosis of pulp tissue is also believed to be a contributory factor, is classified as a periodontal-endodontic lesion (van der Waal 1991).

Horizontal bone loss is characterized by reduction in the height of the alveolar bone in a horizontal direction. It may be localized or generalized based on the regions involved, and usually involves the buccal and lingual cortical plates and the interdental bone (Zaki et al. 2015). Horizontal bone loss is associated with the clinical finding of a suprabony pocket (van der Waal 1991). The amount of radiographic bone loss is also classified according to the 2017 Classification of Periodontal

Diseases as being mild, moderate, severe, or very severe, based on the extent of interproximal bone loss (Lindhe & Lang 2015; van der Waal 1991) (see Chapter 7).

Proximal intrabony defects (focal bone loss) that extend along a root surface apically can be three-walled, where both buccal and lingual cortices are preserved; two-walled, where a buccal or lingual cortex is effaced; or single-walled, where both buccal and lingual cortices are effaced. Vertical bone loss is associated with infrabony pockets (van der Waal 1991). With intraoral 2D projections, the single-walled defect appears lucent and well defined, and the three-walled defect appears hypodense rather than completely lucent, with borders that can appear less well defined (Rams et al. 1995).

Radiographs do not indicate the internal morphology or depth of interdental crater-like defects, as dense cortical facial and lingual plates of interdental bone can obscure destruction of the intervening cancellous bone, and may sometimes appear as vertical defects. An interproximal crater is a trough-like or saucer-shaped defect occurring in the alveolar crest of the interproximal bone. The bony defect has four walls: the buccal and lingual cortical plates, and the roots of two adjacent teeth. The marginal bone of the interproximal crater appears thin (Zaki et al. 2015). To record destruction of the interproximal cancellous bone radiographically, a reduction of 0.5–1 mm in the thickness of the cortical plate is sufficient to permit radiographic visualization of the destruction of the inner cancellous trabeculae (Armitage 2004).

The definitive diagnosis of furcation involvement is made by clinical examination. A large, clearly defined radiolucency in the furcation area is easy to identify; however, root superimposition, caused by anatomic variations or improper radiographic technique, can obscure the radiographic representation of furcation involvement. As a general rule, bone loss is greater than it appears in the radiograph. Diminished radiodensity in the furcation area in which outlines of bony trabeculae are visible suggests furcation involvement. The slightest radiographic change in the furcation area should be investigated clinically, especially if there is bone loss on adjacent roots. Also, whenever there is marked bone loss in relation to a single molar root, it may be assumed that furcation is also involved. Furthermore, a tooth may present marked bifurcation involvement in one film, but appear to be uninvolved in another. Radiographs should thus be taken at different angles to reduce the risk of missing furcation involvement (Armitage 2004).

Utilizing 2D imaging, lucent and relatively well-defined mandibular molar furcations are usually only seen when there is destruction of either the buccal or lingual cortical plates, or both. If one or both of the cortices are preserved, the mandibular molar furcation defect appears as a focal region of varying hypodensity and definition (Rams et al. 1995). 2D radiographic examination for furcation defects of the maxillary molars is rather limited, largely because of the presence of the superimposed shadow of the overlying palatal root (Rams et al. 1995; van der Waal 1991). Early maxillary molar furcation involvement between the mesio-buccal or disto-buccal roots and the palatal root produces a characteristic triangular-shaped radiolucency at the mesial and buccal edges of the tooth (Caton et al. 2018; van der Waal 1991). The identification of a triangular radiographic shadow (furcation arrow) on maxillary molars could be a useful indicator for the presence of a class 2 or 3 furcation involvement, although the absence of the furcation arrow image does not necessarily mean the absence of a bony furcation involvement (Caton et al. 2018). Also, furcation involvement in non-periodontitis cases may be the result of trauma from occlusion and endodontic pathoses due to accessory patent canals communicating with the interradicular space (Hardekopf et al. 1987).

The typical radiographic appearance of a periodontal abscess is a discrete area of radiolucency along the lateral aspect of the root. However, the radiographic picture is often not characteristic, as in the early stages of an acute periodontal abscess when, although it is extremely painful, no radiographic changes may be presented. Lesions in the soft tissue wall of a periodontal pocket are also less likely to produce radiographic changes than those deep in the supporting tissues. Abscesses on the facial or lingual surfaces are obscured by the radiopacity of the root, whereas interproximal lesions are more likely to be visualized radiographically. Radiographs alone, therefore, cannot provide a final diagnosis of a periodontal abscess, but need to be accompanied by careful clinical examination (Armitage 2004).

Trauma from occlusion can produce radiographically detectable changes in the thickness of the lamina dura, morphology of the alveolar crest, width of the PDL space, and density of the surrounding cancellous bone. However, it must be emphasized that radiographic changes are not pathognomonic for trauma from occlusion and must be interpreted in combination with clinical findings, particularly tooth mobility, presence of wear facets, pocket depth, and analysis of occlusal contacts and habits. The injury phase of trauma from occlusion produces a loss of the lamina dura that may be noted in apices, furcations, and marginal areas. This loss of lamina dura results in widening of the PDL space. A generalized or localized widening of the PDL space may be observed in the repair phase of trauma from occlusion, and may also be accompanied by an increased width of the lamina dura, and sometimes by condensation of the perialveolar cancellous bone. More advanced traumatic lesions may result in deep angular bone loss, which, when combined with marginal inflammation, may lead to intrabony pocket formation. In terminal stages, these lesions extend around the root apex, producing a wide, radiolucent periapical image (cavernous lesions). Root resorption may also result from excessive forces on the periodontium, particularly those caused by orthodontic appliances. Although trauma from occlusion produces many areas of root resorption, these areas are usually of a magnitude insufficient to be detected radiographically (Armitage 2004).

Patients presenting with the localized form of aggressive periodontitis are radiographically characterized by severe angular bone loss involving the first molars and the incisors. In many cases there is a virtual absence of local irritants, with the bony lesions being depicted as arch- or saucer-shaped defects (van der Waal 1991; Zaki et al. 2015). The maxillary teeth are involved more than the mandibular teeth and the teeth are involved bilaterally. Apart from the first molars and the incisors, the generalized form involves the canines, the premolars, and the second molars. It is also considered as an extension of the local form (Zaki et al. 2015).

Many locally related factors can influence inflammatory periodontal disease, which may sometimes be identified radiologically. These factors can include the following (Lindhe & Lang 2015; Whaites & Drage 2021):

- Calculus deposits.
- Caries occurring or extending cervically.
- Restorative therapy-related factors, including overhangs, deficiencies, open margins, incorrect contours, and open contacts.
- Root fractures and root resorption.
- Perforations related to endodontic therapy and post preparations.
- Endodontic status in relation to periodontal-endodontic lesions.
- Overerupted opposing teeth.
- Tilted teeth.
- Root approximation.
- Hypercementosis is often idiopathic, but can also be related to increased occlusal loading.
- Increased mobility and/or increased occlusal loading, usually presenting with widened PDL spaces. This widening can involve the entire root or be seen only apically and cervically. A thickened lamina dura is sometimes evident.
- Crown-to-root ratio of a tooth can be observed, which may be relevant to the prognosis of a tooth.

Cone beam computed tomography

Periapical and bitewing radiographs provide information mostly for interdental bone. However, a three-wall defect that preserves the buccal or lingual cortices can be difficult to diagnose, and the buccal, lingual, and furcational periodontal bone levels are hard to evaluate in conventional radiographs (Newman et al. 2019). When three-dimensional (3D) evaluation of the periodontium is indicated, cone beam computed tomography (CBCT) is increasingly becoming the radiographic modality of choice. CBCT avoids the problems of geometric superimposition and unpredictable magnification (Newman et al. 2019). It provides cross-sectional views of the tooth and associated structures, depicting the buccal and lingual/palatal surfaces, including the provision of axial, coronal, and sagittal multiplanar reconstructed images without magnification, thereby offering improved visualization of the morphology of periodontal defects, and thus offers valuable diagnostic information in periodontal evaluation (Acar & Kamburoğlu 2014; Newman et al. 2019).

A key challenge for most clinicians is to evaluate progressive changes in bone levels to monitor advancement of disease. This has been an elusive technique to achieve, largely because of the inability to standardize patient position and image acquisition at the two subsequent time points. Current-day digital image acquisition methods and post-processing programs can help in evaluating changes over time, provided there is standardization of image acquisition at both time points. CBCT may be a useful and more practical clinical tool than digital subtraction radiography for the assessment of changes in periodontal bone over time (Kumar et al. 2015).

Diagnostic applications of cone beam computed tomography for periodontal diseases

- 3D imaging of circumferential bone levels is a potential major advantage in significantly helping the clinician to stage and treat periodontal disease (Mohan et al. 2011). The assessment of regenerative periodontal therapy and bone graft outcomes can also be performed accurately and reliably with CBCT imaging (Eshraghi et al. 2012; Grimard et al. 2009).
- When assessing periodontal bone loss, CBCT has been shown to perform better than digital radiographs in the detection of early furcational defects, particularly in maxillary molars with furcation involvement, three-wall defects, fenestrations, and dehiscence (Newman et al. 2019; Walter et al. 2016). However, the routine use of CBCT for assessing intrabony defects such as one- or two-wall and trough-like defects is not recommended (Newman et al. 2019; Walter et al. 2016). Other authors have concluded that there is not sufficient scientific evidence to support the use of CBCT for the diagnosis and/or treatment planning of intrabony and furcation defects (Nikolic-Jakoba et al. 2016). However, employing CBCT for treatment planning in selected furcation-involved maxillary molars may help to verify the clinical diagnosis and avoid redundant surgical or endodontic interventions (Eshraghi et al. 2012). Studies have reported a high accuracy of CBCT imaging for the analysis of furcation involvement in particularly maxillary molars compared

to probing during clinical examination for the detection of furcation defects (Qiao et al. 2014; Walter et al. 2010).

- Studies have also reported that CBCT images are superior for the detection of apical periodontitis than conventional radiographs (Estrela et al. 2008). Studies have reported that a periapical lesion from endodontic infection might be present without being visible radiographically. To be visible radiographically, a periapical radiolucency should reach nearly 30–50% of bone mineral loss. Lesions confined within the cancellous bone cannot be detected whereas lesions with buccal and lingual cortical involvement produce distinct radiographic areas of rarefaction (Walter et al. 2016). Other conditions, such as apical morphological variations, surrounding bone density, X-ray angulations, and radiographic contrast, also influence radiographic interpretation (Halse et al. 2002). The prevalence of apical periodontitis in endodontically treated teeth, when comparing panoramic and periapical radiographs and CBCT images, has been reported to be 17.6%, 35.3%, and 63.3%, respectively, thus minimizing the possibility of a false-negative diagnosis of apical periodontitis (Estrela et al. 2008).
- Although conflicting views have been reported, bone quality and PDL space have been shown to be better visualized on conventional intraoral radiography (AlJchani 2014; Kumar et al. 2015).
- The use of CBCT imaging around heavily restored teeth may be contraindicated. Beam-hardening artifacts that comprise radiolucent areas and radiopaque lines due to metal artifacts can occur more often in CBCT images. Metal and amalgam restorations cause streaks around materials as well as dark zones that affect the overall quality of the image (Acar & Kamburoğlu 2014).
- CBCT is well suited for imaging highly mineralized structures such as bone or teeth; however, it cannot provide clear images of soft tissues. Nevertheless, soft tissue CBCT (ST-CBCT) is a novel method to visualize and precisely measure distances corresponding to the hard and soft tissues of the periodontium and dentogingival attachment apparatus. Clinicians are able to determine the relationships between gingival margin and facial bone crest, gingival margin and CEJ, and CEJ and facial bone crest. The width of the facial and palatal/lingual alveolar bone and the width of the facial and palatal/lingual gingiva can also be measured. Studies have shown the labial gingival thickness to be moderately associated with the underlying bone thickness measured with CBCT. ST-CBCT can aid clinicians in the planning and execution of procedures with increased predictability (Fu et al. 2010; Januário et al. 2008).

Implementation of cone beam computed tomography in periodontics

While CBCT is a relatively lower radiation dose modality compared to conventional medical computed tomography, the dose is often a key consideration for its judicious use.

The evolution of a lower-dose acquisition mode that images the area of interest using an 180° rotation angle compared to a standard 360° acquisition angle has become a valuable addition for the circumferential evaluation of alveolar bone levels (Mutalik et al. 2020; Tadinada et al. 2017; Yadav et al. 2015). However, CBCT imaging is a higher-dose procedure relative to bitewing radiography, and is also more expensive (Newman et al. 2019; Walter et al. 2016). When compared with conventional radiography, the CBCT radiation dose is equivalent to a full-mouth series and approximately three to seven times the dose of a panoramic radiograph, depending upon the settings used (Katsumata et al. 2009). With all the advantages of 3D imaging, the clinician must however be cognizant of the radiation dose delivered to the patient. The principle of "as low as reasonably achievable" (ALARA) is of the utmost importance and the appropriate field of view and exposure factors must be used to mitigate unnecessary radiation exposure for the patient (Eshragi et al. 2019; Farman 2005; White & Pharoah 2014). No matter how low the dose, it is considered as excessive if it is unlikely to improve the outcomes of the treatment provided. Presently, a lack of studies does not support the use of CBCT imaging as providing either superior short-term or long-term clinical outcomes (Kim et al. 2017; Walter et al. 2010).

In summary, despite the fact that there is rapidly accruing literature on CBCT and its potential diagnostic applications, there are currently insufficient evidence-based guidelines to support its use and implementation for routine periodontal treatment planning (Mandelaris et al. 2017; Walter et al. 2010). Thus, CBCT imaging for periodontal bone evaluation should be considered only for select cases where 2D information is insufficient for diagnostic or treatment planning needs, and it is not recommended for routine evaluation of periodontal bone loss (AlJehani 2014; Eshragi et al. 2019; Newman et al. 2019). Further long-term clinical studies are necessary to establish selection criteria that will help define the conditions and specific indications for the use of CBCT imaging in periodontology to enhance periodontal diagnosis and treatment planning (Feijo et al. 2012). Continued technological advances in CBCT imaging, including higher resolution, reduced imaging artifacts, lower exposure, etc., can promote CBCT usage in the diagnosis and treatment of periodontal diseases (Eshragi et al. 2019).

Future directions

The evolution of artificial intelligence (AI) and advanced post-processing methods in radiographic evaluation open possibilities of better and early detection of periodontal diseases. The use of AI algorithms may enable clinicians to establish and treat the oral and systemic link. Progress in obtaining high-resolution images and incorporation of the fourth dimension (time) in imaging will help in following the disease over time.

REFERENCES

Acar B, Kamburoğlu K. Use of cone beam computed tomography in periodontology. *World J Radiol.* 2014; 6(5):139–147.

AlJehani YA. Diagnostic applications of cone-beam CT for periodontal diseases. *Int J Dent.* 2014; Article ID:865079. doi: 10.1155/2014/865079.

Armitage GC. The complete periodontal examination. *Periodontol 2000.* 2004; 34:22–33.

Bagis N, Kolsuz ME, Kursun S, Orhan K. Comparison of intraoral radiography and cone-beam computed tomography for the detection of periodontal defects: an in vitro study. *BMC Oral Health.* 2015; 15:64.

Bilhan H, Geckili O, Arat Bilhan S et al. The comparison of the precision of different dental radiographic methods in mandibular peri-implantary measurements: an in vitro study. *J Istanb Univ Fac Dent.* 2015; 49(1):1–9.

Caton J, Armitage G, Berglundh T et al. A new classification scheme for periodontal and periimplant diseases and conditions – introduction and key changes from the 1999 classification. *J Clin Periodontol.* 2018; 45(Suppl 20):S1–S8.

Corbet E, Ho D, Lai S. Radiographs in periodontal disease diagnosis and management. *Aus Dent J.* 2009; 54:S27–S43.

Eshraghi T, McAllister N, McAllister B. Clinical applications of digital 2-D and 3-D radiography for the periodontist. *J Evid Based Dent Pract.* 2012; 12:36–45.

Eshraghi VT, Malloy KA, Tahmasbi M. Role of cone-beam computed tomography in the management of periodontal disease. *Dent J.* 2019; 7:57.

Estrela C, Bueno MR, Leles CR, Azevedo B, Azevedo JR. Accuracy of cone beam computed tomography and panoramic and periapical radiography for detection of apical periodontitis. *J Endod.* 2008; 34(3):273–279.

Farman AG. ALARA still applies. *Oral Surg Oral Med Oral Pathol Oral Radiol Endod.* 2005; 100:395–397.

Feijo CV, Lucena JG, Kurita LM, Pereira SL. Evaluation of cone beam computed tomography in the detection of horizontal periodontal bone defects: an in vivo study. *Int J Periodontics Restor Dent.* 2012; 32:e162–e168.

Fu JH, Yeh CY, Chan HL et al. Tissue biotype and its relation to the underlying bone morphology. *J Periodontol.* 2010; 81:569–574.

Grimard BA, Hoidal MJ, Mills MP et al. Comparison of clinical, periapical radiograph, and cone-beam volume tomography measurement techniques for assessing bone level changes following regenerative periodontal therapy. *J Periodontol.* 2009; 80:48–55.

Halse A, Molven O, Fristad I. Diagnosing periapical lesions: disagreement and borderline cases. *Int Endod J.* 2002; 35:703–709.

Hardekopf JD, Dunlap RM, Ahl DR, Pelleu GB. The "furcation arrow." A reliable radiographic image. *J Periodontol.* 1987; 58:258–261.

Januário AL, Barriviera M, Duarte WR. Soft tissue cone-beam computed tomography: a novel method for the measurement of gingival tissue and the dimensions of the dentogingival unit. *J Esthet Restor Dent.* 2008; 20:366–373.

Katsumata A, Hirukawa A, Okumura S et al. Relationship between density variability and imaging volume size in cone-beam computerized tomographic scanning of the maxillofacial region: an in vitro study. *Oral Surg Oral Med Oral Pathol Oral Radiol Endod.* 2009; 107:420–425.

Kim DM, Bassir SH. When is cone-beam computed tomography imaging appropriate for diagnostic inquiry in the management of inflammatory periodontitis? An American Academy of Periodontology best evidence review. *J Periodontol.* 2017; 88(10):979–998.

Kumar T, Puri G, Aravinda K et al. CBCT: a guide to a periodontologist. *SRM J Res Dent Sci.* 2015; 6:48–52.

Lindhe J, Lang NP, eds. *Clinical Periodontology and Implant Dentistry.* Oxford: Wiley-Blackwell; 2015.

Mandelaris GA, Scheyer ET, Evans M. American Academy of Periodontology best evidence consensus statement on selected oral applications for cone-beam computed tomography. *J Periodontol.* 2017; 88(10):939–945.

Miller SC. *Textbook of Periodontia.* Philadelphia, PA: Blackiston; 1950.

Mohan R, Singh A, Gundappa M. Three-dimensional imaging in periodontal diagnosis – utilization of cone beam computed tomography. *J Indian Soc Periodontol.* 2011; 15(1):11–17.

Mutalik S, Tadinada A, Molina MR, Sinisterra A, Lurie A. Effective doses of dental cone beam computed tomography: effect of 360-degree versus 180-degree rotation angles. *Oral Surg Oral Med Oral Pathol Oral Radiol.* 2020; 130(4):433–446.

Newman MG, Takei HH, Klokkevold PR et al. *Newman and Carranza's Clinical Periodontology.* St. Louis, MO: Elsevier Saunders; 2019.

Nikolic-Jakoba N, Spin-Neto R, Wenzel A. Cone-beam computed tomography for detection of intrabony and furcation defects: a systematic review based on a hierarchical model for diagnostic efficacy. *J Periodontol.* 2016; 87:630–644.

Prakash N, KarJodkar FR, Sansare K et al. Visibility of lamina dura and periodontal space on periapical radiographs and its comparison with cone beam computed tomography. *Contemp Clin Dent.* 2015; 6(1):21–25.

Pramod JR. *Textbook of Dental Radiology.* New Delhi: Jaypee Brothers Medical Publishers; 2011.

Qiao J, Wang S, Duan J et al. The accuracy of cone beam computed tomography in assessing maxillary molar furcation involvement. *J Clin Periodontol.* 2014; 41:269–274.

Rams TE, Listgarten MA, Slots J. Utility of radiographic crestal lamina dura for predicting periodontal disease activity. *J Clin Periodontol.* 1995; 21:571.

Shah N, Bansal N, Logani A. Recent advances in imaging technologies in dentistry. *World J Radiol.* 2014; 6(10):794–807.

Tadinada A, Marczak A, Yadav S. Diagnostic efficacy of a modified low-dose acquisition protocol for the preoperative evaluation of mini-implant sites. *Imaging Sci Dent.* 2017; 47(3):141–147.

van der Waal I. Non-plaque related periodontal lesions. An overview of some common and uncommon lesions. *J Clin Periodontol.* 1991; 18:436–440.

Walter C, Schmidt JC, Dula K, Sculean A. Cone beam computed tomography (CBCT) for diagnosis and treatment planning in periodontology: A systematic review. *Quintessence Int.* 2016; 47:25–37.

Walter C, Weiger R, Zitzmann NU. Accuracy of three-dimensional imaging in assessing maxillary molar furcation involvement. *J Clin Periodontol.* 2010; 37:436–441.

Whaites E, Drage N. *Essentials of Dental Radiography and Radiology.* St. Louis, MO: Elsevier; 2021.

White SC, Pharoah MJ. *Oral Radiology: Principles and Interpretation.* St. Louis, MO: Elsevier; 2014.

Yadav S, Palo L, Mahdian M, Upadhyay M, Tadinada A. Diagnostic accuracy of 2 cone-beam computed tomography protocols for detecting arthritic changes in temporomandibular joints. *Am J Orthod Dentofacial Orthop.* 2015; 147(3):339–344.

Zaki HA, Hoffmann KR, Hausmann E, Scannapieco FA. Is radiologic assessment of alveolar crest height useful to monitor periodontal disease activity? *Dent Clin North Am.* 2015; 59(4):859–872.

CHAPTER 13
Periodontal risk assessment

Khalid Almas

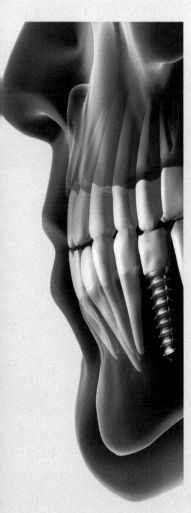

Contents

Learning objectives

- Purposes of oral health risk assessment.
- Risk factors, determinants, indicators, markers/predictors, and local risk factors.
- Clinical relevance of performing periodontal risk assessment.
- Various tools for patient-based periodontal risk assessment.
- Clinical implementation of risk assessment.

Essential Periodontics, First Edition. Edited by Steph Smith and Khalid Almas.
© 2022 John Wiley & Sons Ltd. Published 2022 by John Wiley & Sons Ltd.

Introduction

Periodontal risk assessment is a pragmatic and effective method of categorizing patients, teeth, and sites according to their probability of exhibiting future disease incidence or progression (Trombelli & Farina 2020). From a clinical point of view, the stability of periodontal conditions reflects a dynamic equilibrium between the bacterial challenge and an effective host response. Whenever changes occur in either of these aspects, homeostasis becomes disturbed. Therefore, diagnostic processes must be based on continuous monitoring of multilevel risk profiles. The time intervals between diagnostic assessments should be based on the overall risk profile and the expected benefit for the patient. The use of individual risk profiles to determine the content and frequency of preventive services has been demonstrated to be very cost-effective (Axelsson & Lindhe 1981a, b; Axelsson et al. 1991; Lang & Tonetti 2003).

Oral health risk assessment involves the comprehensive assessment of hereditary, clinical, and lifestyle factors that impact upon the likelihood of developing oral disease, the findings of which are used to support decision-making in planning preventive care for the patient (Chapple & Yonel 2018).

Numerous studies have demonstrated that the host plays a major role in the pathobiology of periodontitis and that risk varies greatly from one individual to another. According to Beck (1998), risk management enables dental care providers to identify patients and populations at increased risk of developing periodontal disease. Identifying risk factors and indicators, as well as undertaking measures that can reduce the risk, can help in maintaining oral health and preventing the onset of any form of periodontal disease. Some risk factors can be modified to reduce the risk of initiation or progression of disease, such as smoking or improved oral hygiene, while other factors cannot be modified, such as genetic factors (Page et al. 2002).

Definitions and terminology

Table 13.1 depicts various definitions and terminologies that are used in general and specific disease risk assessment.

Risk can be identified in terms of risk factors, risk indicators, or risk predictors. A risk factor is thought to be a cause for disease (Table 13.2). It should satisfy two criteria: (i) it is biologically plausible as a causal agent for disease; and (ii) it has been shown to precede the development of disease in prospective clinical studies. Risk factors are biologically related to the occurrence of the disease, but they do not necessarily imply cause and effect, i.e. just because a patient possesses a risk factor does not mean that they will develop the disease. Equally, the absence of a risk factor does not mean that the disease will not develop.

Evidence in the literature points to a direct and significant link between several risk factors and periodontal disease (Pihlstrom 2001). These risk factors may be broadly categorized as:

- *Systemic risk factors* – factors that affect the host response to the plaque biofilm, upsetting the host–microbial balance.
- *Local risk factors* – factors local to the oral cavity, which may influence plaque accumulation or occlusal forces. (Koshi et al. 2012; Timmerman & Van der Weijden 2006).

Risk factors

Tobacco smoking

Substance abuse affects more than one-sixth of the world's population, and the nature of the abuse and the type of addictive substance available to individuals are increasing exponentially. These substances with abusive potential impact both the human immuno-inflammatory system and oral microbial communities (Kumar 2020).

Tobacco smoking is a well-established risk factor for periodontitis (Eke et al. 2016). A direct relationship exists between smoking and the prevalence of periodontal disease. This association is independent of other factors such as oral hygiene or age (Ismail et al. 1983). Studies comparing the response to periodontal therapy in smokers, previous smokers, and non-smokers have shown that smoking has a negative impact on the response to therapy. However, former smokers respond similarly to non-smokers (American Academy of Periodontology 1999).

Smoking is as close as any risk indicator can get to being a true risk factor. It has been estimated that 42% of periodontitis may be attributable to smoking (Tomar & Asma 2000).

Smoking has both local and systemic effects that place patients at greater risk of periodontitis progression:
- Local effects:
  - Reduced tissue vascularity.
  - Impairment of polymorphonuclear leucocyte (PMNL) chemotaxis and function (phagocytosis).
- Systemic effects:
  - Decreased salivary immunoglobulin (Ig)A.
  - Decreased serum IgG.
  - Decreased helper T cells.

Smokers have been shown to have more and deeper pockets (especially palatally), more recession, more bone loss, and increased tooth loss in comparison to non-smokers. Smokers may also experience more bone loss in upper anterior regions than non-smokers (Baharin et al. 2006). Smokers have also been shown to have less marginal bleeding, which can have the effect of masking early critical signs (bleeding gums) of periodontitis. The evidence associating smoking with periodontitis is robust; however, there remains a lack of substantial and sufficiently powered intervention studies that demonstrate improved periodontal outcomes following smoking cessation.

The odds ratios (ORs) for periodontitis in smokers varies between a three- and sevenfold increased relative risk for disease. A dose response exists between smoking and periodontal risk – 10 cigarettes/day increasing risk by 5% and 20/day increasing risk by 10%. Moreover, serum levels of the stable nicotine metabolite cotinine correlate with attachment loss, probing pocket depth, and alveolar crest height.

Table 13.1 Terminology and definitions used in periodontal risk assessments and supportive periodontal therapy.

Terminology	Definition
Risk	The likelihood that a person will get a disease in a specified time period is called risk. The probability of something happening (e.g. suffering from disease/progression) is also known as risk.
Risk factor	The characteristics of a person or their environment that, when present, directly result in an increased likelihood of that person getting the disease, and when absent, directly result in a decreased likelihood (Beck et al. 1995). They have an association with the disease, e.g. for periodontal diseases they are genetics, smoking, stress, and some systemic diseases. Factors that contribute to risk are called risk factors.
Risk markers	Risk markers or predictors that are not causally related to a disease, but their presence is more a consequence of the disease being present. Examples in periodontitis are bleeding on probing, suppuration, tooth mobility, interproximal recession, and evidence of past disease. Risk markers imply the presence of disease and are often used to detect early stages of disease.
True risk factors	Those factors have a causal association; that is, when present, they increase the likelihood of the disease developing, but when they are removed the disease improves, e.g. the oral biofilm.
Putative risk factors	Those factors that are associated with the occurrence of a disease, as observed in cross-sectional studies, e.g. stress or nutritional factors.
Systemic risk factors	Those factors affecting the host response either directly or indirectly. They may be environmental factors (e.g. stress), lifestyle factors (e.g. nutrition or smoking), or those relating to general health (e.g. diabetes status, immunodeficiency, or other conditions such as leucocyte adhesion defects).
Local risk factors	These factors are biofilm retention factors, which may be anatomic in nature (e.g. root grooves, enamel pearls) or relate to poor restoration margins, imbricated teeth, or iatrogenic restorations, and dental appliances affecting the gingival margin.
Modifiable risk factors	These factors can be influenced by the patient or the clinician. They may be systemic or environmental in nature and include smoking cessation, improving diabetes control, improved diet, and reducing biofilm levels through improved oral hygiene, or correction of restorations with subgingival ledges or overhang margins.
Non-modifiable risk factors	Those factors that cannot be influenced by the patient and essentially relate to genetic traits or characteristics.
Risk assessment	The process of predicting an individual's probability of disease. Risk assessment should help clinicians to formulate an effective management plan for a periodontitis patient and to establish the frequency of recall intervals for supportive care.
Risk indicators	A risk indicator is a factor that is biologically plausible as a causative agent for a disease, but has only been shown to be associated with disease in cross-sectional studies. An example of a risk indicator of periodontal disease is the presence of herpes viruses in subgingival plaque.
Risk predictor	A factor that has no current biological plausibility as a causative agent, but has been associated with disease on a cross-sectional or longitudinal basis. For example, the number of missing teeth is a risk predictor for disease, but has little or no plausibility as a causative agent for periodontitis (Koshi et al. 2012).
PRA	Periodontal risk assessment.
Prognostic factors	Factors that increase the likelihood of progression in a previously diseased patient.
PRC	Periodontal risk calculator.
SPT	Supportive periodontal therapy.

The healing response to non-surgical and surgical periodontal therapy is poorer in smokers and maintenance patients who smoke are twice as likely to lose teeth as non-smokers (Chapple et al. 2015). Together, the diverse actions of tobacco smoke create an oxidant-rich, chronic inflammatory environment, promoting pathogen colonization and reducing the repair and remodeling capabilities of cells. In the presence of continued smoking, oral prophylaxis and surgical and non-surgical therapies do little to reverse the virulence of the microbiome, reduce the antigenic burden, or reverse the damage caused by disease (Kumar 2020).

Table 13.2 Various periodontal risk factors, determinants, indicators, and predictors.

Risks	Descriptions
Risk factors	Tobacco smoking Diabetes Pathogenic bacteria and microbial tooth deposits
Risk determinants	Genetic factors Age Sex Socioeconomic status Stress Nutrition
Risk indicators	HIV/AIDS Osteoporosis Infrequent dental visits
Risk markers/ predictors	Previous history of periodontal disease Bleeding on probing
Local risk factors	Iatrogenic (restorations, appliances, crown, and bridge), anatomic (e.g. root grooves), root caries, tooth malignment, false/true pockets, high frenal attachment, mouth breathing, calculus

Diabetes

Epidemiological data demonstrate that the prevalence and severity of periodontitis are significantly higher in patients with type 1 or type 2 diabetes mellitus than in those without diabetes, and that the level of diabetic control is an important variable in this relationship (Elangovan et al. 2019).

There is reportedly a "bi-directional relationship" between diabetes mellitus and periodontitis (Taylor 2001), whereby the presence of one condition adversely affects the other. Severe periodontitis adversely affects glycemic control in diabetes and glycemia in non-diabetes patients, and there is a direct and dose-dependent relationship between periodontitis severity and diabetes complications. Emerging evidence supports an increased risk for diabetes onset in patients with severe periodontitis and mechanisms appear to involve elevated systemic inflammation (acute-phase and oxidative stress biomarkers), resulting from the entry of periodontal organisms and their virulence factors into the circulation (Chapple & Genco 2013).

Pathogenic bacteria and oral biofilm accumulation

It is well documented that the accumulation of bacterial plaque at the gingival margin results in the development of gingivitis and that the gingivitis can be reversed with the implementation of oral hygiene measures (Löe et al. 1965). These studies demonstrate a causal relationship between the accumulation of bacterial plaque and gingival inflammation. However, a causal relationship between *plaque accumulation* and *periodontitis* has been more difficult to establish. Often patients with severe loss

of attachment have minimal levels of bacterial plaque on the affected teeth, indicating that the *quantity* of plaque is not of major importance in the disease process. However, although quantity may not indicate risk, there is evidence that the composition, or *quality*, of the complex plaque biofilm is important (Elangovan et al. 2019).

In terms of quality of plaque, three specific bacteria have been identified as etiological agents for periodontitis: *Aggregatibacter actinomycetemcomitans* (formerly *Actinobacillus actinomycetemcomitans*), *Porphyromonas gingivalis*, and *Tannerella forsythia* (formerly *Bacteroides forsythus*) (Genco et al. 1996). *P. gingivalis* and *T. forsythia* are often found in chronic periodontitis, whereas *A. actinomycetemcomitans* is frequently associated with aggressive periodontitis. Cross-sectional and longitudinal studies support the delineation of these three bacteria as risk factors for periodontal disease. Additional evidence that these organisms are causal agents includes the following (Haffajee & Socransky 1994):

- Their elimination or suppression impacts the success of therapy.
- There is a host response to these pathogens.
- Virulence factors are associated with these pathogens.
- Inoculation of these bacteria into animal models induces periodontal disease.

It is becoming clear from investigations that the plaque composition shifts from a more symbiotic microbial community to one that is more dysbiotic (an imbalance in the relative abundance of microbes leading to disease), composed primarily of anaerobes, as we go from periodontal health to periodontal disease. Certain pathogens (termed *keystone pathogens*) such as *P. gingivalis* play a major role in inducing such a shift, converting commensals into disease-provoking microbes (termed *pathobionts*) (Hajishengallis 2015). Therefore, the quantity of plaque present may not be as important as the quality of the plaque in determining risk for periodontitis.

The evidence for the oral biofilm as a true risk factor for gingivitis is strong, based upon the original experimental gingivitis study of Löe et al. (1965). In this study, volunteers were prevented from toothbrushing for 21 days to allow plaque accumulation. Gingivitis developed and when the biofilm was removed, the gingivitis resolved.

Biofilm accumulation is essential for periodontitis to develop, but as it does not cause periodontitis in all patients, it is regarded as the trigger for disease initiation, but not the sole cause. The amount of biofilm necessary to induce periodontitis, or cause periodontitis progression, varies between patients and, in any individual, the biofilm needs to reach a "threshold" level for disease to occur. Some patients will never develop periodontitis (about 10% of most populations) even if they never brushed, since they are inherently resistant to disease development (Chapple 2015).

The presence of *calculus*, which serves as a reservoir of bacterial plaque, has been suggested as a risk factor for periodontitis. Although the presence of some calculus in healthy individuals receiving routine dental care does not result in a significant loss of attachment, the presence of calculus in other groups of patients, such as those not receiving regular care and those with poorly controlled diabetes, can have a negative impact on periodontal health (Page & Beck 1997).

Risk determinants

Genetic factors

Studies of monozygous twins indicate that genetics may explain about 50% of periodontitis prevalence (Michalowicz et al. 2000). Evidence indicates that genetic differences between individuals may explain why some patients develop periodontal disease and others do not. Studies conducted in twins have shown that genetic factors influence clinical measures of gingivitis, probing pocket depth, attachment loss, and interproximal bone height (Michalowicz et al. 1991a, b, 2000). The familial aggregation seen in localized and generalized aggressive periodontitis also indicates genetic involvement in these diseases (Elangovan et al. 2019).

However, genetics cannot be described as a "true" risk factor, because intervention studies employing gene therapies have not been performed to assess their efficacy in improving periodontal outcomes. Periodontitis is a complex disease and just as it is regarded as being polymicrobial and polyimmune-inflammatory in nature, it can also be regarded as being polygenetic (Chapple et al. 2015).

Kornman et al. (1997) demonstrated that alterations (*polymorphisms*) in specific genes encoding inflammatory cytokines such as interleukin (IL)-1α and IL-1β were associated with severe chronic periodontitis in non-smoking subjects. However, results of other studies have shown a limited association between these altered genes and the presence of periodontitis. Overall, it appears that changes in the IL-1 genes may be only one of several genetic changes involved in the risk for chronic periodontitis. Therefore, although alteration in the IL-1 genes may be a valid marker for periodontitis in defined populations, its usefulness as a genetic marker in the general population may be limited (Kinane & Hart 2003).

Immunological alterations, such as neutrophil abnormalities (Hart et al. 1994), monocytic hyperresponsiveness to lipopolysaccharide stimulation in patients with localized aggressive periodontitis (Shapira et al. 1996), and alterations in the monocyte/macrophage receptors for the Fc portion of antibody (Kinane & Hart 2003; Wilson et al. 1996) also appear to be under genetic control. In addition, genetics plays a role in regulating the titer of the protective immunoglobulin G2 (IgG2) antibody response to *A. actinomycetemcomitans* in patients with aggressive periodontitis (Gunsolley et al. 1997). In addition, epigenetic influences are becoming important in the study of periodontitis. These are the effects of agents such as enzymes produced by bacteria, micronutrients, or oxygen radicals, which are able to modify genes by processes such as methylation, reducing their expression and preventing the gene from working correctly (Chapple et al. 2015).

Age

Both the prevalence and the severity of periodontal disease increase with age (Burt 1994; Eke et al. 2016; Papapanou 1994). It is possible that degenerative changes related to aging may increase susceptibility to periodontitis. However, it is also possible that the attachment loss and bone loss seen in older individuals are the result of prolonged exposure to other risk factors over a person's lifetime, creating a cumulative effect over time. In support of this theory, studies have shown minimal loss of attachment in aging subjects enrolled in preventive programs throughout their lives (Papapanou & Lindhe 1992; Papapanou et al. 1991). Therefore, it is suggested that periodontal disease is not an inevitable consequence of the aging process and that aging alone does not increase disease susceptibility. However, it remains to be determined whether changes related to the aging process, such as medication intake, decreased immune function, and altered nutritional status, interact with other well-defined risk factors to increase susceptibility to periodontitis.

Evidence of loss of attachment may have more consequences in younger patients. The younger the patient, the longer the time for exposure to causative factors. In addition, aggressive periodontitis in young individuals is often associated with unmodifiable risk factors, such as a genetic predisposition to disease (Eke et al. 2016). Therefore, young individuals with periodontal disease may be at greater risk for continued disease as they age.

It is also important to recognize that the population of the developed world is aging, and patients expect to keep their teeth for longer. The World Health Organization has set a target to define successful dentistry as the retention of 20 teeth at 80 years of age. Periodontitis will therefore become more prevalent in older patients (Chapple et al. 2015).

Sex

Surveys conducted in the USA since 1960 demonstrate that men have more loss of attachment than women (US Public Health Service 1965, 1979, 1987). In addition, men have poorer oral hygiene than women, as evidenced by higher levels of plaque and calculus (Abdellatif & Burt 1987; Enwonwu 1972; US Public Health Service 1987). Therefore, sex differences in the prevalence and severity of periodontitis appear to be related to preventive practices rather than any genetic factor.

Socioeconomic status

Gingivitis and poor oral hygiene can be related to lower socioeconomic status (SES) (US Public Health Service 1979). This can most likely be attributed to decreased dental awareness and decreased frequency of dental visits compared with more educated individuals with higher SES. After adjusting for other risk factors, such as smoking and poor oral hygiene, lower SES alone does not result in increased risk for periodontitis.

Stress

The incidence of necrotizing ulcerative gingivitis increases during periods of emotional and physiological stress, suggesting a link between the two (Enwonwu 1972; Shields 1977). Emotional stress may interfere with normal immune function (Ballieux 1991; Sternberg et al. 1992) and may result in increased levels of circulating hormones, which can affect the periodontium (Rose 1980). Stressful life events, such as bereavement and illness, appear to lead to a greater prevalence of periodontal disease (Green et al. 1986), and an apparent association exists between psychosocial factors and risk behaviors such as smoking, poor oral hygiene, and chronic periodontitis (Croucher et al. 1997). Adult patients with periodontitis who are resistant to therapy are more stressed than those who respond to therapy (Axtelius et al. 1998). Individuals with financial strain, distress, depression, or inadequate coping mechanisms have more severe loss of attachment (Genco et al. 1999). Although epidemiological data on the relationship between stress and periodontal disease are limited, stress may be a putative risk factor for periodontitis (Eke et al. 2016).

The evidence for stress per se as a risk factor for periodontitis is weak; however, there is evidence that poor coping strategies may negatively impact upon periodontitis (Wimmer et al. 2002). It has also been demonstrated that patients under financial stress and strain have greater levels of periodontitis, but those who have good coping strategies present with no more disease than unstressed controls. Stress triggers neuroendocrine responses via the hypothalamic–pituitary–adrenal (HPA) axis. This in turn triggers the activation of complement and the release of proinflammatory cytokines.

There is also evidence that certain periodontal pathogens can utilize stress hormones like noradrenaline and adrenaline to acquire iron for growth and virulence (Roberts et al. 2002). Additionally, they appear to produce an auto-inducer of their own growth in response to the same stress hormones (Roberts et al. 2005), indicating that certain periodontal bacteria can take advantage of a stressed host (Chapple et al. 2015).

Nutrition

There is considerable interest in micronutrients as both agonists and antagonists of inflammatory processes (Chapple 2009). Evidence demonstrates that refined carbohydrate intake drives systemic or "meal-induced" inflammation (Monnier et al. 2006).

Several association studies demonstrate that blood levels of certain antioxidant micronutrients are inversely related to periodontitis prevalence; for instance, low vitamin C is estimated to account for 4% of attachment loss seen in certain populations (Chapple & Matthews 2007).

Blood total antioxidants show similar results. To date, there is one intervention study that has demonstrated improved periodontal outcomes following adjunctive use of capsules of dried fruit and vegetable concentrates during non-surgical therapy and follow-up (Chapple et al. 2012). The role of poor nutrition as a risk factor for periodontitis is under-researched at present, but could be significant (Chapple et al. 2015).

Risk indicators

HIV/AIDS

It has been hypothesized that the immune dysfunction associated with HIV infection and AIDS increases susceptibility to periodontal disease (Elangovan et al. 2019). Early reports on the periodontal status of patients with AIDS or those who are HIV seropositive revealed that these patients often had severe periodontal destruction characteristic of necrotizing ulcerative periodontitis (Winkler et al. 1992). More recent reports, however, have failed to demonstrate significant differences in the periodontal status of individuals with HIV infection and healthy controls (Lamster et al. 1994; Swango et al. 1991). The apparent discrepancy in these reports may have been caused by the inclusion of patients with AIDS (versus patients who were exclusively HIV seropositive) in some studies (Eke et al. 2016).

Conflicting results also exist in studies examining the level of immunosuppression and severity of periodontal destruction. Some studies support the observation that as the degree of immunosuppression increases in adults with AIDS, periodontal pocket formation and loss of clinical attachment also increase. Results of other studies have found no relationship between periodontal diseases and HIV/AIDS status. Evidence also suggests that AIDS-affected individuals who practice good preventive oral health measures, including effective home care and seeking appropriate professional therapy, can maintain periodontal health (Stanford & Rees 2003).

Osteoporosis

Osteoporosis has been suggested as another risk factor for periodontitis. Although studies in animal models indicate that osteoporosis does not initiate periodontitis, evidence indicates that the reduced bone mass seen in osteoporosis may aggravate periodontal disease progression (Aufdemorte et al. 1993; Krook et al. 1975). However, reports in humans are conflicting. In a study of 12 women with osteoporosis and 14 healthy women, von Wowern et al. (1994) reported that women with osteoporosis had greater loss of attachment than control subjects. In contrast, Kribbs (1990) examined pocket depth, bleeding on probing, and gingival recession in women with and without osteoporosis. Although the two groups had significant differences in bone mass, no differences in periodontal status were noted. However, it appears that a link may exist between osteoporosis and periodontitis, and additional studies may need to be conducted to determine whether osteoporosis is a true risk factor for periodontal disease (Guers et al. 2003; Kinane 1999). Results from a recent meta-analysis of observational studies showed that osteoporosis is an independent risk factor for periodontitis. This finding may affect the clinical understanding of the etiology of periodontitis in this field and may further enrich the knowledge and means of preventing and controlling osteoporosis (Xu et al. 2021).

Infrequent dental visits

Identifying failure to visit the dentist regularly as a risk factor for periodontitis is controversial (Page & Beck 1997). One study demonstrated an increased risk for severe periodontitis in patients who had not visited the dentist for three or more years, whereas another demonstrated that there was no more loss of attachment or bone loss in individuals who did not seek dental care compared with those who did over a six-year period. However, differences in the ages of the subjects in these two studies may explain the different results. Additional longitudinal and intervention studies are necessary to determine whether infrequency of dental visits is a risk factor for periodontal disease (Elangovan et al. 2019).

Risk markers/predictors

Previous history of periodontal disease

A history of previous periodontal disease is a good clinical predictor of risk for future disease (Page & Beck 1997). Patients with the most severe existing loss of attachment are at greatest risk for future loss of attachment. Conversely, patients currently free of periodontitis have a decreased risk for developing loss of attachment compared with those who currently have periodontitis (Elangovan et al. 2019).

Bleeding on probing

Bleeding on probing is the best clinical indicator of gingival inflammation (Page & Beck 1997). Although this indicator alone does not serve as a predictor for loss of attachment, bleeding on probing coupled with increasing pocket depth may serve as an excellent predictor for future loss of attachment. Lack of bleeding on probing does appear to serve as an excellent indicator of periodontal health (Elangovan et al. 2019).

Local risk factors

Local risk factors may have an important role in the initiation and propagation of periodontal diseases and act by allowing retention of biofilm at the gingival margin, leading to an inflammatory response. A wide range of local factors exists, and management involves removal or modification of the factor along with detailed home-care instruction on subsequent biofilm disruption by the patient (Chapple et al. 2015). Table 13.3 depicts various iatrogenic and anatomic local risk factors that play a role in the initiation and propagation of periodontal diseases.

Clinical relevance

The goal of performing periodontal risk assessment is to develop a more personalized treatment plan for a specific patient, considering the periodontal risk profile of that patient.

Table 13.3 Local iatrogenic and anatomic risk factors.

Iatrogenic	Anatomic
Restorations	Root caries
Appliances	Root grooves
Removable partial dentures	Tooth position/malalignment
Crown/bridge design	False/true pockets
Bridge pontic design	High frenal attachment
	Mouth breathing
	Calculus

Once an at-risk patient is identified and a diagnosis is made, the treatment plan may be modified accordingly.

Continuous risk assessment is a critically important concept, because risk changes throughout the life course and therefore a patient with no apparent disease experience may suffer a major life event, which contributes the final slice in the causal pie to create a "sufficient cause." This could involve, for example, the stress that results from the loss of a loved one or a divorce, which may directly impact upon known neuroendocrine pathways that drive inflammation, or indirectly may result in the neglect of oral hygiene practices and consequently an increased microbial challenge (Chapple 2020).

Kye et al. (2012) have pointed out that, unfortunately, traditional clinical parameters of periodontal disease such as bone and attachment loss are simply cumulative measures of past disease experience and do not necessarily help predict future disease activity or progression. Essentially, risk and disease are distinct concepts, because a high-risk patient may have no disease at a given time point, but that does not mean that they will not develop disease when, for example, they age and immune senescence (a lower efficiency in immune function that arises with aging) starts to emerge. Nevertheless, there is good evidence that the cumulative disease experience of a patient at presentation (now determined by staging and grading of periodontitis) is a strong predictor of future risk of progression, in the absence of clinical interventions aimed at risk factor control, behavior change, and clinical treatment. Moreover, the diagnosis should be documented as a "diagnostic statement" that records the disease type and extent, its stage and grade, and the current activity status (stable, remission, or unstable), and immediately beneath the diagnosis, but part of the diagnostic statement, the relevant risk factors are listed.

For example, a diagnostic statement may appear as:
- *Diagnosis*: Localized periodontitis, stage III, grade B, currently stable.
- *Risk status and risk factors*: High risk; smoking >10 cigarettes/day, high refined sugar intake.

The risk assessment, whether it is performed by using an anecdotal "high," "medium," "low" annotation, or by using a more accurate and objective computer-based tool, is thus embedded in the diagnostic statement (Chapple 2020).

Assessment of the risk level for disease progression in each individual patient enables the practitioner to determine the frequency and extent of professional support required at supportive periodontal therapy (SPT) visits to maintain the attachment levels following active therapy (Trombelli & Farina 2020).

It has been recognized that periodontal risk assessment is a necessary component of all comprehensive dental and periodontal evaluations, as well as part of all periodic dental and periodontal examinations. In a position paper, the American Academy of Periodontology stated that risk assessment may help dental professionals predict the potential for developing periodontal diseases, and allow them to focus on early identification and provide proactive, targeted treatment for patients at risk of progressive/aggressive diseases (American Academy of Periodontology 2008). Similarly, in a recent consensus report, the European Federation of Periodontology supported the usefulness of risk assessment tools, recognizing their validity to capture the complexity of the patient profile, inform clinical decision-making, and communicate potential preventive targets to the patient (Tonetti et al. 2015). The development of a new periodontal classification system that embeds prognostic determination (World Workshop for the Classification of Periodontal Diseases and Conditions; Tonetti et al. 2018), reinforces the importance of risk assessment in the comprehensive patient evaluation. In this respect, the new case definition of periodontitis incorporates a framework for the implementation of a biological grade (risk or actual evidence of progression) of the disease. In the grading system, the patient is assigned a grade A, B, or C (corresponding to slow, moderate, and rapid rate of progression, respectively) depending on direct and indirect evidence of periodontitis progression as well as exposure to true risk factors (smoking and diabetes) (Tonetti et al. 2018).

The arbitrary nature of risk assessment may arise due to the difficulty of including all relevant parameters in an integrated decision. For example, the study by Persson et al. (2003a) showed that individual risk assessment was based almost exclusively on parameters related to disease severity (e.g. radiographic bone levels, periodontal pockets), whereas relevant risk factors (such as diabetes and smoking) were not accounted for in the risk evaluation (Persson et al. 2003a, b).

Periodontal risk assessment

Periodontal risk is multifactorial and risk assessment for patients dictates that those different analytical levels of risk should be employed at different stages of treatment. Thus, multilevel risk assessment is necessary. At the start of treatment, analysis is at the patient level, but as treatment progresses, increasing levels of detail can be employed (Chapple et al. 2015).

Risk assessment should help clinicians to formulate an effective management plan for a periodontitis patient and to establish the frequency of recall intervals for supportive care. Traditionally, periodontitis management and treatment planning have been based on a detailed patient history and examination, but including a risk assessment as a third dimension

will tailor a more appropriate treatment plan for an individual patient (Chapple et al. 2015).

Tools and technologies for patient-based periodontal risk assessment

Observations on the poor accuracy and reproducibility of subjective risk assessment have called for the development of patient-based risk assessment tools, i.e. instruments that include a standardized, composite measure of risk expressing the probability for disease incidence/progression in a specific individual. Such tools aim at obtaining more uniform and accurate information in order to optimize clinical decision-making, improve oral health for patients, and reduce healthcare costs (Lang et al. 2015).

There are different ways of assessing risk, including online tools that offer consistent and accurate scoring and visual biofeedback to patients. This reduces the need for complex therapy, in turn leading to an improvement in oral health with reduced healthcare costs for the patient (Chapple et al. 2015). However, these different assessment tools use different risk factors and algorithms, hence they will not always be in complete agreement (Naga Sai Sujai et al. 2015). Available risk assessment tools are the following:

- *Health Improvement in Dental Practice (HIDEP) system model* (Fors et al. 2001). HIDEP is a computer-based tool. Its model combines preexisting examination methods, risk estimation systems, and treatment suggestions into a new entity. According to HIDEP, the patient is classified as healthy, with a risk ranging between 0S (lowest risk) to 4S (highest risk), or sick, with a disease status ranging between 1 (mild symptoms) and 4 (severe symptoms). In HIDEP, the process links the risk score to prevention/treatment schemes.

- *Periodontal Risk Calculator (PRC)* (in either its original version or as incorporated in broader oral health assessment tools) (Busby et al. 2014; Martin et al. 2010; Page et al. 2002, 2003). The PRC is a web-based tool that was later incorporated into broader oral health risk assessment tools (PreViser; DenPlan Excel/PreViser Patient Assessment [DEPPA]) for calculation of risk related to periodontal disease and other diseases and conditions (e.g. caries, noncarious dental lesions, and oral cancer). According to the PRC, the patient is assigned a risk score ranging from 1 (lowest risk) to 5 (highest risk). Based on the patient risk score and the contribution of each parameter, the system also provides general suggestions on which active interventions may be the most relevant to reduce disease risk.

- *Periodontal Risk Assessment (PRA)* (Lang & Tonetti 2003) and its modifications (Chandra 2007; Lu et al. 2013). The PRA is a spider web-shaped diagram composed of six vectors, each corresponding to a risk factor/indicator. The contribution of each risk factor/indicator to the patient risk is graphically reported on the respective vector (the greater the contribution of the risk factor/indicator, the greater the distance from the center of the diagram). Three concentric areas are identified on the polygon, with different distances from the polygon center. Irrespective of the version of PRA (original or modified), the patient is assigned a low, moderate, or high risk score based on the largest area that has been reached by a predetermined number of vectors. For example, in the original version of the PRA, the patient is assigned a low risk if all parameters are in the low-risk area or, at the most, one parameter is in the moderate-risk area; a moderate risk if at least two parameters are in the moderate-risk area and not more than one parameter is in the high-risk area; and a high risk if at least two parameters are in the high-risk area.

- *PerioRisk* (Trombelli et al. 2009). PerioRisk is based upon five parameters derived from a patient's medical history and clinical recordings. Each parameter is allocated a parameter score (ranging from 0 to 4 for four parameters and from 0 to 8 for one parameter) according to predefined tables. The algebraic sum of the parameter scores is then calculated and relates to a patient risk score between 1 (lowest risk) and 5 (highest risk). Recently, a simplified version of the PerioRisk (which was named SmartRisk) was also proposed and evaluated. Risk profiles of the SmartRisk system were generated by adding the number of cigarettes per day and the number of sites with probing depth ≥5 mm (Trombelli et al. 2017).

- *Dentition Risk System (DRS)* (Lindskog et al. 2010). The DRS is a computer-based, online tool that calculates chronic periodontitis risk for the dentition (level I) and, if an elevated risk is found, prognosticates disease progression tooth by tooth (level II). For patient-based risk calculation, numeric or dichotomous values are assigned to eight systemic predictors and nine local predictors, and then entered into the algorithm after adjustment with relative weights for each factor (unpublished). A risk score related to the dentition (DRS dentition) is then generated as a continuous value.

- *Risk Assessment-Based Individualized Treatment (RABIT)* (Teich 2013). RABIT calculates the risk of periodontitis progression as well as other aspects of oral health according to a series of unpublished parameters and calculation algorithms. In RABIT, the patient is assigned a low, moderate, or high risk, and prevention/treatment schemes are associated with the individual risk score.

Clinical recommendations for the practitioner

Current evidence on periodontal risk assessment supports the following clinical recommendations for oral care providers:

- The use of periodontal risk assessment tools should be considered as a standard of care and should be applied at the first visit (not strictly periodontal, but oral) as well as at the beginning and during SPT. Unfortunately, at present none of the existing tools has been consistently validated for application at both phases. In particular, PRA, PerioRisk, and DRS have been validated only for use after active periodontal therapy; PRC has been validated for use at the first visit; however, contrasting results have been shown when used during SPT.

- Risk scores generated by periodontal risk assessment tools should be used (i) to identify factors with the most relevant impact on individual patient prognosis and then to plan a preventive/treatment regimen targeted on the elimination/control of such factors; and (ii) to quantify and monitor the impact of preventive and treatment interventions on the risk level.

- Risk scores generated by periodontal risk assessment tools should be used to inform the patient regarding his/her disease condition and prognosis, and to motivate the patient for adherence to the suggested preventive/treatment plan (Trombelli & Farina 2020).

Future directions

The concept of precision dentistry as it relates to precision medicine is relatively new to the field of oral health. Precision dentistry is a contemporary, multifaceted, data-driven approach to oral healthcare that uses individual characteristics to stratify similar patients into phenotypic groups. The objective is to provide clinicians with information that will allow them to improve treatment planning and a patient's response to treatment. Providers that use a precision oral health approach would move away from using an "average treatment" for all patients with a particular diagnosis and move toward more specific treatments for patients within each diagnostic subgroup. Precision oral health requires a method or a model that places each individual in a subgroup where each member is the same as every other member in relation to the disease of interest (Beck et al. 2020).

Precision dentistry is a paradigm shift that requires a new way of thinking about diagnostic categories. This approach uses patients' risk factor data (including, but not limited to, genetic, environmental, and health behavioral), rather than expert opinion or clinical presentation alone, to redefine traditional categories of health and disease. The World Workshop on Periodontal Disease Classification has created a new model that uses stages and grading of disease. The model itself seems to work well to create stages that exhibit an increasing risk for tooth loss and grades that also show an increasing risk for tooth loss within each stage. The concept of stages and grading is integral for precision dentistry, because it accounts for the risk of future disease and prognosis as well as enabling the practitioner to use more signs, symptoms, and other associated factors when placing a patient in a diagnostic category (Beck et al. 2020).

It is envisaged that in the foreseeable future, robust risk assessment tools will be available to the general population as part of home care, which will enable preventive management of oral and periodontal diseases.

REFERENCES

Abdellatif HM, Burt BA. An epidemiological investigation into the relative importance of age and oral hygiene status as determinants of periodontitis. *J Dent Res.* 1987; 66:13–18.

American Academy of Periodontology. Position paper: Tobacco use and the periodontal patient. *J Periodontol.* 1999; 70:1419–1427.

American Academy of Periodontology. American Academy of Periodontology statement on risk assessment. *J Periodontol.* 2008; 79(2):202.

Auldemorte TB, Bryan BD, Fox WC et al. Diagnostic tools and biologic markers: animal models in the study of osteoporosis and oral bone loss. *J Bone Miner Res.* 1993; 8(Suppl 2):S529–S534.

Axelsson P, Lindhe J. Effect of controlled oral hygiene procedures on caries and periodontal disease in adults. Results after 6 years. *J Clin Periodontol.* 1981a; 8:239–248.

Axelsson P, Lindhe J. The significance of maintenance care in the treatment of periodontal disease. *J Clin Periodontol.* 1981b; 8:281–294.

Axelsson P, Lindhe J, Nyström B. On the prevention of caries and periodontal disease. Results of a 15-year longitudinal study in adults. *J Clin Periodontol.* 1991; 18:182–189.

Axtelius B, Söderfeldt B, Nilsson A et al. Therapy-resistant periodontitis: psychosocial characteristics. *J Clin Periodontol.* 1998; 25:482–491.

Baharin B, Palmer RM, Coward P, Wilson RF. Investigation of periodontal destruction patterns in smokers and non-smokers. *J Clin Periodontol.* 2006; 33:485–490.

Ballieux RE. Impact of mental stress on the immune response. *J Clin Periodontol.* 1991; 18:427–430.

Beck JD. Risk assessment revisited. *Community Dent Oral Epidemiol.* 1998; 26:220–225.

Beck JD, Koch GG, Offenbacher S. Incidence of attachment loss over 3 years in older adults – new and progressing lesions. *Community Dent Oral Epidemiol.* 1995; 23:291–296.

Beck JD, Philips K, Moss K et al. Advances in precision oral health. *Periodontol 2000.* 2020; 82(1):268–285.

Burt BA. Periodontitis and aging: reviewing recent evidence. *J Am Dent Assoc.* 1994; 125:273–279.

Busby M, Chapple L, Matthews R, Burke FJ, Chapple I. Continuing development of an oral health score for clinical audit. *Br Dent J.* 2014; 216(9):E20.

Chandra RV. Evaluation of a novel periodontal risk assessment model in patients presenting for dental care. *Oral Health Prev Dent.* 2007; 5(1):39–48.

Chapple ILC. Potential mechanisms underpinning the nutritional modulation of periodontal inflammation. *JADA.* 2009; 140:178–184.

Chapple ILC. Risk assessment in periodontal care: the principles. In: ILC Chapple, PN Papapanou (eds), *Risk Assessment in Oral Health. A Concise Guide for Clinical Application.* Cham: Springer Nature; 2020: 77–88.

Chapple ILC, Genco RJ. Diabetes and periodontal diseases: consensus report of the Joint EFP/AAP Workshop on Periodontitis and Systemic Diseases. *J Clin Periodontol.* 2013; 40:106–112.

Chapple ILC, Matthews JB. The role of reactive oxygen and antioxidant species in periodontal tissue destruction. *Periodontol 2000.* 2007; 43:160–232.

Chapple ILC, Milward MR, Ling-Mountford DT et al. Adjunctive daily supplementation with encapsulated fruit, vegetable and berry juice powder concentrates and clinical periodontal outcomes: a double-blind RCT. *J Clin Periodontol.* 2012; 39:62–72.

Chapple ILC, Milward M, Ower P. Periodontal risk-systemic and local risk factors. In: K Eaton, P Ower (eds), *Practical Periodontics.* St. Louis, MO: Elsevier; 2015: 67–79.

Chapple L, Yonel Z. Oral health risk assessment. *Dent Update.* 2018; 45: 841–847.

Croucher R, Marcenes WS, Torres MC et al. The relationship between life-events and periodontitis: a case control study. *J Clin Periodontol.* 1997; 24:39–43.

Eke PI, Wei L, Thornton-Evans GO et al. Risk indicators for periodontitis in US adults: National Health and Nutrition Examination Survey (NHANES) 2009 to 2012. *J Periodontol.* 2016; 87:1174–1185.

Elangovan S, Novak KF, Novak MJ. Clinical risk assessment. In: MG Newman, HH Takei, PR Klokkevold, FA Carranza (eds), *Newman and Carranza's Clinical Periodontology.* Philadelphia, PA: Elsevier; 2019: 2185–2204.

Enwonwu CO. Epidemiological and biochemical studies of necrotizing ulcerative gingivitis and noma (*cancrum oris*) in Nigerian children. *Arch Oral Biol.* 1972; 17:1357–1371.

Fors UG, Sandberg HC. Computer-aided risk management—a software tool for the HIDEP model. *Quintessence Int.* 2001; 32(4):309–320.

Genco R, Kornman K, Williams R et al. Consensus report: periodontal diseases: pathogenesis and microbial factors. *Ann Periodontol.* 1996; 1:926–932.

Genco RJ, Ho AW, Grossi SG et al. Relationship of stress, distress, and inadequate coping behaviors to periodontal disease. *J Periodontol.* 1999; 70:711–723.

Green LW, Tryon WW, Marks B et al. Periodontal disease as a function of life events stress. *J Human Stress.* 1986; 12: 32–36.

Guers NC, Lewis CE, Jeffcoat MJ. Osteoporosis and periodontal disease progression. *Periodontol 2000.* 2003; 32:105–110.

Gunsolley JC, Tew JG, Gooss CM et al. Effects of race, smoking and immunoglobulin allotypes on IgG subclass concentrations. *J Periodontal Res.* 1997; 32:381–387.

Haffajee AD, Socransky SS. Microbial etiological agents of destructive periodontal diseases. *Periodontol 2000.* 1994; 5:78–111.

Hajishengallis G. Periodontitis: from microbial immune subversion to systemic inflammation. *Nat Rev Immunol.* 2015; 15:30–44.

Hart TC, Shapira L, Van Dyke TE. Neutrophil defects as risk factors for periodontal diseases. *J Periodontol.* 1994; 65:521–529.

Ismail AI, Burt BA, Eklund SA. Epidemiologic patterns of smoking and periodontal disease in the United States. *J Am Dent Assoc.* 1983; 106:617–621.

Kinane DF, Hart TC. Genes and gene polymorphisms associated with periodontal disease. *Crit Rev Oral Biol Med.* 2003; 14:430–449.

Kinane DF. Periodontitis modified by systemic factors. *Ann Periodontol.* 1999; 4(1):55–64.

Kornman KS, Crane S, Wang HY et al. The interleukin-1 genotype as a severity factor in adult periodontal disease. *J Clin Periodontol.* 1997; 24:72–77.

Koshi E, Rajesh S, Koshi P, Arunima PR. Risk assessment for periodontal disease. *J Indian Soc Periodontol.* 2012; 16:324–328.

Kribbs PJ. Comparison of mandibular bone in normal and osteoporotic women. *J Prosthet Dent.* 1990; 63:218–222.

Krook L, Whalen JP, Lesser GV et al. Experimental studies on osteoporosis. *Methods Achiev Exp Pathol.* 1975; 7:72–108.

Kumar PS. Interventions to prevent periodontal disease in tobacco-, alcohol-, and drug-dependent individuals. *Periodontology 2000.* 2020; 84:84–101.

Kye W, Davidson R, Martin J, Engebretson S. Current status of periodontal risk assessment. *J Evid Base Dent Pract.* 2012; S1:2–11.

Lamster IB, Begg MD, Mitchell L et al. Oral manifestations of HIV infection in homosexual men and intravenous drug users: study design and relationship of epidemiologic, clinical, and immunologic parameter to oral lesions. *Oral Surg Oral Med Oral Pathol.* 1994; 78:163–174.

Lang NP, Suvan JE, Tonetti MS. Risk factor assessment tools for the prevention of periodontitis progression a systematic review. *J Clin Periodontol.* 2015; 42(Suppl 16):S59–S70.

Lang NP, Tonetti MS. Periodontal risk assessment (PRA) for patients in supportive periodontal therapy (SPT). *Oral Health Prev Dent.* 2003; 1(1):7–16.

Lindskog S, Blomlof J, Persson I et al. Validation of an algorithm for chronic periodontitis risk assessment and prognostication: risk predictors, explanatory values, measures of quality, and clinical use. *J Periodontol.* 2010; 81(4):584–593.

Löe H, Theilade E, Jensen SB. Experimental gingivitis in man. *J Periodontol.* 1965; 36:177–187.

Lu D, Meng H, Xu L et al. New attempts to modify periodontal risk assessment for generalized aggressive periodontitis: a retrospective study. *J Periodontol.* 2013; 84(11):1536–1545.

Martin JA, Page RC, Loeb CF, Levi PA Jr. Tooth loss in 776 treated periodontal patients. *J Periodontol.* 2010; 81(2):244–250.

Michalowicz BS, Aeppli DP, Kuba RK et al. A twin study of genetic variation in proportional radiographic alveolar bone height. *J Dent Res.* 1991a; 70:1431–1435.

Michalowicz BS, Aeppli DP, Virag JG et al. Risk findings in adult twins. *J Periodontol.* 1991b; 62:293–299.

Michalowicz BS, Diehl SR, Gunsolley JC et al. Evidence for a substantial genetic basis for risk of adult periodontitis. *J Periodontol.* 2000; 71:1699–1707.

Monnier L, Colette C, Boniface H. Contribution of postprandial glucose to chronic hyperglycaemia: from the glucose "triad" to the trilogy of "sevens." *Diabetes Metab.* 2006; 32 (Spec2):11–16.

Naga Sai Sujai GV, Triveni VS, Barath S, Harikishan G. Periodontal risk calculator versus periodontal risk assessment. *J Pharm Bioallied Sci.* 2015; 7(Suppl 2):S656–S659.

Page RC, Beck JD. Risk assessment for periodontal diseases. *Int Dent J.* 1997; 47:61–87.

Page RC, Krall EA, Martin J, Mancl L, Garcia RI. Validity and accuracy of a risk calculator in predicting periodontal disease. *J Am Dent Assoc.* 2002; 133:569–576.

Page RC, Martin J, Krall EA, Mancl L, Garcia R. Longitudinal validation of a risk calculator for periodontal disease. *J Clin Periodontol.* 2003; 30(9):819–827.

Papapanou PN. Epidemiology and natural history of periodontal disease. In: NP Lang, T Karring (eds), *Proceedings of the First European Workshop on Periodontology.* London: Quintessence; 1994: n.p. http://www.quintpub.com/display_detail. php3?psku=B8993#.YUAxIJ0zZPY.

Papapanou PN, Lindhe J. Preservation of probing attachment and alveolar bone levels in two random population samples. *J Clin Periodontol.* 1992; 19:583–588.

Papapanou PN, Lindhe J, Sterrett JD et al. Considerations on the contribution of aging to loss of periodontal tissue support. *J Clin Periodontol.* 1991; 18:611–615.

Persson GR, Attstrom R, Lang NP, Page RC. Perceived risk of deteriorating periodontal conditions. *J Clin Periodontol.* 2003; 30(11):982–989.

Persson GR, Mancl LA, Martin J, Page RC. Assessing periodontal disease risk: a comparison of clinicians' assessment versus a computerized tool. *J Am Dent Assoc.* 2003; 134(5):575–582.

Pihlstrom BL. Periodontal risk assessment, diagnosis, and treatment planning. *Periodontol 2000.* 2001; 25:37–58.

Roberts A, Matthews JB, Socransky SS et al. Stress and periodontal diseases: effects of catecholamines on the growth of periodontal bacteria in vitro. *Oral Microbiol Immunol.* 2002; 17:296–303.

Roberts, A, Mathews JB, Socransky SS et al. Stress and periodontal diseases: growth responses of periodontal bacteria to *Escherichia coli* stress-associated autoinducer and exogenous Fe. *Oral Microbiol Immunol.* 2005; 20:47–53.

Rose RM. Endocrine responses to stressful psychological events. *Psychiatr Clin North Am.* 1980; 3:251–257.

Shapira L, Soskolone WA, Van Dyke TF et al. Prostaglandin E2 secretion, cell maturation, and CD14 expression by monocyte-derived macrophages from localized juvenile periodontitis patients. *J Periodontol.* 1996; 67:224–228.

Shields WD. Acute necrotizing ulcerative gingivitis: a study of some of the contributing factors and their validity in an army population. *J Periodontol.* 1977; 48:346–349.

Stanford TW, Rees TD. Acquired immune suppression and other risk factors/indicators for periodontal disease progression. *Periodontol 2000* 2003; 32:118–135.

Sternberg EM, Chrousos GP, Wilder RL et al. The stress response and the regulation of inflammatory disease. *Ann Intern Med.* 1992; 117:854–866.

Swango PA, Kleinman DV, Konzelman JL. HIV and periodontal health: a study of military personnel with HIV. *J Am Dent Assoc.* 1991; 122:49–54.

Taylor GW. Bidirectional interrelationships between diabetes and periodontal diseases: an epidemiological perspective. *Ann Periodontol.* 2001; 6:99–112.

Teich ST. Risk assessment-based individualized treatment (RABIT): a comprehensive approach to dental patient recall. *J Dent Educ.* 2013; 77(4):448–457.

Timmerman MF, Van der Weijden. Risk factors for periodontitis. *Int J Dent Hyg.* 2006; 4:2–7.

Tomar SL, Asma S. Smoking-attributable periodontitis in the United States: findings from NHANES III. National Health and Nutrition Examination Survey. *J Periodontol.* 2000; 71:743–751.

Tonetti MS, Eickholz P, Loos BG et al. Principles in prevention of periodontal diseases: consensus report of group 1 of the 11th European workshop on periodontology on effective prevention of periodontal and peri-implant diseases. *J Clin Periodontol.* 2015; 42(Suppl 16):S5–S11.

Tonetti MS, Greenwell H, Kornman KS. Staging and grading of periodontitis: framework and proposal of a new classification and case definition. *J Clin Periodontol.* 2018; 45(Suppl 20):S149–S161.

Trombelli L, Farina R. Implementation of patient-based risk assessment in practice. In: ILC Chapple, PN Papapanou (eds), *Risk Assessment in Oral Health: A Concise Guide for Clinical Application.* Cham: Springer Nature; 2020: 203–233.

Trombelli L, Farina R, Ferrari S, Pasetti P, Calura G. Comparison between two methods for periodontal risk assessment. *Minerva Stomatol.* 2009; 58(6):277–287.

Trombelli L, Minenna L, Toselli L et al. Prognostic value of a simplified method for periodontal risk assessment during supportive periodontal therapy. *J Clin Periodontol.* 2017; 44(1):51–57.

US Public Health Service. National Institute of Dental Research (NIDR). *Oral health of United States adults: national findings,* NIH Pub No 87-2868, Bethesda, MD: NIDR; 1987.

US Public Health Service. National Center for Health Statistics. Periodontal disease in adults, United States, 1960–1962. PHS Pub No 1000, Series 11, No 12. Washington, DC: US Government Printing Office; 1965.

US Public Health Service. National Center for Health Statistics. Basic data on dental examination findings of persons 1–74 years, United States, 1971–1974. DHEW PHS Pub No 79-1662, Series 11, No 214. Washington, DC: US Government Printing Office; 1979.

von Wowern J, Klausen B, Kollerup G. Osteoporosis: a risk factor in periodontal disease. *J Periodontol.* 1994; 65:1134–1138.

Wilson ME, Kalmar JR. FcγIIa (CD32): a potential marker defining susceptibility to localized juvenile periodontitis. *J Periodontol.* 1996; 76:323–331.

Wimmer G, Janda M, Wieselmann-Penkner K et al. Coping with stress: its influence on periodontal disease. *J Periodontol.* 2002; 73:1343–1351.

Winkler JR, Herrera C, Westenhouse J et al. Periodontal disease in HIV-infected and uninfected homosexual and bisexual men. *AIDS.* 1992; 6:1041 [letter].

Xu S, Zhang G, Guo JF, Tan YH. Associations between osteoporosis and risk of periodontitis: a pooled analysis of observational studies. *Oral Dis.* 2021; 27(2):357–369.

CHAPTER 14
Prognosis and treatment planning for periodontal therapy

Steph Smith

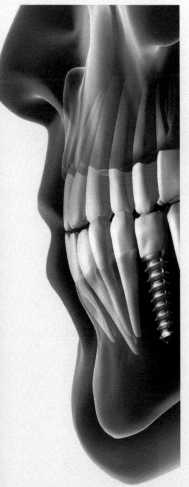

Contents

Learning objectives

- Different types of prognosis.
- Determination of individual and overall prognoses.
- Elements of the McGuire and Nunn, and Kwok and Caton prognosis systems.
- Elements and purposes of treatment planning.
- Sequence and contents of therapeutic modalities in the treatment plan.
- Aspects to consider when deciding to extract teeth.

Essential Periodontics, First Edition. Edited by Steph Smith and Khalid Almas.
© 2022 John Wiley & Sons Ltd. Published 2022 by John Wiley & Sons Ltd.

Prognosis

The four core elements of periodontal care are diagnosis, prognosis, treatment, and supportive periodontal therapy (McGowan et al. 2017). By definition, a prognosis is a prediction of the probable course, duration, and outcome of a disease based on the general knowledge of the multifactorial nature of periodontitis etiopathogenesis, and the presence of risk factors for the disease (Newman et al. 2019). Prognosis is an important part of therapy, however it is a complex task and thus may be significantly more difficult to provide than a diagnosis (McGowan et al. 2017). It is established after the diagnosis is made and before the treatment plan is set, as the assignment of good, long-term prognoses is critical to reliably determining an appropriate restorative treatment plan following periodontal therapy, particularly if major prosthetic reconstruction or placement of dental implants is under consideration (Newman et al. 2019; Nunn et al. 2012). The formation of periodontal prognosis systems has allowed clinicians to better predict the outcome for teeth and has led to better treatment planning and long-term predictable outcomes, and thereby ultimately an improvement in patients' overall oral health (Kwok & Caton 2007; Nguyen et al. 2021). Prognosis can also be influenced by the clinician's previous experience with treatment outcomes (successes and failures) as they relate to a particular case (Newman et al. 2019). It is also used to communicate the probable outcome of disease to both the patient and the clinician involved in their care, so as to establish realistic treatment goals (Kwok & Caton 2007).

Prognosis is commonly expressed as either short term (≤5 years) or long term (>5 years). Determination of prognosis is also a dynamic process and changes with disease activity, because periodontal disease progresses in an episodic manner, and because systemic and local risk factors are not permanent conditions. Therefore, a patient's prognosis does not remain the same (Hamade et al. 2017; Saroch 2019). It is thus advisable that a provisional prognosis be established for a patient until phase 1 therapy is completed and evaluated. If the patient's response to phase 1 therapy is good, with considerable reduction in inflammation and pocket depth, the prognosis may be better than initially assumed before treatment. On the other hand, if the response to phase 1 therapy is not as expected, then the prognosis may be worse than established before (Saroch 2019). Thus, identifying a tooth's prognosis only during the initial appointment does not allow adequate judgment of the probability of tooth survival, as this requires continuous monitoring of potential changes. Determining the prognosis at multiple appointments is also necessary because periodontal destruction does not continually occur at the same rate (Hamade 2017).

An essential element of prognosis is the consideration of individual teeth versus the overall dentition. An overall description of prognosis facilitates communication between professionals and patients. Many general factors such as smoking or diabetes may affect the whole dentition, whereas local factors such as furcation or anatomic defects may affect only individual teeth. Periodontal disease does not progress uniformly throughout the dentition. Some sites, such as those with deep probing depths, molars, and posterior interproximal sites, may behave differently than anterior sites with single-rooted teeth. Other local anatomic factors to consider are for example palatal grooves, cervical enamel projections, enamel pearls, and overhanging restorations. Individual tooth prognosis therefore has to be considered separately to develop a valid treatment plan. This also necessitates that prognosis be considered at both overall and individual levels (Kwok & Caton 2007).

Another aspect to consider is the importance of patient compliance on the maintenance of periodontal health during supportive periodontal therapy (SPT). Advanced periodontal progression is more likely to occur with irregular patient compliance, thereby making provision for an accurate prognosis almost impossible in patients who do not attend their SPT appointments. Any prognosis given to a tooth is thus only valid where the patient returns for all prescribed SPT appointments (McGowan et al. 2017).

Classification of types of prognosis (Saroch 2019)

- *Diagnostic prognosis*: The prognosis of teeth if no treatment is provided. It therefore questions the status of teeth in the future if no treatment is provided for the present periodontal condition.
- *Therapeutic prognosis*: The prognosis of teeth after an appropriate periodontal treatment is provided. The treatment may vary, from primary periodontal treatment to regenerative procedures.
- *Prosthetic prognosis*: The prognosis of teeth for supporting the prosthetic restoration after an appropriate periodontal treatment has been provided. It will also determine whether the prosthesis to be planned shall be therapeutic or detrimental.
- *Individual prognosis*: The prognosis of an individual tooth, based on local and restorative/prosthetic factors that have a direct effect on its prognosis.
- *Overall prognosis*: The prognosis of the teeth based on the sum of various local, systemic, environmental, and other factors that may affect the overall periodontal health of the teeth.

Determination of individual tooth prognosis

Table 14.1 depicts the factors that determine individual tooth prognosis.

Determination of overall prognosis

Table 14.2 depicts the factors that determine the overall prognosis.

Periodontal prognosis systems

McGuire and Nunn

Among the various periodontal prognosis systems, the one most widely used was proposed by McGuire and Nunn in 1996. This system contained a more detailed stratification for individual

Table 14.1 Factors determining individual tooth prognosis.

Remaining bone support	In general, two-thirds to one-half of investing bone is a minimum requirement for a favorable prognosis. However, root length, root form, root shape, and single or multiple roots also have to be considered.
Probing depth	Teeth with shallow pockets have a better prognosis. Complex pockets encompassing multiple root surfaces are a poor prognostic factor. However, deep pockets with adequate bone levels may be amenable to regenerative therapy. Pockets on proximal surfaces have a better prognosis than in furcation areas. Pockets on facial and lingual/palatal surfaces may result in loss of bony plates over convexities of root surfaces. Presence of pseudo-pockets is a good prognostic factor.
Mobility	In general, increased tooth mobility is a poor prognostic factor. If bone loss increases beyond 50%, tooth mobility increases rapidly with each millimeter of bone loss.
Furcation involvement	Furcation involvement is difficult to access and treat and is a poor prognostic factor. In general, a long root trunk, a wide furcation, and a crown fornix near the cementoenamel junction are poor prognostic factors. Other multiple factors should also be considered when establishing prognosis for furcation-involved teeth.
Crown–root ratio	Teeth with short, slender, and tapering roots have a poorer prognosis than teeth with long and broad roots. Multirooted teeth with flared roots have a better prognosis than teeth with close-together or fused roots. A broad occlusal surface is a poor prognostic factor. The center of tooth rotation should also be considered along with the crown–root ratio.
Tooth morphology	Morphological deformities of the root surface such as concavities and grooves jeopardize scaling and root planing procedures. Developmental enamel projections and grooves worsen the prognosis of teeth, as treating periodontal pockets in these areas becomes difficult.
Caries	An increase in number of carious teeth worsens the prognosis. The amount of crown structure lost due to caries is an important prognostic consideration.
Pulpal involvement	Appropriate endodontic treatment can improve the prognosis of a tooth. The more the number of endodontically involved teeth, the worse is the prognosis.
Mucogingival problems	Inadequate width of attached gingiva, recession, high frenal attachment, and presence of periodontal pockets below the mucogingival junction are all related to a poor prognosis.
Number of remaining teeth	The more the number of remaining teeth, the better the prognosis. This is because occlusal forces are distributed adequately among all teeth. If the few remaining teeth have to also support removable or fixed prostheses, the prognosis becomes poorer.
Position and alignment of teeth	Tilted, rotated, or drifting teeth have a worse prognosis compared to well-aligned teeth. Difficult-to-reach areas such as most posterior maxillary and mandibular areas are more difficult to maintain compared to anterior areas.

Source: Adapted from Saroch 2019.

teeth (Kwok & Caton 2007). It consists of five categories: good, fair, poor, questionable, and hopeless. In this system, clinicians assign each tooth to a category based on their ability to control the etiology of disease, attachment loss, presence of furcation involvement, crown/root ratio, and the degree of tooth mobility (McGuire & Nunn 1996). The authors further demonstrated that prognostic values are not stable over time, especially for teeth that are categorized as fair, poor, or questionable. It was shown in their study that only 50% of teeth assigned to one of these three prognoses remained in the same category during subsequent assessments (McGuire 1991). The authors identified possible clinical factors that led to the altering of the initially assigned prognosis. These included smoking, diabetes, probing depth, furcation involvement, and parafunctional habits (McGuire 1991). However, this also did not include teeth that underwent regenerative treatment, such as guided tissue regeneration and the utilization of growth factors around teeth. In periodontitis patients, it is well established that regenerative

procedures on certain defects can lead to bone fill and clinical attachment level gain, and thus improve a tooth's prognosis (Reddy et al. 2015; Reynolds et al. 2015). Table 14.3 depicts the prognosis system of McGuire and Nunn (1996).

Kwok and Caton

Kwok and Caton (2007) proposed a prognosis system based on the prediction of the future stability of the periodontal supporting tissues with treatment of the individual tooth, i.e. on how periodontal disease activity may be suppressed by controlling systemic and local factors (Hamade et al. 2017; Kwok & Caton 2007). These include patient compliance, smoking status, and diabetic conditions as general factors, with deep probing depth, plaque retentive factors, mobility, and trauma from occlusion considered as local factors (Hamada et al. 2017). Table 14.4 depicts the prognosis system of Kwok and Caton (2007).

Table 14.2 Factors determining overall prognosis.

Age	Younger patients have a poorer prognosis compared to older patients. This is because the rate of periodontal destruction is more rapid in younger patients, and rapid bone loss in a short period of time in young patients does not favor good bone reparative capacity.
Medical status	Systemic conditions like uncontrolled diabetes mellitus are associated with a poor periodontal prognosis. Other systemic conditions should also be considered.
Individual tooth prognosis	The individual tooth prognosis should be considered in the overall prognosis, as it is an integral part of the multiple factors that have a direct and indirect relationship with periodontal disease progression.
Complexity of prosthesis	The prognosis is guarded with complex prosthesis compared to a simple prosthesis or none at all.
Rate of disease progression	Past periodontal disease status regarding the rate of disease progression will determine the future status of a tooth. Patients with slow disease progression have a better prognosis. The rate of bone loss in a specific period of time can be determined by past and present radiographic evaluation.
Host response	An inflammatory response consistent with the presence of local factors is a good prognostic marker. A severe response to minimal plaque accumulation indicates a poor prognosis.
Smoking	Smoking is associated with a poor prognosis in periodontally compromised patients. Periodontal disease progression is associated with dose-dependent smoking.
Stress	Emotional stress can modulate the immune system through the neural and endocrine systems. Stress is associated with an adverse prognosis in periodontal disease progression.
Patient cooperation	The patient's participation in the treatment process and extent of compliance with recommendations for maintenance visits are key factors in achieving periodontal therapeutic success.
Economic consideration	Simple periodontic procedures can halt the progression of periodontal diseases, with the prognosis becoming favorable.
Knowledge and ability of dentist	These play a significant role in the overall prognosis. Strict referral protocols should be employed for advanced periodontal treatment. Thereafter, general dentists can proceed with maintenance schedules.

Source: Adapted from Saroch 2019.

Table 14.3 McGuire and Nunn prognosis classification system.

Prognosis	One or more of the following for each category
Good	Control of the etiological factors and enough clinical and radiographical periodontal support to enable the tooth to be maintained by the patient and clinician with proper maintenance.
Fair	Approximately 25% attachment loss as measured clinically and radiographically. Class I furcation involvement. The severity of the furcation involvement would allow adequate maintenance.
Poor	50% attachment loss and class II furcations. The location and degree of the furcations would accommodate proper maintenance, although with difficulty.
Questionable	>50% attachment loss, poor crown–root ratio, class II (not easily accessed) or class III furcation involvement. Class II mobility or more; significant root proximity.
Hopeless	Severe attachment loss, extraction performed or suggested.

Table 14.4 Kwok and Caton prognosis classification system.

Prognosis	Classification
Favorable	Can be stabilized with comprehensive periodontal treatment/maintenance, and with less chance of future breakdown.
Questionable	Influenced by local and/or systemic factors that may or may not be controlled; the periodontium can be maintained with proper care.
Unfavorable	Influenced by local and/or systemic factors that cannot be controlled.
Hopeless	Must be extracted.

Summary

An accurate prognosis for each tooth can provide information on whether proposed periodontal and restorative treatment plans may promise the likelihood of a successful long-term outcome. Prognosis needs to be described at both overall and individual tooth levels (Kwok & Caton 2007). However, in this era of evidence-based dentistry, there is no gold standard for periodontal prognosis tools. Disease progression is affected by many factors, including systemic conditions, local influences, and the practitioner's skill level, thereby making it virtually impossible to establish an absolute prognostic value (Hamada et al. 2017). Determination of prognosis is a dynamic process and, as such, the prognosis initially assigned should be reevaluated after completion of all phases of therapy, including periodontal maintenance (Hamada et al. 2017; Newman et al. 2019). Established prognosis systems can accurately predict the outcome of good and hopeless teeth in the short term (<5 years). However, the long-term (≥5 years) outcome cannot be accurately predicted, especially for teeth with a poor and questionable prognosis, because various factors may create uncertainty in current models (Kwok & Caton 2007; McGuire 1991; McGuire & Nunn 1996). A retrospective study has concluded that the Kwok and Caton prognosis system can predictably determine tooth survivability within a 5-year period. The defined categories of this prognosis system are more reliable than those of other systems in the short term. However, the long-term (>5 years) prediction accuracy of this prognosis system needs further investigation (Nguyen et al. 2021). It should also be remembered that any prognosis given to a tooth is only valid where the patient returns for all prescribed SPT appointments (McGowan et al. 2017).

Treatment planning

The ultimate goal of periodontal therapy is to bring a patient's mouth to a state of health, which is maintained in the long term. A properly formulated treatment plan is paramount to achieving this goal. The treatment plan is thus the blueprint for case management. A treatment plan is a plan for therapy formulated only after a thorough examination has been completed, followed by a diagnosis and the determination of a prognosis, and also includes taking into consideration the needs and desires of the patient. Treatment decisions are based on the prognosis with the purpose of improving that prognosis. It must be recognized that as diagnosis and prognosis will change with treatment, therapeutic needs may also change. As such, the treatment plan must be altered accordingly (Newman et al. 2019).

When a patient presents with medical and systemic problems that may affect periodontal therapy, systemic conditions should be carefully evaluated, because they may require special precautions during the course of periodontal treatment. The tissue response to treatment procedures may be affected, or the preservation of periodontal health may be threatened after treatment is completed. Therefore, the patient's physician should always be consulted in such cases (Newman et al. 2019).

Different patients value esthetics differently, according to their age, gender, profession, and social status. Thus, when formulating a treatment plan, in addition to the restoration of proper function of the dentition, esthetic considerations play an important role. The clinician should carefully evaluate and consider a final esthetic outcome of treatment that will be acceptable to the patient without jeopardizing the basic need of restoring and maintaining periodontal health (Newman et al. 2019).

In complex cases, interdisciplinary consultation with other specialty areas is necessary before a final plan can be made. The opinions of orthodontists and prosthodontists are especially important for the final decision in these patients. Occlusal evaluation and therapy may be necessary during treatment, which may necessitate planning for occlusal adjustment, orthodontics, and splinting. The correction of bruxism and other occlusal habits may also be necessary (Newman et al. 2019).

Sequence of phases of periodontal therapy

Immediately after completion of phase I therapy (Figure 14.1), the patient should be placed on the maintenance phase (phase IV) to preserve the results obtained and prevent any further deterioration and recurrence of disease. While on the maintenance phase, with its periodic evaluation, the patient enters into the surgical phase (phase II) and the restorative phase (phase III) of treatment (Figure 14.2) (Newman et al. 2019).

Table 14.5 outlines the therapeutic modalities in the different phases of the treatment plan.

Extraction of teeth

The removal, retention, or temporary (interim) retention of one or more teeth are important parts of the overall treatment

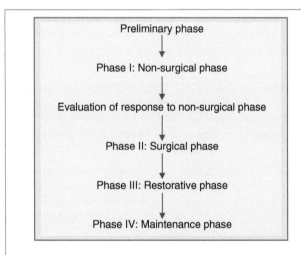

Figure 14.1 Sequence of phases of periodontal therapy.

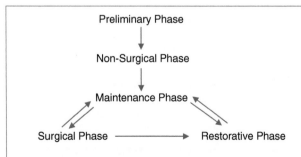

Figure 14.2 Periodic re-evaluation.

Table 14.5 Therapeutic modalities in the treatment plan phases.

Preliminary phase	Treatment of emergencies: • Dental or periapical • Periodontal • Other • Extraction of hopeless teeth and provisional placement if needed (May be postponed to a more convenient time)
Phase I: Non-surgical phase	Plaque control and patient education. • Diet control (in patients with rampant caries) • Removal of calculus and root planing • Correction of restorative and prosthetic irritational factors • Excavation of caries and restoration (temporary or final, depending on whether a definitive prognosis for the tooth has been determined and the location of caries) • Antimicrobial therapy (local or systemic) • Occlusal therapy • Minor orthodontic movement • Provisional splinting and prosthesis
Evaluation of response to non-surgical phase	Rechecking: • Pocket depth and gingival inflammation • Plaque and calculus, caries
Phase II: Surgical phase	• Periodontal surgery: resective, regenerative, mucogingival surgery, esthetic crown lengthening • Preprosthetic surgery: prosthetic crown lengthening, implant site preparation, and implant placement • Extraction of hopeless teeth • Endodontic therapy
Phase III: Restorative phase	• Final restorations • Fixed and removable prosthodontic appliances • Evaluation of response to restorative procedures • Periodontal examination

Phase IV:
Maintenance phase
	Periodic rechecking:
	• Inquiry into new concerns or problems, changes in patient's medical and oral health status
	• Oral hygiene assessment and education
	• Comprehensive periodontal examination
	  • Gingival condition (pockets, inflammation)
	  • Occlusion, tooth mobility
	• Professional maintenance care
	  • Supragingival and subgingival biofilm and calculus removal
	  • Selective scaling and root planing
	• Assessment of recall interval and plan for next visit
	• Other pathological changes

plan. The value of long-term periodontal treatment is measured in years of healthy functioning of the entire dentition and not by the number of teeth retained at the time of treatment. Treatment is directed to establishing and maintaining the health of the periodontium throughout the mouth, rather than attempting spectacular efforts to "tighten loose teeth" (Newman et al. 2019). Teeth on the borderline of a hopeless prognosis do not contribute to the overall usefulness of the dentition. Such teeth become sources of recurrent problems for the patient and detract from the value of the greater service rendered by the establishment of periodontal health in the remainder of the oral cavity. Furthermore, implant replacement of missing teeth

has become a predictable course of therapy. Therefore, attempts to save questionable teeth may jeopardize adjacent teeth and may lead to the loss of bone needed for implant therapy (Newman et al. 2019).

A tooth should be extracted under the following conditions:

- It is so mobile that function becomes painful.
- It can cause acute abscesses during therapy.
- There is no use for it in the overall treatment plan.

In some cases, a tooth can be retained temporarily, postponing the decision to extract until after treatment is completed (Newman et al. 2019).

A tooth in this category can be retained under the following conditions:

- It maintains posterior stops; the tooth can be removed after treatment, when it can be replaced by an implant or another type of prosthesis.
- It maintains posterior stops and may be functional after implant placement in adjacent areas. When the implant is restored, these teeth can be extracted.
- In the anterior aesthetic zone, a tooth can be retained during periodontal therapy and removed when treatment is completed and a permanent restorative procedure can be performed. The retention of this tooth should not jeopardize the adjacent teeth. This approach avoids the need for temporary appliances during therapy.
- Extraction of hopeless teeth can also be performed during periodontal surgery of the adjacent teeth. This approach reduces the number of appointments needed for surgery in the same area.

Summary

It is the dentist's responsibility to advise the patient of the importance of periodontal treatment. However, if treatment is to be successful, the patient must be sufficiently interested in retaining their natural teeth and in maintaining the necessary oral hygiene. Patients who are not particularly perturbed by the thought of losing their teeth are generally not good candidates for periodontal treatment (Newman et al. 2019).

Phase I of the periodontal treatment plan is directed to the elimination of the etiological factors of dental, gingival, and periodontal diseases. When successfully performed, this phase stops the progression of dental and periodontal disease. The surgical and restorative phases include periodontal surgery to treat and improve the condition of the periodontal and surrounding tissues. This may include regeneration of the gingiva and bone for function and aesthetics, placement of implants, and restorative therapy. Following non-surgical periodontal therapy, the patient is placed on periodontal maintenance at regular intervals. Surgical and restorative treatments are scheduled between periodontal recalls (Newman et al. 2019).

Communication of the treatment plan with the patient should be specific, avoiding vague statements and presented with a positive note. Emphasis should be placed on the fact that the important purpose of the treatment is to prevent the other teeth from becoming as severely diseased as the loose teeth that may be scheduled for extraction. Furthermore, the treatment plan should be presented and explained as a unit to the patient. It should be made clear to the patient that dental restorations and prostheses contribute as much to the health of the gingiva as the elimination of inflammation and periodontal pockets (Newman et al. 2019).

REFERENCES

Hamada Y, Kishimoto T, Alqallaf H, John V. Strategies for periodontal risk assessment and prognosis. *J Multidiscip Care.* 2017; Aug. 25. https://decisionsindentistry.com/article/strategies-periodontal-risk-assessment-prognosis.

Kwok V, Caton JG. Commentary: prognosis revisited: a system for assigning periodontal prognosis. *J Periodontol.* 2007; 78(1):2063–2071.

McGowan T, McGowan K, Ivanovski S. A novel evidence-based periodontal prognosis model. *J Evid Base Dent Pract.* 2017; 17(4):350–360.

McGuire MK. Prognosis versus actual outcome: a long-term survey of 100 treated periodontal patients under maintenance care. *J Periodontol.* 1991; 62:51–58.

McGuire MK, Nunn ME. Prognosis versus actual outcome. II. The effectiveness of clinical parameters in developing an accurate prognosis. *J Periodontol.* 1996; 67:658–665.

Newman MG, Takei HH, Klokkevold PR et al. *Newman and Carranza's Clinical Periodontology.* St. Louis, MO: Elsevier Saunders; 2019.

Nguyen L, Krish G, Alsaleh A et al. Analyzing the predictability of the Kwok and Caton periodontal prognosis system: a retrospective study. *J Periodontol.* 2021; 92(5):662–669. doi: 10.1002/JPER.20-0411.

Nunn ME, Fan J, Su X, McGuire MK. Development of prognostic indicators using classification and regression trees (CART) for survival. *Periodontol 2000.* 2012; 58(1):134–142.

Reddy MS, Aichelmann-Reidy ME, Avila-Ortiz G et al. Periodontal regeneration – furcation defects: a consensus report from the AAP Regeneration Workshop. *J Periodontol.* 2015; 86(Suppl 2):S131–S133.

Reynolds MA, Kao RT, Camargo PM et al. Periodontal regeneration – intrabony defects: a consensus report from the AAP Regeneration Workshop. *J Periodontol.* 2015; 86(Suppl 2):S105–S107.

Saroch N. *Periobasics: A Textbook of Periodontics and Implantology.* Solan: Shushrut Publications; 2019. Retrieved from https://periobasics.com/determination-of-prognosis-in-periodontics.

CHAPTER 15
Plaque control for the periodontal patient

Liana Maoil and Qalim Rayman

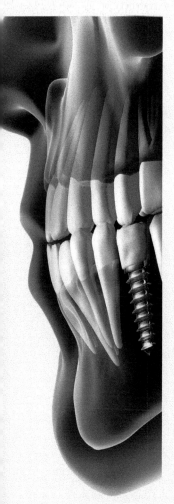

Contents

Learning objectives

- Identify the types of deposits found on tissues of the oral cavity and describe their effect on oral disease progression.
- Explain the importance of daily biofilm removal in order to prevent progression of oral diseases.
- Identify tools, aids, and rinses used to remove and control oral biofilms.
- Compare and contrast the benefits and limitations of power and manual toothbrushes.

Essential Periodontics, First Edition. Edited by Steph Smith and Khalid Almas.
© 2022 John Wiley & Sons Ltd. Published 2022 by John Wiley & Sons Ltd.

Introduction

Periodontal disease and dental caries are biofilm-induced diseases of the oral cavity. Biofilms are complex, communal, three-dimensional arrangements of microbial communities. While most microbes present in oral biofilms are bacteria, yeasts, fungi, protozoa, Archaea, and viruses may also be present (Marsh & Zaura 2017). As biofilms mature, channels allow for circulation of nutrients and provide a system to eliminate wastes. In healthy individuals, biofilms exist harmoniously with the host (*symbiosis*), making important contributions to the normal development and general health of the host. However, this mutually beneficial relationship can falter for a variety of reasons, which include a *dysbiosis*, eventually leading to periodontal disease and dental caries. Additionally, oral bacteria have also been implicated in various systemic diseases. Effective reduction/removal of the biofilm on oral surfaces can prevent the onset of gingivitis and interdental caries, as well as reduce the incidence of systemic disease. For this reason, meticulous daily oral self-care is a critical component of a disease prevention program.

Types of deposits

There are two types of deposits found on tissues in the oral cavity: soft deposit (non-mineralized) and hard deposit (mineralized). Table 15.1 lists and defines the soft and hard deposits (Akcalı & Lang 2018; Thomas & Nakaishi 2006).

Soft deposits, consisting of microbial biofilms, stimulate a host inflammatory response, which, if left unchecked, leads to the destruction of the periodontium. When soft and hard oral tissues (teeth and the tongue) are cleaned regularly, bacteria in biofilms are forced to restart the colonization process. In clean areas, mature biofilms (which are mostly pathogenic) will not be able to develop. Soft deposits can be removed mechanically in a variety of ways by the patient.

Calculus is mineralized (hardened) biofilm. Although there is a positive correlation between the presence of calculus and periodontal disease, no cause–effect relationship has been established. It is believed that the roughened surface of calculus facilitates the adherence and growth of biofilms, which initiates an inflammatory response (Akcalı & Lang 2018). Calculus cannot be removed by a patient at home; it must be removed by an oral healthcare professional in a dental care setting.

Oral hygiene self-care methods

While chemotherapeutics can reduce the microbial load (amount and variety of microorganisms), control of oral biofilms is best achieved by daily manual (physical) disruption. Numerous devices are available to meet an individual's needs and ability.

Toothbrushing

Manual toothbrushes

Ancient civilizations used a "chew stick," a thin twig with a frayed end, to clean their teeth. The predecessors to the modern nylon-bristled toothbrush were made of hog bristles and attached to a handle made of bamboo or bone. Over time, toothbrushes evolved and were made from the softer hair of horses or other animals (https://en.wikipedia.org/wiki/Toothbrush). Today, toothbrushing is the most common method of biofilm removal and technological advancements have allowed researchers to identify qualities that enhance biofilm removal.

Manufacturers vary the size and shape of a toothbrush handle to satisfy patient preferences. The handle may be straight, curved, or offset, and is made of plastic. The head of a toothbrush is made of nylon bristles arranged in specific patterns, designed to enhance plaque removal. Flat-trim toothbrushes place all the bristles at the same length and angle to the brush head. Multilevel toothbrushes have alternating rows of tall and shorter bristles, which may or may not be arranged in separate angles (Figure 15.1). Some manufacturers attach bristles whose ends have been rounded, as opposed to being pointed. This design is gentler on gingival tissues, decreasing damage that may be done by overzealous brushing (Voelker et al. 2013). The bristle diameter determines "strength" and the American Dental Association recommends usage of a soft toothbrush (smaller diameter) (https://www.mouthhealthy.org/en/az-topics/t/toothbrushes). However, toothbrushes currently on the market labeled as "soft" exhibit a range of diameters (Teche et al. 2011). While there is insufficient evidence that one specific toothbrush design is superior to another, several studies have demonstrated that brushes with an angled bristle

Table 15.1 Types of deposits.

Name of deposit	Type of deposit	Definition
Acquired pellicle	Soft deposit	A thin layer of conditioning film composed of bacterial and host products (saliva, gingival crevicular fluid)
Biofilm (plaque biofilm)	Soft deposit	A microbial community housed in a protective matrix that attaches to oral tissues and is capable of initiating a host inflammatory response
Materia alba	Soft deposit	Accumulation of loosely attached microbes and oral debris that appears as a white, cord-like deposit
Food debris	Soft deposit	Food that remains in the oral cavity after eating
Calculus	Hard deposit	Biofilm that has been mineralized (hardened) by calcium phosphate mineral salts present in saliva

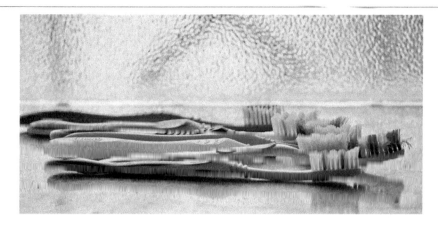

Figure 15.1 Manufacturers vary the shape, number, and configuration of bristles on the head of the toothbrush. Source: PDPics/1363 images/Pixabay.

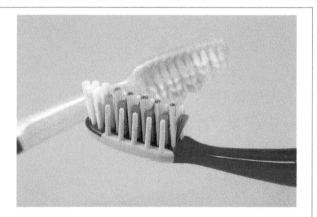

Figure 15.2 Toothbrush heads with varied bristle configurations. Source: Wagner Cesar Munhoz/Flickr.

configuration are more effective at removing plaque (Slot et al. 2012) (Figure 15.2).

Powered toothbrushes

A systematic review carried out by the Cochrane Oral Health Group compared the efficacy of manual and power toothbrushes (PTB) in reducing plaque and gingivitis (Yaacob et al. 2014). Moderate-quality evidence showed that PTBs reduce plaque by 11–21% and gingivitis by 6–11%, compared to manual toothbrushing. PTBs are powered by different modes of action: side-to-side action, counter-oscillation, rotation oscillation, circular, and ultrasonic; the greatest body of evidence indicated rotation oscillation brushes. However, the authors caution that with few trials reporting data over more than a three-month period, it is difficult to ascertain the long-term benefits of PTBs (Figure 15.3).

Techniques of toothbrushing

While a plethora of good scientific evidence supports the removal of oral biofilm to maintain oral health, very little evidence is available to suggest which biofilm removal technique is superior (Claydon 2008). It is recommended that individuals use the technique that produces the best results and is easiest to adopt and perform. Techniques include the Bass/modified Bass (sulcular), Stillman/modified Stillman, Charters, and Fones (circular) methods. Each technique has its indications for use, e.g. the Bass/modified Bass toothbrushing techniques are generally favored for patients who have had periodontitis when using a manual toothbrush. Table 15.2 summarizes toothbrushing techniques and their indications for use.

Regarding frequency, twice-daily brushing for 2 minutes and a systematic pattern are advised (Chapple et al. 2015). Studies conducted regarding toothbrushing habits show that the mean brushing time is 50 seconds and only 10% of that time is spent on the lingual surfaces (Claydon 2008). This underscores the need for improved oral hygiene education.

Tongue cleaning

The ecological diversity of surfaces in the oral cavity allows for the formation of distinct habitats that support the growth of over 700 different types of microorganisms. Mucosal surfaces, teeth, saliva, prosthetic devices, and gingival crevicular fluid create unique environments for the formation of biofilms. While toothbrushing effectively removes biofilm on hard tissues, biofilms form on mucosal surfaces as well, thereby increasing the overall microbial load in the oral cavity. The process of desquamation effectively reduces the microbial load on soft tissues, but the microorganisms found on the tongue differ from those found elsewhere in the oral cavity. This is due to the papillary structure of the tongue and deep fissures that provide niches for microbes to attach to and proliferate. The metabolism of anaerobic, Gram-negative bacteria found on the crevices of the lingual dorsum creates volatile sulfur compounds (VSCs) that cause halitosis (Danser et al. 2003). Tongue coating is also known to contribute to periodontitis and pneumonia in the elderly (Hata et al. 2020; Kishi et al. 2013). For these reasons, it is advised to brush the tongue daily in order to remove biofilms that may become pathogenic and cause oral malodor.

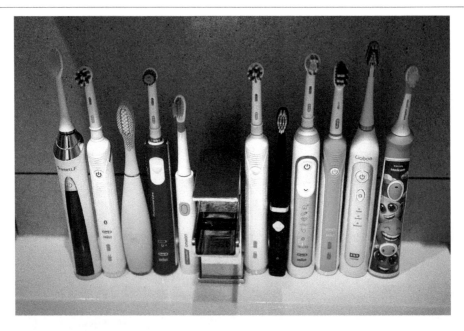

Figure 15.3 Varied powered toothbrushes. Source: Electric Teeth/Flickr.

Table 15.2 Toothbrushing techniques and their indications.

Technique	Description	
Bass (sulcular)/ modified Bass (a roll stroke is added at the end)	Toothbrush filaments are angled *toward* the gingival sulcus at a 45° angle to the long axis of the tooth using gentle pressure. The filaments are then moved horizontally within the sulcus in short, firm, gentle strokes (approx. 3–4 horizontal strokes).	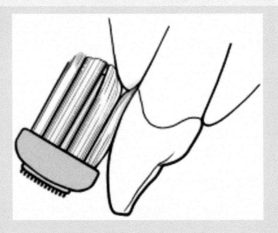 **Figure 15.4** Bass technique.
Stillman/modified Stillman (a roll stroke is added at the end)	Toothbrush filaments are angled toward the gingival margin at a 45° angle to the long axis of the tooth using gentle pressure. Filaments are placed *partly on the cervical portion of teeth and partly on the gingiva*. Short, gentle, horizontal strokes are employed as the brush filaments are moved in an occlusal direction.	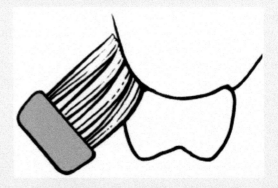 **Figure 15.5** Stillman technique.

Table 15.2 (Continued)

Technique	Description	
Charter	Toothbrush filaments are placed at the gingival margin at a 45° angle and are directed *coronally*. Short, gentle horizontal strokes are employed.	**Figure 15.6** Charter technique.
Fones	Toothbrush filaments are placed on tooth surfaces at a 90° angle. The filaments are then moved across the surface in a short, gentle circular motion.	**Figure 15.7** Fones technique. Source: Shannon Carabajal/United States Airforce.
Roll stroke	Toothbrush filaments are directed apically and rolled in a vertical motion (coronally).	

The tongue may be cleaned by using a toothbrush or a tongue cleaner (also known as a tongue scraper). Manufacturers make scrapers of different shapes and styles using plastic, copper, or stainless steel (Figures 15.8–15.10). The brush or scraper is placed as far back on the tongue as possible and is then pulled forward toward the tip of the tongue. This procedure is then repeated two or more times until the tongue is clean.

Interdental care and embrasure spaces

Selecting the most appropriate interproximal device will be based on efficiency in removing biofilm from the interproximal space and the consistency of the gingival tissues. Anatomic factors also affect the selection of interdental cleaning aids. These include the size and shape of the embrasure, tooth position and alignment, and contour and consistency of the gingival tissues.

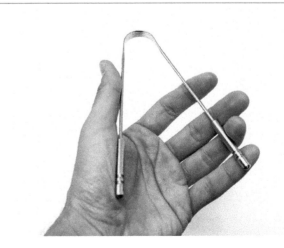

Figure 15.8 Stainless steel tongue scraper. Source: Marco Verch/Flickr.

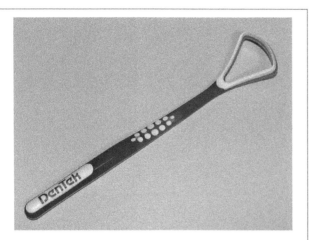

Figure 15.9 A plastic tongue scraper with a handle. Source: Niro5/ Wikimedia Commons.

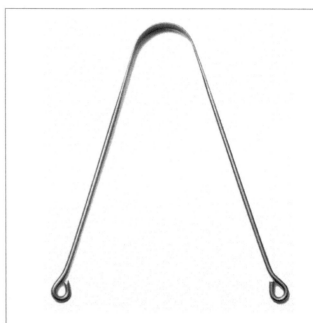

Figure 15.10 A copper tongue scraper.

The interproximal embrasure shape varies from tooth to tooth with no recession and healthy papilla to recession and no papilla. There are three classes of embrasure spaces:

■ Class 1 – No gingival recession with the interdental papilla filling the space.
■ Class II – Moderate papillary recession.
■ Class III – Complete loss of interdental papilla.

Toothbrushes and toothbrush bristles are mostly contoured to directly clean facial/lingual/occlusal surfaces and to reach around line angles, as well as proximal surfaces; however, they are not effective at cleaning interproximal or interdental areas. Removal of plaque biofilm from the interdental areas is important in reducing gingival inflammation and preventing periodontal disease. Periodontal disease most commonly begins in the interproximal col area, which is difficult to clean and is prone to inflammation.

There is a wide variety of interproximal cleaning aids available on the market. When recommending interdental self-care cleaning aids, the dental practitioner should consider the various conditions and risk factors, such as:

■ Probing depths.
■ Contour and consistency of gingival tissues.
■ Size and shape of interproximal areas.
■ Patient's level of dexterity.
■ Patient motivation and preferences.
■ Desired clinical outcome.

Interdental devices

Table 15.3 summarizes various interdental devices and their indications for usage.

Table 15.3 Interdental devices and their indications.	
Dental floss	Dental floss is the most frequently recommended device for cleaning and removing plaque biofilm from interproximal areas with normal gingival contour and embrasure spaces. It has been shown that individuals who floss regularly have less biofilm, gingivitis, bleeding, and calculus (Graves et al. 2015). However, dental floss is only recommended for individuals with class I embrasures with a normal gingival contour. Dental floss is available in unwaxed and waxed forms, and is made of synthetic material such as nylon and polytetrafluoroethylene. Research has shown no difference in clinical outcomes or effectiveness between waxed or unwaxed floss (Ong 1990) (Figure 15.11). If the patient presents with blunted papilla or recession with a class II embrasure space, then dental tape, which is wider and flatter than dental floss, is recommended.
Tufted floss	Tufted floss or textured floss is dispensed as a single strand and is designed to have three continuous segments: a segment of regular dental floss, a spongy or textured surface to clean class II or class III embrasures, and a rigid nylon needle segment for threading beneath fixed bridges or orthodontic appliances (Figure 15.12).
Floss holders	Floss holders are plastic handles that aid in the placement and movement of floss between the teeth. They are designed to assist individuals with compromised dexterity or oral conditions that make them unable to use traditional manual flossing methods. Studies have shown that the floss holder is as effective as manual floss, with increased efficacy regarding patient motivation and compliance (Spolsky et al. 1993) (Figure 15.13).

Table 15.3	(Continued)
Floss threaders	Floss threaders are rigid nylon needle devices with a loop that allows floss to be pulled through the interdental space under the contact point. Floss threaders assist in placing the floss between orthodontic devices, around abutment teeth of a fixed prosthetic bridge, or any other dental device that prevents floss from entering through the contact point (Figure 15.14).
Interdental brushes	Interdental brushes are devices used for class II or class III embrasures and furcations, tooth surfaces adjacent to missing teeth, orthodontic appliances, and proximal areas of abutment teeth. The interdental brush is designed for insertion of a disposable brush in a contra-angled end. The disposable brush is supplied with a cylindrical or cone shape with varying diameters, indicated for different sizes and shapes of embrasures. The brush should fit snugly into the interdental space and never be forced through the embrasure space. The interdental brush is inserted from the buccal side of the mouth and gently moved back and forth (Figure 15.15).
Wood sticks	Wood sticks are triangular-shaped devices usually made of soft wood. The wood stick is placed from the buccal side between the teeth with the flat side down, and applied with a gentle back-and-forth movement. It is recommended to moisten the wood stick prior to usage for comfort and ease of insertion. Wood sticks are used like interdental brushes and must be inserted only if the embrasure space is adequate enough for placement. Recently, plastic versions of this device have been introduced with the advantage of not breaking or splintering (Figure 15.16).
End-tufted brushes	End-tufted brushes are indicated for class II and class III embrasures, difficult-to-reach areas, or around fixed dental appliances. The tufts of the bristles are fixed to the end of a small brush head with a handle, like a standard toothbrush. Tufted brushes are usually not for single usage as is the interdental brush, and are replaced like a toothbrush (Figure 15.17).
Rubber-tip stimulator	Rubber-tip stimulators are primarily designed for gingival stimulation. The rubber tip is attached to the end of a metal or plastic handle and is used to remove plaque biofilm by rubbing it against the exposed tooth surfaces. It is also used to stimulate gingiva and recontour gingival papillae after periodontal therapy (Figure 15.18).

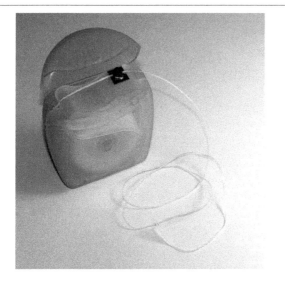

Figure 15.11 Dental floss. Source: Stan Zurek/Wikimedia Commons.

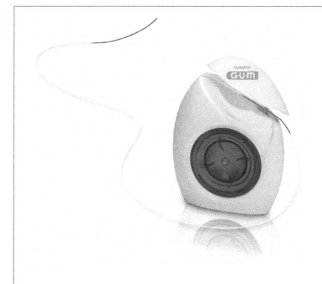

Figure 15.12 Tufted dental floss.

Oral irrigators

An oral irrigator or dental water jet is an effective irrigation device that emits a pulsating lavage with a variable pressure setting. Pulsation and pressure are critical to the effectiveness of the oral irrigator. Research has shown that oral irrigators that produce a pulsating stream reduce plaque biofilm, bleeding, gingivitis, pocket depth, pathogenic microorganisms, and calculus on patients with fixed orthodontic appliances, implants, crowns, and bridges, and individuals undergoing periodontal maintenance programs (Cronin et al. 2005). The

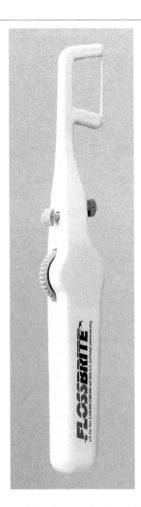

Figure 15.13 Floss holder. Source: Feelfree/Wikimedia Commons.

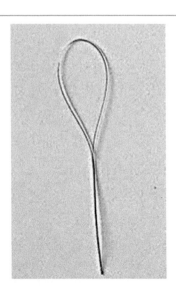

Figure 15.14 Floss threader.

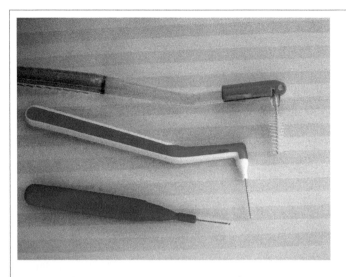

Figure 15.15 Interdental brushes. Source: Hondrej/Wikimedia Commons.

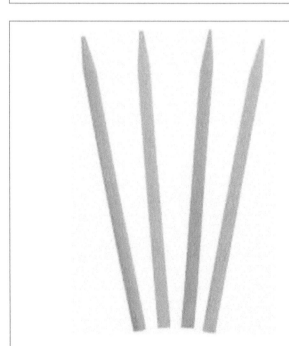

Figure 15.16 Wood sticks.

oral irrigator has been found to be a superior and effective alternative to dental floss in reducing gingival inflammation (Barnes et al. 2005). Water and 0.12% chlorhexidine solution are the most common agents used for subgingival irrigation. The depth of delivery of any solution is dependent on the type of tip that is used. The most common tip is made of hard plastic with a small opening, and is shown to deliver a solution to approximately 50% of the pocket depth (Jahn 2010). Updated tips are available with a soft rubber, latex-free conical shape, which can be used to deliver solutions into deeper periodontal pockets. Patients with orthodontic appliances can use an

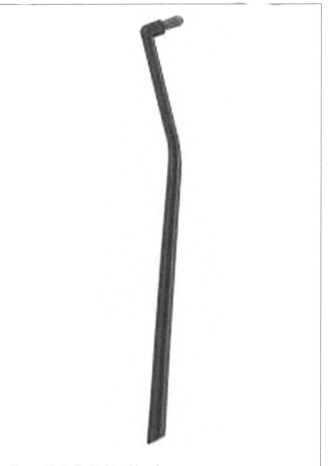

Figure 15.17 End-tuft toothbrush.

irrigation tip in combination with small tufted bristles surrounding the opening (Figure 15.19).

Dentifrices

Dentifrices have long been used as adjuncts to toothbrushing and flossing. They are available as pastes, powders, gels, or liquids and come in a variety of flavors that freshen breath. In addition to flavoring, dentifrices contain surfactants, preservatives, humectants, abrasives, thickening agents, and active ingredients that provide a therapeutic effect.

Fluoride is, by far, the most effective therapeutic ingredient added to dentifrices. The first clinically proven dentifrice was created by Crest® in 1955. Since then, many studies have affirmed fluoride's ability to prevent enamel demineralization and facilitate remineralization of incipient lesions (Walsh et al. 2010). In addition to fluoride, other antimicrobials (tri closan) and desensitizing agents have been added to dentifrices. Evidence for antimicrobials' ability to decrease gingivitis is not as robust as the evidence for fluoride. The addition of potassium nitrate is proven to reduce dentinal hypersensitivity (West et al. 2015). The effectiveness of therapeutic ingredients added to toothpaste can be increased by advising the patient to spit, rather than rinse, after toothbrushing to allow the ingredients to remain in the saliva.

Regarding biofilm removal, addition of a dentifrice does not provide an added effect for the mechanical removal of dental plaque (Valkenburg et al. 2016).

Mouth rinses

For a variety of reasons (including lack of motivation, dexterity, and/or resources), many patients struggle with adherence to oral biofilm control regimens. Additionally, mechanical plaque removal does not eliminate the biofilm that remains on the soft tissues (the lips, buccal mucosa, attached/free gingiva, the tongue, the floor of the mouth, etc.), which comprise approximately 80% of the oral cavity. To remedy these shortcomings, the American Dental Association (ADA) recommends that oral rinses be incorporated into daily oral hygiene practices.

Microbiology

A bacterium is protected from its environment by a membrane on the bacterial wall, the integrity of which is essential to survival of the bacterium. This membrane consists of basic

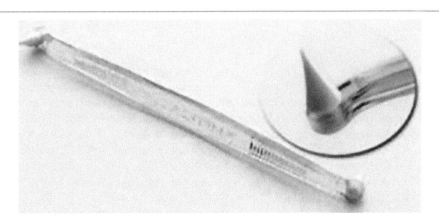

Figure 15.18 Rubber-tip stimulator.

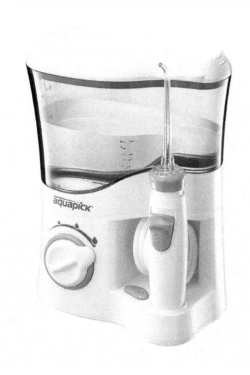

Figure 15.19 Oral irrigator. Source: Qudwh3842/Wikimedia Commons.

compounds such as phospholipids and lipopolysaccharides. The bacterial wall confers rigidity to the organism and differs considerably between Gram-positive and Gram-negative bacteria. This diversity leads to great variation in the potency of antimicrobial agents.

Antimicrobial agents used in oral rinses include essential oils (EOs), bis-biguanides, quaternary ammonium compounds (QACs), phenols, halogens, and oxygenating agents.

Essential oils

Plants contain fragrant components that protect the plant in continually changing internal and external environments. The International Organization for Standardization defines an essential oil as a product made by distillation of these components with either water or steam (http://www.iso.org/iso/home/store/catalogue_tc/catalogue_detail.htm?cs number=51017). EOs are antibacterial, antiviral, antifungal, and antimicrobial, hence their efficacy in combating oral pathogens. They are also known to have anti-inflammatory and antioxidative properties, and few side effects, which add to their ease of use. EOs also possess high specificity (effective against many different bacteria), but low substantivity (duration of antimicrobial action). The active ingredients in Listerine, which has received the ADA Seal of Acceptance, include three EOs: thymol 0.063%, eucalyptol 0.091%, and menthol 0.042%, along with other ingredients (i.e. methyl salicylate 0.0660%) (Asadoorian 2016).

Bis-biguanides

These are a class of chemical compounds, including chlorhexidine (CHX), with strong antibacterial properties. Their mechanism of action is to bind strongly to bacterial cell membranes, increasing the cell permeability, thus initiating leakage of intracellular components. Furthermore, bis-biguanides reduce pellicle formation and hinder the adsorption of bacteria onto the tooth structure. CHX is a broad-spectrum agent effective against Gram-positive and Gram-negative bacteria, fungi, yeasts, and some viruses. It has high substantivity over 7–12 hours after rinsing. It is considered the gold standard, the most potent of all chemotherapeutic agents. Disadvantages include brown staining of the teeth, tongue, and restorations; alteration of taste perceptions; strong, bitter taste; and increased calculus formation (Gunsolley 2006). There is some discrepancy regarding using a dentifrice containing sodium lauryl sulfate (SLS) concurrently with CHX. Some researchers found no difference in efficacy when combining the two and others found that SLS reduced the antimicrobial action of CHX. Without a clear distinction, the recommended procedure has been to use the SLS-containing dentifrice at least 30 minutes and preferably two hours after CHX rinsing.

Quaternary ammonium compounds

QACs irreversibly bind to phospholipids and proteins of the bacterial cell membrane, thereby impairing permeability. The capacity of the bacterial cell to absorb such molecules influences sensitivity; the agent becomes bound to the wall proteins and is thus able to enter and destroy the membrane. Cetylpyridinium chloride is an example of a QAC and it shares some of the adverse effects of CHX, including tooth staining, burning, and increased calculus formation, and does not have high substantivity.

Phenols

Triclosan, a bis-phenyl, is a very effective, broad-spectrum antimicrobial agent. Its judicious use in hospital settings by trained healthcare providers is undisputed. However, it has been implicated in a variety of harmful health effects, including endocrine disruption, impaired muscle contraction, developmental and reproductive toxicity, and carcinogenesis (Halden 2014; Yueh et al. 2014).

Halogens/fluoride

Stannous fluoride has anticariogenic and antibacterial properties. The use of stannous fluoride as an antibacterial is limited due to its instability and side effects. Amine fluoride stabilizes stannous fluoride, and formulations using them in combination are comparable to CHX in reducing oral bacterial accumulations. The negative effects of stannous fluoride include staining and a bitter, metallic taste.

Oxygenating agents

Gram-negative bacteria are highly sensitive to active oxygen. Hydrogen peroxide breaks down into water and oxygen and effectively kills bacteria. Oxygenating agents such as hydrogen peroxide have been used for many years to disinfect oral tissues. Researchers tested Ardox-X, formulated with peroxyborate and specific carriers such as glycerol and cellulose, and reported a significant microbial shift in composition of oral bacterial species such as *Streptococcus* and *Veillonella*. These agents also produce the added benefit of bleaching teeth. Peroxide, however, is unstable and difficult to store, thus limiting its use. Long-term studies have shown a lack of adverse effects to the soft

tissues of the mouth when used in low concentrations (<2%). In high concentrations (>30% solution), soft tissues may exhibit erythema or mucosal sloughing, inflammation, or hyperplasia (Mostajo et al. 2014; Walsh 2000).

A recent systematic review suggests that usage of mouth rinses containing EOs, stannous fluoride, and 0.12% chlorhexidine have demonstrated efficacy in reducing signs of gingival inflammation and gingival bleeding when used as an adjunct to toothbrushing (Araujo et al. 2015; Yueh et al. 2014).

REFERENCES

Akcalı A, Lang NP. Dental calculus: the calcified biofilm and its role in disease development. *Periodontol 2000.* 2018; 76(1);109–115.

Araujo MWB, Charles CA, Weinstein RB et al. Meta-analysis of the effect of an essential oil-containing mouthrinse on gingivitis and plaque. *J Am Dent Assoc.* 2015; 146:610–622.

Asadoorian J. CDHA position paper on commercially available over-the-counter oral rinsing products. *Can J Dent Hyg.* 2016; 50(3):126–139.

Barnes CM, Russell CM, Reinhardt RA, Payne JB, Lyle DM. Comparison of irrigation to floss as an adjunct to toothbrushing: effect on bleeding, gingivitis and supragingival plaque. *J Clin Dent.* 2005; 16(3):71–77.

Chapple IL, Van der Weijden F, Doerfer C et al. Primary prevention of periodontitis: managing gingivitis. *J Clin Periodontol.* 2015; 42: S71–S76.

Claydon NC. Current concepts in toothbrushing and interdental cleaning. *Periodontol 2000.* 2008; 48(1):10–22.

Cronin M, Dembling WZ, Cugini M, Thompson MC, Warren PR. A 30-day clinical comparison of a novel interdental cleaning device and dental floss in the reduction of plaque and gingivitis. *J Clin Dent.* 2005; 16(2):33–37.

Danser MM, Mantilla Gómez S, Van der Weijden GA. Tongue coating and tongue brushing: a literature review. *Int J Dent Hyg.* 2003; 1(3):151–158.

Graves RC, Disney JA, Stamm JW. Comparative effectiveness of flossing and brushing in reducing interproximal bleeding. *J Periodontol.* 1989; 60(5):243–247.

Gunsolley JC. A meta-analysis of six-month studies of antiplaque and anti-gingivitis agents. *J Am Dent Assoc.* 2006; 137:1649–1657.

Halden, R. On the need and speed of regulating triclosan and triclocarban in the United States. *Environ Sci Technol.* 2014; 48(7):3603–3611.

Hata R, Noguchi S, Kawanami T et al. Poor oral hygiene is associated with the detection of obligate anaerobes in pneumonia. *J Periodontol.* 2020; 19(1):65–73.

Jahn CA. The dental water jet: a historical review of the literature. *J Dent Hyg.* 2010; 84(3):114–120.

Kishi M, Ohara-Nemoto Y, Takahashi M et al. Prediction of peri-odontopathic bacteria in dental plaque of periodontal healthy subjects by measurement of volatile sulfur compounds in mouth air. *Arch Oral Biol.* 2013; 58(3):324–330.

Marsh PD, Zaura E. Dental biofilm: ecological interactions in health and disease. *J Clin Periodontol.* 2017; 44(18):S12–S22.

Mostajo MF, van der Reijden WA, Buijs MJ et al. Effect of an oxygenating agent on oral bacteria in vitro and on dental plaque composition in healthy young adults. *Front Cell Infect Microbiol.* 2014; 4:95.

Ong G. The effectiveness of 3 types of dental floss for interdental plaque removal. *J Clin Periodontol.* 1990; 17(7 Pt 1):463–466.

Slot DE, Wiggelinkhuizen L, Rosema NA, Van der Weijden GA. The efficacy of manual toothbrushes following a brushing exercise: a systematic review. *J Dent Hyg.* 2012; 10(3):187–197.

Spolsky VW, Perry DA, Meng Z, Kissel P. Evaluating the efficacy of a new flossing aid. *J Clin Periodontol.* 1993; 20(7):490–497.

Teche FV, Paranhos HF, Motta MF, Zaniquelli O, Tirapelli C. Differences in abrasion capacity of four soft toothbrushes. *Int J Dent Hyg.* 2011; 9(4):274–278.

Thomas JG, Nakaishi LA. Managing the complexity of a dynamic biofilm. *J Am Dent Assoc.* 2006; 137: S10–S15.

Valkenburg C, Slot DE, Bakker EW, Van der Weijden FA. Does dentifrice use help to remove plaque? A systematic review. *J Clin Periodontol.* 2016; 43(12):1050–1058.

Voelker MA, Bayne SC, Liu Y, Walker MP. Catalogue of tooth brush head designs. *J Dent Hyg.* 2013; 87(3):118–133.

Walsh L. Safety issues relating to the use of hydrogen peroxide in dentistry. *Aust Dent J.* 2000; 45(4):257–269.

Walsh T, Worthington HV, Glenny AM et al. Fluoride toothpastes of different concentrations for preventing dental caries in children and adolescents. *Cochrane Database Syst Rev.* 2010; 1:CD007868. doi: 10.1002/14651858.CD007868. pub2.

West NX, Seong J, Davies M. Management of dentine hypersensitivity: efficacy of professionally and self-administered agents. *J Clin Periodontol.* 2015; 42:S256–S302.

Yaacob M, Worthington HV, Deacon SA et al. Powered versus manual toothbrushing for oral health. *Cochrane Database of Syst Rev.* 2014; 17(6):CD002281. doi: 10.1002/14651858. CD002281.pub3.

Yueh M-F, Taniguchi K, Chen S et al. The commonly used antimicrobial additive triclosan is a liver tumor promoter. *Proc Natl Acad Sci U S A.* 2014; 111(48):17200–17205.

CHAPTER 16
Non-surgical periodontal therapy

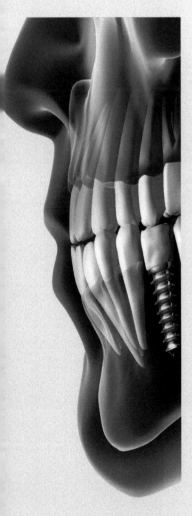

Contents

Essential Periodontics, First Edition. Edited by Steph Smith and Khalid Almas.
© 2022 John Wiley & Sons Ltd. Published 2022 by John Wiley & Sons Ltd.

16.1.1 PERIODONTAL INSTRUMENTS

Khalid Almas and Subraya Bhat

Contents

Learning objectives

- Components and classification of periodontal instruments.
- Usage of various periodontal hand instruments.
- Indications and usage of powered periodontal instruments.
- Advantages and disadvantages of different instrument usages.
- Cleaning and sterilization methods of instruments.

Introduction

Periodontal instruments are designed for specific purposes, such as calculus removal, biofilm removal, and root planing. Because the success of non-surgical periodontal therapy largely depends on the technical skill of the clinician providing treatment, complete knowledge and understanding of periodontal instruments are necessary, including their design, usage, and maintenance.

Classification of periodontal instruments

Periodontal instruments are classified according to the purposes they serve, in both non-surgical and surgical procedures.

Non-surgical instruments

Diagnostic instruments

- Mouth mirror.
- Periodontal probes: used to locate, measure, and mark pockets.
- Explorers: used to locate calculus deposits and caries.

Scaling and root planing instruments

- *For supragingival scaling:*
Sickle scalers, universal scalers, posterior Jacquette scaler, Morse scaler, and others.
- *For subgingival scaling:*
  - Hoe scalers, chisel scalers, and file scalers are used to remove subgingival deposits. Hoe scalers are used for scaling ledges or rings of calculus. Chisel scalers are usually used in the proximal surfaces of anterior teeth (too closely spaced). The chisel scaler is activated with a push motion. The primary function of files is to fracture or crush hard and tenacious calculus. Files are also used sometimes for removal of overhang margins of dental restorations.
  - Curettes are used to plane the root surfaces by removing altered cementum and scraping the soft tissue wall of the pocket.

- Sonic and ultrasonic instruments.
- Rotary instruments.
- Lasers.
- Schwartz periotrievers: a set of two double-ended, highly magnetized instruments designed for the retrieval of broken instrument tips from the periodontal pocket.

Periodontal endoscopes

These are used to visualize deep pockets and furcations during scaling and root planing.

Cleaning and polishing instruments

- Rubber cups, brushes, dental tapes.
- Air-power abrasive system.

Surgical instruments

- Excisional and incisional instruments.
- Surgical curettes and sickles.
- Periosteal elevators.
- Surgical chisel and files.
- Scissors.
- Needle holder.
- Tissue forceps and hemostats.

Components of periodontal instruments

Most periodontal instruments are made of either stainless steel, high carbon steel, or partial titanium and other alloys. Many stainless steel instruments are also now available with titanium nitride or other surface coatings that are not embedded or diffused into the base material (Pattison & Pattison 2013). The parts of each instrument are referred to as the working end (blade), shank, and handle. The instrument handle is that part of the instrument that is held in the hand and connects to one end of the shank. The shank is that part of the instrument that connects the handle to the working end (or blade). See Figure 16.1.1.1.

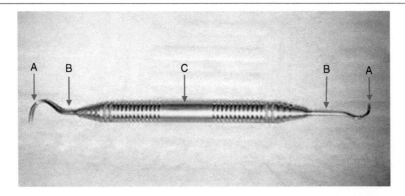

Figure 16.1.1.1 Parts of instruments. (A) Blade; (B) shank; (C) handle.

Periodontal probes

The periodontal probe (Table 16.1.1.1) is used during patient assessment to examine and evaluate the periodontium. It has a long, thin, rod-shaped end (tine), which is calibrated by millimeter markings that are used to measure periodontal pockets and periodontal structures. In cross-section, a probe can be either round or flat, with a blunt, rounded tip. The length and angles of the probe vary widely, as do the measurements marked on the probe. Some probes in color-coded increments for visibility of the measurements (Perio Wise or Perlovac). The periodontal probe is used to measure the depth of the sulcus or pocket, to identify bleeding areas of the sulcular epithelium, to locate the mucogingival junction, and to measure keratinized gingiva or oral lesions.

The pocket depth will vary according to the *probing force* (pressure) applied. Standardized forces should be of approximately 20–25 g (0.2–0.25 N of force); they can be standardized by constant force probes such as electronic probes.

Furcation areas can best be evaluated with the curved, blunt Nabers probe.

There are various factors that may influence the accurate measurement of pocket depths, e.g. operator variation, probing force, probing angulation and position, and the presence of subgingival calculus. Inflammation of gingival and periodontal tissues is one of the major reasons for pocket depth measurement variation. The clinical probing depth does not necessarily correspond precisely to the anatomic (histologically defined) level of the epithelial attachment in inflamed sites, as the probe tends to travel beyond the true attachment level, and in uninflamed sites it tends to stop short of the true level of epithelial attachment (Hughes et al. 2013).

Table 16.1.1.1 Types of periodontal probes.

Probe name	Probe description
Marquis color-coded probe	Calibrations are in 3 mm sections
University of North Carolina 15 probe (UNC-15)	15 mm long probe marked at each millimeter and color coded at the 5th, 10th, and 15th millimeters
University of Michigan "O" probe, with Williams markings	Markings at 1, 2, 3, 5, 7, 8, 9, and 10 mm
Michigan "O" probe	Markings at 3, 6, and 8 mm
World Health Organization (WHO) probe 621	A 0.5 mm ball at the tip, markings at 3.5, 8.5, and 11.5 mm, and color coding from 3.5 to 5.5 mm
Nabers probe	Used for detection of furcation areas, with color-coded markings at 3, 6, 9, and 12 mm

Explorers

Explorers are used to locate subgingival deposits and carious areas and to check the smoothness of the root surfaces after root planing. Explorers are designed with different shapes and angles, and have a variety of uses. They are also called shepherd's hook, straight explorer, curved explorer, or pigtail/cow horn explorer.

Scaling and root planing instruments

Sickle scalers

Sickle scalers have a flat surface and two cutting edges that converge in a sharply pointed tip. The shape of the instrument makes the tip strong so that it will not break off during use. Sickle scalers appear triangular in cross-section. Small, curved sickle scaler blades such as the 204SD can be inserted under ledges of calculus several millimeters below the gingiva. The sickle scaler is used primarily to remove supragingival calculus. Sickle scalers are used with a pull stroke.

The Morse sickle scaler has a very small, miniature blade; it is useful in the mandibular and anterior areas, where there is a narrow, interproximal space. Sickles with straight shanks are designed for use on anterior teeth and premolars. Sickle scalers with contra-angled shanks adapt to posterior teeth.

Curettes

The curette is the instrument of choice for removing deep subgingival calculus, root planing altered cementum, and removing the soft tissue lining the periodontal pocket. Most curettes, especially the new mini-bladed curettes, are smaller and thinner than other hand instruments and permit better tactile sensitivity. Their small size and rounded backs allow them to be inserted more easily under firm tissue and into deep, narrow pockets.

Curettes are finer than sickle scalers and do not have any sharp points or corners other than the cutting edges of the blade. Therefore, curettes can be adapted for and provide good access to deep pockets, with minimal soft tissue trauma. In cross-section, the blade appears semicircular with a convex base. Cutting edges are present on both sides of the blade. Both single- and double-ended curettes are obtainable, depending on the preference of the operator. The curved blade and rounded toe of the curette allow the blade to adapt better to the root surface. There are two basic types of curettes: universal and area specific.

Universal curettes

Universal curettes have cutting edges that may be inserted in most areas of the dentition by altering and adapting the finger rest, fulcrum, and hand position of the operator. The blade size and the angle and length of the shank may vary, but the face of the blade of every universal curette is at a 90° angle (perpendicular) to the lower shank when seen in cross-section from the tip (Pattison & Pattison 2013).

Examples of universal curettes are Barnhart curettes #1-2 and #5-6 and Columbia curettes #13-14, #2R-2L, and #4R-4L. Other popular universal curettes are Younger-Good #7-8, McCall's #17-18, and Indiana University #17-18.

Area-specific (Gracey) curettes

Gracey curettes are representative of area-specific curettes, a set of several instruments designed and angled to adapt to specific anatomic areas of the dentition (Table 16.1.1.2). These curettes and their modifications are probably the best instruments for subgingival scaling and root planing because they provide the best adaptation to complex root anatomy. Gracey curettes also differ from universal curettes in that the blade is not at a 90° angle to the lower shank (Table 16.1.1.3). The term *offset blade* is used to describe Gracey curettes because they are angled approximately 70° from the lower shank. This unique angulation allows the blade to be inserted in the precise position necessary for subgingival scaling and root planing, provided that the lower shank is parallel to the long axis of the tooth surface being scaled (Pattison & Pattison 2013).

Extended-shank curettes or after-five curettes

These are modifications of the standard Gracey curette design. The shank is 3 mm larger, allowing extension into deeper periodontal pockets of 5 mm or more. Other features include a thinned blade with a large diameter and a tapered shank for smoother subgingival insertion or reduced tissue distention.

Mini-bladed curettes

These are modifications of after-five curettes.

Gracey curettes mini-bladed

These are another set of four mini-bladed area-specific curettes.

Langer and mini-Langer curettes

This set of three curettes combines the shank design of the standard Gracey #5-6, 11-12, and 13-14 curettes with a universal blade honed at 90° rather than the offset blade of the Gracey curette.

Quétin furcation curettes

These are specially designed curettes to fit into the roof or floor of the furcation.

Non-surgical periodontal instruments

See Table 16.1.1.4.

Table 16.1.1.2 Double-ended Gracey curettes with their designated areas of use.

Gracey curette	Designated area of use
Gracey #1-2 and #3-4	For anterior teeth
Gracey #5-6	Anterior or premolar teeth
Gracey #7-8	Posterior teeth buccal and lingual surfaces
Gracey #9-10	
Gracey #11-12	Posterior teeth mesial surfaces
Gracey #13-14	Posterior teeth distal surfaces
Additions to the Gracey curettes: Gracey #15-16 and Gracey #17-18	#15-16 is a modification of #11-12; #17-18 is a modification of #13-14, with a shank elongated by 3 mm

Table 16.1.1.3 Distinctions between Gracey and universal curettes.

Features	Gracey curette	Universal curette
Areas of use	Set of many curettes designed for specific areas and surfaces	One curette designed for all areas and surfaces
Cutting edge	One cutting edge used; work is done with the outer edge only	Both cutting edges used, work is done with outer or inner edge
Curvature	Curved in two planes, blade curves up and to the side	Curved in one plane, blades curve up and not to the side
Blind angle	Offset blade, face of blade beveled at 60° to the shank	Not offset, face of the blade beveled at 90° to the shank

Source: Adapted from Pattison & Pattison 2013.

Table 16.1.1.4 Periodontal set (non-surgical kit) – see Figures 16.1.1.2 and 16.1.1.3.

Item #	Item name
1	Mouth mirror with handle (double sided)
2	Explorer Wilken/Tufts
3	Dressing plier
4	Williams probe (Goldman Fox Williams Laser etched probe)
5	Nabers probe
6	Towner-Jacquette scaler 33-415
7	Jacquette scaler 30-33
8	Jacquette scaler 34-35
9	Morse scaler

Table 16.1.1.4 (Continued)

Item #	Item name
10	Gracey curette 1R-2R
11	Gracey curette 3R-4R
12	Gracey curette 5R-6R
13	Gracey curette 7R-8R
14	Gracey curette 9R-10R
15	Gracey curette 11R-11R
16	Gracey curette 13R-14R
17	Younger Good curette YG7-8
18	Columbia curette 13-14
19	Columbia curette 13-14 4R-4L
20	Sharpening stone
21	Aspirating syringe
22	Instruments kit cassette

Surgical periodontal instruments

Macrosurgical instruments

Periodontal surgical instruments are composed of a group of excisional and incisional instruments.

Also included are periodontal knives, interdental knives, and surgical blades (#11, 12D, 15, 15C) and electrosurgery (radiosurgery) equipment. Surgical curettes and sickles, periosteal elevators, surgical chisels and hoes, surgical files, a set of scissors and nippers, and needle holders are commonly used for periodontal surgical procedures (see Tables 16.1.1.5 and 16.1.1.6).

Microsurgical instruments

There are various microsurgical kits available on the market. The kit can also be assembled according to the needs of the clinician (see Figure 16.1.1.7). Allen's specialized surgical kit provides precision micro-instruments specifically designed for today's minimally invasive soft tissue grafting procedures (Figure 16.1.1.8). Surgical applications include soft tissue augmentation, root coverage, vestibular extension, stabilization of mobile marginal tissue, and ridge augmentation.

Power scalers

Ultrasonic and sonic instruments

Ultrasonic and sonic instruments are used for removal of plaque, calculus, scaling, curetting, and stain removal. There are two types of ultrasonic units in common practice (Table 16.1.1.8):

- *Magnetostrictive*: Vibration of the tip is elliptical, hence all the sides can be used. Magnetostrictive ultrasonic inserts generate heat and require water for cooling.

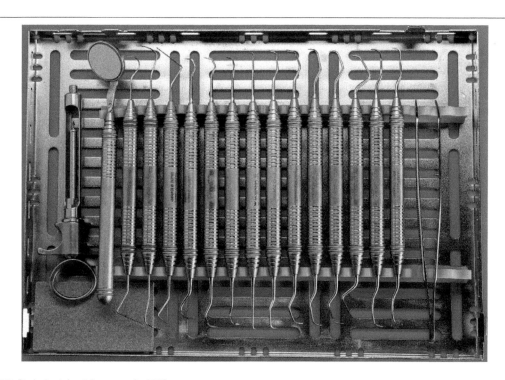

Figure 16.1.1.2 Periodontal set (non-surgical kit).

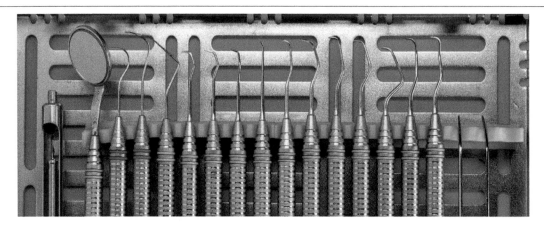

Figure 16.1.1.3 Periodontal set (non-surgical kit).

Table 16.1.1.5 Perio-surgery tray-1 (PS-18) –
see Figure 16.1.1.4.

Item #	Item name
1	Mouth mirror with handle (double sided)
2	Cone burnisher
3	Amalgam plugger/condenser Hollenback
4	Periosteal Pritchard elevator
5	Suture pliers
6	Amalgam carrier
7	Minnesota cheek retractor
8	Aspirating syringe
9	Prichard curette
10	Needle holder (Arruga serrated)
11	Needle holder (carbide caster)
12	Tissue nipper (Goldman Fox)
13	Scissors curved #321
14	Scissors curved #311
15	Kelley's hemostatic straight forceps
16	Sharpening stone
17	Amalgam well
18	Periosteal chisel
19	Instruments kit cassette

- *Piezoelectric*: Pattern of vibration of the tip is linear; only two sides of the tip are active. Ultrasonic vibrations range from 20 000 cycles/sec to 45 000. They operate in a wet field and are attached to water outlets. Sonic and piezoelectric units do not generate heat, but still use water for cooling of frictional heat and for flushing away debris.

The selection of either ultrasonic or hand instrumentation should be determined by the clinician's preference and experience and the needs of each patient (Tables 16.1.1.9 and 16.1.1.10). The success of either treatment method is determined by the time devoted to the procedure and the thoroughness of root debridement. In practice, clinicians typically use a combination of both ultrasonic and hand instrumentation to achieve these aims (Jahn & Jolkovsky 2013).

Magnetostrictive and piezoelectric plastic-tipped ultrasonic inserts are available that do not cause damage to titanium implants (Kwan et al. 1990). In addition, plastic and Teflon-coated sonic scaler tips have been developed for titanium implants for the removal of plaque and subgingival polishing of root surfaces (Kocher et al. 2000, 2001; Ruhling et al. 1994).

The use of ultrasonic and sonic scaling devices has some contraindications. Magnetostrictive devices have been reported to interfere with the function of older cardiac pacemakers (Zappa et al. 1991). In an independent study, a piezoelectric dental scaler produced no electromagnetic interference with defibrillators (Brand et al. 2007). Patients with newer pacemakers can be treated safely; however, a risk may exist if the patient is medically fragile or if electronically defective ultrasonic devices are used (Miller et al. 1998; Trenter & Walmsley 2003; Zappa et al. 1991). Medical consultation is advised when treating patients with such conditions.

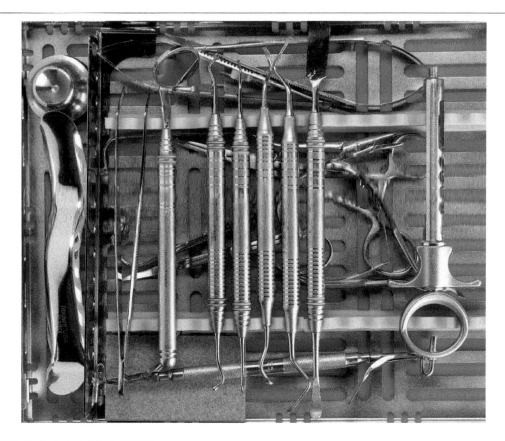

Figure 16.1.1.4 Perio-surgery tray-1 (PS-18).

Item #	Item name
Table 16.1.1.6 Perio-surgery tray-2 (PS-21) – see Figures 16.1.1.5 and 16.1.1.6.	
1	Nabers probe
2	Ochsenbein chisel #1
3	Ochsenbein chisel #2
4	Periodontal file (Schluger)
5	Periodontal file (Sugarman)
6	Gracey curette 1R-2R
7	Gracey curette 3R-4R
8	Gracey curette 5R-6R
9	Gracey curette 7R-8R
10	Gracey curette 9R-10R
11	Gracey curette 11R-12R

Item #	Item name
Table 16.1.1.6 (Continued)	
12	Gracey curette 13R-14R
13	Younger Good curette YG7-8
14	Elevator perio (Glickman) 24G
15	Periodontal knife (Kirkland) 15-16
16	Periodontal knife (Orban) 1-2
17	Blade handle #3
18	Blade handle #5
19	Dressing plier (without lock)
20	Williams probe (Goldman Fox Williams laser etched probe)
21	Explorer Wilken/Tufts
22	Instruments kit cassette

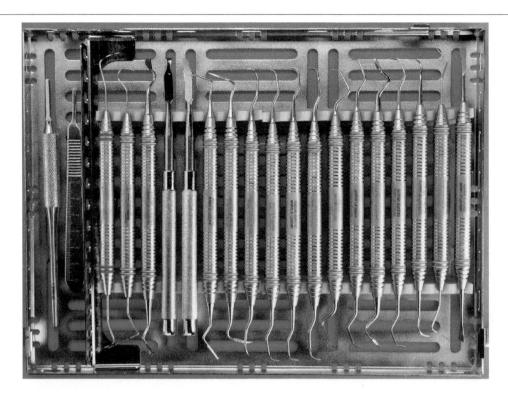

Figure 16.1.1.5 Perio-surgery tray-2 (PS-21).

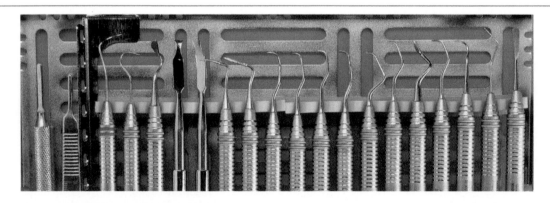

Figure 16.1.1.6 Perio-surgery tray-2 (PS-21).

Table 16.1.1.7 The Allen oral plastic surgery kit (HU-FRIEDY).

16-Instrument Infinity series cassette
Cooke-Waite (CW) aspirating anesthetic syringe
5 straight round scalpel handle
CP-11 color-coded probe
5 Front surface mouth mirror
6 Mirror handle
Allen end-cutting Intrasulcular knife, black line
Arrowhead knife, Everedge®
Modified Allen Orban knife, mini, Everedge
7/8 Younger-Good curette, Everedge
20 Corn suture pliers
Plain straight micro tissue pliers, diamond dusted
Micro Castroviejo perma sharp needle holder
Diamond dusted straight Goldman-Fox perma sharp scissors
Allen periosteal elevator, black line
Allen periosteal elevator, anterior, black line
Allen periosteal elevator, posterior, black line
Immunity steel cup, modified
Allen membrane measurement card

Table 16.1.1.8 Differences between sonic and ultrasonic scalers.

Sonic scalers	Ultrasonic scalers
Attached to a dental unit	Free standing or handheld unit
Need compressed air	Have electric generator
Frequency ranges from 2500 to 6500 cycles/second (Hertz, Hz)	Frequency ranges from 18 000 to 50 000 cycles/second (Hz)
Elliptical or orbital (circular) stroke pattern	Piezoelectric – linear pattern of strokes Magnetostrictive – elliptical or orbital stroke pattern
Tips are universal in design	Variety of tips are available

Source: Adapted from Pattison & Pattison 2013.

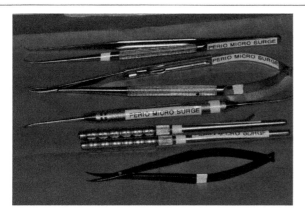

Figure 16.1.1.7 Six most used microsurgical instruments: tissue pliers, needle holder, periosteal elevator, straight microsurgical blade holders, scissors.

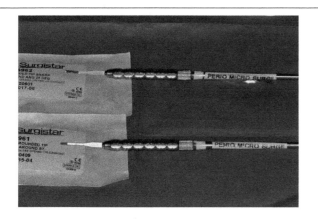

Figure 16.1.1.8 Microsurgical blades with straight blade handles.

Table 16.1.1.9 Advantages and disadvantages of hand instrumentation [3].

Advantages	Disadvantages
Does not produce an aerosol contaminated by microorganisms from the patient and dental unit water lines	Requires proper blade angulation
	Requires sharpening of the blade
Superior tactile sensitivity from the sharp blade on the tooth	Requires heavy lateral pressure for calculus removal, which is tiring for the clinician
Excellent access to deep pockets with mini-bladed curettes	More potential for causing carpal tunnel syndrome or other repetitive motion injuries
Good adaptation to root morphology with mini-bladed curettes	
Does not generate heat and therefore does not require water spray or high-speed evacuation, and better visibility	

Source: Adapted from Pattison 1996.

Aerosols from ultrasonic instrumentation always contain blood and potentially infectious blood-borne and airborne pathogens, and linger in the air for 30 minutes or longer.

Apart from universal precautions and use of personal protective equipment (PPE), direct the patient to rinse for 1 minute with an antimicrobial oral rinse such as 0.12% chlorhexidine to reduce the contaminated aerosol (Veksler et al. 1991; Wilkins 2009).

Table 16.1.1.10 Advantages and disadvantages of ultra-sonic instrumentation.

Advantages	Disadvantages
Instrumentation without pressure	Poor tactile sensation
Highly accessible to reach difficult areas	Aerosols are highly contaminated
Disruption of biofilm by cavitation	Not all handpieces can be autoclaved
Minimal soft tissue damage	Possible risk for patients with pacemakers
Requires less time	Contraindicated in infectious patients
Pocket irrigation is possible	
No sharpening of tips	
Better patient acceptance	
Less tiring for the operator	

Precautions, indications and contraindications for use of mechanized (powered) instruments (*Jahn & Jolkovsky 2013*)

- *Precautions*:
  - Unshielded pacemakers.
  - Infectious diseases: HIV, hepatitis, tuberculosis (active stages).
  - Demineralized tooth surface.
  - Exposed dentin (especially associated with sensitivity).
  - Restorative materials (porcelain, amalgam, gold, composite).
  - Titanium implant abutments unless using special insert (e.g. Quixonic SofTip prophy tips).
  - Children (primary teeth).
  - Immunosuppression from disease or chemotherapy.
  - Uncontrolled diabetes mellitus.
- *Indications*:
  - Supragingival debridement of dental calculus and extrinsic stains.
  - Subgingival debridement of calculus, oral biofilm, root surface constituents, and periodontal pathogens.
  - Removal of orthodontic cement.
  - Gingival and periodontal conditions and diseases.
  - Surgical interventions.
  - Margination (reduces amalgam overhangs).
- *Contraindications*:
  - Chronic pulmonary disease: asthma, emphysema, cystic fibrosis, pneumonia.
  - Cardiovascular disease with secondary pulmonary disease.
  - Swallowing difficulty (dysphagia).

Cleaning and polishing instruments

Rubber cups, bristle brushes, and dental tapes are used with polishing pastes. Dental tapes are used for polishing of proximal surfaces that are inaccessible to larger polishing instruments.

An instrument called a "prophy jet" is specially designed to deliver an air-powered slurry of warm water, abrasive sodium bicarbonate, and air for air-powder polishing. Powder products of aluminum trihydroxide or calcium carbonate are also available, as well as glycine powder, which has fewer abrasive qualities. This system is effective for the removal of extrinsic stains and soft deposits from teeth surfaces.

Condition and sharpness of instruments

Before any instrumentation, all instruments should be inspected to make sure that they are clean, sterile, and in good condition. The working ends of pointed or bladed instruments must be sharp to be effective. Sharp instruments enhance tactile sensitivity and allow the clinician to work more precisely and efficiently. Dull instruments may lead to incomplete calculus removal and unnecessary trauma because of the excess force usually applied to compensate for their ineffectiveness.

Instrument sharpening

It is impossible to carry out periodontal procedures efficiently with dull instruments. A sharp instrument cuts more precisely and quickly than a dull instrument. To do its job at all, a dull instrument must be held more firmly and pressed harder than a sharp instrument. This reduces tactile sensitivity and increases the possibility that the instrument will inadvertently slip, leading to tissue injury. Furthermore, dull instruments may lead to incomplete calculus removal and unnecessary trauma because of excess force applied.

When the instrument is sharp, the cutting edge is a fine line that runs the length of the cutting edge. The cutting edge of a dull curette is rounded. The objective of sharpening is to restore the fine, thin, linear cutting edge of the instrument. This is done by grinding the surfaces of the blade until their junction is once again sharply angular rather than rounded. Ideally, it is best to sharpen instruments after autoclaving and then re-autoclaving them prior to patient treatment.

Advantages of instrument sharpness

- Easier calculus removal.
- Improved stroke control.
- Reduced number of strokes.
- Increased patient comfort.
- Reduced clinician fatigue.

Sharpening stones

Sharpening stones may be quarried from natural mineral deposits or produced artificially. India and Arkansas oilstones are examples of natural abrasive stones (Figure 16.1.1.9). Carborundum, ruby, and ceramic stones are synthetically produced.

- *Mounted rotary stones*: These stones are mounted on a metal mandrel and used in a motor-driven handpiece. They may be cylindrical, conical, or disc shaped.

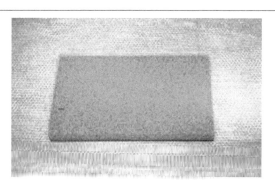

Figure 10.1.1.9 India stone for sharpening instruments.

- *Unmounted stones or sharpening cards*: Unmounted stones come in a variety of sizes and shapes. Some are rectangular with flat or grooved surfaces, whereas others are cylindrical or cone shaped.

Method of sharpening instruments

Sharpening and shaping of instruments should be done according to the manufacturer's guidelines. The instrument is held by a palm grasp and the sharpening stone should form a 100–110° angle with the face of the blade, whereby the 70–80° angle between the face and the lateral surface of the instrument is then automatically preserved (see Figures 16.1.1.10 and 16.1.1.11).

Tactile evaluation of sharpness is performed by drawing the instrument lightly across an acrylic rod known as a "sharpening test stick." A dull instrument will slide smoothly, without "biting" into the surface and raising a light shaving, as a sharp instrument would (Wilkins 2009) (Figure 16.1.1.12).

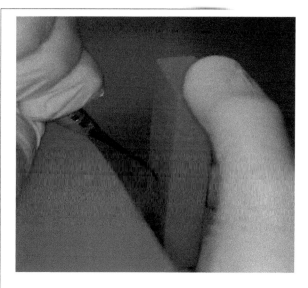

Figure 16.1.1.11 The instrument is stationary and the stone is mobile (moving).

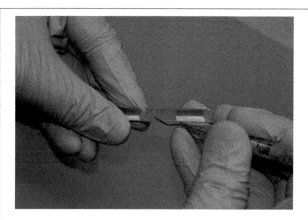

Figure 16.1.1.12 Sharpening test stick.

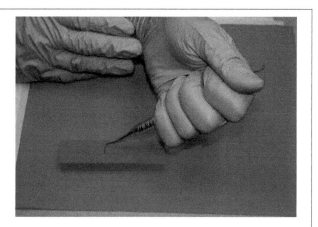

Figure 16.1.1.10 Position of instrument with 110° outer angle and 70° inner angle.

Instrument processing

Care must be taken during instrument processing to ensure that reusable instruments are safely cleaned and sterilized. Manual cleaning (hand scrubbing) is best for instruments that would be damaged if exposed to ultrasonic cleaners (i.e. some handpieces). Ultrasonic cleaners (bath) should mainly be used, which is safer than manual cleaning. The handling of instruments and manual cleaning should be performed with multiple-use utility gloves (heavy rubber or neoprene) and PPE. Instruments should be sterilized if they can be (includes new instruments); otherwise, disposable instruments should be used. During sterilization, instruments must be exposed to all three parameters of sterilization: time, temperature, and presence of steam, as well as weekly spore testing to ensure effective sterilization (Fehrenbach & Weiner 2021) (see Table 16.1.1.11).

Table 16.1.1.11 Commonly used methods of instrument sterilization.

Method	Time	Temperature	Pressure (psi)	Weekly spore testing
Moist heat (steam autoclave): standard	15–20 min	250° F 121° C	15	*Bacillus stearothermophilus*
Moist heat (steam autoclave): quick	3–12 min	270° F 130° C	30	
Chemical vapor (chemiclave)	20 min	270° F 130° C	20–40	*Bacillus stearothermophilus*
Dry heat (oven): standard	1–2 h	320° F 160° C	–	*Bacillus subtilis*
Dry heat (oven): quick	8–12 min	375° F 190° C	–	
Ethylene oxide	10–16 h to 24–48 h	Room temperature	–	*Bacillus subtilis*

SUMMARY

Periodontal instruments are designed for specific purposes, such as calculus removal, biofilm removal, and root planing. The success of periodontal therapy largely depends on the technical skill of the clinician providing treatment, including complete knowledge and understanding of periodontal instruments and of their design and maintenance. For clinical efficacy and predictable outcomes, apart from patient compliance, proper and efficacious use of manual and powered periodontal instruments is mandatory.

REFERENCES

Brand HS, Entjes ML, Nieuw Amerongen AV et al. Interference of electrical dental equipment with implantable cardioverter-defibrillators. *Br Dent J.* 2007; 203(10):577–579.

Fehrenbach MJ, Weiner J. *Saunders Review of Dental Hygiene.* St. Louis, MO: Elsevier; 2021.

Hughes FJ, Seymour KG, Turner W, Shahdad S, Nohl F. Periodontal assessment. In: FJ Hughes et al. (eds), *Clinical Problem Solving in Periodontology and Implantology.* St. Louis, MO: Elsevier; 2013: 3–12.

Jahn CA, Jolkovsky DL. Sonic and ultrasonic instrumentation and irrigation. In: MG Newman, HH Takei, PR Klokkevold, FA Carranza (eds), *Newman and Carranza's Clinical Periodontology.* Philadelphia, PA: Elsevier; 2013: 474–481.

Kocher T, Konig J, Hansen P et al. Subgingival polishing compared to scaling with steel curettes: a clinical pilot study. *J Clin Periodontol.* 2001; 28(2):194–199.

Kocher T, Langenbeck M, Ruhling A et al. Subgingival polishing with a Teflon-coated sonic scaler insert in comparison to conventional instruments as assessed on extracted teeth. *I. Residual deposits. J Clin Periodontol.* 2000; 27(4):243–249.

Kwan J, Zablotsky MH, Meffert RM. Implant maintenance using a modified ultrasonic instrument. *J Dent Hyg.* 1990; 64(9):422.

Miller CS, Leonelli FM, Latham E. Selective interference with pacemaker activity by electrical dental devices. *Oral Surg Oral Med Oral Pathol Oral Radiol Endod.* 1998; 85(1):33–36.

Pattison AM. The use of hand instruments in supportive periodontal treatment. *Periodontol 2000.* 1996; 12:71–89.

Pattison AM, Pattison GL. Scaling and root planing. In: MG Newman, HH Takei, PR Klokkevold, FA Carranza (eds), *Newman and Carranza's Clinical Periodontology.* Philadelphia, PA: Elsevier; 2013: 461–473.

Ruhling A, Kocher T, Kreusch J et al. Treatment of subgingival implant surfaces with Teflon-coated sonic and ultrasonic scaler tips and various implant curettes: an in vitro study. *Clin Oral Implants Res.* 1994; 5(1):19–29.

Trenter SC, Walmsley AD. Ultrasonic dental scaler: associated hazards. *J Clin Periodontol.* 2003; 30(2):95–101.

Veksler AE, Kayrouz GA, Newman MG. Reduction of salivary bacteria by pre-procedural rinses with chlorhexidine 0.12%. *J Periodontol.* 1991; 62(11):649–651.

Wilkins EM. *Clinical Practice of the Dental Hygienist.* Philadelphia, PA: Lippincott Williams & Wilkins; 2009.

Zappa U, Studer M, Merkle A et al. Effect of electrically powered dental devices on cardiac parameter function in humans. *Parodontol.* 1991; 2(4):299–308.

RECOMMENDED FURTHER READING

Darby ML, Walsh MM. *Dental Hygiene Theory and Practice*. St. Louis, MO: Saunders; 2010.

Pattison A, Pattison G, Matsuda S. *Periodontal Instrumentation*. New York: Pearson Education; 2018.

16.1.2 PRINCIPLES OF PERIODONTAL INSTRUMENTATION

Khalid Almas and Subraya Bhat

Contents

Learning objectives

- Purposes and elements of ergonomics in dental practice.
- Patient and clinician positions in periodontal practice.
- Equipment needs to promote ergonomics.
- Correct usage of periodontal instrumentation.
- Usage of periodontal probe, Nabers probe, scalers, and curettes on mandibular and maxillary teeth.

Introduction

The goal of periodontal therapy is to eliminate disease and to restore the periodontium to a state of health, which includes comfort, function, and esthetics that can be maintained adequately by both the patient and the dental professional. Non-surgical therapy aims to control the bacterial challenge characteristic of gingivitis and periodontitis while addressing local risk factors and minimizing the potential impact of systemic factors (Plemons & Eden 2004). The term "nonsurgical therapy" includes the use of oral hygiene self-care, periodontal instrumentation, and chemotherapeutic agents to prevent, arrest, or eliminate periodontal disease.

Periodontal instrumentation performed as part of non-surgical therapy is aimed directly at changing the prevalence of certain periodontal pathogens or reducing the levels of these microorganisms. Whether by direct removal of pathogenic organisms and their byproducts or removal of contributing factors such as calculus and overhanging restorations, the goal is to decrease the quantity of organisms below a critical mass and to alter the composition of the remaining bacterial flora to that associated with health. By this means, equilibrium between the remaining bacterial plaque (oral biofilm) and host response can be reached, resulting in a clinical state of periodontal health (Plemons & Eden 2004).

Ergonomics in periodontal practice

Ergonomics is essentially the science of making things efficient. The science includes the design of products to optimize them for human use, which concentrates on the physical aspects of work and human capabilities such as force, posture, and repetition. This entails designing tools, equipment, work stations, and tasks to fit the job to the worker, and not the worker to the job. Good working ergonomics underlies work capability, efficiency, and a high level of treatment (Figure 16.1.2.1). Failure to apply good working ergonomics can lead to work-related musculoskeletal disorders (Kamat et al. 2018).

Work postures

Patient position (*Kamat et al. 2018*)

For the maxillary arch
- Body: The patient's feet should be at the level of or slightly higher than the tip of their nose.
- Chair back: Almost parallel to the floor for maxillary treatment areas.
- Head: The top of the patient's head should be even with the upper edge of the headrest.
- Headrest: To be adjusted so that the patient's head is in a chin up position, with the patient's nose and chin at the same level

For the mandibular arch
- Body: The patient's feet should be at the level of or slightly higher than the tip of their nose.
- Chair back: To be slightly raised above the parallel position at a 15–20° angle to the floor.
- Head: The top of the patient's head should be even with the upper edge of the headrest.
- Headrest: To be adjusted (slightly raised) so that the patient's head is in a chin-down position, with the patient's chin lower than the nose.

Clinician position

- 7–12:30 o'clock position is preferred for the right-handed operator, and 12:30–5 o'clock for the left-handed operator.
- Sit back on the stool so that body weight is fully supported and back is against the backrest.
- Keep body weight evenly centered on stool.
- Back is straight without being rigid, tilting forward from hips rather than curling the back or hyperextending neck when necessary to get closer.
- Feet flat on floor and height adjusted so thighs are parallel to floor.

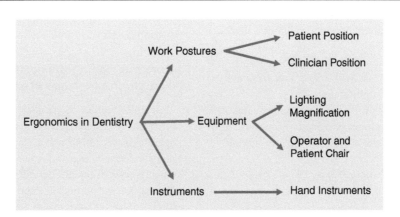

Figure 16.1.2.1 Ergonomic applications in dentistry. Source: Adapted from Das et al. 2018.

- Keep knees and legs apart to create tripod effect between two feet on floor and stool base to give stable seated position.
- Patient's chair height is adjusted to place the mouth at level of clinician's elbows.
- Shoulders should be relaxed and even, neither raised toward the ears nor rotated forward (especially if patient is somewhat upright).
- Upper arm should be kept close to sides, elbows bent, forearms parallel to the floor.
- Arms on a stool allow clinician to rest arms and shoulders between procedures.
- Wrist is held straight (neutral position) as much as possible; other bending of wrist such as pronounced flexion, extension, or deviation to the side should be avoided to prevent excessive stress on the nerves in wrist area.
- Hands should be positioned so that palms are facing inward toward clinician's midline as much as possible and in the same horizontal plane as forearm (neutral position).
- Head should be centered over spine for support; clinician's chin is tilted gently downward for visibility, but head is not tilted to right or left.
- Eyestrain is reduced by having mouth at comfortable focal distance, ~15 in. from clinician's eyes to mouth; clinician may need to consider an eye examination and/or loupes if this is not a comfortable distance.
- Assistant should be at a higher level than operator.

Equipment (Das et al. 2018)

The light source should be in the patient's mid-sagittal plane. Lighting should provide good shadow-free, even, color-corrected illumination to the operating field, so as to provide increased visibility and accessibility to the operator, with the light beam running parallel to the viewing direction.

Dental loupes, operating telescopes, and microscopes are available for magnification systems. Magnification allows a greater working distance, improves neck posture by helping the clinician to prevent leaning forward toward the patient, and provides clearer vision. Under magnification, proprioceptive guidance comes to be of little value, and instead visual guidance is used to accomplish midcourse correction of the hand to accomplish the finest movement with skill and dexterity (Kamat et al. 2018).

The clinician's chair should have adjustable lumbar support, seat height adjustment, adjustable foot rests, wrap-around body support, and seamless upholstery.

The patient chair should promote patient comfort and maximize patient access. This includes pivoting or drop-down armrests, headrest and neck support, and wrist/forearm support.

Instruments (Kamat et al. 2018)

Instrument grasp

The modified pen grasp is the recommended method for holding a periodontal instrument, and requires precise finger placement on the instrument.

Finger rests and fulcrum techniques

A fulcrum is a finger rest used to stabilize the clinician's hand during periodontal debridement. A well-established finger rest is essential for stability, unit control, prevention of injury, patient comfort, and control of length of stroke.

- *Intraoral fulcrum*: The intraoral fulcrum is established when the clinician's dominant hand is stabilized by placing and maintaining the pad of the ring finger on a tooth surface adjacent to or close to the tooth being instrumented.
- *Extraoral fulcrum*: The extraoral fulcrum requires stabilization of the clinician's dominant hand outside the patient's mouth against the cheeks, jaws, and chin, whereby the front or back of the fingers and hand provide the support rather than the tips or pads of the fingers.
- *Reinforced fulcrum*: The non-dominant hand is used for extra support of the instrument (instead of holding the mouth mirror) when scaling with both the intraoral and extraoral fulcrum. The index finger and thumb from the non-dominant hand help support the shank or instrument handle by placing pressure on it during a working stroke, thereby giving additional lateral pressure.

Instrumentation strokes

- Vertical and oblique instrumentation strokes are made in a coronal direction away from the base of the sulcus or periodontal pocket.
- Horizontal instrumentation strokes are used when working around the line angles of a posterior tooth or at the midline of an anterior tooth.
- A calculus removal stroke is used with sickle scalers and universal/area-specific curettes, and is characterized by short, controlled, biting strokes. For each stroke, the working end moves only a few millimeters.
- The root debridement stroke is characterized by a shaving stroke made with light pressure, and the stroke is slightly longer than a calculus removal stroke.

Periodontal probe

Figure 16.1.2.2 depicts examples of probing positions and angulations at various tooth sites.

Factors influencing the accurate measurement of pocket depths (Axtelius et al. 1999)

- *Operator variation*: A small degree of variation (measurement error) is inevitable even when the same experienced operator is repeating measurements. The size of measurement error will increase when comparing measurements taken by two different operators.
- *Probing force*: The pocket depth will vary according to the force applied. Standardized forces should be of approximately 20–25 g (0.2–0.25 N of force).
- *Probe angulation and position*: The probe should be angled along the contour of the root surface. Because the position of

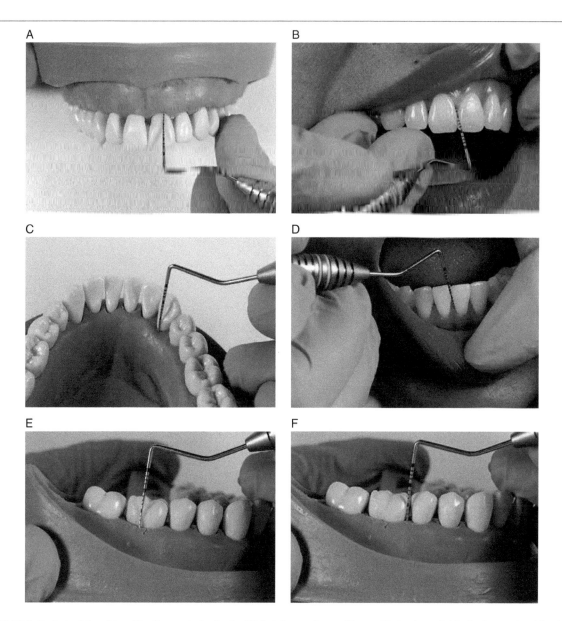

Figure 16.1.2.2 Periodontal probing. Maxillary anterior teeth: (A) facial aspect – working end is kept parallel to the long axis of the tooth; (B) interproximally – probe is slightly tilted (around 15°) to enter the sulcus. Mandibular anterior teeth: (C) lingual aspect – working end is kept parallel to the long axis of the tooth; (D) interproximally – probe is slightly tilted (around 15°) to enter the sulcus. Mandibular posterior teeth: (E) facial aspect – probe is inserted parallel to the long axis of the tooth; (F) interproximally – probe is slightly tilted (around 15°) to enter the sulcus.

each site to be probed is not accurately defined, small variations in position can alter the pocket depth recorded. In clinical studies, accuracy can be improved by using custom-made stents that ensure the probe is used at the same angle and site on each occasion, but this is not feasible for clinical practice.

- *Subgingival calculus*: The presence of subgingival calculus can make it more difficult to get the probe to the base of the pocket.
- *Inflammation*: The clinical probing depth does not necessarily correspond precisely to the anatomic (histologically

defined) level of the epithelial attachment. In inflamed sites, the probe tends to travel beyond the true attachment level, and in uninflamed sites it tends to stop short of the true level of epithelial attachment.

Nabers probe

Figure 16.1.2.3 depicts the use of a Nabers probe to assess the degree of furcation involvement and to classify the lesions accordingly.

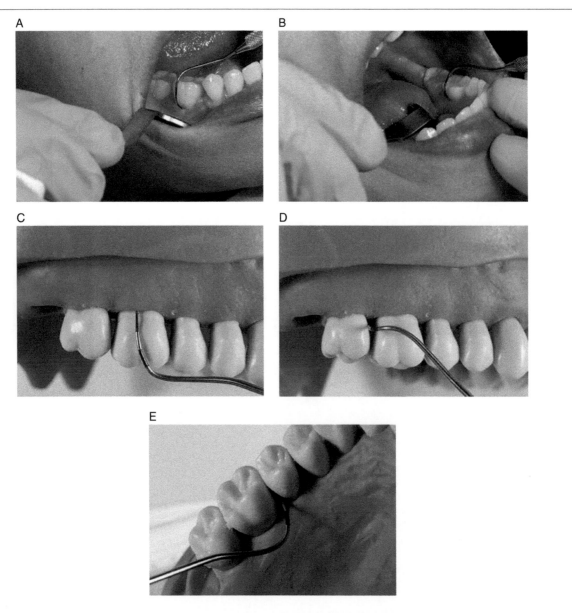

Figure 16.1.2.3 Furcation assessment. Mandibular molars: Nabers probe is inserted in the interradicular area, to follow the curvature of the furcation from the midpoint, (A) buccally and (B) lingually, approximately 5 mm from the cementoenamel junction. Maxillary molars: (C) Nabers probe is inserted along the curvature of tooth buccally; (D) distal furcation is midway between the buccal and palatal aspect, so it can be assessed buccally; (E) mesially the furcation opening is close to the palatal aspect, so the furcation is approached from the palatal aspect.

Scalers/curettes

Figure 16.1.2.4 illustrates the applications of scalers/curettes on anterior maxillary and mandibular teeth. Figure 16.1.2.5 shows the applications of scalers/curettes on posterior maxillary and mandibular teeth.

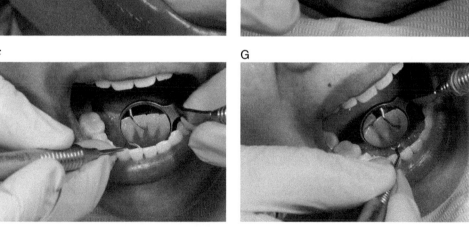

Figure 16.1.2.4 Maxillary anterior facial aspect: finger rest – intraoral, palm up, fourth finger on the incisal edge or surface of the adjacent maxillary teeth. Direct vision. (A) Surfaces away from the operator; (B) surfaces toward the operator. Maxillary anterior palatal aspect: finger rest – intraoral, palm up, fourth finger on the incisal edge or surface of the adjacent maxillary teeth. Indirect vision. (C) Surfaces away from and toward the operator. Mandibular anterior facial aspect: finger rest – intraoral, palm down, fourth finger on the incisal edge or surface of the adjacent mandibular teeth. (D) Surfaces away from the operator and operator position is back; (E) surfaces toward the operator and operator position is front. Mandibular anterior lingual aspect: finger rest – intraoral, palm down, fourth finger on the incisal edge or surface of the adjacent mandibular teeth. Direct or indirect vision. (F) Surfaces away from the operator and operator position is back; (G) surfaces toward the operator and operator position is front.

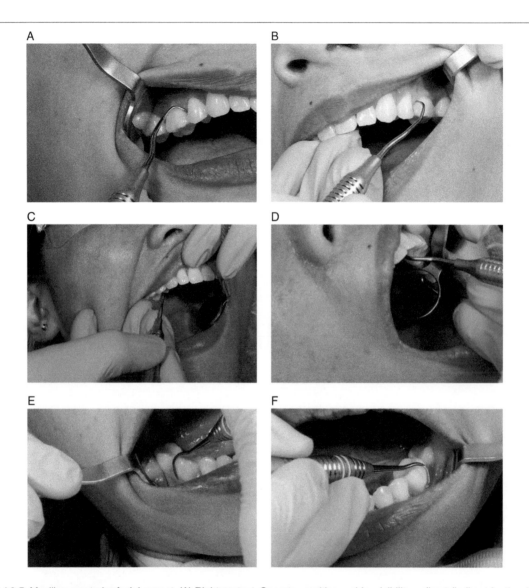

Figure 16.1.2.5 Maxillary posterior facial aspect. (A) Right sextant. Operator position – side; visibility – direct (indirect for the distal surfaces of molars); retraction – mirror or index finger of the non-operating hand; finger rest – extraoral, palm up, back of middle and fourth finger on the lateral aspect of the mandible on the right side of the face. (B) Left sextant. Operator position – back or side; visibility – direct or indirect; retraction – mirror; finger rest – intraoral, palm up, fourth finger on the incisal surface of anterior teeth or occlusal surface of the adjacent teeth. Maxillary posterior palatal aspect. (C) Right sextant. Operator position – side or front; visibility – direct or indirect; retraction – none; finger rest – extraoral, palm up, back of middle and fourth fingers on the lateral aspect of the mandible on the right side of the face. (D) Left sextant. Operator position – front; visibility – direct; retraction – none; finger rest – intraoral, palm down opposite arch, fourth finger on the incisal edge of the mandibular anterior teeth or the facial aspect of mandibular premolars, reinforced with the index finger of the non-operating hand. Mandibular posterior facial aspect. (E) Right sextant. Operator position – side or front; visibility – direct; retraction – mirror or index finger of the non-operating hand; finger rest – intraoral, palm down, fourth finger on the incisal edge or occlusal surface of the adjacent mandibular teeth. (F) Left sextant. Operator position – side or back; visibility – direct or indirect; retraction – mirror or index finger of the non-operating hand; finger rest – intraoral, palm down, fourth finger on the incisal edge or occlusal surface of the adjacent mandibular teeth. Mandibular posterior lingual aspect.

G   H

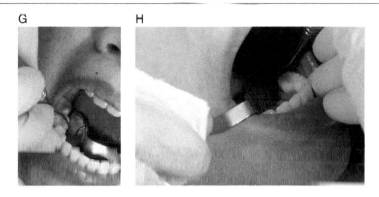

Figure 16.1.2.5 (*Continued*) (G) Right sextant. Operator position – front; visibility – direct or indirect; retraction – mirror retracts the tongue; finger rest – intraoral, palm down, fourth finger on the incisal edge or occlusal surface of the adjacent mandibular teeth. (H) Left sextant. Operator position – front or side; visibility – direct or indirect; retraction – mirror or index finger of the non-operating hand; finger rest – intraoral, palm down, fourth finger on the incisal edge or occlusal or facial surface of the adjacent mandibular teeth.

SUMMARY

A good understanding of ergonomics and how it pertains to periodontal instrumentation is essential for maximizing work capability and efficiency, and for achieving a high level of treatment of periodontal patients. Knowledge of how to apply specific instruments to various tooth surfaces is also pertinent for successful non-surgical treatment of periodontal disease.

REFERENCES

Axtelius B, Söderfeldt B, Attström R. A multilevel analysis of factors affecting pocket probing depth in patients responding differently to periodontal treatment. *J Clin Periodontol.* 1999; 26(2):67–76.

Das H, Motghare V, Singh M. Ergonomics in dentistry: narrative review. *IJADS.* 2018; 4(4):104–110.

Kamat RV, Baburaj MD, Pimple S. Ergonomic considerations in periodontal practice – a mini review. *Acta Scientific Dental Sciences.* 2018; 2(11):153–160.

Plemons JM, Eden BD. Nonsurgical therapy. In: LF Rose (ed.), *Periodontics: Medicine, Surgery and Implants.* Elsevier; 2004: 435–495.

16.1.3 SCALING AND ROOT PLANING

Subraya Bhat and Khalid Almas

Contents

Learning objectives

- Understand the rationale for and objectives of scaling and root planing.
- Understand the indications for scaling and root planing.
- Knowledge of instrumentation, including the instruments to be used for scaling and root planing.
- Understand the challenges of scaling and root planing.
- Understand the therapeutic endpoint and healing following scaling and root planing.

Introduction

Non-surgical periodontal therapy is a fundamental cornerstone in the treatment of periodontal disease. This type of therapy is also known as etiotrophic phase therapy, phase I therapy, or cause-related therapy. The main objective of this phase of periodontal therapy is to eliminate the etiological factors responsible for periodontal disease. Scaling and root planing (SRP; mechanical therapy) forms a major part of this key therapeutic procedure (Kwon et al. 2019).

Mechanical therapy refers to both supragingival and subgingival scaling as well as root planing, debridement of the roots by the meticulous use of hand or power driven scalers to remove plaque, endotoxin, calculus, and other local plaque-retentive factors (Drisko 1998).

Scaling is the process of removal of all surface deposits, plaque, calculus, and other accretions from the tooth surface. This can entail supra- or subgingival scaling, depending upon the procedure being done above or below the gingival tissue (Cobb & Sottosanti 2021).

Root planing is the continuation of subgingival scaling. With recent better understanding of the attachment of deposits to the root surface, which include changes in the concept of endotoxin attachment to the root surface, the procedure has been slightly modified from the original technique, such that several other names have been given for the same procedure, i.e. root surface debridement (RSD), root surface instrumentation (RSI), and root detoxification. RSD entails debridement of the root surface with only a few strokes, without undertaking aggressive instrumentation to remove endotoxins and other root surface irregularities (Cadosch et al. 2003).

Root planing was described as a treatment procedure in the early parts of the twentieth century by Hartzell (1913). In 1953, the use of scalers was described to remove calculus deposits and to smooth the tooth surface by means of removing softened, necrotic cementum (Cadosch et al. 2003).

Definition

Scaling is defined as a process by which biofilm and calculus are removed from both supra- and subgingival tooth surfaces, but no deliberate attempt is made to remove tooth substance along with cementum (Adriaens & Adriaens 2004).

Root planing is defined as the process by which residual embedded calculus and portions of cementum are removed from the root to produce a smooth, hard, and clean surface (Adriaens & Adriaens 2004).

Rationale for scaling and root planing (Lang 1983)

- Plaque, plaque-retentive factors, and calculus are considered to be primary etiological agents of periodontal disease. Removal of these surface deposits is essential to halt the disease process, restore the normalcy of gingival health, and regenerate lost periodontal structure.

- During pocket formation, soft tissue changes and root surface changes occur. Root surface changes include physical changes, chemical changes, and cytotoxic changes. Physical changes that are bound to occur during pocket formation are hypermineralization, demineralization, and root caries formation. These changes cause irregularities on the root surface and act as a trap for plaque formation. In addition to this, the consequential exposure of the root surface to the oral environment leads to the absorption of various chemicals, which also change the physical irritability of the root surface. Further to these changes, endotoxin released by the bacteria adsorb to the root surface and cause endotoxin-related changes in the root surface. Thus, removal of these irregularities is essential to have a plaque-free surface.

- Calculus attachment to the root surface differs from that to the enamel surface. Calculus is frequently embedded in cemental irregularities, and so the removal of this deeply embedded calculus makes root planing essential.

- Removal of the contaminated root surface is a prerequisite for new connective tissue attachment. Root planing prepares the root surface for demineralization and, subsequently, new attachment.

Objectives of scaling and root planing (Cobb 1996)

- Disruption and removal of the subgingival biofilm.
- Removal of plaque-retentive factors such as calculus.
- Conservation of tooth structure (preventing the formation of caries).
- Creation of a biologically acceptable root surface.
- Resolution of inflammation.
- Restoration of health by removing the etiological factors of periodontal disease.
- Obtaining a plaque-free smooth root surface, to prevent the occurrence of periodontal disease, and to assist the individual's daily plaque control measures.
- Preparing the periodontal tissues for periodontal surgical procedures, whenever indicated.

Indications (Lang 1983)

Root planing is considered a definitive mode of periodontal treatment under the following conditions:

- In medically compromised conditions, when periodontal surgeries may be contraindicated.
- For esthetic considerations. One of the disadvantages of periodontal surgical therapy in the esthetic zone is gingival recession. To avoid this unwanted sequela, and as a compromise, SRP is indicated.
- Where the pocket depth is less than 5 mm, with only horizontal bone loss.
- As a routine procedure during phase I therapy where a surgical procedure is later required, so as to get a firm fibrous tissue that can be easily handled in the making of incisions during the surgical procedure.

Lindhe et al. (1982) defined the *critical probing depth* for non-surgical therapy (NST, including SRP) to be 2.9 mm. Sites with probing depths of less than 2.9 mm have been shown to lose clinical attachment as a result of NST. However, at sites with probing depths of more than 2.9 mm, clinical attachment gain will result with NST. On the other hand, when there is a need for access flap therapy, the critical probing depth has been defined to be 4.2 mm. Open flap debridement has been shown to be only beneficial at sites with probing depths above 4.2 mm, while sites with probing depths less than 4.2 mm will result in loss of attachment. SRP should thus not be attempted in cases where pocket depths are less than 3 mm (Lindhe et al. 1982). Looking at the data from both SRP and access flap surgery, another critical probing depth is 5.4 mm. This, in turn, means that flap surgery is indicated predominantly at sites with a probing depth of ‡5.4 mm, while at sites with probing depths between 2.9 mm and 5.4 mm, NST is to be preferred.

Procedure for scaling and root planing (instrumentation)

See Dahiya et al. (2011), Kumar et al. (2015), and Mengel et al. (1997).

Instruments

There are many instruments that can be used. The selection of a specific instrument is largely dependent on the operator's skills. Earlier, the most common instruments used were hoe and chisel scalers. However, a decline in the use of these instruments has been due to the availability of curettes and their modified versions.

Two types of curettes are being used, universal and area-specific curettes (Gracey curettes) (see also Chapter 16.1.1). As the name indicates, a universal curette is a set of one or two instruments used for all the teeth, with modifying finger rests. Area-specific curettes are a set of seven instruments, each being indicated for use in a specific area. As these instruments are in widespread use, further modifications of them have developed, resulting in the availability of extended-shank curettes (shank length extended by 3 mm), also called after-five curettes (for use in pockets of more than 5 mm), mini Gracey curettes (which have an extended shank of 3 mm and the blade size is 50% shorter than regular curettes), and micro-mini-five Gracey curettes. Also available are Langer and mini-Langer curettes, which overcome the disadvantages of both Gracey and universal curettes, since they are a modification of both (combining the shank design of the standard Gracey #5-6, 11-12, and 13-14 curettes with a universal blade honed at 90°).

Sonic and ultrasonic instruments and their modified versions are also used for SRP. Their ease of use and the additional advantages of a lavage effect, less fatigue with hand instrumentation, and less time taken to complete the procedure have made them popular instruments for SRP. Studies comparing hand instrumentation with sonic and ultrasonic instruments have shown similar outcomes with regard to calculus removal, cementum removal, and resultant smooth surfaces. However, the usage of ultrasonic instrumentation always needs to be followed up by final hand instrumentation, which helps remove minute deposits from difficult access areas on the tooth surface. There are newer thin-end ultrasonic scaler systems available to reach deeper probing depths and difficult-to-reach areas.

Innovations in root planing instrumentation

Other than the modification of regular Gracey curettes, other innovations have been made available for use, although they have not gained much popularity. These innovations include the PER-IO-TOR and PER-IO-TOR rotary and VECTOR systems (Mengel et al. 1994; Slot et al. 2008). Endoscopy as an adjunctive to SRP has been utilized in clinical practice. However, studies have not shown any advantages for final clinical outcomes with the usage of endoscopy (Geisinger et al. 2007).

Instrumentation (Zappa et al. 1991)

- SRP is a complex procedure. Subgingival calculus is tenacious and may be deeply embedded within irregularities on the root surface. Furthermore, vision can be obscured by bleeding, movements of instruments cannot be done freely due to the presence of a pocket wall, and dependency upon tactile sensitivity is another challenge.
- Either universal or area-specific curettes are used. Initially the rigid-handle instruments are used, followed by flexible-handle instruments.
- The number of root planing strokes varies. According to an earlier concept, endotoxin attachment was thought to penetrate deep into the cementum, and thus to get a glassy smooth root surface strokes varied from 10 to 70. However, more than 20 strokes are considered to be aggressive, which may also remove much cementum from the root surface. For the removal of cementum, a single brush stroke is considered to be sufficient. However, for the removal of physical irregularities and to create a smoother surface, a slightly increased number of strokes may be necessary. As Mombelli has suggested, "If you think calculus is important, I suggest you leave the room now. I am more interested in living bacteria than petrified ones." Therefore, the presence of a small fleck of calculus, although undesirable, is not said to hinder healing at the cost of cementum. This implies the clinician must limit strokes to 20 for calculus removal. Importance must also be given to the patient's oral hygiene habits and appropriate instructions need to be given.
- If the pocket wall is well distended, ultrasonic and sonic scalers can also be used for subgingival SRP.
- The endpoint of the instrumentation is a surface that is free of calculus (not rough) and smooth, and being conducive to maintenance of a plaque-free area by the patient.
- Adjunctive use of local anesthetic. It is often not required; it may depend upon the patient's pain threshold and tolerance limit. Stoltenberg et al. (2007) compared 20% topical

benzocaine gel to 2% injected lidocaine. Patients experienced less pain with injected anesthesia; however, other patients preferred topical anesthesia due to fear of injection. Transmucosal lidocaine patches have also been shown to provide sufficient anesthesia for therapeutic quadrant SRP procedures (Derman et al. 2014).

Challenge areas for scaling and root planing

See Michaud et al. (2007) and Roussa-Tsoulou et al. (1992).

- Multirooted teeth are considered to be more difficult for SRP compared to single-rooted teeth.
- Furcation areas often do not allow standard Gracey curettes; in these areas, the availability of modified curettes is found to be helpful.
- Distal to the last molar, line angles, and curved surfaces – where adaptation of instruments is found to be difficult.
- Anatomically difficult areas – grooves, furcation ridges, and other similar areas.
- Size of mouth, elasticity of cheeks, range of opening, and dexterity of operator are other challenging factors.

Healing after scaling and root planing (Hughes et al. 1978)

- Day 1 – marked acute inflammation and epithelial migration.
- Day 4–5 – new epithelial attachment (long junctional epithelium).
- Day 14 – clinically healthy gingiva and formation of gingival unit.
- Further remodeling of the tissue occurring for 42–72 days.
- Creeping attachment is a term coined for the coronal shift in the position of the gingival margin. It is commonly observed as a post-surgical phenomenon following a free gingival graft procedure. However, several other procedures also have demonstrated creeping attachment, including SRP. Aimetti et al. (2005) reported a coronal shift of 0.40–0.89 mm. This achieved complete root coverage of 45.83% in 12 months. The authors identified three different factors that help in creeping attachment: initial thick gingiva (thick phenotype), reduction in the convexity of the root, and a plaque-free and flat root surface (Aimetti et al. 2005).

Evaluation of therapeutic success

Factors to consider in relation to whether an SRP procedure has been successful are the following (Cobb 2002):

- *Root smoothness*: Relative smoothness of the root surface is the best immediate clinical indication of adequate instrumentation. Generally, a thin and flexible curette or explorer with good tactile sensitivity, where the working end is curved, permits easy adaptation, and is lengthy enough to extend into a deep pocket.
- *Healing of soft tissue*: Reduction in the signs of gingival inflammation and reduction in probing depth are indications of successful SRP therapy. If areas remain with bleeding after SRP, this may indicate residual calculus.
- *Endpoints*: Hujoel (2004) pointed out the true and surrogate endpoints of SRP. True endpoints are reduction in pain and improved esthetics and efficiency in chewing. Surrogate endpoints include reduced bleeding on probing, pocket closure, attachment gain, and reduced tooth loss.
- *Microbial changes*: Change in biofilm composition is one of the objectives of SRP, which has been reported to result in significant decreases in DNA probe counts of a specific subset of subgingival microbes, including *Porphyromonas gingivalis*, *Bacteroides forsythias*, and *Treponema denticola*. It was also reported that re-emergence of bacteria can occur from the following locations: residual subgingival plaque deposits, radicular dentin or cementum, pocket epithelium or connective tissue, supragingival plaque deposits, subgingival deposits of adjacent teeth, and intraoral soft tissue sites (Cugini et al. 2000).

Unwanted effects (von Troil et al. 2002)

- Root sensitivity occurs in approximately half of patients following subgingival SRP. The intensity of root sensitivity increases for a few weeks following therapy, after which it decreases. Unnecessary excessive root substance loss of cementum is responsible for this.
- There may be root surface exposure and gingival recession can occur due to shrinkage of the pocket wall; it may also be due to inadvertent curettage.
- Root fracture (partial or wall of the root) is possible and pulpitis (often transient) has also been reported following SRP.

Other modes of root surface debridement

Laser therapy, photodynamic therapy, and air polishing are other modes of RSD (Berakdar et al. 2012; Caygur et al. 2017; Schwarz et al. 2003).

SUMMARY

SRP is an integral part of periodontal therapy. All other periodontal procedures follow this non-surgical mode of therapy. Although the understanding of the pathogenesis of periodontal disease has changed, the use of basic instrumentation for this purpose has remained almost the same, with some modifications. Additional modalities of RSD have shown promising results as an adjunct to SRP.

REFERENCES

Adriaens PA, Adriaens LM. Effects of nonsurgical periodontal therapy on hard and soft tissues. *Periodontol 2000.* 2004; 36:121–145.

Aimetti M, Romano F, Peccolo DC, Debernardi C. Non-surgical periodontal therapy of shallow gingival recession defects: evaluation of the restorative capacity of marginal gingiva after 12 months. *J Periodontol.* 2005; 76(2):256–261.

Berakdar M, Callaway A, Eddin MF, Roß A, Willershausen B. Comparison between scaling-root-planing (SRP) and SRP/photodynamic therapy: six-month study. *Head Face Med.* 2012; 8:12.

Cadosch J, Zimmermann U, Ruppert M et al. Root surface debridement and endotoxin removal. *J Periodontal Res.* 2003; 38(3):229–236.

Caygur A, Albaba MR, Berberoglu A, Yilmaz HG. Efficacy of glycine powder air-polishing combined with scaling and root planing in the treatment of periodontitis and halitosis: a randomised clinical study. *J Int Med Res.* 2017; 45(3):1168–1174.

Cobb CM. Clinical significance of non-surgical periodontal therapy: an evidence-based perspective of scaling and root planing. *J Clin Periodontol.* 2002; 29:22–32.

Cobb CM. Non-surgical pocket therapy: mechanical. *Ann Periodontol.* 1996; 1:443–490.

Cobb CM, Sottosanti JS. A re-evaluation of scaling and root planing. *J Periodontol.* 2021. doi: 10.1002/JPER.20-0839.

Cugini MA, Haffajee AD, Smith C, Kent RL Jr, Socransky SS. The effect of scaling and root planing on the clinical and microbiological parameters of periodontal diseases: 12-month results. *J Clin Periodontol.* 2000; 27(1):30–36.

Dahiya P, Kamal R, Gupta R, Pandit N. Comparative evaluation of hand and power-driven instruments on root surface characteristics: a scanning electron microscopy study. *Contemp Clin Dent.* 2011; 2(2):79–83.

Derman SH, Lowden CE, Hellmich M, Noack MJ. Influence of intra-pocket anesthesia gel on treatment outcome in periodontal patients: a randomized controlled trial. *J Clin Periodontol.* 2014; 41(5):481–488.

Drisko CH. Root instrumentation. Power-driven versus manual scalers, which one? *Dent Clin North Am.* 1998; 42(2):229–424.

Geisinger ML, Mealey BL, Schoolfield J, Mellonig JT. The effectiveness of subgingival scaling and root planing: an evaluation of therapy with and without the use of the periodontal endoscope. *J Periodontol.* 2007; 78(1):22–28.

Hartzell TB. The responsibility of the dentist and physician in regard to mouth infections and their relation to constitutional effects. *JAMA.* 1913; 61(14):1270–1275.

Hughes TP, Caffesse RG. Gingival changes following scaling, root planing and oral hygiene—a biometric evaluation. *J Periodontol.* 1978; 49(5):245–248.

Hujoel PP. Endpoints in periodontal trials: the need for an evidence-based research approach. *Periodontol 2000.* 2004; 36:196–204.

Kumar P, Das SJ, Sonowal ST, Chawla J. Comparison of root surface roughness produced by hand instruments and ultrasonic scalers: an invitro study. *J Clin Diagn Res.* 2015; 9(11):ZC56–ZC60.

Kwon T, Salem DM, Levin L. Nonsurgical periodontal therapy based on the principles of cause-related therapy: rationale and case series. *Quintessence Int.* 2019; 50(5):370–376.

Lang NP. Indications and rationale for non-surgical periodontal therapy. *Int Dent J.* 1983; 33(2):127–136.

Lindhe J, Socransky SS, Nyman S, Haffajee A, Westfelt E. "Critical probing depths" in periodontal therapy. *J Clin Periodontol.* 1982; 9(4):323–336.

Mengel R, Buns C, Stelzel M, Flores-de-Jacoby L. An in vitro study of oscillating instruments for root planing. *J Clin Periodontol.* 1994; 21(8):513–518.

Mengel R, Stelzel M, Mengel C, Flores-de-Jacoby L, Diekwisch T. An in vitro study of various instruments for root planing. *Int J Periodontics Restorative Dent.* 1997; 17(6):592–599.

Michaud RM, Schoolfield J, Mellonig JT, Mealey BL. The efficacy of subgingival calculus removal with endoscopy-aided scaling and root planing: a study on multirooted teeth. *J Periodontol.* 2007; 78(12):2238–2245.

Roussa-Tsoulou E, Schug W, Stüben J. Grenzen der Wurzelglättung im Furkationsbereich. Ein mathematischer Vergleich der Krümmungsradien an den Wurzeloberflächen und den Küretten [The limits of root planing in the furcation area. A mathematical comparison of the radii of curvature on the root surfaces and on the curettes]. *Dtsch Zahn Mund Kieferheilkd Zentralbl.* 1992; 80(5):295–298.

Schwarz F, Sculean A, Berakdar M et al. in vivo and in vitro effects of an Er: YAG laser, a GaAlAs diode laser, and scaling and root planing on periodontally diseased root surfaces: a comparative histologic study. *Lasers Surg Med.* 2003; 32(5):359–366.

Slot DE, Koster TJ, Paraskevas S, Van der Weijden GA. The effect of the Vector scaler system on human teeth: a systematic review. *Int J Dent Hyg.* 2008; 6(3):154–165.

Stoltenberg JL, Osborn JB, Carlson JF, Hodges JS, Michalowicz BS. A preliminary study of intra-pocket topical versus injected anaesthetic for scaling and root planing. *J Clin Periodontol.* 2007; 34(10):892–896.

von Troil B, Needleman I, Sanz M. A systematic review of the prevalence of root sensitivity following periodontal therapy. *J Clin Periodontol.* 2002; 29(Suppl 3):173–177; discussion 195–196.

Zappa U, Smith B, Simona C, Graf H, Case D, Kim W. Root substance removal by scaling and root planing. *J Periodontol.* 1991; 62(12):750–754.

16.2 ANTIMICROBIALS IN PERIODONTICS

Subraya Bhat

Contents

Learning objectives

- Rationale for the usage of antibiotics.
- Definitions of various antimicrobial agents.
- Dosages, mechanisms of action, and prescription of systemic antibiotics.
- Principles of therapeutic usage of systemic antibiotics.
- Rationale for the usage of locally delivered drugs.
- Different types of locally delivered drugs.
- Dosages and mechanisms of action of locally delivered drugs.
- Principles of therapeutic usage of locally delivered drugs.

Introduction

The etiopathogenesis of periodontal disease has undergone a paradigm shift. Presently, periodontitis is considered as a proinflammatory bacterial dysbiosis, through the overgrowth of specific, mostly Gram-negative bacteria in dental biofilms (Hajishengallis 2015). Given the major role of the dental biofilm in periodontitis, elimination of the biofilm forms a major part of periodontal therapy. The mechanical removal of the dental biofilm by means of scaling and root planing (SRP) is considered the standard of non-surgical periodontal therapy (Tonetti et al. 2015). However, considering the bacterial etiology, the adjuvant administration of systemic or locally delivered antibiotics to increase the effectiveness of mechanical therapy seems to be clinically relevant (Pretzl et al. 2019).

Therapeutic rationale for antibiotic usage

It has been observed that all cases of periodontitis do not respond favorably to SRP alone. Severe periodontitis and periodontitis that has a rapid progression, or patients with associated risk factors, are considered to have a poor response to SRP (Mombelli et al. 2000). A possible reason for this poor response is a dysbiotic microbiome that does not alter with SRP, and that penetrates deeply into the connective tissues. In such cases, the use of antibiotics is suggested to be helpful in reversing the dental biofilm microbiome from being pathogenic to not pathogenic, or being helpful to the host (Sampaio et al. 2011).

Definitions (Whalen 2018)

- *Anti-infective agent*: a chemotherapeutic agent that acts by reducing the number of bacteria present.
- *Antiseptic*: a chemical antimicrobial agent that stops or slows down the growth of microorganisms. In dentistry it can be used as a topically applied or subgingivally delivered agent, and can be applied to mucous membranes, wounds, or intact dermal surfaces to destroy microorganisms and to inhibit their reproduction or metabolism. Mouth rinses or dentifrices are common examples of this group of medicaments.
- *Disinfectant*: an antimicrobial agent that is generally applied to inanimate surfaces to destroy microorganisms.
- *Antibiotic*: a naturally occurring, semi-synthetic, or synthetic type of anti-infective agent that destroys or inhibits the growth of select microorganisms, generally at low concentrations. They are broadly categorized based on their bacterial action as being either bacteriostatic or bactericidal.
  - *Bacteriostatic antibiotic*: a pharmacological agent that prevents the growth and multiplication of bacteria (e.g. tetracycline and clindamycin).
  - *Bactericidal antibiotic*: an agent that actually kills bacteria (e.g. penicillin and metronidazole)

Systemic antibiotics

The microbial etiology of periodontal disease has opened an avenue for many researchers and clinicians to use systemic antibiotic therapy for the treatment of periodontal disease. The introduction of Koch's postulate and subsequently Socransky's postulates has allowed many clinicians of that era to choose antibiotics as another mode of therapy, just as was done for any other systemic disease of microbial etiology (Ciancio 2000).

- *Tetracycline, minocycline and doxycycline*: Once commonly used for the treatment of periodontal disease, these are presently not used due to bacterial resistance. These broad-spectrum antibiotics have been used for many of their advantages over other antibiotics. They are secreted in gingival crevicular fluid (GCF) in concentrations of up to 2–10 times more than their plasma concentrations. This allows a high drug concentration to be attained in the periodontal pocket. Tetracyclines are also found to be effective in concentrations as low as 2–4 µg/mL in GCF against many periodontal pathogens. In addition to their antibiotic action, they are also used for their host modulatory effect, which includes anti-collagenase and anti-inflammatory properties. Tetracycline was a commonly prescribed antibiotic for the treatment of localized aggressive periodontitis (presently, this classification is no longer used; see Table 16.2.1). In addition to the disadvantage of antibiotic resistance, taking the medication four times a day is a compliance issue with patients. This compliance issue has been overcome by prescribing minocycline (100 mg twice a day) and doxycycline (a loading dose of 100 mg twice a day, followed by 100 mg once a day for 7–10 days) (Caton et al. 2000; Gordon et al. 1981; Sinha et al. 2014).
- *Metronidazole*: This bactericidal antibiotic has been commonly prescribed for anaerobic infections and used in the treatment of acute necrotizing ulcerative gingivitis (ANUG). However, this antibiotic is considered to be ineffective against *Aggregatibacter actinomycetemcomitans* (A.a) when used alone. Its combination with amoxicillin or amoxicillin–clavulanate potassium (Augmentin), or ciprofloxacin, is considered to be the current management protocol for aggressive periodontitis or chronic periodontitis. However, caution is to be taken when prescribing these medications for patients who are on warfarin therapy (due to inhibition of warfarin metabolism and prolonging of its action) and who are consuming alcohol (Antabuse reaction) (Pretzl et al. 2019).
- Amoxicillin/amoxicillin–potassium clavulanate (Augmentin): This semi-synthetic penicillin along with penicillin itself has been commonly used for the treatment of ANUG. However, it was replaced partially by metronidazole. Amoxicillin/Augmentin is considered to be ineffective for the treatment of chronic or aggressive periodontitis when prescribed alone. However, as mentioned above, it is effective when used in combination with metronidazole (Pretzl et al. 2019).
- *Ciprofloxacin*: This is a quinolone, and is the only antibiotic considered to be effective against all strains of A.a. As with amoxycillin, ciprofloxacin is found to be effective when

used In combination with metronidazole for the treatment of localized aggressive periodontitis (Rams et al. 1992).

- *Azithromycin*: This antibiotic is considered for the treatment of periodontitis, due to its presence in tissue specimens from periodontal lesions being significantly higher than that in normal gingiva. It has also been shown to penetrate into fibroblasts and phagocytes in concentrations that are up to 100–200 times greater than the concentrations thereof In the extracellular compartment. This is due to azithromycin being directly transported to sites of inflammation by phagocytes, and then being directly released at these sites. There are only a few studies presently available

using azithromycin, with conflicting results. Furthermore, increased caution is advised in patients with cardiovascular events (O'Rourke 2017).

Table 16.2.1 depicts various systemic antibiotics, including their dosage, mechanisms of action, and their usage in periodontal therapy.

Therapeutic Usage of Systemic Antibiotics

Periodontal diseases are initiated by microorganisms, however, antibiotics are not required to treat all types of periodontal diseases. The first mode of periodontal therapy is mechanical plaque

Table 16.2.1 Usage of antibiotics in periodontal therapy.

Category	Agent	Mechanism of action	Dosage	Specific features	Use in periodontics
Penicillin	Amoxycillin	Bactericidal – targeting cell wall synthesis	500 mg three times a day for 5–7 days	Extended spectrum of antimicrobial activity; excellent oral absorption	Rarely used alone and used along with metronidazole
	Augmentin	Same as above	375 mg or 625 mg twice a day for 5–7 days	Effective against penicillinase-producing microorganisms	Same as above
Tetracyclines	Minocycline	Bacteriostatic – Inhibitors of protein biosynthesis; act upon the conserved sequences of the 16S r-RNA of the 30S ribosomal subunit to prevent binding of t-RNA to the A site	100 mg once a day for 7 days	Effective against broad spectrum of microorganisms; used systemically and applied locally (subgingivally)	Used alone, systemically, or locally delivered
	Doxycycline		200 mg loading dose first day, with 100 mg daily for 7–10 days		
	Tetracycline		250 mg four times daily for 7–10 days (21 days was used earlier)		
Nitroimidazole	Metronidazole, tinidazole, or newer group of drugs	Bactericidal – inhibitors of DNA replication	250 mg or 400 mg twice a day	Effective against anaerobic bacteria	Used alone or in combination with amoxycillin or Augmentin, used locally or systemically
Macrolide	Azithromycin	Primarily bacteriostatic, also bactericidal activity; affects early stage of protein synthesis, namely translocation	500 mg once a day for 3 days or 500 mg on first day followed by 250 mg twice a day for 4 days	Concentrates at sites of inflammation, may absorb inside the bone	Used alone, systemically
Quinolones	Ciprofloxacin	Bactericidal – inhibits DNA replication by inhibiting bacterial DNA topoisomerase and DNA-gyrase	500 mg twice a day for 8 days	Effective against Gram-negative rods; promotes health-associated microflora	Used alone or in combination with metronidazole

control, where the major plaque burden is removed. Thus, in cases of dental biofilm-induced gingivitis and stage I grade A periodontitis, or where progression of disease is slower, mechanical plaque control is sufficient. In cases of ANUG, necrotizing ulcerative periodontitis (NUP), and necrotizing ulcerative stomatitis (NUS), and in periodontitis where progression is severe or there is continuous loss of attachment occurring with efficient mechanical plaque control, then the use of adjunctive antibiotics may be warranted. A periodontal abscess, acute or chronic, requires drainage and may require treatment of the associated osseous defect. If there are associated systemic diseases, like uncontrolled diabetes, then along with controlling the diabetes the adjunct use of antibiotics may be required.

It is clear from several systematic reviews and meta-analyses that the usage of antibiotics as a sole mode of therapy is not advisable. Furthermore, whenever there is a need for an antibiotic, its selection must be based on the consideration of factors including rate of progression of periodontitis, clinical presentation (activity of the disease, including signs and symptoms), and radiographic features. Along with this, in cases and in sites where disease progression is occurring despite good maintenance, then microbiological sampling can be done and resistance to antibiotics can be investigated, which may assist in the choice of antibiotics. The clinician is also required to gather information regarding the medical history of the patient, including the usage of medications, so as to avoid possible drug interactions and adverse side effects (Haffajee et al. 2003; Pretzl et al. 2019).

Local drug delivery

Therapeutic rationale

Regarding the pathogenesis of periodontal disease, which includes a change in the understanding of the progression of the disease, i.e. from a linear progression model to a continuous progression or rapid burst model, the concept has developed that not all periodontal disease sites progress at the same rate. This may vary from tooth to tooth, and from site to site in the same tooth (Nomura et al. 2017; Teles et al. 2018). Microbial composition analyses of different teeth and different sites in the same mouth have shown variations in pathognomic bacterial composition (Mira et al. 2017). Thus, the approach to individual diseased sites has become site specific. Site specificity of the disease process in the true sense, therefore, does not justify the use of systemic antibiotics, as there may also be the possibility of seepage of antibiotics into healthy sites. This change in the model of progression of periodontal disease has prompted the use of locally delivered antibiotics/antiseptics, thereby avoiding unnecessary exposure to these pharmacological agents in healthy sites. In addition to this, a major drawback of systemic antibiotics is unwanted systemic side effects. To overcome this, when antibiotics are delivered to specific sites, then not only is there the complete elimination of unwanted systemic side effects, but also there is a localized rendering of higher concentrations of the antibiotic, achieved with a minimal amount of antibiotic. This is the major rationale for the use of local drug delivery (LDD) antibiotics/antiseptics (Tan et al. 2019).

Classification of local drug delivery

Many classifications have been proposed for LDD. The most common in practice is based upon the release of the active agent within a specific time period (Tan et al. 2019) (see Figure 16.2.1).

In the non-sustained mode of drug delivery (mouthwash and irrigation), there is immediate release of the active agent.

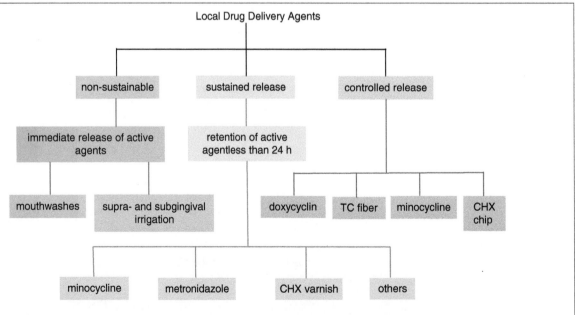

Figure 16.2.1 Local drug delivery agents. CHX, chlorohexidine; TC, tetracycline. Source: Adapted from Tan et al. 2019.

However, there is no sustainability of these agents and they do not show a direct effect on subgingival microorganisms, due to their poor penetration into subgingival areas (Nagarakanti et al. 2015). There are multiple devices available for supra- and subgingival irrigation, mostly designed for daily home use (Jahn 2010). At the other end, sustained-released devices provide a high concentration of the agent into periodontal pockets for a short duration (less than 24 h). Although there may be a fast release of these agents to exert their effects, this may not be acceptable in all cases. In contrast to this, controlled delivery systems deliver the active agent over an extended period of time (more than 24 h) depending upon the formulations used, and in some reports they also retain the minimum inhibitory concentration (MIC) for up to 2 weeks (Liang et al. 2020).

Pharmacotherapeutic agents used in local drug delivery (commercially used preparations)

As used in systemic antibiotic therapy, many antibiotics/antiseptics are being used for LDD. Some of the older formulations are no longer in use because of difficulty in administering them.

- *Tetracycline*: Goodson and colleagues were the first to introduce a controlled-release LDD system, consisting of hollow fibers made of cellulose acetate containing tetracycline. This was followed in 1994 by another product with a fiber system, Actisite® tetracycline fiber (ALZA Corporation, Palo Alto, CA, USA), which became popular since it was a commercially available controlled-release product (Tonetti et al. 1990). However, with the development of newer biodegradable agents, this product, which required a second appointment, was withdrawn from the market in 2003. Periodontal Plus AB is a newer bioresorbable product based on a collagen film system. It is available in vials containing 25 mg fibrillar collagen impregnated with 2 mg tetracycline hydrochloride (Sinha et al. 2014). As was seen with other LDD preparations, a 12-month study utilizing this product showed no clinical benefits over SRP (Reddy et al. 2016).
- *Doxycycline and minocycline*: These are second-generation semi-synthetic derivatives of tetracycline. Doxycycline Atridox is the first Food and Drug Administration (FDA)-approved resorbable doxycycline gel system, available as a two-syringe system of powder and liquid that are mixed together, which forms a thixotropic gel and solidifies upon contact with tissue fluid. Doxycycline levels can remain above 1000 µg/mL for 18 h in the GCF (Stoller et al. 1998). It has also been observed to remain above the MIC for periodontal pathogens (6.0 µg/mL) at local sites for up to 7 days, and 10–20 mg/mL of the drug may still be detected 3–5 days after removal of the polymer. However, in a 12-month study, no clinical benefits were shown when compared to SRP alone (Nguyen et al. 2014).
- *Minocycline*: The use of minocycline has become more popular than tetracycline. Arestin is the first formulation that has been made available in the form of microspheres, and

was approved by the FDA in 2001. The preparation consists of two syringes, one containing 4 mg of 20–60 µm diameter bioresorbable microspheres, equivalent to 1 mg minocycline base, in a polymer (glycolide-lactide) carrier (Vanderkerckhove et al. 1998); the other syringe containing a powder that, when exposed to oral fluids, becomes hydrolyzed, and together with the polymer there is then adherence to the periodontal pocket. This aids in the sustained release of minocycline of about 340 µg per mL through 14 days, exceeding the MIC for periodontopathogens (Williams et al. 2001). However, this drug demands more than one application in a year and, as with the other formulations, a study has failed to show any clinical benefit over a 6-month period when compared to SRP (Killeen et al. 2018). Other commercial preparations in ointment form are used in the UK and Japan, namely Dentomycin and Periocline. Both are in a biodegradable form with minocycline 0.5 mg ointment consisting of 2% minocycline hydrochloride (10 mg minocycline) in a matrix of hydroxyethyl cellulose, aminoalkyl methacrylate, triacetine, and glycerine. A controlled 18-month clinical trial that included repeated administration of the drug did not however show any clinical benefit when compared to SRP alone (Timmerman et al. 1996).

- *Metronidazole*: The popular systemic administration of this drug for the treatment of NUG and other periodontal conditions has led to its usage for LDD. Elyzol is a gel that consists of 40% metronidazole benzoate in an oil-based (glyceryl mono-oleate and sesame oil) mixture that, when injected into the subgingival area, is slowly disintegrated by GCF enzymes into 25% metronidazole (Norling et al. 1992). When applied with a syringe applicator, it initially liquefies at body temperature and then changes into a highly viscous semi-solid state upon contact with GCF. According to Stoltze (1992), this LDD attains a concentration of above 1 µg/mL for up to 36 h in the pocket, with concentrations above the MIC for susceptible periodontopathogens occurring 24 h after administration, without any systemic side effects. However, a study has reported no clinical benefit over SRP alone at 6-month intervals (Hanes & Purvis 2003).
- *Chlorohexidine* (CHX): A gold standard chemical plaque control agent, CHX is used in various formulations, such as irrigation solutions, periodontal dressings, gels, in chip form, and as a varnish. Usage of CHX during subgingival irrigation as an adjunct to SRP has shown no additional benefit (Bonito et al. 2005; Hanes & Purvis 2003). This may be attributed to rapid clearance of the drug despite its properties of substantivity. CHX in chip form, Periochip is an FDA-approved biodegradable controlled-release chip containing 2.5 mg chlorhexidine gluconate in a gelatin matrix. It is easy to insert, and the small chip measures 4.0 mm × 5.0 mm × 0.35 µm. The chip releases chlorhexidine in a bi-phasic manner, with an initial peak of 2007 µg/mL within 2 h in the GCF post insertion, followed by a

maintenance of high concentrations (above 1000 µg/mL) for the following 96 h, with complete biodegradation occurring between 7 and 10 days after insertion (Soskolne et al. 1998). Periocol-CG incorporates 2.5 mg chlorhexidine into a collagen membrane chip derived from freshwater fish. Conflicting results have been reported, with some studies favoring usage of the product together with SRP over a period of 9–12 months, while other studies have reported no clinical benefit when compared to SRP alone (Carvalho et al. 2007; Reddy et al. 2016). Chlo-Site is a xanthan-based chlorhexidine gel containing a combination of 0.5% chlorhexidine digluconate and 1.0% chlorhexidine dihydrochloride. This product has been made available in a saccharide polymer, which increases liquid viscosity, gets adhered to the pocket mucosa, and is released over a period of time (Jain et al. 2013). A systematic review study has however reported contrasting results regarding improvement in bleeding scores and reduction in pocket depths (Tan et al. 2019). Another study has reported limited improvement in clinical outcomes after a 6-month follow-up period (Matesanz et al. 2013). CHX in a varnish form

has mostly been used in caries prevention and has not been studied extensively for the treatment of periodontal disease. Only a few studies are available showing positive results. These include a reduction in the anaerobic bacterial count within the periodontal pocket for up to 3 months with multiple applications (Manikandan et al. 2016).

Table 16.2.2 depicts pharmacotherapeutic agents used in various LDD formulations. The application and duration of usage are according to the manufacturers and related studies.

Figure 16.2.2 depicts the local delivery of drugs by means of fibers, gel, and chip.

Clinical relevance/indications of local drug delivery

Presently, meta-analysis and systematic review studies do not favor the long-term benefits of LDD when used alone. LDD systems offer no advantages as a monotherapy; however, clinical reduction in pocket depths and gain in clinical attachment have been shown when LDD is used in combination with SRP (Smiley et al. 2015). Even though 6-month follow-up studies

Table 16.2.2 Commercially available local drug delivery agents.

Active agent	Commercial preparation	Manufacturer	Dosage	Type of formulation	Application and duration of use
Chlorohexidine (CHX)	Chlo-Site®	Ghimas Company, Casalecchio di Reno, Italy	1.5% CHX	Gel	1 application 15 days' treatment
	Periochip®	Perio Products Ltd, Jerusalem, Israel	2.5 mg CHX gluconate	Chip	1 application 7 days' treatment
	PerioCol®-CG	Eucare Pharmaceuticals Ltd, Chennai, India	2.5 mg CHX gluconate	Chip	1 application 7 days' treatment
	EC40®	Biodent BV, Nijmegen, Netherlands	35% CHX diacetate	Varnish	1 application 7 days' treatment
Doxycycline (DOXY)	Atridox®	Atrix Laboratories, Fort Collins, CO, USA	10% DOXY hyclate	Gel	1 application 7 days' treatment
Metronidazole (MET)	Elyzol®	Dumex, Copenhagen, Denmark	25% MET benzoate	Gel	2 applications 7 days' treatment
Minocycline (MINO)	Arestin®	OraPharma, Inc., Warminster, PA, USA	1 mg MINO hydrochloride	Microspheres	1 application 14 days' treatment
	Dentomycin®	Lederle Dental Division, Gosport, Hampshire, UK	2% MINO hydrochloride	Ointment	3–4 applications 14 days' treatment
	Periocline®	Sunstar Corp., Tokyo, Japan			
Tetracycline (TET)	Periodontal Plus AB™	Advanced Biotech Products, Chennai, India	2 mg TET hydrochloride	Fibers (thread)	1 application 7 days' treatment

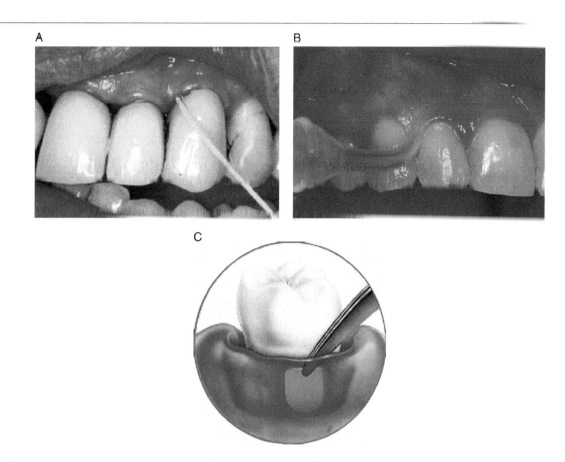

Figure 16.2.2 Local delivery of drugs by means of (A) fibers, (B) gel, and (C) chip.

have shown statistically significant results, their clinical significance needs to be further studied. Despite the above findings, LDD has been suggested for usage in local non-responding or recurrent sites during supportive periodontal therapy, where there is the presence of residual pockets in the esthetic zone where surgery may compromise esthetics or phonetics, and in persistent bleeding pockets at intrabony sites during presurgical preparation. It has also been suggested that LDD is to be used in high-risk groups, such as smokers, diabetics, or in patients showing poor compliance, including those with relative or absolute contraindications to surgical intervention (Chambrone et al. 2016).

Future considerations

The microbial etiology of periodontal disease has prompted the use of systemic and local delivery of antibiotics/antiseptics. Various antibiotics/antiseptics have been investigated, with mixed results. Usage of these agents in combination with other host-modifying agents, antioxidants and probiotics, may be helpful in arresting periodontal disease with better clinical outcomes. Managing periodontal disease in patients with multiple risk factors is a greater challenge, due to these factors influencing the pathogenesis of the disease. Initiating antibiotic/antiseptic therapy in combination with other existing or new therapies needs to be evaluated in future research.

REFERENCES

Bonito A, Lux L, Lohr, K. Impact of local adjuncts to scaling and root planing in periodontal disease therapy: a systematic review. *J Periodontol.* 2005; 76:1227–1236.

Carvalho J, Novak MJ, Mota LF. Evaluation of the effect of subgingival placement of chlorhexidine chips as an adjunct to scaling and root planing. *J Periodontol.* 2007; 78:997–910.

Caton JG, Ciancio SG, Blieden TM et al. Treatment with subantimicrobial dose doxycycline improves the efficacy of scaling and root planing in patients with adult periodontitis. *J Periodontol.* 2000; 71:521–532.

Chambrone L, Vargas M, Arboleda S et al. Efficacy of local and systemic antimicrobials in the non-surgical treatment of smokers with chronic periodontitis: a systematic review. *J Periodontol.* 2016; 87:1320–1332.

Ciancio SG. Antiseptics and antibiotics as chemotherapeutic agents for periodontitis management. *Compend Contin Educ Dent.* 2000; 21:59–62.

Gordon JM, Walker CB, Murphy CJ et al. Tetracycline: levels achievable in gingival crevice fluid and in vitro effect on subgingival organisms. Part I. Concentrations in crevicular fluid after repeated doses. *J Periodontol.* 1981; 52:609–612.

Haffajee AD, Socransky SS, Gunsolley JC. Systemic anti-infective periodontal therapy: a systematic review. *Ann Periodontol.* 2003; 8:115–181.

Hajishengallis G. Periodontitis: from microbial immune subversion to systemic inflammation. *Nat Rev Immunol.* 2015; 15:30–44.

Hanes PJ, Purvis JP. Local anti-infective therapy: pharmacological agents. *A systematic review. Ann Periodontol.* 2003; 8:79–98.

Jahn CA. The dental water jet: a historical review of the literature. *J Dent Hyg.* 2010; 84(3):114–120.

Jain M, Dave D, Jain P et al. Efficacy of xanthan-based chlorhexidine gel as an adjunct to scaling and root planing in treatment of the chronic periodontitis. *J Indian Soc Periodontol.* 2013; 17:439–443.

Killeen AC, Harn JA, Jensen J et al. Two-year randomized clinical trial of adjunctive minocycline microspheres in periodontal maintenance. *J Dent Hyg.* 2018; 92:51–58.

Liang J, Peng X, Zhou X, Zou J, Cheng L. Emerging applications of drug delivery systems in oral infectious diseases prevention and treatment. *Molecules.* 2020; 25(3):516.

Manikandan D, Balaji VR, Niazi TM et al. Chlorhexidine varnish implemented treatment strategy for chronic periodontitis: a clinical and microbial study. *J Pharm Bio Allied Sci.* 2016; 8:S133–S137.

Matesanz P, Herrera D, Echeverría A et al. Randomized clinical trial on the clinical and microbiological efficacy of a xanthan gel with chlorhexidine for subgingival use. *Clin Oral Investig.* 2013; 17:55–66.

Mira A, Simon-Soro A, Curtis MA. Role of microbial communities in the pathogenesis of periodontal diseases and caries. *J Clin Periodontol.* 2017; 44(Suppl 18):S23–S38.

Mombelli A, Schmid B, Rutar A, Lang NP. Persistence patterns of *Porphyromonas gingivalis*, *Prevotella intermedia/nigrescens*, and *Actinobacillus actinomycetemcomitans* after mechanical therapy of periodontal disease. *J Periodontol.* 2000; 71:14–21.

Nagarakanti S, Gunupati S, Chava VK, Reddy BV. Effectiveness of subgingival irrigation as an adjunct to scaling and root planing in the treatment of chronic periodontitis: a systematic review. *J Clin Diagn Res.* 2015; 9(7):6–9.

Nguyen F, Starosta AL, Arenz S et al. Tetracycline antibiotics and resistance mechanisms. *Biol Chem.* 2014; 395:559–575.

Nomura Y, Morozumi T, Nakagawa T et al. Site-level progression of periodontal disease during a follow-up period. *PLoS One.* 2017; 12(12):e0188670.

Norling T, Lading P, Engström S et al. Formulation of a drug delivery system based on a mixture of monoglycerides and triglycerides for use in the treatment of periodontal disease. *J Clin Periodontol.* 1992; 19:687–692.

O'Rourke VJ. Azithromycin as an adjunct to non-surgical periodontal therapy: a systematic review. *Aust Dent J.* 2017; 62(1):14–22.

Pretzl B, Sälzer S, Ehmke B et al. Administration of systemic antibiotics during non-surgical therapy—a consensus report. *Clin Oral Investig.* 2019; 23(7):3073–3085.

Rams TE, Feik D, Slots J. Ciprofloxacin/metronidazole treatment of recurrent adult periodontitis. *J Dent Res.* 1992; 71:319.

Reddy S, Bhowmick N, Singh S et al. A comparison of chlorhexidine and tetracycline local drug delivery systems in management of persistent periodontal pockets—a clinical study. *Int J Appl Dent Sci.* 2016, 2:11–15.

Sampaio E, Rocha M, Figueiredo LC et al. Clinical and microbiological effects of azithromycin in the treatment of generalized chronic periodontitis: a randomized placebo-controlled clinical trial. *J Clin Periodontol.* 2011; 38:838–846.

Sinha S, Kumar S, Dagli N, Dagli RJ. Effect of tetracycline HCl in the treatment of chronic periodontitis—a clinical study. *J Int Soc Prev Community Dent.* 2014; 4:149–153.

Smiley CJ, Tracy SL, Abt E et al. Evidence-based clinical practice guideline on the nonsurgical treatment of chronic periodontitis by means of scaling and root planing with or without adjuncts. *J Am Dent Assoc.* 2015; 146:525–535.

Soskolne WA, Chajek T, Flashner M et al. An in vivo study of the chlorhexidine release profile of the PerioChip in the gingival crevicular fluid, plasma and urine. *J Clin Periodontol.* 1998; 25:1017–1102.

Stoller NH, Johnson LR, Trapnell S, Harrold CQ, Garrett S. The pharmacokinetic profile of a biodegradable controlled-release delivery system containing doxycycline compared to systemically delivered doxycycline in gingival crevicular fluid, saliva, and serum. *J Periodontol.* 1998; 69:1085–1091.

Stoltze K. Concentration of metronidazole in periodontal pockets after application of a metronidazole 25% dental gel. *J Clin Periodontol.* 1992; 19(9):698–701.

Tan OL, Safii SH, Razali M. Commercial local pharmacotherapeutics and adjunctive agents for nonsurgical treatment of periodontitis: a contemporary review of clinical efficacies and challenges. *Antibiotics (Basel).* 2019; 9(1):11.

Teles R, Moss K, Preisser JS et al. Patterns of periodontal disease progression based on linear mixed models of clinical attachment loss. *J Clin Periodontol.* 2018; 45(1):15–25.

Timmerman MF, Van der Weijden GA, Van Steenbergen TJM et al. Evaluation of the long-term efficacy and safety of locally applied minocycline in adult periodontitis patients. *J Clin Periodontol.* 1996; 23:707–716.

Tonetti M, Cugini MA, Goodson JM. Zero-order delivery with periodontal placement of tetracycline loaded ethylene vinyl acetate fibers. *J Periodontal Res.* 1990; 25:243–249.

Tonetti MS, Eickholz P, Loos BG et al. Principles in prevention of periodontal diseases: consensus report of group 1 of the 11th European Workshop on Periodontology on effective prevention of periodontal and peri-implant diseases. *J Clin Periodontol.* 2015; 42(Suppl 16):S5–S11.

Vanderkerckhove BNA, Quirynen M, Van Steenberghe D. The use of locally delivered minocycline in the treatment of chronic periodontitis. A review of the literature. *J Clin Periodontol.* 1998; (11 Pt 2):964–968.

Whalen K. (ed.), *Lippincott Illustrated Reviews: Pharmacology.* Delhi: Wolters Kluwer; 2018.

Williams RC, Paquette DW, Offenbacher S et al. Treatment of periodontitis by local administration of minocycline microspheres: a controlled trial. *J Periodontol.* 2001; 72:1535–1544.

16.3 HOST MODULATION THERAPY

Subraya Bhat and Khalid Almas

Contents

Learning objectives

- Understand the mechanisms of host modulation.
- Understand the role of therapeutic agents.
- Understand the role of agents that promote healing.
- Be aware of current trends.

Introduction

Periodontal disease is a microbially initiated, immuno-inflammatory disease (Bartold & Van Dyke 2013, 2017). A paradigm shift has emerged in the understanding of the pathogenesis of periodontal disease, i.e. from a predominantly microbial-based destruction to an inflammatory-based destruction. This has opened up a gateway for the utilization of pharmacological agents to modify the host response in periodontal therapy (Cekici et al. 2014; Sanz et al. 2017; Van Dyke 2017; Van Dyke & Sima 2020).

Definition

Host modulation therapy (HMT) is a pharmacological strategy targeted to reduce tissue destruction, stabilize, or even regenerate the periodontium, by modifying or down-regulating destructive aspects of the host response (Preshaw 2018). This new mode of periodontal therapeutics was developed almost three decades ago by Golub et al. (1994, 1998).

Therapeutic rationale

The host response in periodontal pathogenesis is a double-edged sword. The fundamental role of the host is to recruit neutrophils, with the consequent arrival of other inflammatory cells, along with the production of antibodies to protect against the microbial attack. The release of anti-inflammatory cytokines, including interleukin IL)-4), IL-10, and transforming growth factor beta (TGF-β), consequently joins this cascade to prevent tissue destruction (Bartold & Van Dyke 2017). In addition, specialized proresolving lipid mediators are generated that are responsible for proactively signaling termination of inflammation (Ebersole et al. 2013) (see Chapter 5.4). However, in susceptible individuals the constant bacterial challenge perpetuates the host response, which disrupts the homeostatic mechanisms between host and microbes, resulting in uncontrolled and increased release of proinflammatory mediators and cytokines, e.g. IL-1, IL-6, tumor necrosis factor-alpha (TNF-α), proteases (e.g. matrix metalloproteinases, MMPs), and prostanoids (prostaglandin E2) (Van Dyke & Sima 2020). This cycle of uncontrolled and increasing inflammation, microbiome changes, and the eventual chronic inflammatory destruction of the periodontal tissues is directly related to a failure of endogenous resolution pathways (Balta et al. 2017; Ramadan et al. 2020; Van Dyke & Sima 2020). Thus, appropriate controlling of mediators of inflammation is considered to be a possible mode of HMT during the non-surgical phase of periodontal therapy.

Since the inception of HMT, several pharmacological agents have been tried in both animal and human studies (Preshaw 2018). Initial reports of the benefits of these agents were derived from patients who were taking these medications for chronic inflammatory and immunological diseases, e.g. rheumatoid arthritis. Results of these studies have shown reduction in the signs of inflammation and periodontal bone loss. The study results have paved the way for many more agents, with mixed clinical outcomes (Feldman et al. 1983; Waite et al. 1981).

Therapeutic agents

Agents used in HMT are broadly divided into two categories: agents preventing destruction (those that down-regulate the destructive aspects of the host response) and agents promoting resolution and healing (those that up-regulate the protective or regenerative responses) (Lane et al. 2005; Serhan 2008, 2014; Van Dyke 2017). Several of these agents are being investigated, with many of them being rejected because of their unwanted systemic side effects. Table 16.0.1 depicts various HMT agents.

Matrix metalloproteinase inhibitors

This therapy is based on the host modulation effect of inhibiting MMPs, which are zinc- and calcium-dependent endopeptidases secreted by polymorphonuclear leukocytes (PMNL), macrophages, fibroblasts, epithelial cells, osteoblasts, and osteoclasts. MMPs destroy extracellular components like collagen, gelatin, laminin, fibronectin, and proteoglycans (Tumuluri 2001). Collagen of various types is an important component of the connective tissue of the periodontium. The host combats the action of these MMPs on collagen by means of producing endogenous MMP inhibitors (MMPIs) like TIMP (tissue inhibitor of metalloproteinase) and alpha-2-macroglobulin (Golub & Lee 2020). MMPIs are used clinically in the USA (approved by the US Food and Drug Administration) and beyond (Canada, Europe), and is commercially available as Periostat, now generic, and Oracea (Golub et al. 1998; Gu et al. 2012). This is the only non-antimicrobial composition of tetracyclines, i.e. doxycycline (also known as sub-antimicrobial-dose doxycycline), that is utilized by periodontists and dermatologists. (Dosage is one tablet twice daily for 3 months.)

Non-antibiotic tetracyclines as host modulators show pleotropic action by displaying extracellular, cellular, and pro-anabolic effects (Golub & Lee 2020). The American Dental Association evidence-based guidelines have supported this adjunctive treatment as safe and effective as a mode of host modulation (Smiley et al. 2015). Several meta-analyses have also supported the efficacy of sub-antimicrobial-dose doxycycline as an adjunct to non-surgical periodontal therapy (Preshaw 2018; Smiley et al. 2015). Further proof of use in periodontal therapy was detailed in an extensive, multicenter, 6-month clinical trial of 180 patients, whereby scaling and root planing combined with systemically administered sub-antimicrobial-dose doxycycline and a topically applied antimicrobial (Atridox®) resulted in a significantly greater clinical improvement compared with scaling and root planing alone (Novak et al. 2008). Another 2-year randomized double-blind placebo-controlled study including 128 postmenopausal women has provided evidence of the safe use and efficacy of prolonged sub-antimicrobial-dose doxycycline therapy, showing decreased bone loss and improved periodontal parameters

Table 16.3.1 Host modulation therapeutic agents.

Agents	Product name	Action	Side effects
Matrix metalloproteinase inhibitors (**MMPIs**)	Periostat® Oracea®	Inhibit MMPs, through extracellular or cellular mechanisms, and also have pro-anabolic effects	Rare (with Periostat there are reports of severe headache, dizziness, blurred vision, nausea, diarrhea, upset stomach, skin rash or itching, vaginal itching or discharge)
Corticosteroids/ non-steroidal anti-inflammatory drugs (NSAIDs)	Indomethacin, naproxen, piroxicam, ibuprofen, flurbiprofen, ketoprofen, meclofenamic acid	Block the COX-1 and COX-2 pathway of the arachidonic acid (AA) cycle, and block the production of prostaglandins and other inflammatory mediators	Gastrointestinal, renal, hepatic, and hemorrhage impairment due to non-selective inhibition of COX-1 and COX-2
Bone-sparing agents	*Oral bisphosphonates:* alendronate, risedronate, etidronate, ibandronate, clodronate, tiludronate *Intravenous bisphosphonates:* pamidronate, zoledronate, clodronate	Inhibit osteoclast activity by inhibiting osteoclast recruitment and adhesion, increase osteoblast numbers by differentiation and decreased release of cytokines by macrophages/ neutrophils	Osteonecrosis of the jaw – bisphosphonate related (ONJ-BR) – medication-related osteonecrosis of the jaw (MRONJ)
Agents promoting resolution and healing	Omega-3 fatty acids containing eicosapentaenoic acid (EPA), resolvin E1 (RvE1)	Reduce neutrophil-mediated tissue damage, increase neutrophil apoptosis, increase lipoxin production (LX4)	No side effects yet established

(Payne & Golub 2011). Another group of drugs, namely chemically modified tetracycline-3 (CMT-3; 6-demethyl 6-deoxy 4-de-dimethylamino tetracycline), also known as COL-3, has been tested in clinical trials on patients with periodontal disease; however, these drugs have not yet been approved by any country (Golub et al. 1998; Novak et al. 2002).

Corticosteroids and non-steroidal anti-inflammatory drugs

The role of arachidonic acid (AA) metabolites (byproducts of the cyclooxygenase and lipoxygenase pathway – prostaglandins, prostacyclin, thromboxane, leukotrienes, and other hydroxy-eicosatetraenoic acids), alone and/or with the other inflammatory mediators like cytokines, is well documented (Tumuluri 2001). Reduction of these AA metabolites has been in focus for decades to prevent the progression of periodontal disease. Systemic non-steroidal anti-inflammatory drugs (NSAIDs), e.g. indomethacin, naproxen, piroxicam, ibuprofen, and flurbiprofen, have been extensively studied for controlling alveolar bone resorption and retarding the progression of periodontal disease (Howell et al. 1991; Nyman et al. 1979; Williams et al. 1987, 1988a). However, due to their adverse effects, including gastrointestinal, renal, hepatic, and hemorrhage impairment due to non-selective inhibition of COX-1 and COX-2 enzymes, the long-term (even for 3 to 6 months) use of these agents has been cautioned against (Serhan 2008;

Velo & Milanino 1990). Moreover, immediate recurrence of disease on cessation of therapy has led to questioning of their regular use for the treatment of periodontitis. To overcome the systemic side effects, topical NSAIDs such as piroxicam, ketoprofen, flurbiprofen, ibuprofen, or meclofenamic acid, administered in the form of ointment, gel or dentifrice, have been used in short-term studies (Kornman et al. 1990; Williams et al. 1988b). These NSAIDs are lipophilic in nature and their quick absorption helps in formulating these agents for topical use. Although reduction of gingival inflammation may be statistically significant, the clinical significance of these studies and the long-term benefits of these agents have not been published (Jeffcoat et al. 1995). Currently, the Food and Drug Administration (FDA) has not approved any NSAID formulation for HMT.

Bone-sparing agents (bisphosphonates)

Bisphosphonates are analogs of pyrophosphate and have a high affinity for calcium phosphate in bone tissue. They inhibit osteoclastic activity by inhibiting osteoclast recruitment and adhesion, increase osteoblast number by differentiation, and decrease the release of cytokines by macrophages/neutrophils. They also possess the property of inhibiting ion-dependent enzyme activity (MMPs) through chelation of cations (Tenenbaum et al. 2002). These agents are commonly used in the treatment of osteoporosis due to their ability to inhibit the loss of bone density and to preserve normal bone turnover. The ability to slow down bone resorption has been utilized in a few clinical studies for the treatment of periodontitis as an adjunct to scaling and root planing (SRP). These studies showed significant/modest improvements in bone levels when evaluated by clinical and radiographic methods (Lane et al. 2005; Rocha et al. 2001; Takaishi et al. 2001). However, their prolonged usage for treatment of periodontitis is cautioned due to their adverse effects, such as osteonecrosis of the jaws (ONJ). The incidence of ONJ has been observed more with intravenous use than with oral use. Currently the FDA has approved bisphosphonates only for the treatment of systemic bone loss (osteoporosis and similar conditions) (Palomo et al. 2007).

Statins

The use of statins (3-hydroxy-3-methylglutarylcoenzyme A, HMG CoA), either synthetic or fermentation-derived (simvastatin, pravastatin, atorvastatin, cerivastatin, fluvastatin, pitavastatin, and rosuvastatin), is recently being tried for their host modulatory effects. This group of drugs influences the production of receptor activator of nuclear factor kappa-B ligand (RANKL) and osteoprotegerin by human gingival fibroblasts to favor bone catabolism under non-inflammatory conditions. The beneficial effects of these drugs when used systemically or as a locally delivered drug for the treatment of chronic periodontitis includes a greater decrease in the gingival index (GI) and probing depths (PD) and more clinical attachment level gain, with significant intrabony defect fills at sites treated with SRP (Petit et al. 2019). However, their routine use in periodontal therapy is still not being recommended.

Other modes of host modulation

There are many host modulating agents that require further studies regarding their usage in routine periodontal therapy. RANK/RANKL/osteoprotegerin modulators, cytokine (immune) modulators, cathepsin k inhibitors, histone deacetylase inhibitors, nitric oxide synthase inhibitors, and the modulation of Toll like receptors (TLRs) are among those that are undergoing research. Many of these agents are in the clinical trial stage and a few of them are being used for systemic conditions, especially cytokine modulators (Mohindra & Nirola 2017).

Agents promoting resolution and healing (proresolving mediators)

In the last decade, a lot of interest has shifted from the active part of inflammation (destructive inflammatory pathway) to the resolution state of inflammation. Once considered as not an important phase of healing, it has now taken the center stage of HMT (Van Dyke 2017). The resolution phase is considered as an active process involving biochemical circuits that actively biosynthesize local mediators with the help of stromal cells, which includes the withdrawal of survival signals, the normalization of chemokine gradients, and the induction of resolution programs that allow infiltrating cells to undergo apoptosis or to exit the inflamed tissue through draining lymphatics (Hasturk et al. 2017). These recognized anti inflammatory and proresolving molecules are lipoxins (LX), resolvins of the E (RvE) and D series (RvD), aspirin-triggered lipoxins (ATL), glucocorticoid-induced annexin-1, melanocortin/nuclear receptor agonists, and hemoxygenase 1. Among these, resolvins have been used in experimental animal models. Resolvins are synthesized from omega 3 polyunsaturated fatty acid (PUFA), eicosa-pantaenoic acid (EPA), and docosahexaenoic acid (DHA). The potential of these agents is due to their inflammatory and immunomodulatory actions, which are in the range of nanogram dosages. The topical application of RvE1 in experimental models of periodontitis in rabbits has been shown to halt the progression of periodontitis, with radiographic evidence of a decreased percentage of bone loss. Present recommendations do not include resolvins for non-surgical periodontal therapy (Hasturk et al. 2007).

Clinical relevance

Many host modulatory agents have been listed and tried. However, to date only one host modulatory agent, namely MMPI (Periostat), has been approved for usage as an adjunct to SRP. SRP in conjunction with Periostat has been suggested due to reduced PDs and gains in clinical attachment loss. The long-term effects of these agents are yet to be evaluated, keeping in mind their unwanted side effects.

Future research

As we better understand the molecular basis of the pathogenesis of periodontal disease, there may be further unfolding of the possible use of newer host modulating agents in its treatment. Many of the newer host modulating agents (chemically modified curcumin, for instance) are under clinical trials for use in systemic disease. Utilizing them together with assessing the risk-to-benefit ratio for the treatment of periodontal disease also needs to be appropriately weighed.

REFERENCES

Balta MG, Loos BG, Nicu EA. Emerging concepts in the resolution of periodontal inflammation: a role for resolvin e1. *Front Immunol.* 2017; 14(8):1682.

Bartold PM, Van Dyke TE. Periodontitis: a host-mediated disruption of microbial homeostasis. Unlearning learned concepts. *Periodontol 2000.* 2013; 62(1):203–217.

Bartold PM, Van Dyke TE. Host modulation: controlling the inflammation to control the infection. *Periodontol 2000*. 2017; 75:317–329.

Cekici A, Kantarci A, Hasturk H, Van Dyke TE. Inflammatory and immune pathways in the pathogenesis of periodontal disease. *Periodontol 2000*. 2014; 64(1):57–80.

Ebersole JL, Dawson DR, Morford LA et al. Periodontal disease immunology: "double indemnity" in protecting the host. *Periodontol 2000*. 2013; 62(1):163–202.

Feldman RS, Szeto B, Chauncey HH, Goldhaber P. Nonsteroidal anti-inflammatory drugs in the reduction of human alveolar bone loss. *J Clin Periodontol*. 1983; 10:131–136.

Golub LM, Lee HM. Periodontal therapeutics: current host-modulation agents and future directions. *Periodontol 2000*. 2020; 82(1):186–204.

Golub LM, Lee HM, Ryan ME et al. Tetracyclines inhibit connective tissue breakdown by multiple non-antimicrobial mechanisms. *Adv Dent Res*. 1998; 12:12–26.

Golub LM, Wolff M, Roberts S et al. Treating periodontal diseases by blocking tissue-destructive enzymes. *J Am Dent Assoc*. 1994; 125:163–169.

Gu Y, Walker C, Ryan ME, Payne JB, Golub LM. Non-antibacterial tetracycline formulations: clinical applications in dentistry and medicine. *J Oral Microbiol*. 2012; 4:19227.

Hasturk H, Kantarci A, Goguet-Surmenian E et al. Resolvin E1 regulates inflammation at the cellular and tissue level and restores tissue homeostasis in vivo. *J Immunol*. 2007; 179(10):7021–7029.

Howell TH, Jeffcoat MK, Goldhaber P et al. Inhibition of alveolar bone loss in beagles with the NSAID naproxen. *J Periodontal Res*. 1991; 26:498–501.

Jeffcoat MK, Reddy MS, Haigh S et al. A comparison of topical ketorolac, systemic flurbiprofen, and placebo for the inhibition of bone loss in adult periodontitis. *J Periodontol*. 1995; 66:329–338.

Kornman KS, Blodgett RF, Brunsvold M, Holt SC. Effects of topical applications of meclofenamic acid and ibuprofen on bone loss, subgingival microbiota and gingival PMN response in the primate *Macaca fascicularis*. *J Periodontal Res*. 1990; 25:300–307.

Lane N, Armitage GC, Loomer P. Bisphosphonate therapy improves the outcome of conventional periodontal treatment: results of a 12-month, randomized, placebo-controlled study. *J Periodontol*. 2005; 76: 1113–1122.

Mohindra K and Nirola A. Host Modulation. Austin *J Dent*. 2017; 4(6):1086.

Novak MJ, Dawson DR, Magnusson I et al. Combining host-modulation and antimicrobial therapy in the management of moderate to severe periodontitis: a randomized multi-center trial. *J Periodontol*. 2008; 79(1):33–41.

Novak MJ, Johns LP, Muller RC et al. Adjunctive benefits of sub-antimicrobial dose doxycycline in the management of severe, generalized, chronic periodontitis. *J. Periodontol*. 2002; 73:762–769.

Nyman S, Schroeder HE, Lindhe J. Suppression of inflammation and bone resorption by indomethacin during experimental periodontitis in dogs. *J Periodontol*. 1979; 50:450–461.

Palomo L, Liu J, Bissada NF. Skeletal bone diseases impact the periodontium: a review of bisphosphonate therapy. *Expert Opin Pharmacother*. 2007; 8:309–315.

Payne JB, Golub LM. Using tetracyclines to treat osteoporotic/osteopenic bone loss: from the basic science laboratory to the clinic. *Pharmacol Res*. 2011; 63(2):121–129.

Petit C, Batool F, Bugueno IM et al. Contribution of statins towards periodontal treatment: a review. *Mediators Inflamm*. 2019; 2019: Article ID 6367402.

Preshaw PM. Host modulation therapy with anti-inflammatory agents. *Periodontol 2000*. 2018; 76:131–149.

Ramadan DE, Hariyani N, Indrawati R, Ridwan RD, Diyatri I. Cytokines and chemokines in periodontitis. *Eur J Dent*. 2020; 14(3):483–495.

Rocha M, Nava LE, Vazquez de la Torre C et al. Clinical and radiological improvement of periodontal disease in patients with type 2 diabetes mellitus treated with alendronate: a randomized, placebo-controlled trial. *J Periodontol*. 2001; 72:204–209.

Sanz M, Beighton D, Curtis MA et al. Role of microbial biofilms in the maintenance of oral health and in the development of dental caries and periodontal diseases. Consensus report of group 1 of the Joint EFP/ORCA workshop on the boundaries between caries and periodontal disease. *J Clin Periodontol*. 2017; 44:S5–S11.

Serhan CN. Controlling the resolution of acute inflammation: a new genus of dual anti-inflammatory and proresolving mediators. *J Periodontol*. 2008; 79:1520–1526.

Serhan CN. Novel pro-resolving lipid mediators are leads for resolution physiology. *Nature*. 2014; 510(7503):92–101.

Smiley CJ, Tracy SL, Abt E et al. Evidence-based clinical practice guideline on the nonsurgical treatment of chronic periodontitis by means of scaling and root planing with or without adjuncts. *J Am Dent Assoc*. 2015; 146(7):525–535.

Takaishi Y, Miki T, Nishizawa Y, Morii H. Clinical effect of etidronate on alveolar pyorrhoea associated with chronic marginal periodontitis: report of four cases. *J Int Med Res*. 2001; 29:355–365.

Tenenbaum HC, Shelemay A, Girard B, Zohar R, Fritz PC. Bisphosphonates and periodontics: potential applications for regulation of bone mass in the periodontium and other therapeutic/diagnostic uses. *J Periodontol*. 2002; 73:813–822.

Tumuluri V. Matrix metalloproteinase regulation in periodontal treatment. *J Periodontol*. 2001; 22:50–57.

Van Dyke TE. Pro-resolving mediators in the regulation of periodontal disease. *Mol Aspects Med*. 2017; 58:21–36.

Van Dyke TE, Sima C. Understanding resolution of inflammation in periodontal diseases: is chronic inflammatory periodontitis a failure to resolve? *Periodontol 2000*. 2020; 82:205–213.

Velo GP, Milanino R. Non-gastrointestinal adverse reactions to NSAID. *J Rheumatol Suppl*. 1990; 20:42–45.

Waite IM, Saxton CA, Young A, Wagg BJ, Corbett M. The periodontal status of subjects receiving non-steroidal anti-inflammatory drugs. *J Periodontal Res.* 1981; 16:100–108.

Williams RC, Jeffcoat MK, Howell I H et al. Indomethacin or flurbiprofen treatment of periodontitis in beagles: comparison of effect on bone loss. *J Periodontal Res.* 1987; 22: 403–407.

Williams RC, Jeffcoat MK, Howell TH et al. Ibuprofen: an inhibitor of alveolar bone resorption in beagles. *J Periodontal Res.* 1988a; 23:225–229.

Williams RC, Jeffcoat MK, Howell TH et al. Topical flurbiprofen treatment of periodontitis in beagles. *J Periodontal Res.* 1988b; 23:166–169.

CHAPTER 17
Periodontal plastic surgery

Steph Smith, Arif Salman and Khalid Almas

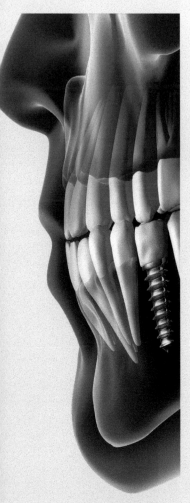

Contents

Essential Periodontics, First Edition. Edited by Steph Smith and Khalid Almas.
© 2022 John Wiley & Sons Ltd. Published 2022 by John Wiley & Sons Ltd.

Learning objectives

- Definition and success criteria for periodontal surgical procedures.
- Indications for different mucogingival surgical procedures.
- Healing of apically repositioned flaps, pedicle flaps, and soft tissue grafts.
- Predisposing factors and causes of gingival recession.
- Prognostic determinants for predicting success of surgical treatment of gingival recession.
- Clinical aspects and treatment modalities for mucosal defects at implants, aberrant frona, and ectopic tooth eruption.
- Surgical options for crown lengthening procedures.
- Prevention of ridge collapse after tooth extraction and soft tissue augmentation procedures for edentulous ridges.

Introduction

Periodontal plastic surgery is defined as surgical procedures performed to prevent or correct anatomic, developmental, traumatic, or disease-induced defects of the gingiva, alveolar mucosa, or bone (Proceedings of the 1996 World Workshop on Periodontics 1996).

The proper selection of a variety of surgical techniques used for solving mucogingival problems must be based on the predictability of success, which is based on specific criteria. These criteria include esthetic considerations of the patient; knowledge of the configuration (anatomy) of the recipient (defect) and donor sites; availability of donor tissue; a surgical site free of biofilm, calculus, and inflammation; an adequate blood supply to the donor tissue; the stability of the grafted tissue to the recipient site; and minimal trauma induced to the surgical site (Takei et al. 2019).

Various soft and hard tissue procedures included within the definition of periodontal plastic surgery are the following (Wennström & Zucchelli 2015):

- Gingival augmentation.
- Root coverage.
- Correction of mucosal defects at implants.
- Crown lengthening.
- Removal of aberrant frenulum.
- Gingival preservation at ectopic tooth eruption.
- Prevention of ridge collapse following tooth extraction.
- Augmentation of the edentulous ridge.

Gingival augmentation

For many years a prevailing concept has existed that the presence of an "adequate" or "sufficient" wide band of keratinized and attached mucosa around the tooth is critical for maintaining gingival health and preventing attachment loss and soft tissue recession. It has been suggested that <1 mm of gingiva may be sufficient (Bowers 1963; Miyasato et al. 1977), while other authors have suggested a minimal apicocoronal height of 2–3 mm of keratinized tissue (Corn 1962; Lang & Löe 1972). Attached gingiva is however considered as important to maintain gingival health in patients with suboptimal plaque control, and a lack of keratinized tissue is considered a predisposing factor for the development of gingival recessions and inflammation (Kim & Neiva 2015). The current consensus, which is based on case series and case reports, is that 2 mm of keratinized tissue and about 1 mm of attached gingiva are desirable around teeth to maintain periodontal health, even though a minimum amount of keratinized tissue is not needed to prevent attachment loss when optimal plaque control is present (Kim & Neiva 2015).

An "inadequate" zone of gingiva has been considered to (Carranza & Carraro 1970; Friedman 1957, 1962; Hall 1981; Matter 1982; Ochsenbein 1960; Ruben 1979):

- Be insufficient to protect the periodontium from injury caused by friction forces encountered during mastication.
- Facilitate subgingival plaque formation because of improper pocket closure resulting from the movability of marginal tissues.
- Favor attachment loss and soft tissue recession because of less tissue resistance to apical spread of plaque-associated gingival lesions.
- Impede proper oral hygiene measures.
- Dissipate the pull on the gingival margin created by the muscles of the adjacent alveolar mucosa.

Histological analysis of the size of the inflammatory cell infiltrate and its extension in an apical direction has been shown to be similar in areas of only a narrow and mobile zone of keratinized tissue, compared to areas with a wide and firmly attached gingiva (Wennström & Lindhe 1983a, b). Even although clinically visible signs of inflammation, such as redness and swelling, may be more frequent in areas with <2 mm of gingiva than in areas with a wider zone of gingiva, the clinical signs do not correspond with the size of the inflammatory cell infiltrate

(Wennström & Zucchelli 2015). Longitudinal studies have furthermore shown that a minimal zone of gingiva may not compromise periodontal health, and that the resistance to continuous attachment loss is not linked to the height (width) of the gingiva (Dorfman et al. 1982; Freedman et al. 1999; Kennedy et al. 1985; Wennström 1987). Gingival health can thus be maintained independent of its dimensions (Wennström & Zucchelli 2015). Both experimental and clinical studies have shown that, in the presence of plaque, areas with a narrow zone of gingiva possess a similar degree of resistance to continuous attachment loss to areas with a wide zone of gingiva (Lindhe & Nyman 1980; Schoo & van der Velden 1985). The conclusion is thus reached that the need for an "adequate" width (in millimeters) of gingiva, or an attached portion of gingiva, for prevention of attachment loss and for maintenance of gingival health is not scientifically supported (Wennström & Zucchelli 2015). Consequently, the presence of a narrow zone of gingiva per se cannot justify surgical intervention (Lang & Karing 1994; Proceedings of the 1996 World Workshop on Periodontics 1996).

However, there are situations in which gingival augmentation procedures may be considered (Wennström & Zucchelli 2015), such as:

- A patient experiencing discomfort during toothbrushing and/or chewing due to interference from a lining mucosa at teeth or implants.
- When orthodontic tooth movement is planned and the final positioning of the tooth can be expected to result in an alveolar bone dehiscence.
- When an increase of the thickness of the covering soft tissue may reduce the risk for development of soft tissue recession.
- An increase of the thickness of the gingiva may also be considered when subgingival restorations are placed in areas with a thin marginal tissue.

Soft tissue augmentation techniques to increase the width of keratinized tissue and attached gingiva are as follows (Thoma et al. 2009; Wennström & Zucchelli 2015):

- An apically repositioned flap/vestibuloplasty (Donnenfeld et al. 1964).
- The use of grafts:
  - Pedicle grafts (Wennström & Zucchelli 2015).
  - Free grafts (see Figures 17.1. and 17.2): autogenous tissue grafts (Edel 1974; Hawley & Staffileno 1970); allogenic graft materials (Harris 2001; McGuire & Nunn 2005; Wei et al. 2000).

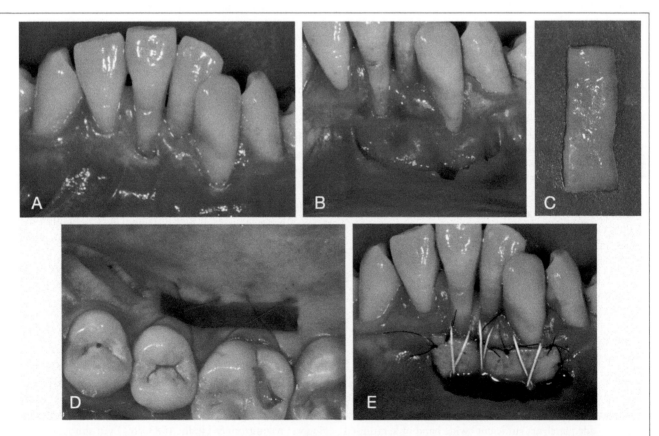

Figure 17.1 Free gingival graft. (A) Baseline picture showing minimal keratinized tissue width and difficulty in brushing #22 and #24. (B) Apically positioned partial-thickness flap to create connective tissue bed at the recipient site. (C) Intermediate-thickness (1 mm) free gingival graft harvested from the palate. (D) Donor site covered with a collagen dressing. (E) Free gingival graft placed at the recipient bed and stabilized with sutures.

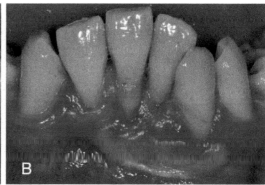

Figure 17.2 Healing of a free gingival graft. (A) Healing of the graft at two weeks. (B) Healing of the graft at eight weeks. Notice an increase in the width and thickness of keratinized gingiva at #22 and #24.

Healing following an apically repositioned flap/vestibuloplasty

An apically repositioned flap procedure includes the elevation of soft tissue flaps and their displacement during suturing in an apical position, often leaving 3–5 mm of alveolar bone denuded in the coronal part of the surgical area (Friedman 1962; Wennström & Zucchelli 2015). The denudation technique includes the removal of all soft tissue within an area extending from the gingival margin to a level apical to the mucogingival junction, leaving the alveolar bone completely exposed (Corn 1962; Wilderman 1964). However, the exposure of alveolar bone produces severe bone resorption with permanent loss of bone height (Costich & Ramfjord 1968). With a split-flap procedure, only the superficial portion of the oral mucosa within the wound area is removed, leaving the bone covered by periosteum (Staffileno et al. 1966). Unless a relatively thick layer of connective tissue is retained on the bone surface with the split-flap procedure, the periosteal connective tissue can undergo necrosis, together with loss of crestal bone height (Costich & Ramfjord 1968). The denudation technique usually results in more bone loss than the split-flap technique (Bohannan 1962a, b). An apically repositioned flap procedure can also result in the same risk for extensive bone resorption as with other denudation techniques (Friedman 1962).

Following a denudation or split-flap technique, the wound area is filled with granulation tissue derived from the periodontal ligament, the tissue of the bone marrow spaces, the retained periosteal connective tissue, and the surrounding gingiva and lining mucosa (Wennström & Zucchelli 2015). The degree of resorption of crestal bone exposes varying amounts of the periodontal ligament tissue in the marginal area, allowing granulation tissue from the periodontal ligament to fill out the coronal portion of the wound. This particular granulation tissue possesses the capability to induce keratinization of the covering epithelium.

However, the results that may be achieved with respect to increasing the gingival width by means of periosteal exposure or denudation of the alveolar bone are unpredictable, including recession of marginal gingiva in the surgical area often exceeding the gain of gingiva obtained in the apical portion of the wound (Carraro et al. 1964). Due to such complications and severe postoperative pain for the patient, the use of these techniques can hardly be justified and such therapeutic methods may thus be deemed inappropriate (Wennström & Zucchelli 2015).

Healing following grafting procedures

Healing of free soft tissue grafts (epithelialized tissue grafts) placed entirely on a connective tissue recipient bed can be divided into three phases (Nobuto et al. 1988; Oliver et al. 1968):

- *Initial phase* (from 0 to 3 days): A thin layer of exudate forms between the graft and the recipient bed and the grafted tissue survives with an avascular plasmatic circulation from the recipient bed. A thick layer of exudate or a blood clot may be detrimental to the plasmatic circulation, resulting in rejection of the graft. The establishment and maintenance of a plasmatic circulation are therefore critical, hence blood between the graft and the recipient site must be removed by exerting pressure against the graft following suturing. During this initial healing phase, the epithelium of the free graft degenerates and is subsequently desquamated.
- *Revascularization phase* (from 2 to 11 days): Anastomoses becomes established between the blood vessels of the recipient bed and those in the grafted tissue, thereby re-establishing circulation in the pre-existing blood vessels of the graft. Simultaneously, a fibrous union is established between the graft and the underlying connective tissue bed. Re-epithelialization of the graft occurs mainly by proliferation of epithelium from adjacent tissues. If a free graft is placed over denuded root surfaces, apical migration of epithelium along the tooth-facing surface of the graft may take place at this stage of healing.

■ *Tissue maturation phase* (from 11 to 42 days): The number of blood vessels in the transplant is gradually reduced, with the vascular system of the graft becoming normal after 14 days. The epithelium gradually matures with the formation of a keratin layer.

Root coverage

Displacement of the soft tissue margin apical to the cementoenamel junction (CEJ) with exposure of the root surface, i.e. marginal tissue recession, is commonly found in populations with high standards of oral hygiene, as well as in populations with poor oral hygiene (Löe et al. 1992; Serino et al. 1994; Susin et al. 2004). In periodontally untreated populations, all tooth surfaces may be affected by soft tissue recession, although the prevalence and severity are more pronounced at single-rooted teeth than at molars (Löe et al. 1992; Miller et al. 1987; Yoneyama et al. 1988).

Longitudinal clinical studies have validated the lack of a relationship between the height of the gingiva and the development of soft tissue recession (Freedman et al. 1999; Schoo & van der Velden 1985; Wennström 1987). Gingival height is not critical for the prevention of marginal tissue recession, but development of a recession will result in loss of gingival height (Freedman et al. 1999; Wennström & Zucchelli 2015). Furthermore, it has been shown that recession sites without attached gingiva might not experience further attachment loss and recession if inflammation is controlled (Dorfman et al. 1982).

The predominant causative factor for the development of recessions, particularly in young individuals, is vigorous toothbrushing, especially associated with tooth malposition and the usage of hard toothbrushes (Checchi et al. 1999; Daprile et al. 2007; Khocht et al. 1993), while periodontal disease may be the primary cause in older adults (Wennström & Zucchelli 2015).

Other local factors associated with marginal tissue recession are:

■ Anatomic factors (which may be inter-related), such as:
 ■ Alveolar bone dehiscences (Bernimoulin & Curilivic 1977; Löst 1984).
 ■ Fenestrations.
 ■ Abnormal tooth position in the arch.
 ■ An aberrant path of eruption of the tooth.
 ■ The shape of the individual tooth (Zucchelli & Mounssif 2015).
■ Improper flossing techniques (Zucchelli & Mounssif 2015).
■ Perioral and intraoral piercing (Zucchelli & Mounssif 2015).
■ Direct trauma associated with class II, division 2 malocclusion (Zucchelli & Mounssif 2015).
■ High muscle attachment and frenal pull (Trott & Love 1966).
■ Plaque and calculus (Susin et al. 2004; Van Palenstein Helderman et al. 1998).

■ Iatrogenic factors related to restorative and periodontal treatment procedures (Lindhe & Nyman 1980; Valderhaug 1980). Subgingivally placed restorations that favor plaque accumulation together with an adjacent thin gingiva are a potential risk for the development of soft tissue recession (Ericsson & Lindhe 1984; Stetler & Bissada 1987).
■ Partial dentures (Zucchelli & Mounssif 2015).
■ Orthodontic treatment. If a tooth is moved exclusively within the alveolar bone, soft tissue recession will not develop. Predisposing alveolar bone dehiscences, which may be induced by uncontrolled facial expansion of a tooth through the cortical plate, can render the tooth liable to the development of soft tissue recession (Karring et al. 1982; Wennström et al. 1987), particularly in areas of a thin gingival phenotype (<0.5 mm) in the presence of plaque-induced inflammation or toothbrushing (Melsen & Allais 2005; Yared et al. 2006). It is the volume (thickness), and not the height of the covering marginal soft tissue (quality), on the pressure side of the tooth during orthodontic tooth movement that is the determining factor for the development of the recession (Wennström & Zucchelli 2015). It has been shown that the integrity of the periodontium can be maintained during orthodontic therapy in areas that have only a minimal zone of gingiva (Coatoam et al. 1981).
■ Herpes simplex virus type 1 – multiple vesicles that rupture, rapidly giving rise to ulcers, whereby toothbrushing is responsible for the evolution of ulcers involving the gingival margin (Zucchelli & Mounssif 2015).

Three different types of marginal tissue recessions may be defined (Wennström & Zucchelli 2015):

■ *Recessions associated with mechanical factors, predominately toothbrushing trauma*: These are usually at sites with clinically healthy gingiva and where the exposed root has a wedge-shaped defect, the surface of which is clean, smooth, and polished.
■ *Recessions associated with localized plaque-induced inflammatory lesions*: These are usually found at teeth that are prominently positioned, including a thin alveolar bone or where bone is absent (bone dehiscence), in addition to a thin gingival phenotype. The inflammatory lesion can engage the entire connective tissue portion of the thin and delicate gingiva, whereby proliferation of epithelial cells from the oral as well as the dentogingival epithelium into the thin and degraded connective tissue may bring about a subsidence of the epithelial surface, which clinically becomes manifest as recession of the tissue margin (Coatoam et al. 1981).
■ *Recessions associated with generalized forms of destructive periodontal disease*: Loss of periodontal support at proximal sites may result in compensatory remodeling of the support at the buccal/lingual aspect of teeth, leading to an apical shift of the soft tissue margin (Serino et al. 1994). An inevitable consequence of the resolution of periodontal lesions following treatment, independent of a non-surgical or a surgical treatment approach, is the apical displacement of the soft tissue margin.

Factors influencing the prognosis of root coverage

Patient-related factors

- Poor oral hygiene.
- Toothbrushing trauma.
- Smokers: showing less improvement in gingival recession, less gain in clinical attachment and more incomplete root coverage (Chambrone et al. 2009).

Tooth-related factors

- The amount/thickness of residual keratinized tissue can be a critical factor when utilizing a coronally advanced flap (CAF). A systematic review found a positive relationship between gingival thickness and clinical outcome, whereby the critical threshold thickness was found to be about 1 mm (Hwang & Wang 2006). Another study demonstrated a flap thickness of >0.8 mm to be a strong predictor of complete root coverage (Baldi et al. 1999).
- The dimensions of the recession defect. Less favorable treatment outcomes have been reported at sites with wide (>3 mm) and deep (≥5 mm) recessions (Holbrook & Ochsenbein 1983; Pini Prato et al. 1992; Trombelli et al. 1995). Recessions with deeper baselines and smaller amounts of apicocoronal keratinized tissue have shown a lower probability for complete root coverage and long-term stability of the gingival margin (Pini Prato et al. 2012); however, other studies have shown that the pretreatment gingival height apical to the recession defect is not correlated to the amount of root coverage that can be obtained (Harris 1994; Romanos et al. 1993).
- The dimension of the interdental papilla. Complete root coverage has been shown to correlate inversely with papilla height, suggesting a greater probability of complete root coverage for thick periodontal phenotypes with short interdental papillae (Olsson & Lindhe 1991). Conversely, papilla height and papilla width have been shown to be significant and positive predictors of root coverage, and a papilla height of ≥5 mm has been shown to be associated with complete root coverage (Haghighati et al. 2009).
- Multiple gingival recessions are more challenging defects compared to single recession defects, as the surgical field is larger with higher anatomic variability that may include prominent roots, shallow vestibules, enamel–root abrasions, and unevenness in residual keratinized tissue. Also, the total number of surgical procedures and the amount of donor tissue that can be obtained from the palate should be considered (Cairo et al. 2011).
- The thickness of the graft in free graft procedures influences the success of root coverage, and a thickness of about 2 mm has been recommended (Borghetti & Gardella 1990).
- Loss of interdental bone. A clinical variable regarded as critical to determine the possible outcome of a root coverage procedure is the level of periodontal tissue support at the proximal sites of the tooth, and this is considered a great

Table 17.1 Miller classification of gingival recession.

Class I	The interdental periodontal support is intact and the gingival recession does not reach the mucogingival line. Complete root coverage can be achieved.
Class II	The interdental periodontal support is intact and the gingival recession reaches the mucogingival line. Complete root coverage can be achieved.
Class III	There is some interdental attachment and bone loss and the gingival recession reaches the mucogingival line. Partial root coverage can be achieved.
Class IV	Bone and attachment loss are so severe that no root coverage can be accomplished.

Source: Adapted from Miller 1985.

Table 17.2 Cairo classification based on the interdental clinical attachment loss measurement.

Recession type 1 (RT1)	Buccal tissue recession with no loss of interproximal attachment.
Recession type 2 (RT2)	Buccal tissue recession associated with loss of interproximal attachment less than or equal to the buccal attachment loss.
Recession type 3 (RT3)	Buccal tissue recession associated with loss of interproximal attachment greater than the buccal attachment loss.

Source: Adapted from Cairo et al. 2011.

limitation for root coverage, thereby affecting the prognosis of gingival recessions. Miller (1985) has classified gingival recessions into four classes, taking into consideration the anticipated root coverage that is possible to obtain with the use of a free gingival graft (Table 17.1).

Evidence suggests that surgical therapeutic approaches are highly predictable for Miller class I and II single-tooth defects. Challenges do however arise when patients present with Miller class III and IV defects, as well as with multiple-tooth gingival recession defects and lingual/palatal mucogingival concerns. Systematic reviews and randomized clinical trials have demonstrated the successful use of subepithelial connective tissue graft (CTG) techniques when treating facial maxillary Miller class I and II single-tooth defects (Richardson et al. 2015).

A simplified classification has been suggested by Cairo et al. (2011), which is a treatment-oriented classification to forecast the potential for final root coverage outcomes, and is based on the clinical assessment of interproximal clinical attachment levels (Table 17.2).

Treatment (technique)-related factors

- Treatment of the exposed root surface prior to surgically treating root coverage:

- The exposed portion of the root should be rendered free from bacterial biofilms. This can be achieved by the use of a rubber cup and a polishing paste (Wennström & Zucchelli 2015).
- Root planing should only be performed in situations where a reduced root prominence would be considered beneficial for graft survival or tissue regeneration, or if shallow root caries has been diagnosed. No differences in terms of root coverage or residual probing depth have been shown between teeth that have been root planed or polished only (Oles et al. 1988; Pini Prato et al. 1999).
- Fillings in the root should preferably be removed (Wennström & Zucchelli 2015).
- Chemical root surface conditioning (root surface demineralization) has been advocated to remove the smear layer, and to facilitate the formation of a new fibrous attachment through exposure of collagen fibrils of the dentin and cementum matrix, thereby allowing subsequent interdigitation of these fibrils with those in the covering connective tissue (Hanes et al. 1985, 1991). Acids that have been used include citric and phosphoric acids, ethylenediaminetetraacetic acid, and tetracycline hydrochloride (Zucchelli & Mounssif 2015). The usage of laser therapy has also been included (Oliveira & Muncinelli 2012). Animal models have shown that these procedures induce cementogenesis and enhance attachment by connective tissue ingrowth (Garrett et al. 1978; Willey & Steinberg 1984). However, in human studies, controlled clinical trials have failed to demonstrate a beneficial effect of acid root biomodification, and the conclusion has been drawn that there is no evidence that root surface biomodification prior to soft tissue root coverage improves the clinical outcome of root coverage procedures (Bouchard et al. 1997; Caffesse et al. 2000; Chambrone et al. 2009; Oliveira & Muncinelli 2012).
- A positive relationship is mandatory between the flap length and the flap base, whereby the flap base should be wide to incorporate as many supraperiosteal vessels as possible (Mörmann & Ciancio 1977).
- Flap tension may be a critical factor during healing. Excessive tension may interfere with the blood supply from supraperiosteal vessels, causing constriction and hindering proper blood support of the gingival graft over the exposed root surface (Willey & Steinberg 1984).

Root coverage surgical procedures

The ultimate goal of a root coverage procedure is complete coverage of the recession defect with a good appearance related to the adjacent soft tissues and minimal probing depth following healing (Zucchelli & Mounssif 2015). The selection of the most suitable surgical technique for treating gingival recessions will furthermore be influenced by the presence of non-carious cervical lesions; the presence of interdental clinical attachment level loss; the presence of buccal displacement of the root; the baseline amount of keratinized tissue apical to exposed roots; and the gingival thickness.

Indications for root coverage procedures are (Wennström & Zucchelli 2015; Zucchelli & Mounssif 2015):

- Esthetic/cosmetic demands.
- Root sensitivity.
- Root abrasion/caries.
- Inconsistency/disharmony of gingival margin.
- Changing the topography of the marginal soft tissue in order to facilitate plaque control.

Factors to consider when selecting the surgical procedure for achieving root coverage are (Wennström & Zucchelli 2015):

- Jaw and tooth position.
- Recession depth and width.
- Tissue thickness and quality apical and lateral to the recession.
- Esthetic demands.
- Patient compliance.

Surgical procedures used in the treatment of recession defects are classified as follows (Lindhe et al. 2008; Richardson et al. 2015; Stefanini et al. 2018; Zucchelli et al. 2014):

- Pedicle soft tissue graft procedures (rotational flap procedures):
  - Laterally sliding flap.
  - Double papilla flap.
  - Oblique rotated flap.
- Free soft tissue graft procedures:
  - Epithelialized graft.
  - Subepithelial CTG.
  - Soft tissue graft substitutes (acellular dermal matrix and xenogeneic collagen matrix materials).
- Advanced flap procedures:
  - Coronally repositioned flap.
  - Semilunar coronally repositioned flap.
  - CAF + subepithelial CTG.
  - Tunnel technique with graft insertion (see Figure 17.3).
  - Modified CAF and tunnel technique.
  - CTG wall technique.
- Regenerative procedures (with barrier membrane and/or recombinant human platelet-derived growth factor and enamel matrix derivative).

Healing following a pedicle graft procedure

Healing can be divided into four stages (Wilderman & Wentz 1965):

- *Adaptation stage* (0–4 days): The surgical flap is separated from the root by a thin fibrin layer. The epithelium covering the transplanted tissue flap starts to proliferate and reaches the tooth surface at the coronal edge of the flap after a few days and proliferating epithelial cells start to make contact with the root surface.
- *Proliferation stage* (4–21 days): Connective tissue invades the fibrin layer from the basal level of the flap, and fibroblasts detectable near the root surface differentiate into

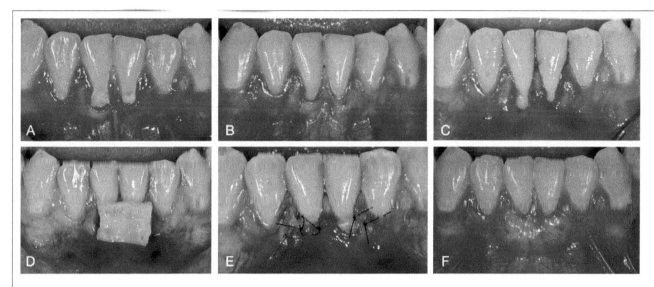

Figure 17.3 Tunnel technique with connective tissue graft. (A) Gingival recession RT1 in #24 and #25, thin periodontal phenotype, and aberrant frenum. (B) Control of gingival inflammation with oral prophylaxis. (C) Modified tunnel preparation. (D) Connective tissue graft harvested from palate. (E) Connective tissue graft inserted into the tunnel and stabilized with sutures. (F) Healing at three months showing complete root coverage, increase in tissue thickness, and apical displacement of frenal attachment.

cementoblasts. Epithelium is detected over the root at the coronal level of the wound, while a thin connective tissue is detectable more apically, even if fibers are not inserted into the root at this stage.

- *Attachment stage* (21–28 days): Fibers are inserted into a layer of new cementum in the apical part of the recession defect.
- *Maturation stage* (1–6 months): An increase and continuous formation of collagen fibers occur in this period, with bundles of collagen fibers becoming inserted into the cementum layer, leading to a variable amount of connective tissue repair coronal to the bone crest and apical to the junctional epithelium. A similar arrangement of fibroblasts and collagen fibers is evident at the level of the crestal alveolar bone.

Evidence evaluated from randomized clinical trials for the treatment of single recessions, without interdental attachment loss, by means of utilizing CTGs and advanced flap procedures, has led to the following conclusions (Tonetti & Jepsen 2014):

- CAF plus CTG is more effective than CAF alone to obtain root coverage.
- CAF plus CTG is more effective than CAF plus guided tissue regeneration.
- The addition of enamel matrix derivative underneath a CAF improves the outcomes of a CAF in terms of complete root coverage.
- Additional research is needed to assess the role of alternatives to autologous soft tissue grafting in combination with CAF.
- Additional research is also needed to identify the optimal surgical design and the need for additional soft tissue grafting (or alternatives) at recessions with interdental attachment loss, and at multiple recessions.

Regarding multiple gingival recessions:

- The tunnel procedure has been shown to be a promising treatment of multiple recessions (Cairo 2017).
- Modified CAF and tunnel approaches have been shown to produce the highest percentages of complete root coverage, and CAF plus CTG procedures appear to achieve the best outcome (Graziani et al. 2014).
- A study has shown that sites treated with CAF plus CTG showed a higher percentage of sites with complete root coverage (52%) compared with sites treated with CAF alone (35%) after a 5-year follow-up period (Pini Prato et al. 2010).
- Another study has shown a stable gingival margin for at least 5 years in sites treated with CAF plus CTG, but an apical relapse of the gingival margin in several sites can occur in sites treated with CAF only (Zucchelli & De Sanctis 2000).

Correction of peri-implant soft tissue defects

A well-functioning soft tissue barrier, which is considered to be necessary for the maintenance of stability and function of a load-carrying dental implant, is regarded as essential for the long-term success rate of implant therapy (Wennström & Zucchelli 2015). Various classifications of peri-implant soft tissue deformities have been proposed (Gamborena & Avila-Ortiz 2021; Suzuki et al. 2012; Zucchelli et al. 2019). However, there exists heterogeneity of implant systems and prosthetic designs, as well as the lack of robust connective tissue attachment of the peri-implant mucosa to implant components. Hence, further clinical research is needed to determine the applicability and reproducibility of these various classifications (Gamborena & Abila-Ortiz 2021).

Peri-implant soft tissue deficiencies and defects can be categorized into three distinct groups (Gamborena & Avila-Ortiz 2021).

Keratinized mucosa width deficiencies

The peri-implant keratinized mucosa width is depicted as the height of keratinized soft tissue that runs in an apico-coronal direction from the mucosal margin to the mucogingival junction (Avila-Ortiz et al. 2020). An amount of peri-implant keratinized mucosa (i.e. <2 mm) has been regarded as being insufficient, and has been associated with difficulty in performing adequate oral hygiene and therefore may be a predisposing factor for the occurrence of inflammatory peri-implant diseases and mucosal recession (Gobbato et al. 2013; Kim et al. 2009; Perussolo et al. 2018).

The importance of the width of keratinized mucosa as being adequate for the success of implant therapy has been questioned. Lining mucosa has been regarded as not providing a sufficient barrier function (Warrer et al. 1995; Zarb & Schmitt 1990). Thus, it has been suggested that keratinized tissue should be created with mucogingival surgical techniques prior to implant placement when not present in adequate amounts (Meffert et al. 1992). A dimension of ≥2 mm of keratinized mucosa at dental implants has also been proposed (Lang & Löe 1972).

However, a systematic review has indicated that with good oral hygiene habits, peri-implant soft tissue health can be maintained even when keratinized mucosa is lacking (Wennström & Derks 2012). There is no evidence for a long-term effect of "inadequate" keratinized mucosa on the development of soft tissue recession, peri-implant bone loss, or implant loss. Furthermore, there is a lack of evidence supporting the concept that grafting procedures aimed at increasing the amount of keratinized mucosa will improve the outcomes of implant therapy (Wennström & Zucchelli 2015).

It has been suggested, however, that patients can experience pain and discomfort during brushing at implant sites facing the lining mucosa, thereby hampering adequate cleaning. In such cases, grafting procedures may be considered to establish a firmer marginal tissue of keratinized mucosa (Wennström & Zucchelli 2015).

Mucosal thickness deficiencies

Peri-implant mucosal thickness is the horizontal dimension of the peri-implant soft tissue, which may or may not be keratinized (Avila-Ortiz et al. 2020). Thin peri-implant mucosa (i.e. <2 mm) may be associated with tissue discoloration caused by mucosal transparency of the underlying implant components (Bressan et al. 2011). Thin peri-implant mucosa may also be a predisposing factor for the development of marginal mucosa defects secondary to peri-implant bone loss (Mailoa et al. 2018).

Peri-implant marginal mucosa defects

Peri-implant marginal mucosa defects (PMMDs) are alterations of the peri-implant soft tissue architecture characterized by an apical discrepancy of the mucosal margin respective to its ideal position, with or without exposure of transmucosal prosthetic components or the implant fixture surface (Gamborena & Avila-Ortiz 2021).

PMMDs may be caused by actual apical migration of the mucosal margin (i.e. recession) as a result of local inflammatory processes, sustained trauma, or iatrogenic dentistry (active pattern); or by progressive marginal mucosa discrepancies respective to the adjacent teeth because of lifelong craniofacial growth (passive pattern); or by a combination of both (Cocchetto et al. 2019; Gamborena & Avila-Ortiz 2021).

PMMDs may predispose for biofilm accumulation and subsequent initiation and/or progression of peri-implant inflammatory diseases, and are also frequently associated with underlying bone dehiscences, keratinized mucosa width, and/or mucosal thickness deficiencies (Berglundh et al. 2018; Isler et al. 2019; Poli et al. 2016).

Surgical considerations for the management of peri-implant soft tissue defects

See Figure 17.4. Current literature regarding the surgical management of single-tooth PMMDs is scant and consists mainly of case reports and prospective case series (Mazzotti et al. 2018). Management of PMMDs may require a purely surgical or a combined surgical–prosthetic approach, including adjustment or complete replacement of the existing prosthesis. Restorative work on adjacent teeth, such as modification of the contact area, may also be indicated to achieve an optimal outcome (Stefanini et al. 2020; Zucchelli et al. 2013).

Prior to any surgical procedure being performed, the depth and width of the PMMD must be considered, as well as the amount of papillary atrophy, keratinized mucosa width, mucosal thickness, and the local inflammatory status. Furthermore, the periodontal status of the adjacent teeth must also be assessed, as severe attachment loss and mucogingival deformities on the adjacent teeth can influence the amount of any predicted peri-implant soft tissue corrections (Gamborena & Avila-Ortiz 2021).

In cases where there is facial PMMD with no interproximal bone or papillary height loss, a bilaminar approach has been recommended, consisting of a CAF, either pedicled or tunneled, in conjunction with a soft tissue graft, even if an underlying bone dehiscence is present. Cases including the presence of unilateral and/or bilateral papillary deficiencies are more demanding to treat, as the more deficient the peri-implant phenotype may be, the more soft tissue augmentation interventions may be necessary. The degree of difficulty is directly related to the extent of interproximal bone loss and the proximity of the implant shoulder to the adjacent tooth, which may result in serious space limitations to recreate an adequate papillary anatomy (Gamborena & Avila-Ortiz 2021).

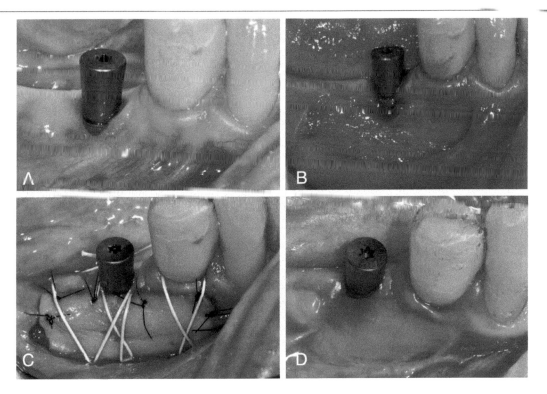

Figure 17.4 Free gingival graft to increase keratinized peri-implant mucosa width. (A) Implant at #28 site showing peri-implant mucosa that is thin, non-keratinized, with initial mucosal recession. (B) Apically positioned partial-thickness flap to create connective tissue bed at the recipient site. (C) Free gingival graft placed at the recipient bed and stabilized with sutures. (D) Healing at eight weeks showing correction of mucosal recession, increase in mucosal thickness, and keratinized mucosa width.

Crown lengthening

Crown-lengthening procedures are performed to improve dentofacial esthetics (excessive gingival display), and for the exposure of sound tooth structure. However, to select the proper treatment approach for crown lengthening, an analysis of the individual case with regard to crown–root–alveolar bone relationships should be done (Wennström & Zucchelli 2015).

Excessive gingival display

In cases with an excessive display of gingiva where the size and shape of the teeth and the location of the gingival margins are normal, the excessive display of gingiva is usually caused by vertical maxillary excess and a long mid-face. In such cases, periodontal crown-lengthening procedures are not the solution, but rather the maxilla must be altered by a major maxillofacial surgical procedure.

In other cases, dentofacial esthetics can be improved by a combination of periodontal and prosthetic treatment measures by modifying/controlling the form of the teeth and interdental papillae as well as the position of the gingival margins and the incisal edges of the teeth (Wennström & Zucchelli 2015).

In young adults, the height of free gingiva may be >1 mm, resulting in a disproportional appearance of the clinical crown, giving the appearance of "small front teeth." In such cases, with an intact periodontium and when the periodontium is of a thin phenotype, full exposure of the anatomic crown can be accomplished by a gingivectomy/gingivoplasty procedure. If the periodontium is of the thick phenotype and there is a bony ledge at the osseous crest, an apically positioned flap procedure should be performed, thus allowing for osseous recontouring.

In patients who do indeed have short anatomic crowns in the anterior section of the dentition, prosthetic measures must be used after resective periodontal therapy to increase the apicocoronal dimension of the crowns:

- In subjects who have normal occlusal relationships and incisal guidance, the incisal line of the front teeth must remain unaltered, but the clinical crowns can be made longer by surgically exposing the root structure and by locating the cervical margins of the restorations apical to the CEJ.
- In subjects who have abnormal occlusal relationships with excessive interocclusal space in the posterior dentition when the anterior teeth are in edge-to-edge contact, the length of the maxillary front teeth can be reduced without inducing posterior occlusal interferences. In addition, the marginal gingiva can be resected or relocated to an apical position before crown restorations are made.

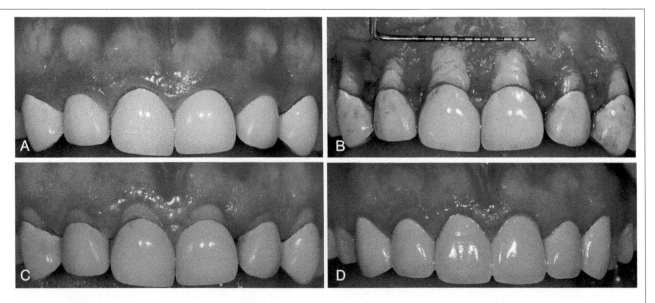

Figure 17.5 Esthetic crown lengthening. (A) Short clinical crowns resulting in an unesthetic smile and a diagnosis of altered active eruption. (B) Apically positioned flap with ostectomy and osteoplasty to achieve a supracrestal tissue attachment. Note the discrepancy between the prosthetic crown margins and cementoenamel junction. (C) Healing at three months exposing the anatomic crowns. (D) New prosthetic crowns to achieve a harmonious smile.

Exposure of sound tooth structure

Crown-lengthening procedures may be required to solve problems such as:

- Inadequate amount of tooth structure for proper restorative therapy.
- Subgingival location of fracture lines.
- Subgingival location of carious lesions.

The techniques used to accomplish crown lengthening include:

- An apically positioned flap procedure including bone resection (see Figure 17.5).
- Forced tooth eruption with or without fiberotomy.

Removal of an aberrant frenulum

A frenum is a mucous membrane fold that contains muscle and connective tissue fibers that attach the lip and the cheek to the alveolar mucosa, the gingiva, and the underlying periosteum (Devishree et al. 2012). Several frena are usually present in the oral cavity, most notably the maxillary labial frenum, the mandibular labial frenum, and the lingual frenum (Priyanka et al. 2013). Their primary function is to provide stability of the upper and lower lips and the tongue (Mintz et al. 2005).

The maxillary labial frenum develops as a post-eruptive remnant of the ectolabial bands that connect the tubercle of the upper lip to the palatine papilla. When the central incisors erupt widely separated, no bone is deposited inferior to the frenum. This results in a V-shaped bony cleft between the two central incisors and an abnormal frenum attachment. An aberrant mandibular labial frenum is associated with a decreased vestibular depth and an inadequate width of attached gingiva (Devishree et al. 2012). Frenal problems occur most often on the facial surface between the maxillary and mandibular central incisors and in the canine and premolar areas. They occur less often on the lingual surface of the mandible.

Classification of labial frenal attachments (Priyanka et al. 2013)

- *Mucosal* – when the frenal fibers are attached up to the mucogingival junction.
- *Gingival* – when the fibers are inserted within the attached gingiva.
- *Papillary* – when the fibers are extending into the interdental papilla.
- *Papilla penetrating* – when the frenal fibers cross the alveolar process and extend up to the palatine papilla.

A pathogenic frenum is characterized by (Devishree et al. 2012; Priyanka et al. 2013):

- Causation of a midline diastema, or if the tissue inhibits the closure of a diastema during orthodontic treatment.
- Being unusually wide or flattened with no apparent zone of attached gingiva, closely attached to the gingival margin. This can cause gingival recession and hinder maintenance of oral hygiene.
- Causing a shift of the interdental papilla with blanching when the frenum is extended.
- Prejudice to the fit or retention of a denture, leading to psychological disturbances to the individual.

Surgical management to remove frenal attachments

See Figure 17.6, Devishree et al. (2012) and Priyanka et al. (2013). A frenectomy is complete removal of the frenum, including its attachment to underlying bone. A frenotomy is relocation of the frenum, usually in a more apical position.

Simple (classical) excision technique

The frenum is engaged with a hemostat, which is inserted into the depth of the vestibule. Incisions are made on the upper and the undersurface of the hemostat until it is free. A narrow elliptic incision around the frenal area down to the periosteum is made, and the fibrous tissue is sharply dissected from the underlying periosteum and soft tissue. The margins of the wound are then gently undermined and re-approximated.

Z plasty

This technique is indicated when there is hypertrophy of the frenum with a low insertion, which is associated with an inter-incisor diastema, and also in cases of a short vestibule. After excision of the fibrous tissue, two oblique incisions of equal length are made in a Z fashion, one at each end of the previous area of excision. By using fine tissue forceps, the submucosal tissues are dissected beyond the base of each flap, into the loose non-attached tissue planes, thereby creating two triangular double-rotation flaps. The flaps are then mobilized and transposed through 90° and sutured to close the initial vertical incision horizontally, i.e. to close the wound along the cut edges of the attached mucoperiosteum and the labial mucosa.

Localized vestibuloplasty with secondary epithelialization

An incision is made through mucosal tissue and underlying submucosal tissue, without perforating the periosteum. A supraperiosteal dissection is completed by undermining the mucosal and submucosal tissue with scissors. After a clean periosteal layer is identified, the edge of the mucosal flap is sutured to the periosteum at the maximal depth of the vestibule and the exposed periosteum is allowed to heal by secondary epithelialization.

Gingival preservation at ectopic tooth eruption (Wennström & Zucchelli 2015)

Surgical intervention is often indicated for ectopically erupted teeth, which have an eruption position facial to the alveolar process. To create a satisfactory width of the gingiva for the permanent tooth, the tissue entrapped between the erupting tooth and the deciduous tooth is usually utilized as donor tissue. Depending on the distance from the donor site (entrapped gingiva) to the recipient site (area located facially–apically to the erupting permanent tooth), three different techniques have been described (Agudio et al. 1985; Pini Prato et al. 2000):

- *Double pedicle graft*: This technique is indicated when the permanent tooth erupts within the zone of keratinized tissue but close to the mucogingival junction. An intrasulcular incision is performed at the deciduous tooth and extended laterally to the gingival crevice of the adjacent teeth and apically to the erupting permanent tooth. The flap is then mobilized apical to the mucogingival line, and the entrapped

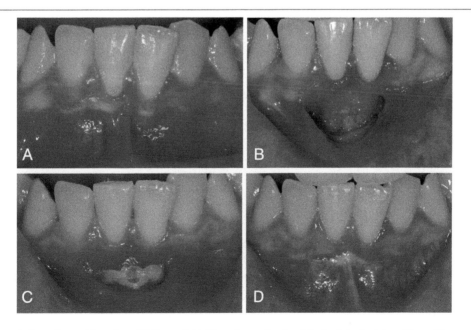

Figure 17.6 Removal of an aberrant frenulum. (A) Lower labial frenulum extending into the interdental papilla making oral hygiene measures difficult for the patient. (B) Complete excision of the frenulum and scoring of the periosteum at the apical region. (C) Healing at one week. (D) Healing at eight weeks showing apical displacement of the frenulum attachment.

gingiva is elevated and transposed for positioning apically to the erupting tooth. Sutures are placed to secure the position of the gingival tissue facial to the erupting tooth.

- *Apically positioned flap*: This technique is indicated when the permanent tooth is erupting apical to the mucogingival junction. Two vertical lateral releasing incisions are made to allow for apical positioning of the keratinized tissue and are extended apically beyond the mucogingival junction. An intrasulcular incision is performed at the deciduous tooth and a partial-thickness flap is elevated beyond the ectopically erupting tooth. The mobilized gingival flap is moved apical to the erupting tooth and secured in position by sutures.
- *Free gingival graft*: This technique is indicated when the tooth is erupting within the alveolar mucosa distant to the mucogingival junction. The entrapped gingiva is removed by a split incision and is utilized as an epithelialized CTG. The free gingival graft is placed at a prepared recipient site facial/apical of the erupting tooth. Suturing is performed to secure close adaptation of the graft to the underlying connective tissue bed.

Prevention of ridge collapse following tooth extraction (Wennström & Zucchelli 2015)

Following extraction of a tooth, the topography of the surrounding soft and hard tissues will be altered (see Figure 17.7):

- *Prevention of ridge collapse due to soft tissue collapse*: Following tooth extraction, the soft tissue margin will collapse and the height of the adjacent papillae will be reduced. This may be prevented by immediate post-extraction placement of an ovate pontic to preserve the outline of the soft tissue ridge, thus supporting the soft tissues. Other procedures include flap elevation for complete soft tissue closure of the extraction sites, and placement of connective tissue grafts over the extraction sites (Borghetti & Gardella 1990; Wennström & Zucchelli 2015).

- *Prevention of ridge collapse due to alveolar bone resorption*: Alveolar bone resorption following tooth extractions can occur due to trauma and/or fracture of the vestibular osseous plate; resorption of the vestibular osseous plate; or the presence of a thin vestibular bone plate. Resorption can be prevented by placement of bone grafts together with the placement of barrier membranes (Becker et al. 1994; Lekovic et al. 1997).

Augmentation of the edentulous ridge

A ridge deformity is directly related to the volume of root structure and associated bone that is missing or has been destroyed (Wennström & Zucchelli 2015). Ridge defects can be divided into three classes (Seibert 1983):

- *Class I*: Loss of buccolingual width but normal apicocoronal height.
- *Class II*: Loss of apicocoronal height but normal buccolingual width.
- *Class III*: A combination of loss of both height and width of the ridge.

A partially edentulous ridge may be considered as a normal ridge, i.e. it has retained the buccolingual and apicocoronal dimensions of the alveolar process; however, there is the absence of the eminences that existed in the bone over the roots, and the interdental papillae are missing. Thus, the smooth contours of the normal ridge can create problems for the restorative dentist. With the utilization of fixed partial dentures, pontics may frequently give the impression that they rest on the top of the ridge rather than emerge from within the alveolar process. Pontics also lack a root eminence. Pontics furthermore will lack marginal gingivae and interdental papillae.

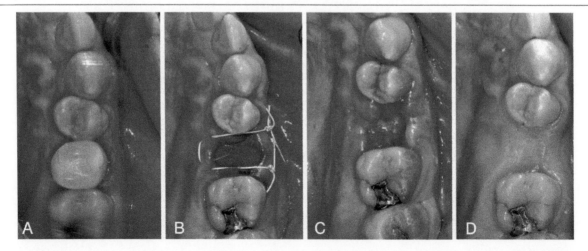

Figure 17.7 Ridge preservation following tooth extraction. (A) Non-restorable #13. (B) Atraumatic extraction followed by grafting with xenograft and covered with a collagen plug. (C) Healing at two weeks. (D) Healing at four months showing adequate maintenance of ridge width and height.

Dark triangles, which interfere with dentofacial esthetics, will also be present in the embrasure area between the pontics and between the abutments and the pontics (Wennström & Zucchelli 2015).

Ridge augmentation procedures should thus be preceded by careful surgical–prosthetic treatment planning so as to obtain optimal esthetic results (Wennström & Zucchelli 2015).

Surgical soft tissue augmentation procedures for edentulous ridges

- Pedicle graft procedure.
- Roll flap procedure.
- Free graft procedures:
  - Pouch graft procedure.
  - Interpositional graft procedure.
  - Onlay full-thickness graft procedure.
  - Combined onlay–interpositional graft procedure.

The pedicle graft procedure is mainly used for correction of a single-tooth ridge defect with minor horizontal and vertical loss (Studer et al. 1997). The roll flap procedure is used in a single-tooth space in the treatment of small to moderate class I ridge defects. Hence, a buccolingual ridge concavity can be converted into a ridge convexity resembling the eminence pro-

duced by the roots of the adjacent teeth (Abrams 1980). The pouch graft technique is used to correct class I defects. However, patients with large-volume defects may have thin palatal tissues, thus hard tissue augmentation may also be needed (Cohen 1994). Interpositional graft procedures are used to correct class I as well as small and moderate class II defects (Seibert 1993). Onlay graft procedures are used in the treatment of large class II and III defects in the apicocoronal plane, i.e. to gain ridge height (Seibert 1983). Combined onlay–interpositional graft procedures are indicated for class III ridge defects where augmentation is required in both vertical and horizontal dimensions (Seibert & Louis 1996).

In general, it is furthermore recommended to moderately overcorrect the ridge in the area of the deformity, thereby allowing for compensation for wound contraction and providing the necessary bulk of tissue within the ridge, which can then be sculpted to its final form. Sculpturing can be done by means of gingivoplasty techniques, whereby adjustments can be made to shape the cervical contour and emergence profile of pontic teeth to match those of the contralateral teeth. This can also be done in combination with reshaping of the tissue-contacting surfaces of the pontic teeth of the provisional prosthesis with autopolymerizing resin (Wennström & Zucchelli 2015).

SUMMARY

The main goal of periodontal plastic surgical procedures is the achievement of an acceptable esthetic outcome. Much study is still needed to compare the esthetic outcome achieved using different surgical procedures. Critical analysis of surgical techniques should guide the evolution toward better clinical methods to ensure the predictability of results. Blood supply is the most significant concern and underlying issue for all decisions regarding the choice of any specific surgical procedure. The formation of a circulation through anastomosis and angiogenesis is crucial to the survival of these therapeutic procedures, as a major complicating factor is the avascular root surface. To obtain optimal esthetic results with ridge augmentation procedures, well-planned surgical–prosthetic treatments are required. As tissue-engineering techniques improve, the success and predictability of mucogingival surgery have the potential to dramatically increase (Stefanini et al. 2018; Takei et al. 2019; Wennström & Zucchelli 2015).

REFERENCES

Abrams L. Augmentation of the residual edentulous ridge for fixed prosthesis. *Compend Contin Educ Dent.* 1980; 1:205–214.

Agudio G, Pini Prato G, De Paoli S, Nevins M. Mucogingival interceptive therapy. *Int J Periodontics Restorative Dent.* 1985; 5:49–59.

Avila-Ortiz G, Gonzalez-Martin O, Couso-Queiruga E, Wang HL. The peri-implant phenotype. *J Periodontol.* 2020; 91:283–288.

Baldi C, Pini-Prato G, Pagliaro U et al. Coronally advanced flap procedure for root coverage. Is flap thickness a relevant predictor to achieve root coverage? A 19-case series. *J Periodontol.* 1999; 70:1077–1084.

Becker W, Becker BE, Caffesse R. A comparison of demineralized freeze-dried bone and autologous bone to induce bone formation in human extraction sockets. *J Periodontol.* 1994; 65:1128–1133.

Berglundh T, Armitage G, Araujo MG et al. Peri-implant diseases and conditions: consensus report of workgroup 4 of the 2017 World Workshop on the classification of periodontal and peri-implant diseases and conditions. *J Periodontol.* 2018; 89(Suppl 1):S313–S318.

Bernimoulin JP, Curilivic Z. Gingival recession and tooth mobility. *J Clin Periodontol.* 1977; 4:208–219.

Bohannan HM. Studies in the alteration of vestibular depth. *I. Complete denudation. J Periodontol.* 1962a; 33:120–128.

Bohannan HM. Studies in the alteration of vestibular depth. II. Periosteum retention. *J Periodontol.* 1962b; 33:354–359.

Borghetti A, Gardella J-P. Thick gingival autograft for the coverage of gingival recession: a clinical evaluation. *Int J Periodontics Restorative Dent.* 1990; 10:217–229.

Bouchard P, Nilveus R, Etienne D. Clinical evaluation of tetracycline HCL conditioning in the treatment of gingival recessions. *A comparative study. J Periodontol.* 1997; 68:262–269.

Bowers GM. A study of the width of attached gingiva. *J Periodontol.* 1963; 34:201–209.

Bressan E, Paniz G, Lops D et al. Influence of abutment material on the gingival color of implant-supported all-ceramic restorations: a prospective multicenter study. *Clin Oral Implants Res.* 2011; 22:631–637.

Caffesse RG, De LaRosa M, Garza M et al. Citric acid demineralization and subepithelial connective tissue grafts. *J Periodontol.* 2000; 71:568–572.

Cairo F. Periodontal plastic surgery of gingival recessions at single and multiple teeth. *Periodontol. 2000.* 2017; 75:296–316.

Cairo F, Nieri M, Cincinelli S, Mervelt J, Pagliaro U. The interproximal clinical attachment level to classify gingival recessions and predict root coverage outcomes: an explorative and reliability study. *J Clin Periodontol.* 2011; 38:661–666.

Carranza FA, Carraro JJ. Mucogingival techniques in periodontal surgery. *J Periodontol.* 1970; 41:294–299.

Carraro JJ, Carranza FA, Albano EA, Joly GG. Effect of bone denudation in mucogingival surgery in humans. *J Periodontol.* 1964; 35:463–466.

Chambrone L, Chambrone D, Pustiglioni FE, Chambrone LA, Lima LA. The influence of tobacco smoking on the outcomes achieved by root-coverage procedures: a systematic review. *J Am Dent Assoc.* 2009; 140:294–306.

Chambrone L, Sukekava F, Araujo MG et al. Root coverage procedures for the treatment of localized recession-type defects. *Cochrane Database Syst Rev.* 2009; 2:CD007161. doi: 10.1002/14651858.CD007161.pub2.

Checchi L, Daprile G, Gatto MR, Pelliccioni GA. Gingival recession and toothbrushing in an Italian School of Dentistry: a pilot study. *J Clin Periodontol.* 1999; 26:276–280.

Coatoam GW, Behrents RG, Bissada NF. The width of keratinized gingiva during orthodontic treatment: its significance and impact on periodontal status. *J Periodontol.* 1981; 52:307–313.

Cocchetto R, Pradies G, Celletti R, Canullo L. Continuous craniofacial growth in adult patients treated with dental implants in the anterior maxilla. *Clin Implant Dent Relat Res.* 2019; 21:627–634.

Cohen ES. Ridge augmentation utilizing the subepithelial connective tissue graft: case reports. *Pract Periodontics Aesthet Dent.* 1994; 6:47–53.

Corn H. Periosteal separation – its clinical significance. *J Periodontol.* 1962; 33:140–152.

Costich ER, Ramfjord SF. Healing after partial denudation of the alveolar process. *J Periodontol.* 1968; 39:5–12.

Daprile G, Gatto MR, Checchi L. The evaluation of buccal gingival recessions in a student population: a 5-year follow-up. *J Periodontol.* 2007; 78:611–614.

Devishree, Gujjari SK, Shubhashini PV. Frenectomy: a review with the reports of surgical techniques. *J Clin Diagn Res.* 2012; 6(9):1587–1592.

Donnenfeld OW, Marks RM, Glickman I. The apically repositioned flap – a clinical study. *J Periodontol.* 1964; 35:381–387.

Dorfman HS, Kennedy JE, Bird WC. Longitudinal evaluation of free gingival grafts. A four-year report. *J Periodontol.* 1982; 53:349–352.

Edel A. Clinical evaluation of free connective tissue grafts used to increase the width of keratinized gingiva. *J Clin Periodontol.* 1974; 1:185–196.

Ericsson I, Lindhe J. Recession in sites with inadequate width of the keratinized gingiva. An experimental study in the dog. *J Clin Periodontol.* 1984; 11:95–103.

Freedman AL, Green K, Salkin LM, Stein MD, Mellado JR. An 18-year longitudinal study of untreated mucogingival defects. *J Periodontol.* 1999; 70:1174–1176.

Friedman N. Mucogingival surgery. *Tex Dent J.* 1957; 75:358–362.

Friedman N. Mucogingival surgery: the apically repositioned flap. *J Periodontol.* 1962; 33:328–340.

Gamborena I, Avila-Ortiz G. Peri-implant marginal mucosa defects: classification and clinical management. *J Periodontol.* 2021; 92(7):947–957.

Garrett J, Crigger M, Egelberg J. Effects of citric acid on diseased root surfaces. *J Periodontal Res.* 1978; 13:155–163.

Gobbato L, Avila-Ortiz G, Sohrabi K, Wang CW, Karimbux N. The effect of keratinized mucosa width on peri-implant health: a systematic review. *Int J Oral Maxillofac Implants.* 2013; 28:1536–1545.

Graziani F, Gennai S, Roldan S et al. Efficacy of periodontal plastic procedures in the treatment of multiple gingival recessions. *J Clin Periodontol.* 2014; 41(Suppl 15):S63–S76.

Haghighati F, Mousavi M, Moslemi N, Kebria MM, Golestan B. A comparative study of two root-coverage techniques with regard to interdental papilla dimension as a prognostic factor. *Int J Periodontics Restorative Dent.* 2009; 29:179–189.

Hall WB. The current status of mucogingival problems and their therapy. *J Periodontol.* 1981; 52:569–575.

Hanes P, O'Brien N, Garnick J. A morphological comparison of radicular dentin following root planing and treatment with citric acid or tetracycline HCl. *J Clin Periodontol.* 1991; 18:660–668.

Hanes P, Polson A, Ladenheim S. Cell and fiber attachment to demineralized dentin from normal root surfaces. *J Periodontol.* 1985; 56:752–765.

Harris RJ. The connective tissue with partial thickness double pedicle graft: the results of 100 consecutively-treated defects. *J Periodontol.* 1994; 65:448–461.

Harris RJ. Clinical evaluation of 3 techniques to augment keratinized tissue without root coverage. *J Periodontol.* 2001; 72:932–938.

Hawley CE, Staffileno H. Clinical evaluation of free gingival grafts in periodontal surgery. *J Periodontol.* 1970; 41:105–112.

Holbrook T, Ochsenbein C. Complete coverage of the denuded root surface with a one-stage gingival graft. *Int J Periodontics Restorative Dent.* 1983; 3:9–27.

Hwang D, Wang HL. Flap thickness as a predictor of root coverage: a systematic review. *J Periodontol.* 2006; 77:1625–1634.

Isler SC, Uraz A, Kaymaz O, Cetiner D. An evaluation of the relationship between peri-implant soft tissue biotype and the severity of peri-implantitis: a cross-sectional study. *Int J Oral Maxillofac Implants.* 2019; 34:187–196.

Karring T, Nyman S, Thilander B, Magnusson I, Lindhe J. Bone regeneration in orthodontically produced alveolar bone dehiscences. *J Periodontal Res.* 1982; 17:309–315.

Kennedy JE, Bird WC, Palcanis KG, Dorfman HS. A longitudinal evaluation of varying widths of attached gingiva. *J Clin Periodontol.* 1985; 12:667–675.

Khocht A, Simon G, Person P, Denepitiya JL. Gingival recession in relation to history of hard toothbrush use. *J Periodontol.* 1993; 64:900–905.

Kim BS, Kim YK, Yun PY et al. Evaluation of peri-implant tissue response according to the presence of keratinized mucosa. *Oral Surg Oral Med Oral Pathol Oral Radiol Endod.* 2009; 107:e24–e28.

Kim DM, Neiva R. Periodontal soft tissue non-root coverage procedures: a systematic review from the AAP Regeneration Workshop. *J Periodontol.* 2015; 86(S2):S56–S72.

Lang NP, Löe H. The relationship between the width of keratinized gingiva and gingival health. *J Periodontol.* 1972; 43:623–627.

Lang NP, Karing T. (ed.), Proceedings of the 1st European Workshop on Periodontology. *Consensus report of session II.* Berlin: Quintessence; 1994: 210–214.

Lekovic V, Kenney EB, Weinlaender M et al. A bone regenerative approach to alveolar ridge maintenance following tooth extraction. Report of 10 cases. *J Periodontol.* 1997; 68:563–570.

Lindhe J, Lang NP, Karring T. Mucogingival therapy. Periodontal plastic surgery. In: E Ermes (ed.), *Clinical Periodontology and Implant Dentistry.* Oxford: Blackwell Munksgaard; 2008: 995–1043.

Lindhe J, Nyman S. Alterations of the position of the marginal soft tissue following periodontal surgery. *J Clin Periodontol.* 1980; 7:525–530.

Löe H, Ånerud Å, Boysen H. The natural history of periodontal disease in man: prevalence, severity, extent of gingival recession. *J Periodontol.* 1992; 63:489–495.

Löst C. Depth of alveolar bone dehiscences in relation to gingival recessions. *J Clin Periodontol.* 1984; 11:583–589.

Mailoa J, Arnett M, Chan HL et al. The association between buccal mucosa thickness and peri-implant bone loss and attachment loss: a cross-sectional study. *Implant Dent.* 2018; 27:575–581.

Matter J. Free gingival grafts for the treatment of gingival recession. A review of some techniques. *J Clin Periodontol.* 1982; 9:103–114.

Mazzotti C, Stefanini M, Felice P et al. Soft-tissue dehiscence coverage at peri-implant sites. *Periodontol 2000.* 2018; 77:256–272.

McGuire MK, Nunn ME. Evaluation of the safety and efficacy of periodontal applications of a living tissue-engineered human fibroblast-derived dermal substitute. I. Comparison to the gingival autograft: a randomized controlled pilot study. *J Periodontol.* 2005; 76:867–880.

Meffert RM, Langer B, Fritz ME. Dental implants: a review. *J Periodontol.* 1992; 63:859–870.

Melsen B, Allais, D. Factors of importance for the development of dehiscences during labial movement of mandibular incisors: a retrospective study of adult orthodontic patients. *Am J Orthod Dentofacial Orthop.* 2005; 127:552–561.

Miller AJ, Brunelle JA, Carlos JP, Brown LJ, Löe H. *Oral Health of United States Adults. National Institute of Dental Research. NIH Publication No. 87-2868.* Bethesda, MD: National Institutes of Health; 1987.

Miller PD. A classification of marginal tissue recession. *Int J Periodontics Restorative Dent.* 1985; 5:8–13.

Mintz SM, Siegel MA, Seider PJ. An overview of oral frena and their association with multiple syndromes and nonsyndromic conditions. *Oral Surg Oral Med Oral Pathol Oral Radiol Endod.* 2005; 99:321–324.

Miyasato M, Crigger M, Egelberg J. Gingival condition in areas of minimal and appreciable width of keratinized gingiva. *J Clin Periodontol.* 1977; 4:200–209.

Mörmann W, Ciancio SG. Blood supply of human gingiva following periodontal surgery. A fluorescein angiographic study. *J Periodontol.* 1977; 48:681–692.

Nobuto T, Imai H, Yamaoka A. Microvascularization of the free gingival autograft. *J Periodontol.* 1988; 59:639–646.

Ochsenbein C. Newer concept of mucogingival surgery. *J Periodontol.* 1960; 31:175–185.

Oles RD, Ibbott CG, Laverty WH. Effects of root curettage and sodium hypochlorite on pedicle flap coverage of localized recession. *J Can Dent Assoc.* 1988; 54:515–517.

Oliveira GHC, Muncinelli EAG. Efficacy of root surface biomodification in root coverage: a systematic review. *J Can Dent Ass.* 2012; 78:c122.

Oliver RG, Löe H, Karring T. Microscopic evaluation of the healing and re-vascularization of free gingival grafts. *J Periodontal Res.* 1968; 3:84–95.

Olsson M, Lindhe J. Periodontal characteristics in individuals with varying form of the upper central incisors. *J Clin Periodontol.* 1991; 18:78–82.

Perussolo J, Souza AB, Matarazzo F, Oliveira RP, Araujo MG. Influence of the keratinized mucosa on the stability of periimplant tissues and brushing discomfort: a 4-year follow-up study. *Clin Oral Implants Res.* 2018; 29:1177–1185.

Pini Prato GP, Baccetti T, Magnani C, Agudio G, Cortellini P. Mucogingival interceptive surgery of buccally-erupted premolars in patients scheduled for orthodontic treatment. I. A seven-year longitudinal study. *J Periodontol.* 2000; 71:172–181.

Pini Prato G, Baldi C, Pagliaro U et al. Coronally advanced flap procedure for root coverage. Treatment of root surface: root planing versus polishing. *J Periodontol.* 1999; 70:1064–1076.

Pini Prato G, Cairo F, Nieri M et al. Coronally advanced flap versus connective tissue graft in the treatment of multiple gingival recessions: a split-mouth study with a 5-year follow-up. *J Clin Periodontol.* 2010: 37: 644–650.

Pini-Prato G, Franceschi D, Rotundo R et al. Long-term 8-year outcomes of coronally advanced flap for root coverage. *J Periodontol.* 2012; 83:590–594.

Pini Prato GP, Tinti C, Vincenzi G et al. Guided tissue regeneration versus mucogingival surgery in the treatment of human buccal gingival recession. *J Periodontol.* 1992; 63:919–928.

Poli PP, Beretta M, Grossi GB, Maiorana C. Risk indicators related to peri-implant disease: an observational retrospective cohort study. *J Periodontal Implant Sci.* 2016; 46:266–276.

Priyanka M, Sruthi R, Ramakrishnan T, Emmadi P, Ambalavanan N. An overview of frenal attachments. *J Indian Soc Periodontol.* 2013; 17:12–15.

Proceedings of the 1996 World Workshop on Periodontics. Consensus report on mucogingival therapy. *Ann Periodontol.* 1996; 1:702–706.

Richardson CR, Allen EP, Chambrone L et al. Periodontal soft tissue root coverage procedures: practical applications. From the AAP Regeneration Workshop. Clin Adv *Periodontics.* 2015; 5:2–10.

Romanos GE, Bernimoulin JP, Marggraf E. The double lateral bridging flap for coverage of denuded root surface: longitudinal study and clinical evaluation after 5 to 8 years. *J Periodontol.* 1993; 64;683–688.

Ruben MP. A biological rationale for gingival reconstruction by grafting procedures. *Quintessence Int.* 1979; 10:47–55.

Schoo WH, van der Velden U. Marginal soft tissue recessions with and without attached gingiva. *J Periodontal Res.* 1985; 20:209–211.

Seibert JS. Reconstruction of deformed, partially edentulous ridges, using full thickness onlay grafts: I. Technique and wound healing. *Compend Contin Educ Dent.* 1983; 4:437–453.

Seibert JS. Treatment of moderate localized alveolar ridge defects: preventive and reconstructive concepts in therapy. *Dent Clin North Am.* 1993; 37:265–280.

Seibert JS, Louis J. Soft tissue ridge augmentation utilizing a combination onlay-interpositional graft procedure: case report. *Int J Periodontics Restorative Dent.* 1996; 16:311–321.

Serino G, Wennström JL, Lindhe J, Eneroth L. The prevalence and distribution of gingival recession in subjects with high standard of oral hygiene. *J Clin Periodontol.* 1994; 21:57–63.

Staffileno H, Levy S, Gargiulo A. Histologic study of cellular mobilization and repair following a periosteal retention operation via split thickness mucogingival surgery. *J Periodontol.* 1966; 37:117–131.

Stefanini M, Marzadori M, Aroca S et al. Decision making in root coverage procedures for the esthetic outcome. *Periodontol 2000.* 2018; 77:54–64.

Stefanini M, Marzadori M, Tavelli L, Bellone P, Zucchelli G. Peri-implant papillae reconstruction at an esthetically failing implant. *Int J Periodontics Restorative Dent.* 2020; 40:213–222.

Stetler KJ, Bissada NB. Significance of the width of keratinized gingiva on the periodontal status of teeth with submarginal restorations. *J Periodontol.* 1987; 58:696–700.

Studer S, Naef, R, Schärer P. Adjustment of localized alveolar ridge defects by soft tissue transplantation to improve mucogingival esthetics: a proposal for clinical classification and an evaluation of procedures. *Quintessence Int.* 1997; 28:785–805.

Susin C, Haas AN, Oppermann RV, Haugejorden O, Albandar JM. Gingival recession: epidemiology and risk indicators in a representative urban Brazilian population. *J Periodontol.* 2004; 75:1377–1386.

Suzuki M, Okawara J, Ogata Y, Classification and treatment plans of peri-implant soft tissue recession at the anterior zone. *J Implant Adv Clin Dent.* 2012; 4:87–92.

Takei HH, Scheyer ET, Azzi RR, Allen EP, Han TJ. Periodontal plastic and aesthetic surgery. In: MG Newman, HH Takei, PR Klokkevold, FA Carranza (eds), *Newman and Carranza's Clinical Periodontology.* Philadelphia, PA: Elsevier; 2019: 3621–3708.

Thoma DS, Benić GI, Zwahlen M, Hämmerle CH, Jung RE. A systematic review assessing soft tissue augmentation techniques. *Clin Oral Implants Res.* 2009; 20(Suppl 4):146–165.

Tonetti MS, Jepsen S. Clinical efficacy of periodontal plastic surgery procedures: consensus report of Group 2 of the 10th European Workshop on Periodontology. *J Clin Periodontol.* 2014; 41 (Suppl. 15):S36–S43.

Trombelli L, Schincaglia GP, Scapoli C, Calura G. Healing response of human buccal gingival recessions treated with expanded polytetrafluoroethylene membranes. *A retrospective report. J Periodontol.* 1995; 66:14–22.

Trott JR, Love B. An analysis of localized recession in 766 Winnipeg high school students. *Dent Pract Dent Rec.* 1966; 16:209–213.

Valderhaug J. Periodontal conditions and caries lesions following the insertion of fixed prostheses: a 10-year follow-up study. *Int Dent J.* 1980; 30:296–304.

Van Palenstein Helderman WH, Lembariti BS, van der Weijden GA, van't Hof MA. Gingival recession and its association with calculus in subjects deprived of prophylactic dental care. *J Clin Periodontol.* 1998; 25:106–111.

Warrer K, Buser D, Lang NP, Karring T. Plaque-induced peri-implantitis in the presence or absence of keratinized mucosa. An experimental study in monkeys. *Clin Oral Implants Res.* 1995; 6:131–138.

Wei P-C, Laurell L, Geivelis M, Lingen MW, Maddalozzo D. Acellular dermal matrix allografts to achieve increased attached gingival. Part 1. A clinical study. *J Periodontol.* 2000; 71:1297–1305.

Wennström JL. Lack of association between width of attached gingiva and development of gingival recessions. A 5-year longitudinal study. *J Clin Periodontol.* 1987; 14:181–184.

Wennström JL, Derks J. Is there a need for keratinized mucosa around implants to maintain health and tissue stability? *Clin Oral Implants Res.* 2012; 23(Suppl 6):136–116.

Wennström JL, Lindhe J. Plaque-induced gingival inflammation in the absence of attached gingiva in dogs. *J Clin Periodontol.* 1983a; 10:266–276.

Wennström JL, Lindhe J. The role of attached gingiva for maintenance of periodontal health. Healing following excisional and grafting procedures in dogs. *J Clin Periodontol.* 1983b; 10:206–221.

Wennström JL, Lindhe J, Sinclair F, Thilander B. Some periodontal tissue reactions to orthodontic tooth movement in monkeys. *J Clin Periodontol.* 1987; 14:121–129.

Wennström JL, Zucchelli G. Mucogingival therapy: periodontal plastic surgery. In: J Lindhe, NP Lang (eds), *Clinical Periodontology and Implant Dentistry.* Oxford: Wiley; 2015: 969–1042.

Wilderman MN. Exposure of bone in periodontal surgery. *Dent Clin North Am.* 1964; 23–26.

Wilderman MN, Wentz FM. Repair of a dentogingival defect with a pedicle flap. *J Periodontol.* 1965; 36:218–231.

Willey R, Steinberg A. Scanning electron microscopic studies of root dentin surfaces treated with citric acid, elastase, hyaluronidase, pronase and collagenase. *J Periodontol.* 1984; 55:592–596.

Yared KFG, Zenobio EG, Pacheco W. Periodontal status of mandibular central incisors after orthodontic proclination in adults. *Am J Orthod Dentofacial Orthop.* 2006; 130.6.e1–e8.

Yoneyama T, Okamoto H, Lindhe J, Socransky SS, Haffajee AD. Probing depth, attachment loss and gingival recession. Findings from a clinical examination in Ushiku, Japan. *J Clin Periodontol.* 1988; 15:581–591.

Zarb GA, Schmitt A. The longitudinal clinical effectiveness of osseointegrated dental implants: the Toronto study. Part III: Problems and complications encountered. *J Prosthet Dent.* 1990; 64:185–194.

Zucchelli G, De Sanctis M. Treatment of multiple recession-type defects in patients with esthetic demands. *J Periodontol.* 2000; 71:1506–1514.

Zucchelli G, Mazzotti C, Mounssif I et al. A novel surgical-prosthetic approach for soft tissue dehiscence coverage around single implant. *Clin Oral Implants Res.* 2013; 24:957–962.

Zucchelli G, Mazzotti C, Tirone F et al. The connective tissue graft wall technique and enamel matrix derivative to improve root coverage and clinical attachment levels in Miller Class IV gingival recession. *Int J Periodontics Restorative Dent.* 2014; 34:601–609.

Zucchelli G, Mounssif I. Periodontal plastic surgery. *Periodontol 2000.* 2015; 68:333–368.

Zucchelli G, Tavelli L, Stefanini M et al. Classification of facial peri-implant soft tissue dehiscence/deficiencies at single implant sites in the esthetic zone. *J Periodontol.* 2019; 90:1116–1124.

CHAPTER 18
Resective periodontal surgery

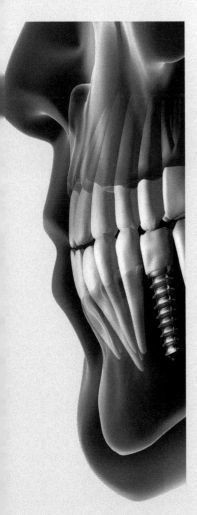

Contents

Essential Periodontics, First Edition. Edited by Steph Smith and Khalid Almas.
© 2022 John Wiley & Sons Ltd. Published 2022 by John Wiley & Sons Ltd.

18.1 GINGIVECTOMY/GINGIVOPLASTY

Arif Salman and Karo Parsegian

Contents

Learning objectives

- Describe the historical and current states of gingivectomy, including the surgical and non-surgical aspects of the procedure.
- Understand the indications and contraindications of gingivectomy using the reported evidence in the literature.
- Identify local, systemic, environmental, and behavioral factors affecting the outcomes of gingivectomy.

Introduction and definition

Gingivectomy is a periodontal surgical procedure aimed at excision of the gingiva to eliminate periodontal pockets. It is usually performed along with gingivoplasty, so as to recontour the gingival margin and create physiological gingival architecture.

As a surgical procedure, gingivectomy was first introduced by Robicsek in 1884, who proposed to perform a straight incision to respect the gingival collar (Stern et al. 1965). Zentler further modified the technique in 1918 by proposing a scalloped incision. The detailed description of the procedure along with armamentarium, gingivectomy indications and contraindications, and adequate postoperative care was first provided by Goldman in 1951, and they have not changed much since then. Gingivectomy is presently not routinely used for the elimination of true periodontal pockets as various other sophisticated flap techniques are available. However, it remains an effective surgical approach when indicated.

Indications and contraindications

Currently acceptable indications for gingivectomy include (Goldman 1946; Levine 1967):

- Elimination of suprabony pockets if the gingiva is firm and fibrotic.
- Gingival enlargement (Mavrogiannis et al. 2006).
- Shallow gingival craters and clefts, commonly observed in cases of necrotizing gingivitis and periodontitis.
- Pericoronal conditions.

- Some cases of altered passive eruption when there is an adequate zone of keratinized gingiva (Mele et al. 2018).

Contraindications (Goldman 1951):

- Inadequate zone of keratinized gingiva and its complete removal as an anticipated outcome of the surgery.
- The presence of bone defects and their access is required as part of the surgery.
- The presence of infrabony pockets.
- Soft and friable gingiva.

Surgical technique

Gingivectomy can be performed using a scalpel, electrosurgery, laser, cryotherapy, and chemical agents (chemosurgery using 5% paraformaldehyde or potassium hydroxide) (Loe 1961; Mavrogiannis et al. 2006; Waite 1965; Wolfsohn 1951). The current chapter is focused on performing gingivectomy using the scalpel (Figures 18.1.1, 18.1.2, and 18.1.3). The technique has been described extensively in the literature (Goldman 1951; Sorrin & Ward 1939).

- Ensure excellent oral hygiene (Stahl et al. 1969) and disinfect the mouth before the procedure, using an antiseptic solution.
- Proper choice of anesthesia (infiltration, interdental). Infiltration anesthesia using 2% lidocaine with 1 : 100 000 epinephrine has been shown to be more effective in terms of surgical time and the amount of blood lost during gingivectomy, compared to inferior alveolar nerve (IAN) block anesthesia using the same anesthetic agent (Hecht & App 1974).

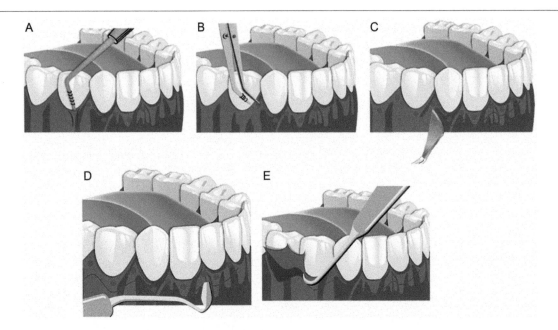

Figure 18.1.1 (A) Probing to determine the depth of suprabony pockets. (B) Pocket marker marking the bleeding points corresponding to the depth of pockets. (C) External bevel incision with Kirkland knife. (D) Interdental incision with Orban knife. (E) Removal of excised gingiva.

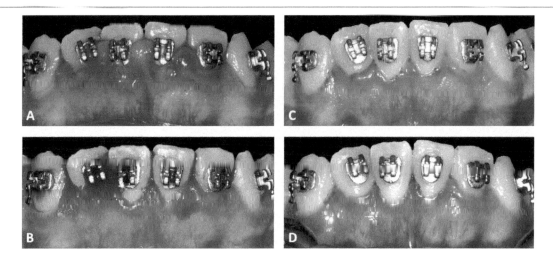

Figure 18.1.2 Inflammatory gingival enlargement during orthodontic therapy treated with external bevel gingivectomy and gingivoplasty using scalpel. (A) Presurgical view showing inflammatory gingival enlargement. (B) External bevel gingivectomy and gingivoplasty performed. (C) Healing at one week. (D) Healing at two weeks shows physiological gingival architecture.

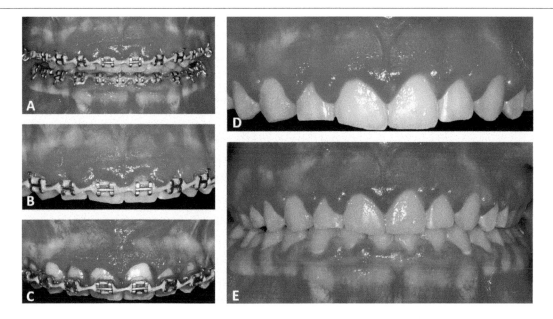

Figure 18.1.3 Inflammatory gingival enlargement during orthodontic therapy treated with internal bevel gingivectomy and gingivoplasty using scalpel. (A, B) Presurgical view showing significant inflammatory gingival enlargement causing difficult access to orthodontic brackets. (C) Internal bevel gingivectomy and gingivoplasty performed with scalpel. (D, E) 10 months postsurgical view at the time of orthodontic brackets removal. Patient has altered passive eruption that needs to be addressed.

- Thorough calculus removal to minimize bleeding and to improve healing and visualization.
- Bone sounding and labeling the depth of periodontal pockets, leaving bleeding points to guide the primary incision line (Figure 18.1.1). The thickness of gingival tissue is an important consideration.
- The primary incision is externally beveled at approximately 45° to the tooth surface, re-creating the normal scalloped gingival morphology. This incision is called an "external bevel incision." The external bevel incision is started apical to the bleeding points marked and directed coronally to a point between the bleeding points and crest of the bone. This incision is usually made with a periodontal knife, called the Kirkland knife. The primary incision is made first on the buccal aspect and then on the lingual aspect. Then, an interdental incision is made with an Orban knife to

separate both buccal and lingual collars of the gingiva, with very little curettage in the interproximal area. Finally, the excised gingiva is removed.

- Thorough removal of remaining calculus and root planing of the root surface.
- Ensure that postoperative bleeding is minimized using gauze, cotton soaked with hemostatic agents, and periodontal packs. Electrosurgical instruments and recently lasers are extremely useful in achieving hemostasis, creating properly festooned gingival margins, and ensuring smooth gingival contours without any tissue tears. Postoperative bleeding after gingivectomy can also be provoked by aspirin (Thomason et al. 1997).

Wound healing following gingivectomy

The healing of soft tissue in the area of the surgery has been described in detail in both animal and human studies.

Animal studies

In a classic study by Engler in 1966, an external bevel incision gingivectomy was performed on Rhesus monkeys, whereby cell proliferation and wound healing dynamics were sequentially studied through a combination of histological and radioautographic techniques (Engler et al. 1966; Ramfjord et al. 1966). Two hours following gingivectomy, the incision surface was covered by a thin fibrinoid in which neutrophils were incorporated. An acute inflammatory reaction had already been established in the connective tissues of the wound margin. In the next few hours, the incision line became sealed with a blood clot and progression of acute inflammation was observed. Thirteen hours after the surgery, there was a band of polymorphonuclear neutrophils covering the wound. This "poly-band" included the superficially degenerated and necrotic connective tissue resulting from the surgical procedure, and also part of the surface blood clot.

Migration and increased synthesis of DNA in epithelial cells started between 12 and 24 hours after surgery and reached a peak activity between 24 and 36 hours. This epithelial cell regeneration and migration started from the wound margin, and reached the tooth surface in 5–6 days, covering a distance of approximately 3 mm at a rate of 0.5 mm per day. These migrating epithelial cells wedged themselves between the "poly-band" and the healing connective tissue. The connective tissue healing started later than the epithelial healing and reached a peak on the third day. Connective tissue healing started 0.3–0.5 mm under the "poly-band," but spread to the rest of the supracrestal tissues after epithelialization of the wound. An upgrowth of this connective tissue of the wound then created a sulcus, which subsequently became epithelialized, and so established a new epithelial attachment. This recreation of the sulcus and epithelial attachment took 3–5 weeks, although the outer surface of the gingiva completely healed and keratinized in 2 weeks. Functional arrangement and collagenous maturation of the gingival connective tissue fibers required 3–5 weeks.

The critical period for complete healing of a gingivectomy wound is between 2 and 5 weeks. For the establishment of a physiological gingival sulcus, meticulous plaque control during this period is important.

Human studies

When performing blade-aided gingivectomy, inflammation has been histologically observed in all samples (Stahl et al. 1968). Clinically, reformation of the gingival contour has been observed around 4 weeks post surgery, and appears to be completed at 8 weeks. Histologically, gingival epithelization was completed at 2 weeks; however, minor inflammation has been observed up to week 8 (Stahl et al. 1969).

The use of periodontal dressing and 0.2% chlorhexidine mouthwashes following the gingivectomy procedure resulted in reduced and clinically insignificant (0.16 mm) differences in probing depth (Addy & Dolby 1976). In this study, an approximately equal proportion of patients preferred either dressing or chlorhexidine.

At 6 months postoperatively, gingivectomy resulted in a greater extent of gingival recession compared to a modified Widman flap procedure (1.9 vs. 1.6 mm, respectively), but no significant differences have been observed in the reduction of deep periodontal pockets (Proestakis et al. 1992).

Reasons for failure of gingivectomy

Levine (1967) described the following reasons that can lead to the failure of gingivectomy.

Prior to surgery

- Poor case selection.
- Poorly controlled systemic conditions that can compromise tissue healing.
- Unreasonable esthetic demands.

During surgery

- Incomplete elimination of the pockets.
- Failure to perform proper gingivoplasty and achieve physiological gingival architecture.
- An irregular and torn gingival margin that can favor the proliferation of granulation tissue.
- Failure to remove calculus and granulation tissue.

After surgery

- Poor patient compliance, oral hygiene, and motivation.
- Failure to address inadequate restorations immediate to the surgical site.

REFERENCES

Addy M, Dolby AE. The use of chlorhexidine mouthwash compared with a periodontal dressing following the gingivectomy procedure. *J Clin Periodontol.* 1976; 3(1):59–65.

Engler WO, Ramfjord SP, Hiniker JJ. Healing following simple gingivectomy. A tritiated thymidine radioautographic study. I. Epithelialization. *J Periodontol.* 1966; 37(4):298–308.

Goldman HM. Gingivectomy; indications, contraindications, and method. *Am J Orthod Oral Surg.* 1946; 32(Oral Surg):323–326.

Goldman HM. Gingivectomy. *Oral Surg Oral Med Oral Pathol.* 1951; 4(9):1136–1157.

Hecht A, App AR. Blood volume lost during gingivectomy using two different anesthetic techniques. *J Periodontol.* 1974; 45(1):9–12.

Levine S. Failures with gingivectomy. *Aus Dent J.* 1967; 12(5):406–410.

Loe H. Chemical gingivectomy effect of potassium hydroxide on periodontal tissues. *Acta Odontol Scand.* 1961; 19:517–535.

Mavrogiannis M, Ellis JS, Thomason JM, Seymour RA. The management of drug-induced gingival overgrowth. *J Clin Periodontol.* 2006; 33(6):434–439.

Mele M, Felice P, Sharma P et al. Esthetic treatment of altered passive eruption. *Periodontol 2000.* 2018; 77(1):65–83.

Proestakis G, Söderholm G, Bratthall G et al. Gingivectomy versus flap surgery: the effect of the treatment of infrabony defects. A clinical and radiographic study. *J Clin Periodontol.* 1992; 19(7):497–508.

Ramfjord SP, Engler WO, Hiniker JJ. A radioautographic study of healing following simple gingivectomy. II. *The connective tissue. J Periodontol.* 1966; 37(3):179–189.

Sorrin S, Ward HL. Gingivectomy: a basic surgical procedure. *J Am Dent Assoc.* 1963; 67:150–151.

Stahl SS, Witkin GL, Dicesare A, Brown R. Gingival healing. I. Description of the gingivectomy sample. *J Periodontol.* 1968; 39(2):106–108.

Stahl SS, Witkin GJ, Heller A, Brown R Jr. Gingival healing. IV. The effects of homecare on gingivectomy repair. *J Periodontol.* 1969; 40(5):264–267.

Stern IB, Everett FG, Robicsek KS. Robicsek—a pioneer in the surgical treatment of periodontal disease. *J Periodontol.* 1965; 36:265–268.

Thomason JM, Seymour RA, Murphy P, Brigham KM, Jones P. Aspirin-induced post-gingivectomy haemorrhage: a timely reminder. *J Clin Periodontol.* 1997; 24(2):136–138.

Waite IM. The present status of the gingivectomy procedure. *J Clin Periodontol.* 1975; 2(4):241–249.

Wolfsohn MD. Modified gingivectomy. *J Periodontol.* 1951; 22(4):212–215.

18.2 PERIODONTAL FLAP SURGERY

Arif Salman and Murugan Thamaraiselvan

Contents

Learning objectives

- Understand the principles of periodontal flap surgery.
- Describe in detail the steps involved in the modified Widman flap.
- Describe in detail the steps involved in the apically repositioned flap.
- Describe in detail the steps involved in the Kirkland flap.
- Describe in detail the steps involved in the papilla preservation flap.

Introduction

Surgical procedures in periodontal therapy involve intentional severing of periodontal tissues for various reasons, like treating periodontal pockets or correcting mucogingival defects. Periodontal flap surgery is one among these surgical procedures that intend to treat periodontal pockets with the aim of eliminating pathological changes in pocket walls, creating an easily maintainable and stable periodontium, and, whenever possible, promoting periodontal regeneration. A periodontal flap is a portion of the gingiva and alveolar mucosa that is surgically separated from the underlying tissues for the purpose of increased visibility and accessibility to the root surface and bone.

Objectives of periodontal flap surgery

Periodontal flap surgery treats periodontal pockets by accomplishing the following objectives:

- To improve accessibility to the root surface that facilitates complete removal of plaque and calculus. As the probing depth increases, accessibility to the roots is impaired with non-surgical therapy. Complete calculus removal with non-surgical therapy is possible only with probing depths that are less than 4 mm (Stambaugh et al. 1981).
- To reduce the pocket depth to a physiological sulcular depth that can be easily maintained plaque free by the patient and the clinician.
- To reshape soft and hard tissues to facilitate and maintain harmonious topography.
- To gain access to deep intrabony defects (≥4 mm) that can be regenerated (Cortellini et al. 1998).

The decision on whether surgery is required for a periodontitis patient can be made at the time of initial treatment planning. However, the final decision is always made at the time of re-evaluation after non-surgical periodontal therapy. Factors like sites with probing depth of ≥5 mm, percentage of bleeding on probing, plaque score, involvement of furcation, presence of deep intrabony defects, tissue response to non-surgical periodontal therapy, and patient compliance should be considered while making the final decision.

The re-evaluation is typically made at least a month after non-surgical periodontal therapy and sometimes even extending to nine months (Badersten et al. 1984). This time frame allows for several advantages, such as:

- Resolution of inflammation resulting in fibrous tissue consistency that is conducive for surgical handling.
- Resolution of inflammation reveals the residual pocket depth, which determines whether periodontal flap surgery is required or not.
- It allows for the patient to get accustomed to the recommended oral hygiene practices that will determine the long-term success of the therapy. A lack of adequate self-performed

plaque control by the patient is a contraindication for flap surgery (Nyman et al. 1977; Rosling et al. 1976).

Thus, it is important to understand that periodontal surgery is an addition to non-surgical periodontal therapy in treating periodontal pockets.

Indications

Periodontal flap surgery is indicated in the following clinical scenarios:

- Moderate to deep periodontal pockets that do not resolve after thorough and adequate non-surgical periodontal therapy (presence of sites with probing depth of ≥ 5 mm after non-surgical periodontal therapy) (Matuliene et al. 2008).
- Correction of bone architecture that may favor recurrence of periodontal disease (presence of craters and negative bone architecture) (Schluger 1949).
- Presence of periodontal pockets in difficult-to-access areas like furcations.
- Exposure of alveolar bone to perform resective/regenerative therapy (presence of intrabony defects of ≥4 mm) (Cortellini et al. 1998).

The use of flap technique to treat periodontal pockets dates back to 1918, which includes the original Widman flap. Following this, several other surgical techniques were developed in the twentieth century. All these flap techniques involve the use of a combination of horizontal and vertical incisions.

Modified Widman flap

This flap technique was described by Ramfjord and Nissle in 1974, for improving access to the root and bone surface. It is the most preferred flap technique when the intention is to reduce the pocket depth and gain attachment. The technique involves the following steps:

The first incision is a scalloped internal bevel incision that is started 0.5–1 mm away from the gingival margin and directed toward the alveolar crest parallel to the long axis of the tooth. This incision eliminates the pocket lining, creates a knife-edge gingival margin, and exposes the connective tissue of the gingiva to be placed against the root surface. The scalloping effect of the incision is exaggerated on the palatal aspect to achieve an optimal interproximal flap closure. If the probing depths are shallow and/or esthetic considerations exist, a crevicular incision can be used.

The second incision, the sulcular or crevicular incision, is started from the base of the pocket and directed toward the alveolar crest. At this stage, through the internal bevel incision, a full-thickness flap is elevated to expose alveolar bone not more than 2–3 mm from the alveolar crest.

This facilitates the placement of the third incision, the interdental incision, which is done on the alveolar crest to detach the diseased pocket lining from the underlying bone, especially over the interdental bone.

Following this, the loosened collar of gingival tissue around the tooth neck is totally detached and removed using a sharp curette. The exposed root surfaces are scaled and planed with ultrasonic scalers and curettes.

Next, the buccal and lingual flaps are adapted to the bone and to each other interproximally. If the adaptation between flaps is incomplete, particularly in the interproximal region, thinning of the flaps and/or osteoplasty of the bone may be necessary to enhance flap adaptation.

Finally, the flaps are sutured interproximally with interrupted sutures. Periodontal dressing may be placed to hold the flaps tightly against the bone. The sutures and dressing are removed after one week, the teeth are polished, and the patient is instructed in oral hygiene.

Apically repositioned flap

New surgical techniques to treat periodontal pockets were introduced in the 1950s and 1960s. During this time, the importance of retaining an adequate zone of keratinized tissue after periodontal surgery was emphasized. The apically repositioned flap was a modification of an original technique called "repositioning the attached gingiva" proposed by Nabers in 1954 and later modified by Ariaudo and Tyrrell in 1957. Friedman in 1962 refined this technique and called it an apically repositioned flap. According to Friedman, the entire complex of gingiva, alveolar mucosa, periosteum, and all the structures within the flap are moved apically and sutured into position so that the margin of the flap just covers the crest of the alveolar bone. In this way, the mucogingival complex forms the new investing tissue while eliminating the pocket. The technique involves the following steps:

First, a scalloped internal bevel incision is made to adequately thin the fibrotic gingiva. The depth of the pockets and the thickness and width of gingiva determine how far this incision will be from the gingival margin. If the keratinized gingiva is minimal and thin, the internal bevel incision will be made close to the gingival margin.

Next, vertical releasing incisions extending beyond the mucogingival junction are made at both ends of the internal bevel incision to facilitate apical repositioning of the flap at the end of surgery. A full-thickness mucoperiosteal flap is reflected beyond the mucogingival junction. The remaining collar of gingiva around the neck of the teeth is removed with curettes and thorough scaling and root planing are performed.

Osseous surgery is next performed to correct interdental craters and negative bone architecture. The goal is to recreate a physiological bone architecture, but at a more apical level. Finally, buccal and lingual flaps are repositioned apically and sutured into position so that the margin of the flap just covers the alveolar crest. A periodontal dressing may be placed. The

sutures and dressing are removed after one week, the teeth polished, and the patient is instructed in oral hygiene. If performed properly, this technique will result in the elimination of pockets, including the preservation of an adequate zone of gingiva.

Kirkland flap

Kirkland in 1931 described a surgical technique called the "modified flap operation" to treat periodontal pockets. The goal of this access flap technique (Figures 18.2.1 and 18.2.2) is to provide access to the root surfaces for proper root debridement. In this technique, no submarginal incisions are utilized, and the flap is returned to its original position at the end of surgery. This minimizes post-surgical gingival recession and is of great value when esthetic considerations are high. The technique involves the following steps:

The surgery is started with a sulcular incision from the base of the pocket to the alveolar crest. This incision is placed both on the buccal and lingual sides and extended mesiodistally as needed. A full-thickness mucoperiosteal flap is reflected, taking care to preserve all the interproximal tissue and to give adequate access to the root surfaces. The roots are scaled and planed. Granulation tissue is removed from the inner aspect of the flap and the flap is returned to its original position and held with interproximal sutures.

Papilla preservation flap

A periodontal pocket in an interdental region can sometimes be seen with a wide interdental space between the teeth. In this case, conventional flap techniques would usually split the wide papilla in the interdental region into buccal and lingual flaps. A papilla preservation flap in turn would preserve the entire papilla without splitting it, and incorporate it into either a buccal or lingual flap. This preserved papilla can help to contain and secure any graft material placed in the intrabony defect and minimize the amount of recession postoperatively. Takei and colleagues introduced the papilla preservation flap technique in 1985. Modifications to the original technique were later introduced by Cortellini and colleagues in 1995 and 1999. These were called the "modified papilla preservation flap" (Figure 18.2.3) and "simplified papilla preservation flap," to be used in conjunction with regenerative therapies. The technique involves the following steps:

A crevicular incision around the tooth with periodontal pockets is made without splitting the interdental papilla. A semilunar incision on one side of the involved papilla is made, starting from the line angle of one tooth to the line angle of the adjacent tooth, connecting the crevicular incisions. The semilunar incision can be done on the buccal or lingual side, depending on whether the papilla is to be included on the

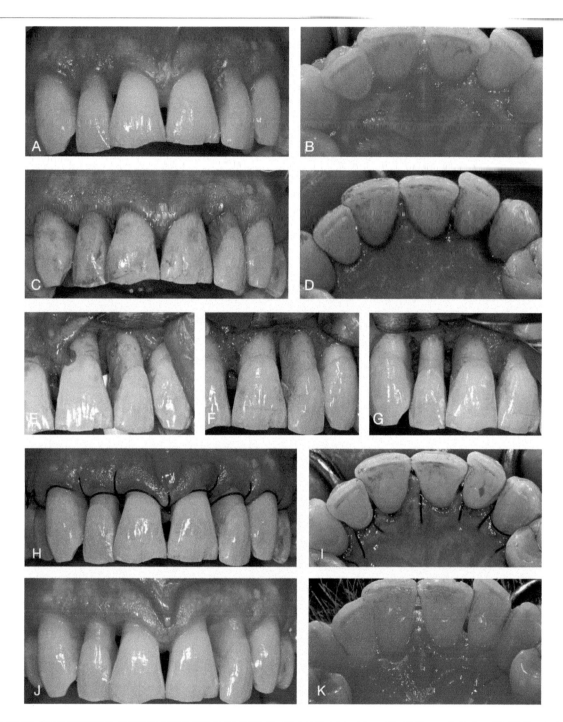

Figure 18.2.1 Deep pockets in maxillary anterior teeth treated with access flap procedure. (A, B) Presurgical view. (C, D) Crevicular incisions placed on the buccal and palatal. (E) Buccal and palatal full-thickness flaps reflected, showing the presence of calculus on the mesial aspect of the maxillary left lateral incisor. (F, G) Teeth scaled and root planed thoroughly. (H, I) Flaps repositioned with continuous sling suture. (J, K) Healing at three months.

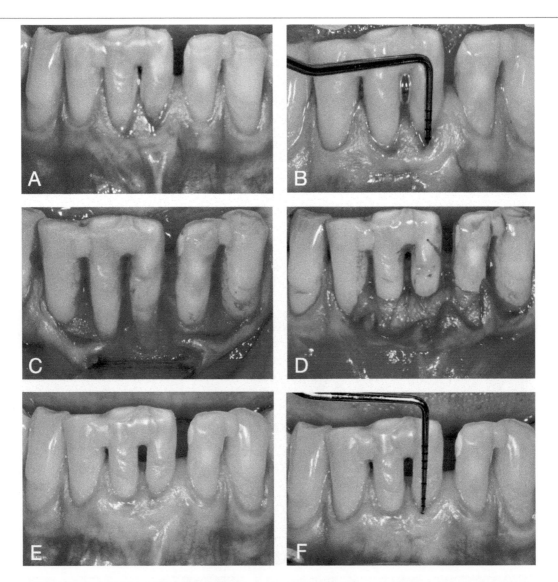

Figure 18.2.2 Deep pocket in mandibular left central incisor with a mucogingival defect treated with access flap procedure and connective tissue graft. (A, B) Presurgical view showing 6 mm pocket on the mid-buccal aspect, with the base of the pocket apical to the mucogingival junction. Also notice the aberrant frenum attachment. (C) Crevicular incision placed, and buccal full-thickness flap reflected. Thorough scaling and root planing performed. (D) A connective tissue graft is harvested from the palate and stabilized at the surgical site to manage the mucogingival defect. (E, F) Healing at six months shows complete resolution of deep pocket and apical displacement of frenal attachment.

lingual or buccal flap respectively. The semilunar incision must be at least 3 mm apical to the margin of the interproximal bony defect. This will ensure that the flap margin is adequately away from the defect to be grafted, and that the graft material will be completely covered by the intact papillary tissue at the time of suturing.

Flap reflection is started after completion of the incisions. A curette and/or interproximal knife is used to free the interdental papilla from the underlying bone. It is important that the interdental papilla is completely free and mobile before proceeding to its reflection. The detached interdental papilla is carefully pushed through the embrasure with a blunt instru-

ment so that the flap can be easily reflected with the papilla intact. Full-thickness buccal and lingual flaps are reflected to enable access to the underlying bony defect.

The roots are scaled and planed. Granulation tissue is completely removed from the bony defect and the bony defect morphology is then assessed. If the defect is a regeneratable one, appropriate graft material is used. Flaps are repositioned and stabilized with cross-mattress sutures. Alternatively, a direct suture of the semilunar incisions can be done as the only means of flap closure. A periodontal dressing may be placed. The sutures and dressing are removed after one week, the teeth are polished, and the patient is instructed in oral hygiene.

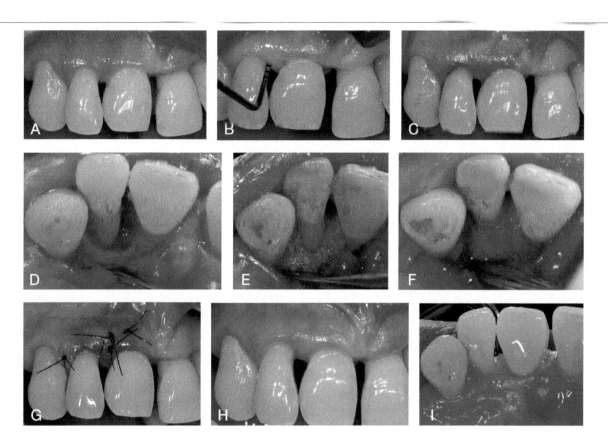

Figure 18.2.3 Deep pocket in maxillary right lateral incisor treated with modified papilla preservation flap procedure. (A, B) Presurgical view showing 8 mm pocket on the mesio-buccal aspect of the maxillary right lateral incisor. Notice the wide interproximal space. (C) Incision design. (D) Full-thickness flap reflected, with the interproximal tissue attached to the palatal flap. Notice the intrabony defect. (E, F) Intrabony defect grafted with an appropriate bone graft and covered with a collagen membrane. (G) Flap repositioned and sutured. (H, I) Healing at nine months with very minimal recession post surgery.

REFERENCES

Ariaudo AA, Tyrell HA. Repositioning and increasing the zone of attached gingiva. *J Periodontol.* 1957; 28:106–110.

Badersten A, Nilveus R, Egelberg J. Effect of nonsurgical periodontal therapy. II. Severely advanced periodontitis. *J Clin Periodontol.* 1984; 11:63–76.

Cortellini P, Carnevale G, Sanz M, Tonetti MS. Treatment of deep and shallow intrabony defects. A multicenter randomized controlled clinical trial. *J Clin Periodontol.* 1998; 25:981–987.

Cortellini P, Pini Prato G, Tonetti M. The modified papilla preservation technique. A new surgical approach for interproximal regenerative procedures. *J Periodontol.* 1995; 66:261–266.

Cortellini P, Pini Prato G, Tonetti, M. The simplified papilla preservation flap. A novel surgical approach for the management of soft tissues in regenerative procedures. *Int J Periodontics Restorative Dent.* 1999; 19:589–599.

Friedman, N. Mucogingival surgery. *The apically repositioned flap. J Periodontol.* 1962; 33:328–340.

Kirkland O. The suppurative periodontal pus pocket; its treatment by the modified flap operation. *J Am Dent Assoc.* 1931; 18:1462–1470.

Matuliene G, Pjetursson BE, Salvi GE et al. Influence of residual pockets on progression of periodontitis and tooth loss: results after 11 years of maintenance. *J Clin Periodontol.* 2008; 35:685–695.

Nabers CL. Repositioning the attached gingiva. *J Periodontol.* 1954; 25:38–39.

Nyman S, Lindhe J, Rosling B. Periodontal surgery in plaque-infected dentitions. *J Clin Periodontol.* 1977; 4:240–249.

Ramfjord SP, Nissle RR. The modified Widman flap. *J Periodontol.* 1974; 45:601–607.

Rosling B, Nyman S, Lindhe J, Jern B. The healing potential of the periodontal tissues following different techniques of periodontal surgery in plaque-free dentitions. A 2-year clinical study. *J Clin Periodontol.* 1976; 3:233–250.

Schluger S. Osseous resection – a basic principle in periodontal surgery. *Oral Surg Oral Med Oral Pathol Oral Radiol Endod.* 1949; 2:3–12.

Stambaugh RV, Dragoo M, Smith DM, Carasali L. The limits of subgingival scaling. *Int J Periodontics Restorative Dent.* 1981; 1(5):30–41.

Takei HH, Han TJ, Carranza FA, Kennedy EB, Lekovic V. Flap technique for periodontal bone implants. *Papilla preservation technique. J Periodontol.* 1985; 56:204–210.

18.3 OSSEOUS RESECTIVE SURGERY

Arif Salman

Contents

Learning objectives

- Understand the principles of osseous resective surgery.
- Understand indications and contraindications of osseous surgery using the reported evidence in the literature.
- Describe in detail the steps involved in osseous surgery.
- Understand the rationale behind the two most commonly utilized osseous surgical approaches, namely the palatal and lingual approaches.

Introduction and definition

Elimination of periodontal pockets is a fundamental objective of periodontal therapy, as it ensures that the natural dentition can be saved and maintained in comfort and function. At the beginning of the twentieth century, gingivectomy was regarded as the treatment of choice to achieve pocket elimination. However, its effectiveness to achieve pocket elimination in all clinical scenarios and to maintain the results in the long term became questionable. Schluger for the first time in 1949 observed that osseous deformities that result as a consequence of periodontal disease are the reason for failure of gingivectomy to achieve pocket elimination, and so presented the concept of osseous surgery. Osseous resective surgery is defined as the surgical removal of a portion of gingiva and reshaping the bone to achieve a physiological architecture of bone (Friedman 1955). Osteoplasty and ostectomy are performed as part of osseous surgery to achieve this. Osteoplasty involves reshaping and removing non-supporting bone around teeth, and ostectomy involves the removal of supporting bone (Friedman 1955).

Objectives

- To eliminate periodontal pockets and to achieve shallow probing depths (≤3 mm) that are well maintainable (Carnevale & Kaldahl 2000).
- To recreate a gingival tissue morphology that enhances good self-performed oral hygiene and periodontal health (Carnevale & Kaldahl 2000).

Rationale

In a healthy periodontium, the interdental bony crest is coronal to the crest of radicular bone on the facial and palatal/lingual root surfaces, and this is called "positive bone architecture" (Ochsenbein & Bohannan 1963). The overlying marginal gingiva also follows the same scalloped pattern. The development of an interproximal pocket leads to a change in this physiological architecture and the resulting osseous defect is most commonly an interdental crater (Figure 18.3.1) (Ochsenbein & Bohannan 1963). A crater is a saucer-shaped buccolingual concavity produced when resorption of the

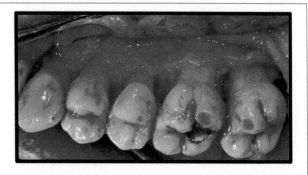

Figure 18.3.1 Interdental craters between posterior teeth.

interdental crestal bone occurs between the buccal and lingual cortical plates. Craters account for almost half of the bony defects seen in periodontitis patients (Vrotsos et al. 1999). The traditional technique of osseous surgery is aimed at eliminating the interdental crater to achieve a physiological bone architecture. It uses both osteoplasty and ostectomy to re-establish the marginal bone morphology around the teeth to resemble "normal bone with a positive architecture," albeit at a more apical position (Carnevale & Kaldahl 2000). Osteoplasty is used to treat buccal and lingual bony ledges or tori, shallow (≤3 mm) lingual or buccal intrabony defects, thick interproximal areas, and incipient furcation involvements that do not necessitate removing supporting bone (Friedman 1955; Ochsenbein 1958). An ostectomy is utilized to treat shallow (1–2 mm deep) to medium (3–4 mm deep) intrabony craters and hemiseptal osseous defects, and to correct negative architecture (Goldman & Cohen 1958; Ochsenbein 1986; Schluger 1949).

Indications and contraindications for osseous surgery

Indications

- Probing depth in the range of 5–8 mm.
- Presence of shallow (1–2 mm deep) to medium (3–4 mm deep) interdental craters.
- Presence of buccal and lingual bony ledges, tori, or buttressing bone formation.
- Incipient furcation involvements that do not necessitate removing supporting bone.
- To treat advanced furcation defects with root resection or hemisection.
- Clinical crown lengthening.

Contraindications

- Sites with very deep pockets (>8 mm probing depth).
- Intrabony defects that can be regenerated (intrabony component ≥4 mm deep).
- Deep craters where defect elimination may lead to opening an uninvolved furcation (≥5 mm deep).
- Sites where aesthetics is of high concern.

Surgical technique

In osseous resective surgery, the approach of eliminating an intrabony crater and its periodontal pocket is to remove the walls of bone that make up the defect, and to place the gingival complex in a more apical position. To achieve the desired physiologically scalloped bone anatomy, reversals in the osseous topography (i.e. when the surface of the facial or lingual radicular bone is in a more coronal position than the interproximal bone) are also corrected. The removal of both supporting bone (ostectomy) and non-supporting bone (osteoplasty) from the involved tooth or adjacent teeth with the utilization of an apically positioned flap is called osseous resective surgery (Carnevale & Kaldahl 2000).

Incision design and flap management

The primary scalloped incision of the apically positioned flap can be intrasulcular or at various distances from the free gingival margin (Figure 18.3.2). The interproximal bone sounding depth and the width of the keratinized gingiva dictate the design and the position of this incision. If there is an adequate width of keratinized gingiva, the distance of the primary incision from the gingival margin is proportional to the differences in the interproximal bone sounding measurements of the adjacent teeth. The apical repositioning of the flap allows the gingival margin to coincide finally with the osseous crest. If the keratinized gingival width is inadequate, the primary incision is placed intrasulcularly. In this case, vertical releasing incisions can facilitate the flap to be repositioned apically at the alveolar crest (Carnevale & Kaldahl 2000).

Following the scalloped incision, a flap is reflected to expose the underlying bone surrounding the teeth. A secondary flap delineated by the scalloped incision is then removed with sulcular and interdental incisions. At this stage, complete removal of granulation tissue and calculus is performed. This will give adequate access to the type of bone defects that are present and to correct them with osteoplasty and ostectomy.

Hard tissue management

Hard tissue management primarily involves elimination of interdental craters, correction of negative bone architecture, and removal of ledges.

Interdental craters

One approach is to remove both walls of bone of an intrabony crater so that the previously apically located base of the defect is now even with the adjacent bone (Goldman & Cohen 1958). With this approach, the removal of the buccal wall of the crater may lead to negative bone architecture that will necessitate the removal of tooth-supporting bone on the buccal. The other approach is to remove only one wall of the crater, mostly the palatal or lingual wall, thereby creating an apical slope of the interproximal bone crest, from a buccal to lingual direction (Figure 18.3.3) (Tibbetts et al. 1976). This is called palatal or lingual ramping. Mandibular molars usually tilt lingually and therefore the lingual furcation as well as the lingual cementoenamel junction are in a more apical location than the corresponding buccal area (Tibbetts et al. 1976). Hence, removal of

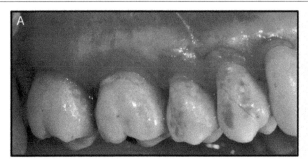
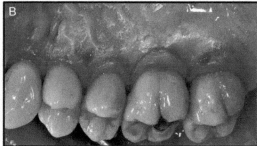

Figure 18.3.2 Primary scalloped and double-scalloped incision. (A) Buccal view; (B) Palatal view.

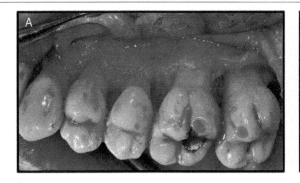
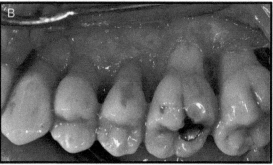

Figure 18.3.3 Palatal ramping and correction of negative architecture. (A) Prior to osteoplasty and ostectomy; (B) After osteoplasty and ostectomy. The ledge seen on the palatal of second molar underwent osteoplasty. The palatal wall of the crater was removed to enable ramping and ostectomy performed on the radicular palatal surfaces to achieve positive architecture.

the lingual wall of the crater may require only minimal radicular bone removal. Similarly, removal of the palatal wall of the crater coupled with marginal bone reduction avoids the possibility of opening an uninvolved buccal furcation (Ochsenbein & Bohannan 1963).

Correction of negative architecture

Negative bony architecture (that is, facial or lingual radicular osseous surfaces being in a more coronal position than the interproximal surface) is often present as a result of periodontitis or when an ostectomy is performed to eliminate the interdental crater. This anatomic situation is the reverse of normal, and its correction is performed by removing the facial and/or lingual bone over the roots to a level where its radicular osseous margin is apical to the interproximal bone level (Figure 18.3.3). This re-creates the physiological scalloped appearance of the alveolus from a facial and/or lingual view (Carnevale & Kaldahl 2000).

Removal of ledges

The alveolar margin may be associated with a ledge, an exostosis, a bony protuberance, or a buttressing bone, which can comprise the physiological form and periodontal maintenance of the area. This abnormally thick bony anatomy over a tooth or several teeth is thinned to a more normal width during osseous resective surgery (Figure 18.3.3) (Carnevale & Kaldahl 2000). Alveolar bone on the facial and lingual aspects of the interproximal region is often removed, by means of creating vertical grooves or interproximal "sluice-ways." However, the created sluice-ways can fill in with bone during healing and remodeling (Moghaddas & Stahl 1980).

Approaches to osseous crater management

Traditional approach

In the early years of osseous surgery, the "buccal approach" was employed to eliminate osseous craters owing to its ease of surgical access. Following a submarginal scalloped incision, a buccal flap was reflected. A secondary flap was next removed with sulcular and interdental incisions. Complete removal of granulation tissue and calculus was then performed. This gave access to the buccal wall of the crater, which was removed along with the adjacent marginal bone. After elimination of the crater, a flap was apically positioned and sutured. Some clinicians advocated the removal of both buccal and lingual walls of the crater, thereby establishing the base of the crater as the new tip of the surgically prepared interdental cone of the bone. Although the buccal approach produced acceptable results, the following concerns were noticed in the long term (Ochsenbein & Bohannan 2000):

- Reverse gingival architecture and subsequent postoperative development of a bulbous interradicular papilla.
- Denudation of buccal radicular surfaces.

- Buccal recession.
- Inadequate buccal embrasure space.

To overcome concerns encountered with the buccal approach, Ochsenbein and Bohannan (2000) proposed a "palatal approach" to osseous surgery in maxillary molars, and Tibbetts et al. (1976) proposed a "lingual approach" to osseous surgery in mandibular molars.

Palatal approach

With the palatal approach, gross reduction of the crater is done from the palatal side and every attempt is made to preserve and maintain bone height on the facial (Figure 18.3.4). However, if osseous problems exist on the buccal aspect, they must be corrected from the buccal. An example is correction of negative bone architecture. There are a few anatomic considerations that make the palatal approach more ideal for osseous surgery (Ochsenbein & Bohannan 2000):

- Palatal bone is usually thicker than buccal bone and most likely presents with cancellous bone. This is beneficial during wound healing as postsurgical bone resorption may be minimal.
- The entire palate is covered by masticatory mucosa and is attached. A scalloping incision can be more pronounced in palatal compared to buccal.
- Variation in tooth form from palatal to buccal has surgical advantages. The removal of the palatal wall of the crater, coupled with marginal bone reduction, avoids the possibility of opening an uninvolved buccal furcation.
- The embrasure space is wider palatally compared to buccal. The wide embrasure space provides easy access to interdental bone.
- The tongue has a cleansing effect on the palatal tissues.

Lingual approach

With the lingual approach, gross reduction of the crater is done from the lingual side and every attempt is made to preserve and maintain bone height on the facial. However, if osseous problems exist on the buccal aspect, they must be corrected from the buccal. An example is correction of negative bone architecture. There are a few anatomic considerations that make the lingual approach more ideal for osseous surgery (Tibbetts et al. 1976):

- Mandibular posteriors usually tilt lingually and therefore the lingual furcation as well as the lingual cementoenamel junction are in a more apical location than the corresponding buccal area.
- Root trunk length of mandibular molars is shorter buccally than lingually.
- Interdental craters are usually located more toward the lingual (directly below the contact area).
- Wider lingual embrasures usually provide more access for surgery.
- On the buccal, a thick shelf of bone and a shallow vestibule accompany the external oblique ridge.

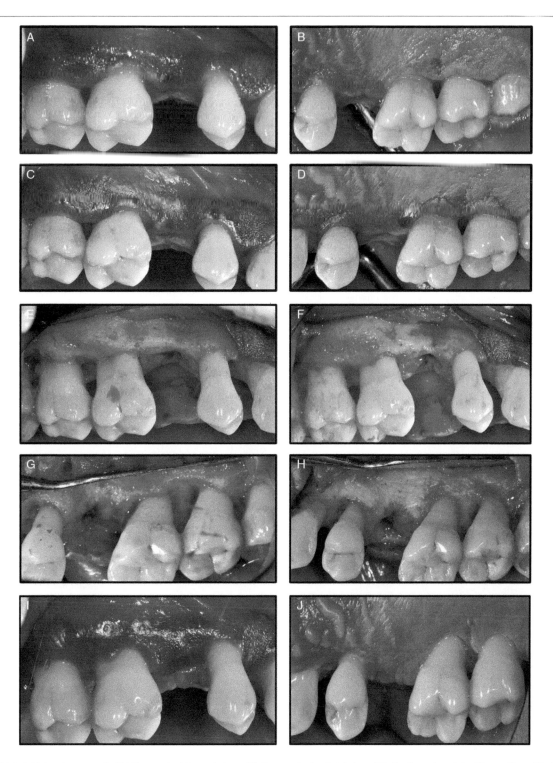

Figure 18.3.4 Palatal approach. (A) Presurgical buccal view; (B) Presurgical palatal view; (C) Scalloped and double-scalloped incision on the buccal; (D) Scalloped incision on the palatal. (E) Prior to osteoplasty and ostectomy on the buccal: ledge, buttressing bone formation, and negative bone architecture seen. (F) After osteoplasty and ostectomy on the buccal. (G) Prior to osteoplasty and ostectomy on the palatal: ledge, interdental crater, and negative bone architecture seen. (H) After osteoplasty and ostectomy on the palatal; crater ramped toward palatal and positive bone architecture achieved. (I) Three-month postsurgical buccal view: notice the open interproximal spaces and apical positioning of the gingival margin. (J) Three-month postsurgical palatal view: notice the open interproximal spaces and apical positioning of the gingival margin.

Healing following osseous surgery

Soft and hard tissue healing following osseous surgery has been widely documented in the literature. The changes in the probing depth, attachment level, and the position of the free gingival margin have been studied.

Soft tissue changes

The magnitude of recession immediately following osseous resective surgery decreases somewhat during the first postoperative year with a coronal shift of the gingival margin (Carnevale & Kaldahl 2000). Osseous resective surgery has been shown to significantly decrease probing depths, with the magnitude of decrease declining longitudinally over time, but never reaching preoperative levels (Carnevale & Kaldahl 2000). Probing depths, clinical attachment levels, and gingival margin locations obtained in the immediate post-healing phase after osseous resective surgery may show some change over time. However, it has been shown long term (5 or 7 years) that these changes are not likely to reach pre-treatment levels (Kaldahl et al. 1996; Townsend-Olsen et al. 1985).

Hard tissue changes

Selipsky (1976), in a classic study, demonstrated that ostectomy performed during osseous resective surgery removed a mean of 0.6 mm of supporting bone height per tooth on a circumferential average. Selipsky (1976) argued that, even though a considerable amount of bone is removed on one surface of the tooth, the average bone reduction per tooth is negligible. In this study, tooth mobility slightly increased after surgery, but returned to pre-treatment levels after one year post surgery.

Importance of plaque control

The patient's ability to remove plaque effectively is an important factor in healing and periodontal stability following osseous surgery. Rosling et al. (1976), in another classic study, demonstrated that, following surgical therapy with osseous recontouring, patients with good plaque control and periodic periodontal maintenance therapy remained stable. On the other hand, Nyman et al. (1977) showed that patients who had poor plaque control and lacked periodontal maintenance therapy had increased probing depths and further loss of attachment over a two-year postsurgical period.

Conclusion

Osseous resective surgery in combination with an apically positioned flap, when properly performed, achieves a physiological bone architecture that allows proper healing of the gingival flap with shallow probing depths, which can be maintained in the long term.

REFERENCES

Carnevale G, Kaldahl WB. Osseous resective surgery. *Periodontol 2000.* 2000; 22:59–87.

Friedman N. Periodontal osseous surgery: osteoplasty and ostectomy. *J Periodontol.* 1955; 26:257–269.

Goldman HM, Cohen DW. The infrabony pocket: classification and treatment. *J Periodontol.* 1958; 29:272–291.

Kaldahl WB, Kalkwarf KL, Patil KD, Molvar MP, Dyer JK. Long-term evaluation of periodontal therapy. I. Response to 4 therapeutic modalities. *J Periodontol.* 1996; 67:93–102.

Moghaddas H, Stahl SS. Alveolar bone remodeling following osseous surgery. *A clinical study. J Periodontol.* 1980; 51:376–381.

Nyman S, Lindhe J, Rosling B. Periodontal surgery in plaque-infected dentitions. *J Clin Periodontol.* 1977; 4:240–249.

Ochsenbein C. Osseous resection in periodontal surgery. *J Periodontol.* 1958; 29:15–26.

Ochsenbein C. A primer for osseous surgery. *Int J Periodontics Restorative Dent.* 1986; 6(1):8–47.

Ochsenbein C, Bohannan HM. The palatal approach to osseous surgery. I. Rationale. *J Periodontol.* 1963; 34(1):60–68.

Rosling B, Nyman S, Lindhe J, Jern B. The healing potential of periodontal tissues following different techniques of periodontal surgery in plaque-free dentitions. A 2-year clinical study. *J Clin Periodontol.* 1976; 3:233–250.

Schluger S. Osseous resection – a basic principle in periodontal surgery. *Oral Surg Oral Med Oral Pathol Oral Radiol Endod.* 1949; 2:3–12.

Selipsky H. Osseous surgery – how much need we compromise? *Dent Clin North Am.* 1976; 20:79–106.

Tibbetts LS Jr, Ochsenbein C, Loughlin DM. Rationale for the lingual approach to mandibular osseous surgery. *Dent Clin North Am.* 1976; 20:61–78.

Townsend-Olsen C, Ammons W, van Belle G. A longitudinal study comparing apically repositioned flaps with and without osseous surgery. *Int J Periodontics Restorative Dent.* 1985; 5:1–33.

Vrotsos JA, Parashis AO, Theofanatos GD, Smulow JB. Prevalence and distribution of bone defects in moderate and advanced adult periodontitis. *J Clin Periodontol.* 1999; 26(1):44–48.

CHAPTER 19

Biomaterials in periodontal regeneration

Nader Hamdan, Zeeshan Sheikh, Haidor Al-Waeli and Michael Glogauer

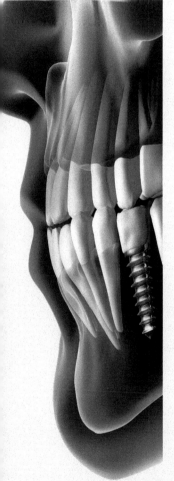

Contents

Learning objectives

- Types of biomaterials used for alveolar bone grafting.
- Definitions, classification, and usage of various types of grafts.
- Examples of osteoconductive and osteoinductive graft materials.
- Various biomaterials used for bone augmentation.
- Definitions and types of barrier membranes used in regeneration procedures.

Essential Periodontics, First Edition. Edited by Steph Smith and Khalid Almas.
© 2022 John Wiley & Sons Ltd. Published 2022 by John Wiley & Sons Ltd.

Introduction

Periodontitis is a chronic multifactorial inflammatory disease associated with bacterial dysbiosis and is characterized by progressive destruction of the tooth-supporting structures (Caton et al. 2018). Periodontal disease is a result of a complex and dynamic interplay of multiple causative factors, including lifestyle, tooth anatomy, systemic diseases, genetics, and the environment. The primary features of periodontitis include the loss of periodontal tissues manifested through clinical attachment loss and radiographic bone loss, and the presence of periodontal pocketing and gingival bleeding (Albandar 2005; Armitage & Cullinan 2010). Various treatment modalities have been investigated to repair/regenerate damaged or lost periodontal tissues (Ramseier et al. 2012). The natural tissues and synthetic bone replacement grafts and barrier membranes used for periodontal regeneration are discussed in this chapter.

Natural tissues and synthetic biomaterials for bone grafting

There are several graft options available that are used for alveolar bone grafting. They are divided into natural transplants (autografts, allografts, and xenografts) and synthetic materials (alloplasts) (see Figure 19.1 and Table 19.1). These graft materials are used because they are either osteogenic, osteoinductive, and/or osteoconductive (Sheikh et al. 2013). Hard tissue substitute materials that are resorbable undergo a process by which they are partially or completely resorbed by macrophages/osteoclasts before bone is deposited by osteoblasts (Sheikh et al. 2015a, b).

Autografts

Autografts are harvested from a donor site in the same individual and transplanted to another site. Autografts are a source of the most osteogenic organic material for grafting; however, donor site morbidity and the limited graft volume that can be obtained are disadvantages (McAllister & Haghighat 2007; Younger & Chapman 1989). Autografts used for dental grafting applications may be of extraoral or intraoral origin (Figure 19.1). Intraoral autograft harvest sites are the spina nasalis, the tuberosity and crista zygomatico-alveolaris from the maxilla, the ramus, retromolar region, and symphysis region in the mandible, as well as bony exostoses and bone harvested from different sites utilizing bone scrapers (Draenert et al. 2014).

Mandibular autografts are commonly used as bone chips, blocks, and milled particles (Misch 1997; Simion et al. 2001). The common extraoral harvest site that offers large amounts of autologous cortical-cancellous bone is the iliac crest, which provides osteoinductive, osteoconductive, and osteogenic potential (Cypher & Grossman 1996). However, root resorption has been found to occur with the use of fresh iliac bone autografts (Dragoo & Sullivan 1973). Cortical autografts have high initial strength, which after around six months of implantation is about 50% weaker than the physiologically normal bone tissue (Wilk, 2004). Conversely, cancellous bone autografts are initially weaker because of their porous structure and gain strength over time (Sheikh et al. 2013). The cancellous autografts revascularize earlier than the cortical grafts around the fifth day after implantation due to their spongy architecture (Sheikh et al. 2013).

Allografts

An allograft is bone (or other tissues) that is transplanted from a genetically non-identical member of a same species to another. These typically come from a donor or cadaver, and are available in larger quantities for use. Allografts (cortical and cancellous) of various particle size ranges are used routinely for bone augmentation procedures (Araujo et al. 2013; Block &

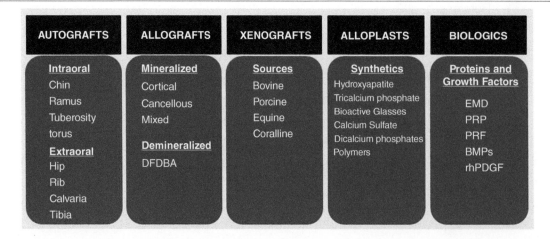

Figure 19.1 Natural tissues, synthetic biomaterial graft options and biologics for periodontal bone regeneration. BMPs, bone morphogenetic proteins; DFDBA, demineralized freeze-dried bone allograft; EMD, enamel matrix derivative; PRF, platelet-rich fibrin; PRP, platelet-rich plasma; rhPDGF, recombinant growth factor.

Table 19.1 Some of the commercially available bone graft materials for periodontal and other maxillofacial applications.

Category	Brand name	Company	Generic name/composition	Source
Allograft	Accell®	Citagenix, Inc., Laval, Canada	Demineralized bone matrix	Human bone
	DBX® Putty	Dentsply Sirona, York, PA, USA	Demineralized bone matrix	Human bone
	DynaBlast®	Keystone Dental, Inc., Burlington, MA, USA	Demineralized and mineralized bone matrix	Human bone
	Grafton®	BioHorizons Implant Systems, Inc., Birmingham, AL, USA	Demineralized bone matrix	Human bone
	MTF® – DFDBA	MTF Biologics, Edison, NJ, USA	Demineralized freeze-dried bone	Human bone
	MTF® – FDBA	MTF Biologics	Freeze-dried bone	Human bone
	OsteoSelect®	Bacterin International, Inc., Belgrade, MT, USA	Demineralized bone matrix	Human bone
	OsteoSponge®	Bacterin International, Inc.	Demineralized bone matrix	Human bone
	Puros®	Zimmer Biomet, Warsaw, IN, USA	Mineralized bone	Human bone
	Raptos®	Citagenix, Inc.	Mineralized/ demineralized bone allograft	Human bone
Xenograft	Biocoral®	Bio Coral Calcium Bone, Saint-Gonnery, France	Coraline calcium carbonate	Marine corals
	Bio-Oss®	Geistlich Pharma AG, Wolhusen, Switzerland	Deproteinized bovine bone mineral	Bovine bone
	Cerabone®	Botiss Biomaterials GmbH, Zossen, Germany	Decalcified freeze-dried bovine bone	Bovine bone
	Endobon®	Zimmer Biomet	Deproteinized bovine bone mineral	Bovine bone
	Gen-Os®	Tecnoss Dental Srl, Turin, Italy	Anorganic porcine bone mineral	Porcine bone
	Interpore 200®	InterPore International, Inc., Irvine, CA, USA	Porous HA	Marine corals
	Osseograft®	Osteomed LP, Glendale, CA, USA	Demineralized bone matrix	Bovine bone
	Osteograf/N®	Dentsply Sirona	Anorganic bovine bone mineral	Bovine bone
Xenograft/ synthetic	PepGen P-15®	Dentsply Sirona	Anorganic bovine bone mineral with a synthetic biomimetic of the 15 amino acid sequence of type I collagen	Bovine bone/ tissue engineering
Alloplast	Ceros®	Thommen Medical (Schweiz) AG, Grenchen, Switzerland	β-TCP	Synthetic
	Cerasorb®	Curasan, Inc., Kleinostheim, Germany	β-TCP	Synthetic
	IngeniOs® β-TCP	Zimmer Biomet	β-TCP	Synthetic
	Macrobone®	Euroteknika Groupe, Sallanches, France	β-TCP	Synthetic
	Vitoss®	Stryker Corp., Kalamazoo, MI, USA	β-TCP	Synthetic

(*Continued*)

Table 19.1 (Continued)

Category	Brand name	Company	Generic name/composition	Source
	Guidor easy-graft®	Collagen Matrix, Inc., Oakland, NJ, USA	In situ hardening β-TCP granules coated with PLGA	Synthetic
	Biogran®	Atek Medical, LLC, Grand Rapids, MI, USA	Bioactive glass	Synthetic
	PerioGlass®	NovaBone Products, LLC, Jacksonville, FL, USA	Bioactive glass	Synthetic
	Capset®	Lifecore Biomedical, Inc., Chaska, MN, USA	CS	Synthetic
	Osteoset®	Wright Medical Group NV, Amsterdam, Netherlands	CS	Synthetic
	Calciresorb 35®	Ceraver, Roissy, France	DCP (65% HA/35% β-TCP)	Synthetic
	Ceraform®	Teknimed, L'Union, France	DCP (65% HA/35% β-TCP)	Synthetic
	Eurobone®	Kasios SAS, L'Union, France	DCP/ dihydrate (brushite) – DCPD	Synthetic
	Cerapatite®	Ceraver	HA	Synthetic
	IngeniOs® HA	Zimmer Biomet	HA	Synthetic
	TransOssatite®	Transysteme JMT implant, Nîmes, France	HA	Synthetic

β-TCP, beta-tricalcium phosphate; CS, calcium sulfate; DCP, dicalcium phosphate; DCPD, dihydrated dicalcic phosphate; DFDBA, demineralized freeze-dried bone allograft; FDBA, freeze-dried bone allograft; HA, hydroxyapatite; PLGA, polylactic-co-glycolic acid.
Source: Adapted from Sheikh et al. 2017a, 2019b.

Degen 2004; Sterio et al. 2013). Allografts are available for periodontal applications as cortical wedges, cortical chips, cortical granules, and cancellous powder, which are prepared as frozen, freeze-dried, mineralized, and demineralized bone (Al Ruhaimi 2001).

Fresh or frozen allografts

Due to the risk of disease transmission, fresh or frozen iliac allografts are not used any more; however, these demonstrate the highest osteoconductive and osteoinductive potential among all allografts (Dias et al. 2016; Macedo et al. 2012). In the past, atrophic maxillary ridges, when grafted with human block grafts of tibia and fresh-frozen chips, showed features representative of mature and compact osseous tissue surrounded by marrow spaces (Contar et al. 2009, 2011).

Mineralized freeze-dried bone allografts

During processing, the freeze-drying distorts the three-dimensional (3D) presentation of the human leucocyte antigens on the surface of graft particles, which affects immune recognition (Friedlaender et al. 1976; Quattlebaum et al. 1988). Freeze-dried bone allografts (FDBAs) are known to be osteoconductive and can be combined with autografts to enhance the osteogenic potential (Committee on Research 2001; Mellonig 2000). These graft tissues are mineralized and used for the treatment of periodontal defects (Blaggana et al. 2014; Kukreja et al. 2014; Markou et al. 2009; Mellonig 1991). Cortical FDBAs demonstrate greater osteoinductive potential due to the growth factors stored in the matrix (Sunitha Raja & Naidu 2008). FDBAs used in combination with absorbable barrier membranes have been used as replacement for autograft blocks for ridge augmentation (Lyford et al. 2003). The use of FDBA blocks for alveolar ridge grafting has shown the presence of vital bone with a lamellar organization (Jacotti et al. 2012; Wallace & Gellin 2010). FDBAs in combination with resorbable barrier membranes can be used as a replacement for autogenous block grafts for ridge augmentation prior to implant placement (Lyford et al. 2003).

Demineralized freeze-dried bone allogeneic grafts

These allografts are demineralized and used alone or in combination with FDBAs and/or autografts (Sheikh et al. 2019b) Demineralized freeze-dried bone allogeneic grafts (DFDBAs) undergo resorption at a quick rate (Hopp et al. 1989; Russell et al. 1997) and often have osteoinductive potential (Mellonig et al. 1981). Demineralization of these grafts exposes bone morphogenetic proteins (BMPs) found in the bone matrix and may activate them. However, there is a high degree of variability in the DFDBAs available for use, with some products having little to no osteoinductive capability (Schwartz et al. 1996). The inductive potential of DFDBAs varies considerably with the donor age. DFDBA samples from donors aged more than 50 years have been shown to have significantly less inductive ability. Furthermore, the inductive capacity of DFDBA varies between batches within the same bone bank (Schwartz et al. 1998). DFDBAs have been shown to produce less vital new bone in comparison to autografts (Scarano et al. 2006).

Xenografts

Xenografts are graft tissues obtained from non-human species and are usually osteoconductive, with limited resorptive potential (McAllister et al. 1999; Thaller et al. 1993). The most used xenograft in periodontal regenerative procedures is deproteinized bovine bone mineral (DBBM) (Sheikh et al. 2015f). DBBM is commercially available bone of bovine origin processed to yield natural bone mineral without the organic elements (Liu et al. 2016). After heat and chemical treatments, the inorganic phase of bovine bone consists mainly of hydroxyapatite (HA), which retains the porous architecture (Jarcho 1981).

Bovine-derived bone graft particles and blocks have been used for alveolar ridge augmentation procedures and intrabony defect filling (Yildirim et al. 2000; Zitzmann et al. 1997). Of particular interest is the use of DBBM as a graft material during direct subantral augmentation (sinus lift) procedures, where dental implants placed in DBBM grafts had survival rates similar to autogenous grafts (Wallace & Froum 2003). Although bovine-derived bone block grafts have high osteoconductive potential, these grafts are brittle and lack toughness. This makes them inherently prone to failure during screw fixation procedures and/or after implantation (Felice et al. 2009; Yildirim et al. 2000).

Bone mineral can be obtained from porcine or equine sources. Porcine bone graft tissue is a porous anorganic bone graft material consisting predominantly of calcium phosphate. It is supplied in granular form and is manufactured with the removal of the organic components from porcine bone (Nannmark & Sennerby 2008; Pearce et al. 2007). The anorganic bone mineral matrix is biocompatible, having an interconnecting macro- and microscopic porous structure that supports the formation and ingrowth of new bone at the implantation site (Nannmark & Sennerby 2008).

The porous microstructure of marine coral has also been used as a template to fabricate porous coralline HA materials (White & Shors 1986). These materials are fabricated from coral being subjected to high temperature under pressurized treatment in the presence of aqueous phosphate solutions (Roy & Linnehan 1974). This converts the coral to calcium HA, while conserving the highly organized, permeable, and interconnecting porous structure with an average pore diameter of 200 μm (Roy & Linnehan 1974; White & Shors 1986).

Some other xenograft materials that are currently being researched include chitosan, red algae, and gussuibu (Cho et al. 2005; Wong & Rabie 2006). Chitosan is a product of the exoskeleton of crustaceans and has shown the ability to stimulate mesenchymal stem cell differentiation into osteoblasts. When chitosan is combined with HA, the osteoconductivity is markedly increased (Cho et al. 2005). Red algae are one of the oldest groups of eukaryotic algae, and can be chemically converted to HA, which is then utilized for grafting bone defects (Ewers 2005) (see Figure 19.2).

Alloplasts

Alloplastic synthetic biomaterials were developed to overcome the inherent disadvantages of autografts and are fabricated in various forms with varying physicochemical properties, and can be both degradable and non-degradable (AlGhamdi et al. 2010; Sheikh et al. 2015a, c, e, f, 2017; Shetty & Han 1991). Alloplasts are usually osteoconductive, without any osteoinductive or osteogenic potential on their own, and have been used extensively for periodontal regeneration (Sheikh et al. 2017a, 2019a, b; Shetty & Han 1991). The most routinely used alloplastic materials are HA, tricalcium phosphate (TCP), and bioactive glasses. Calcium phosphate biomaterials are of great interest to be used as bone replacement graft materials in periodontal regeneration, as they have a similar composition to bone mineral, are osteoconductive, form bone apatite-like material or carbonated HA, and form a very strong bone–calcium phosphate biomaterial interface (Sheikh et al. 2015a, e).

Hydroxyapatite

This is a commonly used calcium phosphate biomaterial for bone regeneration applications due to its having a composition and structure similar to natural bone mineral (Wang et al. 2007). HA-based grafts form a chemical bond directly to bone once implanted (Bagambisa et al. 1993). Synthetic HA is available and used in various forms:

- Porous non-resorbable.
- Solid non-resorbable.
- Resorbable (non-ceramic, porous) (Tevlin et al. 2014).

HA is non-osteogenic and mainly functions as an osteoconductive graft material. HA grafts show slow and limited resorptive potential, depending on the method of formation, the calcium to phosphate ratio, the crystallographic structure, and porosity (Jarcho 1981; Osborn & Newesely 1980). The ability

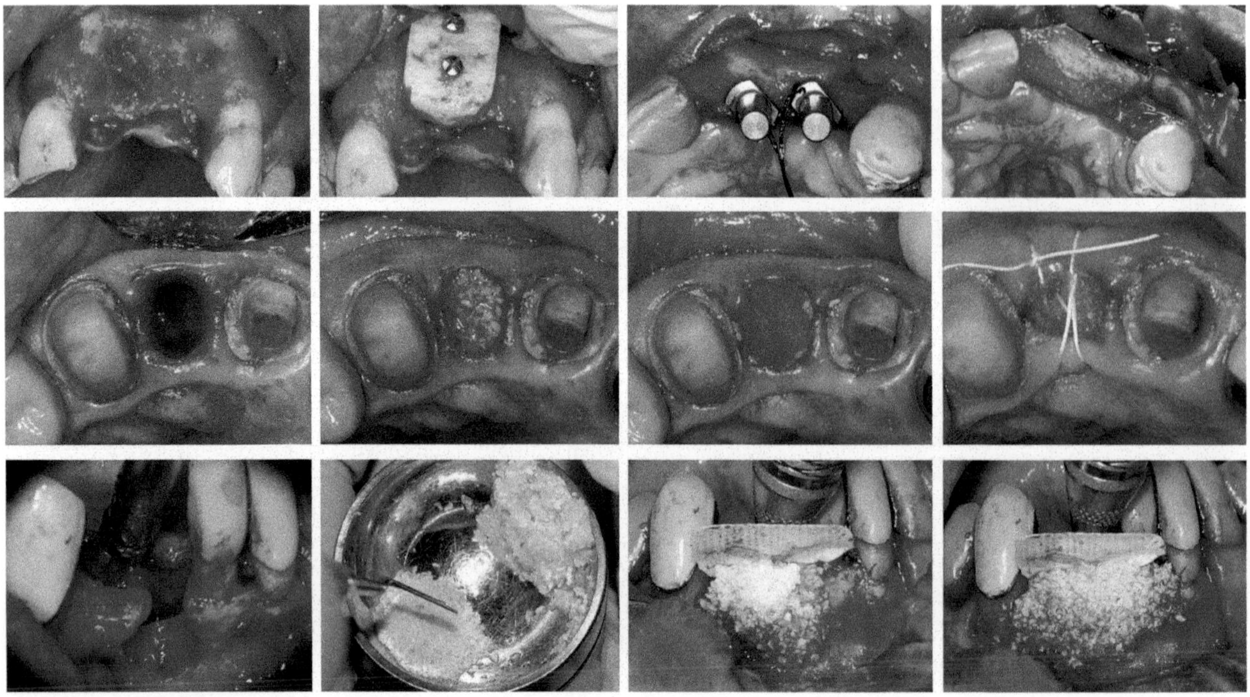

Figure 19.2 Examples of some of the bone graft materials being used intraorally. The top row shows an autogenous block graft harvested from the ascending ramus. The middle row shows deproteinized bovine bone mineral (DBBM) used during a ridge preservation procedure. The bottom row shows a freeze-dried bone allograft (FDBA) being used in conjugation with DBBM to reconstruct a bony defect in the mandible.

of HA to resorb is also heavily dependent upon the processing temperature, with grafts synthesized at high temperatures being highly dense with very limited biodegradability (Klein et al. 1983). These dense grafts are usually used as inert biocompatible fillers (Meffert et al. 1985; Rabalais et al. 1981). At lower temperatures, the particulate HA is porous and undergoes slow resorption (Ricci et al. 1992). Ridge augmentation with HA granules alone (Sugar et al. 1995) or in combination with autografts has been investigated (Small et al. 1993).

Tricalcium phosphate

TCP has been used and extensively investigated as a bone substitute and has two crystallographic forms: α-TCP and β-TCP (Tamimi et al. 2012). β-TCP exhibits good biocompatibility and osteoconductivity and is used commonly as a partially resorbable filler, allowing replacement with newly formed bone (Shetty & Han 1991). In terms of bone regenerative potential, β-TCP grafts have been shown to be similar to autogenous bone, FDBA, DFDBA, and collagen sponge (Nakajima et al. 2007). TCP biomaterials have been used in human clinical studies to repair periapical and marginal periodontal defects, as well as alveolar bony defects (Metsger et al. 1982; Stavropoulos et al. 2010). In addition, studies have reported variable results using β-TCP for alveolar ridge augmentation in vertical and horizontal dimensions (Nyan et al. 2014; Shalash et al. 2013).

Bioactive glasses

These graft materials are composed of silicon dioxide, calcium oxide, sodium oxide, and phosphorus pentoxide (Schepers et al. 1991; Shue et al. 2012). The particle sizes of bioactive glasses (Bioglass) range from 90 to 710 µm and from 300 to 355 µm (Schepers & Ducheyne 1997; Schepers et al. 1991). After implantation of bioactive glass, a silicon-rich gel is formed on the bioactive ceramic surface, with the outer layer serving as a bonding surface for osteogenic cells and collagen fibers (Hall et al. 1999; Xynos et al. 2001). Bioactive glass nanoparticles have been shown to induce cementoblasts to proliferate in an in vivo study (Carvalho et al. 2012). Clinical reports of alveolar ridge grafting performed with bioactive glass reveal bone formation in close contact to the particles (Schepers et al. 1991). However, these do not resorb and limited true periodontal regenerative outcomes based on human histological analysis have been demonstrated (Knapp et al. 2003; Nevins et al. 2000).

Calcium sulfate

Compounds of calcium and sulfates have a compressive strength greater than that of cancellous bone (Moore et al. 2001). A combination of β-TCP and calcium phosphate has been investigated that does not require a membrane, lowers costs, reduces surgical time, and has the potential to treat periodontal intrabony defects (Paolantonio et al. 2008; Sukumar et al. 2011).

A randomized controlled clinical trial over 12 months has shown that the use of calcium sulfate is useful in minimizing post-surgical recession when compared with the use of collagen membranes (Paolantonio et al. 2008; Sheikh et al. 2014, 2017b). The clinical outcome of class II mandibular molar furcation defects has also been shown to be enhanced with the use of a mixture of calcium sulfate and DFDBA (Maragos et al. 2002).

Dicalcium Phosphates

These are acidic calcium phosphates that have a high solubility at physiological pH. Dicalcium phosphate dihydrate (DCPD or brushite) has been investigated for both bone defect repair and vertical bone augmentation applications as injectable cements or as pre-set cement granules (Sheikh et al. 2016a; Tamimi et al. 2009, 2010). It has been demonstrated that injectable brushite cements are capable of regenerating bone in atrophic alveolar ridges, buccal dehiscence defects, and maxillary sinus floor elevation procedures (Gehrke & Famà 2010). Bone growth in the vertical direction obtained with brushite cement granules has been seen to be higher than that obtained with commercially available bovine HA materials (Tamimi et al. 2006). However, brushite grafts after implantation undergo phase conversion to insoluble HA, which ultimately limits their resorption rate and extent (Sheikh et al. 2015g; Tamimi et al. 2012). Brushite can be used as a precursor to the anhydrous form of DCP, i.e. dicalcium phosphate anhydrous, also known as DCPA or monetite. Monetite does not convert to HA after implantation (Sheikh et al. 2015g, 2016a, 2017c; Tamimi et al. 2006, 2008) and resorbs at faster rates compared to brushite cement grafts (Fine et al. 2020; Gbureck et al. 2007; Idowu et al. 2014; Sheikh et al. 2017c; Tamimi et al. 2012). Monetite granules have been compared with commercially available bovine HA (Bio-Oss), and have shown greater resorption and bone formation in extraction sockets (Tamimi et al. 2010).

Polymers

Polymers can be classified based on their origin: natural and synthetic. Natural polymers that have been utilized in the fabrication of bone grafts include polysaccharides (e.g. alginate, argose, chitosan, and hyaluronic acid) and polypeptides (e.g. gelatin and collagen). Natural polymers possess weak mechanical properties and variable or negligible rates of degradation, hence their use is limited as bone grafting materials (Asghari et al. 2017). However, natural polymers play an important role in composite grafts by serving as a polymeric shell capsule that incorporates particles of allografts. Synthetic polymers (e.g. polyglycolic acid, polylactic acid, polyorthoester, and polyanhydride) provide a platform for regulating and controlling the biomechanical properties of scaffolds, and they also serve as drug delivery carriers in tissue engineering applications (Sokolsky-Papkov et al. 2007).

HTR™ Synthetic Bone (Bioplant, Norwalk, CT, USA) is a biocompatible microporous composite made up of polymethylmethacrylate, polyhydroxyethylmethacrylate, and calcium hydroxide. The acronym HTR stands for 'hard tissue replacement' and acceptable clinical results have been achieved in the treatment of intrabony and furcation defects with its use (Yukna 1990, 1994). Histologically, new bone growth has been observed on the particles of this material (Froum 1996; Stahl et al. 1990; Yukna & Greer 1992). This material furthermore possesses hydrophilicity that enhances clotting, and the negative particle charges on the surface allow adherence to bone. Clinically acceptable defect fill and resolution can be achieved, which supports the use of HTR as a biocompatible alloplastic bone substitute (Buck et al. 1989; Murray 1990). Furthermore, polymers have also traditionally been used as barrier membranes in periodontal guided tissue regeneration (GTR) procedures (Murphy & Gunsolley 2003).

Biologics for bone augmentation and periodontal tissue regeneration

Continuous research is being conducted to develop newer strategies and technologies to achieve periodontal regeneration. There has been great interest in using BMPs, enamel matrix derivatives (EMD), platelet-rich plasma (PRP), and, more recently, biomimetic bone anabolic conjugates (mixed with resorbable matrices and/or DBBM) (Sheikh et al. 2015d, 2018, 2019a, b, 2020b). BMPs, through their chemotactic, mitogenic, and differentiating mechanisms, play a crucial role in bone remodeling and demonstrate potent effects on the promotion of periodontal tissue regeneration in acute periodontal wounds, involving new formation of cementum, periodontal ligament (PDL), and bone (Sykaras & Opperman 2003). BMP use has shown promising results for intraoral applications such as sinus augmentation and alveolar ridge preservation (Edmunds et al. 2014; Katanec et al. 2014; Kim et al. 2014; Sheikh et al. 2015d; Shweikeh et al. 2016). The most potent BMPs are BMP 2 and BMP 7 (Giannobile et al. 1998; Rao et al. 2013). Recombinant human osteogenic protein-1 (OP-1) induces new bone formation in vivo, with a specific activity comparable with natural bovine osteogenic protein, and stimulates osteoblast proliferation and differentiation. It has also been demonstrated to be efficient in periodontal regeneration, even in grade III furcation defects (Giannobile et al. 1998). Further in-depth studies are required for the development of delivery systems that can allow for controlled and precise release of BMPs for periodontal regeneration (Sheikh et al. 2015d).

EMDs are purified protein fractions from the enamel layer of developing porcine teeth. It was assumed that these proteins, mostly made of amelogenins, might stimulate cementum deposition and periodontal regeneration (Miron et al. 2016). Several studies have provided human histological evidence of intrabony regeneration associated with EMD therapy (Heijl 1997; Hoffmann et al. 2016). EMD is still present on root surfaces for more than 4 weeks after its application, and early signs of periodontal regeneration can be observed after 2–6 weeks. A review by the American Academy of Periodontology concluded that EMD is generally comparable with DFDBA and GTR therapy in improving clinical parameters in the treatment of intrabony defects (Kao et al. 2015). Increased attachment gain, greater reduction of pocket depths, and higher bone fill have been reported with EMD when compared with open flap debridement (OFD) for the management of infrabony defects. A majority of studies have indicated no additional benefits in either clinical and/or radiographic gains when EMD is used with the addition of graft materials (Guida et al. 2007).

PRP is an autogenous concentration of platelets in a small volume of plasma and is considered to be an extremely rich source of autogenous growth factors such as platelet-derived growth factor (PDGF), transforming growth factor (TGF)-ß, vascular endothelial growth factor (VEGF), epidermal growth factor (EGF), insulin-like growth factor (IGF)-1, and basic fibroblast growth factor (bFGF) (Marx 2004). PRP has been used alone or in combination with autografts and allografts for the treatment of periodontal defects, extraction socket preservation, alveolar ridge augmentation, mandibular reconstruction, sinus floor elevation, and maxillary cleft repair (Plachokova et al. 2008). Results have shown greater volume and denser bone compared to autografts used alone for bone regeneration (Marx et al. 1998). The improvement in the bone healing potential is believed to be due to growth factors being present

in PRP (Plachokova et al. 2008), and several studies have reported positive results from PRP use with bone regeneration (Camargo et al. 2002; Fennis et al. 2004; Kassolis & Reynolds 2005; Lekovic et al. 2003; Nikolidakas 2006). However, PRP does not provide additional benefits in bone formation, nor does it improve implant survival rates in sinus lift cases (Pocaterra et al. 2016). Platelet-rich fibrin (PRF) or leucocyte- and platelet-rich fibrin (L-PRF) is a second-generation PRP wherein autologous platelets and leucocytes are present in a complex fibrin matrix, and has been considered to accelerate the healing of soft and hard tissue. PRF has shown to have little to no effect on the healing, quality, and quantity of bone in vivo (Knapen et al. 2015). However, PRF has been suggested to be efficient in accelerating soft tissue healing, and may have antimicrobial activity (Miron et al. 2017).

rhPDGF-BB, a recombinant form of growth factor, has been shown to enhance periodontal regeneration (bone, PDL, and cementum). Its use has been described as safe and efficient for the treatment of infrabony defects in some studies, especially when combined with synthetic beta-tricalcium-phosphate. However, improvements in clinical parameters are not significantly superior to those of bone-grafted infrabony defects. Linear bone growth continues to improve over 36 months and no membrane is required in this technique (see Figure 19.3).

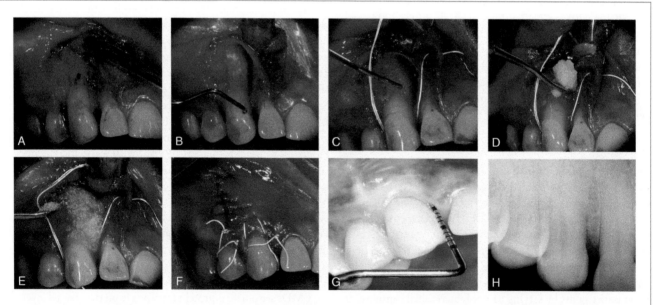

Figure 19.3 An example of the use of enamel matrix derivative (EMD) combined with a beta-tricalcium phosphate bone ceramic (β-TCP) for the management of advanced tissue loss around a single-rooted tooth. (A) Deep osseous defect with subgingival calculus. (B) Root surface thoroughly planed and granulation tissue removed. (C) Root surface was prepared to receive the bone graft with EMD. (D) EMD + β-TCP was incrementally applied against the root surface and into the bony defect. (E) EMD + β-TCP covering the root surface and the bony defect. (F) The flap sutured to its original position. (G) 22 months follow-up shows a stable 4 mm periodontal probing depth and about 1 mm of recession. (H) 9 months post-surgery radiograph showing radiographic defect fill.

Barrier membranes for periodontal guided regenerative applications

Periodontal regeneration utilizing membrane techniques is based on the principle of separation of different tissues by means of the surgical placement of physical barriers (Linde et al. 1993). Soft tissue turnover rate is faster than bone and periodontal tissue formation, and using barrier membranes allows for a defect space to be maintained for regenerating tissues that would otherwise be infiltrated and occupied by epithelial cells (Figure 19.4). If membranes are used in combination with bone grafts, then they also serve to stabilize, contain, and preserve the graft materials (Figure 19.4) (Sheikh et al. 2014). This also results in reducing the rate of graft resorption (Buser et al. 1999; Sheikh et al. 2016b). There are a variety of degradable and non-degradable barrier membranes that have been synthesized for periodontal GTR and guided bone regeneration (GBR) applications (Table 19.2 and Figure 19.4) (Sheikh et al. 2014, 2017b). The general characteristics that must be considered when designing barrier membranes intended for periodontal regeneration are:

- Biocompatibility.
- Cell exclusiveness.
- Space-making ability.
- Tissue integration
- Degradability.
- Adequate mechanical properties.
- Optimal clinical handling characteristics (Dahlin & Linde 1988; Hardwick & Dahlin 1994).

Non-degradable barrier membranes

Materials such as cellulose acetate laboratory filters, silicone sheets, and expanded polytetrafluoroethylene (ePTFE) were the first non-degradable biomaterials used for investigating barrier membranes for regenerative therapy (Sheikh et al. 2014). Although these materials demonstrated some therapeutic potential, limitations such as inability to integrate with surrounding tissue, brittleness, and the need to remove them after a certain period of time limited their clinical usefulness (Aukhil et al. 1983; Magnusson et al. 1988).

The function of non-degradable membranes is temporary, as they maintain their structural integrity upon placement and are later retrieved via surgery. Although this gives the clinician greater control over the length of time the membrane will remain in place, the retrieval procedure increases the risk of

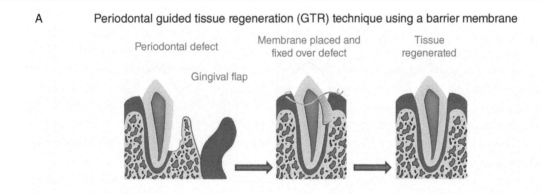

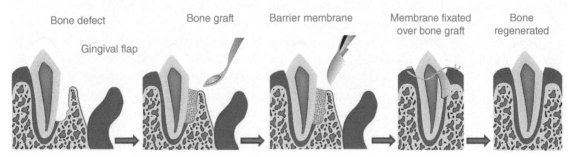

Figure 19.4 (A) Depiction of periodontal guided tissue regeneration (GTR) technique using a barrier membrane. GTR is a surgical procedure that utilizes membranes to regenerate soft tissues. The membrane serves as an occlusive barrier that creates a secluded space around the defect, thus providing an opportunity for the periodontal tissues to regenerate. (B) Depiction of guided bone regeneration (GBR) technique using bone graft and a barrier membrane. In GBR, a membrane is positioned to prevent fibroblastic cells from colonizing an intraosseous wound with bone grafting during healing, while allowing osseous cells to migrate and fill the defect, thus resulting in direct bone regeneration and deposition. Courtesy of Ms. Esraa Khalil.

Table 19.2 Common collagen-based barrier membranes for clinical use.

Membrane	Manufacturer	Constitution	Method of cross-linking	Tissue sources	Resorption time
BioGide®	Geistlich Pharma AG, Wilhusen, Switzerland	Types I and III collagen	None	Porcine (dermis)	24 weeks
BioMend®	Zimmer Biomet, Warsaw, IN, USA	Type I collagen	Formaldehyde	Bovine (tendon)	6–8 weeks
BioMend Extend®	Zimmer Biomet	Type I collagen	Formaldehyde	Bovine (tendon)	18 weeks
Tissue Guide	Koken, Tokyo, Japan	Atelocollagen + tendon collagen	HMDIC	Bovine (tendon + dermis)	4–8 weeks
BioBar®	US Biological, Salem, MA, USA	Type I collagen	N/A	Bovine (tendon)	24–32 weeks
Paroguide®	Gaba Vebas Srl, Rome, Italy	Type I collagen (96%) and chondroitin-4 sulfate (4%)	DPPA	Calf skin	4–8 weeks
Biostite®	Acteon Products, Mérignac, France	Type I collagen (9.5%), chondroitin-4 sulfate (2.5%), and HA (88%)	DPPA	Calf skin	4–8 weeks
Periogen®	Periogen Co., San Diego, CA, USA	Types I and III collagen	Gluteraldehyde	Bovine (dermis)	4–8 weeks
AlloDerm® Regenerative Tissue Matrix (RTM)	BioHorizons Implant Systems, Inc., Birmingham, AL, USA	Type I collagen	None	Human cadavers (skin)	28–36 weeks
Cytoplast® RTM	Osteogenics Biomedical, Lubbock, TX, USA	Type I collagen	N/A	Bovine (tendon)	26–38 weeks

DPPA, diphenylphosphorylazide; HA, hydroxypatite; HMDIC, hexamethylenediiscyanate.
Source: Bunyaratavej & Wang 2001; Sheikh et al. 2017a, 2019a, b; Wang & MacNeil 1998.

surgical site morbidity and leaves the regenerated tissues susceptible to damage and post-surgery bacterial contamination (Tatakis et al. 1999). Membrane exposure due to flap dehiscence during healing is also a frequent post-surgical complication (Murphy 1995). However, in situations such as alveolar ridge augmentation prior to placement of dental implants, it may be desirable for the membrane to retain its functional characteristics long enough for adequate healing to occur, and then to be removed. Hence, in specific situations, a nondegradable membrane can provide predictable performance (Hämmerle & Jung 2003; Hardwick et al. 1995).

Polytetrafluoroethylene (PTFE) is a non-porous, inert and biocompatible fluorocarbon polymer (Sculean et al. 2008). Two non-resorbable barrier membranes that have been commonly used are the ePTFE and high-density polytetrafluoroethylene (dPTFE) membranes. ePTFE has been commonly used in vascular surgeries (Kempczinski et al. 1985) and is fabricated by exposing PTFE to high tensile stresses, which results in expansion and the formation of a porous microstructure

(Bauer et al. 1987). However, ePTFE membranes, due to having a larger pore size (>20 μm), have been known to be more prone to bacterial infection and are no longer used (Sheikh et al. 2014). dPTFE has a smaller pore size (0.3 μm) that does not allow bacterial ingrowth into the graft material if left exposed (Hürzeler & Strub 1994). When there is a clinical requirement that requires larger areas of space maintenance, titanium-reinforced PTFE (Ti-dPTFE/Cytoplast Ti-250) can be used, as it is stiffer due to the central portion of the membrane being reinforced with titanium to prevent collapse (Scantlebury 1993).

Biodegradable barrier membranes

Extensive research has been focused toward developing degradable barrier membranes so that a second surgical procedure for removal is not required. Clinical studies in the early 1990s reported the successful use of degradable membranes for GBR therapy (Hürzeler & Strub 1994; Lundgren et al. 1994;

Nobréus et al. 1997). Both natural and synthetic polymers have been investigated for this purpose, with collagen and aliphatic polyesters being the most studied (Ratner 2004). It is important for the design of a degradable membrane to be such that it maintains its functional characteristics for an adequate healing period. Currently, the most commonly used degradable membranes are made of collagen or polyglycolide and/or polylactide or co-polymers of them (Sheikh et al. 2017b; Simion et al. 1996).

Biodegradable barrier membranes are mostly incapable of maintaining the defect space on their own due to their lack of rigidity, especially when exposed to oral fluids and/or blood. For this reason, these membranes are frequently used in combination with autogenous or synthetic bone graft substitutes (Avera et al. 1996; Parodi et al. 1996), with or without reinforcements, support screws, and pins (Gotfredson et al. 1994).

Natural degradable barrier membranes

Natural degradable barrier membranes are fabricated by utilizing collagen from tissues from human or animal sources (Table 19.2). Collagen is used extensively in biomedical applications and can be acquired from animal intestines, skin, and tendons (Ratner 2004). Collagen has numerous biological properties that are desirable, such as having low immunogenicity, attracting and activating gingival fibroblast cells, and being hemostatic (Bunyaratavej & Wang 2001). Collagen membranes have been shown to stimulate fibroblast DNA synthesis (Lundgren et al. 1994) and osteoblasts show improved adherence to collagen membrane surfaces in comparison to other barrier membrane surfaces (Behring et al. 2008). The biodegradation of collagen membranes is accomplished by endogenous collagenases into carbon dioxide and water (Bunyaratavej & Wang 2001). The degree of cross-linking of collagen fibers directly affects the rate of degradation, with the relationship being inversely proportional (Lee et al. 2001).

BioMend is a biodegradable barrier membrane fabricated from type I collagen derived from bovine Achilles' tendon. The membrane is semi-occlusive, having a pore size of 0.004 μm, and resorbs in 4–8 weeks after implantation. Clinical results have revealed limited clinical effectiveness, which is highly dependent upon the form and size of the defect (Wang & Carroll 2000). To overcome the disadvantage of fast resorption, BioMend Extend was later developed for use in cases that require the membrane to maintain its function longer than BioMend. BioMend Extend has an in vivo stability of around 18 weeks (Li et al. 2013). BioGide is a barrier membrane that resorbs in about 8 weeks and is synthesized from collagen types I and III, which is derived from porcine skin sources (Schliephake et al. 1994).

AlloDerm Regenerative Tissue Matrix (RTM) is a collagen type I membrane derived from human skin (cadavers). The membrane thickness ranges from 0.9 to 1.6 mm and clinical applications include root coverage, gingival augmentation, soft tissue ridge augmentation, and soft tissue augmentation around dental implants (Oh et al. 2003). AlloDerm GBR RTM is manufactured utilizing the same process used for AlloDerm RTM and the membrane thickness ranges from 0.5 to 0.9 mm; it is used for graft protection, containment, and flap extension to achieve adequate primary closure (Lee & Kim 2014).

Paroguide is a collagen type I membrane enriched with chondroitin sulfate. There have been reports of PDL regeneration and alveolar bone regeneration, with no signs of inflammation (Magnusson et al. 1988; Parodi et al. 1996). Cytoplast RTM is synthesized from collagen type I derived from bovine tendon and is a multilayered membrane that takes 20–38 weeks for complete resorption. It has an organized fiber orientation providing good handling and high tensile strength (Vert 1989; Vert et al. 1992).

A collagen membrane cross-linked with diphenolphosphoryl azide, a type I collagen membrane that is derived from calf pericardium, has been investigated for regenerative applications. Although histology reveals a significant inflammatory reaction (Minabe 1991), clinical studies have shown effective tissue regeneration outcomes (Magnusson et al. 1988). Collistat is another collagen type I–derived material that has demonstrated potential for GTR, with the membrane completely resorbing 7 days after implantation (Jepsen et al. 2002). Chitosan is a polysaccharide comprised of co-polymers of glucosamine and N-acetylglucosamine (Kweon et al. 2003). It shows good biocompatibility and degradation appears to have no toxicity (Kumar 2000). In addition, it has bacteriostatic properties, and inhibits the growth of Gram-negative and Gram-positive bacteria such as *Aggregatibacter actinomycetemcomitans* and *Streptococcus mutans* (Xu et al. 2012).

A chitosan-based non-woven barrier membrane has been investigated that has a porous structure and is easy to manipulate (Yeo et al. 2005). It has shown the ability to enhance new bone and cementum formation in surgically created one-wall intrabony defects in beagle dogs (Yeo et al. 2005). Avitene is a microfibrillar hemostatic collagen type I membrane that is derived from bovine corium. Histological evaluation in a clinical study has shown that this membrane was not clinically effective and is difficult to handle during surgery (Tanner et al. 1988) (see Figure 19.5).

Synthetic degradable barrier membranes

The most commonly used biomaterials utilized to fabricate synthetic degradable barrier membranes are the poly-α-hydroxy acids, which include polylactic polyglycolic acid and their co-polymers (Caton et al. 1994). The advantage of using polyhydroxy acids is that they undergo complete hydrolysis to water and carbon dioxide, which allows for complete removal from the implantation site (Vert et al. 1992). However, the degradation rate varies depending on the presence of glycols and lactides in the constitutional makeup (Israelachvili & Wennerström 1996).

Epi-Guide® (Curasan, Inc., Wake Forest, NC, USA) is a porous, three-layered and three-dimensional barrier membrane,

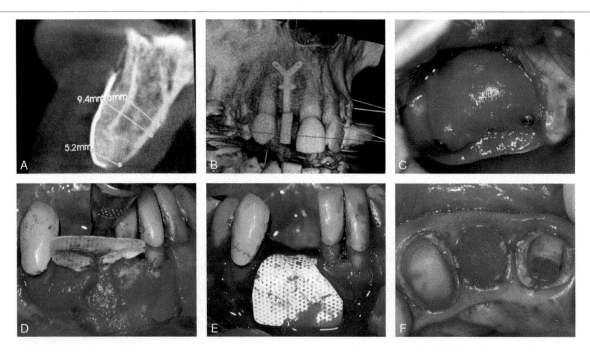

Figure 19.5 Examples of absorbable and non-resorbable barrier membranes used during intraoral guided bone regeneration procedures. (A, B) Cone beam computed tomography scan of the anterior maxilla 5 months after bone augmentation with freeze-dried bone allograft (FDBA) covered with a dense titanium-reinforced polytetrafluoroethylene (dPTFE) membrane. Note the stability of the membrane and the added volume of horizontal bone achieved. (D, E) Application and customization of the titanium-reinforced dPTFE membrane to a bony defect in the mandible. (C, F) Two examples of the application of absorbable collagen membranes.

fabricated from polylactic acid polymers (D, D-L, L polylactic acid), and is completely resorbed in 6–12 months. The three-layered construction of the membrane attracts, traps, and retains fibroblasts and epithelial cells while maintaining space around the defect. Epi-Guide is a self-supporting barrier membrane and can be used in situations without support from bone grafting materials (Parodi et al. 1996; Rapley et al. 1999). Resolut LT® (W.G. Gore & Associates, Inc., Newark, DE, USA) is a barrier membrane made of glycolides and lactic co-polymers and a porous network of polyglycolide fibers that completely resorb in about 5–6 months (Milella et al. 2001; Sculean et al. 2008).

Atrisorb® (Block Drug Corp., Jersey City, NJ, USA) is a barrier membrane that is prepared chair-side during the surgical procedure, because it is made up of a polylactic polymer in a flowable form, dissolved in poly-dl-lactide and a solvent. It is composed 37% of a liquid polymer of lactic acid that is dissolved in 63% N-methyl-2-pyrrolidone, and has a thickness of 600–750 μm. The potential for periodontal regeneration has been investigated in both animal and human class II furcation defects, which have demonstrated favorable regeneration (Coonts et al. 1998). Studies have reported its efficacy in the treatment of periodontal defects (Simion et al. 1996) and it resorbs completely in 6–12 months after implantation (Aurer & Jorgie-Srdjak 2005). Treatment outcomes of GTR were investigated when using Atrisorb in intrabony defects in a 3-year follow-up study (Sakallıoğlu et al. 2007). The results

showed that the outcome of treatment with Atrisorb may be similar to that of OFD (Sakallıoğlu et al. 2007). A randomized controlled clinical trial showed that there was no regeneration when the biodegradable membrane Atrisorb was used in combination with autogenous bone grafts (Nygaard-Østby et al. 2010).

Guidor® (Osteogenics Biomedical, Lubbock, TX, USA) is a double-layered resorbable barrier membrane composed of both polylactic acid and a citric acid ester known as acetyl tributyl-citrate. The external layer of the barrier membrane is designed with rectangular perforations, allowing the integration of the overlying gingival flap. This surface design successfully promotes tissue integration and only limited gingival recession after usage has been reported (Araujo et al. 1998; Simion et al. 1996). Between the internal and external layers, internal spacers are present that create space for tissue ingrowth. The internal layer has smaller circular perforations and outer spacers for maintaining the space between the membrane and the root surface. Studies have shown this membrane to be successful in the treatment of various periodontal defects (Araujo et al. 1998).

Vicryl® periodontal mesh (Ethicon, Inc., Somerville, NJ, USA) is made up of polyglactin 910 fibers that are co-polymers of glycolide and L-lactide, forming a tight woven mesh (Taddei et al. 2002). This barrier membrane has been shown to start resorbing after 2 weeks of implantation and completely resorbs in about 4 weeks (Park et al. 1997). Mempol® (Ethicon, Inc.) is manufactured from polydioxanon (PDS) with a bilayer structure. The first layer is covered with PDS loops 200 μm long to be used on the gingival side and is completely non-permeable (Dörfer et al. 2000; Singh 2013).

Conclusion and future considerations

Extensive research has been carried out over the past few decades for the development of novel biomaterial options for periodontal regenerative applications. Various hard tissue grafts and barrier membranes have been investigated for use in different combinations to promote periodontal regeneration. It is quite evident that the mechanical properties, biological behavior, and biodegradation mechanisms vary among the different biomaterials. To date, there is no ideal biomaterial option or surgical technique that consistently provides perfect clinical results with regard to periodontal regeneration. Further extensive research is required, with a need to focus on improving the biological interfacing between the graft material and the host tissues. Further approaches in the field of periodontal regeneration will rely on a combination of therapies together with the usage of improved biomaterial options.

REFERENCES

Al Ruhaimi KA. Bone graft substitutes: a comparative qualitative histologic review of current osteoconductive grafting materials. *Int J Oral Maxillofac Implants.* 2001; 16(1):105–114.

Albandar JM. Epidemiology and risk factors of periodontal diseases. *Dent Clin North Am.* 2005; 49(3):517–532.

AlGhamdi AS, Shibly O, Ciancio SG. Osseous grafting part II: xenografts and alloplasts for periodontal regeneration—a literature review. *J Int Acad Periodontol.* 2010; 12(2):39–44.

Araujo M, Berglundh T, Lindhe J. GTR treatment of degree III furcation defects with 2 different resorbable barriers. An experimental study in dogs. *J Clin Periodontol.* 1998; 25(3):253–259.

Araujo PP, Oliveira KP, Montenegro SC et al. Block allograft for reconstruction of alveolar bone ridge in implantology: a systematic review. *Implant Dent.* 2013; 22(3):304–308.

Armitage GC, Cullinan MP. Comparison of the clinical features of chronic and aggressive periodontitis. *Periodontol* 2000. 2010; 53:12–27.

Asghari F, Samiei M, Adibkia K, Akbarzadeh A, Davaran S. Biodegradable and biocompatible polymers for tissue engineering application: a review. *Artif Cells Nanomed Biotechnol.* 2017; 45(2):185–192.

Aukhil I, Simpson D, Schaberg T. An experimental study of new attachment procedure in beagle dogs. *J Periodontal Res.* 1983; 18(6):643–654.

Aurer A, Jorgie-Srdjak K. Membranes for periodontal regeneration. *Acta Stomatol Croat.* 2005; 39:107–112.

Avera SP, Stampley WA, McAllister BS. Histologic and clinical observations of resorbable and nonresorbable barrier membranes used in maxillary sinus graft containment. *Int J Oral Maxillofac Implants.* 1996; 12(1):88–94.

Bagambisa FB, Joos U, Schilli W. Mechanisms and structure of the bond between bone and hydroxyapatite ceramics. *J Biomed Mater Res.* 1993; 27(8):1047–1055.

Bauer JJ, Salky BA, Gelernt IM, Kreel I. Repair of large abdominal wall defects with expanded polytetrafluoroethylene (PTFE). *Ann Surg.* 1987; 206(6):765.

Behring J, Junker R, Walboomers XF, Chessnut B, Jansen JA. Toward guided tissue and bone regeneration: morphology, attachment, proliferation, and migration of cells cultured on collagen barrier membranes. *A systematic review. Odontology.* 2008; 96(1):1–11.

Blaggana V, Gill AS, Blaggana A. A clinical and radiological evaluation of the relative efficacy of demineralized freeze-dried bone allograft versus anorganic bovine bone xenograft in the treatment of human infrabony periodontal defects: A 6 months follow-up study. *J Indian Soc Periodontol.* 2014; 18(5):601–607.

Block MS, Degen M. Horizontal ridge augmentation using human mineralized particulate bone: preliminary results. *J Oral Maxillofac Surg.* 2004; 62(9 Suppl 2):67–72.

Buck B, Malinin TI, Brown MD. Bone transplantation and human immunodeficiency virus: an estimate of risk of acquired immunodeficiency syndrome (AIDS). *Clin Orthop Relat Res.* 1989; 240:129–136.

Bunyaratavej P, Wang H-L. Collagen membranes: a review. *J Periodontol.* 2001; 72(2):215–229.

Buser D, Dula K, Hess D, Hirt HP, Belser UC. Localized ridge augmentation with autografts and barrier membranes. *Periodontol* 2000. 1999; 19:151–163.

Camargo PM, Lekovic V, Weinlaender M et al. Platelet-rich plasma and bovine porous bone mineral combined with guided tissue regeneration in the treatment of intrabony defects in humans. *J Periodontal Res.* 2002; 37(4):300–306.

Carvalho SM, Oliveira AA, Jardim CA et al. Characterization and induction of cementoblast cell proliferation by bioactive glass nanoparticles. *J Tissue Eng Regen Med.* 2012; 6(10):813–821.

Caton J, Greenstein G, Zappa U. Synthetic bioabsorbable barrier for regeneration in human periodontal defects. *J Periodontol.* 1994; 65(11):1037–1045.

Caton JG, Armitage G, Berglundh T et al. A new classification scheme for periodontal and peri-implant diseases and conditions—introduction and key changes from the 1999 classification. *J Clin Periodontol.* 2018; 45(Suppl 20):S1–S8.

Cho BC, Chung HY, Lee DG et al. The effect of chitosan bead encapsulating calcium sulfate as an injectable bone substitute on consolidation in the mandibular distraction osteogenesis of a dog model. *J Oral Maxillofac Surg.* 2005; 63(12):1753–1764.

310 / Chapter 19: Biomaterials in periodontal regeneration

Committee on Research, Science and Therapy of the American Academy of Periodontology. Tissue banking of bone allografts used in periodontal regeneration. *J Periodontol.* 2001; 72(6):834–838.

Contar CM, Sarot JR, Bordini J Jr et al. Maxillary ridge augmentation with fresh-frozen bone allografts. *J Oral Maxillofac Surg.* 2009; 67(6):1280–1285.

Contar CM, Sarot JR, da Costa MB et al. Fresh-frozen bone allografts in maxillary ridge augmentation: histologic analysis. *J Oral Implantol.* 2011; 37(2):223–231.

Coonts B, Whitman S, O'Donnell M et al. Biodegradation and biocompatibility of a guided tissue regeneration barrier membrane formed from a liquid polymer material. *J Biomed Mater Res.* 1998; 42(2):303–311.

Cypher TJ, Grossman JP. Biological principles of bone graft healing. *J Foot Ankle Surg.* 1996; 35(5):413–417.

Dahlin C, Linde A, Gottlow J, Nyman S. Healing of bone defects by guided tissue regeneration. *Plast Reconstr Surg.* 1988; 81(5):672–676.

Dias RR, Sehn FP, de Santana Santos T et al. Corticocancellous fresh-frozen allograft bone blocks for augmenting atrophied posterior mandibles in humans. *Clin Oral Implants Res.* 2016; 27(1):39–46.

Dörfer CE, Kim TS, Steinbrenner H, Holle R, Eickholz P. Regenerative periodontal surgery in interproximal intrabony defects with biodegradable barriers. *J Clin Periodontol.* 2000; 27(3):162–168.

Draenert FG, Huetzen D, Neff A, Mueller WE. Vertical bone augmentation procedures: basics and techniques in dental implantology. *J Biomed Mater Res A.* 2014; 102(5):1605–1613.

Dragoo MR, Sullivan HCJ. A clinical and histological evaluation of autogenous iliac bone grafts in humans. Part II. External root resorption. *J Periodontol.* 1973; 44(10):614–625.

Edmunds RK, Mealey BL, Mills MP et al. Maxillary anterior ridge augmentation with recombinant human bone morphogenetic protein 2. *Int J Periodontics Restorative Dent.* 2014; 34(4):551–557.

Ewers R. Maxilla sinus grafting with marine algae derived bone forming material: a clinical report of long-term results. *J Oral Maxillofac Surg.* 2005; 63(12):1712–1723.

Felice P, Marchetti C, Iezzi G et al. Vertical ridge augmentation of the atrophic posterior mandible with interpositional bloc grafts: bone from the iliac crest vs. bovine anorganic bone. Clinical and histological results up to one year after loading from a randomized-controlled clinical trial. *Clin Oral Implants Res.* 2009; 20(12):1386–1393.

Fennis J, Stoelinga P, Jansen J. Mandibular reconstruction: a histological and histomorphometric study on the use of autogenous scaffolds, particulate cortico-cancellous bone grafts and platelet rich plasma in goats. *Int J Oral Maxillofac Surg.* 2004; 33(1):48–55.

Fine N, Sheikh Z, Al-Jaf F et al. Differential response of human blood leukocytes to brushite, monetite, and calcium polyphosphate biomaterials. *J Biomed Mater Res B Appl Biomater.* 2020; 108(1):253–262.

Friedlaender GE, Strong DM, Sell KW. Studies on the antigenicity of bone. I. Freeze-dried and deep-frozen bone allografts in rabbits. *J Bone Joint Surg Am.* 1976; 58(6):854–858.

Froum SJ. Human histologic evaluation of HTR polymer and freeze-dried bone allograft. *A case report. J Clin Periodontol.* 1996; 23(7):615–620.

Gbureck U, Hölzel T, Klammert U et al. Resorbable dicalcium phosphate bone substitutes prepared by 3D powder printing. *Adv Funct Mater.* 2007; 17(18):3940–3945.

Gehrke S, Famà G. Buccal dehiscence and sinus lift cases—predictable bone augmentation with synthetic bone material. *Implants.* 2010; 11:4.

Giannobile WV, Ryan S, Shih MS et al. Recombinant human osteogenic protein-1 (OP-1) stimulates periodontal wound healing in class III furcation defects. *J Periodontol.* 1998; 69(2):129–137.

Gotfredsen K, Nimb L, Hjørting-Hansen E. Immediate implant placement using a biodegradable barrier, polyhydroxybutyrate-hydroxyvalerate reinforced with polyglactin 910. An experimental study in dogs. *Clin Oral Implants Res.* 1994; 5(2):83–91.

Guida L, Annunziata M, Belardo S et al. Effect of autogenous cortical bone particulate in conjunction with enamel matrix derivative in the treatment of periodontal intraosseous defects. *J Periodontol.* 2007; 78(2):231–238.

Hall EE, Meffert RM, Hermann JS, Mellonig JT, Cochran DL. Comparison of bioactive glass to demineralized freeze-dried bone allograft in the treatment of intrabony defects around implants in the canine mandible. *J Periodontol.* 1999;70(5):526–535.

Hämmerle CH, Jung RE. Bone augmentation by means of barrier membranes. *Periodontol 2000.* 2003; 33(1):36–53.

Hardwick R, Dahlin C. Healing pattern of bone regeneration in membrane-protected defects: a histologic study in the canine mandible. *Int J Oral Maxillofac Implants.* 1994; 9(1):13–29.

Hardwick R, Hayes BK, Flynn C. Devices for dentoalveolar regeneration: an up-to-date literature review. *J Periodontol.* 1995; 66(6):495–505.

Heijl L. Periodontal regeneration with enamel matrix derivative in one human experimental defect. *A case report. J Clin Periodontol.* 1997; 24(9 Pt 2):693–696.

Hoffmann T, Al-Machot E, Meyle J, Jervøe-Storm P-M, Jepsen S. Three-year results following regenerative periodontal surgery of advanced intrabony defects with enamel matrix derivative alone or combined with a synthetic bone graft. *Clin Oral Investig.* 2016; 20(2):357–364.

Hopp SG, Dahners LE, Gilbert JA. A study of the mechanical strength of long bone defects treated with various bone autograft substitutes: an experimental investigation in the rabbit. *J Orthop Res.* 1989; 7(4):579–584.

Hürzeler M, Strub J. Guided bone regeneration around exposed implants: a new bioresorbable device and bioresorbable membrane pins. *Practical periodontics and aesthetic dentistry: PPAD.* 1994; 7(9):37–47.

Idown B, Cama G, Deb S, Di Silvio L. in vitro osteoinductive potential of porous monetite for bone tissue engineering. *J Tissue Eng.* 2014; 5:2041731414536572.

Israelachvili J, Wennerström H. Role of hydration and water structure in biological and colloidal interactions. *Nature.* 1996; 379(6562):219–225.

Jacotti M, Wang HL, Fu JH, Zamboni G, Bernardello F. Ridge augmentation with mineralized block allografts: clinical and histological evaluation of 8 cases treated with the 3-dimensional block technique. *Implant Dent.* 2012; 21(6):444–448.

Jarcho M. Calcium phosphate ceramics as hard tissue prosthetics. *Clin Orthop Relat Res.* 1981; 157:259–278.

Jepsen S, Eberhard J, Herrera D, Needleman I. A systematic review of guided tissue regeneration for periodontal furcation defects. What is the effect of guided tissue regeneration compared with surgical debridement in the treatment of furcation defects? *J Clin Periodontol.* 2002; 29(s3):103–116.

Kao RT, Nares S, Reynolds MA. Periodontal regeneration—intrabony defects: a systematic review from the AAP regeneration workshop. *J Periodontol.* 2015; 86(2-s):S77–S104.

Kassolis JD, Reynolds MA. Evaluation of the adjunctive benefits of platelet-rich plasma in subantral sinus augmentation. *J Craniofac Surg.* 2005; 16(2):280–287.

Katanec D, Granic M, Majstorovic M, Trampus Z, Panduric DG. Use of recombinant human bone morphogenetic protein (rhBMP2) in bilateral alveolar ridge augmentation: case report. *Coll Antropol.* 2014; 38(1):325–330.

Kempczinski RF, Rosenman JE, Pearce WH et al. Endothelial cell seeding of a new PTFE vascular prosthesis. *J Vasc Surg.* 1985; 2(3):424–429.

Kim YJ, Lee JY, Kim JE et al. Ridge preservation using demineralized bone matrix gel with recombinant human bone morphogenetic protein-2 after tooth extraction: a randomized controlled clinical trial. *J Oral Maxillofac Surg.* 2014; 72(7):1281–1290.

Klein CP, Driessen AA, de Groot K, van den Hooff A. Biodegradation behavior of various calcium phosphate materials in bone tissue. *J Biomed Mater Res.* 1983; 17(5):769–784.

Knapen M, Gheldof D, Drion P et al. Effect of leukocyte- and platelet-rich fibrin (L-PRF) on bone regeneration: a study in rabbits. *Clin Implant Dent Relat Res.* 2015; 17(Suppl 1):e143–e152.

Knapp CI, Feuille F, Cochran DL, Mellonig JT. Clinical and histologic evaluation of bone-replacement grafts in the treatment of localized alveolar ridge defects. Part 2: Bioactive glass particulate. *Int J Periodontics Restorative Dent.* 2003; 23(2):129–137.

Kukreja BJ, Dodwad V, Kukreja P, Ahuja S, Mehra P. A comparative evaluation of platelet-rich plasma in combination with demineralized freeze-dried bone allograft and DFDBA alone in the treatment of periodontal intrabony defects: a clinicoradiographic study. *J Indian Soc Periodontol.* 2014; 18(5):618–623.

Kumar MNR. A review of chitin and chitosan applications. *React Funct Polym.* 2000; 46(1):1–27.

Kweon D-K, Song S-B, Park Y-Y. Preparation of water-soluble chitosan/heparin complex and its application as wound healing accelerator. *Biomaterials.* 2003; 24(9):1595–1601.

Lee C, Grodzinsky A, Spector M. The effects of cross-linking of collagen glycosaminoglycan scaffolds on compressive stiffness, chondrocyte-mediated contraction, proliferation and biosynthesis. *Biomaterials.* 2001; 22(23):3145–3154.

Lee S-W, Kim S-G. Membranes for the guided bone regeneration. *Maxillofac Plast Reconstr Surg.* 2014; 36(6):239–246.

Lekovic V, Camargo PM, Weinlaender M et al. Effectiveness of a combination of platelet-rich plasma, bovine porous bone mineral and guided tissue regeneration in the treatment of mandibular grade II molar furcations in humans. *J Clin Periodontol.* 2003; 30(8):746–751.

Li S-T, Chen H-C, Lee NS, Ringshia R, Yuen D. A comparative study of Zimmer Biomend® and Biomend® extend™ membranes made at two different manufacturing facilities. *Zimmer Dental White Paper,* 2013.

Linde A, Alberius P, Dahlin C, Bjurstam K, Sundin Y. Osteopromotion: a soft-tissue exclusion principle using a membrane for bone healing and bone neogenesis. *J Periodontol.* 1993; 64(11s):1116–1128.

Liu X, Li Q, Wang F, Wang Z. Maxillary sinus floor augmentation and dental implant placement using dentin matrix protein-1 gene-modified bone marrow stromal cells mixed with deproteinized boving bone: a comparative study in beagles. *Arch Oral Biol.* 2016; 64:102–108.

Lundgren D, Sennerby L, Falk H, Friberg B, Nyman S. The use of a new bioresorbable barrier for guided bone regeneration in connection with implant installation. *Case reports. Clin Oral Implants Res.* 1994; 5(3):177–184.

Lyford RH, Mills MP, Knapp CI, Scheyer ET, Mellonig JT. Clinical evaluation of freeze-dried block allografts for alveolar ridge augmentation: a case series. *Int J Periodontics Restorative Dent.* 2003; 23(5):417–425.

Macedo LG, Mazzucchelli-Cosmo LA, Macedo NL, Monteiro AS, Sendyk WR. Fresh-frozen human bone allograft in vertical ridge augmentation: clinical and tomographic evaluation of bone formation and resorption. *Cell Tissue Bank.* 2012; 13(4):577–586.

Magnusson I, Batich C, Collins B. New attachment formation following controlled tissue regeneration using biodegradable membranes. *J Periodontol.* 1988; 59(1):1–6.

Maragos P, Bissada NF, Wang R, Cole BP. Comparison of three methods using calcium sulfate as a graft/barrier material for the treatment of Class II mandibular molar furcation defects. *Int J Periodontics Restorative Dent.* 2002; 22(5):493–501.

Markou N, Pepelassi E, Vavouraki H et al. Treatment of periodontal endosseous defects with platelet-rich plasma alone or in combination with demineralized freeze-dried bone allograft: a comparative clinical trial. *J Periodontol.* 2009; 80(12):1911–1919.

Marx RE. Platelet-rich plasma: evidence to support its use. *J Oral Maxillofac Surg.* 2004; 62(4):489–496.

Marx RE, Carlson ER, Eichstaedt RM et al. Platelet-rich plasma: growth factor enhancement for bone grafts. *Oral Surg Oral Med Oral Pathol Oral Radiol Endod.* 1998; 85(6):638–646.

McAllister BS, Haghighat K. Bone augmentation techniques. *J Periodontol.* 2007; 78(3):377–396.

McAllister BS, Margolin MD, Cogan AG et al. Eighteen-month radiographic and histologic evaluation of sinus grafting with anorganic bovine bone in the chimpanzee. *Int J Oral Maxillofac Implants.* 1999; 14(3):361–368.

Meffert RM, Thomas JR, Hamilton KM, Brownstein CN. Hydroxylapatite as an alloplastic graft in the treatment of human periodontal osseous defects. *J Periodontol.* 1985; 56(2):63–73.

Mellonig JT. Freeze-dried bone allografts in periodontal reconstructive surgery. *Dent Clin North Am.* 1991; 35(3):505–520.

Mellonig JT. Human histologic evaluation of a bovine-derived bone xenograft in the treatment of periodontal osseous defects. *Int J Periodontics Restorative Dent.* 2000; 20(1):19–29.

Mellonig JT, Bowers GM, Bailey RC. Comparison of bone graft materials. Part I. New bone formation with autografts and allografts determined by Strontium-85. *J Periodontol.* 1981; 52(6):291–296.

Metsger DS, Driskell T, Paulsrud J. Tricalcium phosphate ceramic—a resorbable bone implant: review and current status. *J Am Dent Assoc.* 1982; 105(6):1035–1038.

Milella E, Ramires P, Brescia E et al. Physicochemical, mechanical, and biological properties of commercial membranes for GTR. *J Biomed Mater Res.* 2001; 58(4):427–435.

Minabe M. A critical review of the biologic rationale for guided tissue regeneration. *J Periodontol.* 1991; 62(3):171–179.

Miron RJ, Fujioka-Kobayashi M, Bishara M et al. Platelet-rich fibrin and soft tissue wound healing: a systematic review. *Tissue Eng Part B Rev.* 2017; 23(1):83–99.

Miron RJ, Sculean A, Cochran DL et al. Twenty years of enamel matrix derivative: the past, the present and the future. *J Clin Periodontol.* 2016; 43(8):668–683.

Misch CM. Comparison of intraoral donor sites for onlay grafting prior to implant placement. *Int J Oral Maxillofac Implants.* 1997; 12(6):767–776.

Moore WR, Graves SE, Bain GI. Synthetic bone graft substitutes. *ANZ J Surgery.* 2001; 71(6):354–361.

Murphy KG. Postoperative healing complications associated with Gore-Tex periodontal material. Part I. Incidence and characterization. *Int J Periodontics Restorative Dent.* 1995; 15(4):363–375.

Murphy KG, Gunsolley JC. Guided tissue regeneration for the treatment of periodontal intrabony and furcation defects. *A systematic review. Ann Periodontol.* 2003; 8(1):266–302.

Murray VK. Clinical applications of HTR polymer in periodontal surgery. *Compend Suppl.* 1988(10):S342–S347.

Nakajima Y, Fiorellini JP, Kim DM, Weber HP, Dent M. Regeneration of standardized mandibular bone defects using expanded polytetrafluoroethylene membrane and various bone fillers. *Int J Periodontics Restorative Dent.* 2007; 27(2):151–159.

Nannmark U, Sennerby L. The bone tissue responses to prehydrated and collagenated cortico-cancellous porcine bone grafts: a study in rabbit maxillary defects. *Clin Implant Dent Relat Res.* 2008; 10(4):264–270.

Nevins ML, Camelo M, Nevins M et al. Human histologic evaluation of bioactive ceramic in the treatment of periodontal osseous defects. *Int J Periodontics Restorative Dent.* 2000; 20(5):458–467.

Nikolidakis D, Dolder JVD, Wolke JG, Stoelinga PJ, Jansen JA. The effect of platelet-rich plasma on the bone healing around calcium phosphate–coated and non-coated oral implants in trabecular bone. *Tissue Eng.* 2006; 12(9):2555–2563.

Nobréus N, Attström R, Linde A. Guided bone regeneration in dental implant treatment using a bioabsorbable membrane. *Clin Oral Implants Res.* 1997; 8(1):10–17.

Nyan M, Miyahara T, Noritake K et al. Feasibility of alpha tricalcium phosphate for vertical bone augmentation. *J Investig Clin Dent.* 2014; 5(2):109–116.

Nygaard-Østby P, Bakke V, Nesdal O, Susin C, Wikesjö UM. Periodontal healing following reconstructive surgery: effect of guided tissue regeneration using a bioresorbable barrier device when combined with autogenous bone grafting. A randomized-controlled trial 10-year follow-up. *J Clin Periodontol.* 2010;37(4):366–373.

Oh TJ, Meraw SJ, Lee EJ, Giannobile WV, Wang HL. Comparative analysis of collagen membranes for the treatment of implant dehiscence defects. *Clin Oral Implants Res.* 2003; 14(1):80–90.

Osborn J, Newesely H. The material science of calcium phosphate ceramics. *Biomaterials.* 1980; 1(2):108–111.

Paolantonio M, Perinetti G, Dolci M et al. Surgical treatment of periodontal intrabony defects with calcium sulfate implant and barrier versus collagen barrier or open flap debridement alone: a 12-month randomized controlled clinical trial. *J Periodontol.* 2008; 79(10):1886–1893.

Park YJ, Nam KH, Ha SJ et al. Porous poly (L-lactide) membranes for guided tissue regeneration and controlled drug delivery: membrane fabrication and characterization. *J Control Release.* 1997; 43(2):151–160.

Parodi R, Santarelli G, Carusi G. Application of slow-resorbing collagen membrane to periodontal and peri-implant guided tissue regeneration. *Int J Periodontics Restorative Dent.* 1996; 16(2):174–185.

Pearce A, Richards R, Milz S, Schneider E, Pearce S. Animal models for implant biomaterial research in bone: a review. *Eur Cell Mater.* 2007; 13(1):1–10.

Plachokova AS, Nikolidakis D, Mulder J, Jansen JA, Creugers NH. Effect of platelet-rich plasma on bone regeneration in dentistry: a systematic review. *Clin Oral Implants Res.* 2008; 19(6):539–545.

Pocaterra A, Caruso S, Bernardi S et al. Effectiveness of platelet-rich plasma as an adjunctive material to bone graft: a systematic review and meta-analysis of randomized controlled clinical trials. *Int J Oral Maxillofac Surg.* 2016; 45(8):1027–1034.

Quattlebaum JB, Mellonig JT, Hensel NF. Antigenicity of freeze-dried cortical bone allograft in human periodontal osseous defects. *J Periodontol.* 1988; 59(6):394–397.

Rabalais ML Jr, Yukna RA, Mayer ET. Evaluation of durapatite ceramic as an alloplastic implant in periodontal osseous defects. *I. Initial six-month results. J Periodontol.* 1981; 52(11):680–689.

Ramseier CA, Rasperini G, Batia S, Giannobile WV. Advanced reconstructive technologies for periodontal tissue repair. *Periodontol 2000.* 2012; 59(1):185–202.

Rao SM, Ugale GM, Warad SB. Bone morphogenetic proteins: periodontal regeneration. *N Am J Med Sci.* 2013; 5(3):161–168.

Rapiey J, Nechamkin SJ, Ringeisen TA, Derhaili M, Brekke J. The use of biodegradable polylactic acid barrier materials in the treatment of grade II periodontal furcation defects in humans—part II: a multi-center investigative surgical study. *Int J Periodontics Restorative Dent.* 1999; 19:57–65.

Ratner BD. *Biomaterials Science: An Introduction to Materials in Medicine.* New York: Academic Press; 2004.

Ricci JL, Blumenthal NC, Spivak JM, Alexander H. Evaluation of a low-temperature calcium phosphate particulate implant material: physical-chemical properties and in vivo bone response. *J Oral Maxillofac Surg.* 1992; 50(9):969–978.

Roy DM, Linnehan SK. Hydroxyapatite formed from coral skeletal carbonate by hydrothermal exchange. *Nature.* 1974; 247(5438):220–222.

Russell J, Scarborough N, Chesmel K. Ability of commercial demineralized freeze-dried bone allograft to induce new bone formation. *J Periodontol.* 1997; 68(8):804–806.

Sakallıoğlu U, Yavuz Ü, Lütfioğlu M, Keskiner I, Açıkgöz G. Clinical outcomes of guided tissue regeneration with Atrisorb membrane in the treatment of intrabony defects: a 3-year follow-up study. *Int J Periodontics Restorative Dent.* 2007; 27(1):79–88.

Scantlebury TV. 1982–1992: A decade of technology development for guided tissue regeneration. *J Periodontol.* 1993; 64(11s):1129–1137.

Scarano A, Degidi M, Iezzi G et al. Maxillary sinus augmentation with different biomaterials: a comparative histologic and histomorphometric study in man. *Implant Dent.* 2006; 15(2):197–207.

Schepers E, de Clercq M, Ducheyne P, Kempeneers R. Bioactive glass particulate material as a filler for bone lesions. *J Oral Rehabil.* 1991; 18(5):439–452.

Schepers EJ, Ducheyne P. Bioactive glass particles of narrow size range for the treatment of oral bone defects: a 1–24-month experiment with several materials and particle sizes and size ranges. *J Oral Rehabil.* 1997; 24(3):171–181.

Schliephake H, Neukam F, Hutmacher D, Becker J. Enhancement of bone ingrowth into a porous hydroxylapatite-matrix using a resorbable polylactic membrane: an experimental pilot study. *J Oral Maxillofac Surg.* 1994; 52(1):57–63.

Schwartz Z, Mellonig J, Carnes D Jr et al. Ability of commercial demineralized freeze-dried bone allograft to induce new bone formation. 1996; 67(9):918–926.

Schwartz Z, Somers A, Mellonig J et al. Ability of commercial demineralized freeze-dried bone allograft to induce new bone formation is dependent on donor age but not gender. *J Periodontol.* 1998; 69(4):470–478.

Sculean A, Nikolidakis D, Schwarz F. Regeneration of periodontal tissues: combinations of barrier membranes and grafting materials—biological foundation and preclinical evidence: a systematic review. *J Clin Periodontol.* 2008; 35(s8):106–116.

Shalash MA, Rahman HA, Azim AA et al. Evaluation of horizontal ridge augmentation using beta tricalcium phosphate and demineralized bone matrix: a comparative study. *J Clin Exp Dent.* 2013; 5(5):e253–e259.

Sheikh Z, Abdallah MN, Al-Jaf F et al. Achieving enhanced bone regeneration using monetite granules with bone anabolic drug conjugates (C3 and C6) in rat mandibular defects. *J Biomed Mater Res.* 2020a; 108(6):2670–2680.

Sheikh Z, Abdallah MN, Al-Jaf F et al. Improved bone regeneration using bone anabolic drug conjugates (C3 and C6) with deproteinized bovine bone mineral as a carrier in rat mandibular defects. *J Periodontol.* 2020b; 91(11):1521–1531.

Sheikh Z, Abdallah M-N, Hanafi AA et al. Mechanisms of in vivo degradation and resorption of calcium phosphate-based biomaterials. *Materials.* 2015a; 8(11):7913–7925.

Sheikh Z, Brooks PJ, Barzilay O, Fine N, Glogauer M. Macrophages, foreign body giant cells and their response to implantable biomaterials. *Materials.* 2015b; 8(9):5671–5701.

Sheikh Z, Chen G, Thévenin M et al. A novel anabolic conjugate (c3) in the matrix of dicalcium phosphate onlay block grafts for achieving vertical bone augmentation: an experimental study on rabbit calvaria. *Int J Oral Maxillofac Implants.* 2019a; 34(4):e51–e63.

Sheikh Z, Drager J, Zhang YL et al. Controlling bone graft substitute microstructure to improve bone augmentation. *Adv Healthc Mater.* 2016a; 5(13):1646–1655.

Sheikh Z, Geffers M, Christel T, Barralet JE, Gbureck U. Chelate setting of alkali ion substituted calcium phosphates. *Ceram Int.* 2015c; 41(8):10010–10017.

Sheikh Z, Hamdan N, Abdallah M-N, Glogauer M, Grynpas M. Natural and synthetic bone replacement graft materials for dental and maxillofacial applications. In: Z Khurshid, S Najeeb, MS Zafar, F Sefat (eds), *Advanced Dental Biomaterials*. St. Louis, MO: Elsevier; 2019b: 347–376.

Sheikh Z, Hamdan N, Ikeda Y et al. Natural graft tissues and synthetic biomaterials for periodontal and alveolar bone reconstructive applications: a review. *Biomater Res.* 2017a; 21(1):9.

Sheikh Z, Hamdan N, Javaid MA, Z Khurshid. Barrier membranes for tissue regeneration and bone augmentation techniques in dentistry. In: KP Matilinna (ed.), *Handbook of Oral Biomaterials*. Singapore: Pan Stanford; 2014.

Sheikh Z, Hasanpour S, Glogauer M. Bone grafting. In: E Emami, J Feine (eds), *Mandibular Implant Prostheses*. Cham: Springer; 2018: 155–174.

Sheikh ZA, Javaid MA, Abdallah MN. Bone replacement graft materials in dentistry. In: SZ Khurshid (ed.), *Dental Biomaterials (Principle and Its Application)*. Paramount Publishing; 2013: 74–87.

Sheikh Z, Javaid MA, Hamdan N, Hashmi R. Bone regeneration using bone morphogenetic proteins and various biomaterial carriers. *Materials.* 2015d; 8(4):1778–1816.

Sheikh Z, Khan AS, Roohpour N, Glogauer M, U Rehman I. Protein adsorption capability on polyurethane and modified-polyurethane membrane for periodontal guided tissue regeneration applications. *Mater Sci Eng C Mater Biol Appl.* 2016b; 68:267–275.

Sheikh Z, Najeeb S, Khurshid Z et al. Biodegradable materials for bone repair and tissue engineering applications. *Materials.* 2015e; 8(9):5744–5794.

Sheikh Z, Qureshi J, Alshahrani AM et al. Collagen based barrier membranes for periodontal guided bone regeneration applications. *Odontology.* 2017b; 105(1):1–12.

Sheikh Z, Sima C, Glogauer M. Bone replacement materials and techniques used for achieving vertical alveolar bone augmentation. *Materials.* 2015f; 8(6):2953–2993.

Sheikh Z, Zhang YL, Grover L et al. in vitro degradation and in vivo resorption of dicalcium phosphate cement-based grafts. *Acta Biomater.* 2015g; 26:338–346.

Sheikh Z, Zhang YL, Tamimi F, Barralet J. Effect of processing conditions of dicalcium phosphate cements on graft resorption and bone formation. *Acta Biomater.* 2017c; 53:526–535.

Shetty V, Han TJ. Alloplastic materials in reconstructive periodontal surgery. *Dent Clin North Am.* 1991; 35(3):521–530.

Shue L, Yufeng Z, Mony U. Biomaterials for periodontal regeneration: a review of ceramics and polymers. *Biomatter.* 2012; 2(4):271–277.

Shweikeh F, Hanna G, Bloom L et al. Assessment of outcome following the use of recombinant human bone morphogenetic protein-2 for spinal fusion in the elderly population. *J Neurosurg Sci.* 2016. 60(2):256–271.

Simion M, Jovanovic SA, Tinti C, Benfenati SP. Long-term evaluation of osseointegrated implants inserted at the time or after vertical ridge augmentation. A retrospective study on 123 implants with 1–5-year follow-up. *Clin Oral Implants Res.* 2001; 12(1):35–45.

Simion M, Misitano U, Gionso L, Salvato A. Treatment of dehiscences and fenestrations around dental implants using resorbable and nonresorbable membranes associated with bone autografts: a comparative clinical study. *Int J Oral Maxillofac Implants.* 1996; 12(2):159–167.

Simion M, Scarano A, Gionso L, Piattelli A. Guided bone regeneration using resorbable and nonresorbable membranes: a comparative histologic study in humans. *Int J Oral Maxillofac Implants.* 1996; 11(6):735–742.

Singh AK. GTR membranes: the barriers for periodontal regeneration. *DHR Int J Med Sci.* 2013; 4(1):31–38.

Small SA, Zinner ID, Panno FV, Shapiro HJ, Stein JI. Augmenting the maxillary sinus for implants: report of 27 patients. *Int J Oral Maxillofac Implants.* 1993; 8(5):523–528.

Sokolsky-Papkov M, Agashi K, Olaye A, Shakesheff K, Domb AJ. Polymer carriers for drug delivery in tissue engineering. *Adv Drug Deliv Rev.* 2007; 59(4-5):187–206.

Stahl SS, Froum SJ, Tarnow D. Human clinical and histologic responses to the placement of HTR polymer particles in 11 intrabony lesions. *J Periodontol.* 1990; 61(5):269–274.

Stavropoulos A, Windisch P, Szendröi-Kiss D et al. Clinical and histologic evaluation of granular beta-tricalcium phosphate for the treatment of human intrabony periodontal defects: a report on five cases. *J Periodontol.* 2010; 81(2):325–334.

Sterio TW, Katancik JA, Blanchard SB, Xenoudi P, Mealey BL. A prospective, multicenter study of bovine pericardium membrane with cancellous particulate allograft for localized alveolar ridge augmentation. *Int J Periodontics Restorative Dent.* 2013; 33(4):499–507.

Sugar AW, Thielens P, Stafford GD, Willins MJ. Augmentation of the atrophic maxillary alveolar ridge with hydroxyapatite granules in a Vicryl (polyglactin 910) knitted tube and simultaneous open vestibuloplasty. *Br J Oral Maxillofac Surg.* 1995; 33(2):93–97.

Sukumar S, Drizhal I, Paulusová V, Bukac J. Surgical treatment of periodontal intrabony defects with calcium sulphate in combination with beta-tricalcium phosphate: clinical observations two years post-surgery. *Acta Medica (Hradec Kralove).* 2011; 54(1):13–20.

Sunitha Raja V, Naidu M. Platelet-rich fibrin: evolution of a second-generation platelet concentrate. *Indian J Den Res.* 2008;19(1):42–46.

Sykaras N, Opperman LA. Bone morphogenetic proteins (BMPs): how do they function and what can they offer the clinician? *J Oral Sci.* 2003; 45(2):57–73.

Taddei P, Monti P, Simoni R. Vibrational and thermal study on the in vitro and in vivo degradation of a bioabsorbable periodontal membrane: Vicryl® Periodontal Mesh (Polyglactin 910). *J Mater Sci Mater Med.* 2002; 13(1):59–64.

Tamimi F, Le Nihouannen D, Eimar H et al. The effect of autoclaving on the physical and biological properties of dicalcium phosphate dihydrate bioceramics: brushite vs. monetite. *Acta Biomater.* 2012; 8(8):3161–3169.

Tamimi F, Sheikh Z, Barralet J. Dicalcium phosphate cements: brushite and monetite. *Acta Biomater.* 2012b; 8(2):474–487.

Tamimi F, Torres J, Bassett D, Barralet J, Cabarcos EL. Resorption of monetite granules in alveolar bone defects in human patients. *Biomaterials.* 2010; 31(10):2762–2769.

Tamimi F, Torres J, Kathan C et al. Bone regeneration in rabbit calvaria with novel monetite granules. *J Biomed Mater Res A.* 2008; 87(4):980–985.

Tamimi F, Torres J, Lopez-Cabarcos E et al. Minimally invasive maxillofacial vertical bone augmentation using brushite based cements. *Biomaterials.* 2009; 30(2):208–216.

Tamimi FM, Torres J, Tresguerres I et al. Bone augmentation in rabbit calvariae: comparative study between Bio-Oss (R) and a novel beta-TCP/DCPD granulate. *J Clin Periodontol.* 2006; 33(12):922–928.

Tanner MG, Solt CW, Vuddhakanok S. An evaluation of new attachment formation using a microfibhllar collagen barrier. *J Periodontol.* 1988; 59(8):524–530.

Tatakis DN, Promsudthi A, Wikesjö UM. Devices for periodontal regeneration. *Periodontol 2000.* 1999; 19(1):59–73.

Tevlin R, McArdle A, Atashroo D et al. Biomaterials for craniofacial bone engineering. *J Dent Res.* 2014; 93(12):1187–1195.

Thaller SR, Hoyt J, Borjeson K, Dart A, Tesluk H. Reconstruction of calvarial defects with anorganic bovine bone mineral (Bio-Oss) in a rabbit model. *J Craniofac Surg.* 1993; 4(2):79–84.

Vert M. Bioresorbable polymers for temporary therapeutic applications. *Die Angewandte Makromolekulare Chemie.* 1989; 166(1):155–168.

Vert M, Li S, Spenlehauer G, Guérin P. Bioresorbability and biocompatibility of aliphatic polyesters. *J Mater Sci Mater Med.* 1992; 3(6):432–446.

Wallace S, Gellin R. Clinical evaluation of freeze-dried cancellous block allografts for ridge augmentation and implant placement in the maxilla. *Implant Dent.* 2010; 19(4):272–279.

Wallace SS, Froum SJ. Effect of maxillary sinus augmentation on the survival of endosseous dental implants. *A systematic review. Ann Periodontol.* 2003; 8(1):328–343.

Wang H, Li Y, Zuo Y et al. Biocompatibility and osteogenesis of biomimetic nano-hydroxyapatite/polyamide composite scaffolds for bone tissue engineering. *Biomaterials.* 2007; 28(22):3338–3348.

Wang H-L, Carroll M. Guided bone regeneration using bone grafts and collagen membranes. *Quintessence Int.* 2000; 32(7):504–515.

Wang H-L, MacNeil RL. Guided tissue regeneration. Absorbable barriers. *Dent Clin North Am.* 1998; 42(3):505–522.

White E, Shors E. Biomaterial aspects of Interpore-200 porous hydroxyapatite. *Dent Clin North Am.* 1986; 30(1):49–67.

Wilk, R. Bony reconstruction of the jaws. In: M Miloro, GE Ghali, P Larsen, P Waite (eds), *Peterson's Principles of Oral and Maxillofacial Surgery.* London: Hamilton; 2004: 785–787.

Wong RW, Rabie AB. Effect of Gusuibu graft on bone formation. *J Oral Maxillofac Surg.* 2006; 64(5):770–777.

Xu C, Lei C, Meng L, Wang C, Song Y. Chitosan as a barrier membrane material in periodontal tissue regeneration. *J Biomed Mater Res B Appl Biomater.* 2012; 100(5):1435–1443.

Xynos ID, Edgar AJ, Buttery LD, Hench LL, Polak JM. Gene-expression profiling of human osteoblasts following treatment with the ionic products of Bioglass® 45S5 dissolution. *J Biomed Mater Res.* 2001; 55(2):151–157.

Yeo YJ, Jeon DW, Kim CS et al. Effects of chitosan nonwoven membrane on periodontal healing of surgically created one-wall intrabony defects in beagle dogs. *J Biomed Mater Res B Appl Biomater.* 2005; 72(1):86–93.

Yildirim M, Spiekermann H, Biesterfeld S, Edelhoff D. Maxillary sinus augmentation using xenogenic bone substitute material Bio-Oss in combination with venous blood. A histologic and histomorphometric study in humans. *Clin Oral Implants Res.* 2000; 11(3):217–229.

Younger EM, Chapman MW. Morbidity at bone graft donor sites. *J Orthop Trauma.* 1989; 3(3):192–195.

Yukna RA. HTR polymer grafts in human periodontal osseous defects. I. 6-month clinical results. *J Periodontol.* 1990; 61(10):633–642.

Yukna RA, Greer RO Jr. Human gingival tissue response to HTR polymer. *J Biomed Mater Res.* 1992; 26(4):517–527.

Yukna RA. Clinical evaluation of HTR polymer bone replacement grafts in human mandibular Class II molar furcations. *J Periodontol.* 1994; 65(4):342–349.

Zitzmann NU, Naef R, Scharer P. Resorbable versus nonresorbable membranes in combination with Bio-Oss for guided bone regeneration. *Int J Oral Maxillofac Implants.* 1997; 12(6):844–852.

CHAPTER 20
Periodontal sutures and suturing techniques

Nader Hamdan, Zeeshan Sheikh and Haider Al-Waeli

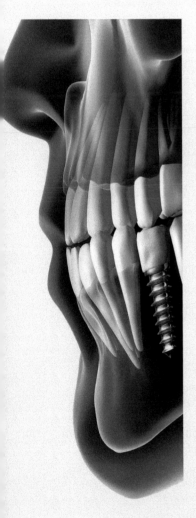

Contents

Learning objectives

- Different types of suture materials.
- Properties of suture materials.
- Principles of suturing and knots.
- Various suturing techniques.
- Suture removal.

Essential Periodontics, First Edition. Edited by Steph Smith and Khalid Almas.
© 2022 John Wiley & Sons Ltd. Published 2022 by John Wiley & Sons Ltd.

Introduction

The main objective of suturing is to position and secure surgical flaps to promote uneventful and optimal healing. When performed with the right materials and technique, the surgical sutures function to approximate flap edges until the wound has healed enough to withstand physiological and functional stresses (Wikesjö et al. 1992). Proper flap adaptation and wound stabilization allow for primary intention healing without development of dead spaces (Silverstein 2005). Suturing also helps to control bleeding/maintain hemostasis, reduce postoperative pain, and prevent bone exposure. The success of a surgical procedure is heavily dependent upon the quality of suturing, which is dependent upon the correct choice of needle type and size, suture type and size, and the proper suturing technique.

Armamentarium

In addition to suture material (needle and attached thread), several instruments are needed for proper suturing (Figure 20.1), which are broadly categorized into the following: soft tissue retractors (Figure 20.1A), flap retractors (Figure 20.1B), flap holders (Figure 20.1C), needle holders (Figure 20.1D), and a blade on a blade holder or scissors for cutting the suture threads (Figure 20.1E).

Suture materials

There are several factors that affect the choice of the three main suturing components: suture material, needle type, and technique employed for suturing. In order to make an informed choice, it is imperative for clinicians not only to ascertain the thickness and the quality of the tissue being sutured, but also to have an in-depth knowledge of the healing process in that particular tissue within that particular site in the oral cavity. The location of intended use in the mouth dictates the ease or difficulty in handling of the materials. Other factors that influence the choice of the suture material include the physical and biological characteristics of the suture material, planned time of suture removal, and cost.

Needles

The surgical needle comprises three main parts: the needle point (tip), the needle body, and the swaged (press-fit) end (Figure 20.2). Some of the ideal properties of the needle include having a suitable length for the intended use/site, e.g. a needle that will be used in the posterior dentate mandible needs to be long enough if the suturing technique used would necessitate passing the needle between the molars; being rigid and strong enough to prevent excessive bending/fracture, especially in thick fibrotic tissues; being sharp enough to penetrate tissues with ease and with minimal trauma to the tissues; being stable when held by the needle holder; having approximately the same diameter as the suture material to minimize tissue trauma; and of course being sterile and corrosion resistant (Moy et al. 1992).

Suture needles are commonly classified based on their radius, shape, and curvature. The most-used needles in dental surgery are 3/8 and 1/2 circle needles (Silverstein 1999). The 3/8 needle rotates on a central axis, allowing for passing the needle from one surface to another in one pass. In contrast, the 1/2 circle needle is useful in more restricted areas (e.g. buccal of the maxillary molars) and for periosteal and mucogingival surgery (Chandran & Subashini 2012; Silverstein 1999, 2005). Suture needles can be either round bodied, conventional cutting, or reverse cutting (Silverstein et al. 2009). In dental surgery, round-bodied needles are not preferred and reverse-cutting suture needles are favoured, as they have an inside concave non-cutting curvature to prevent the needle from tearing through the papillae or surgical flap edges (Silverstein 1999).

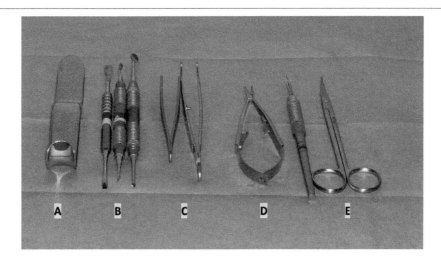

Figure 20.1 Basic suturing armamentarium.

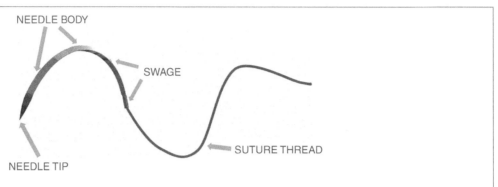

Figure 20.2 Various parts of the surgical needle connected to the suture thread material.

Suture thread

It is crucial to select the specific suture thread and diameter based on the thickness and type of the tissues to be sutured (Silverstein 1999). The suture thread material selection should be based on clear knowledge of the desired outcomes of the surgical procedure and the physical and biological characteristics of the suture thread in relationship to the biological healing processes. It is important for the suture thread and knots to retain sufficient tensile strength to keep the wound edges together until the tissues regain adequate strength. For example, if a suture is to be placed in a tissue that heals rapidly, clinicians may select a resorbable suture that will lose its tensile strength at about the same rate as the tissue gains back its physiological strength (Minozzi et al. 2009). If longer healing times are expected, however, a suture material that retains long-term stability and strength is preferred (Silverstein 2005). In addition, there might be factors that influence the choice of suture material independent of the interplay between the material properties and tissue healing expected, e.g. a patient who lives in a remote area and cannot attend soon for suture removal might need a monofilament (i.e. more hygienic) suture that would not easily accumulate bacteria.

Desired properties of suture threads

The ideal or desired properties of suture materials include being biocompatible and producing no or minimal tissue reaction; able to be used in any tissue type; not supporting bacterial accumulation and growth; being relatively strong (with a high tensile strength) yet with a small diameter to minimize tissue trauma; being easy to handle/manipulate and gliding through the tissues with ease; having good knot security and low elastic memory; not getting adversely affected (mechanically or chemically) by sterilization methods; being easily visualized during the procedure; being absorbable with no toxic or tissue adverse breakdown products; and being affordable and relatively inexpensive (Silverstein et al. 2009; Srinivasulu & Kumar 2014).

Suture size

Surgical threads can be classified based on the diameter of thread used. When compared with a suture made from the same material, the higher the number of zeros, the thinner and more delicate the suture is, with decreased strength (Minozzi et al. 2009). Modern sutures range from #5 (heavy braided suture used in orthopedics) to #11-0 (fine monofilament suture used in ophthalmic surgery). The most-used suture sizes in oral surgery and periodontics are 3-0, 4-0, 5-0, and 6-0. In periodontal surgery, a 5-0 thread diameter is most often used to secure soft tissue grafts and transpositional/sliding pedicle flaps, whereas a 4-0 thread is used to secure most other periodontal mucoperiosteal flaps. A 4-0 thread is also used to secure implant surgical flaps when interrupted sutures, some mattress sutures, and most continuous suture techniques have been performed (Silverstein et al. 2009).

Types of suture material

Practitioners have a varied armamentarium of suture materials from which to select (Figure 20.3). Surgical suture threads can be classified according to resorption, origin, or structure. According to resorption, sutures can be either absorbable or non-absorbable (Figure 20.4); according to origin, sutures may be natural or synthetic (Figures 20.4–20.6); and according to structure, they can be either monofilament or multifilament/braided (Figures 20.5 and 20.6). Monofilament sutures are more difficult to handle as they often have package memory (i.e. they tend to coil) and possess less knot security compared to multifilament sutures. However, monofilament sutures result in less tissue drag, do not wick (absorb fluids along with bacteria), and induce minimal tissue reactions. Conversely, polyfilament suture materials, although having better knot security and being easier to manipulate, tend to wick, cause higher tissue drag, and induce more tissue reaction (Silverstein et al. 2009).

Absorbable sutures

Catgut sutures are natural monofilament materials made by twisting together strands of purified collagen taken from the

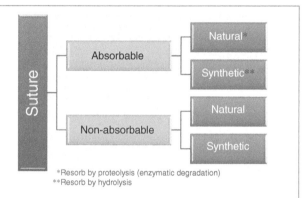

Figure 20.3 Examples of different suture materials that are available on the market.

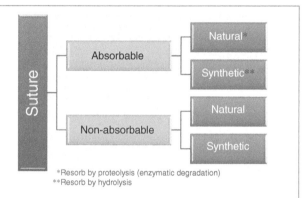

*Resorb by proteolysis (enzymatic degradation)
**Resorb by hydrolysis

Figure 20.4 Classification of suture materials according to absorbability.

small intestine of healthy ruminants (cattle, sheep, goat) or from beef tendon. Catgut sutures are either plain gut or treated with chromic acid salt to form chromic gut sutures. Plain gut sutures lose 50% of their tensile strength within 5–7 days, whereas chromic gut sutures lose 50% tensile strength within 10–14 days in use (Silverstein et al. 2009). Therefore, chromic gut is preferred when it is desired to wait longer for tissues to heal.

Poliglecaprone (e.g. Monocryl®; Ethicon, Inc., Cornelia, GA, USA) is a synthetic monofilament suture material composed of poliglecaprone 25, which is a co-polymer of glycolide and epsilon-caprolactone. Poliglecaprone loses 50% of tensile strength within 7–10 days and is completely absorbed after 91–119 days (Silverstein et al. 2009).

Polyglycan910 (e.g. Vicryl®; Ethicon, Inc.) is a synthetic polyfilament absorbable co-polymer of lactide (a cyclic diester of lactic acid) and glycoside. Polyglycan910 loses 50% of tensile strength within 21 days and is completely absorbed after 56–70 days (Silverstein et al. 2009).

Non-absorbable sutures

Surgical stainless steel is a very strong natural non-absorbable material and has excellent knot security. However, the main disadvantages of steel sutures include difficult handling and cutting easily through tissues, which makes their use extremely traumatic, and current use is mainly limited to hard tissue, i.e. bone applications.

Silk is a natural non-absorbable polyfilament suture that traditionally has been a commonly used material in dentistry and many other surgical fields (Macht & Krizek 1978). The reasons for silk's popularity have been that it is easy to handle, it ties with a stable knot, and it is relatively inexpensive compared with other non-absorbable suture materials currently available. However, silk has several disadvantages. It is non-absorbable and is a multifilament that "wicks" and pulls bacteria and fluids into the wound site (Manor & Kaffe 1982). Therefore, silk should not be the first suture material of choice. It can be used intraorally for very short periods of time, for training purposes, or as an accessory material for tying threads to small components for safety (to prevent accidental swallowing).

Nylon is a non-absorbable synthetic monofilament suture composed of long-chain aliphatic polymers: Nylon 6 and Nylon 6,6. Nylon has pronounced memory and low knot security (Silverstein et al. 2009), which makes it unpopular for intraoral surgical applications.

Polypropylene (e.g. Prolene®; Ethicon, Inc.) is a non-absorbable synthetic monofilament material composed of an isotactic crystalline stereoisomer of polypropylene, a synthetic linear polyolefin. The suture is usually pigmented blue to enhance visibility. It has minimal tissue reactivity and good durability, with higher tensile strength than nylon. However, polypropylene is fragile, has high plasticity, is expensive, and is difficult to handle (Silverstein et al. 2009).

ePTFE (expanded polytetrafluoroethylene; e.g. Gore-Tex®, WL Gore & Associates, Inc., Newark, DE, USA) is a non-absorbable synthetic monofilament suture that is non-wicking, soft and comfortable for patients, has excellent handling properties, and has superior knot security with little or no package memory. In addition, ePTFE is strong and biologically inert, with no expected tissue reaction (Silverstein 2005; Silverstein et al. 2009). All these characteristics make ePTFE sutures ideal for almost every intraoral surgical application. The main

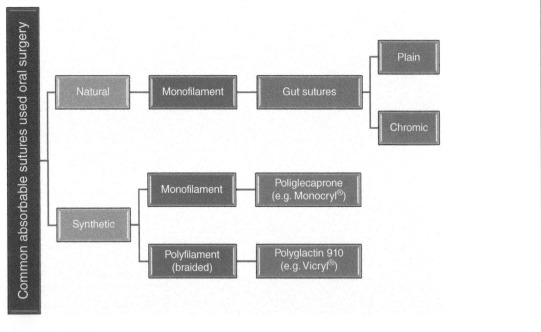

Figure 20.5 Commonly used absorbable sutures.

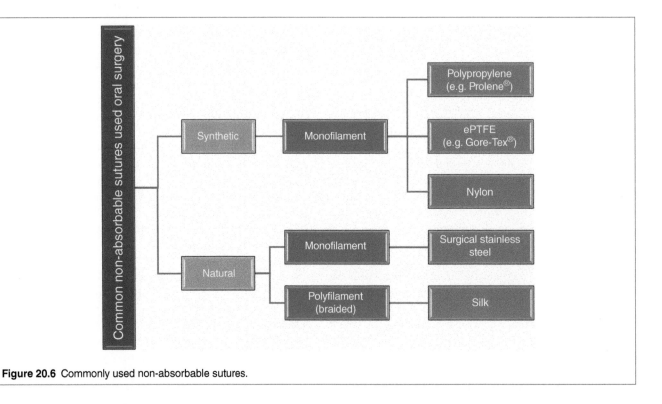

Figure 20.6 Commonly used non-absorbable sutures.

disadvantage of this material is its cost, as it tends to be more expensive than almost all other suture materials.

Suture material absorption

Absorbable/resorbable suture materials are degraded, absorbed, or resorbed via two mechanisms, "proteolysis,"

which is enzymatic degradation, and simple hydrolysis (Silverstein et al. 2009). Natural suture materials of biological origin, such as plain and chromic gut, are gradually digested by intraoral enzymes (Silverstein 2005). In addition, absorbable sutures may also break rapidly in the presence of very low intraoral pH. Therefore, clinicians should select a natural absorbable suture, keeping in view the time required for it to function based on the surgical procedure and expected healing.

Knots

The practice and art of surgical knot tying form an important component of successful suturing. The sutures can be tied either with a simple knot or with a surgeon's knot. The surgeon's knot is commonly employed and comprises two throws in one direction, being tied, and then one throw in the opposite direction and tied. For knot security and to prevent untimely knot untying, it is imperative that the appropriate surgical knot technique be employed for the selected suture material being used. The type of knot that is used for each material is determined by the method by which each type of thread is manufactured (Silverstein et al. 2009). For example, with synthetic resorbable and other non-absorbable synthetic suture materials, a surgeon's knot must be used to prevent knot untying and early loosening (Silverstein 2005).

Principles of suturing

For clinical success of the procedure being performed, it is crucial to follow and adhere to the basic principles of suturing. Some of these principles are:

- Use of good-quality sutures.
- Maintaining excellent visibility when suturing.
- Choosing the appropriate needle (type and size) and suture material (type and size) for the particular procedure performed and the tissues being sutured.
- Minimizing tissue trauma.
- Using the smallest needle and thread possible (less irritating and traumatic to tissues).

- Using the lowest number of sutures to adequately approximate and close the wound margins.
- Suturing in keratinized tissue when possible.
- Piercing the tissues perpendicular to their surface.
- Passing sutures from movable tissue to non-movable tissue and following the curvature of the needle, thereby preventing tissue tearing and knot slippage.
- Taking adequate bites of tissue.
- Ensuring sutures are not too close to incision lines or papillae edge (at least 2–4 mm).
- Stabilizing the tissues well and inserting the needle perpendicular to the surface.
- Placing knots at the buccal side of the incision line and not directly over the incision.
- Ensuring that after final re-contouring and thinning of gingival tissues, the flaps are placed passively in position before suturing.
- Cutting the suture thread at least 3–4 mm away from the knot to prevent knot opening.
- In interdental areas, placing the needle below a level parallel to the cementoenamel junction.
- Flaps being everted and not blanching when tying a suture.
- Not relying on sutures to pull the flap beyond its passive positioning, as tension created on the flap will interfere with blood supply to the gingiva, resulting in necrosis of the marginal portion of the flap and delayed healing.
- Removing any remaining sutures that are no longer needed (Silverstein 1999).

Common suturing techniques

There are several suturing techniques available for clinicians to employ during their surgical procedures (Figure 20.7). The

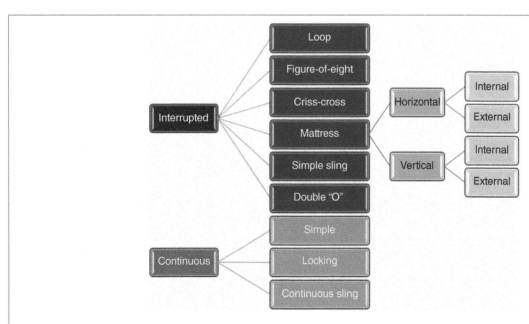

Figure 20.7 Common suturing techniques in oral surgery.

interrupted suture technique is one of the most used and encompasses a few suturing techniques: the simple/loop, the figure-of-eight, the criss-cross, the mattress, and the double "O." The simple/loop suture (Figure 20.8) is routinely used to approximate tension-free, mobile surgical flaps (Silverstein 1999). The simple/loop suture is useful in edentulous ridge areas, for suturing vertical releasing incisions, and for periosteal suturing. The criss-cross suture (Figure 20.9) is useful for extraction socket management, with or without socket grafting being performed. A criss-cross suture is tied by entering the mesial buccal and exiting the distal buccal. The suture is then crossed over the socket and enters the mesial lingual and exits the distal lingual. The suture at the distal lingual is tied to the free end at the mesial buccal, and the knot is positioned toward the buccal.

The figure-of-eight suture (Figure 20.10) is placed similarly to the simple loop suture on the buccal aspect; however, on the lingual aspect, the needle penetrates the outer and not the inner surface of the lingual flap. The figure-of-eight suture is useful when suturing on the lingual aspect of the lower molars, especially in a patient with an active gag reflex or with a large, cumbersome tongue (Silverstein 1999). Both interrupted suture techniques achieve similar results when used for wound closure with tension-free flaps.

Another suturing technique is the mattress technique, a variation of the interrupted suture. This technique is usually used in areas where tension-free flap closure cannot be kept (Silverstein 1999). Mattress suturing techniques are generally used to resist muscle pull, to evert the wound edges, and to adapt the tissue flaps tightly to underlying structures (e.g. bone graft, tissue graft, alveolar ridge, regenerative membrane, or dental implant). Variations of the mattress suture technique are referred to as the vertical, apically or coronally repositioned vertical mattress, vertical sling, and horizontal mattress.

A horizontal mattress suture (Figure 20.11) is tied by penetration of the needle at the mesial buccal apical to the mucogingival junction, and is crossed under the flap to exit at the mesial lingual. The suture then penetrates the tissue at the distal lingual and again crosses under the flap to exit at the distal buccal apical to the mucogingival junction. The suture at the distal buccal is tied to the free end at the mesial buccal. The vertical mattress suture (Figure 20.12) is used for everting flap edges, allows for good placement and stabilization of papillae, and is particularly useful for guided tissue regeneration surgery.

The interrupted suspensory suture is commonly referred to as the simple sling suture (Figure 20.13) and is used when only one side, or one or more papillae of a flap, is independently repositioned to its original position or coronally repositioned. The sling suture technique is especially useful when performing coronally repositioned sliding flaps. For a

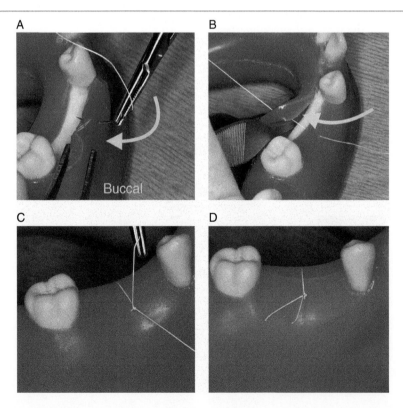

Figure 20.8 Simple suture/loop. (A) Needle inserted from buccal side of the flap 3–4 mm from flap margin. (B) Needle is withdrawn toward the lingual side through the lingual side of the flap. (C) Suture knot made on the buccal side. (D) Suture cut leaving 4–5 mm of suture material to maintain knot stability.

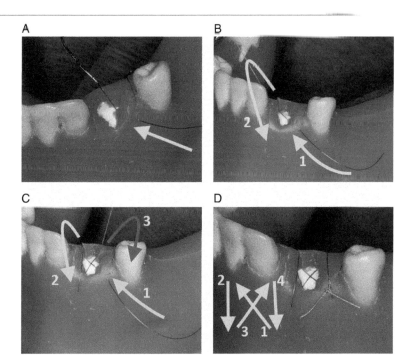

Figure 20.9 The criss-cross suture technique. (A) Needle inserted from buccal side of the flap 3–4 mm from flap margin. (B) Needle withdrawn diagonally across the area to be covered by the criss-cross suture to exit on the lingual side and then brought back toward the buccal. (C) Needle taken diagonally again as in step B and then brought back toward the buccal for making the knot. (D) Final suture.

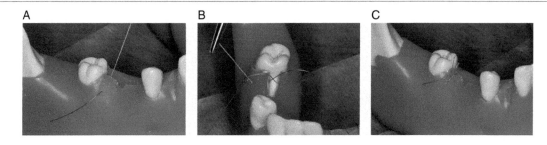

Figure 20.10 Figure-of-eight suture. (A) Needle inserted from buccal side of the flap 3–4 mm from flap margin. (B) Needle withdrawn past the lingual side of the flap and then reinserted from the lingual side and brought on the buccal to form a figure of eight. (C) Suture knot made on the buccal side, leaving 4–5 mm of suture material to maintain knot stability.

sling suture, the needle enters the buccal flaps papilla mesially and is carried lingually around the neck of the tooth or implant to cross over the papilla distally and exiting buccally. The suture is then reinserted from the distal buccal aspect, looped back around the same tooth or implant lingually, and tied with the free end, positioning the knot buccally. With this suture technique, each suture involves a papilla on the mesial and distal of every other tooth using separate ties.

The double "O" suture is an interrupted suturing technique that is utilized to prevent wound opening under expected extreme tension post surgery. The name refers to the fact that this technique is in fact a combination of two loop sutures, one

done at a superficial level and the other done more apical to it (Figure 20.14). The suture is usually started with the needle entering and exiting as if for a loop suture, but placed deep apical to the flap margin, and then instead of tying back on the buccal, the needle is reinserted on the buccal but at a shallower level from the flap margin both on the buccal and lingual, before being taken back to the buccal and tying to form a single knot.

Another variation of a suture technique is called a continuous suture. Simple continuous sutures (Figure 20.15) can be used to attach two surgical flap edges or to secure multiple interproximal papillae of one flap independently of the other flap. The advantage of the continuous suture is that there are

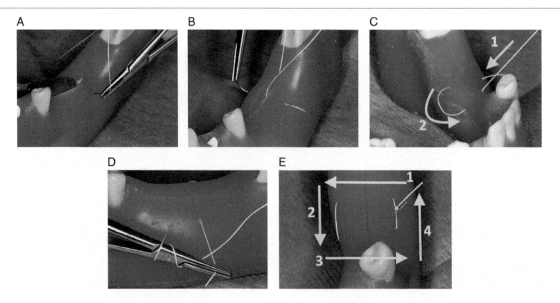

Figure 20.11 Horizontal mattress suture. (A) Needle inserted from buccal side of the flap 4–5 mm from flap margin. (B) Needle withdrawn toward the lingual side through the lingual side of the flap at the same level of the buccal needle entrance. (C) Needle moved horizontally and reinserted from the lingual flap toward the buccal. (D) Needle exits the buccal flap at the same level of the buccal needle insertion, while maintaining similar horizontal displacement as on the lingual side, and then tied on the buccal. (E) Final horizontal mattress suture.

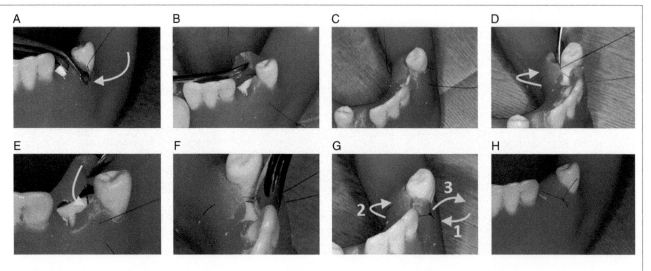

Figure 20.12 Vertical mattress suture. (A) Initially, a simple interrupted suture is started without cutting the suture. (B) Only the short end of the suture is then cut. (C) A series of loops are created by passing the suture from one side to another multiple times. (D) The loops are pulled tight as they are made. (E) Once the final loop is reached, (F, G) it is utilized as if it was the short end of the suture for making the second knot. (H) The loop and the suture line are cut to leave three tails around the second knot.

fewer individual suture ties, decreasing surgical time. However, the crucial disadvantage is that if one knot or loop breaks, the integrity of the entire surgical site will become compromised (Hutchens 1995). Therefore, a variation on the continuous suture technique is the continuous locking suture (Figure 20.16), which provides improved integrity even if a knot breaks or becomes loose, and is used on long-span wounds with moderate tension or when additional hemostasis is desired.

Suture removal

Once the suture materials have been in function, they are removed or replaced when they become broken, loose, and/or if they are not needed any more as the wound reaches adequate strength. The sutures may also be removed if they get infected or cause pathology. Some of the principles associated with suture removal are assessment of the wound for maturity to ensure that the suture can be removed without risking wound

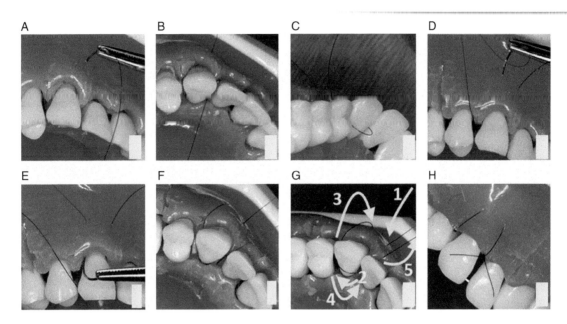

Figure 20.13 Simple sling suture. (A) Needle inserted on the buccal of the tooth. (B) Needle passed from the buccal to the lingual/palatal without engaging the palatal tissues. (C) Needle passed from the lingual/palatal back toward the buccal, forming a loop around the tooth and without engaging the lingual/palatal tissues. (D, E) Needle inserted through the buccal again on a horizontal level similar to the initial entrance and 3–5 mm apart. (F) As in the initial step, needle passed from the buccal to the lingual/palatal side and then back toward the buccal, forming a second loop around the tooth and without engaging the lingual/palatal tissues. (G) The previous steps in sequence. (H) Suture tied on the buccal, pulling the buccal flap coronally.

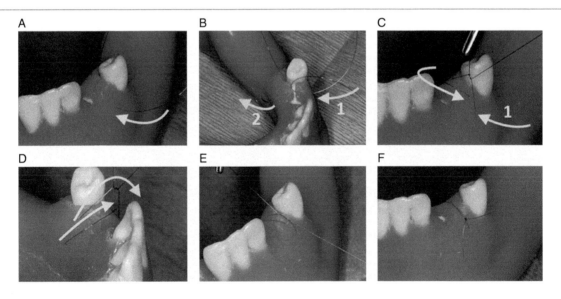

Figure 20.14 Double "O" suture – deep/deep, shallow/shallow. (A) Needle inserted in the buccal flap around 6–8 mm from flap margin (deep). (B) Needle passed through the lingual flap at around the same level of the buccal, 6–8 mm from flap margin (deep). (C, D) Needle inserted in the buccal flap around 3–4 mm from flap margin (shallow) and then passed through the lingual at around the same level (shallow). (E) The two created loops are pulled tight and the suture tied on the buccal. (F) Final knot on the buccal.

opening; the usage of proper sterile suture holders and proper sharp suture scissors; cleaning the suture by flushing with chlorhexidine or normal saline prior to removal; gently holding the suture away from the tissues; cutting one side of the loop as close to the surface as possible to decrease bacterial contamina-

tion; when removing continuous sutures, each section being pulled out and removed individually; and always pulling the suture out gently and smoothly toward the incision line to prevent dehiscence and to check that all suture material has been removed.

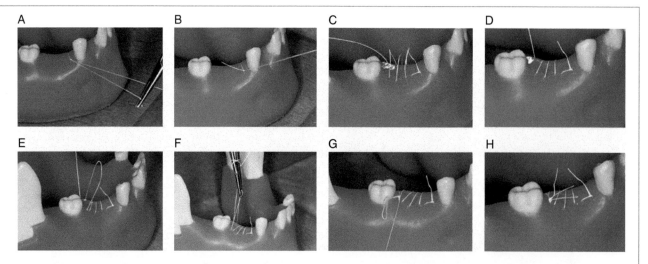

Figure 20.15 Simple continuous suture. (A) Initially, a simple interrupted suture is started without cutting the suture. (B) Only the short end of the suture is then cut. (C) A series of loops are created by passing the suture from one side to another multiple times. (D) The loops are pulled tight as they are made. (E) Once the final loop is reached, (F, G) it is utilized as if it was the short end of the suture for making the second knot. (H) The loop and the suture line are cut to leave three tails around the second knot.

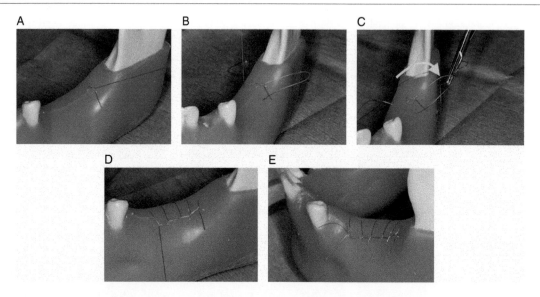

Figure 20.16 Continuous locking suture. (A) Initially, a simple interrupted suture is started and only the short end of the suture is then cut. (B) A loop is created by passing the suture from one side to another without fully pulling the suture. (C) The needle is inserted through the loop and then pulled. The previous steps are repeated and the loops are pulled tight as they are made. (D) Once the final loop is reached, it is utilized as if it was the short end of the suture for making the second knot. (E) The loop and the suture line are cut to leave three tails around the second knot.

Conclusion

Extensive research and evolution in biomaterials technology and processing have allowed for clinicians to have in their armamentarium sutures designed for specific surgical procedures. The ultimate success of any surgical procedure is heavily dependent upon the correct choice of suture material and the technique employed by the surgeon. Recent innovations help to alleviate difficulties previously encountered, and also decrease the potential for postoperative infections and complications. With continued research and establishment of newer fabrication processes, newer and more improved suture materials are expected to be available in the future.

REFERENCES

Chandran LG, Subashini SJ. Modified vertical mattress suturing technique for flap approximation after ramping. *Ann Dent UM.* 2012; 19(1):19–23.

Hutchens LH. Periodontal suturing: a review of needles, materials and techniques. *Postgrad Dent.* 1995; 2(4):1–15.

Macht S, Krizek TJ. Sutures and suturing—current concepts. *J Oral Surg.* 1978; 36(9):710–712.

Manor A, Kaffe IJ. Unusual foreign body reaction to a braided silk suture: a case report. *J Periodontol.* 1982; 53(2):86–88.

Minozzi F, Bollero P, Unfer V, Dolci A, Galli M. The sutures in dentistry. *Eur Rev Med Pharmacol Sci.* 2009; 13(3):217–226.

Moy RL, Waldman B, Hein DW. A review of sutures and suturing techniques. *J Dermatol Surg Oncol.* 1992; 18(9):785–795.

Silverstein LH. *Principles of Dental Suturing: The Complete Guide to Surgical Closure.* Mahwah, NJ: Montage Media Corporation; 1999.

Silverstein LH. Essential principles of dental suturing for the implant surgeon. *Dent Implantol Update.* 2005; 16(1):1–7.

Silverstein LH, Kurtzman GM, Shatz PC. Suturing for optimal soft-tissue management. *J Oral Implantol.* 2009; 35(2):82–90.

Srinivasulu K, Kumar ND. A review on properties of surgical sutures and applications in medical field. *Int J Res Eng Technol.* 2014; 2(2):85–96.

Wikesjö UM, Nilvéus RE, Selvig KA. Significance of early healing events on periodontal repair: a review. *J Periodontol.* 1992; 63(3):158–165.

CHAPTER 21
Periodontal wound healing

Michel V. Furtado Araujo, Farheen Malek, and Steph Smith

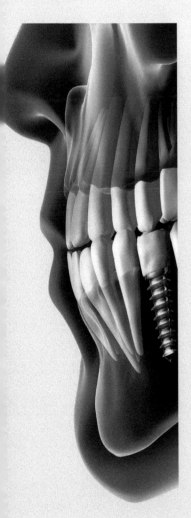

Contents

Learning objectives

- Definitions and possible outcomes of repair and regeneration.
- The biological events occurring in the four phases of periodontal wound repair.
- The principles and reasons for cell extrusion, wound stability, space provision, and primary intention healing during periodontal regeneration.

Essential Periodontics, First Edition. Edited by Steph Smith and Khalid Almas.
© 2022 John Wiley & Sons Ltd. Published 2022 by John Wiley & Sons Ltd.

Introduction

In health, the periodontium maintains the intrinsic characteristics of its constituents. In other words, native or post-treatment periodontal health should be void of inflammatory signs such as bleeding, swelling, or suppuration. Furthermore, attachment and bone levels should be maintained at acceptable levels (Chapple et al. 2018).

The primary objective of any periodontal therapy is to provide a functional, comfortable dentition for the patient's well-being (Zander et al. 1976). Therefore, periodontal treatment components involve eliminating periodontopathogenic bacteria and correcting the defects caused by the bacterial insult (Caton & Greenstein 1994). The most commonly described strategies used in periodontal therapy are new attachment procedures, resective periodontal surgery, and regenerative procedures (Garrett 1996).

The proper identification of healing outcomes following periodontal therapies can only be obtained by histological means. These outcomes do not occur as distinctly separate biological outcomes following reconstruction of the periodontal attachment. For example, periodontal regeneration includes elements of new connective tissue and epithelial attachments (Garrett 1996). Predictability of outcomes following surgical procedures is of fundamental importance in medicine. Because periodontal regenerative procedures are time-consuming and costly, there is increasing interest by clinicians to learn of factors that may impact the clinical outcomes following periodontal reconstructive surgery to provide the best possible service to patients. This goal can only be achieved if the biological aspects of wound healing and regeneration are well understood and considered in treatment planning.

Trauma to the periodontium as a result of surgery, infection, and inflammatory events elicits a biological response in the periodontal tissues. The healing capability of the periodontal tissues is influenced by a variety of biochemical and cellular mechanisms. Although presenting different compositions, the gingiva, root cementum, periodontal ligament, and alveolar bone all respond to trauma or disease by an inflammatory response that invokes the creation of a fibrin matrix. The fibrin network will then allow for the migration of undifferentiated cells for the repair or regeneration of the injured tissues (Figure 21.1).

Patterns of healing of the periodontium

Studies have shown that periodontal procedures can lead to different patterns of healing, which may constitute either repair or regeneration of the periodontium. These patterns are dependent on the four possible cell types that can predominate in the wound site, i.e. epithelial cells, connective tissue cells, bone cells, and periodontal ligament cells (Caton & Greenstein 1994; Froum et al. 1982; Garrett 1996; Newman et al. 2019; Polimeni et al. 2006; Ramseier et al. 2012; Trowbridge & Emling 1997; Wikesjö & Selvig 1999) (Figure 21.2).

Repair

When the damaged tissues (i.e. a periodontal defect) (Figure 21.3) are replaced by structures that do not mimic the function of the original tissues, the process is called "repair." The reduction in probing depths after treatment of severe periodontal suprabony defects is usually due to the formation of a long junctional epithelium (Figure 21.4) and connective tissue repair (Figure 21.5). This connective tissue repair is termed "reattachment."

Periodontal regeneration

Periodontal regeneration is the de novo (new) formation of cementum, a functionally oriented periodontal ligament, alveolar bone, and gingiva (restitutio ad integrum), thus the reconstitution of a new periodontium. Periodontal regeneration can also include elements of new connective tissue and epithelial attachments (Figure 21.6).

The periodontal healing cascade

The environment in which trauma occurs will significantly influence the healing outcome. Oral wound healing is characterized by the fastest healing rate and less scar formation in

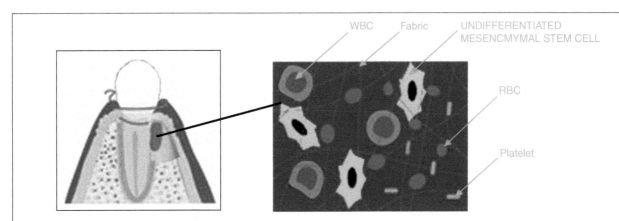

Figure 21.1 Clot as a fibrin network and an environment that facilitates chemotaxis, migration, and differentiation. RBC, red blood cell; WBC, white blood cell. Source: Adapted from John E. Davies BSc, BDS, PhD, DScUnderstanding Peri-Implant Endosseous Healing. http://www.ecf.utoronto.ca/~bonehead.

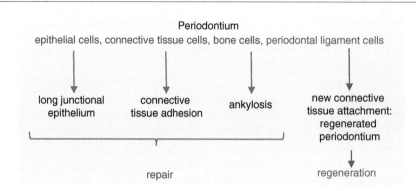

Figure 21.2 The healing pattern that occurs constitutes either repair or regeneration. The downgrowth of epithelial cells results in a long junctional epithelium, the proliferation of connective tissue may result in connective tissue adhesion with/without root resorption, a predominance of bone cells causes ankylosis with/without root resorption, the ingress of periodontal ligament and perivascular cells from the bone can lead to the development of a regenerated periodontium (periodontal regeneration). Source: Adapted from MG Newman, HH Takei, PR Klokkevold et al. Newman and Carranza's Clinical Periodontology. St. Louis, MO: Elsevier Saunders; 2019.

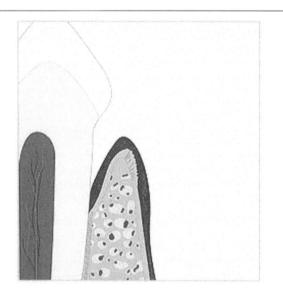

Figure 21.3 Periodontal defect.

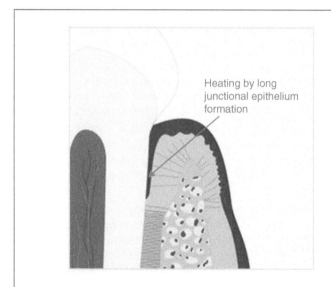

Figure 21.4 Long junctional epithelium.

comparison with cutaneous wound healing (Morand et al. 2017). The periodontal opposing healing interfaces comprise a rigid, non-vascular root surface, a gingival flap composed of connective tissue and epithelium, as well as alveolar bone and periodontal ligament. Cytokines, chemokines, and host-derived enzymes such as matrix metalloproteinases (MMPs) are key regulators of the healing process. Moreover, the levels of their secretion/activity, but also the imbalance with their antagonists/inhibitors, influence wound healing outcome. The resolution of inflammation is initiated by cellular pathways that specifically promote anti-inflammatory and proresolution lipid mediators, such as the lipoxins, resolvins, and protectins that promote the return of homeostasis. Inflammation that occurs at the treated site may influence wound healing and consequently periodontal treatment outcomes, as persistence of infection and inflammation or

dysregulation of mechanisms of the resolution phase at the site will result in chronic inflammation, reducing the healing rate, and lead to tissue fibrosis and more scars (Morand et al. 2017).

In the periodontal compartment, the traumatized interfaces will elicit a cascade of overlapping events/phases. These phases include hemostasis, an inflammatory phase, a proliferation phase, and a remodeling phase. Local trauma causes the rupturing of the vascular network, and in a matter of minutes a blood clot is formed (Clark 1996). This fibrin network allows for the migration of a variety of cells to the injured site. The first inflammatory cells (neutrophils; monocytes) arrive within hours, with the primary goals of disinfecting and "cleaning" the area (Martin 1997). Next, the secretion of local growth factors will attract a second wave of cells (macrophages) that induce damaged tissue remodeling (Clark 1996; Wikesjö & Selvig 1999), while stimulating the proliferation of fibroblasts/

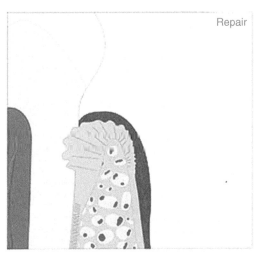

Connective tissue adhesion and root resorption

Figure 21.5 Connective tissue adhesion with/without root resorption.

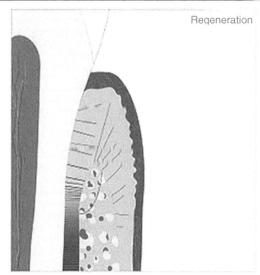

New connective tissue attachment

Figure 21.6 Periodontal regeneration.

endothelial and smooth muscle cells (myofibroblasts). These events will cause wound contraction and create a new vascular grid (angiogenesis) about three days post trauma (Aukhil 2000; Martin 1997). The newly formed lattice of blood vessels will create the conditions for the migration and differentiation of epithelial and mesenchymal stem cells into tissue-specific cells to rebuild the injured tissues to their pre-trauma composition. Within hours of injury, epithelial cells from the basal layer proliferate, migrate through the fibrin clot, and seal the epithelium. At seven days post trauma, some areas already present connective tissue attachment to the injured root surface (Grzesik & Narayanan 2002). Granulation tissue maturation leads to regeneration or repair (scar formation).

Phases of periodontal wound healing

Periodontal wound healing is a highly complex process whereby all the phases require cell-to-cell interactions that are orchestrated by growth factors, cytokines, and extracellular matrix (ECM) components. The healing outcome will depend upon two crucial factors: the availability of required cell types and the release of signals to recruit and stimulate such cells (Grzesik & Narayanan 2002; Morand et al. 2017). These signals include various extracellular matrix components, adhesive proteins, chemotactic factors, growth factors, as well as cytokines. These include tumor necrosis factor alpha (TNF-α), interleukin-1 beta (IL-1β), IL-6, IL-8, transforming growth factor beta (TGF-β), interferon gamma (INF-Υ), complement component C5a (C5a), insulin growth factor (IGF), epidermal growth factor (EGF), platelet-derived growth factor (PDGF), vascular endothelial growth factor (VEGF), fibroblast growth factor (FGF), keratinocyte growth factor (KGF), matrix metalloproteinase (MMP), and bone morphogenetic protein (BMP) (Morand et al. 2017). Figures 21.7–21.10 depict a summary of the wound healing phases with their predominant cells and the main changes of the injured tissue.

Gingival cells extrusion theory

A series of animal models postulated that the periodontal tissue configuration after wound healing is determined by the cells that first populate the root surface (Karring et al. 1980, 1993; Nyman et al. 1980, 1982a, b). Specifically, newly formed connective tissue was found in areas where the periodontal ligament was preserved, in drastic contrast to root surfaces with periodontal disease (Karring et al. 1980, 1993; Nyman et al. 1980). A physical barrier was interposed between the gingival connective tissue and the root surface in a similar defect model, leaving only periodontal ligament cells in charge of rebuilding the defect. The result was new cementum and periodontal ligament formation at six months postoperative (Nyman et al. 1982a, b). This outcome showed that periodontal ligament cells have regenerative capacity, when not impaired by the faster migration of gingival cells to the defect area. This theory is the precursor to guided tissue regeneration (GTR) strategies, where occlusive membranes are used in the reconstruction and augmentation of periodontal and osseous defects (Figures 21.11–21.14).

The importance of primary closure, wound stability, and space provision

Other studies have tested additional factors that affect periodontal healing (Hiatt et al. 1968; Koo et al. 2004a, b; Linghorne & O'Connell 1950; Polimeni et al. 2004a; Polson & Proye 1983; Wikesjö & Nilvéus 1991; Wikesjö et al. 1994). Hiatt et al. (1968) measured the tensile strength of the gingival flap postsurgically. While only a minor increase in strength was found between 3 to 5 days (200g to 340g), a significant difference was evident at two weeks postoperative (>1700 g). Furthermore, stable fibrin clots that efficiently adhered to root

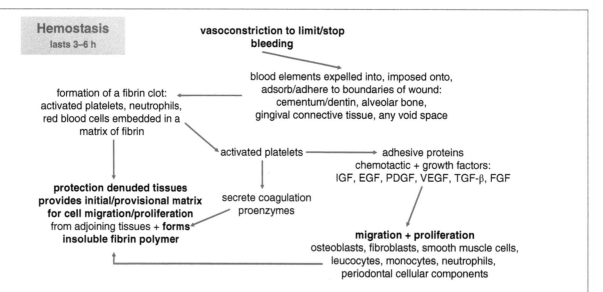

Figure 21.7 Hemostasis. Hemostasis is initiated immediately after initial injury, lasting 3–6 hours. A blood clot constituted by activated platelets, neutrophils, and red blood cells embedded in a matrix of fibrin fills the lesion. Activated platelets secrete coagulation proenzymes to form insoluble fibrin polymers. Activated platelets secrete adhesive proteins, chemotactic and growth factors, inducing the migration and proliferation of various cells into the provisional fibrin matrix. EGF, epidermal growth factor; FGF, fibroblast growth factor; IGF, insulin growth factor; PDGF, platelet-derived growth factor; TGF-β, transforming growth factor beta; VEGF, vascular endothelial growth factor. Courtesy of Dr. Steph Smith.

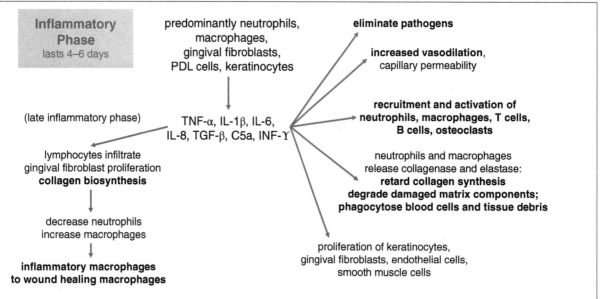

Figure 21.8 Inflammatory phase. The inflammatory phase begins concomitantly with hemostasis and lasts 4–6 days. The predominant cells are neutrophils, macrophages, gingival fibroblasts, PDL cells, and keratinocytes, which secrete various inflammatory cytokines. The main purpose of this phase is to eliminate pathogens, to increase vascular permeability, the recruitment and activation of neutrophils, macrophages, T cells, B cells, and osteoclasts, to retard collagen synthesis and degrade damaged matrix components, and to phagocytose blood cells and tissue debris, including the proliferation of keratinocytes, gingival fibroblasts, endothelial cells, and smooth muscle cells (myofibroblasts). In the later stages of this phase, collagen biosynthesis is initiated together with an increase in the presence of wound healing macrophages. IL, interleukin; INF-ϒ, interferon gamma; PDL, periodontal ligament; TGF-β, transforming growth factor beta; TNF-α, tumor necrosis factor alpha. Courtesy of Dr. Steph Smith.

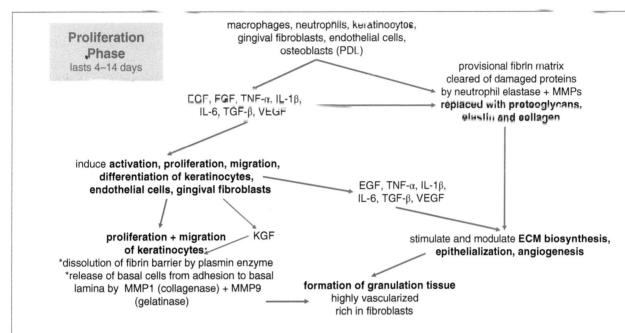

Figure 21.9 Proliferation phase. Recruited cells during the inflammatory phase secrete cytokines, growth factors, and MMPs whereby damaged proteins in the fibrin matrix are replaced with proteoglycans, elastin, and collagen. The activation, proliferation, migration, and differentiation of keratinocytes, endothelial cells, and gingival fibroblasts are also induced, which secrete cytokines and growth factors, leading to the stimulation and modulation of ECM biosynthesis, epithelialization, and angiogenesis. The secretion of keratinocyte growth factor (KGF) by these cells induces the proliferation and migration of keratinocytes. The end result of this phase is the formation of granulation tissue that is highly vascularized and is rich in fibroblasts. ECM, extracellular matrix; EGF, epidermal growth factor; FGF, fibroblast growth factor; IL, interleukin; MMP, matrix metalloproteinase; PDL, periodontal ligament; TGF-β, transforming growth factor beta; TNF-α, tumor necrosis factor alpha; VEGF, vascular endothelial growth factor. Courtesy of Dr. Steph Smith.

surfaces have been shown to prevent the apical migration of gingival cells (Hiatt et al. 1968). Other authors demonstrated that wound mechanical stability (Linghorne & O'Connell 1950) can be enhanced by root surface modification techniques (Baker et al. 2000, 2005; Polson & Proye 1983; Wikesjö et al. 1991) and is one of the main factors that hinder healing by the formation of a long junctional epithelium.

Animal models with critical-size defects (those that do not heal without additional procedures or grafting) were utilized to assess the role of clot formation and stability on periodontal healing (Koo et al. 2004a, b; Wikesjö & Nilvéus 1991; Wikesjö et al. 1994). Test root surfaces were treated with heparin and compared to saline-treated control surfaces. The results showed healing by long junctional epithelium in root surfaces treated with heparin, which indicates that clot formation or adhesion may have been prevented. Conversely, when polymeric implants and membranes were used as stabilizers on the heparin-treated surfaces, healing occurred by the formation of a connective tissue attachment (Haney et al. 1993; Wikesjö & Nilvéus 1990), which indicates that the apical migration of epithelial cells was arrested. Alternatively, fibrin adhesion enhancers such as etching and chelating agents were used on root surfaces to invoke healing by connective attachment (Baker et al. 2000, 2005; Polson & Proye 1983; Wikesjö et al. 1991). The results described herein corroborate that wound stability plays a more critical role in periodontal healing than cell occlusion.

Periodontal healing analyses were employed to compare tissue expanders (Karaki et al. 1984) and rigid, porous membranes to strictly occlusive membranes (Wikesjö et al. 2003a) to evaluate periodontal healing. These investigations showed regeneration with bone (Karaki et al. 1984) and cementum formation and a functionally oriented periodontal ligament when a three-dimensional volume is provided, despite the absence of strict connective tissue occlusion (Wikesjö et al. 2003a). Another study evaluated the combined effects of primary closure, space provision, and occlusive membranes in periodontal healing. The results showed similar regeneration patterns in both porous and occlusive membranes, but the regeneration magnitude was increased in the occlusive barrier group (i.e. increased bone formation). Thus, it could be hypothesized that, although not mandatory, occlusive membranes optimize regeneration in situations where space provision and primary closure are guaranteed (Polimeni et al. 2004b). Conversely, wound failure and membrane exposure were more common in the occlusive membrane group. These results suggest that porous membranes may facilitate flap survival by allowing for vascular growth (Polimeni et al. 2006).

Bone biomaterials were tested as a means to support membranes in periodontal procedures (Polimeni et al. 2004a; Trombelli et al. 1999). While slow-resorbing bone grafts have a possible hindering effect on regeneration (Trombelli et al. 1999), more readily resorbable bone biomaterials have

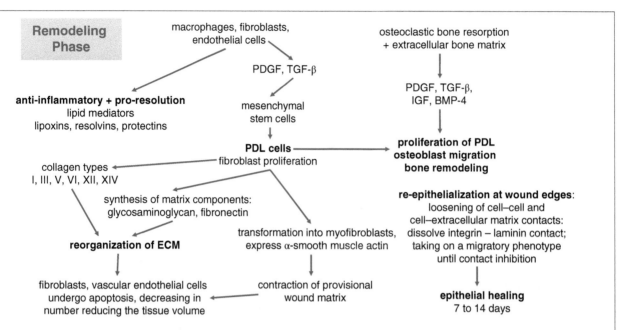

Figure 21.10 Remodeling phase. Remodeling is considered as the long-term final phase of wound healing and is characterized by the development of a new epithelium, elimination of granulation tissue, and ECM remodeling. There is a predominance of anti-inflammatory and proresolution lipid mediators, which are responsible for the resolution of inflammation. Macrophages, fibroblasts, and endothelial cells secrete PDGF and TGF-β, which activate mesenchymal stem cells from the periodontal ligament and stimulate gingival fibroblast proliferation and the synthesis of matrix components such as glycosaminoglycan and fibronectin, as well as the synthesis of different types of collagen. PDGF, TGF-β, IGF, and BMP-4 released from the extracellular bone matrix during osteoclastic bone resorption induce the proliferation and migration of PDL osteoblasts, leading to bone remodeling. Fibroblasts transform into myofibroblasts, causing contraction of the provisional wound matrix. Re-epithelialization at the wound edges takes place by means of epithelial cells taking on a migratory phenotype until contact inhibition occurs, leading to epithelial healing. BMP, bone morphogenetic protein; ECM, extracellular matrix; IGF, insulin growth factor; PDGF, platelet-derived growth factor; PDL, periodontal ligament; TGF-β, transforming growth factor beta. Courtesy of Dr. Steph Smith.

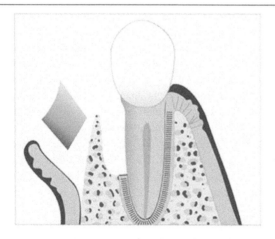

Figure 21.11 Periodontal defect with loss of gingiva, periodontal ligament, and alveolar bone. Membrane/barrier in green.

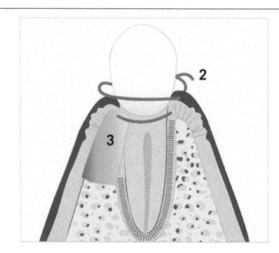

Figure 21.12 Membrane stabilization and primary closure of the defect after debridement, disinfection, and grafting. 2, suture by primary intention; 3, membrane.

enabled improved regeneration when compared to non-grafted sites (Polimeni et al. 2004a). The use of different membranes and various mixtures of bone graft materials has shown the most predictable positive results. For instance, a series of studies corroborated that primary closure and space maintenance

using occlusive membranes over a mix of autogenous and xenograft particulate bone grafts rendered over 5.6 mm in vertical bone gain (Urban et al. 2013). Indeed, occlusive membranes

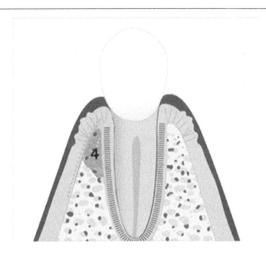

Figure 21.13 Initial healing of the periodontal tissues following guided tissue regeneration. 4, neo-angiogenesis and maturation of periodontal tissues.

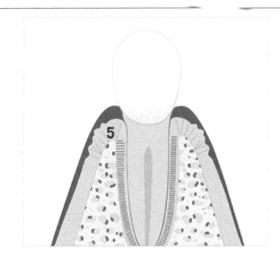

Figure 21.14 Periodontal regeneration. 5, complete restoration of the periodontium following wound stability, volume maintenance, and healing by primary intention.

allied with composite bone grafts (i.e. allogenous, autogenous, recombinant human bone morphogenetic proteins [rhBMPs]) represent the most commonly used strategy (Kim et al. 1998, Polimeni et al. 2004a; Sanz et al. 2004; Trombelli et al. 1999; Wikesjö et al. 1992, 2003b, d).

GTR procedures employing porous membranes were used to compare the effects of space provision in periodontal and peri-implant sites. Results showed a direct correlation between bone regeneration and the initial bone width at teeth and implant defects. In other words, wider initial defects have possibly provided more osteogenic potential for both defect models. However, bone regeneration was more significant in periodontal sites, which could derive from the greater vascular and cellular availability provided by these sites (Polimeni et al. 2004c). The pattern of tissue loss in periodontal bony defects will influence vascularity, wound stability, and closure.

Three- and two-wall defects present more support and vascular sources for healing, while one-wall defects and craters have limited to no ability for regeneration.

Unimpeded healing of periodontal tissues under primary closure largely increases the chances of complete regeneration (Sigurdsson et al. 1994; Wikesjö et al. 2003a, c, d). Inadequate flap design/management and compromised flap nutrition can result in wound site retraction and membrane exposure. These events present serious challenges to proper healing (Sanz et al. 2004; Sigurdsson et al. 1994; Trombelli et al. 1997; Wikesjö et al. 2003a). The exposed and contaminated wound is subjected to an inflammatory reaction, causing the regenerating tissues to undergo necrosis. However, periodontal tissues' maturation may occur if exposed sites are treated early (i.e. within one week postoperative) by membrane removal and primary wound closure (Wikesjö et al. 2003a).

SUMMARY

Findings from the studies described herein are paramount to our understanding of periodontal wound healing. Their value lies mainly in their introduction of three key factors previously poorly understood: (i) wound stability, (ii) space provision, and (iii) primary intention healing. Attaining wound stability, space provision, and primary closure drastically improves regenerative outcomes, even in cases of zero-wall (supra-alveolar) defects that were previously regarded as clinically impossible to regenerate (Sigurdsson et al. 1994; Wikesjö et al. 2003a, c, d). Moreover, these studies highlight the importance of flap design, suturing materials and techniques, and the use of appropriate biomaterials (i.e. membranes, bone grafts, biologic agents) in the stabilization and space provision of the periodontal wound. In an ideal clinical scenario, regeneration would favor a flap design that allows for primary closure and suturing techniques using materials that minimize plaque accumulation and provide passive, mechanical stability for a minimum of two weeks, as well as space provision for at least eight weeks (Kim et al. 1998; Sigurdsson et al. 1994; Wikesjö 2003a, c, d).

REFERENCES

Aukhil I. Biology of wound healing. *Periodontol 2000*. 2000; 22:44–50.

Baker DL, Stanley Pavlow SA, Wikesjö UM. Fibrin clot adhesion to dentin conditioned with protein constructs: an in vitro

proof-of-principle study. *J Clin Periodontol*. 2005; 32(6):561–566.

Baker PJ, Rotch HA, Trombelli L, Wikesjö UM. An in vitro screening model to evaluate root conditioning protocols for periodontal regenerative procedures. *J Periodontol.* 2000; 71(7):1139–1143.

Caton J, Greenstein G. Results of conventional therapeutic techniques for regeneration. In: A Polson (ed.), *Periodontal Regeneration: Current Status and Directions.* Chicago, IL: Quintessence; 1994: 11–20.

Chapple ILC, Mealey BL, Van Dyke TE et al. Periodontal health and gingival diseases and conditions on an intact and a reduced periodontium: consensus report of workgroup 1 of the 2017 World Workshop on the classification of periodontal and peri-implant diseases and conditions. *J Periodontol.* 2018; 89(Suppl 1):S74–S84.

Clark R. Wound repair. Overview and general considerations. In: R. Clark (ed.), *The Molecular and Cellular Biology of Wound Repair.* New York: Plenum Press; 1996: 3–50.

Froum SJ, Coran M, Thaller B et al. Periodontal healing following open debridement flap procedures. I. Clinical assessment of soft tissue and osseous repair. *J Periodontol.* 1982; 53(1):8–14.

Garrett S. Periodontal regeneration around natural teeth. *Ann Periodontol.* 1996; 1(1):621–666.

Grzesik WJ, Narayanan AS. Cementum and periodontal wound healing and regeneration. *Crit Rev Oral Biol Med.* 2002; 13(6):474–484.

Haney JM, Nilvéus RE, McMillan PJ, Wikesjö UM. Periodontal repair in dogs: expanded polytetrafluoroethylene barrier membranes support wound stabilization and enhance bone regeneration. *J Periodontol.* 1993; 64(9):883–890.

Hiatt WH, Stallard RE, Butler ED, Badgett B. Repair following mucoperiosteal flap surgery with full gingival retention. *J Periodontol.* 1968; 39(1):11–16.

Karaki R, Kubota K, Hitaka M et al. Effect of gum-expanding mesh on the osteogenesis in surgical bony defect. *Nippon Shishubyo Gakkai Kaishi.* 1984; 26:516–522.

Karring T, Nyman S, Gottlow J, Laurell L. Development of the biological concept of guided tissue regeneration—animal and human studies. *Periodontol 2000.* 1993; 1:26–35.

Karring T, Nyman S, Lindhe J. Healing following implantation of periodontitis affected roots into bone tissue. *J Clin Periodontol.* 1980; 7(2):96–105.

Kim CK, Cho KS, Choi SH, Prewett A, Wikesjö UM. Periodontal repair in dogs: effect of allogenic freeze-dried demineralized bone matrix implants on alveolar bone and cementum regeneration. *J Periodontol.* 1998; 69(1):26–33.

Koo KT, Polimeni G, Albandar JM, Wikesjö UM. Periodontal repair in dogs: examiner reproducibility in the supraalveolar periodontal defect model. *J Clin Periodontol.* 2004a; 31(6):439–442.

Koo KT, Polimeni G, Albandar JM, Wikesjö UM. Periodontal repair in dogs: analysis of histometric assessments in the supraalveolar periodontal defect model. *J Periodontol.* 2004b; 75(12):1688–1693.

Linghorne WJ, O'Connell DC. Studies in the regeneration and reattachment of supporting structures of the teeth; soft tissue reattachment. *J Dent Res.* 1950; 29(4):419–428.

Martin P. Wound healing—aiming for perfect skin regeneration. *Science.* 1997; 276(5309):75–81.

Morand DN, Davideau J-L, Clauss F et al. Cytokines during periodontal wound healing: potential application for new therapeutic approach. *Oral Dis.* 2017; 23:300–311.

Newman MG, Takei HH, Klokkevold PR et al. *Newman and Carranza's Clinical Periodontology.* St. Louis, MO: Elsevier Saunders; 2019.

Nyman S, Gottlow J, Karring T, Lindhe J. The regenerative potential of the periodontal ligament. An experimental study in the monkey. *J Clin Periodontol.* 1982a; 9(3):257–265.

Nyman S, Karring T, Lindhe J, Plantén S. Healing following implantation of periodontitis-affected roots into gingival connective tissue. *J Clin Periodontol.* 1980; 7(5):394–401.

Nyman S, Lindhe J, Karring T, Rylander H. New attachment following surgical treatment of human periodontal disease. *J Clin Periodontol.* 1982b; 9(4):290–296.

Polimeni G, Koo KT, Qahash M et al. Prognostic factors for alveolar regeneration: effect of a space-providing biomaterial on guided tissue regeneration. *J Clin Periodontol.* 2004a; 31(9):725–729.

Polimeni G, Koo KT, Qahash M et al. Prognostic factors for alveolar regeneration: effect of tissue occlusion on alveolar bone regeneration with guided tissue regeneration. *J Clin Periodontol.* 2004b; 31(9):730–735.

Polimeni G, Koo KT, Qahash M et al. Prognostic factors for alveolar regeneration: bone formation at teeth and titanium implants. *J Clin Periodontol.* 2004c; 31(11):927–932.

Polimeni G, Xiropaidis AV, Wikesjö UM. Biology and principles of periodontal wound healing/regeneration. *Periodontol 2000.* 2006; 41:30–47.

Polson AM, Proye MP. Fibrin linkage: a precursor for new attachment. *J Periodontol.* 1983; 54(3):141–147.

Ramseier CA, Rasperini G, Batia S, Giannobile WV. Advanced reconstructive technologies for periodontal tissue repair. *Periodontol 2000.* 2012; 59(1):185–202.

Sanz M, Tonetti MS, Zabalegui I et al. Treatment of intrabony defects with enamel matrix proteins or barrier membranes: results from a multicenter practice-based clinical trial. *J Periodontol.* 2004; 75(5):726–733.

Sigurdsson TJ, Hardwick R, Bogle GC, Wikesjö UM. Periodontal repair in dogs: space provision by reinforced ePTFE membranes enhances bone and cementum regeneration in large supra-alveolar defects. *J Periodontol.* 1994; 65(4):350–356.

Trombelli L, Kim CK, Zimmerman GJ, Wikesjö UM. Retrospective analysis of factors related to clinical outcome of guided tissue regeneration procedures in intrabony defects. *J Clin Periodontol.* 1997; 24(6):366–371.

Trombelli L, Lee MB, Promsudthi A, Guglielmoni PG, Wikesjö UM. Periodontal repair in dogs: histologic observations of guided tissue regeneration with a prostaglandin E1 analog/methacrylate composite. *J Clin Periodontol.* 1999; 26(6):381–387.

Trowbridge HO, Emling RC. Introduction. In: HO Trowbridge, RC Emling (eds), *Inflammation: A Review of the Process.* Chicago, IL: Quintessence; 1997: 9–10.

Urban IA, Nagursky H, Lozada JL, Nagy K. Horizontal ridge augmentation with a collagen membrane and a combination of particulated autogenous bone and anorganic bovine bone-derived mineral: a prospective case series in 25 patients. *Int J Periodontics Restorative Dent* 2013; 33(3);299–307.

Wikesjö UM, Bogle GC, Nilvéus RE. Periodontal repair in dogs: effect of a composite graft protocol on healing in supraalveolar periodontal defects. *J Periodontol.* 1992; 63(2):107–113.

Wikesjö UM, Claffey N, Nilvéus R, Egelberg J. Periodontal repair in dogs: effect of root surface treatment with stannous fluoride or citric acid on root resorption. *J Periodontol.* 1991; 62(3):180–184.

Wikesjö UM, Kean CJ, Zimmerman GJ. Periodontal repair in dogs: supra-alveolar defect models for evaluation of safety and efficacy of periodontal reconstructive therapy. *J Periodontol.* 1994; 65(12):1151–1157.

Wikesjö UM, Lim WH, Thomson RC, Hardwick WR. Periodontal repair in dogs: gingival tissue occlusion, a critical requirement for GTR? *J Clin Periodontol.* 2003a; 30(7):655–664.

Wikesjö UM, Nilvéus R. Periodontal repair in dogs: effect of wound stabilization on healing. *J Periodontol.* 1990; 61(12):719–724.

Wikesjö UM, Nilvéus R. Periodontal repair in dogs. Healing patterns in large circumferential periodontal defects. *J Clin Periodontol.* 1991; 18(1):49–59.

Wikesjö UM, Selvig KA. Periodontal wound healing and regeneration. *Periodontol 2000.* 1999; 19:21–39.

Wikesjö UM, Xiropaidis AV, Thomson RC et al. Periodontal repair in dogs: space-providing ePTFE devices increase rhBMP-2/ACS-induced bone formation. *J Clin Periodontol.* 2003b; 30(8):715–725.

Wikesjö UM, Xiropaidis AV, Thomson RC et al. Periodontal repair in dogs: rhBMP-2 significantly enhances bone formation under provisions for guided tissue regeneration. *J Clin Periodontol.* 2003c; 30(8):705–714.

Wikesjö UME, Lim WH, Thomson RC et al. Periodontal repair in dogs: evaluation of a bioabsorbable space-providing macro-porous membrane with recombinant human bone morphogenetic protein-2. *J Periodontol.* 2003d; 74(5):635–647.

Zander HA, Polson AM, Heijl LC. Goals of periodontal therapy. *J Periodontol.* 1976; 47(5):261–266.

CHAPTER 22
Supportive periodontal therapy

Tara Taiyeb Ali

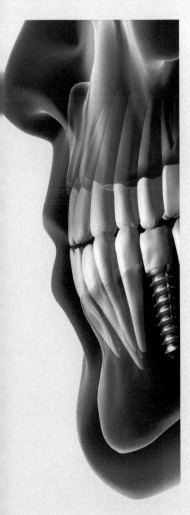

Contents

Learning objectives

- Definition, rationale, and aims of supportive periodontal therapy.
- Causes of recurrence of periodontal disease.
- Aspects of interventional treatment included in supportive therapy.
- Factors determining the classification and scheduling of recall maintenance visits.
- Procedures to be performed during a recall maintenance visit.
- Patient compliance affecting supportive therapy.

Essential Periodontics, First Edition. Edited by Steph Smith and Khalid Almas.
© 2022 John Wiley & Sons Ltd. Published 2022 by John Wiley & Sons Ltd.

Introduction

Periodontitis is a bacterially induced, chronic immuno-inflammatory disease that results in the destruction of the connective tissues and alveolar bone. Active periodontal treatment aims to eliminate or reduce this response, mainly through the removal of dental biofilm deposits. Following the completion of treatment and reduction of inflammation, supportive periodontal therapy (SPT) is implemented to reduce the probability of reinfection and progression of the disease.

The long-term management of periodontal disease requires a routine follow-up program directed at maintaining and improving the outcomes of active treatment as well as preventing the development of new disease or disease recurrence, as detected from clinical trials on the long-term effects of treatment of periodontitis (Isidor & Karring 1986; Kaldahl et al. 1988; Knowles et al. 1979; Lindhe & Nyman 1975, 1984; Nyman et al. 1977; Pihlström et al. 1983; Ramfjord et al. 1968; Rosling et al. 1976; Westfelt et al. 1985). Hence, post-treatment professional maintenance care has become an integral phase of periodontal care. Interceptive professional supportive therapy at regular intervals may, to a certain degree, compensate for the lack of patient compliance with regard to oral hygiene measures. The aim of periodontal therapy is the long-term retention of natural teeth in a healthy, functional, aesthetically acceptable, and painless state (Hirschfeld & Wasserman 1978) by providing supervised control for the patient. The long-term preservation of the dentition is closely associated with the frequency and quality of maintenance therapy.

The 3rd World Workshop of the American Academy of Periodontology (AAP 1998) renamed the maintenance phase as "supportive periodontal therapy" to reflect the need for professional measures to support the patient's efforts to control periodontal infections and to prevent reinfection.

Treatment of active periodontal disease is usually staged. There is insufficient evidence to determine the superiority of different protocols or adjunctive strategies to improve tooth maintenance during SPT. This phase of therapy is instituted following the completion of active periodontal therapy, but it can be used as an interim phase in the treatment planning process. A patient may move from active treatment into SPT and back into active treatment if an exacerbation of the disease is detected (Figure 22.1).

Definition

SPT has been given many names, including periodontal maintenance therapy, recall, and preventive maintenance, which however was changed at the 3rd World Workshop of American Academy of Periodontology (AAP 1998) to SPT. SPT includes therapeutic procedures performed at selected intervals to assist the periodontal patient's individual efforts in maintaining oral health and to control or avoid reinfection.

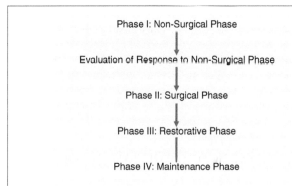

Figure 22.1 Sequence of periodontal treatment.

Rationale

Following completion of treatment and arrest of inflammation, SPT is employed to reduce the probability of reinfection and progression of the disease; to maintain teeth without pain, excessive mobility, or persistent infection in the long term; and to prevent related oral diseases by controlling factors known to contribute to the disease process. The success of SPT has been reported in a number of long-term, retrospective studies (AAP 1998; Lindhe & Nyman 1984).

Aims of supportive periodontal therapy

- To preserve the gingival and periodontal health achieved following the initial and corrective phases of periodontal therapy.
- To prevent or minimize the recurrence and progression of periodontal disease in patients treated for periodontitis.
- To prevent and reduce the incidence of tooth loss by monitoring the dentition, prosthetic replacements, and implants.
- To locate or treat other diseases or conditions found in the oral cavity in a timely manner.
- SPT also increases the probability of recognizing and treating other diseases or conditions found within the oral cavity (Wilson 1996).
- To reinforce proper oral home care.

Causes of recurrence of periodontal disease

- Inadequate subgingival plaque and/or calculus removal.
- Morphology of the dento-gingival unit.
- Improper restorations done or poorly designed prostheses after active periodontal treatment.
- Failure of the patient to comply with periodic recall visits.
- Presence of some systemic diseases that may modify the host response to the dental biofilm.

Intervention in supportive periodontal therapy

Supportive periodontal treatment evolved from traditional dental prophylaxis and at present emphasizes treatment of areas of previous attachment loss and areas where clinical signs of inflammation are found (Wilson 1996). The patient must be informed that SPT is essential to future and long-term control of disease (Kerry 1995).

SPT should include all components of a typical dental recall examination, and importantly should also include periodontal re-evaluation and risk assessment, supragingival and subgingival removal of bacterial plaque and calculus, and retreatment of any sites showing recurrent or persistent disease. A thorough periodontal evaluation, risk assessment, and subsequent treatment, including mechanical debridement of any plaque or calculus deposits, differentiates SPT from routine care.

Maintenance procedures are under the supervision of dentists and include an update of medical and dental histories, extraoral and intraoral soft tissue examination, dental examination, periodontal evaluation, occlusion evaluation, radiographic review, removal of bacterial flora from crevicular and pocket areas, scaling and root planing where indicated, polishing of teeth, and a review of the patient's plaque control efficacy (Cohen 2003).

The best way to determine areas that are losing attachment is still to use a well-organized periodontal charting system. Some computerized systems offer the possibility of easy retrieval and comparison with past findings. No accurate method of identifying disease activity exists, and clinicians rely on the information provided by combining probing pocket depth, bleeding on probing, and sequential attachment measurements. Patients whose disease is progressive may need bacterial culturing and antibiotic therapy in combination with additional mechanical therapy.

Disease does recur in a small number of patients who are identified as high risk or extreme downhill patients, and in the absence of SPT there is a high risk for tooth loss. In patients with advanced periodontally compromised teeth, radiographic and/or microbial monitoring and use of systemic antibiotics as an adjunct to non-surgical SPT can reduce the need for tooth extractions.

Radiographic examination

In patients with less than optimal control of periodontal disease, periapical and/or vertical bitewing radiographs of problem areas every 12–24 months and full-mouth periapicals every 3–5 years are advocated. In cases with satisfactory control of the disease after periodontal treatment, bitewing radiographs are to be taken every 24–36 months and a full-mouth series every 5 years is recommended.

Radiographic perception of periodontal disease progression has a high specificity, but a low sensitivity, with underestimation of the severity of a periodontal defect (Hämmerle et al. 1990). The choice of a reproducible technique like the long cone technique with image receptor holding mechanism, bite block, and an X-ray beam aiming device, as well as the quality of film processing, may assist in reducing some of these shortcomings.

Microbiological monitoring

Microbiological monitoring and antibiotic sensitivity testing can be useful in progressive periodontitis. When the possible causal organisms remain after therapy or if generalized attachment loss continues or recurs, periodic microbial testing is suggested (Slots 1996). When used in these cases, combined with subgingival scaling and root planing, the suitable antibiotic and antimicrobial therapy often produces results superior to scaling and root planing alone (Figure 22.2).

Recall intervals for periodontal maintenance

Periodontitis is a multifactorial disease, with complex interaction between the host and microbial factors, and hence both treatment of disease and successive SPT should be customized in terms of preventive and treatment approaches and frequency. Selection of the recall intervals must be based on the requirements of individual patients.

Studies have indicated that patients who return for regular periodic visits for disease reassessment, scaling, root planing, and oral hygiene reinforcement demonstrate better periodontal health and a better prognosis in the long term than patients who do not return for these appointments (Wilson 1991).

Evidence for a specific recall interval (e.g. every 3 months) for every patient is weak. There are merits in risk-based recommendations because of the difficulties encountered in accurately diagnosing disease activity and predicting disease progression, although the number of well-controlled longitudinal clinical trials is rather limited for patients who have undergone periodontal treatment. However, the significance of controlling risk factors, particularly by reducing bacterial plaque and calculus deposits, is widely accepted.

Clinical parameters may serve as early indicators for new onset or recurrence of the periodontal disease process, i.e. reinfection and progression of periodontal destruction of a previously treated periodontal site. Patients on recall are a varied group depending on their risk factors and response to treatment, and can be categorized according to Merin's classification (Table 22.1) with the suggested recall intervals.

The question of whether the maintenance phase of therapy should be performed by a general practitioner or a specialist should be determined by the amount of periodontal destruction present. Class A recall patients could be maintained by a general dentist, whereas class C patients should be maintained by a specialist. Class B patients can alternate recall visits between a general practitioner and a specialist. The proposed

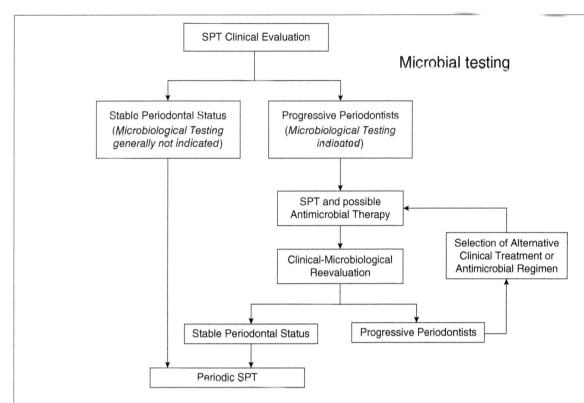

Figure 22.2 Flow chart for microbial testing in supportive periodontal therapy (SPT). Source: Adapted from Slots 1996.

approach is that the patient's disease should dictate whether a general practitioner or a specialist undertakes the maintenance therapy. The recall interval for first-year patients should not be longer than three months in order that the requirements to reinforce oral hygiene techniques, to evaluate closely the results of some periodontal surgical procedures, and to retreat areas overlooked during the initial phase will be more appropriate at this early stage.

Once active periodontal treatment is completed, be it non-surgical and/or surgical, patients with a moderate to high risk must be enrolled into a well-organized recall system, which should provide both continuous risk assessment and adequate supportive care to prevent or reduce progressive loss of attachment (Axelsson & Lindhe 1981a, b; Becker et al. 1984; Cortellini et al. 1994, 1996).

Components of a periodontal maintenance visit

Hancock and Newell (2001) suggest that SPT consists of three parts:

- *Part I: Examination, re-evaluation, and diagnosis.* Approximate time 14 minutes.
  - Update of medical and dental histories and evaluation of patient's risk factors.
  - Assessment of oral hygiene, sites with bleeding on probing (BOP), probing pocket depth (PPD), and clinical

attachment levels; inspection of reinfected sites with pus if any; evaluation of existing reconstructions. Comparison with the baseline data. Vitality testing and diagnostic radiographic evaluation where indicated.

- *Part II: Reinstruction of oral hygiene and treatment.* Approximate time 36 minutes. Motivation, reinstruction of oral hygiene, and instrumentation as necessary, especially in relapse or refractory cases where sites (generalized/localized) with signs of inflammation and active disease are detected. Hence, all the BOP-positive sites and all pockets with a PPD ≥5 mm are carefully re-debrided.

- *Part III: Dental prophylaxis, fluoride application, reporting, and scheduling/referral.* Approximate time 10 minutes. Polishing of full dentition, application of fluorides, and determination of future SPT. Fluorides should be applied in high concentration to replace the fluorides that could have been removed by instrumentation from the surface layers of the teeth and to prevent root surface caries, especially in areas with gingival recession. Future SPT visits should be scheduled based on the patient's risk assessment.

There is no consensus on which treatment regime is most appropriate for the majority of cases, but there is evidence to support the two most common interventions during SPT, namely supragingival and subgingival debridement (Heasman et al. 2002). Relapse or persistent disease, and the degree of control over site- or patient-specific risk factors, may propagate therapeutic measures. Usually, these sites are treated by

Table 22.1 Merin's classification for recall intervals for various classes of recall patients.

Merin classification	Characteristics	Recall interval
First year following periodontal treatment		
First year	First-year patient: routine therapy and uneventful healing	3 months
	First-year patient: difficult case with complicated prosthesis, furcation involvement, poor crown-to-root ratios, or questionable patient cooperation	1–2 months
After first year following periodontal treatment		
Class A	Excellent results well maintained for 1 year or more Patient displays good oral hygiene, minimal calculus, no occlusal problems, no complicated prostheses, no remaining pockets, and no teeth with less than 50% of alveolar bone remaining	6 months to 1 year
Class B	Generally good results maintained reasonably well for 1 year or more, but patient displays some of the following factors: 1. Inconsistent or poor oral hygiene 2. Heavy calculus formation 3. Systemic disease that predisposes to periodontal breakdown 4. Some remaining pockets 5. Occlusal problems 6. Complicated prostheses 7. Ongoing orthodontic therapy 8. Recurrent dental caries 9. Some teeth with less than 50% of alveolar bone support 10. Smoking 11. Positive family history or genetic test 12. More than 20% of pockets bleed on probing	3–4 months (decide on recall interval based on number and severity of negative factors)
Class C	Generally poor results after periodontal therapy and/or several negative factors from the following list: 1. Inconsistent or poor oral hygiene 2. Heavy calculus formation 3. Systemic disease that predisposes to periodontal breakdown 4. Many remaining pockets 5. Occlusal problems 6. Complicated prostheses 7. Recurrent dental caries 8. Periodontal surgery indicated but not performed for medical, psychological, or financial reasons 9. Many teeth with less than 50% of alveolar bone support 10. Condition too far advanced to be improved by periodontal surgery 11. Smoking 12. Positive family history or genetic test 13. More than 20% of pockets bleed on probing	1–3 months (decide on recall interval based on number and severity of negative factors; consider retreating some areas or extracting severely involved teeth)

Source: Adapted from Merin 2002.

subgingival debridement under local anesthesia to accomplish effective removal of microbial deposits. Subgingival debridement is also recommended at sites presenting with PPD greater than 4 mm regardless of signs of inflammation or recurrent disease, as the risk of relapse increases with deeper probing depth measurements.

Patient compliance

Compliance is defined as "the extent to which a person's behaviour coincides with medical or health advice." The periodontal patient must be educated at the onset of periodontal treatment that the long-term success of treatment will depend on the willingness of the patient to adhere to a well-scheduled periodontal maintenance therapy program (Demetriou et al. 1995). Also, as part of SPT, evidence strongly supports the efficacy of professionally delivered counseling regarding tobacco, alcohol, and drug dependency among individuals. Dentists, dental therapists, and dental hygienists are ideally placed to spearhead efforts in supporting behavioral changes and pharmacological support (Kumar 2020). See Appendix 3 regarding counseling on smoking cessation.

As can be expected, a highly compliant patient has been shown to have a better periodontal prognosis compared to non-compliant patients. There are many and varied reasons for non-compliance of patients, the most common ones being personal reasons, financial reasons, psychological reasons, sheer ignorance, and behavioral changes over time (Costa et al. 2011;

Demetriou et al. 1995). It has been noted that the majority of non-compliant patients have more stressful life events and less secure personal relationships, and with the passage of time compliance drops to less than 35% (Wilson et al. 1984).

It has been noted that the more often a patient attends maintenance appointments, the lower the possibility that they would lose teeth (Wilson 1996a; Wilson et al. 1987). Important factors to increase compliance include patient education about the importance of maintenance, simplification of procedures, reminding patients of appointments, record keeping on compliance, providing positive reinforcement, identification of likely non-compliers, and ensuring the dentist's involvement (Wilson 1996b). Patient compliance can be further facilitated by means of reminders, either by telephone calls or mail, to schedule an appointment.

Conclusions

All active periodontal and implant treatment must be followed with periodic supportive periodontal care because of the persistent threat from the dental biofilm. The varied periodontal patient needs that are to be monitored closely on a long-term basis, as well as the interval for recalls, depend on various situations and risk factors. Close monitoring will assist in early detection of progressive or recurrent disease before more advanced periodontal or dental tissue breakdown can occur, thereby facilitating timely interventional treatment. Patients must be well motivated for better compliance with maintenance therapy, as it has been documented that improved periodontal health and decreased progression of periodontal disease can be achieved with long-term SPT.

REFERENCES

American Academy of Periodontology (AAP). Supportive periodontal therapy. *J Periodontol.* 1998; 69(4):502–506.

Axelsson P, Lindhe J. Effect of controlled oral hygiene procedures on caries and periodontal disease in adults. Results after 6 years. *J Clin Periodontol.* 1981a; 8:239–248.

Axelsson P, Lindhe J. The significance of maintenance care in the treatment of periodontal disease. *J Clin Periodontol.* 1981b; 8:281–294.

Becker W, Becker BE, Berg LE. Periodontal treatment without maintenance. A retrospective study in 44 patients. *J Periodontol.* 1984; 55:505–509.

Cohen RE. American Academy of Periodontology. *Position Paper Periodontal Maintenance. J Periodontol.* 2003; 74(9):1395–1401.

Cortellini P, Pini Prato G, Tonetti M. Periodontal regeneration of human infrabony defects. V. Effect of oral hygiene on long term stability. *J Clin Periodontol.* 1994; 21:606–610.

Cortellini P, Pini Prato G, Tonetti M. Long term stability of clinical attachment following guided tissue regeneration and conventional therapy. *J Clin Periodontol.* 1996; 23:106–111.

Costa FO, Miranda Cota LO, Pereira Lages EJ et al. Oral impact on daily performance, personality traits, and compliance in periodontal maintenance therapy. *J Periodontol.* 2011; 82:1146–1154.

Demetriou N, Tsami-Pandi A, Parashis A. Compliance with supportive periodontal treatment in private periodontal practice. A 14-year retrospective study. *J Periodontol.* 1995; 66:145–149.

Hämmerle CHF, Ingold H-P, Lang NP. Evaluation of clinical and radiographic scoring methods before and after initial periodontal therapy. *J Clin Periodontol.* 1990; 17:255–263.

Hancock EB, Newell DH. Preventive strategies and supportive treatment. *Periodontol* 2000. 2001; 25:59–76.

Heasman PA, McCracken GI, Steen N. Supportive periodontal care: the effect of periodic subgingival debridement compared with supragingival prophylaxis with respect to clinical outcomes. *J Clin Periodontol.* 2002; 29(3):163–172.

Hirschfeld L, Wasserman B. A long-term survey of tooth loss in 600 treated periodontal patients. *J Periodontol.* 1978; 49.225–237.

Isidor F, Karring T. Long-term effect of surgical and non-surgical periodontal treatment. A 5-year clinical study. *J Periodontal Res.* 1986; 21:462–472.

Kaldahl WB, Kalkwarf KL, Patil KD, Dyer JK, Bates RE. Evaluation of four modalities of periodontal therapy. Mean probing depth, probing attachment level and recession changes. *J Periodontol.* 1988; 59:783–793.

Kerry GJ. Supportive periodontal treatment. *Periodontol* 2000. 1995; 9:176–185.

Knowles JW, Burgett FG, Nissle RR et al. Results of periodontal treatment related to pocket depth and attachment level. *Eight years. J Periodontol.* 1979; 50:225–233.

Kumar PS. Interventions to prevent periodontal disease in tobacco-, alcohol-, and drug-dependent individuals. *Periodontol* 2000. 2020; 84:84–101.

Lindhe J, Nyman S. The effect of plaque control and surgical pocket elimination on the establishment and maintenance of periodontal health. A longitudinal study of periodontal therapy in cases of advanced disease. *J Clin Periodontol.* 1975; 2:67–79.

Lindhe J, Nyman S. Long-term maintenance of patients treated for advanced periodontal disease. *J Clin Periodontol.* 1984; 11:504–514.

Merin RL. Supportive periodontal treatment. Classification of posttreatment patients. In: MG Newman, HH Takei, FA Carranza (eds), *Carranza's Clinical Periodontology.* Philadelphia, PA: WB Saunders; 2002: 973–974.

Nyman S, Lindhe J, Rosling B. Periodontal surgery in plaque-infected dentitions. *J Clin Periodontol.* 1977; 4:240–249.

Pihlström BL, McHugh RB, Oliphant TH, Ortiz-Campos C. Comparison of surgical and non-surgical treatment of periodontal disease. A review of current studies and additional results after 6½ years. *J Clin Periodontol.* 1983; 10:524–541.

Ramfjord, SP, Nissle RR, Shick RA, Cooper H. Subgingival curettage versus surgical elimination of periodontal pockets. *J Periodontol.* 1968; 39:167–175.

Rosling B, Nyman S, Lindhe J, Jern B. The healing potential of the periodontal tissues following different techniques of periodontal surgery in plaque-free dentitions. *J Clin Periodontol.* 1976; 3:233–250.

Slots J. Microbial analysis in supportive periodontal treatment. *Periodontol* 2000. 1996; 12:56–59.

Westfelt E, Bragd L, Socransky SS et al. Improved periodontal conditions following therapy. *J Clin Periodontol.* 1985; 12:283–293.

Wilson TG Jr. Supportive periodontal treatment: maintenance. *Curr Opin Dent.* 1991; 1:111–117.

Wilson TG Jr. Compliance and its role in periodontal therapy. *Periodontol* 2000. 1996a; 12:16–23.

Wilson TG Jr. A typical supportive periodontal treatment visits for patients with periodontal disease. *Periodontol* 2000. 1996b; 12:24–28.

Wilson TG Jr, Glover ME, Malik AK, Schoen JA, Dorsett D. Tooth loss in maintenance patients in a private periodontal practice. *J Periodontol.* 1987; 58:231–235.

Wilson TG Jr, Glover ME, Schoen J, Baus C, Jacobs T. Compliance with maintenance therapy in a private periodontal practice. *J Periodontol.* 1984; 55:468–473.

CHAPTER 23
Periodontal medicine

Steph Smith

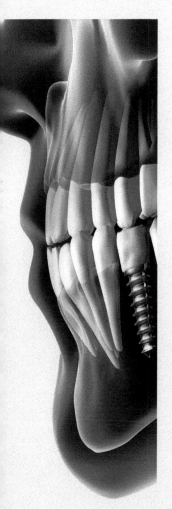

Periodontal medicine is a collective term commonly used to describe how periodontal infection/inflammation may affect extraoral health (Beck et al. 2019). Focal oral infections are defined as infections occurring in different sites of the human body and caused by microorganisms or their products that colonized the oral cavity (Pizzo et al. 2011). Severe periodontitis has been reported to be the sixth most common human disease, affecting an estimated 11.2% of the global adult population, affecting about 45–50% of adults in its mildest forms, and rising to over 60% in people aged >65 years (Global Burden of Disease Study 2013 Collaborators 2015). Severe periodontitis thus represents a significant healthcare, social, and economic burden (Genco & Sanz 2020). Studies have shown increased evidence of epidemiological associations between periodontitis and systemic diseases, such as cardiovascular diseases, diabetes mellitus, metabolic disease and obesity, respiratory disease, preterm delivery, rheumatoid arthritis, and Alzheimer's disease (Monsarrat et al. 2016; Pizzo et al. 2011). Data from epidemiological studies also show evidence of a positive association between periodontal disease and overall cancer risk, and risk of certain specific cancer sites, including cancers of the lung and upper digestive tract (Nwizu et al. 2020). Common risk factors also place individuals at high risk for both periodontitis and systemic diseases, and include environmental risk factors such as tobacco smoking, stress, aging, race or ethnicity, and sex (Li et al. 2000).

In patients with periodontal disease, bacteria have access into connective tissues and the bloodstream. Patients presenting with poor oral health can also induce spontaneous bacteremias during chewing and oral hygiene procedures (Carmona et al. 2002). Dental procedures, including endodontic treatment, periodontal surgery, tooth extraction, scaling, and root planing, can cause oral microorganisms to enter the bloodstream (Carmona et al. 2002). However, the cumulative monthly bacteremia exposure resulting from self-induced oral procedures, such as chewing and toothbrushing, has been shown to be about 1000 times greater than that from a dental extraction (Guntheroth 1984). Furthermore, the periodontium serves as a reservoir of inflammatory cytokines that may also enter the bloodstream, including tumor necrosis factor alpha (TNF-α), interleukin-1 beta (IL-1β), Υ-interferon (IFN-Υ), as well as prostaglandin E2 (PGE2) (Page 1998).

The etiological mechanisms by which oral bacteria may cause systemic diseases are proposed as follows (Monsarrat et al. 2016; Nwizu et al. 2020):

- Gram-negative bacteria can translocate to the bloodstream by breaching the compromised epithelial lining of periodontal pockets, thus causing metastatic infection.
- Circulating exotoxins and endotoxins of periodontal pathogens can cause metastatic injury.
- Pathogens and their toxins can cause metastatic inflammation by means of immunological responses, including the formation of immune complexes, which may give rise to acute and chronic inflammatory reactions at sites of deposition.

Essential Periodontics, First Edition. Edited by Steph Smith and Khalid Almas.
© 2022 John Wiley & Sons Ltd. Published 2022 by John Wiley & Sons Ltd.

REFERENCES

Beck JD, Papapanou PN, Philips KH, Offenbacher S. Periodontal medicine: 100 years of progress. *J Dent Res.* 2019; 98(10):1053–1062.

Carmona IT, Diz Dios P, Scully C. An update on the controversies in bacterial endocarditis of oral origin. *Oral Surg Oral Med Oral Pathol Oral Radiol Endod.* 2002; 93(6):660–670.

Genco RJ, Sanz M. Clinical and public health implications of periodontal and systemic diseases: an overview. *Periodontol 2000.* 2020; 83:7–13.

Global Burden of Disease Study 2013 Collaborators. Global, regional, and national incidence, prevalence, and years lived with disability for 301 acute and chronic diseases and injuries in 188 countries, 1990–2013: a systematic analysis for the Global Burden of Disease Study 2013. *Lancet. 2015*; 386(9995):743–800.

Guntheroth WG. How important are dental procedures as a cause of infective endocarditis? *Am J Cardiol.* 1984; 54(7):797–801.

Li X, Kolltveit KM, Tronstad L, Olsen I. Systemic diseases caused by oral infection. *Clin Microbiol Rev.* 2000; 13(4):547–558.

Monsarrat P, Blaizot A, Kemoun P et al. Clinical research activity in periodontal medicine: a systematic mapping of trial registers. *J Clin Periodontol.* 2016; 43:390–400.

Nwizu N, Wactawski-Wende J, Genco RJ. Periodontal disease and cancer: epidemiologic studies and possible mechanisms. *Periodontol 2000.* 2020; 83:213–233.

Page RC. The pathobiology of periodontal diseases may affect systemic diseases: inversion of a paradigm. *Ann Periodontol.* 1998; 3(1):108–120.

Pizzo G, Guiglia R, Campisi G. Periodontal disease and systemic diseases: interrelationships and interactions. In: SL Yamamoto (ed.), *Periodontal Disease: Symptoms, Treatment and Prevention.* New York: Nova Biomedical Books; 2011: 215–246.

23.1 PERIODONTAL DISEASE, DIABETES, AND OBESITY

Steph Smith

Contents

Learning objectives

- Etiology of type 1 and type 2 diabetes and associated diabetes and periodontal disease prevalences.
- The concept of a bi-directional association between periodontal disease and type 2 diabetes, and the common risk factors involved.
- Understanding the underlying biological mechanisms of the impact of periodontal disease on diabetes.
- Understanding the underlying biological mechanisms of the impact of diabetes on periodontal disease.
- Understanding the various bi-directional associations and pathogeneses between periodontal disease, diabetes, obesity, and dyslipidemia.
- Systemic and oral complications associated with diabetes.
- Management of periodontal patients with diabetes.

Introduction

A close relationship has been suggested among periodontitis, obesity, and type 2 diabetes mellitus (DM), with chronic inflammation being the common denominator. The basic premise underlying this is that proinflammatory cytokines (and/or bacteria and their products) released locally in gingiva may enter the systemic circulation and influence tissues/organs in distant sites. Concurrently, proinflammatory cytokines involved in type 2 DM may reach the gingival environment and aggravate the periodontal condition, resulting in a "bi-directional relationship" between periodontitis and type 2 DM. In addition, adipose cells, especially visceral fat in obese individuals, produce the proinflammatory cytokine tumor necrosis factor-alpha (TNF-α), which induces insulin resistance (IR), thus contributing to the development of type 2 DM in obese subjects. Thus, there is a plausible rationale underlying the association among periodontitis, obesity, and type 2 DM (Watanabe et al. 2008).

DM is a hormonal disease, including changes in carbohydrate, protein, and lipid metabolism. By 2017 it was reported that globally, 425 million adults have diabetes, 50% of whom may still be undiagnosed. The prevalence of diabetes varies among countries, with China, India and the USA having the highest prevalence (Genco & Borgnakke 2020; Watanabe et al. 2008). Hyperglycemia affects one in six pregnancies worldwide, of which 86.4% are reported to be due to gestational diabetes. A large proportion of women with gestational diabetes have been shown to develop diabetes 3–6 years postpartum (Genco & Borgnakke 2020).

Type 1 DM is characterized primarily by an insulin deficiency. It is an organ-specific autoimmune disease including more than 50 type 1 DM susceptibility genes, which causes lymphocytes and other immune cells to destroy pancreatic beta cells (ADA 2010; Boldison & Wong 2016; Graves et al. 2020). The progression of type 1 DM may be enhanced by viruses or environmental toxins inducing insulitis, causing an inflammatory infiltrate in the islets of Langerhans, or by activating the immune system through molecular mimicry of islet autoantigens (Zheng et al. 2018). The prevalence of periodontitis in type 1 diabetics may be increased fourfold compared to normoglycemic controls (Popławska-Kita et al. 2014), and mean clinical attachment loss and bone loss can be twofold higher compared to non-diabetics (Meenawat et al. 2013).

Type 2 DM is characterized by hyperglycemia involving a range of dysfunctions, which include insulin insensitivity combined with insufficient insulin secretion, and excessive or inappropriate glucagon secretion (Biadgo & Abebe 2016). It is related to risk factors such as age, genetics, race, and ethnicity, as well as environmental factors such as diet, physical activity, and smoking. These factors reduce the insulin sensitivity of target organs and affect beta cells that produce insulin (Genco et al. 2020; Kumar et al. 2014). Type 2 DM constitutes 90% of the world's diabetic population, together with a strong genetic component (Genco & Borgnakke 2020). Between 2002 and 2017 a threefold increase was reported in the globally estimated number of adults with type 2 DM. The prevalence increases with age, and 1 in 4 adults aged ≥65 years may be affected by diabetes (Genco et al. 2020).

Diabetes-associated periodontitis should not be regarded as a distinct diagnosis, as no phenotypic characteristics are unique to periodontal disease (PD) in diabetic patients. Diabetes is thus considered an important modifying factor and is to be included in a clinical diagnosis of PD as a descriptor (Jepsen et al. 2018). Furthermore, the level of glycemic control in diabetes influences the grading of periodontitis according to the 2018 classification of PD (Papapanou et al. 2018; Tonetti et al. 2018).

Association between periodontal disease and diabetes

Diabetes and hyperglycemia are associated with more severe PD, edentulism, and tooth loss (Genco & Borgnakke 2020). PD has been recognized as the sixth most frequent complication of diabetes (Loe 1993). Globally, higher levels of PD are seen in populations with poorly controlled DM. Furthermore, it has been reported that over a 10-year period, subjects with DM and PD show a higher mortality rate, both for cardiovascular death and for all-cause mortality, compared with subjects with diabetes alone (Genco et al. 2020). Patients with type 2 DM are 2.8 times more likely to have at least 5 mm clinical attachment loss and 3.4 times more likely to have at least 25% radiographic bone loss, with a fourfold higher risk of severe alveolar bone loss (Genco & Borgnakke 2020; Graves et al. 2020).

PD and diabetes share both modifiable and non-modifiable risk factors. Modifiable risk factors include smoking, excessive alcohol consumption, obesity, physical inactivity, and excessive refined sugar consumption. Non-modifiable risk factors include higher age, male sex, minority race/ethnicity, low socioeconomic status, and genetic predisposition (Genco & Borgnakke 2020).

Bi-directional association between periodontal disease and diabetes

There is an independent bi-directional association between PD and type 2 DM, constituting a vicious cycle that exacerbates both diseases when present in the same patient (Kumar et al. 2014; Mealey 2006; Sanz et al. 2018). Chronic low-grade inflammation involving cells and inflammatory mediators of the immune system is the fundamental underlying mechanism of the pathophysiology in this bi-directional association (Grossi & Genco 1998; Kocher et al. 2018; Nagpal et al. 2015). Local proinflammatory cytokines within the periodontium may enter the bloodstream and impact distant tissues and organs. On the other hand, increased systemic levels of proinflammatory cytokines in diabetic patients can influence local and immune reactions in the periodontium (Grossi & Genco 1998; Nishimura et al. 2003).

Effects of periodontal disease on diabetes

The extent to which PD can influence the course of diabetes is still unclear, including the cellular processes responsible for this relationship (see Figure 23.1.1) (Andersen et al. 2007). Periodontal inflammation may contribute to the onset and persistence of hyperglycemia, which includes the promotion of IR, thereby affecting glycemic control in diabetic patients (Albandar et al. 2018; Zhou et al. 2015). The ulcerated pocket epithelium in the periodontal lesion, as well as the resultant inflammatory increase in vascularity, provides a chronic source of systemic challenge from bacteria and their products, as well as from locally produced inflammatory mediators (Grossi & Genco 1998; Pizzo et al. 2010).

Although inconsistent evidence exists in studies, oral bacteria may also have an impact on diabetes. Studies have not shown a clear difference in the subgingival microflora of PD in DM patients compared with healthy individuals, although differences may exist (Genco et al. 2020; Graves et al. 2020; Madianos & Koromantzos 2018). Periodontopathogens such as *Porphyromonas gingivalis*, *Prevotella intermedia*, *Tannerella forsythia*, *Treponema denticola*, and *Aggregatibacter actinomycetemcomitans* can penetrate the tissues of the periodontium, including a leakage of endotoxins, leading to a bacteremia and an endotoxemia due to lipopolysaccharides (LPS) entering the bloodstream (Pizzo et al. 2010). The intermittent bacteremia and endotoxemia can induce systemic inflammation, thereby enhancing IR, which promotes hyperglycemia (Borgnakke et al. 2013).

Associated immunoinflammatory molecules such as interleukin (IL) 1β, IL-6, tumor necrosis factor (TNF)-α, prostaglandin E2 (PGE2), IL-8, IL-12, and matrix metalloproteinases (MMPs) may also enter the blood circulation. Also, in response to IL-6 and TNF-α, the liver secretes the acute-phase C-reactive protein (CRP). These inflammatory cytokines amplify the cytokine dysregulation associated with diabetes, and interfere with the function of the insulin receptor, leading to IR and altered glucose metabolism (Andersen et al. 2007; Genco et al. 2020; Sun et al. 2011). The metabolic effects of TNF-α include the down-regulation of genes related to normal insulin action and directly affect insulin signaling and glucose transport. IL-6 has been reported to modulate the production of TNF-α and has been associated with IR. IL-1β, in turn, seems to

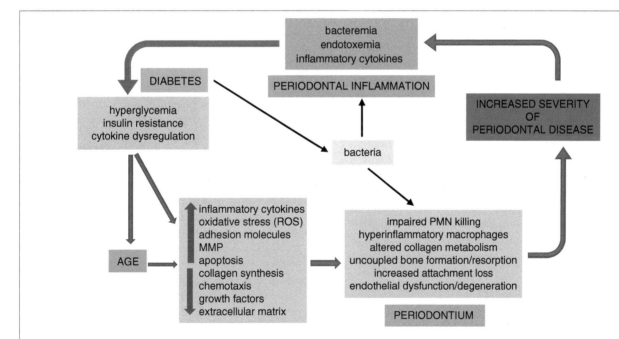

Figure 23.1.1 Bi-directional association between diabetes and periodontal disease. Diabetes is characterized by hyperglycemia, which includes insulin resistance and cytokine dysregulation. In diabetic patients a sustained hyperglycemia affects periodontal tissues directly, by means of alterations of intracellular and molecular pathways, and indirectly by means of advanced glycation end products (AGEs). Cellular alterations include an increase in inflammatory cytokines, oxidative stress, adhesion molecules, matrix metalloproteinases (MMPs), and apoptosis; a decrease in collagen synthesis, chemotaxis, growth factors, and extracellular matrix. This causes the following changes in the periodontium: impaired polymorphonuclear neutrophil (PMN) killing, hyperinflammatory macrophages, altered collagen metabolism, uncoupled bone formation/resorption, increased attachment loss, and endothelial dysfunction/degeneration. This leads to an increased severity of periodontal disease. The associated bacteremia, endotoxins, and immunoinflammatory molecules enter the blood circulation, thereby amplifying the cytokine dysregulation associated with diabetes, including insulin resistance and altered glucose metabolism, thus causing further dysregulation of glycemic control in diabetic patients. Diabetes can alter the bacterial composition to be more pathogenic, and/or enhance a prolonged and greater inflammatory response to bacteria. ROS, reactive oxygen species. Courtesy of Dr. Steph Smith.

participate in the regulation of glucose uptake (Andersen et al. 2007). This then leads to the malfunctioning of various tissues and cells, such as adipocytes, hepatocytes, endothelial cells, and muscle cells, thereby complicating the control of type 2 diabetes in patients with chronic PD (Brownlee 2003; Sun et al. 2011). Increased concentrations of proinflammatory IL-1β cytokines have been shown to be cytotoxic to pancreatic β-cells in animal models of type 1 DM (Brownlee 2003; Sjoholm 1998). Monocytes from diabetic patients have also been shown to produce increased amounts of TNF-α when stimulated with LPS, compared to monocytes from non-diabetic patients (Salvi et al. 2005). TNF-α has been implicated in macrophage-dependent cytotoxicity of pancreatic islets in diabetes (Moller 2000). Chronic infection-induced IR, and thus subsequent poor glycemic control, is considered to be a precursor to active diabetes due to pancreatic β-cell destruction that results from sustained elevations of systemic IL-1β and TNF-α during PD (Moller 2000).

Effects of diabetes on periodontal disease

The severity of PD has been shown to be significantly greater in patients with diabetes (Loe 1993) (Figure 23.1.1). Diabetic patients with poor glycemic control have an increased risk of presenting with deep periodontal pockets, severe attachment loss, and progressive bone loss, compared to well-controlled diabetic patients (Ajita et al. 2013; Guzman et al. 2003). In diabetic patients, a long-term sustained hyperglycemia can affect periodontal tissues in a direct manner, by means of cellular damage through alterations of intracellular and molecular pathways, and indirectly by means of the irreversible non-enzymatic glycation and oxidation of circulating and immobilized proteins and lipids, resulting in the formation of advanced glycation end products (AGEs) (Andersen et al. 2007). AGEs accumulate in diabetic plasma and tissues, including affecting cells of the periodontal tissues (Gharat 2011; Vlassara & Uribarri 2014). This causes a dysregulation of both the innate and adaptive immune systems, including an increase in oxidative stress (Knight et al. 2016; Omori et al. 2008).

Diabetes and periodontal bacteria

Controversy exists as to whether the inflammatory response is enhanced to oral bacteria in diabetics, or whether diabetes alters the bacterial composition so as to increase bacterial pathogenicity, or whether both processes occur (Chapple et al. 2013).

Definitive evidence does show that diabetes alters the inflammatory response to oral bacteria in both type 1 and type 2 DM (Naguib et al. 2004). Animal studies have shown prolonged inflammatory responses, including increased mRNA levels of genes associated with host defense, apoptosis, cell signaling and activity, coagulation/hemostasis, and complement activity (Andriankaja et al. 2012). Infection with *A. actinomycetemcomitans* has been shown to stimulate a 1.5-fold greater increase in TNF-α, a 1.6-fold greater increase in polymorphonuclear neutrophil (PMN) infiltration, and 1.7-fold more bone loss in diabetic rats than normoglycemic rats (Kang et al. 2012).

Inconsistent and contradictory findings have been reported regarding diabetes altering the oral bacterial composition. Animal studies have indicated that the overall effect of diabetes is to reduce oral microbial diversity, with an increase in particular bacteria such as *Proteobacteria* and *Firmicutes*, as well as *P. gingivalis* (Demmer et al. 2017; Xiao et al. 2017). Furthermore, these diabetic oral microbiotas have been found to be more pathogenic when compared to those of normoglycemic controls, by means of inducing more inflammation, including increased PMN accumulation and expression of IL-6, as well as increased expression of receptor activator of nuclear factor kappa-B ligand (RANKL) and osteoclast formation, causing greater bone resorption (Graves et al. 2020) (See also Chapter 5.1).

Advanced glycation end products

As a result of chronic hyperglycemia, advanced glycation end products (AGEs) originate from the irreversible non-enzymatic glycation and oxidation of proteins, lipids, and nucleic acids by the addition of sugars to their polypeptide chain, which alters their structure and functionality (Sczepanik et al. 2020). AGEs accumulate in diabetic plasma and tissues, including affecting cells of the periodontal tissues (Gharat 2011; Vlassara & Uribarri 2014). AGEs cause tissue damage by (i) the intracellular accumulation of AGEs, which alters cytoplasmic and nuclear factors; (ii) the formation of stable abnormal cross-links on collagen, which alters its structure and function; and (iii) interacting with the receptor for advanced glycation end product (RAGE), which leads to cellular signaling, including nuclear factor-κB activation (Sczepanik et al. 2020). When AGEs bind to RAGE, cellular phenotype and function are thus critically impacted, resulting in enhanced inflammation and oxidative stress, which further drive AGE formation and impair tissue repair (Vlassara & Uribarri 2014). Elevated levels of AGEs promote a proinflammatory state by increasing the production of specific cytokines, such as TNF-α, IL-6, IL-1β, and PGE2, which alter oxygen diffusion by changing membrane structure and permeability (Sczepanik et al. 2020). AGEs can also interact with Toll-like receptors (TLRs). Increased expression of TLR2, TLR4, and TLR9 has been observed in gingival tissues of periodontitis patients with diabetes interacting with AGEs, leading to proinflammatory responses (Vlassara & Uribarri 2014). This is manifested in the amplified responses of monocytes, macrophages, neutrophils, endothelial cells, and chondrocytes within the context of inflammatory processes (Sorci et al. 2013), causing a dysregulation of both the innate and adaptive immune systems, including an increase in oxidative stress (Knight et al. 2016; Omori et al. 2008). Box 23.1.1 depicts the effects of AGEs on the production of reactive oxygen species (ROS) during oxidative stress, as well as on the cells and tissues of the periodontium.

Box 23.1.1 Effects of advanced glycation end products on components of the periodontium

Advanced glycation end products and reactive oxygen species

High levels of glucose found in all tissues of diabetic individuals lead to greater production of reactive oxygen species (ROS) generated by both enzymatic (NADPH pathway) and non-enzymatic pathways (polyol pathway) (Fakhruddin et al. 2017). ROS include free radicals, e.g. superoxide and hydroxyl radicals, and non-radical oxygen species, e.g. hydrogen peroxide, reactive lipids, and carbohydrates (Sonnenschein & Meyle 2015). AGE–RAGE (receptor for advanced glycation end product) interaction also elicits the generation of intracellular ROS, whereby evidence suggests that the overproduction of superoxide by the mitochondrial electron transport chain is the unifying underlying pathological condition causing diabetic complications (Brownlee 2003; Sonnenschein & Meyle 2015). ROS subsequently activate mitogen-activated protein kinase and nuclear factor kappa-B signaling, which leads to the production and release of multiple inflammatory factors (Genco & Borgnakke 2020), including intercellular adhesion molecule-1, plasminogen activator inhibitor-1, interleukin (IL)-1β, and monocyte chemoattractant protein-1 (Fukami et al. 2014). Furthermore, AGE-related intracellular glycation of the mitochondrial respiratory chain proteins produce more ROS, which promotes the further formation of AGEs. This causes oxidative stress to become self-supporting and AGEs, which are increased in periodontitis and diabetes, "feed" this process, called "metabolic memory" (Ceriello et al. 2009). ROS may induce cell apoptosis and damage to DNA and structural components of the cells and matrix of the periodontium (Patil et al. 2016). Furthermore, a decline in antioxidant capacity in patients with type 2 diabetes mellitus (DM) and chronic periodontitis may indirectly increase ROS levels and their impact (Genco & Borgnakke 2020).

Advanced glycation end products and inflammatory cells

RAGE-induced cellular signaling in inflammatory cells does not cause inflammation, but rather perpetuates inflammation by promoting phagocyte infiltration as well as causing the amplification of their inflammatory processes, with the consequential release of proinflammatory cytokines and chemokines into various tissues, including the periodontium (Sonnenschein & Meyle 2015). Periodontitis is associated with increased M1 macrophages that enhance inflammation and reduced M2 macrophages (anti-inflammatory) that stimulate repair and reduce inflammation (Zhuang et al. 2018). AGE–RAGE interaction on monocytes and macrophages generates a hyperinflammatory phenotype

of M1 macrophages (Bascones-Martínez et al. 2015; Vlassara & Uribarri 2014; Yan et al. 2010), whereby their activation causes the increased release of proinflammatory cytokines, such as IL-1β, tumor necrosis factor (TNF)-α, IL-6, prostaglandin E2 (PGE2), matrix metalloproteinases (MMPs), and adhesion molecules, as well as inducing a state of enhanced oxidant stress, causing an exacerbated inflammatory response. This causes increased connective tissue destruction of periodontal tissues, including alveolar bone (Gharat 2011; Katz et al. 2005; Yan et al. 2010). Regulatory T cells and M2 macrophages are reduced in diabetic tissues, and are responsible for the secretion of anti-inflammatory factors such as IL-4, IL-10, transforming growth factor-beta, and anti-inflammatory lipid-based mediators. The diminished production of these anti-inflammatory mediators can potentially contribute to greater periodontal inflammation in diabetics (Acharya et al. 2017; Van Dyke 2017).

in vivo diabetes and high levels of in vitro glucose stimulate a greater production of chemokines that induce the recruitment of polymorphonuclear neutrophils (PMNs) in response to a bacterial challenge (Manosudprasit et al. 2017). Other studies have described decreased chemotaxis and reduced phagocytosis of PMNs, including impaired intracellular killing and impaired adherence, thereby preventing the effective removal of bacteria in the periodontal tissues, thus increasing susceptibility to periodontitis (Lazenby & Crook 2010; Manouchehr-Pour et al. 1981; Nagpal et al. 2015). High glucose can elevate protein kinase C activity, leading to neutrophil priming (Karima et al. 2005). Increased PMN retention in periodontal tissues can thus lead to increased periodontal destruction due to continuous secretion of MMPs and an increase in the respiratory burst in PMNs, generating ROS (Preshaw et al. 2012; Taylor et al. 2013). Although PMNs from patients with DM may exhibit a hyper-responsive ROS release, their ability to phagocytose and kill bacteria is paradoxically often impaired (Shetty et al. 2008; Sima & Glogauer 2013). AGE-induced ROS production by PMNs has damaging effects on bone metabolism, leading to impaired bone repair and formation, and also decreases extracellular matrix production (Preshaw et al. 2012).

Dendritic cells modulate adaptive immune responses by activating lymphocytes. Diabetes could potentially affect periodontitis by modulating dendritic cells, causing the increased generation of Th1 or Th17 lymphocytes, as well as reducing the formation of regulatory T cells (Song et al. 2018). Enhanced Th1 or Th17 cytokine expression in diabetics can alter periodontal bone loss (Santos et al. 2010).

Advanced glycation end products and vascular endothelium

RAGE expression on periodontal vascular endothelium induces endothelial dysfunction, causing oxidative stress and vascular injury. Oxidative stress leads to reduced nitric oxide (NO) production and increased NO inactivation, resulting in reduced blood flow in the gingival tissues (Allen et al. 2011; Andersen et al. 2007; Sugiyama et al. 2012). Diabetic angiopathy also includes abnormal growth and impaired regeneration of vessels (Mealey 2006). In hyperglycemic individuals, RAGE-induced oxidation of circulating low-density lipoproteins (LDL) leads to increased oxidant stress within the vasculature, resulting in stimulation of smooth muscle cell proliferation and causing an increase in vessel wall thickness (Genco & Borgnakke 2020). Endothelial dysfunction also leads to the increased release of proinflammatory cytokines, such as IL-1β, TNF-α, and IL-6, as well as the increased expression of adhesion molecules for inflammatory macrophages and other inflammatory cells, causing a resultant increase in periodontal tissue destruction (Gharat 2011; Katz et al. 2005; Yan et al. 2010). AGE-modified collagen also accumulates in blood vessel walls, narrowing the lumen (Vlassara & Bucala 1996). Furthermore, circulating LDL becomes cross-linked to this AGE-modified collagen, causing degenerative vascular changes, including basement membrane (BM) thickening. BM proteins become glycosylated in a hyperglycemic environment, with thickening and changes in their physical properties, including disruption of the BM as well as the collagen fibers within the BM (Position Paper 2000). This interferes with delivery of nutrients and the migration of leucocytes to the periodontium, including impeding oxygen diffusion, antibodies, and elimination of metabolic waste. This leads to increased severity of PD and decreased wound healing (Listgarten et al. 1974; Position Paper 2000; Vlassara & Uribarri 2014).

Advanced glycation end products and collagen metabolism

AGEs cause altered collagen metabolism, which predisposes diabetic patients to periodontal disease (PD), entailing a large reduction in collagen synthesis and the increased degradation of newly synthesized collagen. Increased collagenase activity in type 1 diabetics has been suggested to be as a result of MMP-8 type collagenase secreted from PMNs and fibroblasts (Gharat 2011). Glycosylation of existing collagen comprising glucose-derived cross-links contributes to reduced collagen solubility and turnover rate in patients with diabetes, thereby contributing to delayed wound healing and remodeling of the wound site (Gharat 2011). Increases in levels of highly cross-linked collagen lead to thickening of blood vessel membranes, thereby having deleterious effects on the transport of molecules between the endothelial membrane and tissues. This also leads to increased production of vascular endothelial growth factor (VEGF), further exacerbating problems with both micro- and macrovascular structures (Sczepanik et al. 2020). The AGE-induced inflammatory state of periodontal ligament (PDL) fibroblasts includes secretion of high levels of TNF-α, IL-6, and IL-1β, activation of Toll-like receptors, apoptosis, expression of adhesion molecules, and nuclear factor-kappa B (Polak et al. 2020). Diabetes may also reduce the numbers of PDL fibroblasts and increase apoptosis of these cells (Liu et al. 2013). In gingival fibroblasts, AGEs have been shown to stimulate production of IL-6 and TNF-α by inducing nuclear factor-kappa B (Nonaka et al. 2018). The increased inflammation induces increased production and activation of MMPs and connective tissue destruction, as well as enhanced apoptosis of matrix-producing cells such as fibroblasts, which can then limit repair processes (Pacios et al. 2012). Delayed wound healing may also be attributed to an imbalance in the MMP/MMP-tissue inhibitor of the MMP system, as well as a decreased synthesis of both glycosaminoglycans and collagen (Silva et al. 2008; Willershausen-Zönnchen et al. 1991). The repair of soft tissues in diabetic periodontal tissues is also further limited by reduced anabolic activities linked to diminished growth factor expression (Graves et al. 2020; Pacios et al. 2012). A further hypothesis has been proposed whereby free fatty acid (FFA) interaction (which is due to a hyperlipidemia often associated with diabetes) with membrane-bound receptors and enzyme systems in monocyte cell membranes causes a dysregulation in function, thereby leading to an impaired amplification and transduction of wound healing signals (Iacopino 1995).

Advanced glycation end products and bone metabolism

Type 1 and type 2 DM has a significant impact on bone. Type 1 diabetic patients have been shown to have a 6–7-fold higher fracture risk, and type 2 diabetics a 1.5-fold higher fracture risk (Napoli et al. 2017). Glycation of bone collagen as well as AGE-induced reduction of osteoblastic differentiation and extracellular matrix (ECM) production affect bone turnover, leading to reduced bone formation and diminished mechanical properties of newly formed bone (McCarthy et al. 2001; Mealey 2006). This is attributed to AGE-induced reduction of differentiation of mesenchymal stem cells to osteoblasts as well as increased PDL cell apoptosis (Kanazawa & Sugimoto 2018; Li et al. 2014). Diabetes can enhance the intensity and duration of the inflammatory response in the gingiva and PDL with prolonged osteoclastogenesis (Liu et al. 2006).

The down-regulation of proliferation and differentiation of periodontal osteoblasts, including increased apoptosis, have been shown in animal studies (Andersen et al. 2007). Evidence showing a decrease in matrix-producing cells, including fibroblasts and osteoblasts, occurs due to an increased rate of apoptosis in a hyperglycemic state in response to *Porphyromonas gingivalis* infection (He et al. 2004; Liu et al. 2004; Sima & Glogauer 2013). Animal studies have shown that oral infection leads to nuclear factor kappa B activation in PDL cells, osteoblasts, and osteocytes, leading to increased receptor activator of nuclear factor kappa-B ligand (RANKL) expression, leading to periodontal bone loss. These studies indicate that the key cell types needed for bacteria-induced periodontitis are osteocytes, osteoblasts, and PDL fibroblasts, and suggest that inflammation per se does not induce periodontal bone loss without their involvement (Graves et al. 2020; Pacios et al. 2015).

In uncontrolled DM, an apparent imbalance between RANKL and osteoprotegerin (OPG), which includes the down-regulation of OPG, may be the cause for the inability of diabetic patients to rebuild alveolar bone during progressive PD (He et al. 2004; Sima & Glogauer 2013). RANKL is expressed and secreted as a membrane-bound or soluble ligand, by osteoblasts, fibroblasts, and activated T and B cells (Nagasawa et al. 2007). The binding of RANKL on osteoclastic precursor cells triggers their fusion and differentiation into mature osteoclasts. RANKL can be blocked by its soluble decoy receptor, OPG, thereby preventing osteoclastic bone resorption (Sonnenschein & Meyle 2015). The release of proinflammatory cytokines, such as IL-1, IL-6, and PGE2, by infiltrating inflammatory leukocytes and macrophages causes the up-regulation of RANKL and the down-regulation of OPG expression by osteoblasts, PDL fibroblasts, and gingival fibroblasts (Sonnenschein & Meyle 2015). The uncoupling of bone resorption and bone formation, whereby less reparative bone formation occurs after an episode of resorption, can thus result in net bone loss (Liu et al. 2004). Therefore, the reduced synthesis of glycosaminoglycans and collagen, together with the impairment of macrophage wound healing signaling, as well as the failure of bone formation, can contribute to fewer and shorter periods of quiescence between bursts of progression of disease, resulting in more attachment loss over time (Cullinan & Seymour 2013; Knight et al. 2016; Nagpal et al. 2015).

A self-feeding bi-directional system between periodontitis and diabetes is therefore established, whereby periodontal infection may induce a chronic state of IR, contributing to the cycle of hyperglycemia, non-enzymatic irreversible glycation, and AGE-protein binding and accumulation, thus amplifying the mechanism of diabetic connective tissue degradation, destruction, and proliferation (Li et al. 2000). The end result of this bi-directional association is therefore more severe PD, together with an increased difficulty in the control of blood glucose levels (Grossi & Genco 1998).

Association between periodontitis and obesity

Meta-analysis studies show a statistically significant association between obesity and PD (Andersen et al. 2007; Suvan et al. 2011) (see Figure 23.1.2). These studies have indicated a 50–80% likelihood of periodontitis occurring in obese patients compared to non-obese individuals (Chaffee & Weston 2010; Suvan et al. 2011). Obese patients have been shown to have a 35% increased risk of developing PD when compared to normal-weight patients, this including a higher risk in females compared to males (Gaio et al. 2016; Nascimento et al. 2015). Obese individuals are 2–3 times more likely to suffer from PD independently of traditional risk factors such as age, sex, and cigarette smoking (Suvan et al. 2018). The prevalence of PD is 76% higher among obese individuals aged 18–34 years than in normal-weight individuals (Al-Zahrani et al. 2003).

Adipose tissue is a complex organ affecting whole-body physiology. Adipose tissue dysfunction, rather than the amount of fat mass, has been suggested to be a key factor in the patho-physiology of obesity-related health risk (Albandar et al. 2018). Adipose tissue is a source of bioactive molecules, namely adipokines, e.g. visfatin, leptin, resistin, and adiponectin. Besides insulin sensitivity and energy expenditure, adipokines also regulate inflammatory and wound healing processes. Adiponectin possesses anti-inflammatory characteristics, whereas visfatin, leptin, and resistin exert proinflammatory effects. Obesity causes an increase in the production of proinflammatory adipokines and a decrease in the synthesis of anti-inflammatory adipokines, resulting in a systemic imbalance, and therefore a low-grade inflammatory state (Jepsen et al. 2020).

Limited evidence indicates that the association between periodontitis and obesity is causal in nature, and that this causal relationship is bi-directional (Jepsen et al. 2020) (see Box 23.1.2).

Association between periodontitis, diabetes, and dyslipidemia

The effects of hyperglycemia on PD may be confounded by co-morbidities such as obesity in patients with metabolic syndrome (Andersen et al. Kocher et al. 2018). In addition to obesity and diabetes, dyslipidemia is a clinical condition also associated with PD. It is suggested that dyslipidemia may exist as a link between obesity and periodontitis (Cury et al. 2017; Zuza et al. 2016). Dyslipidemia is characterized by increased serum levels of low-density lipoproteins (LDLs), triglycerides (TRGs), and free fatty acids (FFAs) (Iacopino & Cutler 2000). Hyperlipidemia is furthermore a common risk factor for both diabetes and PD, thereby suggesting a bi-directional

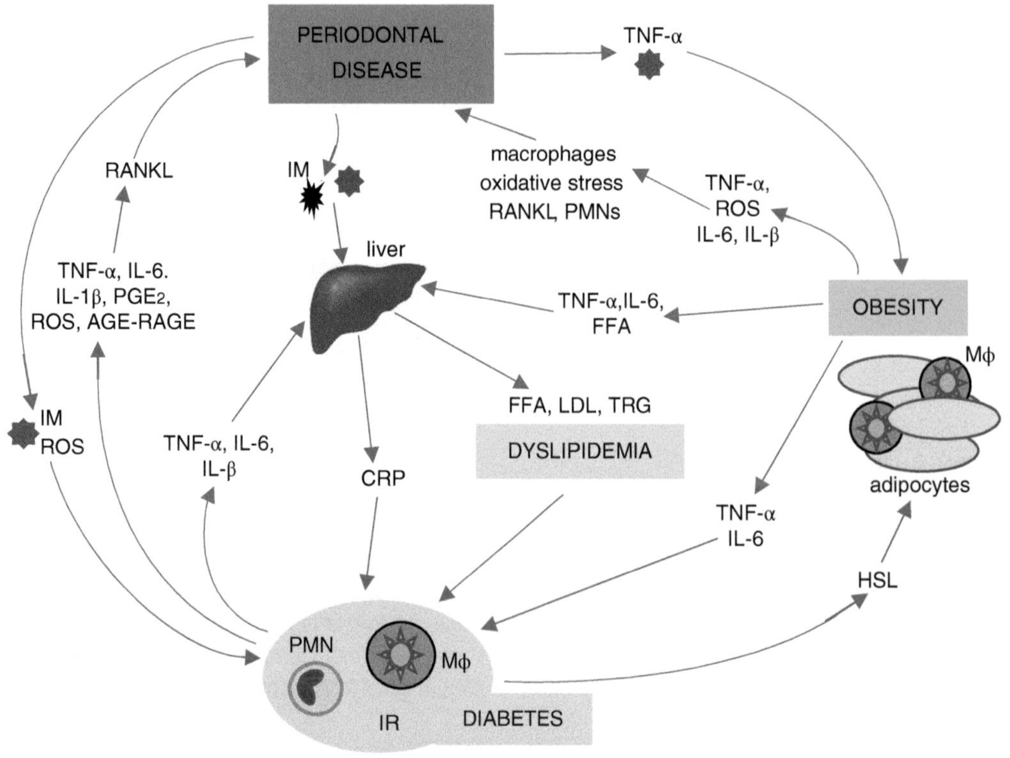

Figure 23.1.2 Association between periodontal disease, diabetes, and dyslipidemia. Bacteremia ✳, lipopolysaccharides ✺ (LPS), as well as serum proinflammatory mediators (IM) associated with periodontal disease (PD) lead to increased hepatic production of free fatty acids (FFA), low-density lipoproteins (LDL), triglycerides (TRG), and/or decreased hepatic TRG clearance (dyslipidemia), as well as hepatic C-reactive protein (CRP), leading to insulin resistance (IR). IM (interleukin [IL]-1β, tumor necrosis factor [TNF]-α) cause IR. Increased dyslipidemia, together with PD-induced serum levels of IL-1β and TNF-α, contribute to IR. Following LPS stimulation of inflammatory phenotype macrophages (Mφ), both Mφ and polymorphonuclear neutrophils (PMN) in diabetic patients that are exposed to a dyslipidemia cause the secretion of elevated levels of IL-1β, IL-6, TNF-α, and prostaglandin E2 (PGE2), and together with AGE–RAGE (advanced glycation end product–receptor for advanced glycation end product) interactions cause increased expression of RANKL (receptor activator of nuclear factor kappa-B ligand), thereby collectively influencing the progression of PD. IL-1β, IL-6, and TNF-α secreted from Mφ also exert effects on lipid metabolism, causing elevated levels of FFA, LDL, and TRG. IR activates hormone-sensitive lipase (HSL), causing the release of stored FFA from adipose cells to reach the liver, leading to further dyslipidemia. PD up-regulates circulating TNF-α, which stimulates Mφ and adipocytes in obese patients to secrete TNF-α and IL-6, thereby increasing IR. Circulating TNF-α from PD also stimulates lipolysis in adipocytes to release FFA, leading to IR. In obese patients, adipocytes and Mφ in adipose tissue secrete TNF-α and IL-6, IL-1 and reactive oxygen species (ROS), leading to the up-regulation of RANKL, fibroblasts to secrete matrix-degrading enzymes, and recruitment of PMNs, thereby exacerbating the progression of pre-existing PD. TNF-α and IL-6 secreted from obese patients also induce hepatic CRP secretion, leading to IR. Courtesy of Dr. Steph Smith.

relationship between hyperlipidemia and diabetes, and between hyperlipidemia and PD (Zhou et al. 2015) (see Figure 23.1.2).

Bi-directional relationship between diabetes and hyperlipidemia

In chronic PD, the associated bacteremia and/or lipopolysaccharide (LPS) endotoxemia, as well as increased serum proinflammatory cytokines, are considered to be insulin antagonists (Iacopino & Cutler 2000). Chronic periodontal infection thus causes cells to become resistant to the action of insulin, thereby inducing IR, resulting in hyperglycemia. Hyperglycemia leads to an increase in insulin production by the pancreas to stimulate glucose uptake by cells, thereby leading to hyperinsulinemia (Iacopino & Cutler 2000; Negrato et al. 2013). Hyperinsulinemia causes abnormalities in lipid metabolism, resulting in hyperlipidemia (Genco & Borgnakke 2020; Moritz & Mealey 2006). Products of chronic PD, including LPS, may also cause inhibition of the hepatic enzyme, lipoprotein lipase, leading to increased hepatic production of FFAs, LDLs, TRGs, and/or decreased hepatic TRG clearance (Feingold et al. 1992; Gylling et al. 2010). Increased serum levels of FFAs, LDLs, and TRGs, as well as PD-induced serum levels of IL-1β and TNF-α, therefore contribute to IR by inhibiting insulin signaling, and may also cause the destruction of pancreatic β-cells, thereby increasing the risk of diabetes (Brownlee 2003; Zhou et al. 2015). In

Box 23.1.2   Bi-directional relationship between periodontitis and obesity

Effects of obesity on the periodontium

Adiponectin is mainly produced by adipocytes. Adiponectin binds to its receptors in gingival fibroblasts and periodontal ligament (PDL) cells. It stimulates fatty acid oxidation, insulin sensitivity, and glucose uptake, causes inhibition of hepatic gluconeogenesis, and exerts anti-inflammatory effects. Adiponectin has been shown to counteract the stimulatory effects of *Porphyromonas gingivalis* on inflammatory cytokine secretion by gingival tissues (Deschner et al. 2014).

Visfatin is predominantly produced by macrophages and adipocytes in adipose tissues. Visfatin induces the production of proinflammatory cytokines and proteases, and also acts as a chemotactic factor. Visfatin has been shown to induce an up-regulation of genes for matrix metalloproteinase (MMP-1) and monocyte chemoattractant protein in PDL cells, and thereby also regulates the migration and infiltration of monocytes, memory T cells, and natural killer cells. It has thus been speculated that visfatin enhances periodontal inflammation, thereby increasing the risk for periodontal disease (PD) or compromised periodontal healing in obese individuals (Deschner et al. 2014).

Leptin is mainly produced by adipose tissue and has been shown to up-regulate the expression of *Prevotella intermedia* lipopolysaccharides (LPS)-induced tumor necrosis factor (TNF)-α production in human macrophages and in PDL cells.

Resistin is mainly secreted by monocytes and macrophages in adipose tissue. It induces the synthesis of proinflammatory cytokines and chemokines, and is linked to insulin resistance (IR) and type 2 diabetes (Deschner et al. 2014).

Obese subjects have a 35% increased chance of developing periodontitis and chronic oxidative stress might be the common link between both conditions (Sczepanik et al. 2020). Obesity is considered to be a modifying factor for periodontal disease through the promotion of a more proinflammatory state, which may increase the susceptibility of obese subjects to pathogenic bacteria and favour a shift toward the progression of periodontitis (Sczepanik et al. 2020).

In obesity, there is an increase in free fatty acids that bind to Toll-like receptors (TLRs), namely TLR2, of immunoinflammatory cells in the periodontium, and chronic exposure of these receptors promotes tolerance. As a consequence of the free fatty acid–induced receptor tolerance, there will be no appropriate response of the immunoinflammatory cells to microbial attack, which then facilitates periodontal destruction (Amar & Leeman 2013). Obesity may thus abate the innate immune response in the periodontium via attenuation of macrophage infiltration

and activation, as well as impairing the systemic immune response, thereby increasing susceptibility to bacterial and viral infections (Dahiya et al. 2012; Huang et al. 2016). Macrophages can show decreased phagocytic function and impaired antigen presentation (Thomas & Apovian 2017). Lymphocyte function and natural killer T-cell activity may also be impaired (Dahiya et al. 2012).

Proinflammatory mediators, such TNF-α, interleukin (IL)-1, IL-6, leptin, and resistin, are elevated in obesity and can inhibit the insulin receptor, which is required for the uptake of glucose from the blood into the cells, causing increased blood glucose levels, leading to hyperglycemia (Fan et al. 2007). Hyperglycemia leads to a hyperinflammatory state, thereby the priming of periodontal tissues, causing an exaggerated response to microbial colonization, and thus finally leading to PD destruction (Sczepanik et al. 2020).

Adipose tissue also secretes plasminogen activator inhibitor (PAI)-1, which initiates agglutination of blood, decreasing blood flow in the periodontium of obese patients, thereby promoting the development of PD (Green & Beck 2017).

Obesity causes the overproduction of reactive oxygen species (ROS) and, together with a reduction of antioxidant capacity, increased levels of circulating ROS may induce gingival oxidative stress and potentiate the onset and/or progression of obesity-induced gingival inflammation, as well as the progression of PD (Green & Beck 2017; Sczepanik et al. 2020; Suvan et al. 2018).

Adipose tissue dysfunction has been associated with an increased number of M1 macrophages, B cells, regulatory B cells, Th1 cells, Th17 cells, polymorphonuclear neutrophils (PMNs), and mast cells (Kanneganti & Dixit 2012). These cells secrete proinflammatory cytokines and chemokines, which can recirculate between adipose tissue, liver, spleen, and blood, thereby contributing to chronic systemic inflammation and insulin resistance (Fan et al. 2007; Thomas & Apovian 2017). The resultant systemic increased inflammatory response, together with an alteration of the oral microbiome, may predispose obese individuals to increased PD (Suvan et al. 2018).

Effects of periodontitis on the expression of adipokines

Gingival fibroblasts have been shown to constitutively express visfatin. This spontaneous expression can be enhanced by *P. gingivalis* and *Fusobacterium nucleatum*, by means of the nuclear factor kappa B and mitogen-activated protein kinase pathways (Damanaki et al. 2014). IL-1β, which is enhanced in PD, also increases the synthesis of visfatin in gingival fibroblasts. Therefore, the local visfatin production in the periodontally diseased gingiva may contribute to enhanced plasma levels of visfatin. *F. nucleatum* and *P. gingivalis* have also been shown to increase the constitutive expression of visfatin in PDL cells (Nogueira et al. 2014). *P. gingivalis* and *Treponema denticola* have also been shown to decrease the constitutive expression of leptin and adiponectin by PDL cells (Deschner et al. 2014).

The local production of visfatin by PDL cells and gingival fibroblasts may therefore represent a pathological mechanism whereby periodontal infections may impact systemic diseases, such as diabetes

mellitus and cardiovascular diseases (Deschner et al. 2014).

Periodontitis-associated low-grade systemic inflammation can inhibit the insulin receptor and its downstream signaling, thereby promoting IR. Consequently, the body tries to compensate for the increased IR by increasing insulin secretion, leading to hyperinsulinemia. Since insulin is an anabolic hormone, which promotes glucose uptake and fat storage, it has been proposed that hyperinsulinemia promotes obesity (Blasco-Baque et al. 2017; Erion & Corkey 2017).

addition, FFAs also inhibit insulin-mediated glucose uptake in muscle cells, leading to hyperglycemia (Penumarthy et al. 2013). In diabetic patients, macrophages of the inflammatory phenotype, which are exposed to FFAs, LDLs, and TRGs following LPS stimulation from *P. gingivalis*, express a suppression in growth factor production, as well as an increased production of proinflammatory cytokines TNF-α, IL-6, and IL-1β, leading to more severe PD. These cytokines also exert effects on lipid metabolism, causing elevated levels of FFA, LDL, and TRG, either by increasing hepatic TRG production and/or decreasing TRG clearance (Gylling et al. 2010; Pizzo et al. 2010).

PMNs exposed to TRGs secrete more IL-1β and also exhibit reduced chemotactic and phagocytic properties (Cury et al. 2017; Iacopino 1995). This imbalance between growth factor production and increased production of proinflammatory cytokines may lead to inability to repair, and increased tissue breakdown in periodontal tissues (Gharat 2011). Furthermore, in diabetic patients, IR affects adipose tissue cells by activating an enzyme, hormone-sensitive lipase (HSL), resulting in the release of stored FFA. This leads to increased amounts of FFAs being delivered from adipose tissue to the liver, giving rise to the hepatic overproduction of LDL and TRG (Pan et al. 1997). A bi-directional relationship between diabetes and hyperlipidemia thus exists, whereby high levels of lipids and/or proinflammatory cytokines contribute to IR by inhibiting insulin signaling or causing the destruction of pancreatic β-cells, leading to hyperglycemia, thereby increasing the risk of diabetes (Zhou et al. 2015). Conversely, IR predisposes a patient to hyperlipidemia (Snipelisky & Ziajka 2012).

Bi-directional relationship between periodontal disease and hyperlipidemia

A bi-directional association exists between PD and dyslipidemia, whereby overweight and obesity may be risk factors for PD (Keller et al. 2015; Zhou et al. 2015). In obesity, the increased concentration of proinflammatory cytokines in adipose tissue, namely IL-1β and others, leads to the recruitment and differentiation of monocytes into M1-type inflammatory macrophages (Donath et al. 2011). M1-type macrophages produce and release additional proinflammatory mediators, such as TNF-α and IL-6 (Pischon et al. 2007; Suresh & Mahendra 2014). TNF-α and IL-6 cause the

up-regulation of RANKL expression, leading to increased osteoclast formation (Wu et al. 2015). TNF-α stimulates fibroblasts to secrete matrix-degrading enzymes. TNF-α also increases the host response to periodontal pathogens by recruitment of PMNs. These effects of TNF-α and IL-6 may then exacerbate the progression of pre-existing PD (Wu et al. 2015). Exacerbated periodontal inflammation further up-regulates circulating TNF-α and, in addition to LPS, stimulates adipose tissue-related monocytes/macrophages and adipocytes to secrete TNF-α and IL-6, thereby increasing IR (Genco et al. 2005; Nishimura et al. 2003). LPS from Gram-negative bacteria harbored in periodontal tissues also triggers the secretion of TNF-α and IL-6 by adipose tissues (Khan et al. 2021; Nishimura et al. 2003). In obese patients, the elevated production of TNF-α and IL-6 increases IR. TNF-α can induce IR at the receptor level by preventing autophosphorylation of the insulin receptor, thereby reducing glucose uptake and use (Nagpal et al. 2015). The increased production of TNF-α, IL-6, and ROS from adipocytes, as well as inflamed periodontal tissues, also stimulates greater hepatic CRP production, which may also increase IR (Chapple et al. 2013; Festa et al. 2000; Thomas & Apovian 2017). Circulating TNF-α from PD also stimulates lipolysis in adipocytes to release FFA, thereby also leading to IR (Feingold et al. 1992). LPS functions in promoting hepatic dyslipidemia and decreases insulin sensitivity, leading to increased obesity and diabetes risk (Feingold et al. 1992; Khan et al. 2021; Nishimura et al. 2003). The release of stored FFA from adipocytes causes decreased cellular glucose uptake, synthesis of glycogen, and glycolysis, and by raising hepatic glucose production all contribute to hyperglycemia and a dysglycemic state (Gylling et al. 2010; Snipelisky & Ziajka 2012). In diabetic patients, elevated levels of IL-1β, IL-6, TNF-α, and PGE2, secreted from PMNs and hyperinflammatory macrophages, together with AGE–RAGE interactions in periodontal tissues, cause increased expression of RANKL, thereby influencing the progression of PD (Deshpande et al. 2010).

General systemic and oral complications associated with diabetes

Complications of DM include acute and chronic complications such as dehydration, poor wound healing, stroke, myocardial infarction, kidney disease, neuropathy, limb ischemia, neurocognitive decline, retinopathy, hyperosmolar coma, and serious foot infections. In the USA, diabetic retinopathy and diabetic kidney disease are reported to be the leading cause of new cases of blindness and kidney failure, respectively (Genco et al. 2020). Delayed wound healing, especially in uncontrolled diabetic patients, is ascribed to hypoxia, dysfunction in fibroblasts and epidermal cells, impaired angiogenesis and neovascularization, high levels of metalloproteases, damage from ROS and AGEs, neuropathy, and multiple levels of decreased host IR (Genco & Borgnakke 2020).

Oral manifestations of diabetes impacting quality of life are probably due to dry mouth, which in turn causes problems with speech, mastication, swallowing, and removable dentures, periodontitis and peri-implantitis, potentially caries, and eventually tooth loss. Medications that patients use for their diabetes can potentially also cause dry mouth. Moreover, candidiasis, fissured tongue, and other oral mucosal lesions are more prevalent in diabetes/hyperglycemia. Hyposalivation, burning mouth, and taste alterations can occur due to diabetic neuropathy (Genco & Borgnakke 2020).

Principles of dental management of periodontal patients with diabetes

Reduction in glycated hemoglobin is an established outcome measure of diabetes treatment and is related to reduction in hyperglycemia, as well as reduction in the numbers of risk of diabetes-associated complications, including retinopathy, kidney disease, and death. Long-term successful periodontal and implant therapy requires proactive coordination of care with the patient's physician so as to ensure proper glycemic control. Special attention should be given to treatment planning and management, especially post treatment. Meta-analysis studies have indicated that effective non-surgical periodontal treatment in people with DM results in a statistically significant reduction in glycated hemoglobin levels within a period of three months. These studies furthermore do not show any significant additional impact of adjunctive antibiotic use on glycemic control. Regular assessment for PD should be done, which includes strict preventive measures for PD.

Patients with PD should receive definitive treatment, including the reduction of periodontal pockets, as well as establishing glycemic control and control of other complications, this being managed in coordination with the patient's physician. Infection

and inflammation associated with PD significantly contribute to the inflammatory burden and negatively impact the efficiency of pharmacological control of type 2 DM, and reduction of this inflammation by rigorous periodontal treatment has been shown to result in better glycemic control. The cumulative impact of continuous and strict periodontal follow-up and maintenance at 2-month intervals following active treatment has been shown to result in an even greater reduction in glycated hemoglobin levels at the end of a 12-month period (Genco et al. 2020). Studies have shown that for each reduction of 1% in glycated hemoglobin levels, there is an associated 25% reduction in risk for certain complications of diabetes, including death, nephropathy, and retinopathy (Genco et al. 2020). The modification of common risk factors, such as smoking and obesity, as well as complete periodontal therapy and regular periodontal maintenance, is imperative for a lifetime of good oral as well as general health (Genco & Borgnakke 2020).

Future considerations

Animal model studies have been very useful for testing a variety of possible biological hypotheses regarding the association between diabetes and PD. These studies have confirmed findings from human studies, and have increased knowledge of the alterations taking place in the diabetic periodontium (Zhou et al. 2015). However, undisputed evidence is still needed to identify the mechanisms involved in these alterations, so as to clarify the impact of PD on the glycemic control of diabetes (Blasco-Baque et al. 2017; Genco & Borgnakke 2020). This includes the risks involved in the development of other diabetic complications (Gharat 2011). Large, randomized, controlled, clinical intervention trials are therefore needed to extend this base of evidence, as well as to establish the potential for management of PD and glycemic control and related complications (Genco et al. 2020; Sanz et al. 2018; Thomas & Apovian 2017). These trials may then establish action protocols that include the multidisciplinary treatment of diabetic patients with PD (Bascones-Martínez et al. 2015).

Obesity and PD are both independently associated with other factors, such as smoking, diet, and insulin sensitivity. Further studies are needed to ascertain the interaction of these factors with the association between obesity and PD (Suvan et al. 2011).

REFERENCES

Acharya AB, Thakur S, Muddapur MV, Kulkarni RD. Cytokine ratios in chronic periodontitis and type 2 diabetes mellitus. *Diabetes Metab Syndr.* 2017; 11(4):277–278.

ADA. Diagnosis and classification of diabetes mellitus. *Diabetes Care* 2010: 33 (Suppl 1):S62–S69.

Ajita M, Karan P, Vivek G, S MA, Anuj M. Periodontal disease and type 1 diabetes mellitus: associations with glycemic

control and complications: an Indian perspective. *Diabetes Metab Syndr.* 2013; 7:61–63.

Al-Zahrani MS, Bissada NF, Borawskit EA. Obesity and periodontal disease in young, middle aged and older adults. *J Periodontol.* 2003; 74:610–615.

Albandar JM, Susin C, Hughes FJ. Manifestations of systemic diseases and conditions that affect the periodontal attachment apparatus: case definitions and diagnostic considerations. *J Clin Periodontol.* 2018; 45(Suppl 20):S171–S189.

Allen EM, Matthews JB, O'Halloran DJ, Griffiths HR, Chapple IL. Oxidative and inflammatory status in Type 2 diabetes patients with periodontitis. *J Clin Periodontol.* 2011; 38:894–901.

Amar S, Leeman S. Periodontal innate immune mechanisms relevant to obesity. *Mol Oral Microbiol.* 2013; 28:331–341.

Andersen CCP, Flyvbjerg A, Buschard K, Holmstrup P. Relationship between periodontitis and diabetes: lessons from rodent studies. *J Periodontol.* 2007; 78:1264–1275.

Andriankaja OM, Galicia J, Dong G et al. Gene expression dynamics during diabetic periodontitis. *J Dent Res.* 2012; 91(12):1160–1165.

Bascones-Martínez A, Muñoz-Corcuera M, Bascones-Ilundain J. Diabetes and periodontitis: a bidirectional relationship. *Medicina Clínica.* 2015; 145(1):31–35.

Biadgo B, Abebe M. Type 2 diabetes mellitus and its association with the risk of pancreatic carcinogenesis: a review. *Korean J Gastroenterol.* 2016; 67(4):168–177.

Blasco-Baque V, Garidou L, Pomié C et al. Periodontitis induced by *Porphyromonas gingivalis* drives periodontal microbiota dysbiosis and insulin resistance via an impaired adaptive immune response. *Gut.* 2017; 66:872–885.

Boldison J, Wong FS. Immune and pancreatic beta cell interactions in type 1 diabetes. *Trends Endocrinol Metab.* 2016; 27(12):856–867.

Borgnakke WS, Ylostalo PV, Taylor GW, Genco RJ. Effect of periodontal disease on diabetes: systematic review of epidemiologic observational evidence. *J Periodontol.* 2013; 84(4-s): S135–S152.

Brownlee M. A radical explanation for glucose-induced beta cell dysfunction. *J Clin Invest.* 2003; 112:1788–1790.

Ceriello A, Ihnat MA, Thorpe JE. Clinical review 2: the "metabolic memory": is more than just tight glucose control necessary to prevent diabetic complications? *J Clin Endocrinol Metab.* 2009; 94:410–415.

Chaffee BW, Weston SJ. Association between chronic periodontal disease and obesity: a systematic review and meta-analysis. *J Periodontol.* 2010; 81:1708–1724.

Chapple IL, Genco R, working group 2 of the joint EFPAAPw. Diabetes and periodontal diseases: consensus report of the Joint EFP/AAP Workshop on Periodontitis and Systemic Diseases. *J Periodontol.* 2013; 84(4 Suppl):S106–S112.

Cullinan MP, Seymour GI. Periodontal disease and systemic illness: will the evidence ever be enough? *Periodontol 2000.* 2013; 62:271–286.

Cury EZ, Santos VR, Maciel SD et al. Lipid parameters in obese and normal weight patients with or without chronic periodontitis. *Clin Oral Investig.* 2017; 22(1):161–167.

Dahiya P, Kamal R, Gupta R. Obesity, periodontal and general health: relationship and management. *Indian J Endocrinol Metab.* 2012; 16(1):88–93.

Damanaki A, Nokhbehsaim M, Eick S et al. Regulation of NAMPT in human gingival fibroblasts and biopsies. *Mediators Inflamm.* 2014; 2014:912821.

Demmer RT, Breskin A, Rosenbaum M et al. The subgingival microbiome, systemic inflammation and insulin resistance: the oral infections, glucose intolerance and insulin resistance study. *J Clin Periodontol.* 2017; 44(3):255–265.

Deschner J, Eick S, Damanaki A, Nokhbehsaim M. The role of adipokines in periodontal infection and healing. *Mol Oral Microbiol.* 2014; 29(6):258–269.

Deshpande K, Jain A, Sharma R et al. Diabetes and periodontitis. *J Indian Soc Periodontol.* 2010; 14:207–212.

Donath MY, Shoelson SE. Type 2 diabetes as an inflammatory disease. *Nat Rev Immunol.* 2011; 11:98–107.

Erion KA, Corkey BE. Hyperinsulinemia: a cause of obesity? *Curr Obes Rep.* 2017; 6:178–186.

Fakhruddin S, Alanazi W, Jackson KE. Diabetes-induced reactive oxygen species: mechanism of their generation and role in renal injury. *J Diabetes Res.* 2017; 2017:8379327.

Fan HQ, Gu N, Liu F et al. Prolonged exposure to resistin inhibits glucose uptake in rat skeletal muscles. *Acta Pharmacol Sin.* 2007; 28:410–416.

Feingold KR, Staprans I, Memon RA et al. Endotoxin rapidly induces changes in lipid metabolism that produce hypertriglyceridemia: low doses stimulate hepatic triglyceride production while high doses inhibit clearance. *J Lipid Res.* 1992; 33:1765–1776.

Festa A, D'Agostino R Jr, Howard G et al. Chronic subclinical inflammation as part of the insulin resistance syndrome: the Insulin Resistance Atherosclerosis Study (IRAS). *Circulation.* 2000; 102:42–47.

Fukami K, Yamagishi SI, Okuda S. Role of AGEs-RAGE system in cardiovascular disease. *Curr Pharm Des.* 2014; 20:2395–2402.

Gaio EJ, Haas AN, Rosing CK et al. Effect of obesity on periodontal attachment loss progression: a 5-year population-based prospective study. *J Clin Periodontol.* 2016; 43:557–565.

Genco RJ, Borgnakke WS. Diabetes as a potential risk for periodontitis: association studies. *Periodontol 2000.* 2020; 83:40–45.

Genco RJ, Graziani F, Hasturk H. Effects of periodontal disease on glycemic control, complications, and incidence of diabetes mellitus. *Periodontol 2000.* 2020; 83:59–65.

Genco RJ, Grossi SG, Ho A, Nishimura F, Murayama Y. A proposed model linking inflammation to obesity, diabetes and periodontal infections. *J Periodontol.* 2005; 76:2075–2084.

Gharat AR. Periodontitis and diabetes—a complex relationship. *Int J Diabetes Dev Ctries.* 2011; 31(3):128–132.

Graves DT, Ding Z, Yang Y. The impact of diabetes on periodontal diseases. *Periodontol 2000.* 2020; 82:214–224.

Green WD, Beck MA. Obesity altered T cell metabolism and the response to infection. *Curr Opin Immunol.* 2017; 46:1–7.

Grossi SG, Genco RJ. Periodontal disease and diabetes mellitus: a two-way relationship. *Ann Periodontol.* 1998; 3:51–61.

Guzman S, Karima M, Wang HY, Van Dyke TE. Association between interleukin-1 genotype and periodontal disease in a diabetic population. *J Periodontol.* 2003; 74:1183–1190.

Gylling H, Hallikainen M, Pihlajamäki J et al. Insulin sensitivity regulates cholesterol metabolism to a greater extent than obesity: lessons from the METSIM Study. *J Lipid Res,* 2010; 51:2422–2427.

He H, Liu R, Desta T et al. Diabetes causes decreased osteoclastogenesis, reduced bone formation, and enhanced apoptosis of osteoblastic cells in bacteria stimulated bone loss. *Endocrinology.* 2004; 145:447–452.

Huang X, Yu T, Ma C et al. Macrophages play a key role in the obesity-induced periodontal innate immune dysfunction via NLRP3 pathway. *J Periodontol.* 2016; 87:1195–1205.

Iacopino AM. Diabetic periodontitis: possible lipid-induced defect in tissue repair through alteration of macrophage phenotype and function. *Oral Dis.* 1995; 1:214–229.

Iacopino AM, Cutler WC. Pathophysiological relationships between periodontitis and systemic disease: recent concepts involving serum lipids. *J Periodontol.* 2000; 71:1375–1384.

Jepsen S, Caton JG, Albandar JM et al. Periodontal manifestations of systemic diseases and developmental and acquired conditions: consensus report of workgroup 3 of the 2017 World Workshop on the classification of periodontal and peri-implant diseases and conditions. *J Clin Periodontol.* 2018; 45(Suppl 20):S219–S229.

Jepsen S, Suvan J, Deschner J. The association of periodontal diseases with metabolic syndrome and obesity. *Periodontol 2000.* 2020; 83:125–153.

Kanazawa I, Sugimoto T. Diabetes mellitus-induced bone fragility. *Intern Med.* 2018; 57(19):2773–2785.

Kang J, de Brito BB, Pacios S et al. *Aggregatibacter actinomycetemcomitans* infection enhances apoptosis in vivo through a caspase-3-dependent mechanism in experimental periodontitis. *Infect Immun.* 2012; 80(6):2247–2256.

Kanneganti TD, Dixit VD. Immunological complications of obesity. *Nat Immunol.* 2012; 13:707–712.

Karima M, Kantarci A, Ohira T et al. Enhanced superoxide release and elevated protein kinase C activity in neutrophils from diabetic patients: association with periodontitis. *J Leukoc Biol.* 2005; 78(4):862–870.

Katz J, Bhattacharyya I, Farkhondeh-Kish F et al. Expression of the receptor of advanced glycation end products in gingival tissues of type 2 diabetes patients with chronic periodontal disease: a study utilizing immunohistochemistry and RT-PCR. *J Clin Periodontol.* 2005; 32:40–44.

Keller A, Rohde JF, Raymond K et al. Association between periodontal disease and overweight and obesity: a systematic review. *J Periodontol.* 2015; 86:766–776.

Khan S, Bettiol S, Kent K et al. Association between obesity and periodontitis in Australian adults: a single mediation analysis. *J Periodontol.* 2021; 92:514–523.

Knight ET, Liu J, Seymour GJ, Faggion CM Jr, Cullinan MP. Risk factors that may modify the innate and adaptive immune responses in periodontal diseases. *Periodontol 2000.* 2016; 71:22–51.

Kocher T, König J, Borgnakke WS, Pink C, Meisel P. Periodontal complications of hyperglycemia/diabetes mellitus: epidemiologic complexity and clinical challenge. *Periodontol 2000.* 2018; 78:59–97.

Kumar M, Mishra L, Mohanty R, Nayak R, Diabetes and gum disease: the diabolic duo. *Diabetes Metab Syndr.* 2014; 8(4):255–258.

Lazenby MG, Crook MA. The innate immune system and diabetes mellitus: the relevance of periodontitis? *A hypothesis. Clin Sci.* 2010; 119:423–429.

Li DX, Deng TZ, Lv J, Ke J. Advanced glycation end products (AGEs) and their receptor (RAGE) induce apoptosis of periodontal ligament fibroblasts. *Braz J Med Biol Res.* 2014; 47(12):1036–1043.

Li X, Kolltveit KM, Leif Tronstad L, Olsen I. Systemic diseases caused by oral infection. *Clin Microbiol Rev.* 2000; 13:547–555.

Listgarten M, Ricker F Jr, Laster L, Shapiro J, Cohen DW. Vascular basement lamina thickness in the normal and inflamed gingiva of diabetics and non-diabetics. *J Periodontol.* 1974; 45:676–684.

Liu J, Jiang Y, Mao J et al. High levels of glucose induces a dose-dependent apoptosis in human periodontal ligament fibroblasts by activating caspase-3 signaling pathway. *Appl Biochem Biotechnol.* 2013; 170(6):1458–1471.

Liu R, Bal H, Desta T et al. Diabetes enhances periodontal bone loss through enhanced resorption and diminished bone formation. *J Dent Res.* 2006; 85(6):510–514.

Liu R, Desta T, He H, Graves D. Diabetes alters the response to bacteria by enhancing fibroblast apoptosis. *Endocrinology.* 2004; 145:2997–3003.

Loe H. Periodontal disease. The sixth complication of diabetes mellitus. *Diabetes Care.* 1993; 16:329–334.

Madianos PN, Koromantzos PA. An update of the evidence on the potential impact of periodontal therapy on diabetes outcomes. *J Clin Periodontol.* 2018; 45(2):188–195.

Manosudprasit A, Kantarci A, Hasturk H, Stephens D, Van Dyke TE. Spontaneous PMN apoptosis in type 2 diabetes and the impact of periodontitis. *J Leukoc Biol.* 2017; 102(6):1431–1440.

Manouchehr-Pour M, Spagnuolo P, Rodman H, Bissada N. Impaired neutrophil chemotaxis in diabetic patients with severe periodontitis. *J Dent Res.* 1981; 60:729–730.

McCarthy AD, Etcheverry SB, Bruzzone L et al. Non-enzymatic glycosylation of a type I collagen matrix: effects on osteoblastic development and oxidative stress. *BMC Cell Biol.* 2001; 2:16–21.

Mealey BL. Periodontal disease and diabetes. A two-way street. *J Am Dent Ass.* 2006; 137(Suppl):26S–31S.

Meenawat A, Punn K, Srivastava V et al. Periodontal disease and type I diabetes mellitus: associations with glycemic control and complications. *J Indian Soc Periodontol.* 2013; 17(5):597–600.

Moller DE. Potential role of TNF-alpha in the pathogenesis of insulin resistance and type 2 diabetes. *Trends Endocrinol Metab.* 2000; 11:212–217.

Moritz A, Mealey B. Periodontal disease, insulin resistance, and diabetes mellitus: a review and clinical implications. *Grand Rounds Oral-Sys Med.* 2006; 2:13–20.

Nagasawa T, Kiji M, Yashiro R et al. Roles of receptor activator of nuclear factor-kappaB ligand (RANKL) and osteoprotegerin in periodontal health and disease. *Periodontol 2000.* 2007; 43:65–84.

Nagpal R, Yamashiro Y, Izumi Y. The two-way association of periodontal infection with systemic disorders: an overview. *Mediators Inflamm.* 2015; 2015:793898.

Naguib G, Al-Mashat H, Desta T, Graves D. Diabetes prolongs the inflammatory response to a bacterial stimulus through cytokine dysregulation. *J Invest Dermatol.* 2004; 123:87–92.

Napoli N, Chandran M, Pierroz DD et al. Mechanisms of diabetes mellitus-induced bone fragility. *Nat Rev Endocrinol.* 2017; 13(4):208–219.

Nascimento GG, Leite FR, Do LG et al. Is weight gain associated with the incidence of periodontitis? A systematic review and meta-analysis. *J Clin Periodontol.* 2015; 42:495–505.

Negrato CA, Tarzia O, Jovanovič L, Chinellato LEM. Periodontal disease and diabetes mellitus. *J Appl Oral Sci.* 2013; 21(1):1–12.

Nishimura F, Iwamoto Y, Mineshiba J et al. Periodontal disease and diabetes mellitus: the role of tumor necrosis factor-α in a two-way relationship. *J Periodontol.* 2003; 74:97–102.

Nogueira AV, Nokhbehsaim M, Eick S et al. Regulation of visfatin by microbial and biomechanical signals in PDL cells. *Clin Oral Investig.* 2014; 18:171–178.

Nonaka K, Kajiura Y, Bando M et al. Advanced glycation end-products increase IL-6 and transforming growth factor-1 expression via RAGE, MAPK and NF-kappaB pathways in human gingival fibroblasts. *J Periodontal Res.* 2018; 53(3):334–344.

Omori K, Ohira T, Uchida Y et al. Priming of neutrophil oxidative burst in diabetes requires preassembly of the NADPH oxidase. *J Leukoc Biol.* 2008; 84:292–301.

Pacios S, Kang J, Galicia J et al. Diabetes aggravates periodontitis by limiting repair through enhanced inflammation. *FASEB J.* 2012; 26(4):1423–1430.

Pacios S, Xiao W, Mattos M et al. Osteoblast lineage cells play an essential role in periodontal bone loss through activation of nuclear factor-kappa B. *Sci Rep.* 2015; 5:16694.

Pan DA, Lillioja S, Kriketos AD et al. Skeletal muscle triglyceride levels are inversely related to insulin action. *Diabetes.* 1997; 46:983–988.

Papapanou PN, Sanz M, Buduneli N et al. Periodontitis: consensus report of workgroup 2 of the 2017 World Workshop on the classification of periodontal and peri-implant diseases and conditions. *J Clin Periodontol.* 2018; 45(Suppl 20):S162–S170.

Patil VS, Patil VP, Gokhale N, Acharya A, Kangokar P. Chronic periodontitis in type 2 diabetes mellitus: oxidative stress as a common factor in periodontal tissue injury. *J Clin Diagn Res.* 2016; 10(4):BC12–BC16.

Penumarthy S, Penmetsa GS, Mannem S. Assessment of serum levels of triglycerides, total cholesterol, high-density lipoprotein cholesterol, and low-density lipoprotein cholesterol in periodontitis patients. *J Indian Soc Periodontol.* 2013; 17:30–35.

Pischon N, Heng N, Bernimoulin JP et al. Obesity, inflammation, and periodontal disease. *J Dent Res.* 2007; 86:400–409.

Pizzo G, Guiglia R, Russo II, Campisi G. Dentistry and internal medicine: from the focal infection theory to the periodontal medicine concept. *Eur J Intern Med.* 2010; 21:496–502.

Polak D, Sanui T, Nishimura F, Shapira L. Diabetes as a risk factor for periodontal disease—plausible mechanisms. *Periodontol 2000.* 2020; 83:46–58.

Popławska-Kita A, Siewko K, Szpak P et al. Association between type 1 diabetes and periodontal health. *Adv Med Sci.* 2014; 59(1):126–131.

Position Paper. Diabetes and Periodontal Diseases. *J Periodontol.* 2000; 71:664-678.

Preshaw PM, Alba AL, Herrera D et al. Periodontitis and diabetes: a two-way relationship. *Diabetologia.* 2012; 55:21–31.

Salvi GE, Collins JG, Yalda B et al. Monocytic TNF-a secretion patterns in IDDM patients with periodontal diseases. *J Clin Periodontol.* 2005; 24:8–16.

Santos VR, Ribeiro FV, Lima JA et al. Cytokine levels in sites of chronic periodontitis of poorly controlled and well-controlled type 2 diabetic subjects. *J Clin Periodontol.* 2010; 37(12):1049–1058.

Sanz M, Ceriello A, Buysschaert M et al. Scientific evidence on the links between periodontal diseases and diabetes: consensus report and guidelines of the joint workshop on periodontal diseases and diabetes by the International Diabetes Federation and the European Federation of Periodontology. *J Clin Periodontol.* 2018; 45:138–149.

Sczepanik FSC, Grossi ML, Casati M et al. Periodontitis is an inflammatory disease of oxidative stress: we should treat it that way. *Periodontol 2000.* 2020; 84:45–68.

Shetty N, Thomas B, Ramesh A. Comparison of neutrophil functions in diabetic and healthy subjects with chronic generalized periodontitis. *J Indian Soc Periodontol.* 2008; 12(2):41–44.

Silva JAF, Lorencini M, Peroni LA et al. The influence of type I diabetes mellitus on the expression and activity of gelatinases (matrix metalloproteinases-2 and-9) in induced periodontal disease. *J Periodontal Res.* 2008; 43:48–54.

Sima C, Glogauer M. Diabetes mellitus and periodontal diseases. *Curr Diab Rep.* 2013; 13:445–452.

Sjoholm A. Aspects of the involvement of interleukin-1 and nitric oxide in the pathogenesis of insulin-dependent diabetes mellitus. *Cell Death Diff.* 1998; 5:461–468.

Snipelisky D, Zlajka P. Diabetes and hyperlipidemia: a direct quantitative analysis. *World J Cardiovasc Dis.* 2012; 2:20–25.

Song L, Dong G, Guo L, Graves DT. The function of dendritic cells in modulating the host response. *Mol Oral Microbiol.* 2018; 33(1):13–21.

Sonnenschein SK, Meyle J. Local inflammatory reactions in patients with diabetes and periodontitis. *Periodontol 2000.* 2015; 69:221–254.

Sorci G, Riuzzi F, Giambanco I, Donato R. RAGE in tissue homeostasis, repair and regeneration. *Biochim Biophys Acta.* 2013; 1833:101–109.

Sugiyama S, Takahashi S-S, Tokutomi F-A et al. Gingival vascular functions are altered in type 2 diabetes mellitus model and/or periodontitis model. *J Clin Biochem Nutr.* 2012; 51:108–113.

Sun W-L, Chen L-L, Zhang S-Z et al. Inflammatory cytokines, adiponectin, insulin resistance and metabolic control after periodontal intervention in patients with type 2 diabetes and chronic periodontitis. *Internal Med.* 2011; 50:1569–1574.

Suresh S, Mahendra J. Multifactorial relationship of obesity and periodontal disease. *J Clin Diagn Res.* 2014; 8: ZE01–ZE03.

Suvan J, D'Aiuto F, Moles DR, Petrie A, Donos N. Association between overweight/obesity and periodontitis in adults. *A systematic review. Obes Rev.* 2011; 12: e381–e404

Suvan JE, Finer N, D'Aiuto F. Periodontal complications with obesity. *Periodontol 2000.* 2018; 78:98–128.

Taylor JJ, Preshaw PM, Lalla E. A review of the evidence for pathogenic mechanisms that may link periodontitis and diabetes. *J Periodontol.* 2013; 84(4 Suppl):S113-S134.

Thomas D, Apovian C. Macrophage functions in lean and obese adipose tissue. *Metabolism.* 2017; 72:120–143.

Tonetti MS, Greenwell H, Kornman KS. Staging and grading of periodontitis: framework and proposal of a new classification and case definition. *J Clin Periodontol.* 2018; 45(Suppl 20):S149–S161.

Van Dyke TE. Pro-resolving mediators in the regulation of periodontal disease. *Mol Aspects Med.* 2017; 58:21–36.

Vlassara H, Bucala R. Recent progress in advanced glycation and diabetic vascular disease: role of advanced glycation end product receptors. *Diabetes.* 1996; 45:(Supp 3):S65–S66.

Vlassara H, Uribarri J. Advanced glycation end products (AGE) and diabetes: cause, effect, or both? *Curr Diab Rep.* 2014; 14(1):453.

Watanabe K, Petro BJ, Shlimon AE, Unterman TG. Effect of periodontitis on insulin resistance and the onset of type 2 diabetes mellitus in zucker diabetic fatty rats. *J Periodontol.* 2008; 79(7):1208–1216.

Willershausen-Zönnchen B, Lemmen C, Hamn G. Influence of high glucose concentrations on glycosaminoglycan and collagen synthesis in cultured human gingival fibroblasts. *J Clin Periodontol.* 1991; 18:190–195.

Wu YY, Xiao E, Graves DT. Diabetes mellitus related bone metabolism and periodontal disease. *Int J Oral Sci.* 2015; 7:63–72.

Xiao E, Mattos M, Vieira GHA et al. Diabetes enhances IL-17 expression and alters the oral microbiome to increase its pathogenicity. *Cell Host Microbe.* 2017; 22(1):120–128.e124.

Yan SF, Ramasamy R, Schmidt AM. The RAGE axis: a fundamental mechanism signaling danger to the vulnerable vasculature. *Circ Res.* 2010; 106:842–853.

Zheng PL, Li ZX, Zhou ZG. Gut microbiome in type 1 diabetes: a comprehensive review. *Diabetes Metab Res Rev.* 2018; 34(7):e3043.

Zhou X, Zhang W, Liu X, Zhang W, Li Y. Interrelationship between diabetes and periodontitis: role of hyperlipidemia. *Arch Oral Biol.* 2015; 60:667–674.

Zhuang Z, Yoshizawa-Smith S, Glowacki A et al. Induction of M2 macrophages prevents bone loss in murine periodontitis models. *J Dent Res.* 2018; 98:200–208.

Zuza EP, Barroso EM, Fabricio M et al. Lipid profile and high-sensitivity C-reactive protein levels in obese and non-obese subjects undergoing non-surgical periodontal therapy. *J Oral Sci.* 2016; 58(3):423–430.

23.2 PERIODONTAL DISEASE AND CARDIOVASCULAR DISEASE

Steph Smith

Contents

Learning objectives

- Fundamentals of endothelial function and activation.
- Components of chronic periodontal disease that target other non-oral organs, such as vascular endothelium.
- Interactions between components of periodontally induced systemic inflammation and vascular endothelium, including periodontal pathogens, outer membrane vesicles, inflammatory cytokines, platelet activation, and the induction and role of autoimmunity.
- Development of the atheromatous lesion.

Introduction

A significant and rather complex association exists between chronic periodontitis (CP) and cardiovascular disease (CVD) (Van Dyke & van Winkelhoff 2013). CP may be considered as an infection that metastasizes, which includes a bacteremia and bacterial infection at non-oral sites (Amar et al. 2003; Van Dyke & van Winkelhoff 2013). This furthermore entails inflammation and inflammatory mediators influencing systemic inflammation, and the activation of innate and adaptive immunity together with systemic consequences (Amar et al. 2003; Bartova et al. 2014). CP thus constitutes a systemic inflammatory stressor that can act as a continuous and independent factor for the increased risk of future atherosclerotic CVD (Papapanou 2015; Tonetti et al. 2013). This includes the plausibility of potential molecular mechanisms linking CP and endothelial dysfunction (ED) associated with subclinical atherosclerosis (Humphrey et al. 2008; Li et al. 2011). Although short-term studies have shown that periodontal interventions result in a reduction in systemic inflammation and ED, appropriate long-term randomized controlled clinical trials are lacking regarding the effectiveness of periodontal interventions in preventing cardiovascular-related clinical events (Papapanou 2015).

The pathognomonic mechanisms of immune dysregulation comprising the elements of CP interacting with vascular endothelial cells (ECs), leading to the formation of atherosclerotic plaques, are complex (Smith 2018). These mechanisms entail low-grade systemic inflammation, including bacteremias, endotoxemias, systemic inflammatory mediators, reactive oxygen species (ROS), and acute-phase reactants generated by CP (Humphrey et al. 2008; Li et al. 2011). Interactions between these elements of CP and ECs cause a shift from normal endothelial function to that of activation, which includes a proinflammatory and prothrombotic state of the endothelium (Gurav 2014). Endothelial activation (dysfunction) is considered as the initial step in the process of atherosclerosis (Schenkein & Loos 2013).

Endothelial function

Vascular endothelium is a multifunctional endocrine organ and is a key regulator of vascular homeostasis (Singh et al. 2002). Normal vascular homeostasis (endothelial function) is regarded as the vascular wall being in a state of quiescence, involving the control of vasomotion; the silencing of cellular processes including the inhibition of inflammation, cellular proliferation, and thrombosis; as well as the inhibition of the uptake of low-density lipoproteins (LDL) (Deanfield et al. 2007; Tousoulis et al. 2012). Endothelial function is modulated by a balance of endothelium-derived vasodilators, especially nitric oxide (NO), and ROS (Higashi et al. 2009) (see Figure 23.2.1).

NO is the principal regulator of vasodilatation (Pober & Sessa 2007). Other functions of NO include the inhibition of vascular smooth muscle cell (SMC) proliferation and platelet activation, and inhibiting the expression of adhesion molecules that mediate leucocyte attachment (anti-inflammatory) (Deanfield et al. 2007; Gurav 2014). NO has a direct effect on leucocytes by preventing their activation to motile forms, thus inhibiting the diapedesis of these cells into the tissues (Pober & Sessa 2007).

ROS are produced in aerobic cells, including SMCs, ECs, and mononuclear cells (Higashi et al. 2009). The subcytotoxic tonal release of ROS is imperative for healthy cell function, acting as signaling molecules to regulate cell physiology, the maintenance of homeostasis, and to promote adaptation to stress (Sena & Chandel 2012). ROS also regulate innate and adaptive immune functions, including early T-cell activation, antiviral, antibacterial, and antiparasitic responses (Kaminski et al. 2010). ROS have potent oxidation ability, and include free radicals such as $O2-$, hydroxyl radical (OH) and NO, and non-free radicals such as hydrogen peroxide (H_2O_2), hypochlorous acid (HOCl) ,and peroxynitrite ($ONOO-$) (Sena & Chandel 2012).

Endothelial activation

Endothelial function can become impaired by an imbalance of the reduced production of NO and the increased/excessive production of ROS, known as oxidative stress. Protective antioxidant mechanisms scavenge ROS in the vasculature, resulting in the inhibition of NO degradation (Higashi et al. 2009). Oxidative stress, however, can overwhelm these defense mechanisms, leading to the oxidization of DNA, protein, carbohydrates, and lipids, as well as accelerated NO degradation (Cai & Harrison 2000; Deanfield et al. 2007). For example, an ROS such as $O2-$ can react with NO to form $ONOO-$, a potent oxidant, which causes the oxidation of co-factor BH4, resulting in a decrease in endothelial nitric oxide synthase (eNOS) levels in ECs (Verma et al. 2000).

Oxidative stress in ECs (endothelial activation), which includes a host defense response, induces the expression of chemokines, inflammatory cytokines, as well as platelet activation, and the up-regulation of adhesion molecules for the purposes of interacting with leucocytes. This promotes leucocyte adhesion and extravasation so as to direct inflammation to specific tissues to remove bacterial pathogens (Gurav 2014; Hansson 2005; Lum & Roebuck 2001) (see Figure 23.2.1).

Endothelial activation also leads to clot formation, platelet activation, adhesion, and aggregation (Yau et al. 2015). Platelets also bind to ECs and to immune cells (monocytes, neutrophils, lymphocytes), and secrete proinflammatory mediators, chemokines, and growth factors (McNicol & Israels 2010). Activated platelets therefore have a major role in the activation and proliferation of the endothelium, by altering the chemotactic and adhesive properties of ECs, contributing also to a procoagulant state (Huo & Ley 2004).

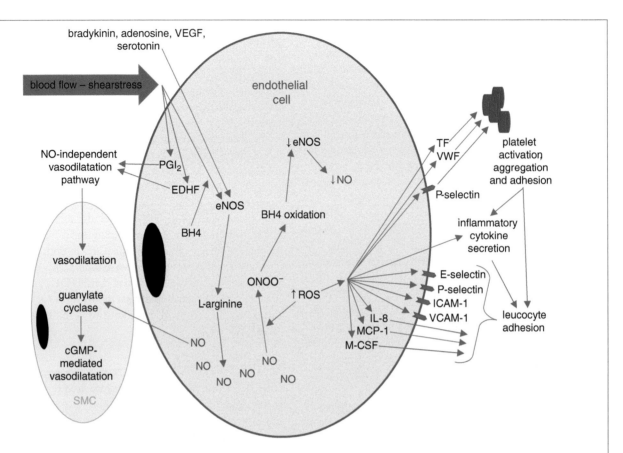

Figure 23.2.1 *Endothelial function* (blue arrows): Laminar shear stress induced by blood flow activates endothelial nitric oxide synthase (eNOS) in the presence of co-factor tetrahydrobiopterin (BH4), which acts upon L-arginine to produce nitric oxide (NO). eNOS is also activated by bradykinin, adenosine, vascular endothelial growth factor (VEGF), and serotonin. NO diffuses to the vascular smooth muscle cells (SMCs) in the medial layer of the vascular wall and activates guanylate cyclase, which leads to cyclic guanosine monophosphate (cGMP)-mediated vasodilatation. Hyperpolarization of vascular SMCs is also mediated by NO-independent pathways, namely by means of the release of endothelium-derived hyperpolarizing factor (EDHF) and prostacyclin (PGI$_2$). *Endothelial activation* (red arrows): During oxidative stress, O2– (an ROS) reacts with NO to form ONOO–, a potent oxidant, causing the oxidation of co-factor BH4, thereby resulting in a decrease in eNOS levels, leading to inhibition of NO production. Excessive ROS leads to the up-regulation of adhesion molecules, such as E-selectin, P-selectin, intercellular adhesion molecules (ICAM)-1, vascular cell adhesion molecule (VCAM)-1 and chemotactic molecules like interleukin (IL)-8, macrophage chemoattractant peptide-1 (MCP-1), and macrophage colony-stimulating factor (M-CSF), thereby promoting leucocyte adhesion and extravasation. Endothelial activation leads to the expression of tissue factor (TF), von Willebrand factor (VWF), and P-selectin, leading to clot formation, platelet activation, adhesion, and aggregation. Activated platelets bind to other platelets, endothelial cells, and immune cells, and secrete inflammatory cytokines. Courtesy of Dr. Steph Smith.

Periodontitis and chronically sustained systemic inflammation

CP is associated with dysbiosis of the commensal species, and it has been hypothesized that subgingival dysbiotic periodontal bacteria are involved in systemic inflammation and subclinical atherogenesis (Pietiäinen et al. 2018) (see Figure 23.2.2). Periodontal tissue destruction causes interruption of the oral sulcular epithelium in the progressively deepening periodontal pocket, resulting in contact between invading periodontal dysbiotic pathogens and the adjacent microvessels (Nanci & Bosshardt 2006; Pietiäinen et al. 2018). Periodontal dysbiotic microbes, lipopolysaccharides (LPS), and inflammatory cytokines from within periodontally infected tissues can

consequently disseminate into the systemic circulation, causing a bacteremia and endotoxemia (LPS) (Gurav 2014; Hayashi et al. 2010; Hirschfeld & Kawai 2015). The extent of the bacteremia depends on the magnitude of the tissue trauma, the bacterial density, and the severity of local inflammation (Wilson et al. 2007), as well as inflammatory cytokines having sufficient concentrations together with their preservation of bioactivity within the circulation (Schenkein & Loos 2013).

In patients with gingivitis or periodontitis, dissemination of bacteria and their products into the systemic circulation through ulcerated periodontal pockets can occur during periodontal therapeutic procedures, toothbrushing, or chewing (Forner et al. 2006). *Porphyromonas gingivalis, Aggregatibacter actinomycetemcomitans, Tannerella forsythia, Prevotella intermedia,* and

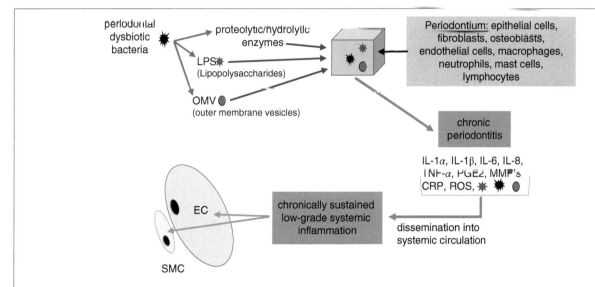

Figure 23.2.2 Periodontitis and chronically sustained systemic inflammation. Chronic periodontitis (CP) entails the infection and invasion of dysbiotic bacteria into the periodontal tissues, with the accompanying release of proteolytic/hydrolytic enzymes, outer membrane vesicles (OMVs), and lipopolysaccharide (LPS) into the periodontal tissues. Resident cells in the periodontium such as fibroblasts, endothelial cells, osteoclasts, epithelial cells, neutrophils, macrophages, lymphocytes, and mast cells consequently react to the bacterial invasion and their products, by releasing reactive oxygen species (ROS) and various proinflammatory products. These host-induced proinflammatory mediators, such as interleukin-1-alpha (IL-1α) and interleukin-1-beta (IL-1β), IL-6, IL-8, tumor necrosis factor-alpha (TNF-α), prostanoids (prostaglandin E2, PGE2), and matrix metalloproteinases (MMPs), as well as C-reactive protein (CRP), ROS, and OMVs, orchestrate host-mediated bone resorption and periodontal tissue destruction. The dissemination of inflammatory mediators, ROS, CRP, LPS, dysbiotic bacteria, and OMV into the bloodstream elicits a state of chronic low-grade systemic inflammation, whereby these products can reach distant organs, leading to bacterial attachment and invasion of various cells, including endothelial cells (EC) and smooth muscle cells (SMC). Courtesy of Dr. Steph Smith.

Fusobacterium nucleatum can also reach distant sites by entering immune cells, such as monocytes/macrophages or dendritic cells in the diseased periodontium. These bacteria have evolved mechanisms to invade and survive within the host cell cytoplasm, where they may gain access to proteins and other key nutrients and also be protected from antimicrobial defense mechanisms present in the extracellular environment (Carrion et al. 2012). These cells may then leave the inflamed tissues and translocate via lymph vessels, enter the circulation, localize, and diapedese into the vascular intima at sites of activated ECs (Carrion et al. 2012; Hayashi et al. 2010). There are thus two modes of invasion of cardiovascular tissues by periodontal pathogens, i.e. a direct route by means of a bacteremia and a conceivable indirect route by means of a phagocyte-mediated bacterial translocation from the periodontal tissues (Carrion et al. 2012; El Kholy et al. 2015). The ensuing bacteremia and endotoxemia can elicit a state of chronic low-grade systemic inflammation, whereby bacteria, endotoxins, and accompanying inflammatory mediators can reach distant organs (Gurav 2014), leading to bacterial attachment and invasion of various cells, including ECs and SMCs (Dorn et al. 2002). This causes the induction and maintenance of inflammation at sites distant from the periodontium (Hayashi et al. 2010; Hirschfeld & Kawai 2015).

A. actinomycetemcomitans, T. forsythia, Treponema denticola, and *P. gingivalis* release outer membrane vesicles (OMVs), which are secreted portions of the bacterial outer membrane, containing constituents of the periplasm and cytoplasm (Ellis et al. 2010; Pietiäinen et al. 2018). Besides being composed of parts of the bacterial membrane, OMVs comprise bacterial proteins, LPS, fatty acids, nucleic acids, peptidoglycan fragments, fimbriae, adhesins, capsule, and species-specific virulence factors, such as cytolethal distending toxin (CDT), leukotoxin (LtxA), and gingipains (Pietiäinen et al. 2018). OMVs facilitate interbacterial interactions such as promoting the growth of co-colonizing pathogens, biofilm formation, and colonization. OMVs are also produced and situated proximally to host cells in the bacterial biofilm, whereby macrophages and dendritic cells that become activated by bacterial OMVs increase the production and expression of proinflammatory mediators, such as tumor necrosis factor-alpha (TNF-α) and interleukin (IL)-12 (Alaniz et al. 2007). OMVs can be present at sites disseminated from direct sites of bacterial colonization, and so deliver active toxins and proteases to degrade host cells (Ellis & Kuehn 2010; Soult et al. 2013). They also actively destroy host defenses, as well as produce an environment that is resistant to antibiotics and antibacterials, this by means of delivery of virulence constituents including proteins, toxins, enzymes, and LPS (Inagaki et al. 2006; Soult et al. 2013). OMVs can attach to, and become internalized into, ECs by endocytosis or via adhesin-receptor mediation, thereby causing internalization of bacterial components, including membrane and cytoplasmic proteins and endotoxin, into the host cell (Alaniz et al. 2007).

C-reactive protein (CRP), which is an acute-phase protein, is primarily synthesized by hepatocytes (Ablij & Meinders 2002). Extrahepatic synthesis of CRP occurs in gingival connective tissues and gingival epithelial cells, where it is constitutively expressed (Lu & Jin 2010). The in vivo activities of CRP are both anti-inflammatory and proinflammatory, whereby inflammatory CRP activates the classical complement cascade, thereby contributing to the clearance of bacteria and damaged cells in inflamed tissues and the bloodstream (Du Clos & Mold 2004; Pietiäinen et al. 2018). With active inflammatory periodontitis, the production of inflammatory CRP in gingival tissues is associated with increased IL-6 activity (Du Clos & Mold 2004). The dissemination into the systemic circulation of elevated numbers of polymorphonuclear neutrophils (PMNs), as well as LPS and IL-6, induces hepatic inflammation, resulting in the further production and release of inflammatory CRP (Devaraj et al. 2009).

Under physiological conditions, low concentrations of ROS production stimulate the growth of fibroblasts and epithelial cells; however, higher concentrations result in tissue injury. This tissue destruction leads to overproduction of lipid peroxides, inflammatory mediators, as well as oxidized proteins. These products further activate macrophages, PMNs, and fibroblasts to generate more ROS, thus forming a vicious circle (Dahiya et al. 2013). Higher ROS levels may be correlated with *P. gingivalis*, *A. actinomycetemcomitans*, *T. forsythia*, *and T. denticola* (Almerich-Silla et al. 2015). Bacterial cells and inflammatory cytokines in gingival tissues cause the recruitment and activation of hyper-responsive neutrophils (PMNs), and, in response to TNF-α, primed PMNs undergo a respiratory burst, releasing O2–, thereby speeding up the production of ROS (Dahiya et al. 2013; Gumus et al. 2016). Inflammation and inflammatory cytokines cause tissue hypoxia, due to an increase in oxygen consumption by invading immune cells (Frede et al. 2007). Hypoxic gingival sulci and diseased periodontal tissues favor proliferation of anaerobic *P. gingivalis*, and expose these tissues to *P. gingivalis* LPS (Gölz et al. 2014). The hypoxia and LPS stimulate up-regulated production of proinflammatory cytokines and ROS in periodontal ligament fibroblasts, especially O2– and hydrogen peroxide (H_2O_2), leading to the activation of macrophages, which secrete MMPs, thus causing tissue and alveolar bone destruction (Frede et al. 2007; Gölz et al. 2014).

P. gingivalis possesses its own protective antioxidants, for example rubrerythrin, providing defense against the oxidative burst of the host (Mydel et al. 2006). Bacteria in the oral cavity and periodontal pockets may consume local tissue antioxidants and suppress ROS detoxification. This then enables the entry of ROS from the periodontal tissues into the bloodstream, inducing circulating oxidative stress (Tomofuji et al. 2009).

Chronic low-grade systemic inflammation is associated with an attenuated total plasma antioxidant capacity in patients with severe CP (Baser et al. 2015), thereby contributing to the promotion of inflammation in the endothelial vascular wall (Gurav 2014).

Chronically sustained systemic inflammation and endothelial activation

Periodontal pathogens and endothelial activation

Periodontal pathogens may either directly disrupt EC function, or indirectly induce the elevated production of inflammatory mediators in the systemic circulation, thereby exacerbating the inflammatory atherosclerotic lesion (Slocum et al. 2016) (see Figure 23.2.3). There is furthermore evidence supporting an association between the gut microbiome and systemic diseases, whereby *P. gingivalis* from the oral microbiome may alter the gut microbiome, resulting in a concurrent increase in gut permeability and systemic proinflammatory cytokines (Arimatsu et al. 2014; Nakajima et al. 2015; Slocum et al. 2016).

It is hypothesized that ED is due to the action of several bacterial species, and not that of a single pathogen (Prasad et al. 2002). The most commonly identified periodontal pathogens are *P. gingivalis* and *A. actinomycetemcomitans*, and species less often identified include *T. forsythia*, *T. denticola*, *P. intermedia*, *Prevotella nigrescens*, *Eikenella corrodens*, *F. nucleatum*, and *Campylobacter rectus* (Chiu 1999). Pathogens such as *Chlamydia pneumoniae*, *Helicobacter pylori*, and *P. gingivalis* have been identified within human atherosclerotic plaques (Latsios et al. 2004).

P. gingivalis is an intracellular pathogen infecting oral epithelial cells, fibroblasts, dendritic cells, macrophages, SMCs, and ECs, where it survives and replicates, leading to a proinflammatory response within these cells (Foey & Crean 2013). The attachment to, as well as EC invasion by, *P. gingivalis* is accomplished by attachment pilli, namely fimbriae (Yoshimura et al. 2009). *P. gingivalis* fimbriae are involved in Toll-like receptors (TLR), namely TLR2- and TLR4-dependent activation of ECs (Khlgatian et al. 2002). Fimbriae, as well as LPS (Zelkha et al. 2010), which are pathogen-associated molecular patterns (PAMPs), interact indirectly with pattern recognition receptors (PRRs) on ECs, namely TLR2 and TLR4 (Hajishengallis et al. 2004). TLR2- and TLR4-dependant activation of ECs by fimbriae requires a co-receptor and an accessory protein (Davey et al. 2008).

Other PRRs important for microbial recognition are soluble cytosolic nucleotide-binding oligomerization domain (NOD1 and NOD2) proteins, which provide an intracellular layer of surveillance and host defense after stimulation of TLRs (Kim et al. 2008).

P. gingivalis ligation and activation of TLRs and NOD1/NOD2 receptors triggers a proinflammatory response, causing the secretion of proinflammatory cytokines in both ECs and

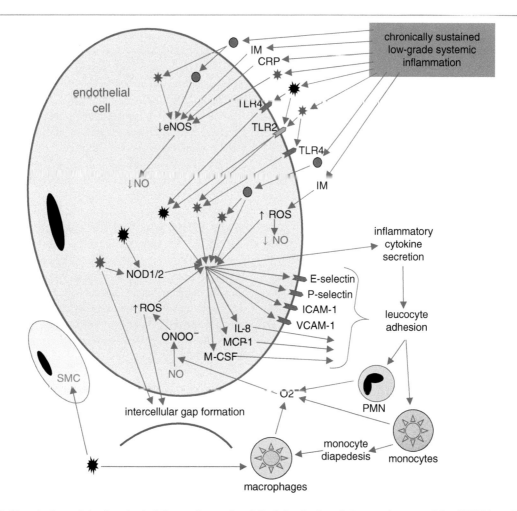

Figure 23.2.3 Chronically sustained systemic inflammation and endothelial activation. Outer membrane vesicles (OMVs) and lipopolysaccharide (LPS) translocated from OMVs, inflammatory mediators (IMs), C-reactive protein (CRP), and bacterial LPS cause a reduction in endothelial nitric oxide synthase (eNOS) expression, leading to decreased nitric oxide (NO). Periodontal bacteria and LPS interact with membrane Toll-like receptor (TLR)2/4 receptors and invade both endothelial cells (ECs) and macrophages. Intracellular bacteria and LPS interact with soluble cytosolic receptors NOD1/2. Ligation and activation of TLRs and NOD1/NOD2 receptors in ECs causes the secretion of proinflammatory cytokines and the up-regulation of adhesion molecules, namely ICAM-1, VCAM-1, MCP-1, E-selectin, and P-selectin, as well as macrophage colony-stimulating factor (M-CSF), thereby initiating the recruitment, attachment, and diapedesis of monocytes. Adherence and internalization of OMVs as well as LPS translocation from OMVs leads to inflammatory cytokine synthesis, adhesion receptor expression, as well as a reduction of eNOS expression. Inflammatory mediators (IMs) from chronic periodontitis (CP) generates ROS in ECs, causing NO degradation. ROS induce the up-regulation of adhesion receptor expression. Adhered and activated leucocytes (polymorphonuclear neutrophils [PMNs] and monocytes/macrophages) release O2–, whereby O2– interacts with endothelial NO, forming ONOO– (ROS). ROS, LPS, and cytokines lead to cell shape change, impaired cell–cell adhesion, adherens junctions, and intercellular junctions, causing intercellular gap formation. *Porphyromonas gingivalis* smooth muscle cell (SMC) infection also triggers SMC proliferation, leading to impairment of endothelial vasomotor function. Courtesy of Dr. Steph Smith.

macrophages (Gibson et al. 2008; Hajishengallis et al. 2004). This inflammatory response in activated ECs and macrophages causes the up-regulation of adhesion molecules, namely intercellular adhesion molecule-1 (ICAM-1), vascular cell adhesion molecule-1 (VCAM-1), monocyte chemoattractant protein-1 (MCP-1), E-selectin, and P-selectin, as well as macrophage colony-stimulating factor (M-CSF), thereby initiating the recruitment, attachment, and diapedesis of monocytes (Chiastikov et al. 2016). *P. gingivalis* SMC infection also triggers

SMC proliferation, leading to impairment of endothelial vasomotor function (Assinger et al. 2011; Nakamura et al. 2008).

Outer membrane vesicles and endothelial activation

The direct recognition, adherence, and internalization of OMVs by ECs trigger an immediate innate and acquired host immune response, leading to the induction and modulation of inflammatory pathways and receptor expression (Ellis &

Kuehn 2010; Jia et al. 2015) (see Figure 23.2.3). LPS is a main vesicular component and the most potent immune-stimulating component of OMVs (Beveridge 1999). LPS translocation from OMVs within ECs, together with other virulence factors in OMVs, such as gingipains and fimbriae, lead to inflammatory cytokine synthesis, namely TNF-α, IL-8, and IL-6 (Kuehn & Kesty 2005). This leads to an increase in ICAM-1 and E-selectin adhesion receptor biosynthesis and expression (Jia et al. 2015), causing the recruitment of leucocytes to activated ECs (Srisatjaluk et al. 1999).

An increased OMV–LPS-mediated TNF-α expression leads to a reduction of eNOS expression. Virulence factors within OMVs also induce the suppression of eNOS expression, at both mRNA and protein levels (Lu et al. 1996).

In addition to having proinflammatory effects, OMVs can have an anti-inflammatory role that benefits the pathogen of origin or that promotes secondary bacterial infections. *P. gingivalis* OMVs can inhibit the up-regulation of major histocompatibility complex (MHC) class II molecules on the surface of interferon (IFN)-γ–stimulated ECs, thus modulating antigen presentation and favoring the survival of the pathogen (Kaparakis-Liaskos & Ferrero 2015).

Inflammatory cytokines, lipopolysaccharides, C-reactive protein, reactive oxygen species, and endothelial barrier dysfunction

Proinflammatory mediators such as TNF-α and IL-6, expressed in CP, reduce the endothelial production of eNOS (Gurav 2014) (see Figure 23.2.3). LPS and LPS-induced TNF-α production cause suppression of eNOS expression by decreasing the half-life of eNOS mRNA, leading to the reduction of NO levels in ECs (Lu et al. 1996; Yoshizumi et al. 1993). Endotoxemia has been identified as a notable cardiometabolic risk factor (Pietiäinen et al. 2018). Although periodontal pathogens may contribute to LPS endotoxemia, the main endogenous origin of LPS endotoxins is presumed to be translocated from the gut microbiota in the small intestine, especially in subjects with increased intestinal permeability (Blum et al. 1997; Giustarini et al. 2009).

The role of inflammatory CRP in the development or progression of atherosclerosis is controversial. CRP is thought to play a role in atherogenesis because of its ability to bind to modified low-density lipoprotein and its effects on endothelial cell function, plaque instability, and thrombosis. High levels of inflammatory CRP may directly impair endothelial function by causing a reduced capacity to activate eNOS mRNA, leading to a reduced production of NO (Gomaraschi et al. 2013; Sproston & Ashworth 2018).

Inflammatory cytokines from periodontal tissues, including macrophages such as TNF-α and IL-1, generate ROS in ECs, whereby oxidative stress then overwhelms endogenous antioxidant defense mechanisms, leading to the oxidization of biological macromolecules, DNA, protein, carbohydrates, and lipids, as well as accelerated NO degradation. ROS leads to the up-regulation of P-selectin, ICAM-1, VCAM-1, and MCP-1,

thereby promoting leucocyte adhesion and extravasation (Gurav 2014; Tonetti et al. 2013).

Activated leucocytes that are adherent to the endothelial cell surface are a major source of ROS. Peripheral blood PMNs from periodontitis patients have been shown to be hyperactive and, regardless of whether they are primed or not, they produce higher levels of unstimulated total and extracellular ROS (Herrera et al. 2020). Stimulation of PMNs by periodontal pathogens by means of the receptors for the fragment crystallizable region of immunoglobulin (Ig)G or TLR consequently induce ROS release from hyper-reactive PMNs (Fredriksson et al. 1998; Matthews et al. 2007).

Studies have shown a link between bone marrow activity, arterial inflammation, and CVD events in humans (Tawakol et al. 2017). A further study has provided supportive evidence that the link between periodontal disease inflammation and arterial inflammation is substantially mediated by heightened hematopoietic activity (up-regulated bone marrow leucopoiesis), leading to the release of monocytes (Ishai et al. 2019). It has thus been further hypothesized that periodontal disease inflammatory cytokines stimulate the release of monocytes from the bone marrow, which are then recruited into the atheroma lesion and, together with periodontal disease cytokine stimulation of macrophages in atherosclerotic lesions, exacerbate atherosclerotic inflammation (Van Dyke et al. 2021).

The adherence of primed PMNs to endothelium, as well as the recruitment of macrophages into the arterial wall, causes the release of O2–, whereby O2– can interact with endothelial NO, forming ONOO–, leading to increased generation of localized vascular oxidative stress, thus forming a vicious circle. ROS such as H_2O_2, as well as LPS, histamine, TNF-α, and IFN-Υ, cause increased intracellular oxidative stress, leading to an overexpression of extracellular matrix proteins and collagen type III by ECs (Dahiya et al. 2013; Lum & Roebuck 2001; Montorfano et al. 2014).

Besides increased oxidative stress, there is also a resultant actin microfilament disruption in ECs. This leads to cell shape change, impaired cell–cell adhesion, adherens junctions, and intercellular junctions, causing intercellular gap formation (Lönn et al. 2018; Lum & Roebuck 2001). ECs thus lose their capacity to function as a selectively permeable barrier due to increased endothelial permeability. This promotes increased filtration of cholesterol-containing LDL particles from the intravascular lumen into the arterial wall, including facilitating leucocyte transmigration into the intima (Nakano et al. 2009; Whitaker et al. 2007). LPS also binds to TLR-4 receptors of T cells, which stimulates MHC class II receptors, leading to activation of T cells with subsequent antibody production, and thus further induced inflammation (Amar et al. 2003).

Platelet activation and endothelial activation

Proinflammatory molecules, such as LPS, TNF-α, IL-1β, thromboxane A2, vascular endothelial growth factor (VEGF), as well as vasoactive histamine, bradykinin, and thrombin, have been shown to activate ECs (Yau et al. 2015). Activated ECs then express tissue factor (TF), von Willebrand factor (VWF), and P-selectin, as well as inflammatory cytokines. This leads to platelet activation, causing clot formation, platelet adhesion, and aggregation (Yau et al. 2015). Platelet adhesion initiates the expression of platelet adhesive receptors, thereby initiating platelet binding to other platelets and to ECs (Huo & Ley 2004; Yau et al. 2015). Activated platelets also secrete proinflammatory mediators, such as chemokines and cytokines, thereby initiating the recruitment and binding of immune cells (monocytes, neutrophils, lymphocytes). Activated platelets therefore have a major role in the activation and proliferation

of the endothelium, which includes the recruitment of leukocytes (Huo & Ley 2004; Yau et al. 2015) (see Figure 23.2.4).

During a CP-induced bacteremia, *Streptococcus mutans*, *A. actinomycetemcomitans*, *Streptococcus sanguinis*, *P. gingivalis*, and *T. denticola* have been shown to activate platelets (Jain et al. 2013), and therefore act synergistically to stimulate platelet adhesion at sites of EC activation, thereby stimulating the migration of inflammatory cells, as well as thrombus formation (Aslam et al. 2006; Huo & Ley 2004; Yau et al. 2015). Both *P. gingivalis* and LPS engage TLR2 and TLR4 receptors on platelets (Shashkin et al. 2008; Yau et al. 2015), inducing platelet neutrophil aggregation, and causing TNF-α release and IL-1

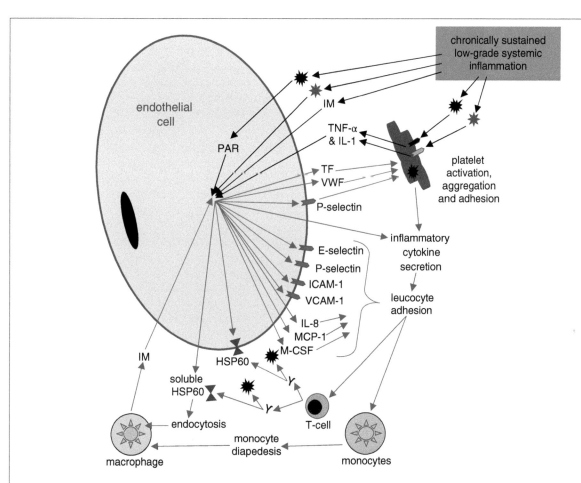

Figure 23.2.4 Platelet activation: Periodontal bacteria activate protease-activated receptor (PAR) and, together with lipopolysaccharide (LPS) and inflammatory mediators (IM), activate endothelial cells (ECs). Periodontal bacteria and LPS interact with Toll-like receptor (TLR)2 and TLR4 on blood platelets, which then secrete tumor necrosis factor (TNF)-α and interleukin (IL)-1. TNF-α and IL-1 activate ECs. Activated ECs secrete tissue factor (TF), von Willebrand factor (VWF), and P-selectin receptors, leading to platelet activation, aggregation, and adhesion. Activated platelets and ECs secrete inflammatory cytokines and adhesion molecules, leading to recruitment of leucocytes. *Porphyromonas gingivalis* can be localized between adherent platelets and be present in engulfment vacuoles of aggregated platelets, enabling them to replicate within platelets and sustain inflammation. Autoimmunity: Stress induction to ECs induces the expression of adhesion molecules on the EC surface, including E-selectin, P-selectin, VCAM-1, ICAM-1, autologous HSP60, as well as inflammatory cytokines. HSP60 are also shed into the circulation as soluble HSP60. The immune system mounts a physiological T-cell–mediated and humoral immune response against autologous HSP60. Antibodies (Υ) against bacterial HSP60 cross-react with autologous HSP60, inducing an autoimmune response, known as molecular mimicry. Activated monocytes and macrophages endocytose soluble HSP60 immune complexes, leading to secretion of inflammatory mediators (IMs), causing stress induction and activation of ECs. Courtesy of Dr. Steph Smith.

synthesis (Blair et al. 2009; Engström et al. 2015). TNF-α and IL-1 lead to the up-regulation and production of TF and VWF in ECs, thereby sustaining EC inflammation (Li et al. 2008; McNicol & Israels 2010; Yau et al. 2015). This suggests a role for platelets in the innate response to bacteremias (Nurden 2011). *P. gingivalis* can be localized on the surface between adherent platelets, as well as be present in engulfment vacuoles of aggregated platelets (Lourbakos et al. 2001; Wick et al. 2014), thereby enabling them to replicate within platelets as well as to sustain inflammation (McNicol & Israels 2010). *P. gingivalis* OMVs containing gingipains activate protease-activated receptors (PARs) in ECs, also inducing the expression of TF and VWF, leading to platelet aggregation (Amberger et al. 1997; Nurden 2011). *P. gingivalis* OMVs can also induce platelet–platelet aggregation (Kaparakis-Liaskos & Ferrero 2015).

Autoimmunity and endothelial activation

Heat-shock proteins (HSPs) are found in several intracellular compartments and function as mediators of protective pathways, including the assembly of polypeptides, and protein translocation across membranes (Xu et al. 2000) (see Figure 23.2.4). Under normal physiological conditions, HSP60 is not expressed on vascular EC surfaces. However, the induction of stress to the EC surface by traditional risk factors for atherosclerosis, as well as infections, causes mitochondrial HSP (autologous HSP60) to be expressed on EC surfaces (Xu et al. 2000). These various stressors also induce the expression of adhesion molecules on the EC surface, including VCAM-1, ELAM-1 (endothelial-leukocyte adhesion molecule 1), and ICAM-1. IL-6 expression is also induced by autologous HSP60 within the EC. Autologous HSP60 itself, furthermore, also induces E-selectin, VCAM-1, and ICAM-1 expression on EC surfaces (Wallin et al. 2002).

Consequently, the immune system mounts a physiological T-cell–mediated and humoral immune response against autologous HSP60. HSP60-reactive T cells induce the initial EC activation in atherosclerosis, comprising autoantibodies against HSP60, whereby the binding of antibodies to the endothelium surface induces an inflammatory autoimmune response. The production of antibodies to HSP60 further accelerates and perpetuates the disease (Xu et al. 2000). HSP60 are also shed into the circulation in a soluble form (Gibson et al. 2008), functioning as potent activators of the innate immune system, leading to activated monocytes and macrophages endocytosing soluble HSP60 (Singh et al. 2002). Activated monocytes and macrophages undergo intracellular signaling, triggering the secretion of proinflammatory cytokines with subsequent activation of ECs (Iacopino & Cutler 2000).

P. gingivalis (HSP60 GroEL), *F. nucleatum* (GroEL), *T. forsythia*, and *A. actinomycetemcomitans* also express HSPs. They have been shown to activate endothelial cells, increase monocyte adhesion and migration, increase foam cell formation, stimulate production of inflammatory cytokines via TLR, and promote coagulation (Deniset & Pierce 2015).

The host with CP also acquires a cellular and humoral immunological response against bacterial HSP60, for example *P. gingivalis* GroEL, as a protective defense against invading periodontal pathogens. *P. gingivalis* GroEL has a strong immunogenic nature; however, it is homologous with host HSP60 (Pober & Sessa 2007). This homology is unrecognizable by host T cells, resulting in the increased risk of antibodies directed against bacterial HSP60 to cross-react with host HSP60 on stressed ECs, thereby inducing an autoimmune response known as molecular mimicry, leading to ED with an ensuing inflammatory cascade (Pietiäinen et al. 2018; Pober & Sessa 2007; Xu et al. 2000).

Various bacteria in plaque biofilms present phosphorylcholine-containing antigens and induce systemic phosphorylcholine IgG immunity. These antibodies cross-react with neoantigens induced as a result of either oxidation or proteolysis of serum lipids, this being another example of molecular mimicry in CVD pathogenesis in periodontitis patients (Meier & Binstadt 2018).

Oxidized low-density lipids (ox-LDL) that are deposited in the intima layer of ECs are chemotactic for monocytes and T cells, whereby macrophages may then present antigenic epitopes of ox-LDL to B cells, inducing the formation of antibodies to ox-LDL. Thus, antibody production to ox-LDL also contributes to an autoimmune pathogenesis of CVD (Maekawa et al. 2011).

Periodontitis and atherosclerotic plaque formation

Atherosclerosis is a multifactorial disease entailing both autoimmune and inflammatory pathogenic mechanisms (see Figure 23.2.5). The first stage of atherosclerotic disease involves fatty streak development, which includes endothelial dysfunction, dyslipidemia, lipoprotein modification and entry within the arterial wall, leucocyte recruitment, and foam cell formation (Amar et al. 2003; Maekawa et al. 2011).

CP-induced low-grade systemic inflammation comprising the systemic dissemination of bacteria, LPS, TNF-α, and IL-1β induces an acute-phase response that includes alterations in lipid metabolism in the liver (Schenkein & Loos 2013). This results in elevated plasma levels of LDL cholesterol, triglycerides (TRG), and omega-6 free fatty acids (FFA) (Miyakawa et al. 2004), as well as a decrease in circulating anti-atherogenic high-density lipoprotein (HDL) cholesterol (Qi et al. 2003). These elevations in serum lipids arise from enhanced hepatic lipogenesis, increased adipose tissue lipolysis, increased synthesis or reduced clearance of TRG, and reduced clearance of LDL due to reductions in lipoprotein lipase activity (Miyakawa et al. 2004).

Periodontal microbes induce free radical ROS production in neutrophils, with subsequent lipid peroxidation. *P. gingivalis* also causes a systemic reduction in antioxidant levels (Brock et al. 2004; Chapple et al. 2007). *P. gingivalis* gingipains can directly aggregate LDLs and, by inducing

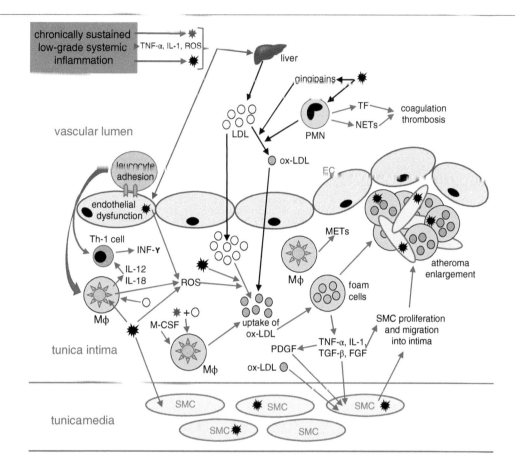

Figure 23.2.5 Elements of atheroma formation. Chronic periodontitis (CP)-induced low-grade systemic inflammation induces endothelial cell (EC) dysfunction as well as a dyslipidemia, causing elevated plasma levels of low-density lipoprotein (LDL) cholesterol. *Porphyromonas gingivalis* gingipains and polymorphonuclear neutrophils (PMNs) oxidize LDL, forming oxidized LDL (ox-LDL). PMNs secrete tissue factor (TF) and together with neutrophil extracellular traps (NETs) induce coagulation and thrombosis. Endothelial dysfunction (ED) causes leucocyte adhesion, increased endothelial permeability, and diapedesis of inflammatory cells. Macrophages (Mϕ) secrete interleukin (IL)-12 and IL-18, inducing Th1 cell differentiation. Th1 cells secrete interferon gamma (IFN)-ϒ, exacerbating atheroma formation. LDLs diffuse into the intima layer. LDLs, inflammatory cytokines (tumor necrosis factor [TNF]-α, IL-1), together with *P. gingivalis* infection of macrophages, cause reactive oxygen species (ROS) production by macrophages. ROS produced from ECs, macrophages, and enzymatic oxidation by *P. gingivalis* cause oxidation of LDLs, forming ox-LDL. Lipopolysaccharide (LPS) binds to LDL, forming LPS-LDL, and together with local macrophage colony-stimulating factor (M-CSF) induces macrophages to up-regulate their expression of scavenger receptors, leading to the uptake of ox-LDLs, resulting in the formation of foam cells. Foam cells secrete IL-1 and TNF-α, which stimulate the local production of platelet-derived growth factor (PDGF) by ECs. TNF-α, IL-1, PDGF, as well as ox-LDLs stimulate smooth muscle cells (SMCs) to proliferate and migrate from the media into the intima. *P. gingivalis* SMC infection triggers SMC proliferation, leading to impairment of endothelial vasomotor function. SMCs synthesize and produce extracellular matrix, and together with foam cells and ECs release cytokines and growth factors, causing further SMC migration and proliferation, thus maintaining inflammation. This leads to further enlargement of the fatty streak (atheromatous plaque), causing restriction of the vascular lumen, leading to tissue ischemia. METs, macrophage extracellular traps. Courtesy of Dr. Steph Smith.

structural modifications in circulating lipoproteins via enzymatic oxidation, also oxidize LDL (Morishita et al. 2013; Nakano et al. 2009). *P. gingivalis*, in the presence of LDL, stimulates macrophages, causing foam cell formation (Kallio et al. 2008). LPS can also bind to LDL, forming LPS-LDL, thereby promoting LDL uptake by macrophages and thus increasing their pro-atherogenic potency (Oorni & Kovanen 2008; Stoll & Bendszus 2006). *P. gingivalis* microorganisms modify LDL not only in the circulation, but also

within the arterial intima (Fentoglua & Bozkurtb 2008). Also, cross-reactive and specific antibodies induced by *P. gingivalis, A. actinomycetemcomitans, T. forsythia*, and *F. nucleatum* have been shown to directly enhance inflammation in the atheroma plaque (Shenkein & Loos 2013). LPS from these bacteria bind to TLR-4 receptors of T cells, which stimulates MHC class II receptors, leading to activation of T cells with subsequent cross-reactive and specific antibody production (Amar et al. 2003).

Increased endothelial permeability as a result of ED allows for entry of LDL into the vessel intima. LDLs then combine with heparin sulfate proteoglycans in the extracellular matrix of the arterial wall (Maekawa et al. 2011; Nakano et al. 2009). This is followed by the oxidation of LDLs (ox-LDL) by ROS produced by ECs (Cai & Harrison 2000; Dahiya et al. 2013; Lum & Roebuck 2001; Montorfano et al. 2014). LDLs interact with macrophages, causing altered gene expression for TNF-α and IL-1β, and, together with *P. gingivalis* infection of macrophages, induce a hyperactive response with consequent increased production of ROS, leading to ox-LDL (Nakano et al. 2009). In response to local M-CSF, phagocytic macrophages up-regulate their expression of scavenger receptors (Falk 2006), leading to the uptake of ox-LDLs, thereby causing the transformation of macrophages into foam cells (Shanahan & Weissberg 1998).

Ox-LDL causes IL-1 and TNF-α cytokine secretion by ECs and SMCs, leading to the increased expression of adhesion molecules, as well as chemoattractant molecules such as MCP-1 as well as IL-8 (Chistiakov et al. 2016; Maekawa et al. 2011). This leads to direct leucocyte migration into the vessel intima, as well as T cells being attracted to the vessel wall (Falk 2006; Wolf 2000). Differentiation of T cells into Th-1 phenotype cells is due to activated macrophages secreting IL-12 and IL-18. Th-1 cells secrete IFN-Y, which exacerbates plaque formation (Tse et al. 2013). Foam cells produce additional inflammatory cytokines and, together with augmented expression of adhesion molecules on the EC surface, further perpetuate the process of atherosclerotic plaque formation (Maekawa et al. 2011).

Foam cells secrete IL-1 and TNF-α, which stimulate the local production of platelet-derived growth factor (PDGF) by ECs (Mesa et al. 2014). The enhanced expression of TNF-α, IL-1, PDGF, as well as ox-LDLs stimulates SMC proliferation and migration from the media into the intima (Falk 2006). *P. gingivalis* SMC infection also triggers SMC proliferation, leading to impairment of endothelial vasomotor function (Assinger et al. 2011; Nakamura et al. 2008). SMCs synthesize and produce extracellular matrix, leading to further progression of atherosclerotic plaque formation (Falk 2006).

With the further progression of the atherosclerotic plaque, foam cells, activated platelets, and ECs release cytokines and growth factors, e.g. TNF-α, IL-1, fibroblast growth factor (FGF), and transforming growth factor (TGF)-β, which further stimulate SMC migration and proliferation (Falk 2006). Foam cells subsequently undergo apoptosis, leaving behind a lipid core in the subendothelial (intimal) region of the artery that contributes to the formation of the atherosclerotic plaque (fatty streak) (Maekawa et al. 2011). SMC activation and cytokine release reinforces and maintains inflammation in the lesion, and the fatty streak evolves into a fibrofatty lesion (Falk 2006). Fibrosis may continue with calcification at later stages, as well as apoptosis of SMCs, leading to the formation of an acellular fibrous capsule that surrounds a lipid-rich core. Further growth can significantly restrict the vessel lumen and impede perfusion, leading to tissue ischemia (Falk 2006).

Studies have documented the presence of neutrophil extracellular traps (NETs), macrophage-derived extracellular traps (METs), mast cell extracellular traps (MCETs), and eosinophil-derived extracellular traps (EETs) in human atherosclerotic plaques and thrombosis (Pertiwi et al. 2019). NETs and METs are most prominent in coronary atherothrombosis, although low numbers of MCETs and EETs can also be identified. NETs appear to dominate in early stages and METs more significantly in late stages of thrombus formation (Pertiwi et al. 2019).

PMNs may contribute to the coagulation process and thrombosis by releasing TF, even in the absence of vascular injury; by releasing neutrophil elastase and cathepsin G (PMN serine proteases), which inactivate the TF pathway inhibitor; and/or by the formation of procoagulant NETs, thereby promoting the coagulation cascade (Mócsai 2013). TF stabilizes clot formation by activating the coagulation cascade and generating thrombin (Pertiwi et al. 2019). NETs have been indicated in various animal studies to be a possible link in the epidemiological association of infection and inflammation with thrombosis (Fuchs et al. 2010). NETs may promote endothelial dysfunction by triggering platelet activation and stimulating thrombus formation on disrupted plaque, by means of providing scaffolds for fibrin deposition (Pertiwi et al. 2019). NET-induced thrombus formation may involve the activation of Factor XII by the negatively charged NET surface, with a direct effect on the stability of the fibrin network (von Brühl et al. 2012).

Death of foam cells leads to extracellular spill of lipids and, consequently, volume expansion of the lipid core. METs contribute to macrophage cell death and thereby to the expansion of lipid-rich atheromatous plaques. A significant number of METs have also been described in perivascular fat tissue around thrombosed plaques (Pertiwi et al. 2019).

In humans, atherosclerotic plaques at high risk for rupture present distinct features, including intense inflammation and oxidative stress, large areas of necrosis composed of apoptotic cells, with thinning and inflammation of the protective fibrous cap (Tabas 2010; Virmani et al. 2006). Rupture of the lipid-rich atherosclerotic plaque is a major cause of major adverse cardiovascular events, resulting in an acute coronary syndrome (Crea & Libby 2017). Upon the rupture of an atherosclerotic plaque, blood coagulation is initiated, followed by the development of an occlusive clot (thrombus) within a blood vessel that further reduces blood flow to distal tissues and organs and restricts the delivery of nutrients and oxygen, resulting in localized tissue and organ necrosis. Large occlusive clots (thrombi) can break off and embolize to form secondary thrombi in distal locations. The process of thrombosis followed by embolism is collectively termed thromboembolism, and is the predominant cause of myocardial infarctions (heart attacks) and strokes (Yau et al. 2015).

Future considerations

Multiple systemic inflammatory mechanisms are commonly shared by the pathogenesis of periodontal diseases and atherosclerotic disease, thereby strongly supporting the association between these two diseases (Herrera et al. 2020). Evidence is still, however, missing on the magnitude of the effect of CP upon CVD, and whether infection and systemic inflammation induced by periodontal diseases can actually trigger the development of atherosclerotic lesions or affect their progression in humans (Herrera et al. 2020). Future studies are required to study the role of bacterial invasion of atheromas and if viruses and fungi are also involved in this process. Studies regarding the impact of the oral microbiome on systemic disease via their interactions with, and alterations of, the gut microbiota can shed further light on the association of CP and systemic disease (Papapanou 2015). Specific research may possibly identify bacterial phenotypes possessing enhanced pathogenic potential, which can influence the composition of the oral microbiome. After entering the circulation, these phenotypes may display specific mechanisms of interaction with endothelium. The development of antimicrobial peptides, which selectively kill specific species of oral bacteria within the oral microbiome, can lead to new approaches in the prevention and modification of CVD (El Kholy et al. 2015; Papapanou 2015).

Specific systemic mediators of inflammation, and their relative importance compared with inflammatory mediators associated with other infections and systemic conditions, such as obesity, need to be evaluated (Schenkein et al. 2020). Recent studies have, however, indicated an independent and significant association between periodontal disease inflammation and atherosclerotic inflammation, which included robust adjustments for disease risk factors that are shared between periodontal disease and atherosclerotic diseases (Fifer et al. 2011; Subramanian et al. 2013). Another study utilizing advanced imaging methods has shown that objectively measured inflammation of the periodontium may predict major adverse cardiovascular events after correction for potential confounders and shared risk factors (Van Dyke et al. 2021).

Scientific evidence has not been able to demonstrate that adequate periodontal therapy is able to reduce the risk for CVD, or the incidence of CVD events in periodontitis patients (Herrera et al. 2020). However, available evidence suggests that periodontal therapy may have an impact on CVD events by means of reducing multiple cardiovascular risk factors (Orlandi et al. 2020). Prospective longitudinal studies incorporating incisive clinical trials to establish a possible causal relationship between CP and CVD, including metabolic disturbances, should be envisaged (Miyakawa et al. 2004; Schenkein & Loos 2013). The identification of more precise risk factors for CVD development, especially at an early age, can lead to enhanced quality of preventive care and treatment of patients at a later age (Amar et al. 2003). The development of prevention programs that focus on monitoring patients with CP in relation to risk factors for CVD development can be greatly beneficial.

REFERENCES

Ablij H, Meinders A. C-reactive protein: history and revival. *Eur J Intern Med*. 2002; 13:412–422.

Alaniz RC, Deatherage BL, Lara JC, Cookson BT. Membrane vesicles are immunogenic facsimiles of *Salmonella typhimurium* that potently activate dendritic cells, prime B and T cell responses, and stimulate protective immunity in vivo. *J Immunol*. 2007; 179:7692–7701.

Almerich-Silla JM, Montiel-Company JM, Pastor S et al. Oxidative stress parameters in saliva and its association with periodontal disease and types of bacteria. *Disease Markers*. 2015; 2015:653537.

Amar S, Gokce N, Morgan S et al. Periodontal disease is associated with brachial artery endothelial dysfunction and systemic inflammation. *Arterioscler Thromb Vasc Biol*. 2003; 23:1245–1249.

Amberger A, Maczek C, Jürgens G et al. Co-expression of ICAM-1, VCAM-1, ELAM-1 and Hsp60 in human arterial and venous endothelial cells in response to cytokines and oxidized low-density lipoproteins. *Cell Stress Chaperones*. 1997; 2:94–103.

Arimatsu K, Yamada H, Miyazawa H et al. Oral pathobiont induces systemic inflammation and metabolic changes associated with alteration of gut microbiota. *Sci Rep*. 2014; 4:4828. doi: 10.1038/srep04828.

Aslam R, Speck ER, Kim M et al. Platelet Toll-like receptor expression modulates lipopolysaccharide-induced thrombocytopenia and tumor necrosis factor-a production in vivo. *Blood*. 2006; 107:637–641.

Assinger A, Buchberger E, Laky M et al. Periodontopathogens induce soluble P-selectin release by endothelial cells and platelets. *Thromb Res*. 2011;127: e20–e26.

Bartova J, Sommerova P, Lyuya-Mi Y et al. Periodontitis as a risk factor of atherosclerosis. *J Immunol Res*. 2014; 2014:636893.

Baser U, Gamsiz-Isik H, Cifcibasi E, Ademoglu E, Yalcin F. Plasma and salivary total antioxidant capacity in healthy controls compared with aggressive and chronic periodontitis patients. *Saudi Med J*. 2015; 36:856–861.

Beveridge TJ. Structures of gram-negative cell walls and their derived membrane vesicles. *J Bacteriol*. 1999; 181:4725–4733.

Blair P, Rex S, Vitseva O et al. Stimulation of Toll-like receptor 2 in human platelets induces a thrombo-inflammatory response through activation of phosphoinositide 3-kinase. *Circ Res*. 2009; 104:346–354.

Blum MS, Toninelli E, Anderson JM et al. Cytoskeletal rearrangement mediates human microvascular endothelial tight junction modulation by cytokines. *Am J Physiol Heart Circ Physiol.* 1997; 273: H286–H294.

Brock GR, Butterworth CJ, Matthews JB, Chapple IL. Local and systemic total antioxidant capacity in periodontitis and health. *J Clin Periodontol.* 2004; 31(7):515–521.

Cai H, Harrison DG. Endothelial dysfunction in cardiovascular diseases. The role of oxidant stress. *Circ Res.* 2000; 87:840–844.

Carrion J, Scisci E, Miles B et al. Microbial carriage state of peripheral blood dendritic cells (DCs) in chronic periodontitis influences DC differentiation, atherogenic potential. *J Immunol.* 2012; 189(6):3178–3187.

Chapple ILC, Brock GR, Milward MR, Ling N, Matthews JB. Compromised GCF total antioxidant capacity in periodontitis: cause or effect? *J Clin Periodontol.* 2007; 34(2):103–110.

Chistiakov DA, Orekhov AN, Bobryshev YV. Links between atherosclerotic and periodontal disease. *Exp Mol Pathol.* 2016; 100(1):220–235.

Chiu B. Multiple infections in carotid atherosclerotic plaques. *Am Heart J.* 1999; 138(5 Pt 2): S534–S536.

Crea F, Libby P. Acute coronary syndromes: the way forward from mechanisms to precision treatment. *Circulation.* 2017; 136:1155–1166.

Dahiya P, Kamal R, Gupta R et al. Reactive oxygen species in periodontitis. *J Indian Soc Periodontol.* 2013; 17:411–416.

Davey M, Liu X, Ukai T et al. Bacterial fimbriae stimulate proinflammatory activation in the endothelium through distinct TLRs. *J Immunol.* 2008; 180:2187–2195.

Deanfield JE, Halcox JP, Rabelink TJ. Endothelial function and dysfunction. *Testing and clinical relevance. Circulation.* 2007; 115:1285–1295.

Deniset JF, Pierce GN. Heat shock proteins: mediators of atherosclerotic development. *Curr Drug Targets.* 2015; 16(8):816–826.

Devaraj S, Singh U, Jialal I. The evolving role of C-reactive protein in atherothrombosis. *Clin Chem.* 2009; 55:229–238.

Dorn BR, Harris LJ, Wujick CT, Vertucci FJ, Progulske-Fox A. Invasion of vascular cells in vitro by *Porphyromonas endodontalis. Int Endod J.* 2002;3 5:366–371.

Du Clos TW, Mold C. C-reactive protein: an activator of innate immunity and a modulator of adaptive immunity. *Immunol Res.* 2004; 30:261–277.

El Kholy K, Genco RJ, Van Dyke TE. Oral infections and cardiovascular disease. *Trends Endocrinol Metab.* 2015; 26(6):315–321.

Ellis TN, Kuehn MJ. Virulence and immunomodulatory roles of bacterial outer membrane vesicles. *Microbiol Mol Biol Rev.* 2010; 74:81–94.

Engström KK, Khalaf H, Kälvegren H, Bengtsson T. The role of *Porphyromonas gingivalis* gingipains in platelet activation and innate immune modulation. *Mol Oral Microbiol.* 2015; 30:62–73.

Falk E. Pathogenesis of atherosclerosis. *J Am Coll Cardiol.* 2006; 18;47(8 Suppl):C7–C12.

Fentoglua O, Bozkurtb FY. The bi-directional relationship between periodontal disease and hyperlipidemia. *Eur J Dent.* 2008; 2:142–149.

Fifer KM, Qadir S, Subramanian S et al. Positron emission tomography measurement of periodontal (18) ffluorodeoxyglucose uptake is associated with histologically determined carotid plaque inflammation. *J Am Coll Cardiol.* 2011; 57:971–976.

Foey AD, Crean S. Macrophage subset sensitivity to endotoxin tolerization by *Porphyromonas gingivalis. PLoS One.* 2013; 8:e67955.

Forner L, Larsen T, Kilian M, Holmstrup P. Incidence of bacteremia after chewing, tooth brushing and scaling in individuals with periodontal inflammation. *J Clin Periodontol.* 2006; 33(6):401–407.

Frede S, Berchner-Pfannschmidt U, Fandrey J. Regulation of hypoxia-inducible factors during inflammation. *Methods Enzymol.* 2007; 435:405–419.

Fredriksson M, Gustafsson A, Åsman B, Bergström K. Hyper-reactive peripheral neutrophils in adult periodontitis: generation of chemiluminescence and intracellular hydrogen peroxide after in vitro priming and FcγR-stimulation. *J Clin Periodontol.* 1998; 25(5):394–398.

Fuchs TA, Brill A, Duerschmied D et al. Extracellular DNA traps promote thrombosis. *Proc Natl Acad Sci U S A.* 2010; 107(36):15880–15885.

Gibson FC 3rd, Ukai T, Genco CA. Engagement of specific innate immune signaling pathways during *Porphyromonas gingivalis* induced chronic inflammation and atherosclerosis. *Front Biosci.* 2008; 13:2041–2059.

Giustarini D, Dalle-Donne I, Tsikas D, Rossi R. Oxidative stress and human diseases: origin, link, measurement, mechanisms, and biomarkers. *Crit Rev Clin Lab Sci.* 2009; 46:241–281.

Gölz L, Memmert S, Rath-Deschner B et al. LPS from *P. gingivalis* and hypoxia increases oxidative stress in periodontal ligament fibroblasts and contributes to periodontitis. *Mediators Inflamm.* 2014; 2014:986264.

Gomaraschi M, Ossoli A, Favari E et al. Inflammation impairs eNOS activation by HDL in patients with acute coronary syndrome. *Cardiovasc Res.* 2013; 100:36–43.

Gumus P, Huseyinalemdaroglu B, Buduneli N. The role of oxidative stress in the interaction of periodontal disease with systemic diseases or conditions. *Oxid Antioxid Med Sci.* 2016; 5:33–38.

Gurav AN. The implication of periodontitis in vascular endothelial dysfunction. *Eur J Clin Invest.* 2014; 44:1000–1009.

Hajishengallis G, Sojar H, Genco RJ, DeNardin E. Intracellular signaling and cytokine induction upon interactions of *Porphyromonas gingivalis* fimbriae with pattern-recognition receptors. *Immunol Investig.* 2004; 33:157–172.

Hansson GK. Inflammation, atherosclerosis, and coronary artery disease. *N Engl J Med.* 2005; 352:1685–1695.

Hayashi C, Gudino CV, Gibson FC 3rd, Genco CA. Review: Pathogen-induced inflammation at sites distant from oral infection: bacterial persistence and induction of cell specific innate immune inflammatory pathways. *Mol Oral Microbiol.* 2010; 25:305–316.

Herrera D, Molina A, Buhlin K, Klinge B. Periodontal diseases and association with atherosclerotic disease. *Periodontol 2000.* 2020; 83:66–89.

Higashi Y, Noma K, Yoshizumi M, Kihara Y. Endothelial function and oxidative stress in cardiovascular diseases. *Circ J.* 2009; 73:411–418.

Hirschfeld J, Kawai T. Oral inflammation and bacteremia: implications for chronic and acute systemic diseases involving major organs. *Cardiovasc Hematol Disord Drug Targets.* 2015; 15:70–84.

Humphrey LL, Fu R, Buckley DI, Freeman M, Helfand M. Periodontal disease and coronary heart disease incidence: a systematic review and meta-analysis. *J Gen Intern Med.* 2008; 23:2079–2086.

Huo Y, Ley KF. Role of platelets in the development of atherosclerosis. *Trends Cardiovasc Med.* 2004; 14:18–22.

Iacopino AM, Cutler CW. Pathophysiological relationships between periodontitis and systemic disease: recent concepts involving serum lipids. *J Periodontol.* 2000; 71(8):1375–1384.

Inagaki S, Onishi S, Kuramitsu HK, Sharma A. *Porphyromonas gingivalis* vesicles enhance attachment, and the leucine-rich repeat BspA protein is required for invasion of epithelial cells by "*Tannerella forsythia.*" *Infect Immun* 2006; 74:5023–5028.

Ishai AT, Osborne MT, El Kholy K et al. Periodontal disease associates with arterial inflammation via potentiation of a hematopoietic-arterial axis. *JACC Cardiovasc Imaging.* 2019; 12(11 Pt 1):2271–2273.

Jain S, Coats SR, Chang AM, Darveau RP. A novel class of lipoprotein lipase-sensitive molecules mediates Toll-like receptor 2 activation by *Porphyromonas gingivalis. Infect Immun.* 2013; 81:1277–1286.

Jia Y, Guo B, Yang W et al. Rho kinase mediates *Porphyromonas gingivalis* outer membrane vesicle-induced suppression of endothelial nitric oxide synthase through ERK1/2 and p38 MAPK. *Arch Oral Biol.* 2015; 60:488–495.

Kallio KAE, Buhlin K, Jauhiainen M et al. Lipopolysaccharide associates with pro-atherogenic lipoproteins in periodontitis patients. *Innate Immun.* 2008; 14(4):247–253.

Kaminski MM, Sauer SW, Klemke CD et al. Mitochondrial reactive oxygen species control T cell activation by regulating IL-2 and IL-4 expression: mechanism of ciprofloxacin-mediated immunosuppression. *J Immunol.* 2010; 184:4827–4841.

Kaparakis-Liaskos M, Ferrero RL. Immune modulation by bacterial outer membrane vesicles. *Nat Rev Immunol.* 2015; 15(6):375–387. doi: 10.1038/nri3837.

Khlgatian M, Nassar H, Chou H-H, Gibson FC, Genco CA. Fimbria-dependent activation of cell adhesion molecule expression in *Porphyromonas gingivalis*-infected endothelial cells. *Infect Immun.* 2002; 70:257–267

Kim YG, Park JH, Shaw MH et al. The cytosolic sensors Nod1 and Nod2 are critical for bacterial recognition and host defense after exposure to Toll like receptor ligands. *Immunity.* 2008; 28:246–257.

Kuehn MJ, Kesty NC. Bacterial outer membrane vesicles and the host-pathogen interaction. *Genes Dev.* 2005; 19:2645–2655.

Latsios G, Saetta A, Michalopoulos NV, Agapitos E, Patsouris E. Detection of cytomegalovirus, *Helicobacter pylori* and *Chlamydia pneumoniae* DNA in carotid atherosclerotic plaques by the polymerase chain reaction. *Acta Cardiol.* 2004; 59:652–657.

Li X, Iwai T, Nakamura H et al. An ultrastructural study of *Porphyromonas gingivalis*-induced platelet aggregation. *Thromb Res.* 2008; 122:810–819.

Li X, Tse HF, Yiu KH, Li LSW, Jin L. Effect of periodontal treatment on circulating CD341 cells and peripheral vascular endothelial function: a randomized controlled trial. *J Clin Periodontol.* 2011; 38:148–156.

Lönn J, Ljunggren S, Klarström-Engström K et al. Lipoprotein modifications by gingipains of *Porphyromonas gingivalis. J Periodont Res.* 2018; 53:403–413.

Lourbakos A, Yuan YP, Jenkins AL et al. Activation of protease-activated receptors by gingipains from *Porphyromonas gingivalis* leads to platelet aggregation: a new trait in microbial pathogenicity. *Blood.* 2001; 97:3790–3797.

Lu JL, Schmiege LM 3rd, Kuo L, Liao JC. Downregulation of endothelial constitutive nitric oxide synthase expression by lipopolysaccharide. *Biochem Biophys Res Commun.* 1996; 225:1–5.

Lu Q, Jin L. Human gingiva is another site of C-reactive protein formation. *J Clin Periodontol.* 2010; 37:789–796.

Lum H, Roebuck KA. Oxidant stress and endothelial cell dysfunction. *Am J Physiol Cell Physiol.* 2001; 280:C719–C741.

Maekawa T, Takahashi N, Tabeta K et al. Chronic oral infection with *Porphyromonas gingivalis* accelerates atheroma formation by shifting the lipid profile. *PLoS ONE.* 2011; 6(5):e20240.

Matthews JB, Wright HJ, Roberts A, Cooper PR, Chapple IL. Hyperactivity and reactivity of peripheral blood neutrophils in chronic periodontitis. *Clin Exp Immunol.* 2007; 147(2):255–264.

McNicol A, Israels SJ. Mechanisms of oral bacteria-induced platelet activation. *Can J Physiol Pharmacol.* 2010; 88:510–524.

Meier LA, Binstadt BA. The contribution of autoantibodies to inflammatory cardiovascular pathology. *Front Immunol.* 2018; 9:911.

Mesa F, Magán-Fernández A, Nikolic D et al. Periodontitis, blood lipids and lipoproteins. *Clin Lipidol.* 2014; 9(2):261–276.

Miyakawa H, Honma K, Qi M, Kuramitsu HK. Interaction of *Porphyromonas gingivalis* with low-density lipoproteins: implications for a role for periodontitis in atherosclerosis. *J Periodontal Res.* 2004; 39(1):1–9.

Mócsai A. Diverse novel functions of neutrophils in immunity, inflammation, and beyond. *J. Exp. Med.* 2013; 210(7):1283–1299.

Montorfano I, Becerra A, Cerro R et al. Oxidative stress mediates the conversion of endothelial cells into myofibroblasts via a TGF-β1 and TGF-β2-dependent pathway. *Lab Invest.* 2014; 94:1068–1082.

Morishita M, Ariyoshi W, Okinaga T et al. *A. actinomycetemcomitans* LPS enhances foam cell formation induced by LDL. *J Dent Res.* 2013; 92(3):241–246.

Mydel P, Takahashi Y, Yumoto H et al. Roles of the host oxidative immune response and bacterial antioxidant rubrerythrin during *Porphyromonas gingivalis* infection. *PLoS Pathog.* 2006; 2:e76. doi: 10.1371/journal.ppat.0020076.

Nakajima M, Arimatsu K, Kato T et al. Oral administration of *P. gingivalis* induces dysbiosis of gut microbiota and impaired barrier function leading to dissemination of enterobacteria to the liver. *PLoS One.* 2015; 10:e0134234.

Nakamura N, Yoshida M, Umeda M et al. Extended exposure of lipopolysaccharide fraction from *Porphyromonas gingivalis* facilitates mononuclear cell adhesion to vascular endothelium via Toll-like receptor-2 dependent mechanism. *Atherosclerosis.* 2008; 196:59–67.

Nakano K, Nemoto H, Nomura R et al. Detection of oral bacteria in cardiovascular specimens. *Oral Microbiol Immunol.* 2009; 264:4–8.

Nanci A, Bosshardt DD. Structure of periodontal tissues in health and disease. *Periodontology* 2000. 2006; 40:11–28.

Nurden AT. Platelets, inflammation and tissue regeneration. *Thromb Haemost.* 2011; 105: S13–S33.

Oorni K, Kovanen PT. Proteolysis of low-density lipoprotein particles by *Porphyromonas gingivalis* microorganisms: a novel biochemical link between periodontitis and cardiovascular diseases? *J Intern Med.* 2008; 263(5):553–557.

Orlandi M, Graziani F, D'Aiuto F. Periodontal therapy and cardiovascular risk. *Periodontol* 2000. 2020; 83:107–124.

Papapanou PN. Systemic effects of periodontitis: lessons learned from research on atherosclerotic vascular disease and adverse pregnancy outcomes. *Int Dent J.* 2015; 65:283–291.

Pertiwi KR, de Boer OJ, Mackaaij C et al. Extracellular traps derived from macrophages, mast cells, eosinophils and neutrophils are generated in a time-dependent manner during atherothrombosis. *J Pathol.* 2019; 247:505–512.

Pietiäinen M, Liljestrand JM, Kopra E, Pussinen PJ. Mediators between oral dysbiosis and cardiovascular diseases. *Eur J Oral Sci.* 2018; 126(Suppl 1):26–36.

Pober JS, Sessa WC. Evolving functions of endothelial cells in inflammation. *Nat Rev Immunol.* 2007; 7:803–815.

Prasad A, Zhu J, Halcox JP et al. Predisposition to atherosclerosis by infections: role of endothelial dysfunction. *Circulation.* 2002; 106(2):184–190.

Qi M, Miyakawa H, Kuramitsu HK. *Porphyromonas gingivalis* induces murine macrophage foam cell formation. *Microb Pathog.* 2003; 35:259–267.

Schenkein HA, Loos BG. Inflammatory mechanisms linking periodontal diseases to cardiovascular diseases. *J Clin Periodontol.* 2013; 40 (Suppl 14):S51–S69.

Schenkein HA, Papapanou PN, Genco RJ, Sanz M. Mechanisms underlying the association between periodontitis and atherosclerotic disease. *Periodontol* 2000. 2020; 83:90–106.

Sena LA, Chandel NS. Physiological roles of mitochondrial reactive oxygen species. *Mol Cell.* 2012; 48(2):158–167.

Shanahan CM, Weissberg PL. Smooth muscle cell heterogeneity: patterns of gene expression in vascular smooth muscle cells in vitro and in vivo. *Arterioscler Thromb Vasc Biol.* 1998; 18:333–338.

Shashkin PN, Brown GT, Ghosh A, Marathe GK, McIntyre TM. Lipopolysaccharide is a direct agonist for platelet RNA splicing. *J Immunol.* 2008; 181:3495–3502.

Singh RB, Mengi SA, Xu Y-J, Arneja AS, Dhalla NS. Pathogenesis of atherosclerosis: a multifactorial process. *Exp Clin Cardiol.* 2002; 7(1):40–53.

Slocum C, Kramer C, Genco CA. Immune dysregulation mediated by the oral microbiome: potential link to chronic inflammation and atherosclerosis (Review). *J Intern Med.* 2016; 280:114–128.

Smith S. Endothelial activation: the basis for the initial association between chronic periodontitis and cardiovascular disease. *Pak Oral Dent J.* 2018; 38(1):3–20.

Soult MC, Lonergan NE, Shah B et al. Outer membrane vesicles from pathogenic bacteria initiate an inflammatory response in human endothelial cells. *J Surg Res.* 2013; 184:458–466.

Sproston NR, Ashworth JJ. Role of C-reactive protein at sites of inflammation and infection. *Front Immunol.* 2018; 9:754.

Srisatjaluk R, Doyle RJ, Justus DE. Outer membrane vesicles of *Porphyromonas gingivalis* inhibit IFN-γ -mediated MHC class II expression by human vascular endothelial cells. *Microb Pathog.* 1999; 27:81–91.

Stoll G, Bendszus M. Inflammation and atherosclerosis: novel insights into plaque formation and destabilization. *Stroke.* 2006; 37(7):1923–1932.

Subramanian S, Emami H, Vucic E et al. High-dose atorvastatin reduces periodontal inflammation: a novel pleiotropic effect of statins. *J Am Coll Cardiol.* 2013; 62:2382–2391.

Tabas I. Macrophage death and defective inflammation resolution in atherosclerosis. *Nat Rev Immunol.* 2010; 10:36–46.

Tawakol A, Ishai A, Takx RA et al. Relation between resting amygdalar activity and cardiovascular events: a longitudinal and cohort study. *Lancet.* 2017; 389(10071):834–845.

Tomofuji T, Irie K, Sanbe T et al. Periodontitis and increase in circulating oxidative stress. *Jpn Dent Sci Rev.* 2009; 45:46–51.

Tonetti MS, Van Dyke TE, Working Group 1 of the Joint EFPaaPW. Periodontitis and atherosclerotic cardiovascular disease: consensus report of the Joint EFP/AAP Workshop on Periodontitis and Systemic Diseases. *J Clin Periodontol.* 2013; 40(Suppl 14):S24–S29.

Tousoulis D, Kampoli AM, Tentolouris C, Papageorgiou N, Stefanadis C. The role of nitric oxide on endothelial function. *Curr Vasc Pharmacol.* 2012; 10:4–18.

Tse K, Tse H, Sidney J, Sette A, Ley K. T cells in atherosclerosis. *Int Immunol.* 2013; 25(11):615–622.

Van Dyke TE, El Kholy K, Ishai A et al. Inflammation of the periodontium associates with risk of future cardiovascular events. *J Periodontol.* 2021; 92:348–358.

Van Dyke TE, van Winkelhoff AJ. Infection and inflammatory mechanisms. *J Clin Periodontol.* 2013; 40(Suppl 14):S1–S7.

Verma S, Lovren F, Dumont AS et al. Tetrahydrobiopterin improves endothelial function in human saphenous veins. *J Thorac Cardiovasc Surg.* 2000; 120:668–671.

Virmani R, Burke AP, Farb A, Kolodgie FD. Pathology of the vulnerable plaque. *J Am Coll Cardiol.* 2006; 47:C13–C18.

von Brühl ML, Stark K, Steinhart A et al. 2012. Monocytes, neutrophils, and platelets cooperate to initiate and propagate venous thrombosis in mice in vivo. *J Exp Med.* 2012; 209:819–835.

Wallin RP, Lundqvist A, Morec SH et al. Heat-shock proteins as activators of the innate immune system. *Trends Immunol.* 2002; 23:130–135.

Whitaker FJ, Thomas IS, Falk JA, Obebe A, Hammond BF. Effect of acetylsalicylic acid on aggregation of human platelets by *Porphyromonas gingivalis. Gen Dent.* 2007; 55:64–69.

Wick, G, Jakic B, Buszko M, Wick MC, Grundtmanet C. The role of heat-shock proteins in atherosclerosis. *Nat Rev Cardiol.* 2014; 11:516–529.

Wilson W, Taubert KA, Gewitz M et al. Prevention of infective endocarditis. *Circulation.* 2007; 116:1736–1754.

Wolf G. Free radical production and angiotensin. *Curr Hypertens Rep.* 2000; 2:167–173.

Xu Q, Schett G, Perschinka H et al. Serum soluble heat shock protein 60 is elevated in subjects with atherosclerosis in a general population. *Circulation.* 2000; 102:14–20.

Yau JW, Teoh H, Verma S. Endothelial cell control of thrombosis. *BMC Cardiovasc Disord.* 2015; 15:130–141.

Yoshimura F, Murakami Y, Nishikawa K, Hasegawa Y, Kawaminami S. Surface components of *Porphyromonas gingivalis. J Periodontal Res.* 2009; 44:1–12.

Yoshizumi M, Perrella MA, Burnett JC Jr, Lee ME. Tumor necrosis factor downregulates an endothelial nitric oxide synthase mRNA by shortening its half-life. *Circ Res.* 1993; 73(1):205–209.

Zelkha SA, Freilich RW, Amar S. Periodontal innate immune mechanisms relevant to atherosclerosis and obesity. *Periodontology 2000.* 2010; 54:207–221.

23.3 PERIODONTAL DISEASE AND CHRONIC OBSTRUCTIVE PULMONARY DISEASE

Steph Smith

Contents

Learning objectives

- Origins and determinants of the pulmonary microbiome.
- Knowledge of prevalence, risk, and genetic factors regarding the association between pulmonary disease (PD) and chronic obstructive pulmonary disease (COPD).
- Understanding the pathogenic mechanisms underlying the association of PD with COPD.
- Understanding the role of smoking in the association of PD and COPD.
- Knowledge of the pathogenic effects of smoking in PD and COPD.
- Knowledge of the effects of COPD medications on the periodontium.

Introduction

Chronic obstructive pulmonary disease (COPD) is a generic term that includes the pathological subtypes of emphysema, chronic bronchitis, and small airways disease. They are distinct entities, although they can occur together in the same patient (Ramesh et al. 2016). COPD is characterized by chronic obstruction to airflow due to narrowing of the airways, with the excess production of sputum resulting from chronic bronchitis and/or emphysema (Peter et al. 2013; Scannapieco 2014). It was predicted to have become the third most common cause of death and the fourth most important disease leading to disability by the year 2020 (Zhou et al. 2011).

The prevalence of COPD is between 5% and 25% in adults aged 40 years or older in various countries (Buist et al. 2007; Mannino et al. 2006). COPD prevalence is influenced by aging, location, smoking status, and occupational exposures (Buist et al. 2007). The prevalence of periodontal disease (PD) is higher among those with COPD compared to non-COPD controls (Lopez-de-Andrés et al. 2018). COPD patients present with a worse periodontal health status, including deeper periodontal pockets, higher levels of clinical attachment loss, more inflammation and gingival bleeding, worse oral hygiene, and a lower number of remaining teeth (Deo et al. 2009; Parashar et al. 2018; Shi et al. 2018).

A significant association has been suggested between poor periodontal health and an increase in the severity of reduced respiratory function in COPD (Peter et al. 2013; Scannapieco 2014; Winning et al. 2019; Zhou et al. 2011). However, other review studies have indicated only a weak association between COPD and PD (Azarpazhooh & Leake 2006).

A biologically plausible link, although speculative, may exist between PD and COPD involving a similar progressive chronic inflammatory mechanism (Fujita & Nakanishi 2007); however, no direct evidence for a causal relationship between PD and COPD has been shown (Garcia et al. 2001). Both these conditions share significant confounding risk factors, such as age, smoking, smoking status, and smoking pack-years (Hobbins et al. 2017; Mojon 2002; Peter et al. 2013; Shi et al. 2018). Second-hand smoke, childhood respiratory infections, air pollution, male sex, genetic factors, and heredity are among other risk factors for COPD (Azarpazhooh & Leake 2006; Scannapieco et al. 2003; Usher & Stockley 2013). Additional risk factors identified are diabetes and low socioeconomic status (Gershon et al. 2012; Usher & Stockley 2013). The most significant risk factor for COPD is prolonged cigarette smoking (Scannapieco 2014), this being dose-dependent, whereby "heavy" smokers may be twice as likely to be affected compared to "light" smokers (Usher & Stockley 2013). PD has also been suggested to be a significant and independent risk factor for COPD (Katancik et al. 2005; Scannapieco et al. 2001; Shi et al. 2018; Usher & Stockley 2013; Zeng et al. 2012).

The oral and pulmonary microbiome

The oropharyngeal microbiome has been suggested to be the likely origin of the pulmonary microbiome, this being ascribed to the topological continuity of the microbiome from the oral cavity to the lower respiratory tract (Mammen et al. 2020). In healthy people, variations in the lung microbiome are dependent on the steady transmission of bacteria from the more abundant oropharynx reservoir microbiome, followed by entry of bacteria into the lungs via regular micro-aspirations of the oral microbiome (Dickson et al. 2017; Mammen et al. 2020). However, the lung microbiome is of much less abundance, with less diversity and representation compared to the oral microbiome, this being due to the transient, but not resident, passage of oral microbiome–related flora that are subsequently removed by lung defense mechanisms (Charlson et al. 2011; Huffnagle et al. 2016). Certain bacteria may also be represented in higher abundance in the airway microbiome, likely due to a selective advantage in replication among particular bacteria taxa in the lung microenvironment (Morris et al. 2013). This can be ascribed to variations in innate immunity, adaptive immunity, and physical anatomic properties of the lung, as well as bacterial metabolic processes, leading to specific bacterial taxa thriving in a particular lung region (Sze et al. 2012). In health, therefore, the composition of the oral microbiome may thus influence the lung microbiome. However, oral microbiome dysbiosis can lead to translocation of bacteria and their metabolites, resulting in modulation of the host immune response, and thus determine the outcomes of host–pathogen interactions within the lung (Kumar 2017; Mammen et al. 2020).

Pathogenic mechanisms of the association between periodontal disease and chronic obstructive pulmonary disease (see Figure 23.3.1)

Genetic factors

Smoking is a widely accepted risk factor for developing COPD; however, COPD only affects a minority of smokers, whereby there is an implication that intrinsic and genetic factors may play a greater role than the effect of smoking (Yu et al 2016). A complex interaction of environmental and genetic factors may increase the risk of susceptibility to COPD in patients with PD (Azarpazhooh & Leake 2006; Laine et al. 2012; Scannapieco et al. 2003; Yu et al. 2016). Toll-like receptors (TLRs) form a bridge between innate and acquired immunity, and play a role in pathogenesis in both PD and COPD (Yu et al. 2016). TLRs recognize pathogen-associated molecular patterns (PAMPs) such as lipopolysaccharide (LPS) in Gram-negative bacteria (Yoshimura et al. 2002). The interaction of TLR4 with LPS induces the production of inflammatory cytokines such as interleukin (IL)-1, IL-6, and tumor necrosis factor alpha (TNF-α), which mediate innate immune and inflammatory responses, resulting in destruction of the periodontium

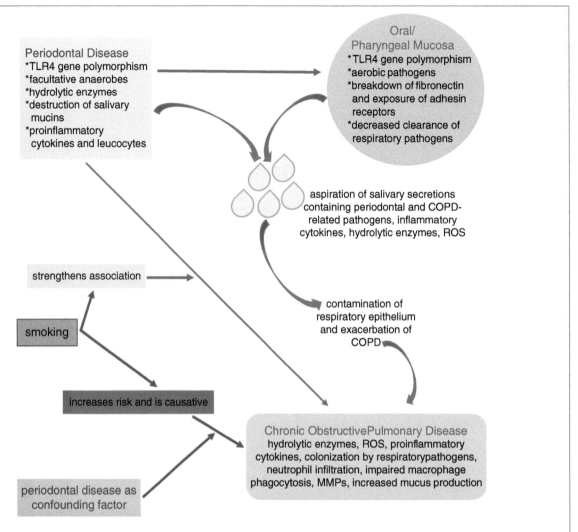

Figure 23.3.1 Periodontitis and chronic obstructive pulmonary disease. Periodontal bacteria and components of periodontal disease affect the oral mucosa and respiratory bacterial attachment. As a result, salivary excretions containing periodontal and chronic obstructive pulmonary disease (COPD)-related pathogens, inflammatory cytokines, hydrolytic enzymes, and reactive oxygen species (ROS) are aspirated and contaminate respiratory epithelium and also cause exacerbation of existing COPD. Periodontal disease is a risk factor for COPD development, and smoking strengthens this association. Smoking is a major causative factor of COPD and periodontal disease is considered as a confounding factor in the association between smoking and COPD. Courtesy of Dr. Steph Smith.

(Yu et al. 2016). The TLR4 rs11536889 C allele is associated with moderate and severe PD (Fukusaki et al. 2007). LPS increases TLR4 mRNA expression in respiratory epithelium, which is associated with the severity of COPD (MacRedmond et al. 2007; Pace et al. 2011). TLR4 gene rs1927907 polymorphism also has a common role in the pathophysiology of PD and COPD (Mammen et al. 2020). TLR4 gene polymorphism may thus partly explain the susceptibility to COPD (MacRedmond et al. 2007; Yu et al. 2016).

Exacerbation of chronic obstructive pulmonary disease

COPD patients experience episodes of exacerbations, including cough, fever, and the elevated production of sputum,

causing the impairment of mucociliary clearance. This impairment increases the host's vulnerability to infection, whereby viral or bacterial microorganisms can cause exacerbations (Mackay & Hurst 2013; Wedzicha et al. 2014). Viral and bacterial infections are not only responsible for acute exacerbations of COPD, but also amplify and perpetuate already established chronic inflammation in stable COPD (Brusselle et al. 2011). Periodontopathogens and PD-related inflammatory cytokines induce systemic inflammation (Mojon 2002; Scannapieco et al. 2003), and thus potentially influence the course of COPD by indirectly contributing to induced inflammatory alterations of the respiratory epithelium characterized in COPD (Bansal et al. 2013; Peter et al. 2013). This may be achieved through dental plaque serving as a reservoir for respiratory pathogens, or by periodontopathogens and their products exacerbating airway inflammation (Brook & Frazier 2003; Paju & Scannapieco 2007; Peter et al. 2013; Wang et al. 2009).

Bacterial etiology of periodontal disease and chronic obstructive pulmonary disease

The majority of pulmonary diseases are caused by aerobic bacteria that are found in the oral flora (Morris & Sewell 1994). These include *Pseudomonas aeruginosa*, *Haemophilus influenzae*, *Streptococcus pneumoniae*, *Moraxella catarrhalis*, and *Staphylococcus aureus* (Domenech et al. 2013). Oral bacteria can influence the pathogenicity of respiratory pathogens involved in lower airway infection (Li et al. 2014; Pan et al. 2009). Facultative anaerobes responsible for PD, such as *Aggregatibacter actinomycetemcomitans*, *Fusobacterium nucleatum*, *P. aeruginosa*, *Porphyromonas gingivalis*, and *Prevotella* species, have been isolated from infected lungs (Ramesh et al. 2016; Taylor et al. 1994). *Eikenella corrodens*, *F. necrophorum*, *Bacteroides gracilus*, *B. oralis*, and *B. buccae* have also been identified (Chen et al. 1995). Exacerbations of COPD may however be the result of a more polymicrobial etiology (Scannapieco 2014). For example, *P. gingivalis* has been detected with *P. aeruginosa* in the trachea of patients with acute exacerbations of COPD (Tan et al. 2014). *P. gingivalis* promotes the ability of *P. aeruginosa* to invade respiratory epithelial cells and modulates the apoptosis-inducing ability of *P. aeruginosa* (Li et al. 2014). Normally, rapid apoptosis of infected epithelial cells leads to effective clearance of *P. aeruginosa* (Cannon et al. 2003); however, the co-invasion with both bacteria leads to a transient inhibition of apoptosis. This then provides bacteria with an intracellular niche, including the opportunity to proliferate and establish infection (Hajishengallis 2015). It is thus possible that the accumulation of PD-associated bacteria may increase the risk for COPD in susceptible individuals, by directly inducing airway injury, including the subsequent exacerbation and progression of COPD (Peter et al. 2013; Scannapieco 2014).

Bacteria, inflammation, and mucosal surfaces

Lower respiratory tract infections, including the exacerbation of COPD, depend on the initial colonization of microbial pathogens on oral/pharyngeal surfaces (Peter et al. 2013). Proteolytic periodontopathogens as well as various hydrolytic enzymes contained in saliva cause mucosal surface alterations, which include breakdown of fibronectin from epithelial cell surfaces (Wikström & Linde 1986; Zambon et al. 1985). Consequently, exposure of adhesin receptors on mucosal epithelium fosters increased adhesion and colonization by respiratory bacterial pathogens (Gibbons et al. 1990). Hydrolytic enzymes from periodontopathogens may alter or destroy protective domains of salivary mucins (Scannapieco 1994), thereby decreasing the ability of mucins to bind and clear respiratory pathogens, such as *H. influenzae*, from the oral cavity (Davies et al. 1995). Inflammatory cytokines released from cells of the

diseased periodontium and leucocytes can alter the expression of cell adhesion molecules on epithelial cell surfaces, thereby inducing the adherence of respiratory pathogens (Reddi et al. 1996). COPD-related pathogens, together with PD-associated bacteria, are then shed into the salivary secretions. Inflammatory products of PD, including hydrolytic enzymes and proinflammatory cytokines, are also released into the saliva (Peter et al. 2013; Ramesh et al. 2016).

These salivary secretion contents can contaminate the distal portions of the respiratory tree, inducing inflammatory alterations of the respiratory epithelium (Peter et al. 2013). This includes the release of hydrolytic enzymes and reactive oxygen species (ROS), resulting in damaged epithelium becoming more susceptible to colonization by respiratory pathogens (Peter et al. 2013; Ramesh et al. 2016; Scannapieco 1999). Contamination by bacteria and their products induces the release of proinflammatory cytokines, such as IL-8, resulting in recruitment and infiltration of neutrophils into the respiratory epithelium. *A. actinomycetemcomitans* is a stronger stimulant in the production of proinflammatory cytokines from epithelial cells when compared with *P. gingivalis* (Scannapieco 1999; Wang et al. 2009). Thus, in the initiation of a host inflammatory response in the lungs, whereby a bacterial challenge from PD is involved, PD can contribute to the exacerbation of COPD (Peter et al. 2013).

Association between smoking, periodontal disease, and chronic obstructive pulmonary disease

Smoking is a major risk and causative factor in the development of COPD (Geijer et al. 2006; Harland et al. 2018; Lokke et al. 2006), with around 80% of COPD patients being current or previous smokers (Mannino et al. 2006). Cigarette smoke (CS) contains chemical components that are in either gaseous or particulate phase (Witschi 2005). These components have cytotoxic, mutagenic, carcinogenic, or antigenic properties (Ding et al. 2008). Passive or active inhalation of CS results in the rapid dissolution of especially particulate phase substances into oral and respiratory epithelium, including fluids and the systemic uptake thereof (Lee et al. 2012).

Smoking compromises epithelial-mediated innate immunity by stimulating mucin release by goblet cells and has a destructive effect on ciliated cells. Smoking also suppresses beta-defensin-2 production, an antimicrobial peptide secreted by gingival epithelial cells (Håkansson et al. 1996; Khair et al. 1996; Lee et al. 2012). Alterations in innate defenses induced by inhalational exposure to tobacco smoke allow particular pathogenic bacteria and other commensal organisms from the micro-aspirated oral microbiome to persevere and flourish in the airways. In an attempt to clear pathogenic bacteria, aberrant signaling occurs when bacteria interact via pathogen recognition receptors on airway epithelial and immune cells, leading to chronic inflammation (Mammen et al. 2020). Subsequently, the inflammation provokes further derangements in innate immune mechanisms, causing lung epithelium to be more susceptible to the colonization of respiratory pathogens, resulting in bacterial persistence and proliferation (Håkansson et al. 1996; Khair et al. 1996; Lee et al. 2012). Consequently, this leads to a vicious cycle of successive rounds of increasing microbiome dysbiosis with subsequent anomalous inflammation, even after the cessation of a primary insult such as smoking (Mammen & Sethi 2016, 2017). Studies have also revealed the role of new strains of bacterial acquisition in the etiology of exacerbations of COPD (Sethi & Murphy 2008).

Increased tissue destruction is observed whereby CS activates innate immune cells, including epithelial cells, neutrophils, and macrophages, leading to activation of adaptive immune responses. This includes T-helper (Th1 and Th17) CD4+ T cells, CD8+ cytotoxicity, and B-cell responses (Brusselle et al. 2011; Hobbins et al. 2017; Johanssen et al. 2014), as well as the induction of proinflammatory cytokine release, together with destructive mediators. This includes C-reactive protein (CRP), IL-8, TNF-α, and matrix metalloproteinases (MMPs) (Barnes & Celli 2009; Sethi & Murphy 2008; Sinden & Stockley 2010).

Macrophages are the first line of cellular defense against smoking (Laskin et al. 2011). CS exposure causes an increase in the number of, as well as morphological changes and impaired phagocytic function of, alveolar macrophages (Arnson et al. 2010; Takeuchi et al. 2001). Following toxicant exposure, the increased generation of ROS, IL-1, TNFα, proteases, and bioactive lipids by alveolar M1 macrophage phenotypes can induce or amplify tissue injury (Laskin et al. 2011). TNFα and IL-1 up-regulate adhesion molecule and chemokine production by endothelium, thereby promoting accumulation of inflammatory cells in lung tissues. TNFα and IL-1 also induce the release of proinflammatory mediators including IL-6, platelet-activating factor, prostaglandins, and MMPs (Laskin et al. 2011). The production of cysteine proteinases and MMPs degrades the supporting matrix of lung parenchyma, contributing to emphysema (Shapiro 1999). Macrophages exhibit increased levels of IL-4 and IL-13 secretion, thereby worsening mucus production (Byers & Holtzman 2011). In chronic lung diseases, such as COPD and idiopathic pulmonary fibrosis, a skewing toward M2 macrophage phenotype has been described (Laskin et al. 2011). Neutrophils in smoker COPD patients show enhanced proteolytic enzyme activity from MMPs, neutrophil elastase, cathepsin G, and protease-3, as well as increased ROS production, which destroys the extracellular matrix, causing direct collateral lung tissue damage (Arnson et al. 2010; Noguera et al. 2001; Usher & Stockley 2013).

Host cells in COPD patients are exposed to large amounts of oxidants and free radicals contained in CS, air pollutants, and bacteria (Neofytou et al. 2012; Usher & Stockley 2013). Oxidative stress occurs in both COPD and PD and is thus implicated in the pathophysiology of both (Usher & Stockley 2013). Endogenous producers of ROS in the lungs are macrophages and neutrophils responding to these environmental insults, bacteria, and their products (Laskin et al. 2011;

Loukides et al. 2011; Weiss 1989). ROS damage the tissues of the lungs, making them more susceptible to proteolytic degradation (Usher & Stockley 2013). They also act as triggers for the further generation of ROS to be released from respiratory, immune, and inflammatory cells, thereby amplifying the inflammatory response and tissue injury (Laskin et al. 2011; Usher & Stockley 2013).

Smoking is also an important risk factor for the development of PD (Harland et al. 2018; Moimaz et al. 2009; Ojima et al. 2006). PD is also recognized as a predominantly chronic neutrophilic inflammatory disorder, with neutrophil granules and enzymes (such as elastase and MMPs), as well as ROS production implicated in the pathogenesis of the disease (Ramesh et al. 2016; Stockley 2002; Trivedi et al. 2015). Patients with PD have more systemic inflammation than those who are healthy (Fredriksson et al. 1999; Noack et al. 2001). However, COPD exacerbation is also associated with elevated systemic inflammation (Groenewegen et al. 2008). Therefore, the combination of PD and smoking may have an interactive effect during the development and exacerbation of COPD, whereby PD is associated with even greater systemic inflammation in smokers with COPD (Zeng et al. 2012). A significant association between smoking and COPD is seen in patients with PD, and a weaker association in those without PD (Harland et al. 2018; Zeng et al. 2012). It is thus suggested that PD strengthens the association between smoking and COPD through systemic inflammation (Harland et al. 2018). Furthermore, PD is more strongly associated with smoking, and less strongly with COPD (Harland et al. 2018), therefore suggesting that the role of smoking in the etiology of both PD and COPD is an important confounding factor in the relationship between PD and COPD (Bergström et al. 2013; Holtfreter et al. 2013; Hyman & Reid 2004).

Medications and chronic obstructive pulmonary disease

Medications used for COPD treatment may contribute to worse periodontal health in COPD patients. Glucocorticoid, salbutamol, and tiotropium bromide are commonly used drugs. The side effects of these drugs include inhibition of bone formation and suppression of calcium absorption, leading to osteoporosis and loss of alveolar bone (Bouvard et al. 2013; Sousa et al, 2017). Salbutamol and tiotropium bromide may cause the reduction of salivary flow and dry mouth, thereby negatively influencing periodontal health (Keating 2012; Ryberg & Johansson 1995).

Future considerations

Randomized controlled interventional studies are needed to validate the relationship between PD, smoking, and COPD (Harland et al. 2018; Peter et al. 2013). Microbiome studies of lower airway samples from patients with COPD exacerbations may reveal the presence of specific oral species along with expected pathogens (Scannapieco 2014). Other research possibilities may involve therapeutic alterations of the lung microbiome by changing the oral microbiome. This may include the addition of beneficial microbiota or depletion of harmful ones (Mammen et al. 2020). The

mechanism of periodontal therapy and the effects thereof on COPD, which may include decreasing systemic and local inflammatory stimuli as well as the frequency of exacerbations, should be further studied (Mammen et al. 2020; Shi et al. 2018).

REFERENCES

Arnson Y, Shoenfeld Y, Amital H. Effects of tobacco smoke on immunity, inflammation and autoimmunity. *J Autoimmun.* 2010; 34(3): J258–J265

Azarpazhooh A, Leake JL. Systematic review of the association between respiratory diseases and oral health. *J Periodontol.* 2006; 77(9):1465–1482.

Bansal M, Khatri M, Taneja V. Potential role of periodontal infection in respiratory diseases—a review. *J Med Life.* 2013; 6(3):244–248.

Barnes PJ, Celli BR. Systemic manifestations and comorbidities of COPD. *Eur Respir J.* 2009; 33(5):1165–1185.

Bergström J, Cederlund K, Dahlén B et al. Dental health in smokers with and without COPD. *PLoS One.* 2013; 8(3):e59492. doi: 10.1371/journal.pone.0059492.

Bouvard B, Gallois Y, Legrand E, Audran M, Chappard D. Glucocorticoids reduce alveolar and trabecular bone in mice. *Joint Bone Spine.* 2013; 80:77–81.

Brook I, Frazier HE. Immune response to *Fusobacterium nucleatum* and *Prevotella intermedia* in the sputum of patients with acute exacerbation of chronic bronchitis. *Chest.* 2003; 124(3):832–833.

Brusselle GG, Joos GF, Bracke KR. New insights into the immunology of chronic obstructive pulmonary disease. *Lancet.* 2011; 378(9795):1015–1026.

Buist AS, McBurnie MA, Vollmer WM et al. International variation in the prevalence of COPD (the BOLD Study): a population-based prevalence study. *Lancet.* 2007; 370(9589):741–750.

Byers DE, Holtzman MJ. Alternatively activated macrophages and airway disease. *Chest.* 2011; 140(3):768–774.

Cannon CL, Kowalski MP, Stopak KS, Pier GB. *Pseudomonas aeruginosa*-induced apoptosis is defective in respiratory epithelial cells expressing mutant cystic fibrosis transmembrane conductance regulator. *Am J Respir Cell Mol Biol.* 2003; 29(2):188–197.

Charlson ES, Bittinger K, Haas AR et al. Topographical continuity of bacterial populations in the healthy human respiratory tract. *Am J Respir Crit Care Med.* 2011; 184(8):957–963.

Chen AC, Liu CC, Yao WJ, Chen CT, Wang JY. *Actinobacillus actinomycetemcomitans* pneumonia with chest wall and subphrenic abscess. *Scand J Infect Dis.* 1995; 27(3):289–290.

Davies J, Carlstedt I, Nilsson AK et al. Binding of *Haemophilus influenzae* to purified mucins from the human respiratory tract. *Infect Immun.* 1995; 63(7):2485–2492.

Deo V, Bhongade ML, Ansari S, Chavan RS. Periodontitis as a potential risk factor for chronic obstructive pulmonary disease: a retrospective study. *Indian J Dent Res.* 2009;20(4):466–470.

Dickson RP, Erb-Downward JR, Freeman CM et al. Bacterial topography of the healthy human lower respiratory tract. *MBio.* 2017; 8(1):e02287-16.

Ding YS, Zhang L, Jain RB et al. Levels of tobacco-specific nitrosamines and polycyclic aromatic hydrocarbons in mainstream smoke from different tobacco varieties. *Cancer Epidemiol Biomarkers Prev.* 2008; 17(12):3366–3371.

Domenech A, Puig C, Marti S et al. Infectious etiology of acute exacerbations in severe COPD patients. *J Infect.* 2013; 67(6):516–523.

Fredriksson MI, Figueredo CM, Gustafsson A, Bergstrom KG, Asman BE. Effect of periodontitis and smoking on blood leukocytes and acute-phase proteins. *J Periodontol.* 1999; 70(11):1355–1360.

Fujita M, Nakanishi Y. The pathogenesis of COPD: lessons learned from in vivo animal models. *Med Sci Monit.* 2007; 13(2):19–24.

Fukusaki T, Ohara N, Hara Y, Yoshimura A, Yoshiura K. Evidence for association between a Toll-like receptor 4 gene polymorphism and moderate/severe periodontitis in the Japanese population. *J Periodontal Res.* 2007; 42(6):541–545.

Garcia RI, Nunn ME, Vokonas PS. Epidemiological associations between periodontal diseases and chronic obstructive pulmonary disease. *Ann Periodontol.* 2001; 6(1):71–77.

Geijer RM, Sachs AP, Verheij TJ et al. Incidence and determinants of moderate COPD (GOLD II) in male smokers aged 40–65 years: 5-year follow up. *Br J Gen Pract.* 2006; 56(530):656–661.

Gershon AS, Dolmage TE, Stephenson A, Jackson B. Chronic obstructive pulmonary disease and socioeconomic status: a systematic review. *COPD.* 2012; 9:216–226.

Gibbons RJ, Hay DI, Childs WC, Davis G. Role of cryptic receptors (cryptitopes) in bacterial adhesion to oral surfaces. *Arch Oral Biol.* 1990; 35(Suppl):S107–S114.

Groenewegen KH, Postma DS, Hop WC et al. Increased systemic inflammation is a risk factor for COPD exacerbations. *Chest.* 2008; 133(2):350–357.

Hajishengallis G. Periodontitis: from microbial immune subversion to systemic inflammation. *Nat Rev Immunol.* 2015; 15(1):30–44.

Håkansson A, Carlstedt I, Davies J et al. Aspects on the interactions of *Streptococcus pneumoniae* and *Haemophilus influenzae* with human respiratory tract mucosa. *Am J Resp Crit Care Med.* 1996; 154: S187–S191.

Harland J, Furuta M, Takeuchi K, Tanaka S, Yamashita Y. Periodontitis modifies the association between smoking and chronic obstructive pulmonary disease in Japanese men. *J Oral Sci.* 2018; 60(2):226–231.

Hobbins S, Chappl IL, Sapey E, Stockley RA. Is periodontitis a comorbidity of COPD or can associations be explained by shared risk factors/behaviors? *Int J Chron Obstruct Pulmon Dis.* 2017; 12:1339–1349. doi: 10.2147/COPD.S127802.

Holtfreter B, Richter S, Kocher T et al. Periodontitis is related to lung volumes and airflow limitation: a cross-sectional study. *Eur Respir J.* 2013; 42(6):1524–1535.

Huffnagle GB, Dickson RP, Lukacs NW. The respiratory tract microbiome and lung inflammation: a two-way street. *Mucosal Immunol.* 2016; 10(2):299–306.

Hyman JJ, Reid BC. Cigarette smoking, periodontal disease: and chronic obstructive pulmonary disease. *J Periodontol.* 2004; 75(1):9–15.

Johannsen A, Susin C, Gustafsson A. Smoking and inflammation: evidence for a synergistic role in chronic disease. *Periodontol* 2000. 2014; 64(1):111–126.

Katancik JA, Kritchevsky S, Weyant RJ et al. Periodontitis and airway obstruction. *J Periodontol.* 2005; 76(Suppl 11):2161–2167.

Keating GM. Tiotropium bromide inhalation powder: a review of its use in the management of chronic obstructive pulmonary disease. *Drugs.* 2012; 72:273–300.

Khair OA, Davies RJ, Devalia JL. Bacterial induced release of inflammatory mediators by bronchial epithelial cells. *Eur Respir J.* 1996; 9(9):1913–1922.

Kumar PS. From focal sepsis to periodontal medicine: a century of exploring the role of the oral microbiome in systemic disease. *J Physiol.* 2017; 595(2):465–476.

Laine ML, Crielaard W, Loos BG. Genetic susceptibility to periodontitis. *Periodontol* 2000. 2012; 58(1):37–68.

Laskin DL, Sunil VR, Gardner CR, Laskin JD. Macrophages and tissue injury: agents of defense or destruction? *Annu Rev Pharmacol Toxicol.* 2011; 51:267–288.

Lee J, Taneja V, Vassallo R. Cigarette smoking and inflammation: cellular and molecular mechanisms. *J Dent Res.* 2012; 91(2):142–149.

Li Q, Pan C, Teng D et al. *Porphyromonas gingivalis* modulates *Pseudomonas aeruginosa*-induced apoptosis of respiratory epithelial cells through the STAT3 signaling pathway. *Microbes Infect.* 2014; 16(1):17–27.

Lokke A, Lange P, Scharling H, Fabricius P, Vestbo J. Developing COPD: a 25 year follow up study of the general population. *Thorax.* 2006; 61(11):935–939.

Lopez-de-Andrés A, Vazquez-Vazquez L, Martinez-Huedo MA et al. Is COPD associated with periodontal disease? A population-based study in Spain. *Int J Chron Obstruct Pulmon Dis.* 2018; 13:3435–3445.

Loukides S, Bakakos P, Kostikas K. Oxidative stress in patients with COPD. *Curr Drug Targets.* 2011; 12(4):469–477.

Mackay AJ, Hurst JR. COPD exacerbations: causes, prevention, and treatment. *Immunol Allergy Clin North Am.* 2013; 33(1):95–115.

MacRedmond RE, Greene CM, Dorscheid DR, McElvaney NG, O'Neill SJ. Epithelial expression of TLR4 is modulated in COPD and by steroids, salmeterol and cigarette smoke. *Respir Res.* 2007; 8:84. doi: 10.1186/1465-9921-8-84.

Mammen MJ, Scannapieco FA, Sethi S . Oral-lung microbiome interactions in lung diseases. *Periodontol* 2000. 2020; 83:234–241.

Mammen MJ, Sethi S. COPD and the microbiome. *Respirology.* 2016; 21(4):590–599.

Mammen M, Sethi S. Microbiome in chronic lung diseases. *Barcelona Respir Netw Rev.* 2017; 3:102–120.

Mannino DM, Watt G, Hole D et al. The natural history of chronic obstructive pulmonary disease. *Eur Respir J.* 2006; 27(3):627–643.

Moimaz SA, Zina LG, Saliba O, Garbin CA. Smoking and periodontal disease: clinical evidence for an association. *Oral Health Prev Dent.* 2009; 7(4):369–376.

Mojon P. Oral health and respiratory infection. *J Can Dent Assoc.* 2002; 68(6):340–345.

Morris A, Beck JM, Schloss PD et al. Comparison of the respiratory microbiome in healthy nonsmokers and smokers. *Am J Respir Crit Care Med.* 2013; 187(10):1067–1075.

Morris JF, Sewell DL. Necrotizing pneumonia caused by mixed infection with *Actinobacillus actinomycetemcomitans* and *Actinomyces israelii*: Case report and review. *Clin Infect Dis.* 1994; 18(3):450–452.

Neofytou E, Tzortzaki EG, Chatziantoniou A, Siafakas NM. DNA damage due to oxidative stress in chronic obstructive pulmonary disease (COPD). *Int J Mol Sci.* 2012; 3(12):16853–16864.

Noack B, Genco RJ, Trevisan M et al. Periodontal infections contribute to elevated systemic C-reactive protein level. *J Periodontol.* 2001; 72(9):1221–1227.

Noguera A, Batle S, Miralles C et al. Enhanced neutrophil response in chronic obstructive pulmonary disease. *Thorax.* 2001; 56(6):432–437.

Ojima M, Hanioka T, Tanaka K, Inoshita E, Aoyama H. Relationship between smoking status and periodontal conditions: findings from national databases in Japan. *J Periodontal Res.* 2006; 41(6):573–579.

Pace E, Giarratano A, Ferraro M et al. TLR4 upregulation underpins airway neutrophilia in smokers with chronic obstructive pulmonary disease and acute respiratory failure. *Hum Immunol.* 2011; 72(1):54–62.

Paju S, Scannapieco FA. Oral biofilms, periodontitis and pulmonary infections. *Oral Dis.* 2007; 13(6):508–512.

Pan Y, Teng D, Burke AC, Haase EM, Scannapieco FA. Oral bacteria modulate invasion and induction of apoptosis in HEp-2 cells by *Pseudomonas aeruginosa*. *Microb Pathog.* 2009; 46(2):73–79.

Parashar P, Parashar A, Saraswat N et al. Relationship between respiratory and periodontal health in adults: a case-control study. *J Int Soc Prev Community Dent.* 2018; 8(6):560 564.

Peter KP, Mute BR, Doiphode SS et al. Association between periodontal disease and chronic obstructive pulmonary disease: a reality or just a dogma? *J Periodontol.* 2013; 84(12):1717–1723.

Ramesh A, Varghese SS, Jayakumar ND, Malaiappan S. Chronic obstructive pulmonary disease and periodontitis – unwinding their linking mechanisms. *J Oral Biosci.* 2016; 58(1):23–26.

Reddi K, Wilson M, Nair S, Poole S, Henderson B. Comparison of the pro-inflammatory cytokine stimulating activity of the surface-associated proteins of periodontopathic bacteria. *J Periodont Res.* 1996; 31(2):120–130.

Ryberg M, Johansson I. The effects of long-term treatment with salmeterol and salbutamol on the flow rate and composition of whole saliva in the rat. *Arch Oral Biol.* 1995; 40:187–191.

Scannapieco FA. Saliva-bacterium interactions in oral microbial ecology. *Crit Rev Oral Biol Med.* 1994; 5(3–4):203–248.

Scannapieco FA. Role of oral bacteria in respiratory infection. *J Periodontol.* 1999; 70(7):793 802.

Scannapieco FA. Individuals with chronic obstructive pulmonary disease (COPD) may be more likely to have more severe periodontal disease than individuals without COPD. *J Evid Base Dent Pract.* 2014; 14(2):79–81.

Scannapieco FA, Bush RB, Paju S. Association between periodontal diseases and risk for nosocomial bacterial pneumonia and chronic obstructive pulmonary disease: a systematic review. *Ann Periodontol.* 2003; 8(1):54–69.

Scannapieco FA, Wang B, Shiau HJ. Oral bacteria and respiratory infection: effects on respiratory pathogen adhesion and epithelial cell proinflammatory cytokine production. *Ann Periodontol.* 2001; 6(1):78–86.

Sethi S, Murphy TF. Infection in the pathogenesis and course of chronic obstructive pulmonary disease. *N Engl J Med.* 2008; 359(22):2355–2365.

Shapiro SD. The macrophage in chronic obstructive pulmonary disease. *Am J Respir Crit Care Med.* 1999; 160(5 Pt 2):S29–S32.

Shi Q, Zhang B, Xing H et al. Patients with chronic obstructive pulmonary disease suffer from worse periodontal health—evidence from a meta-analysis. *Front Physiol.* 2018; 9:33. doi: 10.3389/fphys.2018.00033.

Sinden NJ, Stockley RA. Systemic inflammation and comorbidity in COPD: a result of "overspill" of inflammatory mediators from the lungs? *Review of the evidence. Thorax.* 2010; 65(10):930–936.

Sousa LH, Moura EV, Queiroz AL et al. Effects of glucocorticoid-induced osteoporosis on bone tissue of rats with experimental periodontitis. *Arch Oral Biol.* 2017; 77:55–61.

Stockley RA. Neutrophils and the pathogenesis of COPD. *Chest.* 2002; 121(Suppl 5): 151S–155S.

Sze MA, Dimitriu PA, Hayashi S et al. The lung tissue microbiome in chronic obstructive pulmonary disease. *Am J Respir Crit Care Med.* 2012; 185(10):1073–1080.

Takeuchi M, Nagai S, Nakajima A et al. Inhibition of lung natural killer cell activity by smoking: the role of alveolar macrophages. *Respiration.* 2001; 68(3):262–267.

Tan L, Wang H, Li C, Pan Y. 16S rDNA-based metagenomic analysis of dental plaque and lung bacteria in patients with severe acute exacerbations of chronic obstructive pulmonary disease. *J Periodont Res.* 2014; 49(6):760–769.

Taylor J, Pike R, Imamura I, Potempa J. The role of proteolytic enzymes in the development of pulmonary emphysema and periodontal disease. *Am J Respir Crit Care Med.* 1994; 150(6 Pt 2): S143–S146.

Trivedi S, Lal N, Mahdi AA, Singh B, Pandey S. Association of salivary lipid peroxidation levels, antioxidant enzymes, and chronic periodontitis. *Int J Periodontics Restorative Dent.* 2015; 35(20): e14–e19.

Usher AK, Stockley RA. The link between chronic periodontitis and COPD: a common role for the neutrophil? *BMC Med.* 2013; 11:241. doi: 10.1186/1741-7015-11-241.

Wang Z, Zhou X, Zhang J et al. Periodontal health, oral health behaviours, and chronic obstructive pulmonary disease. *J Clin Periodontol.* 2009; 36(9):750–755.

Wedzicha JA, Singh R, Mackay AJ. Acute COPD exacerbations. *Clin Chest Med.* 2014; 35(1):157–163.

Weiss SJ. Tissue destruction by neutrophils. *N Engl J Med.* 1989; 320(6):365–376.

Wikström M, Linde A. Ability of oral bacteria to degrade fibronectin. *Infect Immun.* 1986; 51(2):707–711.

Winning L, Patterson CC, Cullen KM et al. Chronic periodontitis and reduced respiratory function. *J Clin Periodontol.* 2019; 46(3):266–275.

Witschi H. Carcinogenic activity of cigarette smoke gas phase and its modulation by beta-carotene and N-acetylcysteine. *Toxicol Sci.* 2005; 84(1):81–87.

Yoshimura A, Kaneko T, Kato Y, Golenbock DT, Hara Y. Lipopolysaccharides from periodontopathic bacteria *Porphyromonas gingivalis* and *Capnocytophaga ochracea* are antagonists for human toll-like receptor 4. *Infect Immun.* 2002; 70(1):218–225.

Yu H, Lin M, Wang X, Wang S, Wang Z. Toll-like receptor 4 polymorphism is associated with increased susceptibility to chronic obstructive pulmonary disease in Han Chinese patients with chronic periodontitis. *J Oral Sci.* 2016; 58(4):555–560.

Zambon JJ, Nakamura M, Slots J. Effect of periodontal therapy on salivary enzyme activity. *J Periodont Res.* 1985; 20(6):652–659.

Zeng X-T, Tu M-L, Liu D-Y et al. Periodontal disease and risk of chronic obstructive pulmonary disease: a meta-analysis of observational studies. *PLoS One.* 2012; 7: e46508. doi: 10.1371/journal.pone.0046508.

Zhou X, Wang Z, Song Y, Zhang J, Wang C. Periodontal health and quality of life in patients with chronic obstructive pulmonary disease. *Respir Med.* 2011; 105(1):67–73.

23.4 PERIODONTAL DISEASE AND ADVERSE PREGNANCY OUTCOMES

Steph Smith

Contents

Learning objectives

- Knowledge and understanding of existing discrepancies in the literature regarding the risk and association of periodontal disease with adverse pregnancy outcomes.
- Immunological aspects of pregnancy.
- Understanding the proposed pathogenic mechanisms underlying the effects of periodontitis on adverse pregnancy outcomes.
- Understanding the proposed pathogenic mechanisms underlying the effects of pregnancy on periodontal disease.
- The effect of periodontal treatment on adverse pregnancy outcomes.

Introduction

Adverse pregnancy outcomes include preterm birth (PTB) and low birth weight (LBW). PTB occurs at the gestational age of less than 37 weeks, and LBW includes newborns weighing less than 2500 g at birth (Fogacci et al. 2018). An estimated 9.6% of annual worldwide births (approximately 15 million) are preterm, which is the leading cause of neonatal mortality, morbidity, and developmental loss (Beck et al. 2010; Goldenberg et al. 2008). The highest rates of PTB are in Africa (11.9%) and North America (10.6%), and the lowest rates are in Europe (6.2%) (Beck et al. 2010). About one-third of all PTBs are caused by preterm labor, another one-third caused by premature rupture of membranes (PROM), and the remaining cases may due to pregnancy complications, such as preeclampsia (Bobetsis et al. 2006).

Results of studies on the relationship between maternal periodontitis, PTB, and LBW are controversial and inconclusive (Fogacci et al. 2018). This may be ascribed to various systematic reviews incorporating studies with different methodological designs and representing bias that can affect the reliability of outcomes. This includes heterogeneity of criteria to define periodontitis (Corbella et al. 2016; Wang et al. 2013). Nevertheless, reports of studies have shown that insufficient evidence exists to identify periodontitis as a risk factor for PTB and, conversely, a significant association between periodontitis and LBW has been described (Teshome & Yitayeh 2016; Wang et al. 2013). Of the multiple risk factors for PTB, maternal infection has consistently been identified, and systematic and evidence-based reviews have suggested that periodontitis may be a potential risk factor for PTB and LBW (Ren & Du 2017). Studies have indicated that pregnant women with periodontitis can be 2–7 times more likely to experience PTB or deliver a LBW infant (Offenbacher et al. 1996; Scannapieco et al. 2003; Xiong et al. 2006). Systematic reviews of epidemiological studies have concluded that maternal periodontitis is modestly associated with adverse pregnancy outcomes independent of known confounders (Ide & Papapanou 2013). Inconsistency among other studies means however that there is no clarification on whether periodontal disease plays any causal role in PB and/or LBW (Scannapieco et al. 2013; Wang et al. 2013). Studies have furthermore suggested that the strength of the association between periodontitis and PTB incidence is higher when the severity of periodontitis is increased (Gomes-Filho et al. 2007; Manau et al. 2008). The association between generalized periodontitis and PTB has also been found to be higher compared to the association between localized periodontitis and PTB (Nabet et al. 2010). Periodontitis has also been found to be associated with preeclampsia and PROM (Pattanashetti et al. 2013; Ren & Du 2017; Stadelmann et al. 2015). Studies have also shown associations between periodontal disease and PTB in pregnant females who are young, have pre-pregnancy obesity, as well as being HIV infected (Lee et al. 2014; Ren & Du 2017; Usin et al. 2016).

Adverse pregnancy outcomes are also an important public health problem, which includes significant social and financial implications. The offspring of complicated pregnancies may have to face multiple lifelong challenges, such as respiratory distress, impaired motor skills, cognitive and intellectual impairment, learning difficulties, and cardiovascular and metabolic disorders (Bobetsis et al. 2020).

Immunology of pregnancy

During pregnancy, at the maternal–fetal interface, mixing of maternal and fetal cells occurs, which includes the chronic exposure of foreign antigens to the mother's immune system (Poole & Claman 2004). The fetus carries external DNA obtained from the father and hence acts as an allograft (La Rocca et al. 2014). To prevent immunological rejection of the fetus, physiological alterations occur in the immune system during pregnancy. This is partly due to changes in progesterone, estrogen, and chorionic gonadotropin during pregnancy (Armitage 2013).

A major alteration is the partial dampening of the mother's cell-mediated immune responses associated with T-helper-1 (Th1) and Th17 lymphocytes, as these cells secrete interleukin-2 (IL-2), interferon-gamma (INF-γ), and tumor necrosis factor alpha (TNF-α), which promote cellular immunity (Armitage 2013; Jamieson et al. 2006; Sykes et al. 2012). Simultaneously, this is augmented by antibody-mediated immune responses by Th2 and T-regulatory lymphocytes, which promote replication and stimulation of antibody-producing B-cells Stimulated Th2 cells produce IL-4, IL-5, and IL-10, which suppress cell-mediated immune responses (Jamieson et al. 2006; Poole & Claman 2004). T-regulatory cells suppress antigen-specific immune responses that are important for maternal immunological tolerance of the presence of fetal antigens (Schumacher et al. 2007; Sykes et al. 2012).

An overall effect of this alteration of the Th1–Th2 balance is increased susceptibility to pathogens, such as viruses (Söderström et al. 2003) and other intracellular pathogens, including *Listeria monocytogenes* (Southwick & Purich 1996) and *Plasmodium falciparum* (Fievet et al. 2002).

Deactivation of neutrophils also occurs at the maternal–fetal interface where fetal-derived trophoblasts come into contact with maternal neutrophils (Petty et al. 2006). Deactivation results in a significant reduction in myeloperoxidase (El-Maallem & Fletcher 1980), respiratory burst activities (Tsukimori et al. 2006), and phagocytosis (Maltzer & Silva 1980).

Pathogenic mechanisms of adverse pregnancy outcomes

Pregnancy-induced immunological modifications can increase susceptibility to a number of infections during pregnancy, including periodontal disease; and periodontal infections, at least in some populations, can increase the risk of adverse pregnancy outcomes. These interactions may indicate a possible bi-directional relationship between pregnancy and periodontal disease; however, no clear evidence of this relationship exists, as contradictory findings are reported in the literature (Armitage 2013; Ide & Papapanou 2013).

Periodontitis, PTB, and LBW share multiple risk factors, including socioeconomic status, alcohol and/or drug abuse, smoking, poor general health, and genetic factors (Wang et al. 2013). An increased risk of adverse pregnancy outcomes has been found to be related to poor oral health (Corbella et al. 2012). LBW is also more likely to be associated with maternal periodontitis (Oliveira et al. 2011; Saddki et al. 2008; Toygar et al. 2007). Genetic factors may be involved in altering the immune response against bacteria. Polymorphisms in pro-inflammatory genes associated with the production of IL-1β and IL-6 have been associated with PTB (Moura et al. 2009). Specific polymorphisms of prostaglandin E receptor 3, which is associated with the inflammatory response, have been described to be significantly related to both periodontitis treatment failure and spontaneous PTB (Blasco-Blaque et al. 2017; Jeffcoat et al. 2014).

Two mechanisms have been proposed describing the relationship between periodontal infection and adverse pregnancy outcomes, including a direct pathway (infectious) and an indirect pathway (immune/inflammatory) (Figuero et al. 2020; Puertasa et al. 2018; Sanz & Kornman 2013). The direct pathway includes oral microorganisms or their components invading the fetal–placental unit via hematogenous dissemination, or microorganisms in an ascending route via the genitourinary tract. The indirect pathway is mediated by inflammatory mediators locally produced in periodontal tissues, directly affecting the fetal–placental unit, or circulating to the liver and thus increasing systemic inflammation (Figuero et al. 2020). Both pathways ultimately lead to an inflammatory process and/or in combination with suppression of local growth factors in the fetal–placental unit (Puertasa et al. 2018) (see Figure 23.4.1).

Direct pathways

Urogenital tract infections

- A placental and fetal membrane microbiome exists in the absence of histopathological signs of infection (Aagaard et al. 2014; Steel et al. 2005). The main pathogenic pathway suggested to cause PTB is intra-amniotic infection (Goldenberg et al. 2008; Romero et al. 2015). Vaginal dysbiosis during the early stages of pregnancy has been indicated to double the risk of PTB (Puertasa et al. 2018). An ascending pathway of infection from the urogenital tract microbiome is considered as the main route causing a placental microbiome dysbiosis (Agger et al. 2014).
- Dysbiosis of the urogenital tract is characterized by a decrease in *Lactobacillus* species and proliferation of anaerobic bacteria. *Gardnerella vaginalis*, *Chlamydia trachomatis*, *Mycoplasma hominis*, *Ureoplasma urealyticum*, *Prevotella* spp., *Candida* spp., *Gonorrhea* spp., and *Treponema* spp. have been cited as causative organisms (Aagaard et al. 2014; Agger et al. 2014).

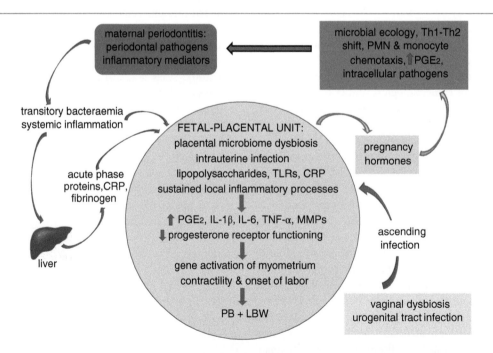

Figure 23.4.1 Association between periodontal disease and adverse pregnancy outcomes. CRP, C-reactive protein; IL, interleukin; LBW, low birth weight; MMP, matrix metalloproteinase; PB, preterm birth; PGE2, prostaglandin 2; PMN, polymorphonuclear neutrophil; TLR, Toll-like receptor; TNF, tumor necrosis factor. Courtesy of Dr. Steph Smith

- Microbial-induced preterm labor is mediated by an inflammatory process. Microorganisms and their products are sensed by Toll-like receptors (TLRs), inducing the production of cytokines, chemokines, prostaglandins, and proteases, leading to parturition (Romero et al. 2015).

Periodontal infections

Studies show a moderate overall association between periodontal infections and adverse pregnancy outcomes. Inconsistent findings may however be due to variations in susceptibility between populations that are based on complex genetic and environmental differences (Armitage 2013; Vergnes & Sixou 2007; Xiong et al. 2007).

- The oral microbiome containing commensal and pathogenic organisms may act as a reservoir for putative placental pathogens. In periodontitis, pathogenic subgingival microorganisms are located in intimate contact with the ulcerated epithelium of periodontal pockets (Figuero et al. 2020). The translocation of pathogenic bacteria to the bloodstream can cause a transitory bacteremia, enabling the establishment of a metastatic infection at the fetal–placental unit (Bobetsis et al. 2020), thereby reaching and crossing the placental barrier and amniotic fluid (Liang et al. 2018; Steel et al, 2005; Xi et al. 2015). Oral bacteria may normally be present in the placenta; however, placental levels of oral pathogens depend largely on the maternal periodontal status (Blanc et al. 2015). Pregnant patients with pregnancy-associated gingivitis, a condition that affects 30–75% of the pregnant population, can also lead to a frequent transient dental bacteremia (Barak et al. 2003). There is nevertheless controversy over the prevalence of the occurrence of bacteremia, which can range from 0% to 53%, due to scaling and root planing or toothbrushing procedures. This may be ascribed to differences in the periodontal condition of the subjects who were evaluated (Figuero et al. 2020).

- *Porphyromonas gingivalis*, *Fusobacterium nucleatum*, *Campylobacter rectus*, and *Bergeyella* sp. are the bacterial species that have been described to be the most strongly associated with adverse pregnancy outcomes (Madianos et al. 2013; Sanz & Kornman 2013).

- *Porphyromonas gingivalis* has been detected in human placental tissues, umbilical cord, and amniotic cavity (Liang et al. 2018). A cohort study indicated the detection of *P. gingivalis* in the placenta to be related to PTB, whereby *P. gingivalis* was detected within the villous mesenchyme in the preterm group, but not in the term group (Hasegawa-Nakamura et al. 2011; Vanterpool et al. 2016). in vitro and animal studies have shown *P. gingivalis* lipopolysaccharides (LPS) to induce the production of IL-6 and IL-8 via TLR2 in chorion-derived cells, and to increase expression levels of IL-8, TNF-α, and COX-2 in extravillous trophoblast cells in a nuclear factor kappa B (NF-κB)-dependent manner (Ao et al. 2015; Hasegawa-Nakamura et al. 2011). Endotoxin from Gram-negative bacteria may enter the circulation at high enough levels to stimulate the amnion to produce inflammatory mediators, such as prostaglandin E2 (PGE2), which is a potent inducer of labor (Klebanoff & Searle 2006). Studies utilizing murine models have shown that *P. gingivalis* induces degeneration and apoptosis of trophoblasts and endothelial cells, as well as necrosis and detachment of the placenta from the uterus (Ao et al. 2015; Katz et al. 2009; León et al. 2007; Liang et al. 2018). Studies have also shown that periodontal pathogens (or their antigens) may cross the placenta and reach the developing fetus in high enough levels to stimulate the fetus to produce immunoglobulin (Ig)M antibody against these bacteria (Boggess et al. 2005, 2006).

- *Bergeyella* is a common oral species that is normally absent in the vaginal flora, and is thus a strong marker of oral–utero transmission. Studies have identified *Bergeyella* sp. in the amniotic fluid and cord blood of different cohorts with PTB, as well as in neonatal sepsis (Figuero et al. 2020; Han et al. 2006; Wang et al. 2013).

- *F. nucleatum* is frequently associated with adverse pregnancy outcomes, yet is absent in the normal vaginal flora (Vander Haar et al. 2018). It is one of the most prevalent species in intrauterine infection, and is associated with 10–30% PTB (Hill 1998). *F. nucleatum* has been detected in a wide variety of placental and fetal compartments associated with adverse pregnancy outcomes, including amniotic fluids, fetal membranes, cord blood, and neonatal gastric aspirates, either as the sole infectious agent or in mixed infections (Figuero et al. 2020). *F. nucleatum* colonization is mediated by its unique adhesin, FadA (Han et al. 2005). FadA binds to vascular endothelial-cadherin, causing loosening of the tight junction and allowing bacteria to penetrate through the endothelium. It has been postulated that FadA plays an essential role in systemic dissemination of oral bacteria and in colonization in the placenta (Ikegami et al. 2009).

- Other oral bacteria also reported to be present in the placenta and amniotic fluid are *Aggregatibacter actinomycetemcomitans*, *Tannerella forsythia*, *Treponema denticola*, *Eikenella corrodens*, *Parvimonas micra*, and *Capnocytophaga* spp., and these have also been reported to be at significantly higher levels in preterm deliveries compared to term births (Kostadinov & Pinar 2005; León et al. 2007; Ren & Du 2017). *E. corrodens*, *F. nucleatum*, and *P. gingivalis* have been shown to be associated with uterine hypercontractility, cervical dilatation, and rupture of the membranes, leading to PTB (Blanc et al. 2015; Madianos et al. 2013; Wang et al. 2013).

- Periodontal infections may also play a part in the multifactorial etiology of preeclampsia. This complication is characterized by hypertension, peripheral edema, and proteinuria. Failure to control these physiological abnormalities can lead to eclampsia, in which convulsions, coma, and death of the mother may occur (Oettinger-Barak et al. 2005; Riché et al. 2002).

- Chronic periodontal infections may thus contribute to the burden of risk for initiating and/or sustaining inflammatory processes occurring in the fetal–placental unit (Ebersole et al. 2014). It must be noted, however, that it is the inflammatory response at the placenta that is responsible for triggering PTB. Accordingly, periodontal treatment should be initialized before pregnancy to reduce the periodontal pathogen burden in the gingival sulcus; and during pregnancy to prevent increases in proinflammatory mediators in both the subgingival and placental environment (Puertasa et al. 2018; Thinkhamrop et al. 2015).

Indirect pathways

Immune/inflammatory mechanisms

- Inflammatory signaling controls normal parturition (Papapanou 2015). Hormonal changes toward the end of pregnancy induce proinflammatory cytokine release in the tissue, which in turn initiates production of prostaglandins in the myometrium, which leads to the contraction of the uterus (Sakowicz 2018). The onset of labor involves a switch of the myometrium from a quiescent to a contractile state. This is accompanied by a shift in signaling between anti-inflammatory and proinflammatory pathways. During pregnancy, progesterone maintains uterine quiescence by repressing the expression of proinflammatory genes (Romero et al. 2015). As pregnancy progresses, amniotic fluid levels of PGE2 and inflammatory cytokines, including TNF-α and IL-1β, IL-6 and IL-8, steadily increase until a critical threshold level is reached (Papapanou 2015). At term, progesterone catabolism also occurs. Increased expression of inflammatory cytokines, chemokines, and increased protease activity (matrix metalloproteinases [MMP]-8 and MMP-9) induces rupture of the amniotic sac membranes, uterine contraction, cervical dilation, and delivery (Papapanou 2015; Romero et al. 2015). However, premature elevation of these inflammatory molecules in the amniotic sac walls or myometrium may thus induce a premature onset of labor (Papapanou 2015).

- It is hypothesized that the physiological cascades initiating parturition can also be activated by inflammatory mediators produced and disseminated from the periodontal region (Stadelmann et al. 2013). Patients with severe periodontitis can have significantly increased levels of locally produced IL-1β, IL-6, IL-17, PGE2, and TNF-α proinflammatory mediators, which can enter the systemic circulation and induce an acute-phase response in the liver that is characterized by an increased level of C-reactive protein (CRP) and fibrinogen (Patil & Desai 2013). Increased CRP levels can enhance the risk of cardiovascular disease, cerebrovascular accidents, as well as preterm LBW infants (Genco & Van Dyke 2010; Park et al. 2013; Souccar et al. 2010). These inflammatory cytokines, including periodontitis-related PGE2, may promote labor activation through enhanced placental and chorion–amnion production of PGE2 (Cetin et al. 2012; Perunovic et al. 2016).

- Thus, local inflammatory mediators produced in periodontal tissues, causing elevated systemic inflammation associated with maternal periodontitis, may reach the placenta and induce production of other inflammatory cytokines and/or acute-phase proteins by local immune cells, placenta, chorion, decidua, and trophoblast, which act at the fetal–placental unit, thereby inducing cervical ripening and uterine contraction, eventually leading to an increased risk for PTB (Mesa et al. 2016; Puertasa et al. 2018). As a response to the elevated influx of proinflammatory cytokines, such as TNF-α and IL-1β, an aberrant extracellular matrix degradation induced by matrix metalloproteinases can also induce early membrane ruptures (Cockle et al. 2007; Sykes et al. 2012).

- LPS produced by Gram-negative periodontal bacteria stimulate local macrophages via TLR4 activation, and via TLR2 in chorion-derived cells, to secrete IL-1β, IL-6, TNF-α, PGE2, as well as transcription factors, causing a change from anti-inflammatory to proinflammatory signals (Mendelson 2009; Romero et al. 2015). This in turn leads to diminished progesterone receptor functioning and to the activation of genes related to changes from quiescence to contractility in the myometrium, resulting in the onset of labor (Goldenberg et al. 2008; Mendelson 2009; Romero et al. 2015).

- An aberrant shift has furthermore been observed in cytokine profiles in the peripheral blood, placenta, and umbilical cord of preeclamptic women with a diminished Th2 and T-regulatory activity in relation to Th1 and Th17 functions (Peixoto et al. 2016; Vargas-Rojas et al. 2016).

- Pathogenic pathways between periodontal infection and an immune inflammatory response in the fetal–placental unit ultimately lead to resultant adverse pregnancy outcomes (Puertasa et al. 2018). Local inflammation at the maternal–fetal interface, rather than systemic inflammation, thus plays an etiopathogenic role in PTB (Wei et al. 2010).

Impact of pregnancy on plaque-induced periodontal infections

During pregnancy, significant fluctuations occur in the levels of progesterone and estrogen. Periodontal cell subsets have receptors for these hormones, rendering periodontal tissues a possible target (Guncu et al. 2005).

There seems to be widespread consensus that the severity and extent of gingival inflammation increase during pregnancy (Armitage 2013; Moss et al. 2005). A specific localized inflammatory lesion, i.e. pregnancy granuloma, appears in 0.2–9.6% of pregnant women, whereas a more generalized inflammatory lesion, referred to as pregnancy gingivitis, is more common and affects more than a third of pregnant women (Bhaskar & Jacoway 1966; Gürsoy et al. 2013). The inflammation can occur concurrently with gingival tenderness, profuse bleeding, and an increase in probing depths. Increased probing depths are due to inflammation-induced swelling of the gingiva in a coronal direction, with no permanent loss of clinical attachment (Gürsoy et al. 2008; Tilakaratne et al. 2000). However, in patients who present with chronic periodontitis prior to becoming pregnant, progression of periodontitis can and does occur (Gürsoy et al. 2008; Lieff et al. 2004).

The mechanisms responsible for increased gingival inflammation during pregnancy are not fully understood, but perturbations in neutrophil function, modifications in cellular and humoral immunity, hormone-induced changes in cellular physiology, and local effects on microbial ecology may all play important roles in the overall process (Armitage 2013). Reduction in phagocytosis and bactericidal activities of peripheral neutrophils in pregnant individuals is quite likely related to the increase in gingival inflammation observed during gestation (Maltzer & Silva 1980; Tsukimori et al. 2006).

Estrogen and progesterone changes associated with pregnancy have been shown to have an effect on the composition of the subgingival microbiota (Kornman & Loesche 1980; Yokoyama et al. 2008). Various studies have described a diverse array of periodontitis-associated subgingival bacterial pathogens, including *Prevotella intermedia, Bacteroides species, Campylobacter, Treponema denticola, Staphylococcus aureus, F. nucleatum, Pseudomonas aeruginosa, Haemophilus influenzae*, and *A. actinomycetemcomitans* (Armitage 2013).

in vitro studies have found that sex hormones, such as estradiol, can reduce neutrophil chemotaxis, and progesterone can enhance chemotaxis of both neutrophils and monocytes (Miyagi et al. 1992, 1993). Sex hormones also have an effect on the in vitro production of proinflammatory mediators such as PGE2 by endotoxin-stimulated monocytes (Miyagi et al. 1993). Furthermore, due to the immunological changes associated with pregnancy, which include an increased susceptibility to intracellular pathogens, the survival of locally invasive *P. intermedia, P. gingivalis*, and *A. actinomycetemcomitans* is enhanced during pregnancy (Armitage 2013) (see Figure 23.4.1).

Effect of periodontal treatment on adverse pregnancy outcomes

The preventive effectiveness of periodontal treatment for PTB is influenced by the diagnostic criteria of periodontitis, the microbial community composition, severity of disease, treatment strategy, treatment efficiency, and whether treatment occurred during the pre-pregnancy period or during the first or second trimester of pregnancy (Ren & Du 2017). Reports from systematic reviews are contradictory. Various reviews have reported the risks of perinatal outcomes to be potentially reduced by periodontal treatment in pregnant women (Schwendicke et al. 2015; Shah et al. 2013). High-quality randomized controlled trials have reported no evidence to support that non-surgical periodontal therapy during pregnancy may alter the incidence of PTB, LBW, and preeclampsia.

However, there is limited evidence of a positive effect of periodontal treatment in decreasing PTB and LBW rates in women at high risk of adverse pregnancy outcomes (Bobetsis & Madianos 2017). Non-surgical periodontal treatment during pregnancy has been shown to be effective in reducing the increased amount of periodontal inflammation associated with pregnancy (Yalcin et al. 2002). Randomized controlled trials have shown that non-surgical periodontal therapy during the second trimester of gestation is safe (López et al. 2005). Studies have also shown a significant reduction in the levels of IL-1β, IL-6, IL-10, and IL-12 in gingival crevicular fluid during pregnancy (Corbella et al. 2016; Penova-Veselinovic et al. 2015). Other reviews have suggested that periodontal treatment does not efficiently reduce the incidence of PTB (Boutin et al. 2013; Chambrone et al. 2011; Michalowicz et al. 2013). Furthermore, subjects refractory to periodontal treatment have been shown to be significantly more likely to have PTB (Ren & Du 2017). Nevertheless, the potential association of periodontal disease with adverse pregnancy outcomes is most important for healthcare providers. The scientific community has a responsibility to inform patients as well as clinicians, and thus to provide clinical guidelines for better interprofessional management of pregnant women (Bobetsis et al. 2020). Oral health maintenance however remains an imperative part of preventive care that is both effective and safe throughout pregnancy, and should be supported before and during pregnancy (Ren & Du 2017).

Future considerations

Data supporting the theories described of circulating microbes together with their by-products causing metastatic injury by initiating an inflammatory response at the fetal–placental unit mainly originate from animal studies. Thus, the validity of these findings needs to be proven in humans (Bobetsis et al. 2020). In order to obtain more solid evidence of the association of periodontitis with adverse pregnancy outcomes, higher-quality longitudinal clinical trials are needed. These studies should include combining several immune markers together with clinical and microbiological data so as to define the exact biological mechanisms between periodontal diseases and adverse pregnancy outcomes (Bobetsis et al. 2020). There is also the need for randomized controlled trials to standardize methodological criteria and to utilize more precise and universally accepted diagnostic criteria for categorical assessments of periodontal definitions and status (Liang et al. 2018; Puertasa et al. 2018). These studies should include multicenter studies with a large number of participants (Ren & Du 2017). Future intervention trials should also include an evaluation of the effectiveness of periodontal treatment as part of the study design. If this variable is not included in the analysis, it is impossible to draw valid conclusions regarding the putative causal link between periodontal infections and risk of adverse pregnancy outcomes (Armitage 2013).

REFERENCES

Aagaard K, Ma J, Antony KM et al. The placenta harbors a unique microbiome. *Sci Transl Med.* 2014; 6:237ra65.

Agger WA, Siddiqui D, Lovrich SD et al. Epidemiologic factors and urogenital infections associated with preterm birth in a midwestern U.S. population. *Obstet Gynecol.* 2014; 124:969–977.

Ao M, Miyauchi M, Furusho H, et al. Dental infection of *Porphyromonas gingivalis* induces preterm birth in mice. *PLoS One.* 2015; 10(8):e137249.

Armitage GC. Bi-directional relationship between pregnancy and periodontal disease. *Periodontol 2000.* 2013; 61:160–176.

Barak S, Oettinger-Barak O, Oettinger M et al. Common oral manifestations during pregnancy: a review. *Obstet Gynecol Surv.* 2003; 58(9):624–628.

Beck S, Wojdyla D, Say L et al. The worldwide incidence of preterm birth: a systematic review of maternal mortality and morbidity. *Bull World Health Organ.* 2010; 88(1):31–38.

Bhaskar SN, Jacoway JR. Pyogenic granuloma—clinical features, incidence, histology, and result of treatment: report of 242 cases. *J Oral Surg.* 1966; 24(5):391–398.

Blanc V, O'Valle F, Pozo E et al. Oral bacteria in placental tissues: increased molecular detection in pregnant periodontitis patients. *Oral Dis.* 2015; 21:905–912.

Blasco-Baque V, Garidou L, Pomie C et al. Periodontitis induced by *Porphyromonas gingivalis* drives periodontal microbiota dysbiosis and insulin resistance via an impaired adaptive immune response. *Gut.* 2017; 66(5):872–885. doi: 10.1136/gutjnl-2015-309897.

Bobetsis YA, Barros SP, Offenbacher S. Exploring the relationship between periodontal disease and pregnancy complications. *J Am Dent Assoc.* 2006; 137:7S–13S.

Bobetsis YA, Graziani F, Gürsoy M, Madianos PN. Periodontal disease and adverse pregnancy outcomes. *Periodontol 2000.* 2020; 83:154–174.

Bobetsis YA, Madianos PN. Treating periodontal disease during pregnancy. European Federation of Periodontology report; 2017. Retrieved August 2020 from http://www.efp.org/publications/projects/oral health and pregnancy/reports/treating-perio-disease.pdf.

Boggess KA, Beck JD, Murtha AP, Moss K, Offenbacher S. Maternal periodontal disease in early pregnancy and risk for a small-for-gestational-age infant. *Am J Obstet Gynecol.* 2006; 194:1316–1322.

Boggess KA, Moss K, Madianos P et al. Fetal immune response to oral pathogens and risk of preterm birth. *Am J Obstet Gynecol.* 2005; 193:1121–1126.

Boutin A, Demers S, Roberge S et al. Treatment of periodontal disease and prevention of preterm birth: systematic review and meta-analysis. *Am J Perinatol.* 2013; 30(7):537–544.

Cetin I, Pileri P, Villa A et al. Pathogenic mechanisms linking periodontal diseases with adverse pregnancy outcomes. *Reprod Sci.* 2012; 19(6):633–641.

Chambrone L, Pannuti CM, Guglielmetti MR, Chambrone LA. Evidence grade associating periodontitis with preterm birth and/or low birth weight, II: a systematic review of randomized trials evaluating the effects of periodontal treatment. *J Clin Periodontol.* 2011; 38(10):902–914.

Cockle JV, Gopichandran N, Walker JJ, Levene MI, Orsi NM. Matrix metalloproteinases and their tissue inhibitors in preterm perinatal complications. *Reprod Sci.* 2007; 14(7):629–645.

Corbella S, Taschieri S, Del Fabbro M et al. Adverse pregnancy outcomes and periodontitis: a systematic review and meta-analysis exploring potential association. *Quintessence Int.* 2016; 47(3):193–204.

Corbella S, Taschieri S, Francetti L, De Siena F, Del Fabbro M. Periodontal disease as a risk factor for adverse pregnancy outcomes: a systematic review and meta-analysis of case–control studies. *Odontology.* 2012; 100:232–240.

Ebersole JL, Holt SC, Cappelli D. Periodontitis in pregnant baboons: systemic inflammation and adaptive immune responses and pregnancy outcomes in a baboon model. *J Periodontal Res.* 2014; 49(2):226–236.

El-Maallem H, Fletcher J. Impaired neutrophil function and myeloperoxidase deficiency in pregnancy. *Br J Haematol.* 1980; 44:375–381.

Fievet N, Tami G, Maubert B et al. Cellular immune response to *Plasmodium falciparum* after pregnancy is related to previous placental infection and parity. *Malar J.* 2002; 1:16.

Figuero E, Han YW, Furuichi Y. Periodontal diseases and adverse pregnancy outcomes: mechanisms. *Periodontol 2000.* 2020; 83:175–188.

Fogacci MF, Cardoso E de OC, Barbirato D da S, de Carvalho DP, Sansone C. No association between periodontitis and preterm low birth weight: a case–control study. *Arch Gynecol Obstet.* 2018; 297:71–76.

Genco RJ, Van Dyke TE. Prevention: reducing the risk of CVD in patients with periodontitis. *Nat Rev Cardiol.* 2010; 7(9):479–480.

Goldenberg RL, Culhane JF, Iams JD, Romero R. Epidemiology and causes of preterm birth. *Lancet.* 2008; 371(9606):75–84.

Gomes-Filho IS, Cruz SS, Rezende EJ et al. Exposure measurement in the association between periodontal disease and prematurity/low birth weight. *J Clin Periodontol.* 2007; 34(11):957–963.

Guncu GN, Tozum TF, Caglayan F. Effects of endogenous sex hormones on the periodontium—review of literature. *Aust Dent J.* 2005; 50(3):138–145.

Gürsoy M, Gürsoy UK, Sorsa T, Pajukanta R, Kononen E. High salivary estrogen and risk of developing pregnancy gingivitis. *J Periodontol.* 2013; 84(9):1281–1289.

Gürsoy M, Pajukanta R, Sorsa T, Könönen E. Clinical changes in periodontium during pregnancy and postpartum. *J Clin Periodontol.* 2008; 35:576–583.

Han YW, Ikegami A, Bissada NF et al. Transmission of an uncultivated *Bergeyella* strain from the oral cavity to amniotic fluid in a case of preterm birth. *J Clin Microbiol.* 2006; 44(4):1475–1483.

Han YW, Ikegami A, Rajanna C et al. Identification and characterization of a novel adhesin unique to oral fusobacteria. *J Bacteriol.* 2005; 187(15):5330–5340.

Hasegawa-Nakamura K, Tateishi F, Nakamura T et al. The possible mechanism of preterm birth associated with periodontopathic *Porphyromonas gingivalis. J Periodontal Res.* 2011; 46(4):497–504.

Hill GB. Preterm birth: associations with genital and possibly oral microflora. *Ann Periodontol.* 1998; 3(1):222–232.

Ide M, Papapanou PN. Epidemiology of association between maternal periodontal disease and adverse pregnancy outcomes – systematic review. *J Periodontol.* 2013; 84(4 Suppl):S181–S194.

Ikegami A, Chung P, Han YW. Complementation of the fadA mutation in *Fusobacterium nucleatum* demonstrates that the surface-exposed adhesin promotes cellular invasion and placental colonization. *Infect Immun.* 2009; 77(7):3075–3079.

Jamieson DJ, Theiler RN, Rasmussen SA. Emerging infections and pregnancy. *Emerg Infect Dis.* 2006; 12:1638–1643.

Jeffcoat MK, Jeffcoat RL, Tanna N, Parry SH. Association of a common genetic factor, PTGER3, with outcome of periodontal therapy and preterm birth. *J Periodontol.* 2014; 85(3):446–454.

Katz J, Chegini N, Shiverick KT, Lamont RJ. Localization of *P. gingivalis* in preterm delivery placenta. *J Dent Res.* 2009; 88:575–578.

Klebanoff M, Searle K. The role of inflammation in preterm birth – focus on periodontitis. *Br J Obstet Gynaecol.* 2006; 113(Suppl 3):43–45.

Kornman KS, Loesche WJ. Direct interaction between estradiol and progesterone with *Bacteroides asaccharolyticus* and *Bacteroides melaninogenicus. Infect Immun.* 1982; 35:256–263.

Kostadinov S, Pinar H. Amniotic fluid infection syndrome and neonatal mortality caused by *Eikenella corrodens. Pediatr Dev Pathol.* 2005; 8:489–492.

La Rocca C, Carbone F, Longobardi S, Matarese G. The immunology of pregnancy: regulatory T cells control maternal immune tolerance toward the fetus. *Immunol Lett.* 2014; 4(1 Pt A):41–48.

Lee HJ, Jun JK, Lee SM et al. Association between obesity and periodontitis in pregnant females. *J Periodontol.* 2014; 85(7):224–231.

León R, Silva N, Ovalle A et al. Detection of *Porphyromonas gingivalis* in the amniotic fluid in pregnant women with a diagnosis of threatened premature labor. *J Periodontol.* 2007; 78:1249–1255.

Liang S, Ren H, Guo H et al. Periodontal infection with *Porphyromonas gingivalis* induces preterm birth and lower birth weight in rats. *Mol Oral Microbiol.* 2018; 33:312–321.

Lieff S, Boggess KA, Murtha AP et al. The oral conditions and pregnancy study: periodontal status of a cohort of pregnant women. *J Periodontol.* 2004; 75:116–126.

López NJ, Da Silva I, Ipinza J, Gutierrez J. Periodontal therapy reduces the rate of preterm low birth weight in women with pregnancy-associated gingivitis. *J Periodontol.* 2005; 76(11 Suppl):2144–2153.

Madianos PN, Bobetsis YA, Offenbacher S. Adverse pregnancy outcomes (APOs) and periodontal disease: pathogenic mechanisms. *J Clin Periodontol.* 2013; 40: S170–S180.

Maltzer MC, Silva J Jr. in vitro defects of phagocyte chemotaxis during pregnancy. *J Clin Microbiol.* 1980; 11:170–173.

Manau C, Echeverria A, Agueda A, Guerrero A, Echeverria JJ. Periodontal disease definition may determine the association between periodontitis and pregnancy outcomes. *J Clin Periodontol.* 2008; 35(5):385–397.

Mendelson CR. Minireview: fetal–maternal hormonal signaling in pregnancy and labor. *Mol Endocrinol.* 2009; 23:947–954.

Mesa F, Pozo E, O'Valle F et al. Relationship between periodontal parameters and plasma cytokine profiles in pregnant woman with preterm birth or low birth weight. *Clin Oral Investig.* 2016; 20:669–674.

Michalowicz BS, Gustafsson A, Thumbigere-Math V, Buhlin K. The effects of periodontal treatment on pregnancy outcomes. *J Clin Periodontol.* 2013; 40(Suppl 14):S195–S208.

Miyagi M, Aoyama H, Morishita M, Iwamoto Y. Effects of sex hormones on chemotaxis of human peripheral polymorphonuclear leukocytes and monocytes. *J Periodontol.* 1992: 63:28–32.

Miyagi M, Morishita M, Iwamoto Y. Effects of sex hormones on production of prostaglandin E2 by human peripheral monocytes. *J Periodontol.* 1993; 64:1075–1078.

Moss KL, Beck JD, Offenbacher S. Clinical risk factors associated with incidence and progression of periodontal conditions in pregnant women. *J Clin Periodontol.* 2005; 32:492–498.

Moura E, Mattar R, de Souza E et al. Inflammatory cytokine gene polymorphisms and spontaneous preterm birth. *J Reprod Immunol.* 2009; 80(1–2):115–121.

Nabet C, Lelong N, Colombier ML et al. Maternal periodontitis and the causes of preterm birth: the case–control Epipap study. *J Clin Periodontol.* 2010; 37(1):37–45.

Oettinger-Barak O, Barak S, Ohel G et al. Severe pregnancy complication (preeclampsia) is associated with greater periodontal destruction. *J Periodontol.* 2005; 76:134–137.

Offenbacher S, Katz V, Fertik G et al. Periodontal infection as a possible risk factor for preterm low birth weight. *J Periodontol.* 1996; 67:1103–1113.

Oliveira AM, de Oliveira PA, Cota LO et al. Periodontal therapy and risk for adverse pregnancy outcomes. *Clin Oral Investig.* 2011; 15:609–615.

Papapanou PN. Systemic effects of periodontitis: lessons learned from research on atherosclerotic vascular disease and adverse pregnancy outcomes. *Int Dent J.* 2015; 65(6):283–291.

Park CW, Yoon BH, Park JS, Jun JK. An elevated maternal serum C-reactive protein in the context of intra-amniotic inflammation is an indicator that the development of amnionitis, an intense fetal and AF inflammatory response are likely in patients with preterm labor: clinical implications. *J Matern Fetal Neonatal Med.* 2013; 26(9):847–853.

Patil VA, Desai MH. Effect of periodontal therapy on serum C-reactive protein levels in patients with gingivitis and chronic periodontitis: a clinicobiochemical study. *J Contemp Dent Pract.* 2013; 14(2):233–237.

Pattanashetti JI, Nagathan VM, Rao SM. Evaluation of periodontitis as a risk for preterm birth among preeclamptic and non-preeclamptic pregnant women – a case control study. *J Clin Diagn Res.* 2013; 7(8):1776–1778.

Peixoto AB, Araujo Junior E, Ribeiro JU et al. Evaluation of inflammatory mediators in the deciduas of pregnant women with pre-eclampsia/eclampsia. *J Matern Fetal Neonatal Med.* 2016; 29(1):75–79.

Penova-Veselinovic B, Keelan JA, Wang CA, Newnham JP, Pennell CE. Changes in inflammatory mediators in gingival crevicular fluid following periodontal disease treatment in pregnancy: relationship to adverse pregnancy outcome. *J Reprod Immunol.* 2015; 112:1–10.

Perunovic N, Rakic MM, Nikolic LI et al. The association between periodontal inflammation and labor triggers (elevated cytokine levels) in preterm birth: a cross-sectional study. *J Periodontol.* 2016; 87(3):248–256.

Petty HR, Kindzelskii AL, Espinoza J, Romero R. Trophoblast contact deactivates human neutrophils. *J Immunol.* 2006; 176:3205–3214.

Poole JA, Claman HN. Immunology of pregnancy. Implications for the mother. *Clin Rev Allergy Immunol.* 2004; 26:161–170.

Puertasa A, Magan-Fernandezb A, Blancc V et al. Association of periodontitis with preterm birth and low birth weight: a comprehensive review. *J Matern Fetal Neonatal Med.* 2018; 31:(5):597–602.

Ren H, Du M. Role of maternal periodontitis in preterm birth. *Front Immunol.* 2017; 8:139. doi: 10.3389/fimmu.2017.00139.

Riché EL, Boggess KA, Lieff S et al. Periodontal disease increases the risk of preterm delivery among preeclamptic women. *Ann Periodontol.* 2002; 7:95–101.

Romero R, Dey SK, Fisher SJ. Preterm labor: one syndrome, many causes. *Science.* 2015; 345(6198):760–765.

Saddki N, Bachok N, Hussain NH, Zainudin SL, Sosroseno W. The association between maternal periodontitis and low birth weight infants among Malay women. *Community Dent Oral Epidemiol.* 2008; 36:296–304.

Sakowicz A. The role of NFκB in the three stages of pregnancy: implantation, maintenance and labour; a review article. *BJOG.* 2018; 125(11):1379–1387.

Sanz M, Kornman K. Working Group 3 of Joint EFPAAPw. Periodontitis and adverse pregnancy outcomes: consensus report of the Joint EFP/AAP Workshop on Periodontitis and Systemic Diseases. *J Clin Periodontol.* 2013; 40:S164–S169.

Scannapieco FA, Bush RB, Paju S. Periodontal disease as a risk factor for adverse pregnancy outcomes. *A systematic review. Ann Periodontol.* 2003; 8:70–78.

Schumacher A, Wafula PO, Bertoja AZ et al. Mechanisms of action of regulatory T cells specific for paternal antigens during pregnancy. *Obstet Gynecol.* 2007; 110:1137–1145.

Schwendicke F, Karimbux N, Allareddy V, Gluud C. Periodontal treatment for preventing adverse pregnancy outcomes: a meta- and trial sequential analysis. *PLoS One.* 2015; 10(6):e129060.

Shah M, Muley A, Muley P. Effect of nonsurgical periodontal therapy during gestation period on adverse pregnancy outcome: a systematic review. *J Matern Fetal Neonatal Med.* 2013; 26(17):1691–1695.

Söderström A, Norkrans G, Lindh M. Hepatitis B virus DNA during pregnancy and postpartum: aspects of vertical transmission. *J Gastroenterol Hepatol.* 2003; 35:814–819.

Souccar NM, Chakhtoura M, Ghafari JG, Abdelnoor AM. Porphyromonas gingivalis in dental plaque and serum C-reactive protein levels in pregnancy. *J Infect Dev Ctries.* 2010; 4(6):362–366.

Southwick FS, Purich DL. Intracellular pathogenesis of listeriosis. *N Engl J Med.* 1996; 334:770–776.

Stadelmann P, Alessandri R, Eick S et al. The potential association between gingival crevicular fluid inflammatory mediators and adverse pregnancy outcomes: a systematic review. *Clin Oral Invest.* 2013; 17(6):1453–1463.

Stadelmann PF, Eick S, Salvi GE et al. Increased periodontal inflammation in women with preterm premature rupture of membranes. *Clin Oral Investig.* 2015; 19(6):1537–1546.

Steel JH, Malatos S, Kennea N et al. Bacteria and inflammatory cells in fetal membranes do not always cause preterm labor. *Pediatr Res.* 2005; 57:404–411.

Sykes L, MacIntyre DA, Yap XJ, Teoh TG, Bennett PR. The Th1:Th2 dichotomy of pregnancy and preterm labour. *Mediators Inflamm.* 2012; 2012: 96 7629.

Teshome A, Yitayeh A. Relationship between periodontal disease and preterm low birth weight: systematic review. *Pan Afr Med J.* 2016; 24:215. doi: 10.11604/pamj.2016.24.215.8727.

Thinkhamrop J, Hofmeyr GJ, Adetoro O et al. Antibiotic prophylaxis during the second and third trimester to reduce adverse pregnancy outcomes and morbidity. *Cochrane Database Syst Rev.* 2015; 6:CD002250. doi: 10.1002/14651858.CD002250.pub2.

Tilakaratne A, Soory M, Ranasinghe AW et al. Periodontal disease status during pregnancy and 3 months post-partum, in a rural population of Sri-Lankan women. *J Clin Periodontol.* 2000; 27:787–792.

Toygar HU, Seydaoglu G, Kurklu S, Guzeldemir E, Arpak N. Periodontal health and adverse pregnancy outcome in 3,576 Turkish women. *J Periodontol.* 2007; 78:2081–2094.

Tsukimori K, Fukushima K, Komatsu H, Nakano H. Neutrophil function during pregnancy: is nitric acid production correlated with superoxide production? *Am J Reprod Immunol.* 2006; 55:55–105.

Usin MM, Menso J, Rodriguez VI et al. Association between maternal periodontitis and preterm and/or low birth weight infants in normal pregnancies. *J Matern Fetal Neonatal Med.* 2016; 29(1):115–119.

Vander Haar EL, So J, Gyamfi-Bannerman C, Han YW. *Fusobacterium nucleatum* and adverse pregnancy outcomes: epidemiological and mechanistic evidence. *Anaerobe.* 2018; 50:55–59.

Vanterpool SF, Been JV, Houben ML et al. *Porphyromonas gingivalis* within placental villous mesenchyme and umbilical cord stroma is associated with adverse pregnancy outcome. *PLoS One.* 2016; 11(1):e146157.

Vargas-Rojas MI, Solleiro-Villavicencio H, Soto-Vega E. Th1, Th2, Th17 and Treg levels in umbilical cord blood in preeclampsia. *J Matern Fetal Neonatal Med.* 2016; 29(10):1642–1645.

Vergnes J-N, Sixou M. Preterm low birth weight and maternal periodontal status: a meta-analysis. *Am J Obstet Gynecol.* 2007; 196:135.e1–135.e7.

Wang X, Buhimschi CS, Temoin S et al. Comparative microbial analysis of paired amniotic fluid and cord blood from pregnancies complicated by preterm birth and early-onset neonatal sepsis. *PLoS One.* 2013; 8:e56131.

Wang Y-L, Jui-DerLiou J-D, Pan W-L. Association between maternal periodontal disease and preterm delivery and low birth weight. *Taiwan J Obstet Gynecol.* 2013; 52(1):71–76.

Wei SQ, Fraser W, Luo ZC. Inflammatory cytokines and spontaneous preterm birth in asymptomatic women: a systematic review. *Obstet Gynecol.* 2010; 116:393–401.

Xiong X, Buekens P, Fraser W, Beck J, Offenbacher S. Periodontal disease and adverse pregnancy outcomes: a systematic review. *Br J Obstet Gynaecol.* 2006; 113:135–143.

Xiong X, Buekens P, Vastardis S, Yu SM. Periodontal disease and pregnancy outcomes: state-of-the-science. *Obstet Gynecol Surv.* 2007; 62:1086–1089.

Yalcin F, Basegmez C, Isik G et al. The effects of periodontal therapy on intracrevicular prostaglandin E2 concentrations and clinical parameters in pregnancy. *J Periodontol.* 2002; 73:173–177.

Yokoyama M, Hinode D, Yoshioka M et al. Relationship between *Campylobacter rectus* and periodontal status during pregnancy. *Oral Microbiol Immunol.* 2008; 23:55–59.

Zi MY, Longo PL, Bueno-Silva B, Mayer MP. Mechanisms involved in the association between periodontitis and complications in pregnancy. *Front Public Health.* 2015; 2:290.

23.5 PERIODONTAL DISEASE AND RHEUMATOID ARTHRITIS

Steph Smith

Contents

Learning objectives

- Generation of citrullinated proteins, under both physiological and pathological conditions, including the role of neutrophils during periodontal disease.
- Possible correlations of dysbiotic periodontal microbiota with rheumatoid arthritis.
- The role of *Porphyromonas gingivalis* in the generation of citrullinated proteins and the priming of autoimmunity.
- The role of genetics in rheumatoid arthritis, the generation of anti-citrullinated protein autoantibody, the formation of immune complexes, and the role of smoking.
- Mechanisms of bone loss in rheumatoid arthritis patients with periodontal disease.
- Usage of medications and potential therapeutic difficulties in treating rheumatoid arthritis in periodontal disease patients.

Introduction

Rheumatoid arthritis (RA) is an autoimmune disease, whereby chronic synovial inflammation, together with the destruction of cartilage and bone, results in deformity and functional disability, especially seen in the small joints of the hands and feet (Sotorra-Figuerola & Gay-Escoda 2017). It is the most common autoimmune disease affecting the synovium of the joints, with the prevalence in the worldwide population reaching up to 1% (Manoil et al. 2021). Further development of the disease can include more severe extra-articular complications such as interstitial pneumonia or rheumatoid vasculitis (Turesson 2013). The age of onset is usually between 40 and 50 years old, though it can occur at any age, with women three times more likely to be affected than men (de Souza et al. 2016).

Not everyone who has RA manifests periodontitis, and not everyone with periodontal disease (PD) manifests with RA. Presently, a causal relationship between RA and PD seems unlikely; however, animal studies have demonstrated a biological plausibility for a more feasible association in a subset of susceptible RA patients (Bartold & Lopez-Oliva 2020). Numerous clinical and epidemiological studies have indicated an association between RA and PD (Rutger 2012). Compared to the general population, subjects with PD are at an increased risk of developing RA, and vice versa (Bartold & Lopez-Oliva 2020; Koziel et al. 2014). People with RA are almost twice as likely to have PD than those without RA (Demmer et al. 2011). The clinical course of PD in RA patients has been described to be more severe, this being independent of age, sex, ethnicity, or smoking history, compared to non-RA individuals (Koziel et al. 2014). PD has also been indicated to be a possible factor in the initiation and maintenance of the autoimmune inflammatory response that occurs in RA (Lundberg et al. 2010).

Pathogenesis

Citrullinated autoantigens in periodontal disease

Studies have shown a commonality of pathogenesis between RA and PD, linking patients with PD to an increased susceptibility to the development of RA (Araújo et al. 2015; Kaur et al. 2013). To date, the exact etiopathology of RA remains largely elusive (Manoil et al. 2021). The loss of tolerance to citrullinated proteins in genetically susceptible individuals has been described as the hallmark of the pathogenesis of RA, characterized by the triggering of an autoimmune response to citrullinated proteins (Arend & Firestein 2012; Konig et al. 2015). Citrullinated proteins are generated under physiological conditions, and are essential for many physiological processes, including terminal differentiation of the epidermis (profilaggrin and keratin), brain development (myelin basic protein), and the regulation of gene expression via chromatin remodeling (Wang et al. 2009). Protein citrullination is carried out by peptidylarginine deiminase-2 and peptidylarginine deiminase-4 (PAD) enzymes, which target internal arginine substrates (Bartold & Lopez-Oliva 2020), by converting the amino acid peptidylarginine into the amino acid peptidylcitrulline, resulting in a structural protein modification (Koziel et al. 2014). In people with RA this process becomes overactive, resulting in hypercitrullination and the abnormal accumulation of citrullinated proteins (Konig et al. 2016).

However, citrullination also occurs during pathological inflammatory conditions, including excessive cellular apoptosis, necrosis, and netosis, such as in PD (Araújo et al. 2015). Netosis is characterized by the release and externalization of decondensed chromatin fibers, containing hypercitrullinated histones, as well as the release of granule-derived (antimicrobial) proteins (Wang et al. 2009). Extracellular trap formation by neutrophils (netosis) is dependent on neutrophil PAD citrullination, leading to alterations in intra- and intermolecular interactions of proteins that possess internal arginine residues for their structure (Konig et al. 2015; Leech & Bartold 2015). These proteins include filaggrin, vimentin, collagen type II, and alpha-enolase. PAD activity is thus responsible for alterations in the three-dimensional architecture of these modified peptides, leading to the generation of a new range of autoantigenic anticyclic citrullinated peptides, thereby serving as autoantigens (Knight et al. 2012; Konig et al. 2016; van Venrooij & Pruijn 2014).

Periodontal bacteria and rheumatoid arthritis

The mucosal surfaces of periodontal pockets have been suggested to be sites of RA disease initiation, underpinning the hypothesis of an association between RA and periodontitis (Brusca et al. 2014). This postulate suggests that dysbiotic microbiota of periodontitis generate some of the initial antigens that further cause the adaptive immune system to cross-react with host epitopes (Brusca et al. 2014). In general, there is considerable variation among studies correlating subgingival microbiota with RA (Manoil et al. 2021). Studies have identified *Porphyromonas gingivalis* as contributing to the generation of autoantibodies in RA (du Teil Espina 2019). The genera *Prevotella* and *Leptotrichia* have also been associated with new-onset RA, and the species *Anaeroglobus geminatus* has been reported to positively correlate with autoantibodies and rheumatoid factor antibodies in RA patients (Scher et al. 2012). Another study has identified several periodontal taxa to be differentially abundant in the gingival crevicular fluid (GCF) of RA patients as detached bacteria, compared to control groups that included *P. gingivalis, Leptotrichia, Megasphaera*, and *A. geminatus* (Manoil et al. 2021). *Aggregatibacter actinomycetemcomitans* (A.a) has also been shown to trigger hypercitrullination in neutrophils, resulting in a spectrum of citrullinated proteins detected in GCF that closely resembles the one detected in the synovial fluid of RA patients (Konig et al. 2016). A.a causes hypercitrullination by secretion of leukotoxin A (LtxA), which pokes holes in neutrophils as a self-defense strategy to kill host immune cells. A study has demonstrated that almost half of patients with RA have evidence of infection with A.a compared with 11% of healthy individuals (Konig et al. 2016). However, high LtxA-producing A.a strains are usually more associated with localized aggressive periodontitis, whose association with RA, thus far, remains unclear (Manoil et al. 2021).

Porphyromonas gingivalis and citrullination

Porphyromonas gingivalis, which is strongly associated with PD, has been hypothesized to play a primary role in the initiation and maintenance of the autoimmune inflammatory responses that occur in RA (Wegner et al. 2010). *P. gingivalis* is unique in its expression of a bacterial PAD, namely *P. gingivalis* peptidylarginine deiminase (PPAD) (McGraw et al. 1999). PPAD is detected in the outer membrane fractions as well as in a secreted form of enzyme (McGraw et al. 1999; Quirke et al. 2014). *P. gingivalis* is the only bacterium known to express a PAD enzyme that can cause the citrullination of both bacterial and host proteins (de Souza et al. 2016). PPADs are also co-localized with arginine-specific gingipains in the outer membrane of *P. gingivalis* (Quirke et al. 2014), whereby these gingipains cleave protein chains, for example in filaggrin, fibrinogen, fibrin, collagen type II, vimentin, and α-enolase. The peptides generated by these gingipains lead to the exposure of C-terminal arginines, which are then rapidly citrullinated by PPAD (McGraw et al. 1999; Wegner et al. 2010). This is in contrast to its homolog human peptidylarginine deiminase-2 and peptidylarginine deiminase-4, as human peptidylarginine deiminase targets internal arginine substrates (Bartold & Lopez-Oliva 2020).

Other studies have also suggested that *P. gingivalis* PPAD itself undergoes autocitrullination, including the citrullination of 7 out of 18 arginines in the PPAD polypeptide chain (Quirke et al. 2014). This autocitrullination, although not proven to occur in vivo, may provide a plausible pathway in which *P. gingivalis* can present neoepitopes to the immune system in susceptible individuals, such as human leukocyte antigen (HLA)-DRB1 carriers (Rosenstein et al. 2004). Thus, PPAD, as a citrullinated bacterial protein itself, may then possibly be ascribed to be a potent antigen that may break the tolerance to citrullinated host proteins, whereby *P. gingivalis* infection can uniquely prime the immune response in RA, due to the appearance of PPAD autocitrullinated antigens (de Souza et al. 2016; Koziel et al. 2014; Quirke et al. 2014).

However, a further study has shown another unique antibody population, namely anti-PPAD antibodies, which are not part of the generation of autoantibodies against citrullinated proteins (Konig et al. 2015). These anti-PPAD antibodies in RA have been shown to not target citrullinated PPAD, but are rather exclusively directed against the unmodified enzyme, thereby causing the clearance of PPAD. Anti-PPAD antibodies may thus decrease the survival of *P. gingivalis*, and therefore have a protective role for PD in RA. By implication, then, PPAD autocitrullination is not the underlying mechanism linking *P. gingivalis*–associated PD and RA (Konig et al. 2015).

Nevertheless, RA-associated pathology is dependent on PPAD activity, which, either directly or indirectly (via the enhancement of inflammatory reactions and the release of host PADs), leads to the generation of citrullinated autoantigens, thus stimulating the production of anti-citrullinated protein autoantibodies (ACPAs). In this context, therefore, within a chronic inflammatory environment such as PD, in which the immune system is stimulated by bacteria-derived products such as lipopolysaccharides (LPS), fimbriae, and peptidoglycans, it has been suggested that the pathological citrullination of proteins in periodontal tissues by PPAD breaks immune tolerance to citrullinated proteins and peptides, thereby priming autoimmunity in a subset of patients with RA (Klareskog et al. 2009; Rutger 2012).

Genetics and anti-citrullinated protein autoantibody in susceptible individuals

Host cell and bacterial PAD activity, together with the loss of tolerance to generated autoantigenic citrullinated proteins in the tissues of genetically susceptible individuals, has been shown to initiate the generation of ACPAs in the synovia, and therefore the subsequent development of RA (Klareskog et al. 2009; Konig et al. 2015; Leech & Bartold 2015). Genetic factors have been shown to account for 50% of the risk of RA development, involving a shared epitope in HLA class II, which is associated with the production of ACPA (Araújo et al. 2015; van de Stadt et al. 2011). ACPAs are highly specific markers for the diagnosis of RA, and precede the onset of clinical disease by years (van de Stadt et al. 2011). This may be explained by the fact that low-avidity ACPAs may be found in both healthy subjects and RA patients and, as ACPA avidity maturation increases over time, the onset of clinical disease then occurs (Suwannalai et al. 2012; van de Stadt et al. 2011).

RA is characterized by the production of multiple autoantibodies, the most characteristic being rheumatoid factor (RF) antibody and ACPAs against autoantigens commonly expressed within synovial joints and alternative sites (Boissier et al. 2012; McInnes & Schett 2011). RF is produced by B cells in the synovial membrane and has been indicated to be responsible for the more aggressive destruction seen in joints (Scott 2012); however, other studies have stated that ACPA-positive RA is characterized by a more severe disease course (van Venrooij & Pruijn 2014). ACPAs and citrullinated autoantigens form immune complexes that then stimulate the inflammatory process, whereby the continuous production of immune complexes results in chronic inflammation, which is characteristic for RA (Konig et al. 2015; Manivelavan & Vijayasamundeeswari, 2012).

Smoking and rheumatoid arthritis

Smoking has been suggested to be the most recognized environmental trigger in genetically susceptible individuals, causing increased levels of the PAD enzyme (Di Giuseppe et al. 2014). Meta-analysis studies of gene–environmental interactions between smoking and shared epitopes showed that smoking interacts with HLA-DRB1 SE genes, and thereby increases the risk of ACPA expression in patients with RA (Lee et al. 2009). Smoking has been identified as a risk factor only for ACPA-positive and not for ACPA-negative RA (Klareskog et al. 2011). PAD activity may thus be imperative in initiating and sustaining autoimmunity in ACPA-positive RA (Konig et al. 2016).

Periodontal disease, rheumatoid arthritis, and bone loss

RA is an inflammatory autoimmune disease, while PD is an immunoinflammatory disease of bacterial origin. A correlation between PD and RA has been shown, whereby the mechanisms for the development of inflammation and tissue damage in RA have similarities with that which occurs during the pathogenesis of chronic PD (Araújo et al. 2015). In the periodontal lesion that precedes the RA lesion, citrullination of proteins by endogenous inflammation or by exogenous *P. gingivalis* citrullination leads to the production of autoantibodies to citrullinated proteins. These autoantibodies may then cross-react with cartilage components (autoimmunity to self-antigens) (Bartold & Lopez-Oliva 2020).

Studies have furthermore suggested the possibility of periodontal bacteria (either whole or DNA) translocating from the periodontal tissues to the synovium, where they may exacerbate the inflammatory processes occurring within rheumatoid joints (Bartold & Lopez-Oliva 2020). These bacteria include *P. gingivalis*, *Prevotella intermedia*, *Prevotella melaninogenica*, *T. forsythia*, and *A. actinomycetemcomitans* (Témoin et al. 2012).

Both RA and PD diseases represent a significant dysregulation of the inflammatory response (Bartold & Lopez-Oliva 2020). PAD enzymes, citrullinated proteins, and ACPA have been found in periodontal tissues, and *P. gingivalis* and antibodies to *P. gingivalis* have been found in the serum and synovial fluid of patients with RA (Klareskog et al. 2011). The inflammatory lesion of RA is characterized by the accumulation of leucocytes in the synovial membrane and fluid, including inflammatory mediators such as prostaglandin E2 (PGE2), tumor necrosis factor-alpha (TNF-α), interleukin-1β (IL-1β), IL-6, IL-12, IL-17, IL-18, and IL-33 (Martinez-Martinez et al. 2009). These inflammatory cytokines also induce osteoclastogenesis by increasing the expression of receptor activator of nuclear factor kappa B (NF-κB) ligand (RANKL), as well as reduce osteoprotegerin production in osteoblasts and stromal cells (McInnes & Schett 2011; Nakashima et al. 2000). T-helper 17 (Th17) cells associated with innate immunity against *P. gingivalis* have been indicated to be more osteoclastic than Th1 and Th2 cells, and IL-17 secreted from Th17 cells strongly contributes to bone destruction, as seen in RA (Gümüs et al. 2013).

Treatment of rheumatoid arthritis and periodontal disease

Periodontitis has a high prevalence, and thus may represent an important modifiable factor for RA incidence and severity. Therefore, if this is proven, treatment of periodontitis could present direct benefits for patients with RA. However, larger studies are required to determine the effect of non-surgical periodontal treatment on clinical indicators of RA (Bartold & Lopez-Oliva 2020).

Animal models have shown a bi-directional association between RA and PD, therefore treatments for RA could potentially influence the clinical manifestation of PD. Most treatments for RA involve the use of host-modifying drugs, whereby their usage is emerging as an important area of investigation for the adjunct treatment of PD (Preshaw 2018). Disease-modifying antirheumatic drugs such as TNF-α inhibitors, IL-6 receptor inhibitor, and anti–B lymphocyte therapies have been shown in various studies to have beneficial effects on the periodontal tissues of RA patients (Han & Reynolds 2012; Kobayashi et al. 2014; Mayer et al. 2013). There are however limited data to suggest that these agents can reduce local production of inflammatory cytokines and periodontal inflammation in RA patients with PD, and thus more larger studies are needed (Bartold & Lopez-Oliva 2020). Furthermore, these therapies, such as TNF-α inhibitors, have the potential to significantly suppress biological defense mechanisms, thereby allowing PD to worsen. This may then lead to sustained gingival inflammation and infection, hampering the treatment response in RA (Savioli et al. 2012). The long-time treatment of RA with disease-modifying antirheumatic drugs, such as immune system depressants, including glucocorticoids and methotrexate, may also affect the oral cavity, including impaired saliva secretion, oral ulceration, and candidiasis, as well as PD (Deeming et al. 2005).

REFERENCES

Araújo VMA, Matos-Melo I, Lima V. Relationship between periodontitis and rheumatoid arthritis: review of the literature. *Mediators Inflamm.* 2015; 1:1–15.

Arend WP, Firestein GS. Pre-rheumatoid arthritis: predisposition and transition to clinical synovitis. *Nat Rev Rheumatol.* 2012; 8:573–586.

Bartold PM, Lopez-Oliva I. Periodontitis and rheumatoid arthritis: an update 2012–2017. *Periodontol 2000.* 2020; 83:189–212.

Boissier MC, Semerano L, Challal S, Saidenberg-Kermanac'h N, Falgarone G. Rheumatoid arthritis: from autoimmunity to synovitis and joint destruction. *J Autoimmun.* 2012; 39:222–228.

Brusca SB, Abramson SB, Scher JU. Microbiome and mucosal inflammation as extra-articular triggers for rheumatoid arthritis and autoimmunity. *Curr Opin Rheumatol.* 2014; 26:101–107.

de Souza S, Bansal RK, Galloway J. Rheumatoid arthritis – an update for general dental practitioners. *Br Dent J.* 2016; 10:667–673.

Deeming GMJ, Collingwood J, Pemberton MN. Methotrexate and oral ulceration. *Br Dent J.* 2005; 98:83–85.

Demmer RT, Molitor JA, Jacobs DR Jr, Michalowicz BS. Periodontal disease, tooth loss and incident rheumatoid arthritis: results from the First National Health and Nutrition Examination Survey and its epidemiological follow-up study. *J Clin Periodontol.* 2011; 38:998–1006.

Di Giuseppe D, Discacciati A, Orsini N, Wolk A. Cigarette smoking and risk of rheumatoid arthritis: a dose-response meta-analysis. *Arthritis Res Ther.* 2014; 16:R61. doi: 10.1186/ar4498.

du Teil Espina M, Gabarrini G, Harmsen HJM et al. Talk to your gut: the oral-gut microbiome axis and its immunomodulatory role in the etiology of rheumatoid arthritis. *FEMS Microbiol Rev.* 2019; 43:1–18.

Gümüş P, Buduneli E, Basak B et al. Gingival crevicular fluid, serum levels of receptor activator of nuclear factor-κb ligand, osteoprotegerin, and interleukin-17 in patients with rheumatoid arthritis and osteoporosis and with periodontal disease. *J Periodontol.* 2013; 84:1627–1637.

Han JY, Reynolds MA. Effect of anti-rheumatic agents on periodontal parameters and biomarkers of inflammation: a systematic review and meta-analysis. *J Periodont Impl Sci.* 2012; 42(1):3–12.

Kaur S, White S, Bartold PM. Periodontal disease and rheumatoid arthritis: a systematic review. *J Dent Res.* 2013; 92:399–408.

Klareskog L, Catrina AI, Paget S. Rheumatoid arthritis. *Lancet.* 2009; 373:659–672.

Klareskog L, Malmstrom V, Lundberg K, Padyukov L, Alfredsson L. Smoking, citrullination and genetic variability in the immunopathogenesis of rheumatoid arthritis. *Sem Immunol.* 2011; 23:92–98.

Knight JS, Carmona-Rivera C, Kaplan MJ. Proteins derived from neutrophil extracellular traps may serve as self-antigens and mediate organ damage in autoimmune diseases. *Front Immunol.* 2012, 3:380.

Kobayashi T, Okada M, Ito S et al. Assessment of interleukin-6 receptor inhibition therapy on periodontal condition in patients with rheumatoid arthritis and chronic periodontitis. *J Periodontol.* 2014; 85(1):57–67.

Konig MF, Abusleme L, Reinholdt J et al. *Aggregatibacter actinomycetemcomitans*-induced hypercitrullination links periodontal infection to autoimmunity in rheumatoid arthritis. *Sci Transl Med.* 2016; 8(369):369ra176.

Konig MF, Paracha AS, Moni M et al. Defining the role of *Porphyromonas gingivalis* peptidylarginine deiminase (PPAD) in rheumatoid arthritis through the study of PPAD biology. *Ann Rheum Dis.* 2015; 74:2054–2061.

Koziel J, Mydel P, Potempa J. The link between periodontal disease and rheumatoid arthritis: an updated review. *Curr Rheumatol Rep.* 2014; 16:408–414.

Lee KS, Chung JH, Choi TK et al. Peripheral cytokines and chemokines in Alzheimer's disease. *Dement Geriatr Cogn Disord.* 2009; 28:281–287.

Leech MT, Bartold PM. The association between rheumatoid arthritis and periodontitis. *Best Pract Res Clin Rheumatol.* 2015; 29:189–201.

Lundberg K, Wegner N, Yucel-Lindberg T, Venables PJ. Periodontitis in RA—the citrullinated enolase connection. *Nat Rev Rheumatol.* 2010; 6:727–730.

Manivelavan D, Vijayasamundeeswari CK. Anti-cyclic citrullinated peptide antibody: an early diagnostic and prognostic biomarker of rheumatoid arthritis. *J Clin Diagn Res.* 2012; 6:1393–1396.

Manoil D, Bostanci N, Mumcu G et al. Novel and known periodontal pathogens residing in gingival crevicular fluid are associated with rheumatoid arthritis. *J Periodontol.* 2021; 92:359–370.

Martinez-Martinez RE, Abud-Mendoza C, Patiño-Marin N et al. Detection of periodontal bacterial DNA in serum and synovial fluid in refractory rheumatoid arthritis patients. *J Clin Periodontol.* 2009; 36: 1004–1010.

Mayer Y, Elimelech R, Balbir-Gurman A, Braun-Moscovici Y, Machtei EE. Periodontal condition of patients with autoimmune diseases and the effect of anti–tumor necrosis factor-alpha therapy. *J Periodontol.* 2013; 84(2):136–142.

McGraw WT, Potempa J, Farley D et al. Purification, characterization, and sequence analysis of a potential virulence factor from *Porphyromonas gingivalis*, peptidylarginine deiminase. *Infect Immun.* 1999; 67:3248–3256.

McInnes IB, Schett G. The pathogenesis of rheumatoid arthritis. *N Engl J Med.* 2011; 365:2205–2219.

Nakashima T, Kobayashi Y, Yamasaki S et al. Protein expression and functional difference of membrane-bound and soluble receptor activator of NF-kappaB ligand: modulation of the expression by osteotropic factors and cytokines. *Biochem Biophys Res Commun.* 2000; 275:768–775.

Preshaw PM. Host modulation therapy with anti-inflammatory agents. *Periodontol 2000.* 2018; 76(1):131–149.

Quirke A-M, Lugli EB, Wegner N et al. Heightened immune response to autocitrullinated *Porphyromonas gingivalis* peptidylarginine deiminase: a potential mechanism for breaching immunologic tolerance in rheumatoid arthritis. *Ann Rheum Dis.* 2014; 73:263–269.

Rosenstein ED, Greenwald RA, Kushner LJ et al. Humoral immune response to oral bacteria provides a stimulus for development of rheumatoid arthritis. *Inflammation.* 2004; 28(6):311–318.

Rutger PG. Rheumatoid arthritis and periodontitis – inflammatory and infectious connections. Review of the literature. *J Oral Microbiol.* 2012; 4:11829–11845.

Savioli C, Ribeiro AC, Fabri GM et al. Persistent periodontal disease hampers anti–tumor necrosis factor treatment response in rheumatoid arthritis. *J Clin Rheumatol.* 2012; 18(4):180–184.

Scher JU, Ubeda C, Equinda M et al. Periodontal disease and the oral microbiota in new-onset rheumatoid arthritis. *Arthritis Rheum.* 2012; 64:3083–3094.

Scott DL. Biologics-based therapy for the treatment of rheumatoid arthritis. *Clin Pharmacol Ther.* 2012; 91:30–43.

Sotorra-Figuerola D, Gay-Escoda C. Relation of rheumatoid arthritis and periodontal disease. *JSM Arthritis.* 2017; 2:1020–1023.

Suwannalai P, van de Stadt LA, Radner H et al. Avidity maturation of anti-citrullinated protein antibodies in rheumatoid arthritis. *Arthritis Rheum.* 2012; 64:1323–1328.

Témoin S, Chakaki A, Askari A et al. Identification of oral bacterial DNA in synovial fluid of patients with arthritis with native and failed prosthetic joints. *J Clin Rheumatol.* 2012; 18(3):117–121.

Turesson C. Extra-articular rheumatoid arthritis. *Curr Opin Rheumatol.* 2013; 25:360–366.

van de Stadt LA, de Koning MII, van de Stadt RJ et al. Development of the anti–citrullinated protein antibody repertoire prior to the onset of rheumatoid arthritis. *Arthritis Rheum.* 2011; 63:3226–3233.

van Venrooij WJ, Pruijn GJM. How citrullination invaded rheumatoid arthritis research. *Arthritis Res Ther.* 2014; 16:103.

Wang Y, Li M, Stadler S et al. Histone hypercitrullination mediates chromatin decondensation and neutrophil extracellular trap formation. *J Cell Biol.* 2009; 184:205–213.

Wegner N, Wait R, Sroka A et al. Peptidylarginine deiminase from *Porphyromonas gingivalis* citrullinates human fibrinogen and α-enolase: implications for autoimmunity in rheumatoid arthritis. *Arthritis Rheum.* 2010; 62:2662–2672.

23.6   PERIODONTAL DISEASE AND ALZHEIMER'S DISEASE

Steph Smith

Contents

Learning objectives

- Prevalence of Alzheimer's disease as part of dementia.
- Characteristics of patients with Alzheimer's disease.
- Pathology and pathogenesis of Alzheimer's disease, including the amyloid cascade, inflammatory and pathogen hypotheses.
- Role of periodontal disease in pathogenesis of Alzheimer's disease, including the central and peripheral mechanisms.
- How Alzheimer's disease affects patients' oral health, and suggested principles of therapy.

Introduction

It is estimated that 47 million people live with dementia worldwide, within which approximately 60–80% of dementia cases are attributable to Alzheimer's disease (AD) (Prince et al. 2013). The prevalence of dementia is expected to increase such that there will be over 100 million by 2050 (Brookmeyer et al. 2007). AD is estimated to affect 10–15% of those older than 65 years of age and 20% of those older than 80. Female patients account for two-thirds of all cases of AD (Kocaelli et al. 2002; Lane et al. 2018). It is a progressive neurodegenerative disorder, characterized by irreversible cognitive and physical deterioration (Honjo et al. 2009).

Features of Alzheimer's disease

Patients with AD can present with preclinical, mild, moderate, and severe AD. AD is a continuum in which the first pathological change occurs decades before the onset of dementia. The AD continuum has three stages: preclinical AD, prodromal AD, and AD dementia. Preclinical AD is characterized by the presence of AD-specific pathology, but no symptomatology. Prodromal AD is defined by the presence of clinical signs of mild cognitive impairment and the presence of AD-specific pathology. AD dementia has overt dementia and AD-specific pathology (Kamer et al. 2020). The most common sign of AD development is an elderly patient presenting with insidious, progressive problems associated with episodic memory (Lane et al. 2018). Patients with preclinical AD appear normal, but thereafter various signs and symptoms may be associated with the progression in severity of the disease. These may include, to mention a few, memory loss, confusion about the location of familiar places, shortened attention span, problems recognizing friends and family members, repetitive statements or movement, mood and personality changes, and increased anxiety. In the more severe forms of the disease, symptoms may include weight loss, seizures, increased sleeping, and lack of bladder and bowel control. In end-stage AD, death is often the result of other illnesses, whereby aspiration pneumonia has been described to frequently be the cause (Lakham 2017).

Pathology of Alzheimer's disease

The pathognomonic lesions of AD are characterized by senile or neuritic plaques, neurofibrillary tangles, inflammation, and neuronal degeneration.

The extracellular senile plaques are composed of fibrillar beta-amyloid (β-amyloid) filaments. They are surrounded by dystrophic neuritis, reactive astrocytes, and activated glial cells, and are associated with proinflammatory molecules.

The neurofibrillary tangles (tau tangles) are intraneuronal bundles of filaments, the main component of which is aggregates of hyperphosphorylated tau protein. Tau is a crucial component of the neuronal cytoskeleton and its hyperphosphorylation leads to the disassembly of microtubules and neuronal dysfunction.

The neuronal loss occurs mainly in the hippocampus and in entorhinal and temporoparietal cortices, leading to brain atrophy (Kamer et al. 2020).

Pathogenesis of Alzheimer's disease

The cause of AD is unclear (Kocaelli et al. 2002), however about 70% of AD risk has been shown to be attributable to genetic factors (Grimaldi et al. 2000; Lane et al. 2018). Various hypotheses have been suggested to explain the initiation and pathogenic processes in AD, including the amyloid cascade, inflammatory, and pathogen hypotheses (Kamer et al. 2020).

Amyloid cascade hypothesis

The amyloid precursor protein is a transmembrane glycoprotein, and although its primary function is not known, it has been implicated as a regulator of synapse formation and neural plasticity (Turner et al. 2003). The amyloid precursor protein undergoes proteolysis via alternative pathways, leading to the formation of β-amyloid, and is produced in neurons, astrocytes, and glial cells (Wang et al. 2017). β-amyloid is also produced peripherally in various organs, including the adrenal gland, kidney, heart, liver, spleen, pancreas, muscles, and in cells of blood lineage and endothelial cells. Of β-amyloid produced in the peripheral compartment, 90% is attributed to platelets (Roher et al. 2009).

β-amyloid has also been shown to exhibit biological similarity to the cathelicidin-related antimicrobial peptide LL37, being antimicrobial against viruses, bacteria, and fungi. Initially its production is beneficial by impairing deleterious microbial effects; however, as it accumulates, it becomes pathogenic (Eimer et al. 2018; Moir et al. 2018; Soscia et al. 2010).

The accumulation of amyloid in the brain is a function of its production and clearance. Amyloid clearance occurs both in the brain and in the peripheral compartment through complex processes, including enzymatic degradation, phagocytosis, and direct transport of β-amyloid between the central and peripheral compartments. The efflux of β-amyloid from the brain to the peripheral compartment occurs via the blood–brain barrier, blood–cerebrospinal fluid barrier, interstitial fluid bulk flow, and glymphatic–lymphatic pathways (Tarasoff-Conway et al. 2015). The influx of β-amyloid to the brain might occur at the level of circumventricular organs where the endothelial cells lack tight junctions, or at the level of the blood–brain barrier where the transport of peripheral amyloid to the brain is mediated via binding to the receptor for advanced glycation end products (Deane 2012). A disturbed equilibrium between influx and efflux may lead to brain amyloidosis. The amyloid fibrillar form of β-amyloid is the primary component of amyloid plaques found in the brains of AD patients. The accumulation of β-amyloid initiates a multistep cascade, ultimately leading to neuronal degeneration and dementia (Kamer et al. 2020).

Inflammatory hypothesis

Sources of central or peripheral inflammatory conditions can cause or contribute to neuroinflammation. The peripheral administration of lipopolysaccharides in animal models has been shown to induce the activation of astrocytes in the hippocampus and cerebral cortex by increasing the expression of amyloid precursor protein, leading to production of amyloid-$\beta42$ and the phosphorylation of tau. In turn, β-amyloid can stimulate the glial production of cytokines (Clark & Vissel 2015; Lee et al. 2008). Activated astrocytes and glial cells may then produce proinflammatory cytokines, such as tumor necrosis factor-alpha (TNF-α), interleukin-1 beta (IL-1β), IL-2, IL-6, IL-18, and C-reactive protein (CRP) (Lai et al. 2017). This inflammation within the central nervous system is thought to play a pivotal role in AD (Kronfol & Remick 2000). Studies have linked polymorphisms in the IL-1 gene family to periodontal disease (PD) and AD, whereby these polymorphisms may reflect a hyperinflammatory genotype being a trait common to people with PD and people with dementia (Grimaldi et al. 2000; McDevitt et al. 2000; Yucesoy et al. 2006). These inflammatory mediators thus maintain a vicious cycle firstly by stimulating brain cells, and secondly by activating pathways leading to (i) Alzheimer's disease-specific pathology, (ii) synaptic dysfunction, (iii) blood–brain barrier permeability, (iv) neurodegeneration, and (v) cognitive dysfunction (Clark & Vissel 2015; Kamer et al. 2008; Perry et al. 2007). Disruption of the blood–brain barrier can lead to increased permeability to cytokines, microbes, and their products, such as lipopolysaccharides (LPS) (Banks 2015). Inflammation can also impact β-amyloid clearance. Peripheral administration of LPS can increase brain influx and decrease brain efflux of β-amyloid (Jaeger et al. 2009).

Pathogen hypothesis

Microbial agents act mainly through inflammatory mechanisms to trigger AD pathology and cognitive dysfunction. Thus, the pathogen hypothesis is closely linked to the inflammatory hypothesis (Zhan et al. 2018). Animal and human studies have implicated gut and oral dysbiosis in AD (Kamer et al. 2015). Spirochetes associated with AD have been shown to be derived from the oral cavity (Miklossy et al. 1994). Other microbes include *Chlamydophila pneumoniae*, *Helicobacter pylori*, *Toxoplasma gondii*, *Treponema denticola*, and *Porphyromonas gingivalis* (Kamer et al. 2020; Miklossy et al. 1994; Riviere et al. 2002). Diverse pathological effects induced by dysbiosis can include LPS co-localized with amyloid-$\beta42$ in amyloid plaques and with amyloid-$\beta40$ around vessels in brain tissues, microglia activation, modulation of nutrition and immune systems, enhanced production of neurotransmitters and bacterial metabolic products, and altered neuronal communications (Kamer et al. 2020).

Herpesviruses have also been implicated in AD pathogenesis. These include herpes simplex virus type 1 and type 2, varicella-zoster virus, human herpesviruses 6A and 7, cytomegalovirus, and Epstein–Barr virus (Kamer et al. 2020). It has been proposed that herpesviruses migrate to the brain early in life, where they remain latent. They can then be reactivated periodically, inducing brain inflammation and subsequent pathology (Itzhaki 2018). Studies have shown that herpesviruses cause changes in several transcriptional regulators linked to modulators of amyloid precursor protein metabolism (Readhead et al. 2018).

In addition to inflammatory mechanisms, pathogens may act directly by producing neurotoxins, inhibiting the production of neuronal structure and stimulating β-amyloid (Lukiw et al. 2018; Zhao & Lukiw 2018).

Periodontal disease and pathogenesis of Alzheimer's disease

A possible link between PD and AD has been described (Abbayya et al. 2015). Evidence for the role of PD in AD pathogenesis comes from animal, in vitro, and clinical studies (Kamer et al. 2020). PD can affect each stage of AD pathogenesis through potentially different mechanisms. During the early stages of AD, PD can affect multiple pathogenic processes: β-amyloid production, β-amyloid clearance, tau phosphorylation, synapse and neuronal functioning, neurotransmission, and immune responses. As AD progresses, the PD inflammatory and bacterial burdens can further affect these processes, but they might also contribute to irreversible damage, such as neurodegeneration and neuronal loss. PD can occur before the onset of AD-specific pathology and accordingly has the potential to be causal (Kamer et al. 2020).

PD, with its inflammatory, bacterial, and viral burdens, can contribute to AD pathogenesis by affecting multiple central and peripheral processes (Kamer et al. 2020). The salient pathophysiological feature common to both diseases is a chronic inflammatory response, whereby PD is also considered to be one of the probable risk factors for AD (Abbayya et al. 2015; Kamer et al. 2008).

Central processes

Proinflammatory cytokines secreted in the periodontal tissues, including IL-1β, IL-6, IL8, TNF-α, and CRP, can enter the systemic circulation, reach the brain, and enter the cerebral regions (Kamer et al. 2008; Lee et al. 2009). Inflammatory molecules can access the brain at the level of the blood–brain interface in areas where the blood–brain barrier is permeable, i.e. the circumventricular organs, through fenestrated capillaries of the blood–brain barrier, by use of specific transporters, via routes of cerebrospinal fluid egress, by increases in blood–brain barrier permeability, and by neuronal routes (de Leon et al. 2017; Pan & Kastin 2003; Romeo et al. 2001). LPS bind to MD2 receptors and this complex binds to Toll-like receptors (TLRs), thus triggering a multistep signal transduction with an increase in cytokines. Chronic stimulation of neuronal endings by LPS may result in damage to neurons, and induce glia and astrocytic activation. Systemic LPS can increase systemic expression of cytokines, and centrally in the hippocampus (Hasegawa-Ishii et al. 2017). Leptomeningeal cells respond to peripheral inflammatory molecules, including LPS. Bacteria and inflammatory molecules can activate brain endothelial or leptomeningeal cells to transduce activating signals to the brain (Liu et al. 2013; Wu et al. 2005). Thereafter, a peripheral signal is transduced to the brain and is amplified, resulting in increased brain inflammation (Liu et al. 2013; Wu & Nakanishi 2014).

Pathogens, their LPS, and other virulence factors enter the brain using mechanisms similar to those of inflammatory molecules. Chronic inflammation can increase the permeability of the blood–brain barrier by damaging the tight junctions, which may result in the entry of microbes into the brain (Wu et al. 2008). Spirochetes, and particularly *T. denticola*, may utilize branches of the trigeminal nerve to reach the brain (Miklossy et al. 1994; Riviere et al. 2002). *T. denticola* has been found in cerebrospinal fluid, brain tissue, trigeminal ganglia, and the pons (Riviere et al. 2002). A study has suggested that *Porphyromonas gingivalis* may provide the mechanistic link between PD and AD (Kamer et al. 2020). *P. gingivalis* DNA has been identified in the cerebrospinal fluid and saliva of individuals with mild to moderate cognitive impairment, clinically diagnosed as having probable AD (Dominy et al. 2019). *P. gingivalis* has been identified in the brain of AD patients, where they utilize TLR4 and possibly TLR2 (Dominy et al. 2019). Various studies have shown that PD-derived bacterial species, including *P. gingivalis*, are associated with increases in hippocampus and cortical expression of amyloid-β42 and amyloid-β40, and are thus able to induce neuroinflammation, brain pathology, neurodegeneration, and cognitive impairment (Kamer et al. 2020). Toxic proteases from *P. gingivalis*, i.e. gingipains, although localized throughout the brain, have been shown to be most prominent in regions associated with memory, such as the hippocampus (Ryder 2020). Gingipains have been shown to correlate with tau and ubiquitin pathology, including being co-localized with neurons, and to be in association with tau tangles and intracellular β-amyloid (Ryder 2020), as well as with an increased production of components of amyloid plaques (Dominy et al. 2019). Gingipains have also been described as neurotoxic, causing neuroinflammation, and to cause damage to neurons in the hippocampus (Dominy et al. 2019).

Once in the brain, periodontal bacteria that are rich in LPS or their products are capable of stimulating cytokine production. These cytokines, periodontal bacteria, and LPS may then act on already primed glial cells, resulting in an amplified reaction and possible progression of AD (Lee et al. 2009; Romeo et al. 2001).

Aging brain is characterized by a chronic, low-grade proinflammatory state that confers a priming characteristic to cells, whereby the priming of microglia results in exaggerated responses to consequent inflammatory stimuli. The consequences of PD can thus be accompanied by memory impairment as a result of neuronal loss and inhibition of acetylcholine

(Cunningham et al. 2005; Oue et al. 2013; Santoro et al. 2018). An additional mechanism by which subgingival bacteria can impact AD pathology is through gut dysbiosis (Xue et al. 2020).

Peripheral processes

In addition to the central effects of PD affecting AD patients, an alternative hypothesis has been suggested to explain the effect of PD on peripheral amyloid. This includes inflammatory molecules and bacterial products associated with PD potentially increasing the synthesis of peripheral amyloid and enhancing its transport into the brain (Kamer et al. 2020).

Amyloid precursor protein has been found to be mainly localized in macrophages of gingival connective tissues (Kubota et al. 2014). In inflamed gingival tissues, the level of neprilysin, a β-amyloid–degrading enzyme, is also increased, suggesting active regulation of β-amyloid in inflamed gingival tissue. Studies thus support the supposition that PD enhances production or reduces clearance of β-amyloid locally, which could contribute to its increased systemic levels (Nezu et al. 2017). Furthermore, periodontal inflammatory and bacterial products may contribute to the increase in production of plasma β-amyloid, perhaps by platelet activation (Papapanagiotou et al. 2009).

In addition to bacteria, sites with progressive PD have been shown to be more likely to be associated with reactivated cytomegalovirus and herpes simplex virus type 1 viruses, compared with periodontally stable sites that contain latent viruses (Li et al. 2017; Saygun et al. 2005). Considering the evidence linking herpesviruses to AD pathogenesis, it is conceivable that herpesviruses associated with PD may play a role in AD (Slots 2019).

Alzheimer's disease and dental health

The number of AD-affected persons is expected to double or triple by the year 2050 (Forsyth & Ritzline 1998). Oral dysfunctions such as sucking reflex or involuntary oral movements can limit dental functioning in AD patients, especially affecting the stability of dentures (Shimazaki et al. 2001). Significant dental problems have been shown to result from a progressive diminution in oral self-care, resulting in more gingival plaque, bleeding, and calculus, compared with age- and gender-matched adults (Kieser et al. 1999; Ship 1992). AD patients taking medications may also have decreased salivary secretion (Ship et al. 1990). Dental professionals will therefore face a greater burden of maintaining and preserving dental health in older patients with dementia. The emphasis is thus on the importance of anticipating future oral decline in treatment planning, as well as instituting aggressive preventive measures (such as the use of topical fluoride and chlorhexidine), including frequent recall visits, and daily oral hygiene (Kocaelli et al. 2002). Addressing inflammatory, infectious, and dysbiotic conditions is now emphasized by the AD research community (Rogers 2018). However, note should be taken of the fact that sooner or later any dental care may become unmanageable and no longer be practicable (Chung & Cummings 2000).

Future studies

Studies on gingipain inhibitors may provide a promising approach to the treatment of both PD and AD. The results of the Food and Drug Administration clinical trials presently being performed to assess the effects of gingipain inhibitors on periodontitis and AD may provide more definitive evidence of these effects (Ryder 2020).

REFERENCES

Abbayya K, Puthanakar NY, Naduwinmani S, Chidambar YS. Association between periodontitis and Alzheimer's disease. *N Am J Med Sci.* 2015; 7:241–246.

Banks WA. The blood–brain barrier in neuroimmunology: tales of separation and assimilation. *Brain Behav Immun.* 2015; 44:1–8.

Brookmeyer R, Johnson E, Ziegler-Graham K, Arrighi HM. Forecasting the global burden of Alzheimer's disease. *Alzheimers Dement.* 2007; 3(3):186–191.

Chung JA, Cummings JL. Neurobehavioral and neuropsychiatric symptoms in Alzheimer's disease: characteristics and treatment. *Neurol Clin.* 2000; 18:829–846.

Clark IA, Vissel B. Amyloid beta: one of three danger-associated molecules that are secondary inducers of the proinflammatory cytokines that mediate Alzheimer's disease. *Br J Pharmacol.* 2015; 172(15):3714–3727.

Cunningham C, Wilcockson DC, Campion S, Lunnon K, Perry VH. Central and systemic endotoxin challenges exacerbate the local inflammatory response and increase neuronal death during chronic neurodegeneration. *J Neurosci.* 2005; 25(40):9275–9284.

de Leon MJ, Li Y, Okamura N et al. Cerebrospinal fluid clearance in Alzheimer disease measured with dynamic PET. *J Nucl Med.* 2017; 58(9):1471–1476.

Deane RJ. Is RAGE still a therapeutic target for Alzheimer's disease? *Future Med Chem.* 2012; 4(7):915–925.

Dominy SS, Lynch C, Ermini F et al. Porphyromonas gingivalis in Alzheimer's disease brains: evidence for disease causation and treatment with small-molecule inhibitors. *Sci. Adv.* 2019; 5(1): eaau3333. doi: 10.1126/sciadv.aau3333.

Eimer WA, Vijaya Kumar DK, Navalpur Shanmugam NK et al. Alzheimer's disease-associated beta-amyloid is rapidly seeded by *Herpesviridae* to protect against brain infection. *Neuron.* 2018; 100:1527–1532.

Forsyth E, Ritzline PD. An overview of the etiology, diagnosis, and treatment of Alzheimer disease. *Phys Ther.* 1998; 78:1325–1331.

Grimaldi LM, Casadei VM, Ferri C et al. Association of early-onset Alzheimer's disease with an interleukin-1alpha gene polymorphism. *Ann Neurol.* 2000; 47(3):361–365.

Hasegawa-Ishii S, Shimada A, Imamura F. Lipopolysaccharide initiated persistent rhinitis causes gliosis and synaptic loss in the olfactory bulb. *Sci Rep.* 2017; 7(1):11605.

Honjo K, van Reekum R, Verhoeff NP. Alzheimer's disease and infection: do infectious agents contribute to progression of Alzheimer's disease? *Alzheimers Dement.* 2009; 5(4):348–360.

Itzhaki RF. Corroboration of a major role for herpes simplex virus type 1 in Alzheimer's disease. *Front Aging Neurosci.* 2018; 10:324.

Jaeger LB, Dohgu S, Sultana R et al. Lipopolysaccharide alters the blood–brain barrier transport of amyloid beta protein: a mechanism for inflammation in the progression of Alzheimer's disease. *Brain Behav Immun.* 2009; 23(4):507–517.

Kamer AR, Craig RG, Niederman R, Fortea J, de Leon MJ. Periodontal disease as a possible cause for Alzheimer disease. *Periodontol 2000.* 2020; 83:242–271.

Kamer AR, Dasanayake AP, Craig RG et al. Alzheimer's disease and peripheral infections: the possible contribution from periodontal infections, model and hypothesis. *J Alzheimers Dis.* 2008; 13(4):437–449.

Kamer AR, Pirraglia E, Tsui W et al. Periodontal disease associates with higher brain amyloid load in normal elderly. *Neurobiol Aging.* 2015; 36(2):627–633.

Kieser J, Jones G, Borlase G, MacFadyen E. Dental treatment of patients with neurodegenerative disease. *N Z Dent J.* 1999; 95:130–134.

Kocaelli H, Yaltirik M, Yargic LI, Özbas H. Alzheimer's disease and dental management. *Oral Surg Oral Med Oral Pathol Oral Radiol Endod.* 2002; 93:521–524.

Kronfol Z, Remick DG. Cytokines and the brain: implications for clinical psychiatry. *Am J Psychiatry.* 2000; 157(5):683–694.

Kubota T, Maruyama S, Abe D et al. Amyloid beta (A4) precursor protein expression in human periodontitis-affected gingival tissues. *Arch Oral Biol.* 2014; 59(6):586–594.

Lai KSP, Liu CS, Rau A et al. Peripheral inflammatory markers in Alzheimer's disease: a systematic review and meta-analysis of 175 studies. *J Neurol Neurosurg Psychiatry.* 2017; 88(10):876–882.

Lakhan SE. Alzheimer disease. Drugs & Diseases – Neurology. *Medscape.* 2017. doi: emedicine.medscape.com/article/1134817.

Lane CA, Hardy J, Schott JM. Alzheimer's disease. *Eur J Neurol.* 2018; 25:59–70.

Lee JW, Lee YK, Yuk DY et al. Neuro-inflammation induced by lipopolysaccharide causes cognitive impairment through enhancement of beta-amyloid generation. *J Neuroinflammation.* 2008; 5:37.

Lee KS, Chung JH, Choi TK et al. Peripheral cytokines and chemokines in Alzheimer's disease. *Dement Geriatr Cogn Disord.* 2009; 28:281–287.

Li F, Zhu C, Deng FY et al. Herpesviruses in etiopathogenesis of aggressive periodontitis: a meta-analysis based on case–control studies. *PLoS One.* 2017;12(10):e0186373.

Liu Y, Wu Z, Zhang X et al. Leptomeningeal cells transduce peripheral macrophages inflammatory signal to microglia in response to *Porphyromonas gingivalis* LPS. *Mediators Inflamm.* 2013; 2013:407562.

Lukiw WJ, Cong L, Jaber V, Zhao Y. Microbiome derived lipopolysaccharide (LPS) selectively inhibits neurofilament light chain (NFL) gene expression in human neuronal-glial (HNG) cells in primary culture. *Front Neurosci.* 2018; 12:896.

McDevitt MJ, Wang HY, Knobelman C et al. Interleukin-1 genetic association with periodontitis in clinical practice. *J Periodontol.* 2000; 71(2):156–163.

Miklossy J, Kasas S, Janzer RC, Ardizzoni F, Van der Loos H. Further ultrastructural evidence that spirochaetes may play a role in the aetiology of Alzheimer's disease. *NeuroReport.* 1994; 5(10):1201–1204.

Moir RD, Lathe R, Tanzi RE. The antimicrobial protection hypothesis of Alzheimer's disease. *Alzheimers Dement.* 2018; 14(12):1602–1614.

Nezu A, Kubota T, Maruyama S et al. Expression of neprilysin in periodontitis-affected gingival tissues. *Arch Oral Biol.* 2017; 79:35–41.

Oue H, Miyamoto Y, Okada S et al. Tooth loss induces memory impairment and neuronal cell loss in APP transgenic mice. *Behav Brain Res.* 2013; 252:318–325.

Pan W, Kastin AJ. Interactions of cytokines with the blood–brain barrier: implications for feeding. *Curr Pharm Des.* 2003; 9(10):827–831.

Papapanagiotou D, Nicu EA, Bizzarro S et al. Periodontitis is associated with platelet activation. *Atherosclerosis.* 2009; 202(2):605–611.

Perry VH, Cunningham C, Holmes C. Systemic infections and inflammation affect chronic neurodegeneration. *Nat Rev Immunol.* 2007; 7:161–167.

Prince M, Bryce R, Albanese E et al. The global prevalence of dementia: a systematic review and meta-analysis. *Alzheimers Dement.* 2013; 9(1):63–75.

Readhead B, Haure-Mirande JV, Funk CC et al. Multiscale analysis of independent Alzheimer's cohorts finds disruption of molecular, genetic, and clinical networks by human herpesvirus. *Neuron.* 2018; 99(1):64–82.

Riviere GR, Riviere KH, Smith KS. Molecular and immunological evidence of oral *Treponema* in the human brain and their association with Alzheimer's disease. *Oral Microbiol Immunol.* 2002; 17(2):113–118.

Rogers J. Principles for central nervous system inflammation research: a call for a consortium approach. *Alzheimers Dement.* 2018; 14(11):1553–1559.

Roher AE, Esh CL, Kokjohn TA et al. Amyloid beta peptides in human plasma and tissues and their significance for Alzheimer's disease. *Alzheimers Dement.* 2009; 5(1):18–29.

Romeo HE, Tio DL, Rahman SU, Chiappelli F, Taylor AN. The glossopharyngeal nerve as a novel pathway in immune-to-brain communication: relevance to neuroimmune surveillance of the oral cavity. *J Neuroimmunol.* 2001; 2:91–100.

Ryder MI. Porphyromonas gingivalis and Alzheimer disease: recent findings and potential therapies. *J Periodontol.* 2020; 91(Suppl 1):S45–S49.

Santoro A, Spinelli CC, Martucciello S et al. Innate immunity and cellular senescence: the good and the bad in the developmental and aged brain. *J Leukoc Biol.* 2018; 103(3):509–524.

Saygun I, Kubar A, Ozdemir A, Slots J. Periodontitis lesions are a source of salivary cytomegalovirus and Epstein–Barr virus. *J Periodontal Res.* 2005; 40(2):187–191.

Shimazaki Y, Soh I, Saito T et al. Influence of dentition status on physical disability, mental impairment, and mortality in institutionalized elderly people. *J Dent Res.* 2001; 80:340–345.

Ship JA. Oral health of patients with Alzheimer's disease. *J Am Dent Assoc.* 1992; 123(1):53–58.

Ship JA, DeCarli C, Friedland RP, Baum BJ. Diminished submandibular salivary flow in dementia of Alzheimer type. *J Gerontol Med Sci.* 1990; 45:61–66.

Slots J. Focal infection of periodontal origin. *Periodontol 2000.* 2019; 79(1):233–235.

Soscia SJ, Kirby JE, Washicosky KJ et al. The Alzheimer's disease-associated amyloid beta-protein is an antimicrobial peptide. *PLoS One.* 2010; 5(3):e9505–e9515.

Tarasoff-Conway JM, Carare RO, Osorio RS et al. Clearance systems in the brain—implications for Alzheimer disease. *Nat Rev Neurol.* 2015; 11(8):457–470.

Turner PR, O'Connor K, Tate WP, Abraham WC. Roles of amyloid precursor protein and its fragments in regulating neural activity, plasticity and memory. *Prog Neurobiol.* 2003; 70(1):1–32.

Wang J, Gu BJ, Masters CL, Wang YJ. A systemic view of Alzheimer disease – insights from amyloid-beta metabolism beyond the brain. *Nat Rev Neurol.* 2017; 13(11):703.

Wu Z, Nakanishi H. Connection between periodontitis and Alzheimer's disease: possible roles of microglia and leptomeningeal cells. *J Pharmacol Sci.* 2014; 126(1):8–13.

Wu Z, Tokuda Y, Zhang XW, Nakanishi H. Age-dependent responses of glial cells and leptomeninges during systemic inflammation. *Neurobiol Dis.* 2008; 32(3):543–551.

Wu Z, Zhang J, Nakanishi H. Leptomeningeal cells activate microglia and astrocytes to induce IL-10 production by releasing pro-inflammatory cytokines during systemic inflammation. *J Neuroimmunol.* 2005; 2:90–98.

Xue L, Zou X, Yang XQ et al. Chronic periodontitis induces microbiota-gut-brain axis disorders and cognitive impairment in mice. *Exp Neurol.* 2020; 326:113176.

Yucesoy B, Peila R, White LR et al. Association of interleukin-1 gene polymorphisms with dementia in a community-based sample: the Honolulu-Asia Aging Study. *Neurobiol Aging.* 2006; 27(2):211–217.

Zhan X, Stamova B, Sharp FR. Lipopolysaccharide associates with amyloid plaques, neurons and oligodendrocytes in Alzheimer's disease brain: a review. *Front Aging Neurosci.* 2018; 10:42.

Zhao Y, Lukiw WJ. Bacteroidetes neurotoxins and inflammatory neurodegeneration. *Mol Neurobiol.* 2018; 55(12):9100–9107.

CHAPTER 24

Autoimmune disorders affecting the periodontium

Mabi Singh and Adriane Kilar

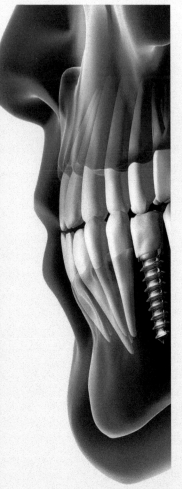

Contents

Learning objectives

- Awareness of autoimmunity affecting the periodontium.
- Oral clinical appearance of autoimmune disorders affecting the oral cavity.
- Differential diagnosis of various oral autoimmune disorders.
- Various pharmacological agents that can be used for treatment.
- Rationale of treatment of oral lesions with an autoimmune pathogenesis.

Essential Periodontics, First Edition. Edited by Steph Smith and Khalid Almas.
© 2022 John Wiley & Sons Ltd. Published 2022 by John Wiley & Sons Ltd.

Introduction

The relationship between autoimmunity and pathogenesis of periodontal disease resulting in destructive periodontitis was first described by Brandtzaeg and Kraus in 1965. This process involves the formation of a localized hypersensitivity reaction complex. The exact cause and mechanism of the initiation of autoimmunity are still unknown, but factors including environmental and infectious agents, e.g. viruses, yeasts, and bacteria (exogenous antigens) in a genetically susceptible individual, are considered possible etiological factors for the initiation and progression of local inflammatory responses in human adult periodontitis (Hirsch et al. 1988). Autoimmune diseases are more prevalent in women than in men and may occur at any age.

The oropharyngeal, gastrointestinal, and respiratory mucosa have a similar fate as the oral mucosa. T lymphocytes are believed to be responsible for the maintenance and integrity of the oral mucosa. Oral microbiota can act as antigenic agents and cross-reactivity may lead to the breakdown of the mucosa, causing ulcerations. In periodontal disease, Gram-negative microorganisms in periodontal pockets promote the production of systemic autoantibodies (Berglundh et al. 2002), resulting in elevated serum containing greater amounts of serum-derived proteins and immunological contents in the gingival crevicular fluid of active disease sites (Ebersole & Capelli 1994; Ebersole et al. 1982, 1987; Genco et al. 1974). As a response to dysbiotic microbiota, the production of these autoantibodies can lead to the destruction of periodontal tissue (Hajishengallis 2014). Periodontal disease may also activate autoantigens against collagen type 1. Aggressive and chronic periodontitis may have different kinds of autoimmune activity with varying degrees of tissue destruction.

Since autoimmune diseases may have manifestations in the oral cavity before other organ systems (Mays et al. 2012), oral healthcare providers have the initial responsibility of diagnosing and managing interdisciplinary care for these patients. Oral discomfort, pain, and compromised oral hygiene may be associated with many autoimmune conditions. Inflammation (classic sign), erythema, gingival recession, and painful ulcerations seen with autoimmune diseases can lead to the exacerbation of a periodontal condition. Furthermore, oral sensitivity to food and drinks as well as difficulty in eating and swallowing may persist, which can disrupt the pleasure of eating, cause a change in diet, and ultimately affect a person's nutritional health, thus decreasing overall quality of life.

The treatment of individual diseases depends upon the severity of the conditions and the response by the individual. Periodontitis associated with systemic autoimmune conditions may not respond to conventional treatments. Treatment includes clinical monitoring; the use of steroids through topical application, systemic use, or local site injections; the use of steroids for immune modulation and suppression; the use of antibiotics such as azathioprine, cyclophosphamide, fluocinonide, and dapsone; the use of retinoids; and the use of other medications such as benzocaine, viscous lidocaine, (hydroxy) chloroquine, and light therapy.

Autoimmune disorders affecting the periodontium

Aphthous ulcerations

Aphthous ulcerations are characterized by the breakdown in the continuity of the mucosa, especially the non-keratinized mucosa. The pathogenesis of aphthous ulceration is not clear, but bacterial involvement with *Streptococcus sanguinis* (Barile et al. 1963) and *S. mitis* (Hoover & Greenspan 1983; Narikawa et al. 1995), along with predisposing factors such as genetic susceptibility, local trauma and irritation, stress, hormonal changes, exposure to pharmaceutical agents, tobacco, and deficiencies of iron, vitamin B12, or folic acid have been frequently proposed. The possible autoimmune process involves the production of proinflammatory cytokines.

Aphthous ulcers tend to be more prevalent in the younger population and recurrent aphthous ulcerations usually occur at different sites. Burning and itchiness occur during the prodromal phase, followed by vesicle formation. Thereafter one or more lesions occur with a central yellowish ulcerated fibrinous area and an erythematous halo. Minor aphthous ulcers (less than a centimeter in diameter) are the most common type and usually heal without scarring in about 1–2 weeks. Major aphthous ulcers are larger than 1 cm in diameter, are more painful and take longer to heal, and heal with scarring. Herpetiform aphthous ulcers present as multiple, clustered lesions that are smaller (1–3 mm), and may include gingival involvement.

Healing is usually spontaneous or self-limiting, thus not requiring any treatment, but may be delayed in areas with increased mobility or may need extensive systemic treatment. Any ulceration lasting more than two weeks should be biopsied. The symptomatic pain and discomfort with stimuli could demand topical anaesthetics and even topical steroids (ointments, creams) of various strengths. The usage of antiseptics and antibiotic mouthwashes will help in reducing secondary infections and in faster healing of the ulcerations. In severe cases, immunomodulation with, e.g., colchicine, pentoxifylline, dapsone, or thalidomide may be required. Low-level and other forms of laser therapy have been used to treat aphthous ulcerations in the oral cavity.

Behçet's disease

Behçet's disease is a chronic and immunologically mediated inflammatory condition, with the oral mucosa being the first site to manifest symptoms similar to recurrent aphthous ulcerations (>95%). Recurrence of the ulceration occurs, especially in the vaginal, vulva, ocular (uveitis, conjunctivitis), and skin areas.

Behçet's disease is a rare systemic vasculitis with significant neutrophil infiltration, endothelial cell swelling, and fibrinoid necrosis, which is diagnosed with exclusion of other diseases on clinical presentation. In contrast to autoimmune disorders, Behçet's disease has clinical features that are mostly autoinflammatory, which places the disease at the crossroads between autoimmune and autoinflammatory syndromes (Pineton de Chambrun et al. 2012). Endothelial dysfunction has been established in Behçet's disease. Inflammatory cells within the lesions mostly include neutrophils, CD4(+) T cells, and cytotoxic cells (Houman et al. 2014). Herpes simplex virus-1 and *Streptococcus* spp. have been postulated, with no pathognomonic laboratory findings (Greco et al. 2018).

The mild form of Bechet's disease may not need treatment, but moderate to severe conditions may need analgesics, anti-inflammatory medications, and even topical corticosteroids or mouthwashes. Systemically, colchicine, tacrolimus (also topical), and prednisone have been used for treatment. The resistant or severe form of Behçet's disease has been treated with immunosuppression, e.g. azathioprine, cyclosporine, cyclophosphamide, rituximab, dapsone, thalidomide, etc., with varied success.

Crohn's disease

Crohn's disease can occur in any population of any age, but it is mostly observed in the second decade of life and has strong familial aggregations. It effects the mucosal lining, from the oral cavity to the anus. The oral lesions may present as indurated tag-like lesions, cobblestoning, mucogingivitis, deep linear ulcerations, and aphthous stomatitis (Lankarani et al. 2013).

Overactivation of the mucosal immune system can be caused by predisposing genetic factors and dysbiosis of gut microbiota. Antigen from the normal commensal bacterial flora and T cells cross-react to cause inflammation (Greenberg et al. 2005).

Topical anesthetic, e.g. viscous lidocaine, and corticosteroids, e.g. triamcinolone 0.1%, dexamethasone elixir, are used for symptomatic treatment along with non-steroidal anti-inflammatory drugs (NSAIDs). Refractory lesions are treated with systemic steroids and the intralesional injection of steroids.

Scleroderma (systemic sclerosis) and CREST syndrome

Scleroderma is characterized by the accumulation of connective tissue on the skin, leading to thickening of the skin, resulting in microstomia, xerostomia, and limiting function of many other organs. Fibrosis of the muscles of the temporomandibular joint alters the degree of opening of the mouth (peusdoankylosis). Restricted opening of the oral cavity can lead to difficulty or failure to provide and receive dental care by the dentist and the patient. Many patients also have strictures on their hands, which can lead to a compromise in manual dexterity. This in turn can cause a decrease in the ability to maintain adequate oral hygiene. A slowly progressive form of systemic scleroderma, CREST syndrome, is characterized by calcinosis cutis, Raynaud's phenomenon, esophageal involvement, sclerodactyly, and telangiectasia (Stanford et al. 1999).

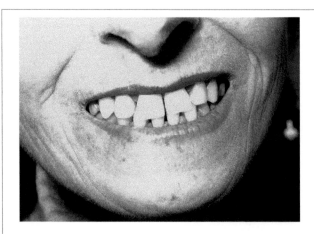

Figure 24.1 Scleroderma. Courtesy of Dr. Athena Papas.

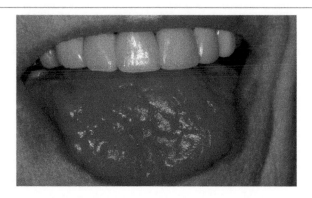

Figure 24.2 Scleroderma affecting the tongue. Courtesy of Dr. Athena Papas.

Clinically, there can be foci of severe gingival recession due to fibrous strictures and attached gingiva stripping, prominent lingual and buccal mucosal crenations, and loss of tongue mobility with fibrotic induration (Eversole et al. 1984). The widening of the periodontal ligament results in various degrees of mobility of teeth. Fibrosis decreases the blood supply, so no bleeding may be observed.

Radiographically, a uniform widening of the periodontal ligament space, especially around the posterior teeth, and varying degrees of bone resorption in the mandible are noted (Martin 1994). Furthermore, due to the limited opening of the mouth and the tense skin, bitewing and periapical radiographs are difficult to capture, so panoramic and cone beam images may be indicated (see Figures 24.1 and 24.2).

Oral lichen planus

Oral lichen planus (OLP) is an autoimmune condition affecting the skin, the mucus membrane of the oral cavity, the genitals, and the scalp. These lesions can occur anywhere in the oral cavity, including the buccal mucosa, gingiva, periodontium, tongue, floor of the mouth, and even the palate. OLP can occur with other autoimmune conditions such as Sjögren's syndrome, where there is a 30% higher chance of occurrence. OLP can present in a variety of forms. Six subtypes of lesions have been described: white, flat, popular, lacy (reticular), red inflamed, ulcerated, or a combination of these. The lacy pattern with Wickham's striae is the most common form (Andreasen 1968). Oral discomfort and pain can range from mild to severe (see Figures 24.3 and 24.4).

The etiology is unknown, but has been linked to allergies to dental materials, cell-mediated hypersensitivity, drugs (e.g. angiotensin-converting enzyme [ACE] inhibitors, beta-blockers, nifedipine), and stress. In OLP, there is migration of cytotoxic CD8+ T lymphocytes into the epithelium, inducing apoptosis of basal keratinocytes (Kurago 2016). OLP has been associated with numerous systemic connotations, such as metabolic syndrome, diabetes mellitus, hypertension, thyroid diseases, psychosomatic ailments, chronic liver disease, gastrointestinal diseases, and genetic susceptibility to cancer (Hasan et al. 2019).

The chance of OLP transforming into malignant lesions such as oral squamous cell carcinoma (OSCC) is higher in women than in men. In a seven-year prospective study, the development of OSCC was seen in areas of OLP (0.36%/year) and the standardized incidence ratio for OSCC was significantly higher in women – 27.0 (95% confidence interval [CI] 11.2–64.8) – than in men – 11.2 (95% CI 3.6–34.9) (Bombeccari et al. 2011). In a retrospective study of OLP, a malignant transformation rate of 1.9% was observed (Ingafou et al. 2006).

It should be emphasized that the management and treatment for OLP are not curative, but involve the reduction of inflammation and improving the quality of life affected by the associated symptoms. Non-symptomatic OLP should be watched on a frequent basis. Mild to moderate OLP is treated with topical corticosteroids, e.g. clobetasol, fluocinonide, dexamethasone elixir; topical calcineurin inhibitors, e.g. tacrolimus, pimecrolimus; and intralesional triamcinolone acetonide injection. Severe cases of OLP are managed with oral prednisone, tapered for 3–6 weeks, and retinoids, e.g. acitretin.

Pemphigus vulgaris

Even though "pemphigus vulgaris" (PV) is suggestive of a (vulgaris) common (pemphix) blistering condition, this autoimmune disease is not very common. It is the most common variant of pemphigus (80%) and is more prevalent in older and middle-aged males, even though it can occur at any age. Studies found that periodontal status is worse in PV patients and that PV might contribute to the development and/or progression of periodontitis (see Figures 24.5 and 24.6).

Direct immunofluorescence studies are positive for immunoglobulin (Ig)G in the intercellular region (Lamey et al. 1992). When PV does not respond to topical steroids, e.g. clobetasol, betamethasone, triamcinolone acetonide, and cyclosporine, systemic corticosteroids, e.g. prednisone and prednisolone, may be used along with immunosuppressives,

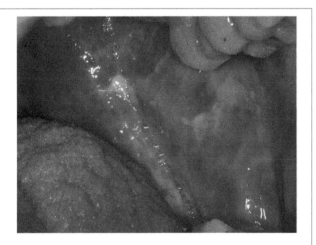

Figure 24.3 Oral lichen planus.

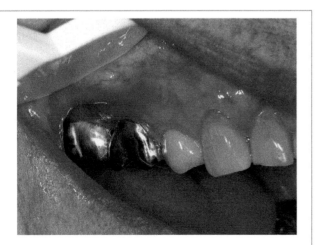

Figure 24.4 Oral lichen planus on posterior maxillary gingiva

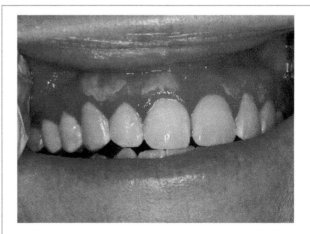

Figure 24.5 Pemphigus vulgaris affecting the maxillary gingiva. Courtesy of Dr. Mark Lerman.

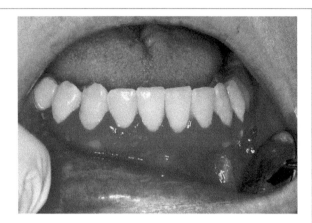

Figure 24.6 Pemphigus vulgaris affecting the mandibular gingiva. Courtesy of Dr. Mark Lerman.

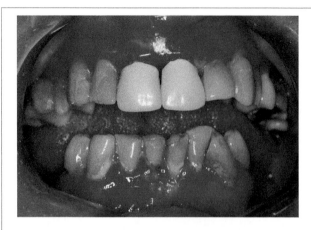

Figure 24.7 Mucous membrane pemphigoid. Courtesy of Dr. Mark Lerman.

e.g. azathioprine, mycophenolate, cyclophosphamide, and cyclosporine. Low-dose methotrexate and antibacterial (dapsone) and anti-inflammatory drugs may also be used.

Mucous membrane pemphigoid

Mucous membrane pemphigoid (MMP), also called cicatricial pemphigoid, is a mucous membrane–dominated autoimmune subepithelial blistering disease that is caused by autoantibodies against various autoantigens in the basement membrane zone (Kamaguchi & Iwata 2019). MMP may appear as PV or erosive/ulcerative lichen planus. A positive Nikolsky sign, present in MMP, is the result of the separation at the basement membrane when pressure is applied to the surface. The definitive diagnosis consists of a perilesional punch biopsy for histopathological studies with H & E staining and direct immunofluorescence (DIF), from healthy tissue relatively distant from the lesion. DIF studies of the diseased and peri-diseased tissue may indicate the presence of IgG, IgA, and/or C3 in the epithelial basement membrane zone.

The disease distribution pattern may vary. It may be limited to the oral cavity or may involve the oral, ocular, esophageal mucosa, and skin. In the oral cavity MMP can present as inflammation, gingivitis, and blistering lesions that can lead to mucosal scarring. It occurs most frequently on the gingiva, buccal mucosa, and the hard and soft palate. It presents with desquamation, erosion, ulcerations, tenderness, pain, and bleeding. Patients can experience sensitivity to food and great discomfort. Brushing is reduced due to the pain and fear of gingival bleeding. This can lead to increased plaque accumulation and plaque-induced gingivitis, as well as the initiation of carious lesions, especially at the gingival third of the teeth (see Figure 24.7).

With low-risk MMP when only the oral mucosa is involved, moderate- to high-potency topical corticosteroids, tacrolimus and cyclosporins, are used for the treatment. Antibiotics, e.g. tetracycline HCl, dapsone, and nicotinamide (vitamin B3), may be useful in treating MMP.

Severe cases of MMP are treated with higher doses of systemic prednisone with or without immunosuppression, e.g. azathioprine.

Sjögren's syndrome

Sjögren's syndrome is an autoimmune disease that primarily affects perimenopausal women, with a ratio of 9:1 for women and men, and affects the exocrine glands. Sjögren's syndrome is diagnosed by the presence of autoantibodies, anti-SSA (Ro), or the biopsy of the minor salivary glands with lymphocytic infiltration of more than 50. A multicenter study evaluating 155 primary Sjögren's syndrome patients found a 12% prevalence of associated oral lesions of autoimmune etiology, which included lichen planus, aphthous stomatitis, chronic ulcerative stomatitis, and lesions of systemic connective tissue disease, with a wide range (7.3–21.2%) found between practices (Likar-Manookin et al. 2013).

The bulk fluid saliva is lost, which alters the oral microenvironment, resulting in inflammation, infection, and the subjective perception of dryness. Multiple studies, however, have shown that the parameters that indicate periodontitis (e.g. pocket depth >5 mm, plaque index, and gingival index) are lower in these patients. Gingival crevicular fluid inflammatory markers are not found in Sjögren's syndrome patients (Özçaka et al. 2018). A population-based study found that patients with periodontal disease have approximately a 50% increased risk of subsequent Sjögren's syndrome. An immune-mediated inflammatory response may contribute to this association (Lin et al. 2019). However, systematic reviews and meta-analysis studies have not found a relationship between Sjögren's syndrome and periodontal diseases (de Goés Soares et al. 2018; Maarse et al. 2019). Sjögren's syndrome patients' clinical attachment loss, gingival index, periodontal pocket depths, and periodontal index were found to be all comparable to control group levels (Maarse et al. 2019). However, due to salivary hypofunction, the oral

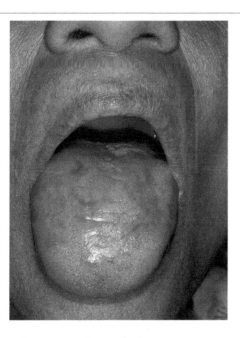

Figure 24.8 Sjögren's syndrome affecting the tongue.

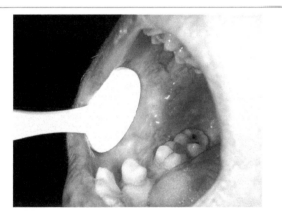

Figure 24.9 Sjögren's syndrome of the buccal mucosa.

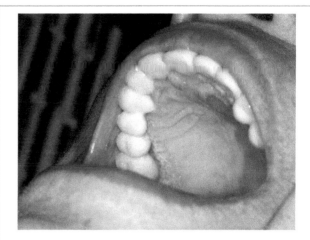

Figure 24.10 Sjögren's syndrome of the palate.

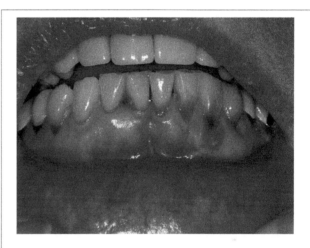

Figure 24.11 Sjögren's syndrome affecting gingival architecture.

mucosa may have a glassy appearance and the normal gingival architecture may be changed (see Figures 24.8–24.11).

Systemic lupus erythematosus

Systemic lupus erythematosus (SLE) is a chronic, progressive, and cell-mediated autoimmune disease that can affect multiple organs due to the deposition of immune complexes. Antinuclear antibodies (ANA) and anti-DNA antibodies are detected in the serum. Ulcerations (Rhodus & Johnson 1990; Tsokos 2011), periodontal disease (Nesse et al. 2010), plaques (honeycomb and keratotic) (Chi et al. 2010), erythema, and candidiasis can also be observed. However, meta-analysis studies have shown significant associations between periodontitis, bleeding on probing, clinical attachment loss, and SLE, although no statistical differences were found in individual measurements of periodontitis, such as probing depth or clinical attachment loss, between SLE cases and controls (Rutter-Locher et al. 2017; Zhong et al. 2020).

Even though the management of SLE is multidisciplinary, symptomatic oral lesions are best managed with topical corticosteroids, e.g. triamcinolone. In more severe cases, potent pharmacological agents, e.g. clobetasol and betamethasone, are used. Tacrolimus and immunomodulatory agents, e.g. hydroxychloroquine, are administered for severe and refractory conditions.

Table 24.1 depicts various autoimmune disorders affecting the periodontium, their clinical presentation, and their differential diagnosis.

Rationale of treatment

Oral healthcare providers encounter numerous autoimmune lesions that manifest in the oral cavity and periodontium, which do not respond to regular periodontal treatment. These

Table 24.1 Autoimmune disorders affecting the periodontium.

Oral lesions	Clinical presentation	Differential diagnosis
Aphthous ulcers	1. Minor 2. Major 3. Herpetiform	Behçet's disease Crohn's disease Systemic lupus erythematosus, ulcerative lichen planus Linear IgA bullous dermatosis, Wegener's granulomatosis Viral infections
Behçet's disease	Recurrent aphthous-like lesions in the oral and genital mucosa	Recurrent aphthous ulcerations Viral infections, Reiter's syndrome, systemic lupus erythematosus, Stevens–Johnson syndrome, inflammatory bowel disease, sarcoidosis
Crohn's disease	Indurated tag-like lesions, cobblestoning, mucogingivitis, deep linear ulceration, aphthous stomatitis	Behçet's disease Crohn's disease Recurrent aphthous ulcerations
Systemic lupus erythematosus	Painless ulcerations	Recurrent aphthous ulcerations Behçet's disease
Oral lichen planus	Reticular Erosive Ulcerative	Recurrent ulcerative stomatitis Erythematous candidiasis Frictional hyperkeratosis Lichenoid reactions Systemic lupus erythematosus Pemphigus Mucus membrane pemphigoid
Pemphigus vulgaris	Mild Moderate Severe Painful blistering Ulcerations	Oral lichen planus Systemic lupus erythematosus
Mucus membrane pemphigoid	Erosive, vesicular, bullous, ulcerative lesions High risk: Ocular, genital, nasopharyngeal, esophageal, and laryngeal mucosal involvement	Lichen planus Herpes Contact mucositis Erythema multiforme Stevens–Johnson syndrome
Sjögren's syndrome	Low risk: Only oral mucosa and skin Xerostomia Gingival recession	Rheumatoid arthritis Systemic lupus erythematosus Chronic active hepatitis
Systemic sclerosis	Severe gingival recession, attached gingiva stripping, lingual and buccal mucosal notching	Sjögren's syndrome

lesions, at times, may not require treatment if asymptomatic or, depending upon the extent of the disease, may require specific treatment for an unspecified time period. Most of the drugs used in treating the lesions are "off-label" drugs designed for skin lesions. Because the clearance of these drugs from the site of application in the oral cavity is fast or diluted due to saliva, the effective dosage may be hard to attain. Also, the immunological attack in the mucosal tissue, as seen with oral lichen planus, occurs below the permeability layer, requiring the medications to penetrate deeper into the tissue. So, it is vital that the cell should be retentive and receptive via an intracellular route. Furthermore, the change in the physical characteristics of the mucosa when ulcerated or eroded causes the permeability barrier to be reduced or lost and may result in enhanced drug delivery (Sankar et al. 2011).

The lesions of the oral cavity are not treated if asymptomatic, for example in OLP, but still need to be observed regularly. Delivery of chemical antimicrobials may help in preventing secondary infections and aid in faster healing. As an initial line of treatment, topical corticosteroids with varied potency (e.g. clobetasol, betamethasone, fluocinonide, triamcinolone acetonide in the form of a cream, gel, lotion, and mouthwash) can be used. There is no cure for autoimmune conditions, so in order to improve quality of life it is important to decrease or control the disease activity. The pharmacological agents may lessen the severity or recurrences, but the disease may still arise. The local delivery of topical steroids is the first line of therapy for mucosal lesions and tends to have lesser side effects, such as adrenal suppression. However, sustained and long-term usage may cause dysbiosis in the oral cavity and give rise to fungal infections. The uncontrolled and refractory conditions may demand intralesional injection of corticosteroids, systemic agents with immunosuppressives, e.g. azathioprine and colchicine, or high doses of systemic corticosteroids such as prednisolone. Stimulation of T cells and suppression of TNF-α production can be achieved by thalidomide. Antibacterial agents, e.g. dapsone (sulfones), have been used to manage various oral lesions. Due to the serious side effects of pharmaceutical agents, their risks and benefits should be weighed.

Conclusion

Normal periodontal parameters may be exacerbated to a diseased status by the development or advancement of the periodontal condition due to systemic autoimmune diseases. The conditions of the periodontium do not improve by means of normal periodontal maintenance procedures and can cause significant distress to the provider and the patient. Recognition of the underlying medical condition and appropriate treatment are needed to maximize the periodontal and systemic outcome. These periodontal conditions cannot be ameliorated entirely, but can be controlled significantly to minimize pain and discomfort, and to improve the overall quality of life for the patient.

REFERENCES

Andreasen JO. Oral lichen planus. 1. A clinical evaluation of 115 cases. *Oral Surg Oral Med Oral Pathol.* 1968; 25(1):31–42.

Barile MF, Graykowski EA, Driscoll EJ, Riggs DB. L Form of bacteria isolated from recurrent aphthous stomatitis lesions. *Oral Surg Oral Med Oral Pathol.* 1963; 16:1395–1402.

Berglundh T, Liljenberg B, Tarkowski A, Lindhe J. The presence of local and circulating autoreactive B cells in patients with advanced periodontitis. *J Clin Periodontol.* 2002; 29:281–286.

Bombeccari GP, Guzzi G, Tettamanti M et al. Oral lichen planus and malignant transformation: a longitudinal cohort study. *Oral Surg Oral Med Oral Pathol Oral Radiol Endod.* 2011; 112(3):328–334.

Brandtzaeg P, Kraus FW. Autoimmunity and periodontal disease. *Odontol Tidskr.* 1965; 30(73):281–393.

Chi AC, Neville BW, Krayer JW, Gonsalves WC. Oral manifestations of systemic disease. *Am Fam Physician.* 2010; 82(11):1381–1388.

de Goés Soares L, Rocha RL, Bagordakis E. et al. Relationship between Sjögren syndrome and periodontal status: a systematic review. *Oral Surg Oral Med Oral Pathol Oral Radiol.* 2018; 125(3):223–231.

Ebersole JL, Cappelli D. Gingival crevicular fluid antibody to *A. actinomycetemcomitans* in periodontal disease. *Oral Microbiol Immunol.* 1994; 9:335–344.

Ebersole JL, Taubman MA, Smith DJ et al. Human serum antibody responses to oral microorganisms IV. Correlation with homologous infection. *Oral Microbiol Immunol.* 1987; 2:53–59.

Ebersole JL, Taubman MA, Smith DJ, Socransky SS. Humoral immune responses and diagnosis of human periodontal disease. *J Periodontal Res.* 1982; 17:478–480.

Eversole LR, Jacobsen PL, Stone CE. Oral and gingival changes in systemic sclerosis (scleroderma). *J Periodontol.* 1984; 55(3):175–178.

Genco RJ, Mashimo PA, Krygier G, Ellison S. Antibody-mediated effects on the periodontium. *J. Periodontol.* 1974; 45:330–337.

Greco A, De Virgilio A, Ralli M et al. Behçet's disease: new insights into pathophysiology, clinical features and treatment options. *Autoimmun Rev.* 2018; 17(6):567–575.

Greenberg GR, Fedorak RN, Thomson ABR. First principles of gastroenterology. In: ABR Thomson, EA Shaffer (eds), *Inflammatory Bowel Disease.* Toronto: Janssen-Ortho; 2005: 307–356.

Hajishengallis G. Immunomicrobial pathogenesis of periodontitis: keystones, pathobionts, and host response. *Trends Immunol.* 2014; 35(1):3–11.

Hasan S, Ahmed S, Kiran R et al. Oral lichen planus and associated comorbidities: an approach to holistic health. *J Family Med Prim Care.* 2019; 8(11):3504–3517.

Hirsch HZ, Tarkowski A, Miller EJ et al. Autoimmunity to collagen in adult periodontal disease. *J Oral Pathol.* 1988; 17(9–10):456–459.

Hoover CI, Greenspan JS. Immunochemical comparison of cell-wall antigens of various viridans streptococci, including strain 2A2 + 3 hot from recurrent oral aphthous ulceration in man. *Arch Oral Biol.* 1983; 28:917–922.

Houman MH, Bel Feki N. Physiopathologie de la maladie de Behçet [Pathophysiology of Behçet's disease]. *Rev Med Interne.* 2014; 35(2):90–96.

Ingafou M, Leao JC, Porter SR, Scully C. Oral lichen planus: a retrospective study of 690 British patients. *Oral Dis.* 2006; 12(5):463–468.

Kamaguchi M, Iwata H. The diagnosis and blistering mechanisms of mucous membrane pemphigoid. *Front Immunol.* 2019; 10:34.

Kurago ZB. Etiology and pathogenesis of oral lichen planus: an overview. *Oral Surg Oral Med Oral Pathol Oral Radiol.* 2016; 122(1):72–80.

Lamey PJ, Rees TD, Binnie WH et al. Oral presentation of pemphigus vulgaris and its response to systemic steroid therapy. *Oral Surg Oral Med Oral Pathol.* 1992; 74(1):54–57.

Lankarani KB, Sivandzadeh GR, Hassanpour S. Oral manifestation in inflammatory bowel disease: a review. *World J Gastroenterol.* 2013; 19(46):8571–8579.

Likar-Manookin K, Stewart C, Al-Hashimi I et al. Prevalence of oral lesions of autoimmune etiology in patients with primary Sjögren's syndrome. *Oral Dis.* 2013; 19(6):598–603.

Lin CY, Tseng CF, Liu JM et al. Association between periodontal disease and subsequent Sjögren's syndrome: a nationwide population-based cohort study. *Int J Environ Res Public Health.* 2019; 16(5):771.

Maarse F, Jager DHJ, Alterch S et al. Sjögren's syndrome is not a risk factor for periodontal disease: a systematic review. *Clin Exp Rheumatol.* 2019; 37(Suppl 118):225–233.

Martin SG. Immunological diseases. In: AL Malcolm, JB Vernon, SG Martin (eds), *Burkitt's Oral Medicine Diagnosis and Treatment.* Philadelphia, PA: JB Lippincott; 1994: 580.

Mays JW, Sarmadi M, Moutsopoulos NM. Oral manifestations of systemic autoimmune and inflammatory diseases: diagnosis and clinical management. *J Evid Based Dent Pract.* 2012; 12(3 Suppl):265–282.

Narikawa S, Suzuki Y, Takahashi M et al. *Streptococcus oralis* previously identified as uncommon *Streptococcus sanguis* in Behcet's disease. *Arch Oral Biol.* 1995; 40:685–690.

Nesse W, Dijkstra PU, Abbas F et al. Increased prevalence of cardiovascular and autoimmune diseases in periodontitis patients: a cross-sectional study. *J Periodontol.* 2010; 81(11):1622–1628.

Özçaka Ö, Alpöz E, Nalbantsoy A, Karabulut G, Kabasakal Y. Clinical periodontal status and inflammatory cytokines in primary Sjögren's syndrome and rheumatoid arthritis. *J Periodontol.* 2018; 89:959–965.

Pineton de Chambrun M, Wechsler B, Geri G, Cacoub P, Saadoun D. New insights into the pathogenesis of Behçet's disease. *Autoimmun Rev.* 2012; 11(10):687–698.

Rhodus NL, Johnson DK. The prevalence of oral manifestations of systemic lupus erythematosus. *Quintessence Int.* 1990; 21(6):461–465.

Rutter-Locher Z, Smith TO, Giles I, Sofat N. Association between systemic lupus erythematosus and periodontitis: a systematic review and meta-analysis. *Front Immunol.* 2017; 8:1295.

Sankar V, Hearnden V, Hull K et al. Local drug delivery for oral mucosal diseases: challenges and opportunities. *Oral Dis.* 2011; 17:(Suppl 1):73–84.

Stanford TW Jr, Peterson J, Machen RL. CREST syndrome and periodontal surgery: a case report. *J Periodontol.* 1999; 70(5):536–541.

Tsokos GC. Systemic lupus erythematosus. *N Engl J Med.* 2011; 365(22):2110–2121.

Zhong HJ, Xie HX, Luo XM, Zhang EH. Association between periodontitis and systemic lupus erythematosus: a meta-analysis. *Lupus.* 2020; 29(10):1189–1197.

CHAPTER 25
Periodontal and medical emergencies

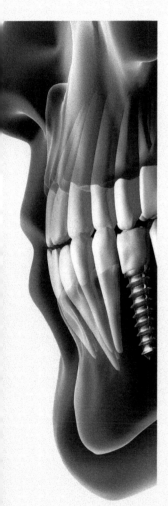

Contents

Essential Periodontics, First Edition. Edited by Steph Smith and Khalid Almas.
© 2022 John Wiley & Sons Ltd. Published 2022 by John Wiley & Sons Ltd.

25.1 MANAGEMENT OF PERIODONTAL EMERGENCIES

Subraya Bhat and Khalid Almas

Contents

Learning objectives

- Understand how to manage an acute periodontal abscess and a gingival abscess.
- Understand the management of acute pericoronitis and a pericoronal abscess.
- Understand the management of necrotizing periodontal diseases.
- Understand how to manage tooth mobility as a functional and aesthetic need.

Introduction

Periodontal emergencies form a major part of dental emergencies. If these conditions are not attended to and treated in a timely manner, then there may be irreversible consequences, including tooth extraction. Acute periodontal conditions include gingival abscess, periodontal abscess, pericoronitis, and pericoronal abscess. There are also other conditions like necrotizing periodontal diseases (NPDs), including necrotizing gingivitis (NG), necrotizing periodontitis (NP), and necrotizing stomatitis (NS), which require emergency treatment (American Academy of Periodontology 2000; Herrera et al. 2000; Papapanou et al. 2018). These conditions may also progress to more severe forms, such as noma (Novak 1999).

For the case definitions, classification, and pathophysiology of NPDs, according to the 2017 World Workshop on the Classification of Periodontal and Peri-Implant Diseases and Conditions (Papapanou et al. 2018), see Chapter 7. For the case definition and classification of periodontal abscess in periodontitis and non-periodontitis patients, according to the 2017 World Workshop on the Classification of Periodontal and Peri-Implant Diseases and Conditions, including the pathophysiology, etiology, and clinical features (Papapanou et al. 2018), see Chapter 10.2.1.

Management of periodontal abscess in the periodontitis patient

Before carrying out any emergency treatment, it is essential to differentiate a periodontal abscess from a gingival abscess and a peri-apical abscess. It is also important to be aware of any associated systemic disease, like diabetes mellitus. In patients with uncontrolled diabetes mellitus, it is suggested that 1 g amoxicillin is given prior to any treatment, followed by the initiation of abscess drainage (Herrera et al. 2000).

Treatment by means of abscess drainage (Marquez 2013)

Through the gingival sulcus

This is the common mode of drainage of periodontal abscess.
1 Anaesthetize the area – local infiltration.
2 Introduce a curette inside the sulcus, identifying the proper cutting edge (in case of Gracey or area-specific curettes), supporting the outer portion of the gingiva with the pad of the finger, and ensure there is support throughout the drainage procedure to ensure soft tissue integrity.
3 Slowly expand the pocket entrance and drain the abscess, where pus gets extruded out.
4 Following this, curette the lateral wall of the pocket until the localized swelling is reduced and the surface flattens to the normal level.
5 Debride the root surface and ensure that all the deposits are eliminated.

6 Irrigate the pocket with saline.
7 Apply pressure to control the bleeding.
Once the abscess is drained, there is usually no need for antibiotic therapy. However, when it is required to be prescribed (when host immunity is compromised), selected antibiotics should be prescribed for 3–5 days (see Chapter 10.2.1).

Incision and drainage

Not all cases require incision and drainage. However, in certain cases (when an abscess is associated with a complex pocket, when there is a pointed abscess, if the pocket entrance is narrow, or if the lesion is sufficiently large, pin-pointed and fluctuating), then incision and drainage are done.
1 Anaesthetize the area – local infiltration.
2 Use a #15 blade to drain the abscess.
3 Recognize the abscess pointed area and make a vertical incision, exactly at this area.
4 Drain the pus.
5 Curette the area thoroughly.
6 Irrigate the area with saline.
7 Apply pressure and control the bleeding.
If there is a need for antibiotic therapy, then this is to be prescribed as mentioned before. The patient should be recalled after 3–5 days for follow-up. After that, if required, surgical treatment is carried out as per underlying osseous changes. If the abscessed tooth shows advanced attachment loss and its prognosis is poor, extraction should be recommended as the course of action.

Management of periodontal abscess in the non-periodontitis patient (Herrera et al. 2018)

An acute gingival abscess may occur following impaction of a toothbrush bristle, apple core, fish bone, or similar things. A gingival abscess can be differentiated from periodontal abscess in that it occurs in the area where the gingiva was previously healthy. Along with this, a proper history is to be taken to find out the associated etiological factors.

Treatment (Marquez 2013):
1 Anaesthetize the area – local infiltration.
2 With a curette, enter the sulcus and drain the pus out.
3 Following that, curette the area thoroughly.
4 Look for the presence of etiological factors as mentioned above.
5 Irrigate the area with saline, and discharge the patient.
6 Antibiotic is *not* required.
7 Analgesics, if required, can be prescribed until the pain subsides.
8 Review the patient after a week and, if required, incision and drainage of the abscess can be done in the same manner as for a periodontal abscess.

Management of acute pericoronitis and pericoronal abscess (Dhonge et al. 2015; Wehr et al. 2019)

Pericoronitis is defined as inflammation of the overlying gingiva associated with infection in the soft tissues surrounding a partially erupted tooth. Mandibular third molars are most commonly affected. This pathological condition is most prevalent in young adults, although patients of any age group may present with pericoronal inflammation.

Pericoronitis is triggered by an accumulation of food debris beneath the operculum that overlaps and surrounds the partially erupted tooth, which propagates an ecological niche for a tremendous variety of polymicrobial flora, mainly consisting of anaerobic pyogenic bacteria.

Treatment of pericoronitis (Dhonge et al. 2015):

1 Anaesthetize the area.
2 Flush the area with warm water to remove debris and exudate after elevating the flap gently from the tooth with a scaler.
3 In cases of presence of pus that is unable to drain thoroughly with elevation of the flap or if a pericoronal abscess is evident, make an anteroposterior incision with a #15 blade to establish thorough drainage, followed by irrigation with saline.
4 Antibiotic can be prescribed if there is lymphadenopathy, which is suggestive of systemic spread of infection. The antibiotic of choice would be the same as that for periodontal abscess.
5 Give oral hygiene instructions to the patient and advice 0.12% chlorhexidine mouthwash/warm saltwater rinse twice a day.
6 After the acute symptoms have subsided, make a determination as to whether the tooth is to be retained or extracted. This decision is governed by the likelihood of further eruption into a good functional position.

Management of necrotizing periodontal diseases (Atout & Todescan 2013; Herrera et al. 2018)

NPDs include a group of diseases progressively involving the gingiva (NG), periodontal tissues (NP), and soft tissues (NS) (Papapanou et al. 2018).

With the severity of infection and different rates of the progression of the disease, in the present classification NPDs can be observed in chronically, severely compromised patients in both adults and children (HIV patients/severely malnourished), and in temporarily and/or moderately compromised patients in both gingivitis and periodontitis patients. (See Chapter 7 for the Classification of Necrotizing Periodontal Diseases.)

Though the overall treatment approach remains the same, the prognosis varies and highly depends upon the underlying systemic condition (HIV/treatment of malnutrition). Removal of the necrotic pseudomembrane is to be done at the first visit (Atout & Todescan 2013; Todescan & Nizar 2013).

1 Under local anaesthesia, debride a small area.
2 Keep ready small cotton pellets.

3 These pellets can either be dipped in hydrogen peroxide 3% or chlorhexidine 0.12%.
4 Each time, select a small area to remove the necrotic pseudomembrane. Thereafter, discard the cotton pellets. With every new area, use a new cotton pellet.
5 Control the bleeding.
6 Provide the patient with specific oral hygiene instructions (to use a soft or supersoft toothbrush), and to use a prescription antibacterial mouthwash: chlorhexidine 0.12% twice daily.
7 Control pain with analgesics: ibuprofen 400–600 mg 3 times daily.
8 Patient counseling should include instruction about proper nutrition, oral care, appropriate fluid intake, and smoking cessation.
9 Antibiotics are necessary only if the patient is immunocompromised (e.g. AIDS, leukemia, cyclic neutropenia) or in case of systemic involvement like fever, malaise, and lymphadenopathy. For any signs of systemic involvement, the recommended antibiotics are amoxicillin, 250 mg 3 times daily for 7 days and/or metronidazole, 250 mg 3 times daily for 7 days.
10 Assess treatment outcomes within 24 hours, then every other day until signs and symptoms are resolved and gingival health and function are restored.
11 Once healing is ensured, carry out gingival examination to see if there are any residual interdental soft tissue craters, which are more susceptible to further clinical attachment loss; evaluate possible surgical treatment of these areas.
12 Follow up with a comprehensive periodontal evaluation after complete resolution of the acute condition.
13 Observe sites that are non-responsive to treatment, which is characterized by recurrence and/or progressive destruction of the gingival and periodontal attachment. Examine these areas thoroughly to see causes for the non-resolution. These can include factors that cause irritation, incomplete debridement, inaccurate diagnosis, patient noncompliance, and/or underlying systemic conditions.
14 Additional therapy and/or medical/dental consultation may also be indicated for non-responding patients. These conditions may tend to recur; therefore, frequent periodontal maintenance visits and meticulous oral hygiene are necessary.
15 In cases of NP, management is almost the same as that above. However, sequestrum formation (necrotic bone) is to be identified and removed, which is a hindrance for healing and causes progression of the disease process.

Tooth mobility and splinting (Watkins & Hemmings 2000)

Tooth mobility is not an emergency; however, it is a functional and esthetic need. Patients may experience it as an emergency treatment need.

All mobile teeth are not indicated for splinting. Before splinting the tooth, the causes for tooth mobility should be recognized. If there is trauma from occlusion, then coronoplasty or occlusal adjustment should be planned, and a time period should be allowed for the response of the periodontal tissue. Once the traumatic occlusion force is eliminated, tooth mobility may reduce and function can revert to normal.

If tooth mobility (grade I to grade II according to the Miller tooth mobility index) is due to loss of alveolar bone, then along with other periodontal non-surgical and surgical procedures, splinting (temporary or provisional) is advised.

Materials available that are used for splinting include orthodontic wires, 0.4 mm or 0.016 in., and fiber-reinforced materials – commercially available: Ribbond® (Seattle, WA, USA), Interlig® (Angelus, Londrina, Brazil), and Dentapreg® (Sarasota, FL, USA) (Foek et al. 2013; Strassler & Brown 2001; Strassler et al. 1999).

Before the splinting procedure is to be done, a working model or cast can be prepared. The teeth to be splinted are measured and the appropriate length of wire (or fiber) is adapted to the surface of the teeth to ensure proper adaptation while using it in the oral cavity.

Splinting procedure (Strassler & Brown 2001):

1 Rubber dam can be used to keep a dry field.
2 Place wedges in the interdental spaces as necessary, so that the spaces to be cleaned are not filled with composite. If you are working without wedges, be careful not to block these spaces with composite.
3 Clean the teeth – all surfaces of the teeth to be splinted are thoroughly polished with a slurry of pumice and water using a rotating brush, then rinsed and dried with air.
4 Measure the fiber using a periodontal probe or dental floss, then cut the fiber and saturate it with bonding agent (or orthodontic wire).
5 Acid etching – apply 37% phosphoric acid to the interproximal and lingual surfaces to be bonded with an applicator tip for 30 seconds. Rinse with water and dry. A lightly frosted appearance can be seen.
6 Use a hand instrument to place a small amount of composite onto the lingual surfaces (but not cured).
7 Apply bonding agent, lightly blow it with air, and cure it to all etched surfaces.
8 Then cover the bonded strip incrementally with flowable composite, resulting in a smooth surface by using a gloved finger, press the strip into the uncured composite, and then cure it into place. Finish and then evaluate the occlusion.

SUMMARY

In a general dental practice or specialty practice, knowledge and skilled management of periodontal emergencies are essential. The timely relief of pain and restoration of function to normalcy will lead to reassurance and gaining of confidence in a patient, which also has the potential to impact overall health.

REFERENCES

American Academy of Periodontology. Parameter on acute periodontal diseases. *J Periodontol.* 2000; 71(5 Suppl):863–866.

Atout RN, Todescan S. Managing patients with necrotizing ulcerative gingivitis. *J Can Dent Assoc.* 2013; 79:d46.

Dhonge RP, Zade RM, Gopinath V, Amirisetty R. An insight into pericoronitis. *Int J Dent Med Res.* 2015; 1(6):172–175.

Foek DL, Yetkiner E, Ozcan M. Fatigue resistance, debonding force, and failure type of fiber-reinforced composite, polyethylene ribbon-reinforced, and braided stainless steel wire lingual retainers in vitro. *Korean J Orthod.* 2013; 43(4):186–192.

Herrera D, Retamal-Valdes B, Alonso B, Feres M. Acute periodontal lesions (periodontal abscesses and necrotizing periodontal diseases) and endo-periodontal lesions. *J Clin Periodontol.* 2018; 45:S78–S94.

Herrera D, Roldan S, Sanz M. The periodontal abscess: a review. *J Clin Periodontol.* 2000; 27(6):377–386.

Marquez IC. How do I manage a patient with periodontal abscess? *J Can Dent Assoc.* 2013; 79:d8.

Novak MJ. Necrotizing ulcerative periodontitis. *Ann Periodontol.* 1999; 4:74–78.

Papapanou PN, Sanz M, Buduneli N et al. Periodontitis: consensus report of workgroup 2 of the 2017 World Workshop on the Classification of Periodontal and Peri-Implant Diseases and Conditions. *J Clin Periodontol.* 2018; 45(Suppl 20):S162–S170.

Strassler HE, Brown C. Periodontal splinting with a thin high-modulus polyethylene ribbon. *Compend Contin Educ Dent.* 2001; (8):696–700.

Strassler HE, Haeri A, Gultz JP. New-generation bonded reinforcing materials for anterior periodontal tooth stabilization and splinting. *Dent Clin North Am.* 1999; 43(1):105–126.

Todescan S, Nizar R. Managing patients with necrotizing ulcerative periodontitis. *J Can Dent Assoc.* 2013; 79:d44.

Watkins SJ, Hemmings KW. Periodontal splinting in general dental practice. *Dent Update.* 2000; 27(6):278–285.

Wehr C, Cruz G, Young S, Fakhouri WD. An insight into acute pericoronitis and the need for an evidence-based standard of care. *Dent J (Basel).* 2019; 7(3):88.

25.2 MANAGEMENT OF MEDICALLY COMPROMISED PATIENTS

Subraya Bhat and Khalid Almas

Contents

Learning objectives

- Identification of particular systemic conditions that require modification in dental/periodontal treatment.
- Knowledge of patient medications and their impact on dental/periodontal treatment.
- Understanding precautions to be taken for specific systemic diseases or conditions.

Introduction

Periodontal and systemic diseases or conditions are interrelated. Understanding the systemic disease background of dental patients is essential, as periodontal disease can be aggravated in the presence of certain systemic diseases or conditions, e.g. diabetes. Knowledge of oral manifestations of systemic diseases may help in diagnosing underlying systemic conditions, e.g. desquamative gingivitis in dermatoses. With certain systemic conditions, alteration or modification of dental treatment and/or precautions may have to be taken prior to starting dental treatment, e.g. bleeding disorders or Infective endocarditis. Periodontal disease may also act as a risk factor for systemic disease, e.g. diabetes or cardiovascular accident (CVA).

Dental/periodontal treatment in hypertensive patients

One of the most common medically compromised conditions to be encountered is hypertension. Periodontitis is also considered to be a possible novel risk factor for hypertension (Muñoz Aguilera et al. 2020). The definition of hypertension includes a systolic blood pressure (SBP) of 140 mmHg or a diastolic blood pressure (DBP) of ≥90 mmHg, or any person being currently prescribed antihypertensive medicine for the purpose of managing hypertension. In addition, hypertension is defined as blood pressure readings elevated on at least two occasions with or without provocation (Li et al. 2021; Unger et al. 2020). Table 25.2.1 depicts the blood pressure and its associated levels of risk.

The dental management of hypertensive patients is depicted in Tables 25.2.2.and 25.2.3.

Other cardiovascular diseases: ischemic heart disease, congestive heart failure

See also Chapter 25.3.

Management of patients with cardiovascular implantable electronic devices

Pacemakers (PMs), implantable cardioverter defibrillators (ICDs), or cardiac resynchronization therapy (CRT) devices are considered to be life prolonging and life saving (Raatikainen et al. 2017). Electromagnetic interference (EMI) is well known to affect the normal function of cardiovascular implantable electronic devices (CIEDs). Electrical equipment in the dental clinic, including ultrasonic and sonic scaling cleaning devices, piezoelectric units, electrosurgery units, and electric pulp testers, as well as some electronic noises, may alter the electromagnetic field of CIEDs, causing oversensing, pacing inhibition, asynchronous pacing, or inappropriate ICD shocks (Yerra & Reddy 2007). Newer devices usually possess protective mechanisms; however, caution is recommended and patients with CIEDs are commonly advised to avoid close and frequent contact with electronic instruments that might be sources of EMI (Niu et al. 2020). Automatic cardioverter defibrillators can get activated without warning when certain arrhythmias occur, which may cause a sudden movement of the patient in the dental chair (Niu et al. 2020).

Management of patients with cardiovascular accident (stroke)

There are two types of stroke: ischemic stroke, which is caused by a blockage (thrombo-embolism); and hemorrhagic stroke, which is caused by the rupture of a blood vessel. If patients experience such in the dental chair, the dentist has to recognize it and take immediate action by applying the FAST rule:

- *Face*: Does one side of the face droop?
- *Arm*: If a person holds both arms out, does one drift downward?
- *Speech*: Is their speech abnormal or slurred?
- *Time*: It's time to call 911 and get to the hospital if any of these symptoms are present.

Table 25.2.1 Blood pressure and associated levels of risk.

Other risk factors, HMOD, or disease	High–normal SBP 130–139 DBP 85–89		Grade 1 SBP 140–159 DBP 90–99		Grade 2 SBP ≥160 DBP ≥100	
No other risk factors	Low		Low	Moderate		High
1 or 2 risk factors	Low		Moderate	High		
≥3 risk factors	Low	Moderate	High	High		
HMOD, CKD grade 3, diabetes mellitus, CVD	High		High	High		

Example based on a 60-year-old male patient. Categories of risk will vary according to age and sex.
CKD, chronic kidney disease; CVD, cardiovascular disease; DBP, diastolic blood pressure; HMOD, hypertension-mediated organ damage; SBP, systolic blood pressure. Adapted from Unger et al. 2020.

Table 25.2.2 Classification and dental management of hypertensive patients.

Classification	Systolic	Diastolic	Dental treatment modification/additional requirement
Normal	≤120	≤80	No changes in dental treatment. **Additional requirement**: Monitor every dental visit.
Pre-hypertensive	120–139	80–89	No changes in dental treatment. **Additional requirement**: Monitor BP at each appointment.
Stage I	140–159	90–99	No changes in dental treatment; minimize stress. **Additional requirements**: a. Monitor BP at each appointment. b. Inform patient of findings and medical consultation or referral.
Stage II	≥160	≥100	a. If systolic BP is <180 mmHg and diastolic is <110 mmHg, perform selective dental care (i.e. routine examination, prophylaxis, restorative non-surgical endodontics, and periodontics); minimize stress. b. If systolic BP ≥180 mmHg or diastolic ≥100 mmHg, give immediate medical consultation or referral and perform emergency dental care only (to alleviate pain, bleeding, infection); minimize stress. **Additional requirements**: a. Monitor BP at each appointment. b. Inform patient of findings and medical consultation or referral.

Source: Adapted from Malamed 2014b; Southerland et al. 2016.

Table 25.2.3 Procedure to be followed to assess and manage the hypertensive patient.

- The first dental office visit should include two BP readings spaced at least 10 minutes apart, which are averaged and used as a baseline.
- The preferred time to do a dental procedure is the morning; however, evidence indicates that BP usually increases around awakening and peaks at mid-morning. It is now suggested to do the procedure in the afternoon, when BP is lower.
- Use of local anesthesia (LA) with epinephrine – concentrations of 1:80 000 significantly affect systolic blood pressure (SBP) and diastolic blood pressure (DBP), as well as affect the heart rate. Similarly, 1:100 000 concentrations can exacerbate SBP and heart rate. Although 1:200 000 exacerbates the heart rate, it is comparatively less than that with previous concentrations. The recommendation is to use 1:200 000 for LA.
- Maximum dosing for adults with questionable uncontrolled hypertension and/or cardiovascular disease is 0.04 mg, totaling two or four cartridges depending on the epinephrine concentration present in the cartridges.
- LA with epinephrine in patient taking non-selective β-blockers (e.g. propranolol, nadolol) – this can elevate BP in a patient with severe hypertension and bradycardia, producing a dangerous decrease in vascular perfusion and possibly causing death.
- If SBP is >180 mmHg or DBP is >110 mmHg and patient requires incision and drainage, caution is required, as excessive bleeding can occur with elevated BP. If the surgical field is small, such as periodontal abscess, bleeding can be adequately controlled.
- Postural hypotension – a decline of ≥20 mmHg in SBP, and/or a decline of ≥10 mmHg in DBP, or an increase of ≥20 beats/ minute in pulse rate, and abrupt symptoms of cerebral ischemia (syncope) following postural change from a supine to an upright position. In prevention, schedule dental appointments 30–60 minutes after the ingestion of meals and medications. Ensure profound anesthesia. Upon completion of procedures, allow at-risk patients to assume an upright position gradually over 2 minutes.
- Antihypertensive medication side effects and dental treatment – depression, which may affect the patient's oral hygiene practice and compliance; nausea, oral dryness, lichenoid drug reactions, and gingival overgrowth (due to calcium channel blockers).
- See also Table 25.2.1.

Source: Adapted from Malamed 2014b; Southerland et al. 2016.

Periodontal treatment (except for an emergency) should not be performed for 6 months. After 6 months, periodontal therapy can be performed, *but* with short appointments and less stress. Profound LA with minimal effective dose of LA agents. Concentrations of epinephrine greater than 1:100 000 are contraindicated. Light conscious sedation and supplemental oxygen are helpful. Monitoring of anticoagulants and BP need to be done prior to treatment (Fatahzadeh & Glick 2006).

Infective endocarditis prevention: dental treatment considerations

Antibiotic prophylaxis has been recommended prior to dental procedures in patients at risk of infective endocarditis (IE) for over half a century. Recent international guidelines have restricted (Europe and the USA) or recommended against (UK) this practice due to lack of evidence. IE is a potentially life-threatening disease of the heart valves or endocardium, which is caused by bacteria and other microorganisms. From a periodontal point of view, α-hemolytic streptococci (e.g. *Streptococcus viridans*), other non-streptococcal organisms like *Eikenella corrodens*, *Aggregatibacter actinomycetemcomitans*, and *Capnocytophaga*, are often found in the periodontal pocket and are also considered to be causes of IE (Carinci et al. 2018).

In 2017, the American Heart Association (AHA) and the American College of Cardiology (ACC) published a focused update to their previous guidelines on the management of valvular heart disease. The subset of diseases that require IE prophylaxis was narrowed and presented as in Box 25.2.1 (American Dental Association 2017).

Table 25.2.4 depicts the single-dose regimen to be taken 30–60 minutes before a procedure is to be performed.

Management of patients with hemorrhagic disorders

Bleeding is the most common complication seen in the dental surgery. To avoid the complication during and after the dental surgical procedure, it is essential to know the underlying causes/presence of systemic disease.

Bleeding disorders are classified as coagulation disorders and platelet disorders (thrombocytopenic purpuras or non-thrombocytopenic purpuras). It is essential to take a proper history to rule out underlying systemic diseases. A history should include the history of bleeding after previous surgery or trauma, past and current drug history (anticoagulants, aspirin, and other non-steroidal anti-inflammatory drugs, NSAIDs), history of bleeding problems among relatives, and illnesses associated with potential bleeding problems (jaundice, ecchymosis, spider telangiectasia, hemarthrosis, petechiae, hemorrhagic vesicles, spontaneous gingival bleeding, and gingival hyperplasia) (Halpern et al. 2020).

Hemophilia

Hemophilia is an inherited coagulation disorder involving a deficiency of factor VIII and IX. Hemophilia A is inherited as an autosomal X-linked recessive trait, and is characterized by a deficiency of factor VIII. It affects both males and females. Patients with a factor VIII activity level of less than 50% are considered to be carriers. This is a common type of hemophilia, affecting close to 85% of all cases of hemophilia (incidence 1:5000 live male births). Hemophilia B is characterized by a deficiency of factor IX (incidence 1:30 000 live male births) (Srivastava et al. 2020).

This bleeding disorder can be classified based on the percentage of factor deficiency (Table 25.2.5).

Precautions for the treatment of a hemophiliac patient are outlined in Box 25.2.2.

Consideration of local anesthetics in hemophiliac patients

Factor VIII should be corrected prior to the administration of an inferior alveolar block, as hematoma formation can lead to life-threatening blockage of the adjacent airway. An

---

Box 25.2.1 Conditions/diseases requiring antibiotic prophylaxis

Key recommendations
1. Prosthetic cardiac valves, including transcatheter-implanted prostheses and homograft.
2. Prosthetic material used for cardiac valve repair, such as annuloplasty rings and chords.
3. Previous infective endocarditis.
4. Unrepaired cyanotic congenital heart disease or repaired congenital heart disease, with residual shunts or valvular regurgitation at the site of or adjacent to the site of a prosthetic patch or prosthetic device.
5. Cardiac transplant with valve regurgitation due to a structurally abnormal valve.

Additional considerations
With the discretion of the treating physician and severity of the condition, the following list also needs to be kept in mind (American Dental Association 2017):

- Patients with previous late artificial joint infection.
- Increased morbidity associated with joint surgery (wound drainage/hematoma).
- Patients undergoing treatment of severe and spreading oral infections (cellulitis).
- Patient with increased susceptibility for systemic infection.
- Congenital or acquired immunodeficiency.
- Patients on immunosuppressive medications.
- Diabetics with poor glycemic control.
- Patients with systemic immunocompromising disorders (e.g. rheumatoid arthritis, lupus erythematosus).
- Patient in whom extensive and invasive procedures are planned.
- Prior to surgical procedures in patients at a significant risk for medication-related osteonecrosis of the jaw.

Table 25.2.4 Prophylactic antibiotic regimens.

Situation	Agent	Adults	Children
Oral	Amoxicillin	2 g	50 mg/kg
Unable to take oral medication	Ampicillin	2 g IM or IV	50 mg/kg IM or IV
	Or cefazolin or ceftriaxone	1 g IM or IV	50 mg/kg IM or IV
Allergic to penicillins or ampicillin – oral	Cephalexin φ δ *Or*	2 g	50 mg/kg
	Clindamycin *Or*	600 mg	20 mg/kg
	Azithromycin or clarithromycin	500 mg	15 mg/kg
Allergic to penicillins or ampicillin and unable to take oral medication	Cefazolin or ceftriaxone δ *Or* Clindamycin	1 g IM or IV	50 mg/kg IM or IV
		600 mg IM or IV	20 mg/kg IM or IV

IM, intramuscular; IV, intravenous. Φ Or other first- and second-generation oral cephalosporin in equivalent adult or pediatric dosage. δ Cephalosporins should not be used in individuals with a history of anaphylaxis, angioedema, or urticaria with penicillins or ampicillin.
Antibiotic Prophylaxis 2017 Update – American Heart Association and American College of Cardiology focused update of the 2014 AHA/ADA Guideline for Management of Patients with Valvular Disease. https://www.aae.org/specialty/wp-content/uploads/sites/2/2017/06/aae_antibiotic-prophylaxis-2017update.pdf.

Table 25.2.5 Classification of hemophilia.

Severity	Serum level of factors	Bleeding severity
Mild	0.05–0.35 IU/mL or 5–35%	No spontaneous bleeding; delayed bleeding after trauma or surgery or dental extraction
Moderate	0.01–0.05 IU/mL or 1–5%	Bleeding into joints and muscles, with minor trauma and bleeding after surgery
Severe	≤0.01 IU/mL or <1%	Spontaneous joint, muscle, and internal bleeding; excessive bleeding after surgery

aspirating syringe should always be used. LA with epinephrine (vasoconstrictor) should be used to ensure prolonged action and vasoconstriction. Buccal infiltration anesthesia, with 4% articaine hydrochloride (1:100 000 epinephrine), shows better results than 2% lidocaine hydrochloride and is preferred over inferior alveolar nerve block. Intrapulpal, intraligamentary, and infiltration are also considered to be safer, and these do not require the adjustment of factor VIII concentrate (Malamed 2014a).

Supragingival scaling in hemophiliac patients

Treatment of patients with mild hemophilia can be done with the use of topical tranexamic acid mouthwash (15–25 mg/kg), applied 2 hours before the dental procedure and continued 4 times daily for 3–4 days. Alternatively, oral administration of

---

Box 25.2.2   Precautions to be taken when treating a hemophiliac patient

- A detailed medical and dental history is to be taken.
- Previous history of episodes of bleeding if any, and how it was controlled.
- Medication history of patients.
- Measure the level of factor VIII in patients with hemophilia A prior to any invasive dental procedures.
- It is recommended that the patient's level of factor VIII should be between 50% and 75% prior to minor oral and periodontal surgery, but if any major surgeries are planned the level should be between 75% and 100%.
- Local hemostatic agents if required to be kept ready during the treatment.
- Need to use hemostatic – if mouthwash, it is to be used one hour before the procedure (tranexamic acid mouthwash with a concentration of 15–25 mg/kg and to be repeated 4 times a day for 7–10 days; or oral administration of tablets, 1 g, 3 times a day for 7–10 days).
- There may be a mobility issue with these patients, due to bleeding to the joints and joint problems thereafter. A wheelchair facility may be necessary.
- Preventive strategy – in a known hemophiliac patient, it is better to control the caries and reduce the plaque from the beginning so that complications related to this are reduced. This minimizes dental treatment and bleeding complications.

Source: Adapted from Srivastava et al. 2020.

tablets 1 g, 1 hour before the procedure and continued 2–3 times a day for 3–4 days, can also be used. Local hemostatic measures need to be kept ready in case they are required. However, in patients with moderate to severe hemophilia, replacement of factor prior to the procedure is a must. Replacement can include factor concentrate, recombinant factor VIII, activated prothrombin complex concentrate, and factor eight inhibitor bypassing activity (FEIBA) (Khyati et al. 2016).

Liver diseases and bleeding

Most coagulation factors are synthesized and removed by the liver. Any changes in liver function are going to affect the clotting mechanism, especially in long-term alcohol abusers or those with chronic hepatitis. Coagulation can also be impaired by vitamin K deficiency, often caused by malabsorption syndromes or due to prolonged antibiotic administration, which alters the intestinal microflora that produce vitamin K. Laboratory tests may be required to determine bleeding and coagulation cascades, including hospitalization, if surgery is required. The international normalized ratio (INR; prothrombin time, PT) should be less than 2.0; however, in the case of a small surgical area, an INR of less than 2.5 is usually safe. Note should be taken that the platelet count should be more than 80 000/mm^3 (Khyati et al. 2016).

Thrombocytopenic purpura

Thrombocytopenia is defined as a platelet count of less than 100 000/mm^3. Purpuras are hemorrhagic diseases characterized by extravasation of blood into the tissues under the skin or mucosa, producing spontaneous petechiae (i.e. small red patches) or ecchymoses (i.e. bruises). In leukemia, with the pancytopenia, thrombocytopenic purpura can become a major issue. Bleeding caused by thrombocytopenia can be seen with idiopathic thrombocytopenic purpuras, radiation therapy, myelosuppressive drug therapy (e.g. chemotherapy), leukemia, or infections (Golla et al. 2004).

Periodontal therapy modifications with thrombocytopenia

Scaling and root planing are usually safe unless the platelet count is less than 60 000/mm^3. No surgical procedure should be performed unless the platelet count is greater than 80 000/mm^3. Platelet transfusion may be required before surgery. Surgical technique should be as atraumatic as possible. Local hemostatic measures should be applied (Israels et al. 2006).

Management of patients on anticoagulant/antiplatelet agent therapy

The medical history of such patients should be reviewed, especially patients with prosthetic heart valves, history of myocardial infarction (MI), CVA, thromboembolism, deep-vein thrombosis (DVT), pulmonary embolism (PE), non-valvular

atrial fibrillation (NVAF), and cardiac arrhythmia. These medications may also be prescribed for other systemic diseases, such as COVID-19, for short durations. Table 25.2.6 depicts a classification of newer and older anticoagulants and antiplatelet agents.

Awareness of terminologies of newer anticoagulant therapies is essential, such as vitamin K antagonists (VKA), single antiplatelet therapy (SAPT), dual antiplatelet therapy (DAPT), direct oral anticoagulants (DOAC), and novel oral antiplatelet therapy (NOAC).

Direct-acting oral anticoagulants

These agents differ from traditional oral anticoagulant therapy (i.e. warfarin) in that they are targeted in action; are given as fixed doses; have more predictable pharmacokinetics and shorter half-lives; require little to no routine monitoring; and have fewer drug or food interactions. A 2015 consensus guideline from the European Heart Rhythm Association (updating 2013 guidelines) (Abayon et al. 2016) suggests that interventions not necessarily requiring discontinuation of the newer anticoagulants include extraction of 1–3 teeth, periodontal surgery, abscess incision, or implant positioning. In 2018 a systematic review reported a similar guideline. However, the authors recommended the need for caution and modifications according to the needs of the individual (Fortier et al. 2018).

Older anticoagulants

It was previously recommended that the anticoagulant is discontinued for 2–3 days prior to periodontal treatment (i.e. the clearance half-life of warfarin is 36–42 hours), and that the INR is checked on the day of therapy. If the INR is within the acceptable target range, the procedure could be done, and

Table 25.2.6 Anticoagulant and antiplatelet therapeutic agents.

Drug class	Drug name
Anticoagulants	Warfarin (Coumadin®)
Antiplatelet agents	Clopidogrel (Plavix®), ticlopidine (Ticlid®), prasugrel (Effient®), ticagrelor (Brilinta®), aspirin
Direct-acting oral anticoagulants (direct thrombin inhibitor and factor Xa inhibitors)	Dabigatran (Pradaxa®), rivaroxaban (Xarelto®), apixaban (Eliquis®), edoxaban (Savaysa®)

Coumadin, Plavix, Eliquis: Bristol-Myers Squibb, Princeton, NJ, USA. Ticlid: Roche Laboratories, Inc., Nutley, NJ, USA. Effient: Lilly Medical, Indianapolis, IN, USA. Brilinta: AstraZeneca, Cambridge, UK. Pradaxa: Boehringer Ingelheim Pharmaceuticals, Inc., Ridgefield, CT, USA. Xarelto: Bayer AG, Leverkusen, Germany. Savaysa: Daiichi Sankyo, Inc., Basking Ridge, NJ, USA. Source: Adapted from American Dental Association 2020.

the anticoagulant was resumed immediately after treatment. However, the latest review and recommendations from the Clinical Practice Statement from the American Academy of Oral Medicine (2016) has determined that moderately invasive oral surgery (defined as "uncomplicated tooth extraction") is safe with an INR of 3.5, with some experts stating that it is safe up to 4.0. However, it is essential that careful technique, complete wound closure, and pressure to minimize hemorrhage are applied. Use of oxidized cellulose, microfibrillar collagen, topical thrombin, and tranexamic acid should be considered for persistent bleeding (American Dental Association 2020).

Single or dual antiplatelet therapy

The American Heart Association, the American College of Cardiology, the Society for Cardiovascular Angiography and Interventions, the American College of Surgeons, and the American Dental Association published a consensus opinion about drug-eluting stents and antiplatelet therapy (e.g. aspirin, clopidogrel, ticlopidine). They have stated that, given the importance of antiplatelet medications for post-stent implantation in minimizing the risk of stent thrombosis, medications should not be discontinued prematurely during dental treatment. A 2020 systematic review and meta-analysis evaluated the incidence of bleeding after minor oral surgery in patients on dual antiplatelet therapy (aspirin plus another antiplatelet agent) compared with single-agent therapy or no antiplatelet therapy, and found clinically similar rates of bleeding across the three groups. However, if there is co-morbidity like liver impairment or alcoholism, kidney failure, thrombocytopenia, hemophilia, or other hematological disorders, or patients currently receiving a course of cytotoxic medication (e.g. cancer chemotherapy), then these recommendations may have to be altered according to a physician's consultation (Dézsi et al. 2017).

Management of agranulocytosis – cyclic neutropenia and granulocytopenia

Granulocytopenia is defined as a reduced number of blood granulocytes, namely neutrophils, eosinophils, and basophils. The term granulocytopenia is often used synonymously with neutropenia and, in that sense, is again confined to the neutrophil lineage alone. Agranulocytosis (lack of granulocytes) is a condition in which the absolute neutrophil count (ANC) is less than 100 neutrophils per microliter of blood, and when the granulocyte (neutrophil) count is between 100 and 1500 per microliter of blood, the term "granulocytopenia" or "neutropenia" is used. Due to this, there is increased susceptibility to infection, including periodontal destruction (Nualart Grossmus et al. 2007).

Severely affected teeth should be extracted. Periodontal treatment should be done during periods of disease remission (in cyclic neutropenia). Treatment should be as conservative as

possible while reducing potential sources of systemic infection. Oral hygiene instruction should include chlorhexidine rinses twice daily. Scaling and root planing should be performed carefully under antibiotic protection (Nualart Grossmus et al. 2007).

Management of the diabetic patient

Diabetes is a complex metabolic disorder characterized by persistent hyperglycemia, which may be due to diminished insulin production/secretion, impaired insulin action/resistance to peripheral action of insulin, or a combination of both (American Diabetes Association 2014). A dentist should always remember the diagnostic criteria, carry out tests in the dental clinic at the first visit, and refer the patient for further laboratory tests (American Diabetes Association 2020). Patients often do not disclose the proper status of their diabetes to the dentist; therefore, it is essential that the dentist asks key questions to find out the exact diabetes status of the patient (Box 25.2.3).

- *If a patient is suspected of having undiagnosed diabetes*: Rule out acute orofacial infection or severe dental infection; if present, provide emergency care immediately. Establish the best possible oral health through non-surgical debridement of plaque and calculus, and provide oral hygiene instruction. Refer the patient to a physician.
- *If a patient is known to have diabetes*: The primary test used to assess glycemic control in a known diabetic individual is the glycated hemoglobin (Hb) assay. Two tests are available, the HbA1 and HbA1c assays; the HbA1c is used more

---

Box 25.2.3 Key questions a dentist may want to ask a patient with diabetes

- How old were you when you were diagnosed with diabetes and what type of diabetes do you have? How long has it been since the diagnosis?
- What medications do you take?
- How do you monitor your blood sugar levels?
- How often do you see your doctor about your diabetes? When was your last visit to the doctor?
- What was the most recent HbA1c (A1c) result?
- Do you ever have episodes of very low (hypoglycemia) or very high blood sugar (hyperglycemia)?
- Do you ever find yourself disoriented, agitated, and anxious for no apparent reason?
- Do you have any mouth sores or discomfort?
- Does your mouth feel dry?
- Do you have any other medical conditions related to your diabetes, such as heart disease, high blood pressure, history of stroke, eye problems, limb numbness, kidney problems, delays in would healing, history of gum disease? Please describe.

Source: Adapted from American Dental Association 2019.

Table 25.2.7 HbA1c levels and corresponding estimated average glucose.

A1c	Estimated average glucose (eAG)	
%	mg/dL	mmol/L
6	126	7
6.5	140	7.8
7	154	8.6
7.5	169	9.4
8	183	10.1
8.5	197	10.9
9	212	11.8
9.5	226	12.6
10	240	13.4

Source: Adapted from American Diabetes Association 2020.

often. This test provides an accurate measure of the average blood glucose concentrations over the preceding 2–3 months. The HbA1c is also defined as "estimated average glucose" or eAG. If the HbA1c reading falls between 4% and 6%, it is considered normal; if it is less than 7%, good diabetes control; if it is between 7% and 8%, it is considered to be moderate diabetic control; if it is more than 8%, then action is suggested to control the diabetes. A chairside glucometer often gives the readings in mg/dL, which can be converted by using a chart (American Diabetes Association 2020). Table 25.2.7 is a chart that relates the HbA1c level to the eAG in mg/dL and mmol/L.

Management of the diabetic patient with periodontal disease

Diabetes mellitus is considered to be have a two-way relationship with periodontitis. If diabetes mellitus is not controlled, it may have an impact on the periodontal health. If periodontitis is not controlled, it may have an impact on the diabetes status. Thus, controlling both is of equal importance.

Scaling and root planing in the diabetic patient

Periodontal infection can worsen glycemic control and should be managed aggressively, which includes mechanical debridement to remove local factors followed by oral hygiene instructions. HbA1c of less than 10% should be established before surgical treatment is performed (American Dental Association 2019; Davies et al. 2018).

Periodontal surgical procedures

In a patient with poorly controlled diabetes, it is better to postpone surgical treatment until the diabetes is under control. If glycemic control has been good and on the particular day of surgery shows a slightly higher number, the surgical procedure may be done. However, with procedures of long duration, the glucose level should be regularly monitored. If a patient becomes hypoglycemic during the procedure, it can be detected early, so as to avoid the severe complications that can arise from hypoglycemic shock (Davies et al. 2018; Jain et al. 2020).

Post-surgically, it is necessary to take care of the patient, especially regarding medication usage. Patients usually avoid eating food after a surgical procedure. The regular intake of normal units of insulin or oral hypoglycemic drugs may thus put them at risk of developing hypoglycemia. Dentists should therefore guide their patients about this and have their physician adjust any dosing as deemed necessary (Jain et al. 2020).

Infectious diseases

All standard infection controls for infectious diseases need to be followed (hepatitis, HIV, and COVID-19). For COVID-19 patients, special protocol guidelines as specified by the World Health Organization are to be followed. Use as many disposable covers as possible, covering light handles, drawer handles, and bracket trays. Headrest covers should also be used. All disposable items (e.g. gauze, floss, saliva ejectors, masks, gowns, and gloves) should be placed in a one-lined waste basket. After treatment, these items and all disposable covers should be bagged, labeled, and disposed of following proper guidelines for biohazardous waste. Aseptic technique should be followed at all times. Minimize aerosol production by not using ultrasonic instrumentation, air syringes, or high-speed handpieces, as saliva contains a distillate of the virus. Pre-rinsing with chlorhexidine gluconate for 30 seconds is highly recommended. When the procedure is completed, all equipment should be scrubbed and sterilized. If an item cannot be sterilized or disposed of, it should not be used (Centers for Disease Control and Prevention 2020, 2021).

In addition, in the case of hepatitis patients, bleeding is likely, during or after treatment, therefore the PT and bleeding time should be measured prior to initiating treatment.

Medication-related osteonecrosis of the jaw

Medication-related osteonecrosis of the jaw (MRONJ) is defined as the "adverse drug reaction described as the progressive destruction and death of bone that affects the mandible and maxilla of patients exposed to the treatment with medications known to increase the risk of disease, in the absence of a previous radiation treatment." This term has replaced bisphosphonate-related osteonecrosis of the jaw (BRONJ), since necrosis has been observed in cases utilizing other medications besides bisphosphonates, such as those with antiangiogenic activity, e.g. bevacizumab, aflibercept, inhibitors of tyrosine kinases, and mTOR inhibitors (Di Fede et al. 2018).

Most studies on oral and systemic bisphosphonates have concluded that the risk for individuals treated with oral bisphosphonates for a period of less than three years appears to be minimal or zero. Regular use of oral bisphosphonates for a period greater than three years suggests a risk profile that increases with time and length of use. Similarly, individuals treated with high-potency, nitrogen-containing bisphosphonates, especially those administered intravenously for cancer treatment (e.g. zoledronate), appear to be at greater risk for MRONJ than individuals taking oral bisphosphonates for prevention and treatment of osteoporosis (Campisi et al. 2019).

Regarding prevention and diagnosis, the Italian Society of Oral Pathology and Medicine consensus was built and discussed in detail. They have put forward a good practice protocol related to MRONJ (Box 25.2.4) (Campisi et al. 2020).

Periodontal treatment and MRONJ

Physicians usually refer patients for dental evaluation before initiating treatment with bisphosphonates and other related drugs. Teeth with a questionable prognosis or which require extraction need to be extracted and the socket should be allowed to heal. Invasive treatment such as extractions, periodontal surgery, implant surgery, and bone augmentation procedures should be avoided in patients on intravenous bisphosphonate therapy (Di Fede et al. 2018).

Management of patients with immunosuppression and chemotherapy

Immunosuppressed or patients on chemotherapy are at risk for infection, where even minor periodontal infections can become life threatening. This is especially the case in cancer patients and in those who are undergoing bone marrow transplantation. Dental evaluation of these patients prior to initiation of therapy is commonly done. All necessary treatment should be completed prior to starting immuno/chemotherapy. Patients should be guided regarding oral hygiene, which includes the usage of chlorohexidine in especially those undergoing chemotherapy, where there is a high chance of mucositis. Furthermore, in patients on chemotherapy, all periodontal treatment should be done prior to the start of the chemotherapy cycle when white blood cell counts are relatively high (white blood cell count above 2000/mm^3, with an absolute granulocyte count of 1000–1500/mm^3) (Ptasiewicz et al. 2020).

Box 25.2.4 Practices at risk of inappropriateness and good practices

Clinical diagnosis of MRONJ

- Evaluate not only the intake of bisphosphonate drugs (current or past), but also further pharmacological therapies (e.g. other antiresorptive agents, or drugs with antiangiogenic activity) and perform a thorough physical examination and medical history, together with targeted radiological examinations (confirmed).
- Perform jawbone biopsies only if there is a suspicion of metastases in cancer patients (confirmed).
- Take into the account not only the presence of exposed necrotic bone, but considering also other clinical signs and first/second-level imaging (confirmed).
- Consider that the symptom "pain" may not always be present in MRONJ cases, especially in the early stages (confirmed).
- Consider that some cases of MRONJ can arise from the presence of dental-periodontal diseases or spontaneously, without any relation to invasive dental procedures (confirmed).

Radiological diagnosis of MRONJ

- Evaluate clinically and radiologically any local risk factors for MRONJ (i.e. dental/endo-periodontal diseases) for preventive dental screening in patients, remarkably cancer ones, who are candidates for therapies at higher risk of MRONJ; sometimes, MRONJ could manifest like dental/endo-periodontal disease, or a worsening of a pre-existent disease (updated).
- Perform radiological exams in all cases of dental/ endo-periodontal diseases in patients at risk of MRONJ (confirmed).
- Reserve the indication for the execution of radiological exams of the second level (e.g. computed tomography, CT) to patients at MRONJ risk only in the presence of ascertained clinical or radiological signs compatible with MRONJ (confirmed).
- Always specify the diagnostic hypothesis when prescribing radiological exams of any level (X-ray panoramic, CT) in patients at MRONJ risk (confirmed).
- Do not delay in prescribing radiological exams to investigate any clinical signs of possible MRONJ, independent of the presence of bone exposure or fistulas (updated).
- Always integrate the clinical check-up with the appropriate imaging exams for the diagnosis of MRONJ (confirmed).
- Prescribe radiological exams for bone diseases without contrast medium for diagnosis of MRONJ (confirmed).
- Set up the MRONJ treatment after defining its extension and severity also by targeted imaging (confirmed).
- Use targeted imaging (i.e. CT every 6 months) to monitor MRONJ during follow-up after conservative and/ or surgical treatment (updated).

Source: Adapted from Campisi et al. 2020.

Management of patients with renal diseases

Patients with renal failure and those who are on dialysis need to be treated with care because of the involved complications, which can include hypertension, anemia, risk of bleeding, and infection. Along with this, medication prescribed for their treatment may have an impact on periodontal treatment.

Patients with renal failure are categorized as stage I to stage V depending upon associated factors. In stage I–III patients, periodontal treatment does not require any changes to the periodontal treatment protocol. However, stages IV and V require precautions to be followed. Periodontal treatment is targeted at maintaining good oral hygiene and preventing the infection. Any questionable teeth should be extracted early. Medications (antibiotics and analgesics) that are nephrotoxic should not be prescribed. Patients on hemodialysis are prone to hepatitis, prolonged hemorrhage, and anemia. Screening for hepatitis should be done regularly. To avoid complications of bleeding, it is advisable that periodontal treatment be done on the day after dialysis, when the effects of heparinization have subsided. If the shunt or fistula is placed in the arm, BP readings should be taken from the other arm. Patients with leg shunts should avoid sitting with the dependent leg for longer than one hour. If the appointment lasts longer, the patient should be given rest and allowed to walk to relieve the pressure on the shunt. Furthermore, in these patients, signs of uremic stomatitis may be seen in the oral cavity as white patches. In such cases, patients need to be referred to oral medicine for proper treatment to be followed (Miyata et al. 2019; Sabharwal et al. 2018).

SUMMARY

Recognizing medical conditions/systemic disease and understanding their management and influence on dental/periodontal treatment is of prime importance in preparation for possible complications that can arise during and after periodontal treatment. Required laboratory tests can be ordered in advance to assist in decisions regarding modification in treatment and follow-up, which will relieve the stress on the dentist. Dental patients often fail to understand the importance of disclosing their medical conditions and treatment under progress, because they are unaware of the impact of systemic disease or medication on dental/periodontal disease and its treatment. A well-designed questionnaire answered by the patient and later reconfirmed by the dentist helps to prepare the patient appropriately for dental treatment.

REFERENCES

Abayon M, Kolokythas A, Harrison S, Elad S. Dental management of patients on direct oral anticoagulants: case series and literature review. *Quintessence Int.* 2016; 47(8):687–696.

American Dental Association. Oral health topics: antibiotic prophylaxis prior to dental procedures. ADA; 2017. http://www.ada.org/en/member-center/oral-health-topics/antibiotic-prophylaxis.

American Dental Association. Oral health topics: diabetes. ADA; 2019. https://www.ada.org/en/member-center/oral-health-topics/diabetes.

American Dental Association. Oral health topics: Oral anticoagulant and antiplatelet medications and dental procedures. ADA; 2020. https://www.ada.org/en/member-center/oral-health-topics/oral-anticoagulant-and-antiplatelet-medications-and-dental-procedures.

American Diabetes Association. Diagnosis and classification of diabetes mellitus. *Diabetes Care.* 2014; 37(Suppl 1):S81–S90.

American Diabetes Association. 2. Classification and diagnosis of diabetes: standards of medical care in diabetes—2020. *Diabetes Care.* 2020; 43(Suppl 1):S14–S31.

Campisi G, Bedogni A, Bertoldo F et al. Proceedings of the closed round table and Italian consensus on the medication-related osteonecrosis of jaws (MRONJ) at the Symposium of Italian Society of Oral Pathology and Medicine (SIPMO) Ancona, 20 October 2018—part III. *Front Physiol.* 2019; 10.

Campisi G, Mauceri R, Bertoldo F et al. Medication-related osteonecrosis of jaws (MRONJ) prevention and diagnosis: Italian consensus update 2020. *Int J Environ Res Public Health.* 2020; 17(16):5998.

Carinci F, Martinelli M, Contaldo M et al. Focus on periodontal disease and development of endocarditis. *J Biol Regul Homeost Agents.* 2018; 32(2 Suppl 1):143–147.

Centers for Disease Control and Infection. COVID-19. CDC; 2020. https://www.cdc.gov/coronavirus/2019-ncov/index.html.

Centers for Disease Control and Infection. Infection control. CDC; 2019. https://www.cdc.gov/infectioncontrol/index.html.

Davies MJ, D'Alessio DA, Fradkin J et al. Management of hyperglycaemia in type 2 diabetes, 2018. A consensus report by the American Diabetes Association (ADA) and the European Association for the Study of Diabetes (EASD). *Diabetologia.* 2018; 61(12):2461–2498.

Dézsi CA, Dézsi BB, Dézsi AD. Management of dental patients receiving antiplatelet therapy or chronic oral anticoagulation: a review of the latest evidence. *Eur J Gen Pract.* 2017; 23(1):197–202.

Di Fede O, Panzarella V, Mauceri R et al. The dental management of patients at risk of medication-related osteonecrosis of the jaw: new paradigm of primary prevention. *Biomed Res Int.* 2018; 2018:1–10.

Fatahzadeh M, Glick M. Stroke: epidemiology, classification, risk factors, complications, diagnosis, prevention, and medical and dental management. *Oral Surg Oral Med Oral Pathol Oral Radiol Endod.* 2006; 102(2):180–191.

Fortier K, Shroff D, Reebye UN. Review: an overview and analysis of novel oral anticoagulants and their dental implications. *Gerodontology.* 2018; 35(2):78–86.

Golla K, Epstein JB, Cabay RJ. Liver disease: current perspectives on medical and dental management. *Oral Surg Oral Med Oral Pathol Oral Radiol Endod.* 2004; 98(5):516–521.

Halpern LR, Adams DR, Clarkson E. Treatment of the dental patient with bleeding dyscrasias: etiologies and management options for surgical success in practice. *Dent Clin North Am.* 2020; 64(2):411–434.

Israels S, Schwetz N, Boyar R, McNicol A. Bleeding disorders: characterization, dental considerations and management. *J Can Dent Assoc.* 2006; 72(9):827.

Jain A, Chawla M, Kumar A et al. Management of periodontal disease in patients with diabetes – good clinical practice guidelines: a joint statement by Indian Society of Periodontology and Research Society for the Study of Diabetes in India. *J Indian Soc Periodontol.* 2020; 24(6):498–524.

Khyati C, Triveni MG, Gopal R et al. Dental considerations in a patient with haemophilia. *J Haemophilia Prac.* 2016 Jan; 3(1):51–54.

Li G, Hu R, Zhang X. The impact of the 2020 International Society of Hypertension global hypertension practice guidelines on the prevention and control of hypertension in China. *Hypertens Res.* 2021; 6:1–2.

Malamed SF. *Handbook of local anesthesia.* Amsterdam: Elsevier Health Sciences; 2014a.

Malamed SF. *Medical emergencies in the dental office.* Amsterdam: Elsevier Health Sciences; 2014b.

Miyata Y, Obata Y, Mochizuki Y et al. Periodontal disease in patients receiving dialysis. *Int J Mol Sci.* 2019; 20(15):3805.

Muñoz Aguilera E, Suvan J, Buti J et al. Periodontitis is associated with hypertension: a systematic review and meta-analysis. *Cardiovasc Res.* 2020; 116(1):28–39.

Niu Y, Chen Y, Li W, Xie R, Deng X. Electromagnetic interference effect of dental equipment on cardiac implantable electrical devices: a systematic review. *Pacing Clin Electrophysiol.* 2020; 43(12):1588–1598.

Nualart Grollmus ZC, Morales Chávez MC, Silvestre Donat FJ. Periodontal disease associated to systemic genetic disorders. *Med Oral Patol Oral Cir Bucal.* 2007; 12(3):211–215.

Ptasiewicz M, Pawłowicz AK, Tymczyna-Borowicz B. Chemotherapy and oral health in leukemic patients. *Pol J Environ Stud.* 2020; 29(5):3263–3271.

Raatikainen MJP, Arnar DO, Merkely B et al. A decade of information on the use of cardiac implantable electronic devices and interventional electrophysiological procedures in the European Society of Cardiology countries: 2017 report from the European Heart Rhythm Association. *Europace.* 2017; 19:ii1–ii90.

Sabharwal A, Gomes-Filho IS, Stellrecht E, Scannapieco FA. Role of periodontal therapy in management of common complex systemic diseases and conditions: an update. *Periodontol 2000.* 2018; 78(1):212–226.

Southerland JH, Gill DG, Gangula PR et al. Dental management in patients with hypertension: challenges and solutions. *Clin Cosmet Investig Dent.* 2016; 8:111.

Srivastava A, Santagostino E, Dougall A et al. WFH guidelines for the management of hemophilia. *Haemophilia.* 2020; 26:1–58.

Unger T, Borghi C, Charchar F et al. 2020 International Society of Hypertension global hypertension practice guidelines. *Hypertension.* 2020; 75(6):1334–1357.

Yerra L, Reddy PC. Effects of electromagnetic interference on implanted cardiac devices and their management. *Cardiol Rev.* 2007; 15:304–309.

25.3   MEDICAL EMERGENCIES IN THE DENTAL OFFICE

Steph Smith

Contents

Learning objectives

- Identification of medical emergencies that may occur in a dental practice.
- Recognition of symptoms of specific medical conditions.
- Knowledge of warning signs that can occur before a medical emergency.
- Knowledge of the appropriate measures and treatment to be administered.
- Essential medications that should be kept in an in-office emergency kit.

Introduction

Medical emergencies can happen in the dental office, possibly threatening a patient's life and hindering the delivery of dental care. Early recognition of medical emergencies begins at the first sign of symptoms (Boyd 2013; Reed 2010).

Visible physical symptoms, such as sweating, paleness, fatigue, change in respiratory rate, or vomiting, should be addressed as soon as they are evident. Some symptoms, such as nausea, chest pain, elevated blood pressure, or irregular pulse, may not be evident unless the patient is asked or special equipment is used. This is why vital signs should be recorded at the beginning of the appointment, and repeated within five minutes if the readings are irregular (Boyd 2013).

This section gives a brief review of some of the commonly encountered medical emergencies in the dental office, including their common manifestations (a) and potential treatments (b) (Boyd 2013; Reed 2010).

Hyperventilation

(a) Severe anxiety or fear of the dentist can trigger hyperventilation, which includes an increased respiratory rate that can be difficult for the patient to control. During the rapid breaths, excessive levels of carbon dioxide are released. Symptoms such as tingling and numbness may occur, and the patient may become apprehensive. If breaths continue to remain uncontrolled, spasms or fainting may occur. Usually, hyperventilation-induced syncope will typically result in a normal respiratory rate and the patient can regain consciousness.

(b) Hyperventilation is the only emergency seen in the dental office when oxygen delivery is contraindicated. A paper bag for breathing should be avoided, because this can cause elevated carbon dioxide levels. Communicate with the patient so that they are aware of their breathing speed, and then verbally coach them into slower breaths, one at a time.

Obstruction

(a) Foreign objects, such as dental supplies, equipment, appliances, or restorations, may find their way into the patient's airway. If obstruction is partial, the patient is able to speak and will begin coughing, but if obstruction is complete, the patient can become cyanotic and clasp the hands across the throat, which is the universal sign for choking. A complete blockage can lead to a life-threatening situation if the object is not removed.

(b) If a patient begins to choke, remove all foreign objects from their mouth immediately. Allow the patient to forcefully cough, which will hopefully open the airway. If the person is unable to talk, cough, or gasp, indicating a completely blocked airway, then abdominal thrusts should be performed until the foreign object is dislodged (Heimlich maneuver). If the patient is unconscious, contact emergency medical services (EMS). Lay the patient flat on the floor. Open the airway using a head-tilt, chin-lift maneuver. Perform a finger sweep if the object can be seen. Never perform a blind finger sweep, because this can cause the object to become lodged deeper. Perform appropriate steps of cardiopulmonary resuscitation (CPR) based on the patient's oxygen flow and pulse.

Loss of consciousness, fainting, syncope

(a) Fainting may be the cause of more than half of all dental office emergencies, due to drug use, seizures, drop in blood sugar, anxiety, or low blood pressure in the brain.

(b) The easiest and least invasive way to increase blood flow to the brain is to place the patient in a supine position. Vasovagal syncope in the dental office is often caused by anxiety, which needs to be addressed. For some patients, this may mean that the dentist simply needs to take more time explaining the dental procedure to them, thus allaying their fears. Other patients may need nitrous oxide or anti-anxiety medication. Some patients who get up too quickly after reclining can experience syncope and should be helped to get up slowly. Most people typically become alert within one minute after fainting. If not, then there is most likely a more serious underlying condition.

Diabetic syncope/hypoglycemia

(a) Most hypoglycemia will only occur in type 1 diabetics (insulin dependent), but it can also occur in type 2 diabetics who are taking hypoglycemic medication. If type 1 diabetics gives themselves an insulin injection but do not eat afterward, they may experience hypoglycemia and have a fainting episode. Before fainting, people may experience dizziness, confusion, diaphoresis (sweating), and tachycardia and feel faint. They also may complain of a headache or behave strangely. It is also possible that in rare circumstances, a hypoglycemic diabetic may experience stroke- or seizure-like symptoms.

(b) If the patient is still conscious, place them in a comfortable position and give them something to eat that contains sugar, such as juice, soda, or cake icing. If the patient is unconscious, they should be placed in a supine position and be given an injection to raise the blood sugar. If unconscious, they should typically regain consciousness within 60 seconds. If the patient has not regained consciousness within 60 seconds, then there is likely a serious underlying condition. Begin initiating basic life support steps as necessary, and EMS should also be notified. If the patient has extremely elevated blood pressure, they may be experiencing a cardiovascular attack instead of diabetic syncope. To avoid diabetic emergencies in the office, it is best to schedule these patients first thing in the morning, after they have eaten a full meal.

Asthma attack

(a) Asthma affects people of all ages and causes a response that tightens the airways. Aerosols in the treatment area or fear of dental treatment may trigger an attack in some people. Patients with this type of respiratory distress, also known as acute bronchospasm, typically will want to sit upright. Symptoms of an asthma attack include coughing, wheezing, and trouble breathing. Patients may also feel pressure in their chest and begin to appear cyanotic.

(b) Put the person into an upright position. Examine the airway to check for swelling or obstruction and record the patient's vitals. Conscious patients can administer their own drugs (usually albuterol) through their inhaler, and then be given oxygen. If they recover in a timely manner, treatment can be continued. If the patient has persistent symptoms and requires a second dose of albuterol, then treatment should be delayed until another day. Should the patient become unconscious, a bronchodilator (albuterol) and parenteral epinephrine should be delivered while also activating EMS.

Allergic reactions

(a) Symptoms of an allergic reaction may include hives, rash, itchiness, swelling, intestinal distress, trouble breathing, redness of the skin, anaphylaxis, and loss of consciousness. Anaphylaxis includes constriction of the airway and reduction in air flow, and can cause a patient to lose consciousness and go into distress from the lack of oxygen.

(b) A mild allergic reaction that results in minor symptoms typically only calls for the patient to be made comfortable and the delivery of an antihistamine such as diphenhydramine, via intramuscular or intravenous injection. The patient should be watched to ensure that more serious symptoms do not become evident, and that vital signs are appropriate. Patients experiencing severe reactions such as anaphylaxis and loss of consciousness must be placed in a supine position, their airways opened, and evaluated for breathing. They must be given a dose of epinephrine, delivered in their thigh or upper arm. Epinephrine is extremely effective because it prevents further histamine release and helps reverse histamine-caused conditions. EMS must be notified if the patient is experiencing a severe allergic reaction, and the patient should be placed on positive pressure oxygen if not breathing, followed by the monitoring of vital signs.

Seizures

(a) Patients experiencing a seizure in your office most likely have a medical history of seizures or epilepsy. Seizures are caused by erratic electrical activity in the brain. These electrical signals can spread over the brain and stimulate areas that control other things, such as muscle control. Some patients can tell when they are about to experience a seizure, which is called an "aura." The aura usually involves strange smells, sounds, sensations, or hallucinations, and can give them a chance to prepare for the seizing event. Generalized seizures affect both sides of the brain and result in unconsciousness. Partial seizures are localized to a specific portion of the brain. Consciousness may or may not be lost. They do not last long, but may spread and cause a generalized seizure. With status epilepticus, an ongoing, continuous seizure can occur for a prolonged duration. After seizing, patients will typically be fatigued or confused.

(b) Seizing patients should have the immediate area freed of equipment or foreign objects that they could come into contact with and possibly harm themselves. All instruments and supplies must be removed from the patient's mouth to prevent aspiration or trauma. Do not restrain the patient. Do not attempt to prop the patient's mouth open in any way or give rescue breaths. Most of the time it is only necessary to monitor the patient and have someone drive them home, but if the seizure is severe, it will be necessary to call EMS.

Cardiovascular arrest and chest pain

(a) Chest pain, cardiac arrest, or other forms of tightness in the chest are cause for alarm. If a patient is experiencing chest pain, they will usually inform the dentist. The discomfort may not necessarily be a sharp, painful feeling, but the person may instead feel as if their chest is being squeezed or under pressure, or experience a tightness or constriction. Classic heart attack symptoms usually include chest pain or pressure; shortness of breath; pain or numbness through the arms, shoulders, jaw, neck, back, or upper abdomen; nausea; and perspiration.

(b) The difficulty for the dentist is the differential diagnosis of chest pain, whereby angina pectoris and acute myocardial infarction (AMI) are the two most likely cardiac problems in a conscious patient who is exhibiting chest pain in the dental office. Pain that is not severe or an elevated blood pressure may be angina pectoris instead of an AMI. Elevation in blood pressure may be a response to the pain being experienced from angina pectoris. If the pain continues through the left side of the body, such as the arm, or blood pressure falls sharply below what the patient's normal baseline value is, then the patient is likely experiencing an AMI. If the heart has been injured, it is less efficient, resulting in a decreased cardiac output and subsequent drop in blood pressure. In such instances, the EMS should be contacted. If the patient has never experienced this type of feeling before, the dentist should treat the patient as if it were an AMI and then EMS should be contacted immediately for transfer to a hospital as quickly as possible. The patient may be given a single dose of aspirin, and then a dose of nitroglycerine from an emergency kit can be administered every five minutes. Some first-time nitroglycerine users may experience low blood pressure, so placing them in a supine position can help them relax. The patient may also be placed on a 50:50 nitrous oxide and oxygen delivery. An unconscious patient experiencing a cardiovascular attack may exhibit spontaneous breathing. Check the patient's vital signs and initiate CPR if necessary, until the paramedics arrive and take over the situation.

Stroke

(a) Known as a cerebrovascular accident (CVA), strokes typically occur in adults with high blood pressure or hardening of the arteries caused by a buildup of plaque within them. Blood clots also are a common cause of stroke, and when the episode occurs, the symptoms are visible almost immediately. Most of the time these episodes are short-lived, but it is possible that they will continue for a lengthy period. Smaller strokes (transient ischemic attacks) are a sign that a more severe attack may be on its way. Symptoms of stroke include trouble walking; problems talking or understanding what others are saying; partial paralysis of the face, arm, or leg; difficulty seeing with one or both eyes; and headache.

(b) Contact EMS immediately if you suspect your patient is experiencing a stroke. Lay the patient on their side and remove all instruments or other objects from the person's mouth to prevent aspiration. If necessary, you may utilize the suction to prevent the patient from inhaling material or large quantities of saliva and blood. It is very common for the patient to lose control of some muscles or the face, so work to keep the person comfortable and calm while waiting for paramedics.

Bleeding disorder

(a) When significant blood loss occurs, it can quickly become an emergency situation. Severe bleeding may be caused by the patient taking blood thinners close to the time of their treatment, aspirin use, trauma to orofacial blood vessels during surgical procedures, or surgical procedures, such as sinus lifts, dental implants, and extractions.

(b) Patients who hemorrhage should be positioned upright to reduce blood flow to the head. Most of the time, firm pressure and care to the local area of bleeding will be enough to control the blood flow. Patients who take blood thinners should have treatment needs addressed with their physician. Do not instruct the patient to discontinue medication on their own. If the bleeding is caused by a traumatic injury from a fall (caused by loss of consciousness or accident), quickly apply pressure to the area. Conscious, spontaneously ventilating patients who are bleeding profusely are treated most commonly with local measures only. Pressure to the affected site, with or without suturing, addresses the problem adequately in most cases. It is not likely that bleeding will be severe enough to need a tourniquet in a dental setting, but should you find that it does, apply steady pressure while EMS is notified.

Essential emergency drugs

- *Epinephrine*: Epinephrine is used for emergencies with allergic reactions, respiratory distress, and cardiovascular emergencies. This injectable drug is easily delivered through a preloaded syringe or pen-type device. Most people with severe food allergies will keep a device such as an EpiPen with them in the event of an exposure. Epinephrine should be given to asthmatic patients who do not respond to albuterol during an attack.

- *Diphenhydramine/histamine blocker*: Histamine blockers may be preferred in patients with a milder allergic reaction. Orally administered antihistamines are appropriate for mild allergic responses. Injectable antihistamines are for more serious reactions, such as when a patient is experiencing anaphylaxis.

- *Sugar/glucose*: This is for diabetic patients who are experiencing hypoglycemia from an insulin imbalance. It can be in the form of juice, cake icing, or soda and should be given to a patient only if they are conscious.

- *Nitroglycerine*: In the form of a spray or tablet, nitroglycerine is used on patients who are experiencing sharp chest pain and have a history of angina attacks. Patients who take nitroglycerine should bring their medication with them to their appointment, but people with undiagnosed conditions may experience symptoms of a heart attack and need to have nitroglycerine administered to them. The dosage can be given every five minutes with a total of three dosages. Most nitroglycerine has a shelf life of only three months after it has been opened.

- *Aspirin*: A minimal, single dose of 162 mg aspirin should be given to heart attack victims. It can also be accompanied by nitroglycerine. Pills should be chewed and then swallowed by the patient.

- *Bronchodilator/albuterol*: This is used when asthmatic patients experience an asthma attack or exhibit symptoms of anaphylaxis. It is the first medicine of choice for patients who are experiencing bronchospasm.

From the moment a patient begins having health troubles until the paramedics arrive, there is a crucial window of time where the dental care provider is responsible for the patient's care and well-being. Identifying the warning signs of medical-related emergencies is essential (Boyd 2013). Prompt recognition and efficient management of medical emergencies by a well-prepared dental team can increase the likelihood of a satisfactory outcome (Boyd 2013; Reed 2010).

Proper precautions should be taken to eliminate medical episodes while the patient is under the dentist's care. Up-to-date medical records, health history screenings, and vital signs should be recorded at every single appointment. Familiarity with the patient's medical profile aids immensely in recognition; knowing what to expect and what to look for promotes a faster response. Neglecting to ask patients about medications they are taking, record their blood pressure and pulse, or document blood sugar levels can place both patients and dental team members in a dangerous situation (Boyd 2013).

Regardless of the specific type of medical emergency, they are best managed in basically the same way: positioning of the patient; accessing and assisting the patient's circulation, airway, and breathing; and providing definitive treatment. Definitive treatment consists of differential diagnosis, drugs, and defibrillation with an automated external/external defibrillator (Boyd 2013; Reed 2010). All dental healthcare providers should be trained and regularly updated in the administration of basic life support, in the form of CPR. Until 2010, most healthcare providers called a memory aid for these actions the emergency ABCs, because the guidelines called for the sequence to be airway, breathing, and circulation assessments. However, the American Heart Association changed this basic life support sequence by placing circulation before airway or breathing checks. So, the memory aid has become known as "CAB" instead of "ABC" (Boyd 2013) Furthermore, by being aware of precursors and risks that make patients susceptible to emergencies, one can refer them to medical services in a timely manner (Boyd 2013).

SUMMARY

REFERENCES

Boyd S. Chapter 6: Medical emergencies in the dental office. Dental.EliteCME.com; 2013. https://s3.amazonaws.com/EliteCME_WebSite_2013/f/pdf/DFL04EDI18.pdf.

Reed KL. Basic management of medical emergencies. *JADA*; 2010; 141:205–245.

CHAPTER 26
Halitosis

David G. Gillam

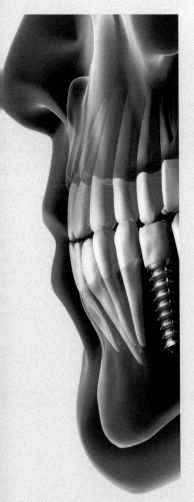

Contents

Learning objectives

- Terminology used to describe and diagnose halitosis.
- Intra-oral and extra-oral causes of halitosis, including the role of microorganisms.
- Methods to clinically evaluate patients with halitosis.
- Treatment needs and various aspects of the management of halitosis.

Essential Periodontics, First Edition. Edited by Steph Smith and Khalid Almas.
© 2022 John Wiley & Sons Ltd. Published 2022 by John Wiley & Sons Ltd.

Introduction

Oral malodor or, more correctly, halitosis is defined as having offensive bad breath causing personal discomfort to those affected, as well as having an impact on their self-confidence, social interactions, and quality of life (QoL). Malodor may originate from both oral and non-oral sources. Historically the condition has been reported in most cultures, sexes, and ethnicities, and numerous treatments have been recommended to resolve the problem (Porter & Scully 2006; Scully & Greenman 2012; Seemann et al. 2014; Winkel 2008). This chapter focuses on the problem of halitosis and its diagnosis, assessment, and management.

Prevalence of halitosis

The actual prevalence of oral malodor is unclear due to the highly sensitive nature of the problem and as such depends on subjective self-estimation. The prevalence or self-perception of halitosis may vary among racially diverse groups, but would appear to range from 8% to 75.1% depending on the location of the study (Porter & Scully 2006; Rayman & Almas 2008; Youngnak-Piboonratanakit & Vachirarojpisan 2010). According to some estimates the condition is ranked as the third most frequent reason following dental caries and periodontal diseases for individuals seeking dental advice and treatment (Loesche & Kazor 2002).

Terminology used to diagnose halitosis

The consensus from an international workshop has suggested that the term "halitosis" be used, which includes all examples of "real halitosis," thus allowing for examples of sources of both intra- and extra-oral halitosis (Seemann et al. 2014). Table 26.1 outlines the terminology used to define and characterize halitosis (Scully & Greenman 2012).

Causes of halitosis

Table 26.2 depicts the intra-oral and extra-oral causes of halitosis (Porter & Scully 2006; Scully & Greenman 2012).

Microorganisms associated with halitosis

The oral microbiome contains ≥700 bacterial species forming complex biofilms in both supra- and subgingival plaque (as in health and periodontal disease), as well as in tongue coatings in both children and adults (Ren et al. 2016; Scully & Greenman 2012; Suzuki et al. 2015). Members of the indigenous microflora, which include Gram-positive and Gram-negative species as well as proteolytic obligate anaerobes, contribute to the production of halitosis (Aylıkcı & Colak 2013; Persson et al. 1990; Porter & Scully 2006). Anaerobic bacteria metabolize and degrade organic substances such as amino acids, and produce volatile sulfur compounds (VSCs) such as hydrogen sulfide (H_2S), methyl mercaptan (CH_3SH), and dimethyl sulfide (CH_3SCH_3) (Scully & Greenman 2012;

Table 26.1 Terminology used to define halitosis.

Term used	Definition	
Halitosis	Any disagreeable odor of unspired air regardless of origin	
Bad breath	Lay term for halitosis	
Genuine halitosis	Breath malodor that can be verified objectively	
	Physiologic halitosis, also termed transient halitosis	Morning breath or lifestyle malodors
	Pathologic halitosis	Subclassified into oral and extra-oral
Oral malodor	Pathologic halitosis originating from the oral cavity	Foetor oris
Extra-oral malodor	Pathologic halitosis originating from outside the oral cavity	Foetor ex-oris
Pseudo-halitosis	Breath malodor that cannot be verified objectively. Patients initially think that they have malodor but without objective evidence. Patients eventually accept that they do not have malodor	
Halitophobia	Breath malodor that cannot be verified objectively. Patients persist in believing that they have malodor despite evidence to the contrary, i.e. monosymptomatic delusional hypochondriasis	

Source: Scully and Greenman 2012, with permission of John Wiley & Sons.

Suzuki et al. 2015; Tonzetich 1977). Other reported odiferous compounds include volatile aromatic compounds and amines (such as indole, skatole, pyridine, picoline, urea); short/medium-chain fatty acids or organic acids (propionic acid, butyric acid, acetic acid, valeric acid, isovaleric acid, esanoic acid); alcohols (methanol, ethanol, propanol); volatile alphatic compounds (cyclopropane, cyclobutene, pentane); and aldehydes and ketones (acetaldehyde, acetone, benzophenone, acetophenone) (Campisi et al. 2011; Scully & Greenman 2012; Suzuki et al. 2015; Tonzetich 1977).

Clinical evaluation of halitosis

Patient history

A halitosis-related questionnaire or a visual analog scale (VAS) can be used to identify the areas in the patient's lifestyle behaviors, medical and dietary history, smoking and drinking habits, etc., to determine the extent and severity of the problem (Nandlal et al. 2016; Seemann et al. 2014; Winkel 2008).

Table 26.2 Causes of halitosis.

Intra-oral causes	
Tongue biofilm coating	Poor oral hygiene, soft diet, smoking
Plaque-related gingival and periodontal disease	Gingivitis, periodontitis, acute necrotizing ulcerative gingivitis, pericoronitis, abscesses
Ulceration	Systemic disease (inflammatory/ infectious disorders, cutaneous, gastrointestinal, and hematological disease), malignancy, local causes, aphthae, drugs
Hyposalivation	Drug therapy, Sjögren's syndrome, cancer therapy
Wearing dental appliances	Poor oral hygiene, candidosis
Dental conditions	Food packing, dental abscesses
Bone diseases	Dry socket, osteomyelitis, osteonecrosis, malignancy
Extra-oral causes	
May include underlying medical conditions that would require further medical consultation originating from respiratory system (with a microbiological etiology); gastrointestinal tract; metabolic disorders (blood borne); drugs (blood borne); and psychogenic causes	

Source: Adapted from Porter & Scully 2006; Scully & Greenman 2012.

In light of the vast range of intra- and extra-oral causes, referral to medical colleagues for further investigation may be more appropriate when more systemic causes are suspected (Scully & Greenman 2012).

Clinical detection

Two main methods have been recommended: (i) an organoleptic/hedonic (subjective) measurement, which is a sensory test scored on the clinician's perception of a patient's breath odor; and (ii) an instrumental (objective) measurement based on the detection of VSCs (Seemann et al. 2014; Winkel 2008). These two methods are also used to evaluate the efficacy of dental products designed to treat oral malodor in clinical studies where a panel of trained malodor judges may be used to assess the "strength" of the breath detected at various time points during the study (Quirynen et al. 2002; Rosenberg 2005; Seemann et al. 2014; Slot et al. 2015; Winkel 2008).

Organoleptic measurement

The initial organoleptic assessment should take place in the morning and the patient should be given prior instructions (before the appointment), which include (Seemann et al. 2014):

- No smoking.
- Avoid using fragrances and other masking products.
- No antibiotic treatment prior to the appointment (at least 3–6 weeks).
- No eating or drinking in the morning prior to the oral examination.
- Avoid any tongue cleaning for 24 hours before the breath assessment.

There are several recommended organoleptic scales that can be used by a clinician, ranging from a simple "yes/no" response to more complex scales that are employed by trained and experienced "odor judges" in clinical studies.

Other simple tests have also been suggested, such as a saliva odor test, which is similar to the lick test where the patient licks the wrist, and after 10 seconds (to allow the wrist to dry) the clinician will be able to give a score for the degree of malodor (Kapoor et al. 2016). Some investigators have recommended either taking tongue scrapings from the dorsum of the tongue to assess the odor, or using a tongue scoring system such as the Winkel tongue coating index (WTCL) to determine the amount of coating present (Aylıkcı & Colak 2013; Kapoor et al. 2016; Winkel 2008).

The advantages of organoleptical scoring are that it is relatively inexpensive and specialist equipment is not required, and following training a clinician should be able to detect a wide range of odors from the oral cavity (Kapoor et al. 2016).

Instrumental measurement

This uses calibration instruments such as a Halimeter® (Interscan Corporation, Chatsworth, CA, USA) (Figure 26.1), or a portable gas chromatography device (OralChroma™, Abilit Corporation, Osaka, Japan) (Figure 26.2) or CHM-2

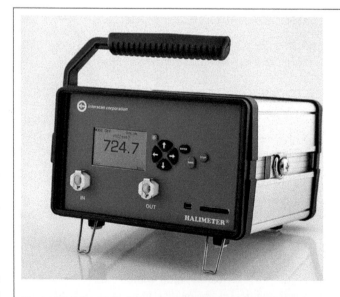

Figure 26.1 Example of a portable sulfide monitor (Halimeter).

(OralChroma™, Nissha FIS, Inc., Osaka, Japan) (Figure 26.3) (Kupaan et al. 2016; Porter & Scully 2006; Rosenberg 2005; Scully & Greenman 2012; Seemann et al. 2014; Winkel 2008). Both instruments are used to detect sulfide and are very reliable, although they may not be suitable for general clinical practice.

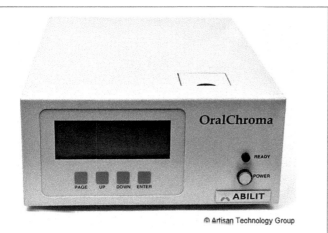

Figure 26.2 Example of an OralChroma instrument.

Table 26.3 Classification of halitosis treatment needs and related management.

Treatment need	Management
TN1	Explanation of halitosis and instructions for oral hygiene, including tongue cleaning and use of additional measures such as mouth rinsing, etc. (Treatment of intra- and extra-oral halitosis, pseudo-halitosis, and halitophobia.)
TN2	Professional prophylaxis and treatment of oral pathological condition (mainly periodontitis) if present. (Treatment of intra-oral halitosis.)
TN3	Referral to a physician, medical specialist, or interdisciplinary halitosis specialist. (Treatment for extra-oral halitosis.)
TN4	Explanation of examination data, further professional instruction, education, and reassurance. (Treatment for pseudo-halitosis.)
TN5	Referral to a clinical psychologist, psychiatrist, or other psychological specialist. (Treatment for halitophobia.)

Source: Adapted from Seemann et al. 2014.

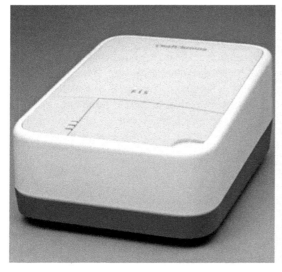
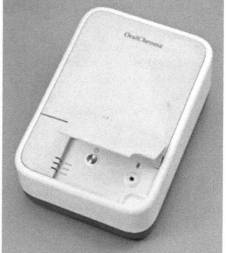

Figure 26.3 Example of a CHM-2 OralChroma instrument.

Management of halitosis

There are extensive recommendations for the treatment of halitosis (Bollen & Beikler 2012; Herman et al. 2018; Lu et al. 2014). Table 26.3 depicts the classification of treatment needs (TN) for patients with halitosis in general dental practice, together with the management thereof (Seemann et al. 2014).

- The management of halitosis is cause related and the onus is on the individual to eat and drink sensibly, avoiding smoking, drugs, and food that may initiate oral malodor. The importance of good oral hygiene practices, including toothbrushing, flossing, and reducing the tongue coating, should be encouraged and reinforced by the clinician (Scully & Greenman 2012).
- Patient education and counseling individuals who may be self-conscious and embarrassed about their perceived

Table 26.4 Adjunctive products used in treatment of halitosis.

Chemical agents	• Chlorhexidine (CHX) (0.12%; 0.2%) • Cetylpyridinium chloride (CPC) (0.05%) • Zinc chloride (ZnCl) (Zn2+ ion) (0.14% Zn2+ ion) • Triclosan (0.03%) (no longer incorporated into dental products) • Stannous (0.45%) and sodium fluoride • Hydrogen peroxide (H_2O_2) • Chlorine dioxide (ClO_2) (0.1%) • Combination of CHX + CPC + Zn or ZnCl + CPC
Natural botanical extracts	• Actinidine • Hinokitiol • Eucalyptus extract (essential oils) • Green tea • Magnolia bark extract and pericarp extract of garcinia mangostana L • Salivary components (lactoferrin and lactoperoxidase)
Probiotic bacteria	• *Lactobacillus salivarius* • *Lactobacillus reuteri* • *Weissella cibaria* • *Streptococcus salivarius*
Halitosis counteractive (cosmetic non-pharmacological products)	• Chewing gum • Parsley • Mint • Cloves • Fennel seeds
Antibiotics	• One-week course of metronidazole 200 mg, three times daily

Source: Adapted from Scully & Greenman 2012; Suzuki et al. 2015.

halitosis should be incorporated into subsequent management strategies (Lenton et al. 2014; Rayman & Almas 2008). A QoL questionnaire such as the Halitosis Associated Life-quality Test (HALT) (Agostinho et al. 2019; Kizhner et al. 2011) or VAS scores (Nandlal et al. 2016) may be utilized to evaluate the impact and severity on the QoL of patients, as well as to identify behaviors that may be implicated in causation. These measures may also be useful for monitoring the problem during treatment. Usage of the P-LI-SS-IT System (Permission, Limited Information, Specific Suggestions and Intensive Therapy) has also been recommended for counseling with a view to changing patients' behavior (Lenton et al. 2014).

■ The management of halitosis is generally in response to existing conditions within the oral cavity, such as patients with tongue coatings, periodontal disease, dental caries, etc. (Ademovski et al. 2016; Seemann et al. 2014). The evidence for the adjunctive use of formulated toothpastes and antimicrobial mouthrinses or using a tongue scraper for the treatment of halitosis is, however, generally unclear (Slot et al. 2015). Various dental products that meet the safety and efficacy criteria for helping to reduce halitosis have a recognized "seal of approval" from several professional bodies, such as the American Dental Association (Pham & Nguyen 2018; Wozniak 2005). Table 26.4 depicts various adjunctive products used in toothpastes and mouthrinses.

SUMMARY

Most patients who seek medical or dental help for halitosis generally have causes that are intra-oral in nature, and this can be successfully treated by a general dental practitioner. Where the source of the malodor is extra-oral, then the individual may be referred to a medical or psychiatric colleague, depending on the initial diagnosis.

Clinicians should emphasize that poor oral hygiene and tongue coating are major contributors to halitosis. A management strategy for the individual patient should thus also

include education of the patient and addressing specific lifestyle behaviors, including smoking and diet, as well as counseling and motivation.

Professional supportive care that includes non-surgical periodontal therapy can be reinforced by the adjunctive use of oral care products such as toothpastes and mouthwashes. Furthermore, it is essential to monitor the patient over time to determine whether the problem has been minimized or resolved.

REFERENCES

Adedapo CE, Martoneron C, Persson GR et al. The effect of periodontal therapy on intra-oral halitosis: a case series. *J Clin Periodontol.* 2016; 43:445–452.

Agostinho AC, de Sousa KG, de Freitas CN et al. Translation, transcultural adaptation and validation of the halitosis associated life-quality test for use in Brazilian adolescents. *Pesquisa Brasileira em Odontopediatria e Clínica Integrada.* 2019; 19:e3807.

Aylıkcı BU, Colak H. Halitosis: from diagnosis to management. *J Nat Sci Biol Med.* 2013; 4(1):14–23.

Bollen CM, Beikler T. Halitosis: the multidisciplinary approach. *Int J Oral Sci.* 2012; 4:55–63.

Campisi G, Musciotto A, Di Fede O et al. Halitosis: could it be more than mere bad breath? *Intern Emerg Med.* 2011; 6:315–319.

Herman S, Lisowska G, Herman J et al. Genuine halitosis in patients with dental and laryngological etiologies of mouth odor: severity and role of oral hygiene behaviors. *Eur J Oral Sci.* 2018; 126:101–109.

Kapoor U, Sharma G, Juneja M et al. Halitosis: current concepts on etiology, diagnosis and management. *Eur J Dent.* 2016; 10(2):292–300.

Kizhner V, Xu D, Krespi YP. A new tool measuring oral malodor quality of life. *Eur Arch Otorhinolaryngol.* 2011; 268(8):1227–1232.

Lenton PA, Majerus G, Bakdash B. *Counseling and treating bad breath patients: a step-by-step approach. Crest® Oral-B® at dentalcare.com.* Continuing Education Course, revised August 2014.

Loesche WJ, Kazor C. Microbiology and treatment of halitosis. *Periodontal 2000.* 2002; 28:256–279.

Lu H-X, Tang C, Chen X et al. Characteristics of patients complaining of halitosis and factors associated with halitosis. *Oral Diseases.* 2014; 20:787–795.

Nandlal B, Shahikumar P, Avinash BS et al. Malodor reductions and improved oral hygiene by toothbrushing and mouthrinsing. *Indian J Dent Res.* 2016; 27:42–47.

Persson S, Yaegaki K, Matsuo T et al. The formation of hydrogen sulfide and methyl mercaptan by oral bacteria. *Oral Microbiol Immunol.* 1990; 5:195–201.

Pham TAV, Nguyen NTX. Efficacy of chlorine dioxide mouthwash in reducing oral malodor: a 2-week randomized, double-blind, crossover study. *Clin Exp Dent Res.* 2018; 4:206–215.

Porter SR, Scully C. Oral malodour (halitosis). *BMJ.* 2006; 333:632–635.

Quirynen M, Zhao H, van Steenberghe D. Review of the treatment strategies for oral malodour. *Clin Oral Investig.* 2002; 6(1):1–10.

Rayman S, Almas K. Halitosis among racially diverse populations: an update. *Int J Dent Hyg.* 2008; 6:2–7.

Ren W, Xun Z, Wang Z et al. Tongue coating and the salivary microbial communities vary in children with halitosis. *Sci Rep.* 2016; 6:24481. doi: 10.1038/srep24481.

Rosenberg M. Odor measurements using instruments and other laboratory tests (GC, GCMS, Halimeter, Sensors, HPLC, OK2KISS, BANA etc.). *Oral Dis.* 2005; 11:122–123.

Scully C, Greenman J. Halitology (breath odour: aetiopathogenesis and management). *Oral Dis.* 2012; 18:333–345.

Seemann R, Conceicao MD, Filippi A et al., Halitosis management by the general dental practitioner—results of an international consensus workshop. *J Breath Res.* 2014; 8:017101.

Slot DE, De Geest S, van der Weijden FA et al. Treatment of oral malodour. Medium-term efficacy of mechanical and/or chemical agents: a systematic review. *J Clin Periodontol.* 2015; 42(Suppl 16):S303–S316.

Suzuki N, Yoneda M, Hirofuji T. Evidence-based control of oral malodor. In: MS Virdi (ed.), *Emerging Trends in Oral Health Sciences and Dentistry.* London: IntechOpen; 2015: 801–816.

Tonzetich J. Production and origin or oral malodor: a review of mechanisms and methods of analysis. *J Periodontol.* 1977; 48:13–20.

Winkel EG. Halitosis control. In: NP Lang, T Karring, J Lindhe (eds), *Clinical Periodontology and Implant Dentistry.* Oxford: Blackwell; 2008: 1325–1340.

Wozniak WT. The ADA guidelines on oral malodor products. *Oral Dis.* 2005;111 (Suppl 1):7–9.

Youngnak-Piboonratanakit P, Vachirarojpisan T. Self-perceived oral malodor in Thai dental patients. *J Dent.* 2010; 7(4):196–204.

CHAPTER 27
Interdisciplinary periodontics

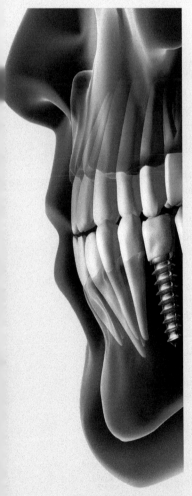

Contents

Essential Periodontics, First Edition. Edited by Steph Smith and Khalid Almas.
© 2022 John Wiley & Sons Ltd. Published 2022 by John Wiley & Sons Ltd.

27.1 THE PERIODONTICS–RESTORATIVE RELATIONSHIP

Ajay K. Dhingra, Sejal R. Thacker, Farheen Malek and Steph Smith

Contents

Learning objectives

- The concept and factors influencing the periodontal–restorative interface, and its relation to restorative procedures.
- Concepts of supracrestal attachment and ferrule effect.
- Definition and purposes of a crown lengthening procedure, including restorative and esthetic indications for crown lengthening.
- Restorative preparations needed prior to surgery.
- Indications, contraindications, and various techniques for crown lengthening surgery.
- Techniques for gingival augmentation procedures.

Introduction

All restorative therapy should be planned and performed with due consideration to periodontal health and maintenance. Knowledge of biological principles pertaining to the periodontal tissues will enable the clinician to predict responses to restorative therapy (Cook & Lim 2019). Every restoration adds burden to the periodontal tissues. Even a perfectly adapted restorative margin, depending on the characteristics of the restorative material, can act as a potential plaque-accumulating surface. A poorly contoured restoration can interfere with oral hygiene measures, thereby enhancing periodontal breakdown as well as recurrent caries at the interface (Heschl et al. 2013; Litonjua et al. 2012).

The periodontal–restorative interface

In order to maintain periodontal health and to achieve optimal esthetics, the clinician should have a clear understanding of the physiology of the dentogingival complex. This will ensure conservation of the integrity of this complex and provide long-term success to treatment rendered.

The dentogingival complex

The dentogingival complex encompasses a relationship between the crest of the alveolar bone surrounding a tooth, the connective tissue attachment, the epithelial attachment, and the sulcus depth (Cook & Lim 2019; Gargiulo et al. 1961; Vacek et al. 1994). The supracrestal attachment ("biological width") has two components: the connective tissue and the epithelial attachment, coronal to the alveolar bone crest.

On average this dimension measures about 2 mm (Gargiulo et al. 1961; Ingber et al. 1977; Vacek et al. 1994) (see Figure 27.1.1). Taking into account 2 mm of supracrestal tissue and 1 mm of sulcus depth, a mean distance of 3 mm between the restorative margins and crest of the bone is considered a safe distance that will significantly reduce the risk of periodontal attachment loss (Ong et al. 2011). Table 27.1.1 depicts the relationship of the components of the dentogingival complex, as well as their clinical significance.

Human and animal studies have shown that impingement of the supracrestal attachment can negatively influence periodontal health, including chronic inflammation as well as crestal bone resorption (Günay et al. 2000; Parma-Benfenali et al. 1985). A new position of the restorative margin with respect to the most apical point of the gingival marginal scallop can be achieved by performing a crown lengthening procedure. This procedure involves surgical apical positioning of the entire complex. It thus exposes more crown structure, thereby ensuring a stable and predictable long-term exposure of the desired amount of tooth structure.

Factors influencing the periodontal–restorative interface

The factors that influence the periodontal–restorative interface are as follows:

Periodontal phenotype

See also Chapter 10.3. Determination of the periodontal phenotype is necessitated for assessing therapy outcomes in periodontal and implant therapy, prosthodontics, and

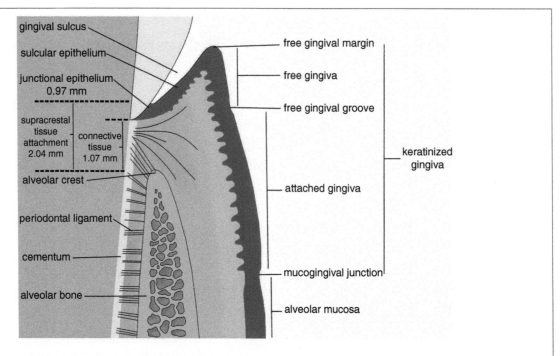

Figure 27.1.1 The periodontium. Courtesy of Dr. Abdulqader Alhammadi.

Table 27.1.1 Relationship of components of the dentogingival complex.

Dentogingival component	Location	Dimension	Clinical significance
Histological sulcus	Gingival margin to the epithelial attachment	0.69–1.34 mm	May differ from the clinical sulcus depth
Epithelial attachment	Distance from coronal to apical portion of the attachment	0.97–1.14 mm	The most variable component
Connective tissue attachment	Distance from epithelial attachment to crest of alveolar bone	0.77–1.07 mm	The most consistent component

Source: Adapted from Cook & Lim 2019.

orthodontics (Cortellini & Bissada 2018). Three categories of periodontal phenotypes have been classified (Zweers et al. 2014):

- *Thin scalloped phenotype* is associated with slender triangular crowns, a subtle cervical convexity, interproximal contacts being close to incisal edges, a narrow zone of keratinized tissue (KT), clear thin delicate gingiva, and relatively thin alveolar bone.
- *Thick flat phenotype* is associated with square-shaped tooth crowns, pronounced cervical convexity, large interproximal contacts located more apically, a broad zone of KT, thick fibrotic gingiva, and comparatively thick alveolar bone.
- *Thick scalloped phenotype* is associated with thick fibrotic gingiva, slender teeth, a narrow zone of KT, and pronounced gingival scalloping.

To diagnose the periodontal phenotype, a periodontal probe can be used to determine the visual detection thereof through the gingival sulcus. Visual detection of the probe is associated with a thin periodontal phenotype, and the inability to visualize the probe is associated with a thick/average periodontal phenotype (Ingber et al. 1977; Kan et al. 2012).

Alveolar crest position

Bone sounding can enable the clinician to locate the position of the alveolar bone crest in relation to the gingival margin and the cementoenamel junction (CEJ) (Cook & Lim 2019). A relationship between the CEJ and the crest of the alveolar bone shows variation as follows (Cook et al. 2011; Kois 1996; Machado 2014):

- *Normal crest*: The midfacial alveolar crest is 3 mm and the proximal alveolar crest is 3–4.5 mm apical to the CEJ (in 85% of cases).
- *High crest*: The midfacial alveolar crest is less than 3 mm and the proximal alveolar crest is 3 mm apical to the CEJ (in 2% of cases).
- *Low crest*: The midfacial alveolar crest is greater than 3 mm and the proximal alveolar crest is greater than 4.5 mm apical to the CEJ (in 13% of cases).

Position of the gingival margin

Ideal gingival esthetics is associated with the gingival margins of the maxillary central incisors and canines (Springer et al. 2011). Two categories of ideal gingival esthetics have been suggested, i.e., strong and soft (Machado 2014). In the strong configuration, the gingival margins of the maxillary center incisors, lateral incisor, and canines coincide on a horizontal plane. In the soft configuration, the gingival margins of the maxillary central incisors and canines coincide, whereas the gingival margin of the lateral incisors is slightly inferior (0.5 to 1.0 mm) to this horizontal line (Machado 2014; Springer et al. 2011).

Placement of the restorative margin

The ideal location for restorative margin placement is slightly coronal to the CEJ (Cook & Lim 2019). Supragingival margin placement is the preferred option to maintain periodontal health. However, margin location may be influenced by esthetics, retention and resistance of restorations, root caries, the position of the CEJ, and the presence of recession (Cook & Lim 2019; Valderhaugw & Birkeland 1976). Over a period of 5 years, 68% of subgingival margins may become equal-gingival or supragingival due to gingival recession. Subgingival placement of margins may also be associated with greater loss of attachment of up to 1.2 mm, compared to supragingival margin placement with a loss of attachment of 0.6 mm (Donaldson 1973; Valderhaugw & Birkeland 1976). These factors will play an important role in individualizing the patients' restorative and periodontal treatment. For example:

- In patients with a thick/average periodontal phenotype, the alveolar crest is located closer to the CEJ (Cook et al. 2011), thus subgingival margin placement may increase the risk for biological width impingement.
- In patients with a thin periodontal phenotype, whereby the distance from a normal crest position usually increases, the alveolar crest position will be more apically positioned to the CEJ. The placement of a subgingival margin in this instance may then result in postoperative recession (Cook & Lim 2019).

Gingival retraction

Soft tissue management of tooth-borne restorations includes the production of acceptable restorative margins being recorded in a good impression without causing irreparable damage to the periodontal tissues (Benson et al. 1986). Gingival retraction techniques can result in mechanical and/or chemical trauma to the gingival tissues, which may trigger an inflammatory response. Often the injury is self-limiting and reversible, or the injury can lead to recession. The length of time of gingival displacement should be kept minimal, as prolonged displacement may jeopardize the ability for adequate healing (Cook & Lim 2019; de Gennaro et al. 1982; Harrison 1961; Ruel et al. 1980). The utilization of gingival retraction cords and varying cord techniques, as well as cordless displacement materials, offers different advantages and disadvantages (Chiche & Pinault 1994). The double cord technique has the potential to induce more gingival trauma, especially in a thin phenotype (Baba et al. 2014). Cordless displacement materials may cause less damage as they generate less pressure, but the amount and duration of gingival displacement may be less than when utilizing retraction cords (Bennani et al. 2012; Chandra et al. 2016).

Provisional restorations, restorative material selection, and inflammation

A common occurrence associated with provisional restorations is inflammation and recession of the free gingival margin, which may also be time dependent (Donaldson 1973, 1974). This may be attributed to poor contour, marginal adaptation, and surface roughness of the provisional restoration, irrespective of the material utilized; all these factors contribute to plaque accumulation (Dragoo & Williams 1982; Waerhaug & Zander 1957). Periodontal inflammation associated with provisional treatment can be expected to be reversible, provided that provisional restorations are smooth, well-fitting, properly contoured, as well as being utilized over a short time span, thereby inducing a minimal amount of gingival irritation (Chiche 1990; Dragoo & Williams 1982).

Materials used for fixed dental restorations may exhibit differing gingival responses, this being attributed to their variations in plaque accumulation (Heschl et al. 2013; Litonjua et al. 2012). Also, in patients with true metal allergies, despite limited evidence zirconia-based restorations may be an option (Gokcen-Rohlig et al. 2010). However, other studies have shown no statistical difference in plaque and gingival inflammation levels between non-treated teeth and teeth with full-coverage restorations (Morris 1989). Patient compliance, including personal oral hygiene and periodontal maintenance, has been shown to be more influential with regard to periodontal health than restorative material selection (Konradsson et al. 2007; Litonjua et al. 2012). Also, in most instances the quality of the fit and finish of the restoration rather than the material itself, even if placed subgingivally, is far more applicable with regard to gingival health (Richter & Ueno 1973).

Crown lengthening

Periodontal intervention by means of surgery is often indicated to enhance the longevity of a prosthesis, i.e. as related to restorative function and/or esthetics, as well as to promote oral hygiene maintenance. This can be achieved via soft and/or hard tissue reduction in a process called crown lengthening. Crown lengthening is defined as "A surgical procedure designed to increase the extent of supragingival tooth structure, primarily for restorative purposes, by apically positioning the gingival margins with or without the removal of supporting bone" (AAP Connect 2021).

Restorative indications for crown lengthening

During tooth preparation for direct or indirect restorations, margins may have to be extended subgingivally, so they rest on sound tooth structure, or to gain retention/resistance form, or for esthetics. Extending margins too deep into the sulcus without management of the dentogingival complex will jeopardize the surrounding periodontal health. Hence, from a restorative point of view, crown lengthening surgeries are indicated to:

- Relocate margins of restorations that are impinging on the biological width.
- Increase clinical crown height lost due to caries, fracture, or wear.
- Access subgingival caries.
- Access a perforation in the coronal third of the root.
- Attain a ferrule effect while maintaining a favorable crown to root ratio.

The ferrule is the 360° subgingival collar of the restoration surrounding the parallel walls of the dentin extending coronal to the margin of the preparation, as far as possible beyond the gingival seat of the core, and thereby completely surrounding the perimeter of the cervical part of the tooth (Sorensen & Engelman 1990). Placing a ferrule around a preparation provides resistance against dislodgement and protects the remaining tooth structure against fracture (Jotkowitz & Samet 2010). An abutment is considered to be most resistant to fracture if it provides 1.5–2.0 mm of tooth structure above the estimated margin, for the ferrule effect to provide fracture resistance (Akkayan 2004; Juloski et al. 2012). In carious teeth with loss of significant tooth structure, a foundation restoration, such as post and core, may be required for added intracanal retention. Foundation restorations facilitate occlusal forces becoming concentrated at the interface between the root and the post, resulting in cement fatigue and displacement of the post and core, or tooth fracture (Wagenberg et al. 1989) (Figure 27.1.2). However, studies have shown that the presence of a 1.5–2.0 mm height of tooth structure above the gingiva, the ferrule, is important for preventing fractures of carious teeth (Al-Wahadni & Gutteridge 2002; Ferrari et al. 2012). Crown lengthening procedures become necessary to provide the needed ferrule effect, and also allow the forces of occlusion to be transferred to the bone and to avoid fracture of the tooth (Gegauff 2000) (Figure 27.1.3).

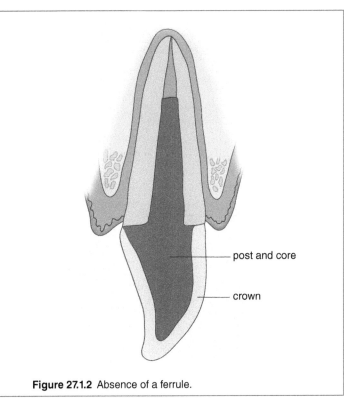

Figure 27.1.2 Absence of a ferrule.

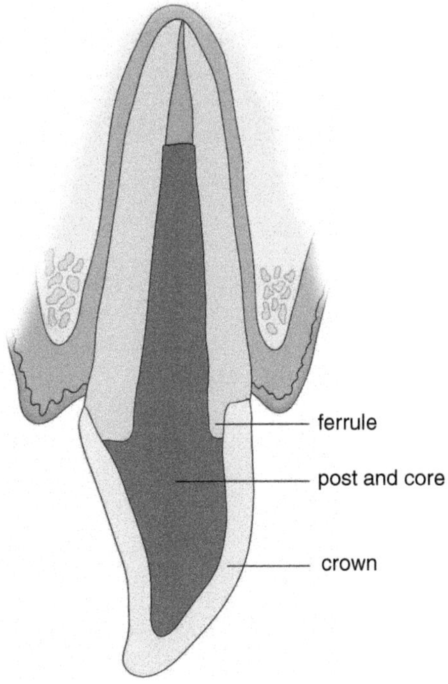

Figure 27.1.3 Ferrule effect after crown lengthening.

Esthetic indications for crown lengthening

Excessive gingival display

A smile is considered beautiful, attractive, and healthy when there is a balance between the shape and symmetry of lips, teeth, and gingiva. However, when showing a significant amount of gingival mucosa (more than 3 mm) during normal speech and smile, the condition is termed a "gummy smile" (Silberberg et al. 2009). A high smile line accentuates this situation. Possible etiological factors for excessive gingival display include altered passive eruption, plaque-induced or drug-induced hyperplasia, short clinical crowns, vertical maxillary excess, a short and hyperactive upper lip, or a combination of these clinical situations (Dolt & Robbins 1997; Levine & McGuire 1997). Altered passive eruption occurs when the dentogingival junction is located close to the CEJ, involving a more coronal periodontium, with the gingival margins slightly covering the coronal limits of the dental crown. When the gingival margin occupies a much more incisal position, it gives rise to short clinical crowns (Alpiste-Illueca 2011; Coslet et al. 1977) (Figure 27.1.4).

Uneven gingival contours

The gingival margins over maxillary anterior teeth have a specific location in the normal dentition. However, certain situations, for example crown fractures and supra-eruption of teeth, can cause uneven gingival contours, including disruption of the gingival zeniths of maxillary teeth, thereby affecting the esthetic balance between teeth and gingiva (Figure 27.1.5). The position of the gingival margins can be surgically altered with or without adjunctive prosthodontic therapy to achieve optimum esthetics.

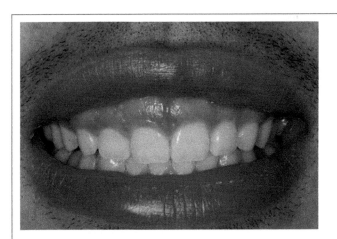

Figure 27.1.4 Excessive gingival display: combination of short upper lip, vertical maxillary excess, and altered eruption.

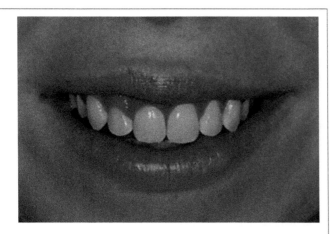

Figure 27.1.5 Uneven gingival zeniths in a patient with an average smile line.

Drug-induced gingival hyperplasia

Over 20 drugs have been associated with gingival overgrowth as a side effect (Dongari-Bagtzoglou 2004). The most common types of drugs include phenytoin, amlodipine, and cyclosporin A. For gingival hyperplasia patients, a thorough medical history and a list of medications are necessary to determine the cause.

Contraindications for crown lengthening

- Active inflammation or periodontal disease.
- Vertical maxillary excess.
- Poor crown/root ratio.
- Compromised adjacent osseous tooth support.
- Exposure of furcation areas in case of short root trunk followed by crown lengthening.
- Non-restorable tooth.
- Aesthetic concerns in the anterior region.
- Anatomic concerns, including root proximity, large torus, maxillary sinus, ascending ramus, proximity of a neurovascular bundle.

Crown lengthening procedures

Prior to the surgical procedure, the following restorative steps should be first undertaken wherever indicated in this sequence: (i) caries control; (ii) endodontic treatment; and (iii) post and core placement with temporization. Thereafter, surgical crown lengthening can be performed, followed by healing and placement of the final restoration.

Crown lengthening can be done using one of the following procedures (see Chapters 17 and 18).

Gingivectomy

A gingivectomy is indicated in cases presenting with gingival excess due to drug-induced gingival overgrowth; or cases presenting with altered passive eruption when it is determined that the osseous level is appropriate, whereby the distance from the alveolar bone crest to the gingival margin is greater than 3 mm, including an adequate zone of attached gingiva to be remaining after surgery (Dolt & Robbins 1997).

Apically positioned flap

An apically positioned gingival flap with bone recontouring can be performed in the following cases:

- Esthetic crown lengthening, when diagnostic procedures have revealed osseous levels to be approximating the CEJ in altered passive eruption cases.
- Functional crown lengthening is indicated for restorative reasons (Figure 27.1.6). However, it is contraindicated in single anterior teeth in the esthetic zone (Lindhe & Lang 2015). As a general rule, at least 4 mm of the sound tooth structure must be exposed at the time of surgery. This will ensure adequate space from the alveolar bone crest, so as to accommodate for ferrule effect and the supracrestal attachment (Lindhe & Lang 2015).

During healing of the apically positioned flap, there is usually rebound of tissue or coronal displacement of the gingival margin. This is mainly due to tissue bridging and also depends on flap repositioning after osseous recontouring, with respect to the newly created bone crest level (Deas et al. 2004; Marzadori et al. 2018). Precise surgical technique, adequate osseous reduction, and positioning of the flap about 3–4 mm coronal to the bone crest can reduce post-surgical tissue rebound (Deas et al. 2004; Marzadori et al. 2018).

It is recommended to wait 6 weeks for healing of the soft tissues in a non-esthetic zone before placing a final restoration. However, in the esthetic zone the healing time should be 3–6 months, so as to allow adequate maturity and stability of the tissues prior to proceeding with a final restoration (if restorations are indicated) (Brägger et al. 1992; Lanning et al. 2003; Marzadori et al. 2018).

Forced tooth eruption

Orthodontic tooth movement utilizing moderate eruptive forces can be used to erupt teeth in adults, whereby the entire attachment apparatus will move in unison with the tooth (Ingber 1976; Lindhe & Lang 2015). Once the tooth has reached its intended position and has stabilized, a full-thickness flap is elevated and bone recontouring is performed to expose sound root structure (Lindhe & Lang 2015). Alternatively, fiberotomy can be performed using a scalpel at 7–10 day intervals during the forced eruption to sever the supracrestal tissue fibers, thereby preventing the attachment apparatus from moving coronally. This will then eliminate the need for surgical entry and bone recontouring (Kozlovsky et al. 1988).

Gingival augmentation for restorative purposes

A band of 2–3 mm of attached gingiva around the tooth is required for the long-term success of subgingival restorations

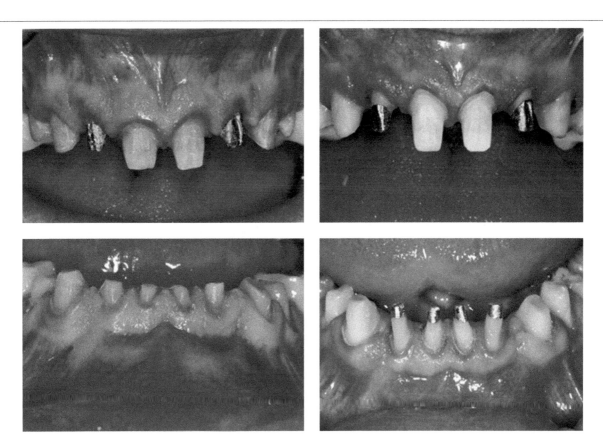

Figure 27.1.6 Apically positioned flap for functional crown lengthening to achieve crown height for retention, ferrule effect, and space for supracrestal attachment.

(Barone et al. 1998). Sites presenting with a lack of, or with a minimal zone of, attached gingiva are indicated for gingival augmentation procedures, so as to increase the zone of attached gingiva and the vestibular depth for hygiene maintenance. These procedures are not only indicated for teeth planned with subgingival restorations, but also in edentulous patients planned for removable or implant-supported prosthesis. Attached gingiva and increased vestibular depth can be obtained by performing one of the following procedures:

■ *Denudation technique* includes the removal of all soft tissue within the area extending from the gingival margin to a level apical to the mucogingival junction, leaving the alveolar bone exposed. Healing may result in increased height of attached gingiva, but also in severe morbidity and loss of bone height (Lindhe & Lang 2015).

■ *Periosteal retention technique* is similar but involves a partial-thickness flap elevation and exposure of the periosteum covering the bone. However, bone loss, although less, may also be a consequence (Lindhe & Lang 2015; Staffileno et al. 1966).

■ *Grafting procedures* utilize free autografts or allografts to increase the width of keratinized tissue (Harris 2001; Sullivan & Atkins 1968).

See also Chapter 17.

REFERENCES

AAP Connect. Glossary of Periodontal Terms. AAP; 2021. https://members.perio.org/libraries/glossary?ssopc=1.

Akkayan B. An in vitro study evaluating the effect of ferrule length on fracture resistance of endodontically treated teeth restored with fiber-reinforced and zirconia dowel systems. *J Prosthet Dent.* 2004; 92(2):155–162.

Al-Wahadni A, Gutteridge DL. An in vitro investigation into the effects of retained coronal dentine on the strength of a tooth restored with a cemented post and partial core restoration. *Int Endod J.* 2002; 35(11):913–918.

Alpiste-Illueca F. Altered passive eruption (APE): a little-known clinical situation. *Med Oral Patol Oral Cir Bucal.* 2011; 16(1):e100–e104.

Baba N, Goodacre CJ, Jekki R et al. Gingival displacement for impression making in fixed prosthodontics: contemporary principles, materials, and techniques. *Dent Clin North Am.* 2014; 58:45–68.

Barone R, Clauser C, Grassi R, Merli M, Prato GP. A protocol for maintaining or increasing the width of masticatory mucosa around submerged implants: a 1-year prospective study on 53 patients. *Int J Periodontics Restorative Dent.* 1998, 18(4):377–387.

Bennani V, Aarts JM, He LH. A comparison of pressure generated by cordless gingival displacement techniques. *J Prosthet Dent.* 2012; 107:388–392.

Benson BW, Bonberg TJ, Hatch RA et al. Tissue displacement methods in fixed prosthodontics. *J Prosthet Dent.* 1986; 55:175–181.

Brägger U, Lauchenauer D, Lang NP. Surgical lengthening of the clinical crown. *J Clin Periodontol.* 1992; 19(1):58–63.

Chandra S, Singh A, Gupta KK et al. Effect of gingival displacement cord and cordless systems on the closure, displacement, and inflammation of the gingival crevice. *J Prosthet Dent.* 2016; 115(2):177–182.

Chiche G. Improving marginal adaptation of provisional restorations. *Quintessence Int.* 1990; 21:325–329.

Chiche GJ, Pinault A. Impressions for the anterior dentition. In: GJ Chiche, A *Pinault, Esthetics of Anterior Fixed Prosthodontics.* Chicago: Quintessence; 1994: 161–176.

Cook DR, Mealey BL, Verrett RG et al. Relationship between clinical periodontal biotype and labial plate thickness: an in vivo study. *Int J Periodontics Restorative Dent.* 2011; 31:344–354.

Cook R, Lim K. Update on perio-prosthodontics. *Dent Clin N Am.* 2019; 63:157–174.

Cortellini P, Bissada NF. Mucogingival conditions in the natural dentition: narrative review, case definitions, and diagnostic considerations. *J Clin Periodontol.* 2018; 45(Suppl 20):S190–S198.

Coslet JG, Vanarsdall R, Weisgold A. Diagnosis and classification of delayed passive eruption of the dentogingival junction in the adult. *Alpha Omegan.* 1977; 70(3):24–28.

de Gennaro GG, Landesman HM, Calhoun JE et al. A comparison of gingival inflammation related to retraction cords. *J Prosthet Dent.* 1982; 47:384–389.

Deas DE, Moritz AJ, McDonnell HT, Powell CA, Mealey BL. Osseous surgery for crown lengthening: a 6-month clinical study. *J Periodontol.* 2004; 75(9):1288–1294.

Dolt AH, Robbins JW. Altered passive eruption: an etiology of short clinical crowns. *Quintessence Int.* 1997; 28(6):363–372.

Donaldson D. Gingival recession associated with temporary crowns. *J Periodontol.* 1973; 44:691–696.

Donaldson D. The etiology of gingival recession associated with temporary crowns. *J Periodontol.* 1974; 45:468–471.

Dongari-Bagtzoglou A, Research, Science and Therapy Committee, American Academy of Periodontology. Drug-associated gingival enlargement. *J Periodontol.* 2004; 5(10):1424–1431.

Dragoo MR, Williams GB. Periodontal tissue reactions to restorative procedures, part II. *Int J Periodontics Restorative Dent.* 1982; 2:34–45.

Ferrari M, Vichi A, Fadda GM et al. A randomized controlled trial of endodontically treated and restored premolars. *J Dent Res.* 2012; 91:S72–S78.

Gargiulo AW, Wentz FM, Orban B. Dimensions and relations of the dentogingival junction in humans. *J Periodontol.* 1961; 32(3):261–267.

Gegauff AG. Effect of crown lengthening and ferrule placement on static load failure of cemented cast post-cores and crowns. *J Prosthet Dent.* 2000; 84(2):169–179.

Gokcen-Rohlig B, Saruhanoglu A, Cifter ED et al. Applicability of zirconia dental prostheses for metal allergy patients. *Int J Prosthodont.* 2010; 23:562–565.

Günay H, Seeger A, Tschernitschek H, Geurtsen W. Placement of the preparation line and periodontal health – a prospective 2-year clinical study. *Int J Periodontics Restor Dent.* 2000; 20(2):171–181.

Harris RJ. Gingival augmentation with an acellular dermal matrix: human histologic evaluation of a case—placement of the graft on bone. *Int J Periodontics Restorative Dent.* 2001; 21(1):69–75.

Harrison JD. Effect of retraction materials on the gingival sulcus epithelium. *J Prosthet Dent.* 1961; 11:514–521.

Heschl A, Haas M, Haas J et al. Maxillary rehabilitation of periodontally compromised patients with extensive one-piece fixed prostheses supported by natural teeth: a retrospective longitudinal study. *Clin Oral Investig.* 2013; 17:45–53.

Ingber JS. Forced eruption: part II. A method of treating non-restorable teeth—periodontal and restorative considerations. *J Periodontol.* 1976; 47(4):203–216.

Ingber JS, Rose LF, Coslet JG. The "biologic width"—a concept in periodontics and restorative dentistry. *Alpha Omegan.* 1977; 70(3):62–65.

Jotkowitz A, Samet N. Rethinking ferrule – a new approach to an old dilemma. *Br Dent J.* 2010; 209(1):25–33.

Juloski J, Radovic I, Goracci C, Vulicevic ZR, Ferrari M. The ferrule effect: a literature review. *Int Endod J.* 2012; 38(1):11–19.

Kan JY, Morimoto T, Rungcharassaeng K, Roe P, Smith DH. Gingival biotype assessment in the esthetic zone: visual versus direct measurement. *Int J Periodontics Restorative Dent.* 2010; 30:237–243.

Kois J. The restorative-periodontal interface: biological parameters. *Periodontol 2000.* 1996; 11:29–38.

Konradsson K, Claesson R, van Dijken JW. Dental biofilm, gingivitis and interleukin-1 adjacent to approximal sites of a bonded ceramic. *J Clin Periodontol.* 2007; 34:1062–1067.

Kozlovsky A, Tal H, Lieberman M. Forced eruption combined with gingival fiberotomy. A technique for clinical crown lengthening. *J Clin Periodontol.* 1988; 15(9):534–538.

Lanning SK, Waldrop TC, Gunsolley JC, Maynard JG. Surgical crown lengthening: evaluation of the biological width. *J Periodontol.* 2003; 74(4):468–474.

Levine RA, McGuire M. The diagnosis and treatment of the gummy smile. *Compend Contin Educ Dent.* 1997; 18(8):757–762.

Lindhe J, Lang NP (ed.), *Clinical Periodontology and Implant Dentistry*. Oxford: Wiley-Blackwell; 2015.

Litonjua LA, Cabanilla LL, Abbott LJ. Plaque formation and marginal gingivitis associated with restorative materials. *Compend Contin Educ Dent.* 2012; 33:6–10.

Machado AW. 10 commandments of smile esthetics. *Dental Press J Orthod.* 2014; 19:136–157.

Marzadori M, Stefanini M, Sangiorgi M et al. Crown lengthening and restorative procedures in the esthetic zone. *Periodontol 2000.* 2018; 77:84–92.

Morris HF. Veterans Administration Cooperative Studies Project No 147. Part VIII: plaque accumulation on metal ceramic restorations cast from noble and nickel-based alloys. A five-year report. *J Prosthet Dent.* 1989; 61:543–549.

Ong M, Tseng S-C, Wang H-L. Crown lengthening revisited. *Clin Adv Periodontics.* 2011; 1(3):233–238.

Parma-Benfenali S, Fugazzoto PA, Ruben MP. The effect of restorative margins on the postsurgical development and nature of the periodontium. Part I. *Int J Periodontics Restorative Dent.* 1985; 5(6):30–51.

Richter WA, Ueno H. Relationship of crown margin placement to gingival inflammation. *J Prosthet Dent.* 1973; 30:156–161.

Ruel J, Schuessler PJ, Malament K et al. Effect of retraction procedures on the periodontium in humans. *J Prosthet Dent.* 1980; 44:508–515.

Silberberg N, Goldstein M, Smidt A. Excessive gingival display – etiology, diagnosis and treatment modalities. *Quintessence Int.* 2009; 40(10):809–818.

Sorensen JA, Engelman MJ. Ferrule design and fracture resistance of endodontically treated teeth. *J Prosthet Dent.* 1990; 63(5):529–536.

Springer NC, Chang C, Fields HW et al. Smile esthetics from the layperson's perspective. *Am J Orthod Dentofacial Orthop.* 2011; 139:91–101.

Staffileno H, Levy S, Gargiulo A. histologic study of cellular mobilization and repair following a periosteal retention operation via split thickness mucogingival flap surgery. *J Periodontol.* 1966; 37(2):117–131.

Sullivan HC, Atkins JH. Free autogenous gingival grafts. 1. Principles of successful grafting. *Periodontics.* 1968; 6(1):5–13.

Vacek JS, Gher ME, Assad DA et al. The dimensions of the human dentogingival junction. *Int J Periodontics Restorative Dent.* 1994; 14:154–165.

Valderhaugw J, Birkeland JM. Periodontal conditions in patients 5 years following insertion of fixed prostheses. *J Oral Rehabil.* 1976; 3:237–243.

Waerhaug J, Zander HA. Reaction of gingival tissues to self-curing acrylic restorations. *J Am Dent Assoc.* 1957; 54:760–768.

Wagenberg BD, Eskow RN, Langer B. Exposing adequate tooth structure for restorative dentistry. *Int J Periodontics Restorative Dent.* 1989; 9(5):322–331.

Zweers J, Thomas RZ, Slot DE, Weisgold AS, Van der Weijden GA. Characteristics of periodontal biotype, its dimensions, associations and prevalence: a systematic review. *J Clin Periodontol.* 2014; 41:958–971.

27.2 THE PERIODONTAL–ORTHODONTIC RELATIONSHIP

Achint Utreja and Feras Al Khatib

Contents

Learning objectives

- Review the impact of fixed and removable orthodontic appliances on oral microbial flora.
- Present underlying biological changes in the periodontium during orthodontic tooth movement.
- Illustrate the common adjunctive periodontal procedures in orthodontic patients.
- Review supplemental periodontal procedures to accelerate orthodontic treatment.

Introduction

Orthodontic treatment is indicated in dental patients with malocclusion to establish a functional and esthetic occlusion. Orthodontic tooth movement occurs in response to an externally applied mechanical force to a tooth or group of teeth. The force or sustained pressure results in a cascade of biological events in the surrounding periodontal tissues, including the cementum, periodontal ligament (PDL), alveolar bone, and gingiva. Conventional wisdom suggests that the establishment of a harmonious occlusal relationship is important for promoting and maintaining the health of the periodontium. The proponents of this theory attribute a high prevalence of periodontal disease, particularly at later stages in life, to untreated malocclusion and therefore recommend orthodontic correction of all malocclusions. On the other hand, orthodontic treatment, due to its long duration, often leads to adverse effects on the periodontium, thus increasing the risk of periodontal tissue breakdown. This can be more concerning in adult patients, as the incidence of periodontal disease also increases with age (Guo et al. 2016). With an increasing number of adult patients seeking orthodontic treatment, these factors play an important role in the overall success of the treatment plan.

Periodontal clinical examination of the orthodontic patient

Potential candidates for comprehensive orthodontic treatment must undergo a thorough dental and periodontal exam. Control of the disease phase, including dental caries as well as treatment of periodontal disease, takes precedence and should be addressed before initiating orthodontic treatment. Failure to detect and treat active periodontal disease can lead to further destruction of the periodontium (Proffit 2013) This is particularly concerning if the esthetic zone is involved.

A detailed clinical examination, supplemented with radiographs, is the first step toward an accurate diagnosis and thorough treatment plan. The following should be assessed carefully during the clinical examination:

- General appearance of the gingival tissue (color, inflammation, gingival biotype, etc.).
- Oral hygiene and the presence of plaque on tooth surfaces.
- Presence of supra- or subgingival calculus.
- Mobility of the teeth.
- Frenum attachments.
- Areas of mucogingival defects or gingival recession.
- Bleeding on probing.
- Pocket depth of more than 5 mm.

Bone loss can be detected on bitewings and panoramic radiographs. These should be taken as part of the patient's orthodontic records. A comparison with previous radiographs, if available, can help in evaluating the status of periodontal disease (Johal & Ide 1999).

Based on the clinical and radiographic findings, the proper intervention should be ascertained. Accumulation of plaque at multiple intraoral sites often indicates inadequate home care and/or poor toothbrushing technique. If not associated with other problems, this can be addressed by patient education. Prior to the placement of any orthodontic appliance, all plaque and calculus should be removed, and the patient must be able to demonstrate compliance with oral hygiene instructions. Soft tissue concerns such as frenum attachment and gingival recession are covered later in this chapter. The periodontal clinical examination performed before orthodontic treatment is crucial for diagnosing periodontal concerns and recommending treatment interventions. Bleeding on probing and pocket depths >5 mm are both signs of active periodontal disease, indicating immediate referral to a periodontist. It also guides the clinician in deciding the optimal recall interval required to maintain good oral health during orthodontic treatment (Johal & Ide 1999). After the pathology is treated, the patient should be in maintenance before orthodontic treatment is initiated.

Orthodontic tooth movement and the periodontium

The application of sustained pressure or force on a tooth or group of teeth results in orthodontic tooth movement (OTM). This clinically visible change is accompanied by cellular and molecular changes in the periodontal tissues surrounding mechanically "loaded" teeth. The underlying biological response depends on the characteristics of the externally applied force, such as its duration, magnitude, and frequency (Cattaneo et al. 2008; Henneman et al. 2008). The periodontal tissues, PDL, and alveolar bone are key to this process. The PDL is *compressed* and the alveolar bone undergoes resorption in the direction of the OTM (Krishnan & Davidovitch 2009). In the opposite direction to the OTM, the PDL is under *tension* and alveolar bone is deposited. This leads to an overall remodeling of both the mineralized and non-mineralized component tissues of the periodontium.

Bone remodeling during orthodontic tooth movement

The sequence of biological events during OTM closely resembles an inflammatory response. Orthodontic forces stimulate chemical messengers, which in turn activate specialized progenitor cells in the alveolar bone and PDL. The proliferation and differentiation of these quiescent cells form the basis of periodontal remodeling during OTM.

The continuous replacement of bone tissue by remodeling is essential for its maintenance in both health and disease. Bone turnover is best described using the *bone remodeling cycle*, in which key constituent cells are responsible for orchestrating resorption followed by deposition (Crockett et al. 2011). Osteoblasts are bone-forming cells that produce the organic bone matrix and regulate its mineralization (Karsenty et al. 2009). Osteoclasts are exocrine cells that dissolve bone mineral and enzymatically degrade extracellular matrix (ECM) proteins (Teitelbaum 2007). Osteocytes are mature, post-mitotic osteoblasts that become embedded in the bone matrix, and perform endocrine and mechano-sensing functions (Bonewald & Johnson 2008).

Osteoblast regulation

The differentiation of osteoblasts is regulated by the expression of key transcription factors. Local as well as systemic bone formation is regulated by crosstalk between various cell signaling pathways, particularly the transforming growth factor-beta (TGF-β)/bone morphogenetic protein (BMP) (Cao & Chen 2005), wingless (Wnt) (Karner & Long 2017), Hedgehog, Notch, and fibroblast growth factor (FGF) pathways (Chen et al. 2012). In the BMP signaling pathway, *Smad* proteins control the expression of Runt-related transcription factor 2 (Runx2)/core binding factor alpha1 (Cbfa1) (Ducy 2000) – a transcription factor that is an indispensable regulator of osteoblast differentiation. During OTM, cells on the tension and compression sides sequentially express osteoblast marker proteins as they differentiate (Holland et al. 2019). This change from precursor cells to mature osteoblasts is termed *osteoblast lineage progression* and is a hallmark feature of bone remodeling in all tissues, including the PDL and alveolar bone.

Inflammatory mediators during orthodontic tooth movement

Previously the biology of OTM was limited to visualizing histological changes in the surrounding periodontium (Reitan 1967). Research advances in osteoimmunology, however, have led to significant interest in the role of cytokines in bone remodeling (Jiang et al. 2015). Application of orthodontic forces to a tooth results in vascular changes that are similar to those seen during acute inflammation in other body tissues (Tompkins 2016). Altered blood microcirculation in the PDL leads to localized ischemia as well as areas of vasodilation. Although these changes are temporary, they are essential for the activation and release of downstream chemical messengers.

Proinflammatory cytokines

During OTM, cytokines are commonly measured in the gingival crevicular fluid (GCF). Analysis and comparisons have been done of the levels of proinflammatory cytokines in orthodontic patients undergoing short- and long-duration OTM (Ren et al. 2007). After 24 hours of force application, the levels of interleukins (IL)-1β, -6, and tumor necrosis factor (TNF)-α have been shown to be significantly increased, whereas IL-8 levels are increased after 1 month. All levels returned close to baseline values after the initial spurt in OTM, indicating that these proinflammatory mediators are more important in the early stages of OTM compared to later stages (Ren et al. 2007). Other studies have described a significantly increased expression of IL-1β on the tension side of the PDL after 24 hours of orthodontic loading (Tsuge et al. 2016). These studies thus showed that the early reaction on the tension side comprises an immediate inflammatory response, followed by rapid recovery and remodeling of the PDL and alveolar bone (Tsuge et al. 2016).

Orthodontic tooth movement and periodontal disease

Adult orthodontics may be required either to correct a malocclusion or to be a component of an inter/multidisciplinary dental treatment plan. Individuals with moderate to severe periodontitis often present with malpositioning of teeth such as pathological migration (Figure 27.2.1), and thus require orthodontic intervention. However, comprehensive or limited orthodontic treatment in these patients should always be approached with extreme caution, which includes a complete understanding of the involved benefits and risks. Similar to the early phase of OTM, proinflammatory cytokines including IL-1β and TNF-α are increased during periodontal disease (Cochran 2008). The effect of OTM in the presence of periodontitis has been shown to exacerbate periodontal breakdown by means of up-regulating proinflammatory cytokines (Boas Noguiera et al. 2013), thus highlighting the importance of orthodontic diagnoses and treatment planning in adult patients with a compromised periodontal status or questionable prognosis.

Biomechanical considerations

The "center of resistance" (C^{Res}) is defined as a point located on the long axis of a tooth, at which an externally applied force produces pure translation of the tooth without any rotation (Nanda & Tosun 2010). For a single-rooted tooth with a healthy periodontium, the C^{Res} is 24–35% of the distance from the alveolar bone crest to the root apex. Factors that affect the location of C^{Res} include the number, morphology, and length of the root as well as the level of the alveolar bone crest (Nanda & Tosun 2010). The C^{Res} is located more apical in instances of resorption of the tooth root or alveolar bone, with a direct correlation noted between the severity of bone loss and the apical migration of C^{Res} (Proffit 2013). Clinically, this

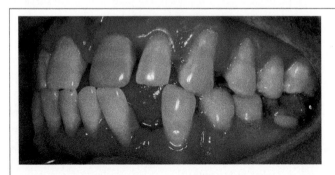

Figure 27.2.1 Pathological tooth migration as a common sequela of severe periodontitis.

implies that when the same amount of orthodontic force is applied, teeth with reduced periodontal support tend to tip more compared to teeth with a normal periodontium.

Microbial flora and orthodontic appliances

Dental plaque is a key etiological factor in the development of gingivitis and periodontitis. Malocclusion, particularly severe dental crowding that includes significant overlapping between teeth, affects an individual's ability to maintain oral hygiene. Orthodontic treatment addresses this issue; however, fixed orthodontic appliances further compromise the maintenance of oral hygiene. The design of contemporary orthodontic brackets incorporates various undercuts that can provide a niche for plaque accumulation. The placement and bonding of brackets on tooth surfaces may incorporate excess composite resin or "flash" that is not completely removed from around the brackets. This resin is not only unsightly, but also provides additional surfaces for microorganisms to colonize (Figure 27.2.2). Additionally, elastomeric ligatures that are routinely used to secure the archwire in the bracket slot provide another surface for the adhesion of microorganisms. Thus, daily good oral hygiene practice to minimize plaque accumulation is imperative during orthodontic treatment. Severe side effects such as white spot lesions can result if this is not strictly enforced (Figure 27.2.3).

Quantifying plaque accumulation

Analysis of dental plaque accumulation during orthodontic treatment provides a useful estimate of oral hygiene maintenance. Studies have found that the original Silness and Loë plaque index is the most preferred method to monitor oral hygiene compliance (Al-Anezi & Harradine 2012). However,

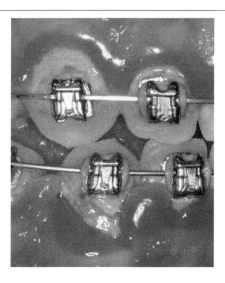

Figure 27.2.2 Excess composite resin and plaque accumulation seen around orthodontic brackets.

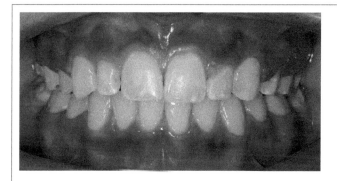

Figure 27.2.3 White spot lesions depicted as areas of demineralization of enamel.

continued advances in technology warrant the use of digital measurements such as those on standardized photographs. These are likely to be more valid and reproducible than categorical indices.

Microbiological and clinical changes

The microbiological changes in periodontal tissues due to orthodontic treatment can be correlated with the clinical findings from the initial periodontal examination. Dental plaque accumulation is usually associated with gingival inflammation and increased pocket probing depths. Research indicates that both microbiological and clinical parameters increase after the placement of fixed orthodontic appliances (Ristic 2007). These changes have been shown to be transient, with peak values noted around 3 months after initiation of orthodontic treatment. Damage to periodontal tissues is prevented, as the values tend to be closer to baseline levels at 6 months (Ristic 2007).

The immediate changes in microbial and clinical parameters following the initiation of orthodontic treatment can be due to the patient's inability to maintain proper oral hygiene. Furthermore, research has indicated that within 3 months after the removal of orthodontic appliances, a significant reduction in periodontal probing depths, bleeding on probing, and GCF flow can be observed, thus indicating improvement (van Gastel et al. 2011). These parameters may still remain significantly higher than baseline values, however, with a reported continued trend for a decrease in parameters for up to 2 years after orthodontic treatment (Ghijselings et al. 2014). This partial reversal of parameters has been ascribed to the increased presence of salivary levels of selected periodontal pathogens (*Aggregatibacter actinomycetemcomitans*, *Fusobacterium nucleatum*, *Porphyromonas gingivalis*, *Prevotella intermedia*, and *Tannerella forsythia*), even after the removal of orthodontic appliances (Kim et al. 2016).

Clear aligners and the periodontium

Comprehensive orthodontic treatment can be accomplished with either fixed appliances or removable appliances such as aligners. Offering a "clear" alternative to the conventional orthodontic armamentarium (bands, brackets, and wires), aligners have lately gained widespread acceptance, particularly among adult patients. As these plastic trays are removable, oral hygiene is easier to maintain when compared to fixed appliances, which includes an improvement in periodontal health indices during clear aligner treatment (Rossini et al. 2015). However, other studies comparing the short- and long-term effects of clear aligners and orthodontic brackets, utilizing the plaque index, gingival index, and periodontal bleeding index, have shown no difference in oral hygiene levels between aligners and brackets after 18 months of orthodontic treatment (Chhibber et al. 2018). Overall, based on limited evidence, clear aligners do not appear to offer a definitive periodontal advantage over conventional fixed appliances.

Orthodontic retention and the periodontium

Successful orthodontic treatment can be divided into two phases: active treatment with appliances and retention of the final occlusal outcome. Relapse or the tendency of the teeth to move back toward their pre-treatment position can be prevented with retainers. There is considerable variation in the selection of a retention protocol and the appropriate retainer. Retainers are categorized as either fixed or removable. Fixed retention does not depend on patient compliance, but can adversely affect periodontal health, as maintaining oral hygiene becomes challenging (Al-Moghrabi et al. 2016). A study over a four-year period compared fixed and removable retainers on the stability of orthodontic treatment outcomes and periodontal health, by assessing gingival inflammation, calculus and plaque levels, clinical attachment levels, and bleeding on probing. The study showed that both types of retainers were associated with gingival inflammation and plaque accumulation (Al-Moghrabi et al. 2018).

Periodontal considerations for the orthodontic patient

Impacted teeth

A tooth is considered impacted when its eruption is significantly delayed beyond the normal range of its appearance in the oral cavity. Impacted teeth can be associated with ankylosis, root resorption of adjacent teeth, and dentigerous cysts. Besides upper and lower third molars, other frequently impacted teeth are maxillary canines followed by mandibular second premolars. Orthodontic treatment plans for managing impacted teeth often require periodontal surgery to expose or uncover the tooth. An attachment is bonded to the tooth during the surgical procedure to allow the orthodontist to move the tooth to its desired position in the dental arch (Figure 27.2.4). Soft and hard tissue preservation with minimal trauma is an important consideration when planning and performing the surgical exposure. Poor management can lead to gingival recession and loss of attachment around the tooth after it reaches its final position.

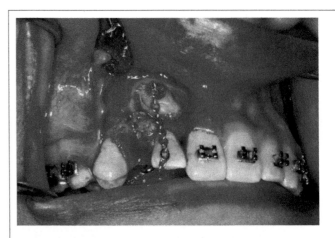

Figure 27.2.4 Exposure of impacted maxillary canine with attachment of a metal chain to apply orthodontic forces.

Surgical procedure

The location of the impacted tooth must be determined using cone beam computed tomography (CBCT), or alternatively two-dimensional panoramic and occlusal radiographs can be used. This procedure is necessary to ensure that sufficient space is available in the arch to accommodate the planned eruption.

The tooth should always erupt through attached gingiva. Laser or electrosurgery can be considered in cases where the tooth is positioned labially and covered only with gingival mucosa. If the tooth is more apically positioned, a flap should be reflected so as to enable reattachment of the attached gingiva around the crown of the tooth (Graber et al. 2017; Proffit 2013). Less gingival recession, attachment loss, and gingival inflammation can be expected if only 4–5 mm of the most apical portion of the crown is exposed instead of exposing the entire crown (Boyd 1984). It is crucial not to expose the tooth beyond its cementoenamel junction to protect the periodontal fibers, so as to avoid loss of attachment or ankylosis (Kohavi et al. 1984).

Palatally impacted maxillary canines can be exposed using either a closed or an open technique. In the closed technique, a flap is reflected and an attachment is bonded to the tooth crown. The tissues are then sutured in place, leaving only a part of the bonded attachment exposed in the oral cavity. In the open technique, the palatal mucosa over the tooth crown is removed, leaving it exposed. Research indicates no resulting differences in gingival recession and attachment loss when comparing the two clinical procedures. However, the treatment time is shorter with the open technique. This can be attributed to increased tissue resistance in the closed technique (Cassina et al. 2018; Parkin et al. 2017; Sampaziotis et al. 2018).

Mandibular frenum

A mandibular labial frenum with a high insertion creates a mucogingival defect, often accompanied by an inadequate zone of attached gingiva. In this situation, the loss or detachment of keratinized tissue is caused by the movement of the marginal gingiva (Graber et al. 2017). A frenectomy is indicated to address this issue.

Maxillary midline frenum

A low maxillary frenum insertion may interfere with mesial migration of the central incisors, and can also lead to ectopic eruption of the lateral incisors and/or canines (Figure 27.2.5). Indications for a frenectomy procedure as well as the timing thereof are controversial, i.e. whether it should be performed before or after closing the diastema (Graber et al. 2017; Proffit 2013). The clinician should thus determine the need and timing of the procedure after considering all patient-related factors. Indications are to delay the frenectomy until the space is closed orthodontically (Proffit 2013). A thick fibrous frenum is likely to interfere with orthodontic space closure, or if the frenum becomes traumatized/causes pain then a frenectomy is recommended before attempting orthodontic space closure (Graber et al. 2017). Diastemas caused by low frenum attachments should be distinguished from those due to physiological spaces that exist before the eruption of the permanent canines. Large midline diastemas attributed to thick fibrous tissue, leaving insufficient space for the permanent canines, should be considered for a frenectomy so as to facilitate the mesial migration of the upper incisors (Graber et al. 2017; Proffit 2013). However, an unwarranted surgical procedure can cause unnecessary trauma and prevent the space from closing.

Permanent retention in the form of a bonded fixed retainer is recommended after closing a maxillary midline diastema, as there is a need for long-term retention due to a high possibility of relapse after orthodontic treatment (Graber et al. 2017; Proffit 2013). Another complication of this procedure is the appearance of a dark triangle because of a lack of interdental papilla (Figure 27.2.6). This can be addressed with interproximal reduction (IPR) to move the contact point between the incisors more apically. The smaller the distance between the

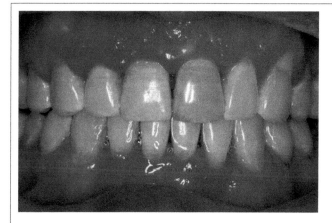

Figure 27.2.6 A dark triangle following maxillary midline diastema closure.

contact point of the incisors and the alveolar crest, the more likely it is that the interdental papilla will form (Chang 2009; Chen et al. 2010).

Gingival recession

Controversy exists pertaining to extraction versus non-extraction orthodontic treatment. Non-extraction and dental arch expansion treatment have led to an increased interest in the association between OTM and gingival recession. Evidence suggests that OTM is not a major risk factor for the development of gingival recession, neither does it cause gingival recession (Gebistorf et al. 2018; Morris et al. 2017). On the contrary, other studies have described the prevalence of recession increasing with age, as well as over time, after orthodontic treatment (Renkema et al. 2013). This includes an increased prevalence of both labial (buccal) and lingual (palatal) gingival recession during orthodontic treatment, with further increases during the long-term post-treatment period (Gebistorf et al. 2018). Overall, the gingival phenotype, i.e. the thickness of the soft and hard tissues in the facio-palatal dimension, is an important factor in determining the likelihood of gingival recession. A thin-scalloped phenotype has a higher prevalence of gingival recession compared to a thick phenotype (Angeregg et al. 1995; De Rouck et al. 2009; Kois 2004; Koke et al. 2003; Olsson & Lindhe 1991). Furthermore, there is consensus that gingival recession is likely when teeth are pushed outside their alveolar housing.

Proclination of lower incisors

Increased inclination or proclination of the mandibular incisors has traditionally been considered a risk factor for the development of gingival recession. However, clinical studies including children and adolescents have found no correlation between lower incisor proclination during orthodontic treatment and gingival recession (Morris et al. 2017). Studies analyzing gingival recession 32 years after orthodontic treatment

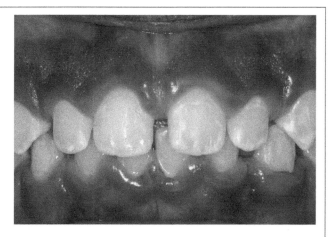

Figure 27.2.5 Prominent maxillary labial frenum contributing to a midline diastema.

with the Herbst appliance have found minor recession in some patients. This was primarily associated with bodily displaced and crowded anterior teeth, but no correlation was found to post-treatment tooth inclination (Pancherz & Bjerklin 2014).

Maxillary expansion

The utilization of self-ligating brackets and clear aligners in contemporary orthodontics relies on arch development and expansion to relieve crowding, thus avoiding dental extraction(s). However, gingival recession has been found to be inevitable when the maxillary arch is expanded. Correlations have been described between the severity of maxillo-mandibular transverse skeletal discrepancies and the susceptibility of developing gingival recession and periodontal disease (Anzilotti & Balakrishnan 2002). The likelihood of moving teeth beyond the housing alveolar process increases in patients with a large mandible and small maxilla, thus predisposing these patients to gingival recession (Anzilotti & Balakrishnan 2002). Expansion with palatal expanders decreases the thickness of the buccal plate and increases the thickness of the palatal plate, even though studies have concluded that maxillary expansion and gingival recession have a weak positive correlation (Morris et al. 2017). Furthermore, no significant difference in gingival recession has been shown to occur when comparing rapid and slow palatal expansion (Bastos et al. 2019; Greenbaum & Zachrisson 1982).

Computed tomography has been used to evaluate periodontal changes after maxillary expansion with tooth tissue–borne and tooth-borne expanders (Garib et al. 2006). Usage of tooth-borne expanders has been shown to increase palatal plate thickness as well as cause a greater reduction of the alveolar crest around the first premolar. Molars and premolars with thinner buccal bone plates have shown a greater degree of dehiscence formation when used as anchorage teeth for rapid palatal expanders (Garib et al. 2006). In addition to tipping, tissue-borne expanders have shown significant dehiscences in the first premolar area (Garib et al. 2006). Other studies have concluded that bone-borne expanders produce more skeletal effects and less tipping of the teeth when compared to tissue-borne expanders (Lin et al. 2015). Thus, bone-borne expanders are recommended when treating cases with severe skeletal discrepancies, multiple missing teeth, advanced periodontal problems, and in skeletally mature individuals (Graber et al. 2017).

Surgically assisted rapid maxillary expansion (SARME) has been described to be associated with significant recession in the molar and premolar areas after the procedure (Jensen et al. 2015; Sendyk et al. 2018). However, other studies have indicated that SARME does not contribute to significant changes in periodontal health and attachment levels after a SARME procedure (Jensen et al. 2015).

Gingival hyperplasia

Mild to moderate gingival enlargement is commonly seen in orthodontic patients, particularly in individuals being treated

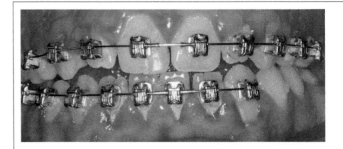

Figure 27.2.7 Gingival hyperplasia during orthodontic treatment.

with fixed appliances (Figure 27.2.7). This situation is usually reversible without permanent damage to the periodontium, and the enlargement tends to disappear after removal of the orthodontic appliances. Gingivectomy is not indicated during orthodontic treatment unless the enlargement interferes with OTM (Eid et al. 2014). However, if gingival enlargement persists after the completion of orthodontic treatment and following the removal of fixed appliances, the patient must be referred to a periodontist for gingivectomy.

Periodontal adjuncts to accelerate orthodontic tooth movement

Comprehensive orthodontic treatment can be time-consuming, and surveys of adult patients have shown a preferable treatment time lasting 6–12 months (Uribe et al. 2014). Shorter treatment times are beneficial for maintaining oral hygiene and promoting periodontal health. To achieve shorter treatment times, incorporation of the biological response of the periodontium to orthodontic forces have been suggested. This includes exogenous cytokines, corticotomy, piezocision, and micro-osteoperforation.

Exogenous cytokines

The local administration of exogenous cytokines to further mediate bone remodeling has been attempted to increase the rate of OTM (Gurton et al. 2004; Kale et al. 2004; Sekhavat et al. 2002). To avoid unwanted side effects, injected chemicals should be localized to the site of tooth movement. However, due to the short half-life of cytokines, the clinical relevance of this procedure becomes rather limited.

Corticotomy

Endogenous cytokine levels can be increased in the periodontium by localized trauma. Periodontally accelerated osteogenic orthodontics (PAOO) involves reflecting a full-thickness muco-periosteal flap, decorticating the buccal and lingual sides of the alveolar bone, and adding particulate bone graft material under the periosteum (Cano et al. 2012; Frost 1983; Wilcko et al. 2001). A transient osteopenia and increased cytokine levels are suggested to be responsible for the increased rate of OTM

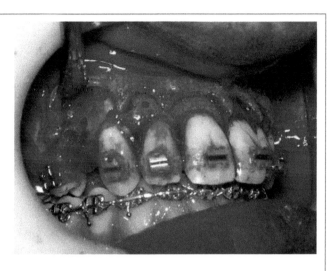

Figure 27.2.8 The corticotomy procedure.

(Figure 27.2.8). Corticision is a variant of this procedure that does not require reflection of a mucoperiosteal flap (Park 2016).

Piezocision

Advocated as a minimally invasive technique, piezocision combines micro-incisions and decortications made by a piezotome (vibrating knife). A mucoperiosteal flap is not reflected (similar to corticision); instead, an incision is made in the buccal gingiva (Dibart et al. 2009).

Micro-osteoperforation

Micro-osteoperforation is less invasive than either corticotomy or piezocision as no flaps or incisions are required. The procedure includes perforating the gingiva and alveolar bone with a disposable stainless steel screw at three locations adjacent to a tooth or group of teeth (Alikhani et al. 2013).

SUMMARY

Comprehensive orthodontic treatment poses challenges in the maintenance of periodontal health. Factors contributing to this are the bulk of the orthodontic appliances as well as the prolonged duration of orthodontic treatment. The initial biological response to orthodontic forces is inflammatory in nature, followed by tissue remodeling. Thus, the periodontal clinical examination, particularly in adults with a documented history of poor oral health, is critical during orthodontic treatment planning.

Clear aligners offer an alternative to conventional fixed appliances, but there is limited evidence that they are more "periodontal tissue friendly." Similarly, high-quality evidence to support the use of periodontal adjuncts to accelerate the rate of OTM is lacking.

REFERENCES

Guo L, Feng Y, Guo HG, Liu BW, Zhang Y. Consequences of orthodontic treatment in malocclusion patients: clinical and microbial effects in adults and children. *BMC Oral Health.* 2016; 16(1):112.

Proffit, W.R. (2013). *Contemporary Orthodontics.* St. Louis, Mo.: Elsevier/Mosby.

Johal A, Ide M. Orthodontics in the adult patient, with special reference to the periodontally compromised patient. *Dent Update.* 1999; 26(3):101-4, 6-8.

Cattaneo PM, Dalstra M, Melsen B. Moment-to-force ratio, center of rotation, and force level: a finite element study predicting their interdependency for simulated orthodontic loading regimens. *Am J Orthod Dentofacial Orthop.* 2008; 133(5):681-689.

Henneman S, Von den Hoff JW, Maltha JC. Mechanobiology of tooth movement. *Eur J Orthod.* 2008; 30(3):299-306.

Krishnan V, Davidovitch Z. On a path to unfolding the biological mechanisms of orthodontic tooth movement. *J Dent Res.* 2009; 88(7):597-608.

Crockett JC, Rogers MJ, Coxon FP, Hocking LJ, Helfrich MH. Bone remodelling at a glance. *J Cell Sci.* 2011; 124(Pt 7):991-998.

Karsenty G, Kronenberg HM, Settembre C. Genetic control of bone formation. *Annu Rev Cell Dev Biol.* 2009; 25:629-648.

Teitelbaum SL. Osteoclasts: what do they do and how do they do it? *Am J Pathol.* 2007; 170(2):427-435.

Bonewald LF, Johnson ML. Osteocytes, mechanosensing and Wnt signaling. *Bone.* 2008; 42(4):606-615.

Cao X, Chen D. The BMP signaling and in vivo bone formation. *Gene.* 2005;357(1):1-8.

Karner CM, Long F. Wnt signaling and cellular metabolism in osteoblasts. *Cell Mol Life Sci.* 2017; 74(9):1649-1657.

Chen G, Deng C, Li YP. TGF-beta and BMP signaling in osteoblast differentiation and bone formation. *Int J Biol Sci.* 2012; 8(2):272-288.

Ducy P. Cbfa1: a molecular switch in osteoblast biology. *Dev Dyn.* 2000; 219(4):461-471.

Holland R, Bain C, Utreja A. Osteoblast differentiation during orthodontic tooth movement. *Orthod Craniofac Res.* 2019; 22(3):177-182.

Reitan K. Clinical and histologic observations on tooth movement during and after orthodontic treatment. *Am J Orthod.* 1967; 53(10):721-745.

Jiang C, Li Z, Quan H, et al. Osteoimmunology in orthodontic tooth movement. *Oral Dis.* 2015; 21(6):694-704.

Tompkins KA. The osteoimmunology of alveolar bone loss. *Connect Tissue Res.* 2016; 57(2):69-90.

Ren Y, Hazemeijer H, de Haan B, Qu N, de Vos P. Cytokine profiles in crevicular fluid during orthodontic tooth movement of short and long durations. *J Periodontol.* 2007; 78(3):453-458.

Tsuge A, Noda K, Nakamura Y. Early tissue reaction in the tension zone of PDL during orthodontic tooth movement. *Arch Oral Biol.* 2016; 65:17-25.

Cochran DL. Inflammation and bone loss in periodontal disease. *J Periodontol.* 2008; 79(8 Suppl):1569-1576.

Boas Nogueira AV, Chaves de Souza JA, Kim YJ, Damiao de Sousa-Neto M, Chan Cirelli C, Cirelli JA. Orthodontic force increases interleukin-1beta and tumor necrosis factor-alpha expression and alveolar bone loss in periodontitis. *J Periodontol.* 2013; 84(9):1319-1326.

Nanda, R.S., Tosun, Y. (2010). *Biomechanics in Orthodontics: Principles and Practice.* Hanover Park, IL: Quintessence Pub. Co.

Al-Anezi SA, Harradine NW. Quantifying plaque during orthodontic treatment. *Angle Orthod.* 2012; 82(4):748-753.

Ristic M, Vlahovic Svabic M, Sasic M, Zelic O. Clinical and microbiological effects of fixed orthodontic appliances on periodontal tissues in adolescents. *Orthod Craniofac Res.* 2007; 10(4):187-195.

van Gastel J, Quirynen M, Teughels W, Coucke W, Carels C. Longitudinal changes in microbiology and clinical periodontal parameters after removal of fixed orthodontic appliances. *Eur J Orthod.* 2011; 33(1):15-21.

Ghijselings E, Coucke W, Verdonck A, et al. Long-term changes in microbiology and clinical periodontal variables after completion of fixed orthodontic appliances. *Orthod Craniofac Res.* 2014; 17(1):49-59.

Kim K, Jung WS, Cho S, Ahn SJ. Changes in salivary periodontal pathogens after orthodontic treatment: An in vivo prospective study. *Angle Orthod.* 2016; 86(6):998-1003.

Rossini G, Parrini S, Castroflorio T, Deregibus A, Debernardi CL. Periodontal health during clear aligners treatment: a systematic review. *Eur J Orthod.* 2015; 37(5):539-543.

Chhibber A, Agarwal S, Yadav S, Kuo CL, Upadhyay M. Which orthodontic appliance is best for oral hygiene? A randomized clinical trial. *Am J Orthod Dentofacial Orthop.* 2018; 153(2):175-183.

Al-Moghrabi D, Pandis N, Fleming PS. The effects of fixed and removable orthodontic retainers: a systematic review. *Prog Orthod.* 2016; 17(1):24.

Al-Moghrabi D, Johal A, O'Rourke N, et al. Effects of fixed vs removable orthodontic retainers on stability and periodontal health: 4-year follow-up of a randomized controlled trial. *Am J Orthod Dentofacial Orthop.* 2018; 154(2):167-174.

Graber, L.W., Vanarsdall, R.L., Vig, K.W.L. et al. (2017). *Orthodontics: Current Principles and Techniques.* St. Louis, Missouri: Elsevier.

Boyd RL. Clinical assessment of injuries in orthodontic movement of impacted teeth. *II. Surgical recommendations. Am J Orthod.* 1984; 86(5):407-418.

Kohavi D, Becker A, Zilberman Y. Surgical exposure, orthodontic movement, and final tooth position as factors in periodontal breakdown of treated palatally impacted canines. *Am J Orthod.* 1984; 85(1):72-77.

Sampaziotis D, Tsolakis IA, Bitsanis E, Tsolakis AI. Open versus closed surgical exposure of palatally impacted maxillary canines: comparison of the different treatment outcomes-a systematic review. *Eur J Orthod.* 2018; 40(1):11-22.

Parkin N, Benson PE, Thind B, Shah A, Khalil I, Ghafoor S. Open versus closed surgical exposure of canine teeth that are displaced in the roof of the mouth. *Cochrane Database Syst Rev.* 2017; 8:CD006966.

Cassina C, Papageorgiou SN, Eliades T. Open versus closed surgical exposure for permanent impacted canines: a systematic review and meta-analyses. *Eur J Orthod.* 2018; 40(1):1-10.

Chang LC. Effect of bone crest to contact point distance on central papilla height using embrasure morphologies. *Quintessence Int.* 2009; 40(6):507-513.

Chen MC, Liao YF, Chan CP, Ku YC, Pan WL, Tu YK. Factors influencing the presence of interproximal dental papillae between maxillary anterior teeth. *J Periodontol.* 2010; 81(2):318-324.

Gebistorf M, Mijuskovic M, Pandis N, Fudalej PS, Katsaros C. Gingival recession in orthodontic patients 10 to 15 years posttreatment: A retrospective cohort study. *Am J Orthod Dentofacial Orthop.* 2018; 153(5):645-655.

Morris JW, Campbell PM, Tadlock LP, Boley J, Buschang PH. Prevalence of gingival recession after orthodontic tooth movements. *Am J Orthod Dentofacial Orthop.* 2017; 151(5):851-859.

Renkema AM, Fudalej PS, Renkema A, Kiekens R, Katsaros C. Development of labial gingival recessions in orthodontically treated patients. *Am J Orthod Dentofacial Orthop.* 2013; 143(2):206-212.

Olsson M, Lindhe J. Periodontal characteristics in individuals with varying form of the upper central incisors. *J Clin Periodontol.* 1991; 18(1):78-82.

Kois JC. Predictable single-tooth peri-implant esthetics: five diagnostic keys. *Compend Contin Educ Dent.* 2004; 25(11):895-896.

De Rouck T, Eghbali R, Collys K, De Bruyn H, Cosyn J. The gingival biotype revisited: transparency of the periodontal probe through the gingival margin as a method to discriminate thin from thick gingiva. *J Clin Periodontol.* 2009; 36(5):428-433.

Anderegg CR, Metzler DG, Nicoll BK. Gingiva thickness in guided tissue regeneration and associated recession at facial furcation defects. *J Periodontol.* 1995; 66(5):397-402.

Koke U, Sander C, Heinecke A, Muller HP. A possible influence of gingival dimensions on attachment loss and gingival recession following placement of artificial crowns. *Int J Periodontics Restorative Dent.* 2003; 23(5):439-445.

Pancherz H, Bjerklin K. Mandibular incisor inclination, tooth irregularity, and gingival recessions after Herbst therapy: a 32-year follow-up study. *Am J Orthod Dentofacial Orthop.* 2014; 146(3):310-318.

Anzilotti, C.V.R., Balakrishnan, M. (2002). *Expansion and Evaluation of Post-Retention Gingival Recession. Thesis.* Philadelphia: University of Pennsylvania.

Greenbaum KR, Zachrisson BU. The effect of palatal expansion therapy on the periodontal supporting tissues. *Am J Orthod.* 1982; 81(1):12-21.

Bastos R, Blagitz MN, Aragon M, Maia LC, Normando D. Periodontal side effects of rapid and slow maxillary expansion: A systematic review. *Angle Orthod.* 2019; 89(4):651-660.

Garib DG, Henriques JF, Janson G, de Freitas MR, Fernandes AY. Periodontal effects of rapid maxillary expansion with tooth-tissue-borne and tooth-borne expanders: a computed tomography evaluation. *Am J Orthod Dentofacial Orthop.* 2006; 129(6):749-758.

Lin L, Ahn HW, Kim SJ, Moon SC, Kim SH, Nelson G. Tooth-borne vs bone-borne rapid maxillary expanders in late adolescence. *Angle Orthod.* 2015; 85(2):253-262.

Sendyk M, Sendyk WR, Pallos D, Boaro LCC, Paiva JB, Rino Neto J. Periodontal clinical evaluation before and after surgically assisted rapid maxillary expansion. *Dental Press J Orthod.* 2018; 23(1):79-86.

Jensen T, Johannesen LH, Rodrigo-Domingo M. Periodontal changes after surgically assisted rapid maxillary expansion (SARME). *Oral Maxillofac Surg.* 2015; 19(4):381-386.

Eid HA, Assiri HA, Kandyala R, Togoo RA, Turakhia VS. Gingival enlargement in different age groups during fixed Orthodontic treatment. *J Int Oral Health.* 2014; 6(1):1-4.

Tsichlaki A, Chin SY, Pandis N, Fleming PS. How long does treatment with fixed orthodontic appliances last? A systematic review. *Am J Orthod Dentofacial Orthop.* 2016; 149(3):308-318.

Uribe F, Padala S, Allareddy V, Nanda R. Patients', parents', and orthodontists' perceptions of the need for and costs of additional procedures to reduce treatment time. *Am J Orthod Dentofacial Orthop.* 2014; 145(4 Suppl):S65-73.

Gurton AU, Akin E, Sagdic D, Olmez H. Effects of PGI2 and TxA2 analogs and inhibitors in orthodontic tooth movement. *Angle Orthod.* 2004; 74(4):526-532.

Kale S, Kocadereli I, Atilla P, Asan E. Comparison of the effects of 1,25 dihydroxycholecalciferol and prostaglandin E2 on orthodontic tooth movement. *Am J Orthod Dentofacial Orthop.* 2004; 125(5):607-614.

Sekhavat AR, Mousavizadeh K, Pakshir HR, Aslani FS. Effect of misoprostol, a prostaglandin E1 analog, on orthodontic tooth movement in rats. *Am J Orthod Dentofacial Orthop.* 2002; 122(5):542-547.

Cano J, Campo J, Bonilla E, Colmenero C. Corticotomy-assisted orthodontics. *J Clin Exp Dent.* 2012; 4(1):e54-59.

Frost HM. The regional acceleratory phenomenon: a review. *Henry Ford Hosp Med J.* 1983; 31(1):3-9.

Wilcko WM, Wilcko T, Bouquot JE, Ferguson DJ. Rapid orthodontics with alveolar reshaping: two case reports of decrowding. *Int J Periodontics Restorative Dent.* 2001; 21(1):9-19.

Park YG. Corticision: A flapless procedure to accelerate tooth movement. *Front Oral Biol.* 2016; 18:109-117.

Dibart S, Sebaoun JD, Surmenian J. Piezocision: a minimally invasive, periodontally accelerated orthodontic tooth movement procedure. *Compend Contin Educ Dent.* 2009; 30(6):342-344, 6, 8-50.

Alikhani M, Raptis M, Zoldan B, et al. Effect of micro-osteoperforations on the rate of tooth movement. *Am J Orthod Dentofacial Orthop.* 2013; 144(5):639-648.

CHAPTER 28

Fundamentals of dental implants

Brittany Camenisch, Nehal Almehmadi, Pratishtha Mishra and Mohanad Al-Sabbagh

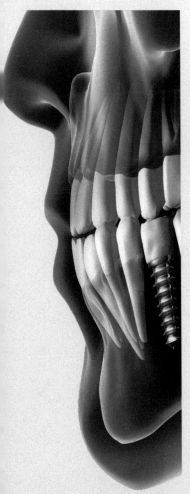

Contents

Learning objectives

- Highlight the process of osseointegration.
- Review different types of implant material.
- Overview of implant design.
- Concepts of implant surface modification (macro-, micro-, and nanosurface).

Essential Periodontics, First Edition. Edited by Steph Smith and Khalid Almas.
© 2022 John Wiley & Sons Ltd. Published 2022 by John Wiley & Sons Ltd.

Introduction

The success of the first titanium dental implant revolutionized its use for the partial or complete replacement of the dentition (Adell et al. 1981). The implant is placed in the jawbone and allowed to heal for a period of time to allow the implant to integrate with bone. A dental prosthesis is then attached to the implant to restore function and esthetics. A wide range of biomaterials and designs have been used to fabricate dental implants and supporting dental prostheses.

Three main types of dental implants have historically been used: endosseous, subperiosteal, and transosseous implants. An *endosseous implant* is a type of implant that is inserted inside the bone to anchor the prosthetic tooth replacement. A *subperiosteal implant* is fabricated out of a direct impression of a surgically exposed surface of the jawbone, and subsequently seated and fixed onto the jawbone underneath the periosteum. It was a popular treatment modality for the rehabilitation of completely edentulous patients in the 1970s. A *transosseous implant* is an implant that extends all the way through the anterior portion of the mandibular jawbone and is fixated on both sides of the mandible. It was used for severely atrophic mandibles to avoid complicated ridge augmentation procedures.

A *root form endosseous implant* is the most common type of dental implant used since the Brånemark discovery of osseointegration in the 1980s. In order to improve the treatment outcome and to enhance osseointegration, endosseous implants underwent a series of modifications. The modification of endosseous implants included biomaterial composition, geometrical design, and surface topography. Many different titanium endosseous implant systems are available with different shapes and surface treatments (Figure 28.1).

Several advantages exist when missing teeth are replaced with dental implants, including high predictable outcome and patient satisfaction. There are no absolute contraindications for placing a dental implant; however, certain patient-related factors may decrease the likelihood of osseointegration (Diz et al. 2013). Relative contraindications for implant placement include cognitive decline, American Society of Anesthesiology Patient Status IV or higher, or medical conditions that affect the lifespan of the patient (Kullar & Miller 2019).

Osseointegration

The success of a dental implant depends mainly on successful osseointegration (Smeets et al. 2016). Osseointegration is the "direct structural and functional connection between living bone and the surface of a load carrying implant" (Albrektsson & Johansson 2001; Branemark 1985; Schroeder 1976). The continued success of osseointegration is dependent upon the ability to maintain the integrity of the structural connection after functional forces are applied to the implant (Ogle 2015).

Biology of osseointegration

When an implant is placed into the alveolar bone, a series of healing events are provoked to allow for new bone formation, including necrosis followed by resorption of traumatized bone around the implant (Berglundh et al. 2003). According to Davies (1998), peri-implant bone healing has three phases: osteoconduction, de novo bone formation, and bone remodeling. *Osteoconduction* is defined as the apposition of bone onto a surface or scaffold (Albrektsson & Johansson 2001). *De novo bone formation* is the formation of a mineralized matrix on the implant surface similar to that present in natural bone (Baksh & Davies 2000). *Bone remodeling* is the lifelong process of continued bone removal and deposition. During the osseointegration process, bone formation around the implant surface is achieved by two processes. Contact osteogenesis is the direct formation of new bone on the implant surface, while distant osteogenesis is the process by which new bone is formed on the pre-existing bone (Davies 1998).

Several factors influence the formation of the bone–implant interface. These include not only implant-related factors, such as material, shape, topography, and surface chemistry, but also mechanical loading, surgical technique, and patient variables (e.g. bone quality and quantity) (Puleo & Nanci 1999).

Timeline of osseointegration

Mechanical (primary) stability of an implant at the time of placement is considered one of the most important factors for successful osseointegration. Any motion between the implant and the surrounding bone is a risk factor for early implant loss,

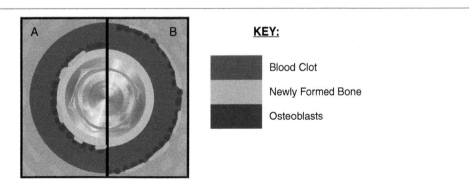

Figure 28.1 A cross-sectional schematic drawing of an implant. (A) Contact osteogenesis involves the formation of new bone directly onto the implant by osteoblasts. (B) Distance osteogenesis involves newly formed bone deposited onto pre-existing bone by osteoblasts.

especially during the early healing phase (Berglundh et al. 2003). After the endosseous implant is placed, biological (secondary) stability steadily replaces primary mechanical stability. This transition to biological stability occurs during the early stages of wound healing due to newly formed bone at the implant site (Berglundh et al. 2003). Schwartz and Boyan (1994) describe the events involved in bone apposition around the implant in humans. Serum proteins adhere to the implant surface immediately after implantation. During the first three days, mesenchymal cells attach to and proliferate on the surface of the implant. Osteoid is produced by the sixth day, followed by complete calcification of the matrix by the second week. Remodeling of newly formed bone takes place in the third week (Schwartz & Boyan 1994).

Factors affecting osseointegration

The occurrence of osseointegration is dependent on the interaction between the implant and the host. Several factors may influence or inhibit osseointegration (Figure 28.2). Once an implant is integrated, the continued success of osseointegration is also dependent on mechanical and biological factors (Ogle 2015).

Methods to assess osseointegration

Several methods have been used to clinically validate osseointegration. These include but are not limited to implant mobility test, radiographic film, and sound analysis (using a metal instrument to tap on the implant and assess the transmitted sound) (Albrektsson & Jacobsson 1987). Presently, more diagnostic tools are used to assess implant stability, like resonance frequency

analysis (RFA), which is used as a diagnostic test for long-term implant success (Al-Sabbagh et al. 2019; Meredith 1998).

Dental implant components

Dental implants are surgical replacements of the tooth. Endosteal implants are the most common type of dental implant used. The endosteal implant with the attached prosthesis typically comprises three components, which are connected to each other. The implant portion that corresponds to the tooth root is referred to as the implant, implant body, or fixture, while the abutment corresponds to the prepared part of the tooth on which the crown is fixed (via cement or screw retention). The abutment is attached to the implant fixture by an abutment screw (Figure 28.3).

The primary goal of the dental implant is to act as the root of a tooth that supports the prosthetic replacement of a tooth or teeth. However, the anatomy and characteristics of dental implants are different than those of a tooth root (Figure 28.4).

Implant biomaterials

The desirable characteristics of an implant material include biocompatibility, low modulus of elasticity (similar to bone), mechanical strength, high ductility, and high corrosion resistance. Dental implants are made from a variety of materials: titanium, titanium alloys, or zirconium.

Titanium

Titanium is a porous, corrosion-resistant, and biocompatible material, which makes it ideal for clinical use. There are four

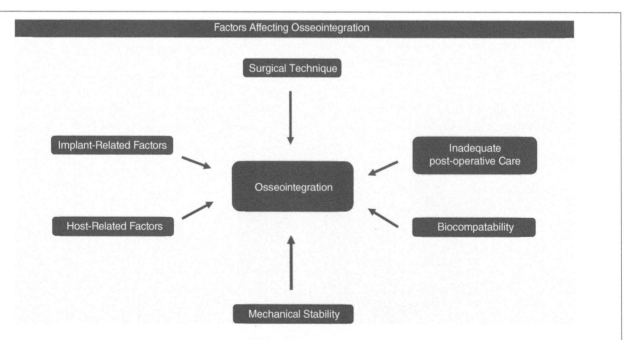

Figure 28.2 Factors affecting osseointegration. Primary stability, implant characteristics, and biological response of the host bone are factors that affect the process of osseointegration.

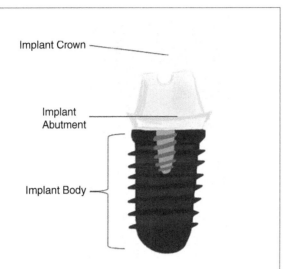

Figure 28.3 Components and structural characteristics of a restored dental implant. The primary components for implants consist of three components: implant crown, abutment, and implant body.

grades of commercially pure titanium (cpTi) based on purity and processing techniques. These grades differ in corrosion resistance, ductility, and mechanical strength. CPTi grade 4 is readily used in implant dentistry due to high strength and elastic modulus (Table 28.1). Titanium alloys have also been introduced to improve strength and elastic modulus (Abdel-Hady Gepreel & Niinomi 2013). Titanium–aluminum 6%–vanadium 4% (Ti-6Al-4V), known as grade 5 titanium, is commonly used to manufacture implants. However, grade 5 titanium has drawbacks, such as the release of vanadium and aluminum that could cause type IV allergic reactions and neurological disorders, respectively (Abdel-Hady Gepreel & Niinomi 2013).

Alumina ceramics

Attempts to counteract some of the esthetic and biological problems related to titanium have led to the introduction of ceramic implants. Initially, ceramic implants were made with alumina (Al_2O_3), which is an inert, corrosion-resistant, non-absorbable, and hard material. The surface of alumina ceramic implants could be modified into porous alumina. In addition, alumina ceramics can be combined with bioglass and hydroxyapatite to create a surface conducive to osseointegration (Camilo et al. 2017). Alumina implants have been totally replaced with zirconia implants due to their low fracture toughness.

Zirconia

The versatility of zirconia as a restorative material in dentistry has resulted in its utilization in implant dentistry. Some key physical properties of zirconia that distinguish it from titanium or titanium alloys include high flexural and compressive strength and fracture toughness (Andreiotelli et al. 2009). However, it is sensitive to shear and tensile stresses (Osman et al. 2013). The angle between the axis of the implant and biting force vector on the implant is directly proportional to the level of shear stresses (Gahlert et al. 2012; Osman et al. 2013, 2014). As these forces increase, it increases the likelihood of fracture of the zirconia implant.

Integration of zirconia implants after placement has been demonstrated to be harmonious with surrounding hard and soft tissue. In fact, research has demonstrated that the peri-implant bone volume density was superior when comparing integrated zirconia implants versus titanium ones (Gahlert et al. 2009). Various surface modifications of zirconia implants can improve osteoblast cell attachment, differentiation, and bone-to-implant contact (Depprich et al. 2008). Data published between 2006 and 2011 found that the survival rates of zirconia implants ranged from 74 to 98% after 12–56 months (Depprich et al. 2014). Another study reported that survival rates of titanium implants ranged from 97 to 100% after 3–10.4 years, showing that titanium implants had a marginally better survival rate than zirconia implants (Koller et al. 2011).

Dental implant topography

Implant design is fundamental to the osseointegration process. The evolution of macro- and microscopic features of implants has increased the predictability and success of implant therapy.

Implant macro-topography

The macro-topography of an implant is determined by its visible geometry, which is typically measured using the metric scale. The macroscopic features of an implant include size, shape, design, and type (Figure 28.5).

Implant size

The size of an implant is described in terms of the implant diameter (width) and height (length). Implant height corresponds to the portion of the implant imbedded in bone. It is typically measured from the apex of the implant to either the implant platform for bone-level implants, or the apical end of the smooth collar for tissue-level implants. Implant width corresponds to the largest diameter of the fixture (including threads if they are present) (Figure 28.6).

The length and diameter of implants play important roles in implant primary stability, a parameter used to predict success of osseointegration (Albrektsson 1983). Increasing implant length and width significantly improves implant primary stability in areas with reduced bone quality. There is no consensus in the dental literature on millimetric measurements that clearly categorize implant length and diameter. For instance, Christensen considered a 3.3 mm diameter implant as a standard diameter (Gleiznys et al. 2012), while the same diameter has been referred to as a small or narrow diameter in other studies (Al-Nawas et al. 2012; Ioannidis et al. 2015; Romanos

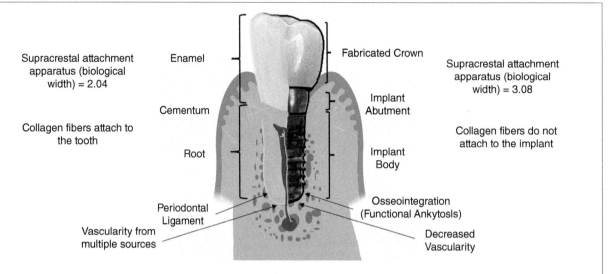

Figure 28.4 Comparison of a dental implant and the tooth. Dental implants are intimately connected to the bone via functional ankylosis. Unlike a dental implant, the tooth is attached to the bone via the periodontal ligament (PDL). The PDL serves to protect and support the tooth. The supracrestal attachment apparatus (biological width) around a tooth and implant is different, as is the attachment of the collagen fibers. A more detailed list of the differences between tooth and implant is given in this schematic. The attachment of the surrounding collagen fibers and sources of vascularity also differ between an implant and a tooth.

Table 28.1 Physical properties of the five grades of titanium. The yield strength is the amount of stress placed on a metal, where permanent deformation occurs. The yield strength of grade 5 titanium is substantially larger than other commercially pure titanium. It also has the highest elastic modulus, which measures the resistance of the material to elastic deformation. Objects with high modulus of elasticity stretch very little when they are pulled. Clinically, grade 5 is used for orthopedic surgery, where the strength of the alloy is imperative for success.

Alloy	Elastic modulus/GPa	Yield strength/MPa	Density/gcm^{-3}
CpTi Grade 1	102	170	4.5
CpTi Grade 2	102	275	4.5
CpTi Grade 3	102	380	4.5
CpTi Grade 4	104	483	4.5
Ti-6Al-4V (Grade 5)	113	795	4.4

CpTi, commercially pure titanium; GPa, gigapascal; MPa, megapascal; Ti-6Al-4V, titanium–aluminum 6%–vanadium 4%.
Source: Adapted from Nicholson 2020.

et al. 2018). A classification scheme for implant length and diameter was proposed by Al-Johany et al. (2017) based on a total of 85 studies (Figure 28.7).

Implant shape

The shape of the endosteal implant body is either cylindrical or tapered (Figure 28.8). Cylindrical implants are parallel-walled implants that have an equal diameter along the entire length of the implant body. Although less primary stability is frequently reported when using cylindrical implants, a recent systematic review and meta-analysis reported no significant differences in the detection of implant failure rates between cylindrical and tapered implants (Atieh et al. 2018). The stability of cylindrical implants measured by the implant stability quotient (ISQ) has been shown to increase over time as osseointegration progresses (Rokn et al. 2011).

Tapered implants mimic the form of a tooth root, with the implant diameter gradually converging toward the apex. The tapered walls compress the bone laterally during insertion and distribute occlusal forces more favorably toward the apex and adjacent bone, making tapered implants the preferred choice for immediate implant placement or loading (Glauser et al. 2004; Morris et al. 2004). Because of their design, tapered implants are indicated in soft bone or in sites with anatomic limitations.

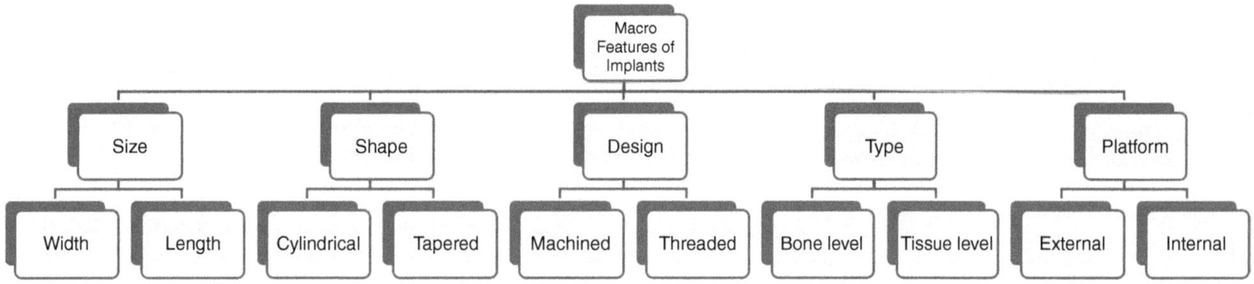

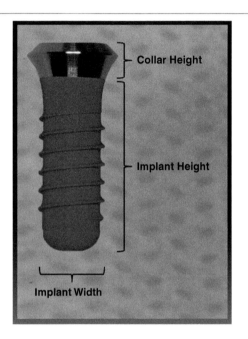

Figure 28.5 Macroscopic implant topography. The visible features of an implant are known as the macroscopic features. Differences in size, shape, design, and type lead to wide variations in available dental implants.

Figure 28.6 A tissue-level (collared) implant. The implant height is the distance between the apex of the implant and the apical end of the smooth collar.

Implant design

Implants with a threaded design have replaced non-threaded implants due to their increased surface area and increased bone-to-implant contact (BIC). The increased BIC allows for increased primary stability and reduced micromovement, which are central in the osseointegration process (Sennerby & Meredith 2008; Steigenga et al. 2003; Watzak et al. 2005). Thread designs vary according to thread geometry, which includes thread shape, width, depth, pitch, and lead. The geometry of the thread design dictates the primary stability and stress distribution during osseointegration and thenceforward.

Thread shape

The implant thread shape is determined by the angle formed between the implant wall and the body of the thread (face angle) as well as the thread thickness (Boggan et al. 1999). Thread shape plays an important role in implant primary stability and load distribution, and various shapes exist in order to increase the surface area and BIC. Variations in shape allow for force distribution to the surrounding bone, thus limiting implant micromovement and preventing early implant failure (Szmukler-Moncler et al. 1998). Variations in face angle and

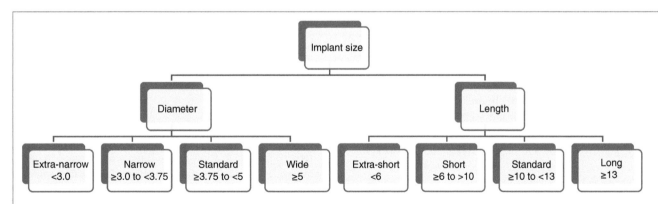

Figure 28.7 A classification scheme for implant size. The classification for implant diameter can be divided into extra narrow, narrow, standard, and wide. The implant length classification includes extra short, short, standard, and long. This classification was proposed by Al-Johany et al. 2017.

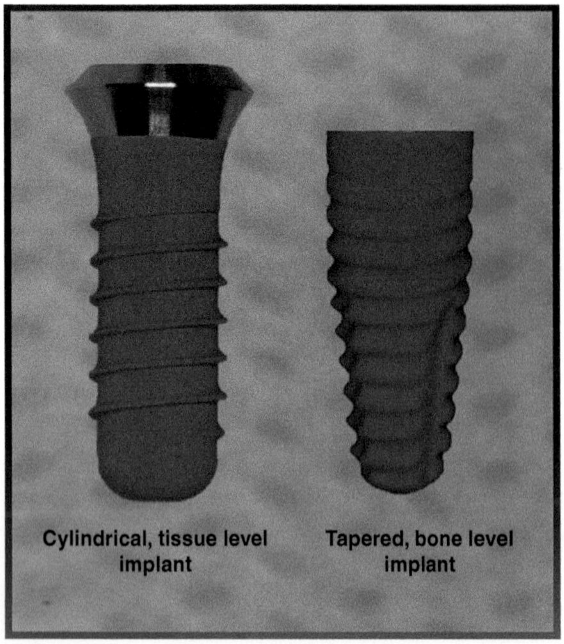

Figure 28.8 Implant shape and type. Shapes of dental implants include cylindrical and tapered design. Tissue level and bone level are the two categories of implant type.

thread thickness have led to the five commonly used implant thread shapes: square, V-shape, buttress, reverse buttress, and spiral threads (Figure 28.9). Data from finite element analysis has shown that the square thread design has the most favorable stress distribution (Chun et al. 2002; Eraslan & Inan 2010). The square thread design also provides the best primary stability in an immediate loading situation (Chang et al. 2012).

Thread depth and width

Thread depth is defined as the distance from the thread crest to the body of the implant, while thread width is measured from the superior end to the inferior end of the same thread (Misch 1999). Implants with reduced thread depth are generally easier to insert without the need for bone tapping. However, deeper threads increase BIC and consequently promote implant primary stability (Lee et al. 2015; Menini et al. 2020). Studies have shown that thread depth reduces peak stresses within the bone more significantly than thread width (Ao et al. 2010; Kong et al. 2008). To date, there is no consensus on an optimum thread depth and width values, and the ideal thread depth and width dimensions may vary depending on other geometric aspects of implant threads (Figure 28.10).

Thread pitch and lead

Thread pitch and lead are important geometric factors that determine BIC, stress distribution, and primary stability. Thread pitch is the distance between the crests of two adjacent threads measured at the same side of the implant axis (Goldstein

et al. 2020; Misch et al. 2006). It could be as narrow as 0.5 mm or as wide as 2.4 mm. The smaller the pitch on an implant length, the greater the number of threads and hence the more BIC. Implants with smaller pitch should be selected when primary stability is a concern (Orsini et al. 2012). Thread lead is the axial distance of implant body inserted in bone in one turn. Thread lead could be single, double, triple, or more, depending on the number of threads that run parallel to each other. Although multiple lead allows for faster implant insertion, single-lead implants have superior stability (Ma et al. 2007).

Crest module

The implant neck, also known as the crestal module or implant collar, is the most coronal portion of the implant body. The micro- and macro-design of the implant neck plays a role in maintaining crestal bone levels by the favorable distribution of stresses and transmission of compressive forces (Quirynen et al. 1992; Shimada et al. 2007). Divergent, straight, or convergent profiles are the three macro-designs of the implant crestal module, whereas the micro-design may include smooth, rough, or micro-grooved implant necks. Implants with smooth and polished crest modules have been designed to control plaque accumulation. However, a parallel smooth crest module results in shear forces that are detrimental to the crestal bone region, leading to increased bone loss (Goswami 2009; Hänggi et al. 2005; Hermann et al. 2001).

An additional negative factor that might cause crestal bone resorption around smooth implant necks that are inserted below the bone crest is the lack of mechanical stimulation of the bone. The concept of bone stimulation led to the introduction of micro-threading of the implant collar to transmit compressive forces to the crestal bone, and thus to minimize crestal bone resorption (Hansson 1999).

Studies have found that crestal bone loss was significantly less around implants with micro-threaded collar designs compared to smooth collar designs (Goswami 2009; Norton 1998). These findings are in concurrence with a recent systematic review and meta-analysis comparing marginal bone loss around implants with different collar designs. Micro-threaded rough-surfaced neck implants showed the lowest marginal bone loss compared to implants with polished or rough-surfaced non-micro-threaded neck implants (Koodaryan & Hafezeqoran 2016).

Implant types

Dental implants are commercially available with regard to two different levels in relation to the bone crest: tissue level and bone level. The neck of tissue-level implants has a smooth titanium collar that is positioned above the bone crest at the time of implant placement (Figure 28.6), whereas the entire body of a bone-level implant is seated within the bony housing. The main advantage of using tissue-level implants is conceivably to prevent crestal bone loss by positioning the

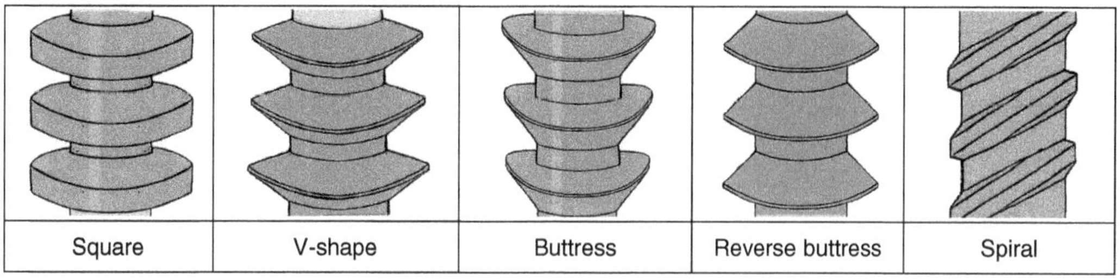

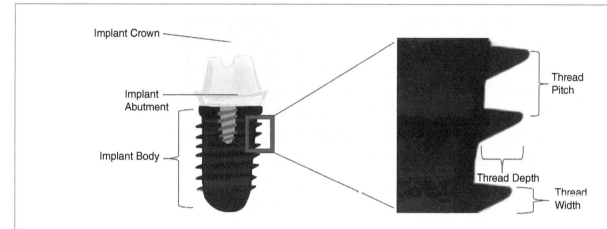

Figure 28.9 Different implant thread shapes. Source: Adapted from Abuhussein et al. 2010.

Figure 28.10 Dental implant thread geometry. The implant body can be non-threaded or threaded. This threaded implant shows the structural geometry of dental implant threads, including thread depth, width, and pitch.

implant/abutment interface (micro-gap) coronal to the bone crest. However, tissue-level implants require more interocclusal distance and provide less vertical clearance for a proper prosthetic emergence profile.

Platform

The design of the implant platform has evolved to improve mechanical retention of the abutment/crown, and the biological stability of surrounding crestal bone. Implant–abutment connection and platform switching are the two major modifications that have been incorporated into the implant platform design.

Implant–abutment connection

The abutment is the piece that connects the implant-supported prosthesis to the implant body. Different types of connections exist between the abutment and the implant (Table 28.2). Initial abutment–implant connections were composed of an external hex with a butt joint. An *external connection (hex)* extends coronal to the implant platform. Abutment screw loosening is a common occurrence with external connections due to adverse tipping forces. Consequently, the search for a better form of connection led to the development of an internal con-

nection that moved the connection to inside the implant body. The butt joint connection has since evolved into slip-fit and friction-fit joints. The internal connections have different shapes: octagonal, hexagonal, cone screw, cylinder hex, spline, tri-channel, and cam tube.

Platform switching

Peri-implant crestal bone loss has been commonly observed around implants after abutment connection (Albrektsson et al. 1986). It was believed that the micro-gap in the implant–abutment interface is a factor that causes such bone loss (Ericsson et al. 1995).

The platform switching (PLS) concept was introduced to reposition the micro-gap horizontally away from the outer edge of the implant and the surrounding bone toward the central axis of the implant (Gardner 2005; Lazzara & Porter 2006). The incorporation of PLS into the implant facilitates the preservation of crestal bone and associated supracrestal attachment apparatus (biological width) around the neck of the implant (Hermann et al. 2007).

According to the most recent systematic review and meta-analysis by Hsu et al. (2017), PLS may have an indirect protective effect on peri-implant hard tissue outcomes, suggesting

Table 28.2 Types of dental implant–abutment mating surface, fit, and shape.

Mating surface	Nature of fit	Shape	
• Slip	• Slip friction	• Hexagonal	• Hex
• Butt joint	• Friction fit	• Cone hex	• Cam tube
		• Cam	• Cone (conical) screw
		• Octagonal	• Spline
		• Cylinder	• Pin/slot

that bone resorption is decreased with thick soft tissues at baseline. Another systematic review conducted by Gupta and coworkers (2019) compared marginal bone loss outcome around platform-switched implants to those around non-platform-switched implants. The systematic review suggested that platform-switched implants result in less marginal bone resorption.

Implant micro-topography

Microscopic modification of implant surfaces was incorporated to optimize osseointegration that takes place at the interface between the implant and surrounding tissue (Smeets et al. 2016). Surface characteristics such as topography, wettability, and coatings contribute to the biological processes by mediating direct interaction with host osteoblasts (Dohan Ehrenfest et al. 2010; Esposito et al. 2014; Junker et al. 2009). Altering the surface topography of an implant can greatly improve the stability of an implant (Simon & Watson 2002).

Modification of the micro-topography of implant surfaces (measured on a 1–100 micrometer scale) is achieved through manufacturing processes such as machining, acid etching, anodization, sandblasting, grit blasting, and different coating procedures, so as to increase BIC (Dohan Ehrenfest et al. 2010; Kohles et al. 2004). The micro-topography of the implant surface has been proposed to act at the cellular level of osseointegration (Albrektsson & Wennerberg 2004), while the nano-topography (1–100 nm) of an implant surface is thought to influence cell–implant interactions at both cellular and protein levels (Mendonça et al. 2008).

Implant surface energy is enhanced by increasing surface roughness and altering surface chemistry (Coelho et al. 2015). Thus, changes in nano-topography exert their influence at a physical, chemical, and biological level (Junker et al. 2009), which results in increased adhesion of osteoblasts and potentially promotes osseointegration (Webster & Ejiofor 2004). Surface irregularities can be produced through ablative/subtractive procedures or additive procedures (Table 28.3).

Ablative/subtractive procedures

■ *Titanium oxide–blasted and acid-etched implants*: The surface texture achieved is a result of two subtractive, consecutive manufacturing steps. The micro-scale surface roughness is produced by titanium oxide blasting. The next etching

Table 28.3 Manufacturing procedures for the micro-modifications of an implant surface.

Ablative/subtractive procedures	Additive procedures
Sand blasting	Plasma spraying
Acid etching	Electrophoretic deposition of
Sandblasting and acid	hydroxyapatite
etching	Sputter deposition
Anodizing	Sol gel coating
Laser peening	Pulsed laser deposition
	Biomimetic precipitation

Source: Adapted from Parekh et al. 2012.

step with hydrofluoric acid forms the nanostructure of the implant (Coelho et al. 2015).

■ *Sandblasted and acid-etched (SLA)*: The SLA approach to implant surface modification is considered the gold standard in the implant industry. The implant surface is sandblasted by using aluminum oxide particles (250–500 μm) and then etched by acidic solution of specific concentration. The average surface roughness (Ra) of the treated implant surface is 1.5 μm (Szmukler-Moncler et al. 2004).

■ *Anodization*: The crystallinity of the titanium oxide layer and the micro-structure of the implant surface are produced by the process of anodization (Lazzara et al. 1999). The bone growth into the pores of the implant surface created by anodization results in mechanical interlocking and biochemical bonding, which are the two proposed mechanisms that explain osseointegration after anodization (Jungner et al. 2005).

■ *Shot peening/laser peening*: The shot peening process (Pypen et al. 1997) involves blasting the implant surface with spherical particles to form small indentations. On the other hand, laser peening involves the use of a high-intensity laser beam with nanosecond pulses ranging from 10 to 30 ns. The laser beam strikes a protective layer of paint on the surface of the implant. These implants exhibit small pores and a honeycomb surface pattern (Gaggl et al. 2000).

Additive procedures

A variety of additive methods to implant surfaces exist to enhance osseointegration. Among the initially implemented additive surface modifications was the coating of implant surfaces with layers of calcium phosphate, mainly composed of hydroxyapatite (HA) (Weinlaender et al. 1992). It is well recognized that calcium phosphate coatings have led to better initial clinical success rates compared to uncoated titanium implants (Morris et al. 2000; Weinlaender et al. 1992). HA coating creates both chemical and mechanical bonds to the surrounding bone (Sykaras et al. 2000).

- *Plasma-sprayed HA*: Plasma spraying (PS) utilizes thermal spray technology that uses a device to melt and deposit a coating material at a high velocity onto a substrate. Commercially available PS coatings are reported to have a thickness of greater than 30 μm (Ong & Chan 2000). Adhesion of HA to titanium is purely mechanical and can be enhanced by a roughened implant surface (Hermann et al. 2001). Shortcomings of PS include poor bond strength between coatings and titanium implant surfaces. Moreover, variations between commercial vendors of HA coatings play a critical role in the outcome achieved using HA-coated implants (Wennerberg et al. 1993).

- *Electrophoretic deposition of HA*: Electrophoretic deposition (EPD) is a process in which liquid-suspended colloidal particles migrate under the influence of an electrical field and get deposited onto a countercharged electrode (Lavenus et al. 2010; Meng et al. 2006). The advantages of EPD include low cost, a high deposition rate achieved using simple methodology, and the ability to tightly control the thickness of the coatings, which results in a uniform coating thickness in most challenging objects such as threaded implants (Meng et al. 2006). EPD can generate a coating thickness ranging from <1 to >500 μ thick (Meng et al. 2006). The major disadvantage of EPD is the need for post-deposition high heat treatment (at least 1200 °C) to densify the coating, which, in turn, negatively affects the interfacial strength between the metal and the coating (Lee et al. 2000; Meng et al. 2006).

Surface wettability

Surface wettability or hydrophilicity of implants plays a role in osseointegration. It has been proposed that surface hydrophilicity can maintain the function and conformation of proteins, while hydrophobicity might induce conformational stresses that denature proteins (Terheyden et al. 2012). Protein adsorption is enhanced by hydrophilicity of implant surfaces, which in turn promotes osteogenic cellular attachment, migration, differentiation, and maturation along the implant surface, thereby accelerating osseointegration (Zhao et al. 2005).

Conventional titanium oxide has low surface energy due to absorbed atmospheric hydrocarbons and carbonates that occur during implant storage (Zhao et al. 2005). In an attempt to improve the surface hydrophilicity, implants are rinsed and stored in isotonic saline solution (Figure 28.11) (Zhao et al. 2005). The maintenance of high surface energy is achieved by keeping a hydroxylated/hydrated surface that limits contamination with

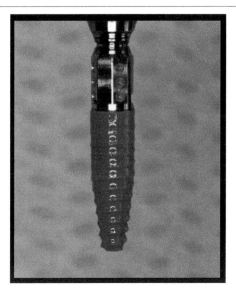

Figure 28.11 Implant stored in isotonic solution to prevent contamination of atmospheric carbonates and hydrocarbons, thereby maintaining surface hydrophilicity.

hydrocarbons and carbonates from the air (Schwarz et al. 2009). Stadlinger et al. (2009) proposed an alternative method to improve the wettability of implant surfaces by applying hydroxide ion solution (Gao et al. 2013). To date, clinical trials on the outcomes of hydrophilic implants are scarce.

Photofunctionalization of implant surfaces with ultraviolet (UV) treatment enhances bioactivity and osseointegration by altering the titanium dioxide on the implant surface (Gao et al. 2013). UV treatment promotes implant surface energy and wettability by reducing contaminating surface hydrocarbon (Altmann et al. 2013; Funato et al. 2013; Minamikawa et al. 2014; Park et al. 2013). Even though data on the clinical performance of photofunctionalized dental implants are too limited to draw a solid conclusion, it appears that UV treatment restores the surface energy of titanium implants, consequently promoting early bone deposition during osseointegration.

Future trends

In an effort to meet the increasing demand for rapid loading of dental implants, bioactive surface coatings have been extensively researched to optimize implant surface micro-topography. Surface coatings should resist disintegration or displacement during implant insertion (Hägi et al. 2010). Biomaterial research has been focusing on three clinical goals (Smeets et al. 2016):

- Promotion of interaction between implant and natural cascades of osseointegration to optimize the implant.
- Improvement of implant neck design to enhance peri-implant soft tissue response and integration.
- Reduction of peri-implantitis rate by designing implant surfaces that impede bacterial adhesion and colonization.

Research focusing on dental implant surface modifications with HA and nanocomposite coatings, growth factors, extracellular proteins, peptides, messenger molecules, and drugs is currently being conducted (Smeets et al. 2016). In summary, pre-clinical studies have shown promising histomorphometry and biomechanical properties of newly investigated implant coatings. However, clinical studies are needed to validate the superior effect of the new coatings compared to currently available implant surface micro-topography.

REFERENCES

Abdel-Hady Gepreel M, Niinomi M. Biocompatibility of Ti-alloys for long-term implantation. *J Mech Behav Biomed Mater.* 2013; 20:407–415.

Abuhussein H, Pagni G, Rebaudi A, Wang H-L. The effect of thread pattern upon implant osseointegration. *Clin Oral Implants Res.* 2010; 21(2):129–136.

Adell R, Lekholm U, Rockler B, Brånemark PI. A 15-year study of osseointegrated implants in the treatment of the edentulous jaw. *Int J Oral Surg.* 1981; 10(6):387–416.

Al-Johany SS, Al Amri MD, Alsaeed S, Alalola B. Dental implant length and diameter: a proposed classification scheme. *J Prosthodont.* 2017; 26(3):252–260.

Al-Nawas B, Brägger U, Meijer HJA et al. A double-blind randomized controlled trial (RCT) of Titanium-13Zirconium versus Titanium Grade IV small-diameter bone level implants in edentulous mandibles—results from a 1-year observation period. *Clin Implant Dent Relat Res.* 2012; 14(6):896–904.

Al-Sabbagh M, Eldomiaty W, Khabbaz Y. Can osseointegration be achieved without primary stability? *Dent Clin North Am.* 2019; 63(3):461–473.

Albrektsson T. Direct bone anchorage of dental implants. *J Prosthet Dent.* 1983; 50(2):255–261.

Albrektsson T, Jacobsson M. Bone-metal interface in osseointegration. *J Prosthet Dent.* 1987; 57(5):597–607.

Albrektsson T, Johansson C. Osteoinduction, osteoconduction and osseointegration. *Eur Spine J.* 2001; 10(2):S96–S101.

Albrektsson T, Wennerberg A. Oral implant surfaces: part 1—review focusing on topographic and chemical properties of different surfaces and in vivo responses to them. *Int J Prosthodont.* 2004; 17(5):536–543.

Albrektsson T, Zarb G, Worthington P, Eriksson AR. The long-term efficacy of currently used dental implants: a review and proposed criteria of success. *Int J Oral Maxillofac Implants.* 1986; 1(1):11–25.

Altmann B, Kohal R-J, Steinberg T et al. Distinct cell functions of osteoblasts on UV-functionalized titanium- and zirconia-based implant materials are modulated by surface topography. *Tissue Eng Part C Methods.* 2013; 19(11):850–863.

Andreiotelli M, Wenz HJ, Kohal RJ. Are ceramic implants a viable alternative to titanium implants? A systematic literature review. *Clin Oral Implants Res.* 2009; 20(Suppl 4):32–47.

Ao J, Li T, Liu Y et al. Optimal design of thread height and width on an immediately loaded cylinder implant: a finite element analysis. *Comput Biol Med.* 2010; 40(8):681–686.

Atieh MA, Alsabeeha N, Duncan WJ. Stability of tapered and parallel-walled dental implants: a systematic review and meta-analysis. *Clin Implant Dent Relat Res.* 2018; 20(4):634–645.

Baksh D, Davies JE. Design strategies for 3-dimensional in vitro bone growth in tissue-engineering scaffolds. In: JE Davies (ed.), *Bone Engineering.* Toronto: em squared; 2000: 488–495.

Berglundh T, Abrahamsson I, Lang NP, Lindhe J. De novo alveolar bone formation adjacent to endosseous implants: a model study in the dog. *Clin Oral Implants Res.* 2003; 14(3):251–262.

Boggan RS, Strong JT, Misch CE, Bidez MW. Influence of hex geometry and prosthetic table width on static and fatigue strength of dental implants. *J Prosthet Dent.* 1999; 82(4):436–440.

Branemark P-I. *Tissue-Integrated Prostheses: Osseointegration in Clinical Dentistry.* Batavia, IL: Quintessence; 1985.

Camilo CC, Silveira CAE, Faeda RS et al. Bone response to porous alumina implants coated with bioactive materials, observed using different characterization techniques. *J Appl Biomater Funct Mater.* 2017; 15(3):e223–e235.

Chang P-K, Chen Y-C, Huang C-C et al. Distribution of micromotion in implants and alveolar bone with different thread profiles in immediate loading: a finite element study. *Int J Oral Maxillofac Implants.* 2012; 27(6):e96–e101.

Chun HJ, Cheong SY, Han JH et al. Evaluation of design parameters of osseointegrated dental implants using finite element analysis. *J Oral Rehabil.* 2002; 29(6):565–574.

Coelho PG, Jimbo R, Tovar N, Bonfante EA. Osseointegration: hierarchical designing encompassing the macrometer, micrometer, and nanometer length scales. *Dent Mater.* 2015; 31(1):37–52.

Davies J. Mechanisms of endosseous integration. *Int J Prosthodont.* 1998; 11(5):391–401.

Depprich R, Naujoks C, Ommerborn M et al. Current findings regarding zirconia implants. *Clin Implant Dent Relat Res.* 2014; 16(1):124–137.

Depprich R, Ommerborn M, Zipprich H et al., Behavior of osteoblastic cells cultured on titanium and structured zirconia surfaces. *Head Face Med.* 2008; 4:29.

Diz P, Scully C, Sanz M. Dental implants in the medically compromised patient. *J Dent.* 2013; 41(3):195–206.

Dohan Ehrenfest DM, Coelho PG, Kang B-S, Sul Y-T, Albrektsson T. Classification of osseointegrated implant surfaces: materials, chemistry and topography. *Trends Biotechnol.* 2010; 28(4):198–206.

Eraslan O, Inan O. The effect of thread design on stress distribution in a solid screw implant: a 3D finite element analysis. *Clin Oral Investig.* 2010; 14(4):411–416.

Ericsson I, Persson LG, Berglundh T et al. Different types of inflammatory reactions in peri-implant soft tissues. *J Clin Periodontol.* 1995; 22(3):255–261.

Esposito M, Ardebili Y, Worthington HV. Interventions for replacing missing teeth: different types of dental implants. *Cochrane Database Syst Rev.* 2014; (7):CD003815. doi: 10.1002/14651858.CD003815.pub4.

Funato A, Yamada M, Ogawa T. Success rate, healing time, and implant stability of photofunctionalized dental implants. *Int J Oral Maxillofac Implants.* 2013; 28(5):1261–1271.

Gaggl A, Schultes G, Müller WD, Kärcher H. Scanning electron microscopical analysis of laser-treated titanium implant surfaces—a comparative study. *Biomaterials.* 2000; 21(10):1067–1073.

Gahlert M, Burtscher D, Grunert I, Kniha H, Steinhauser E. Osseointegration of zirconia and titanium dental implants: a histological and histomorphometrical study in the maxilla of pigs. *Clin Oral Implants Res.* 2009; 20(11):1247–1253.

Gahlert M, Burtscher D, Grunert I, Kniha H, Steinhauser E. Failure analysis of fractured dental zirconia implants. *Clin Oral Implants Res.* 2012. 23(3):287–293.

Gao Y, Liu Y, Zhou L et al. The effects of different wavelength UV photofunctionalization on micro-arc oxidized titanium. *PLoS One.* 2013; 8(7):e68086.

Gardner DM. Platform switching as a means to achieving implant esthetics. *N Y State Dent J.* 2005; 71(3):34–37.

Glauser R, Sennerby L, Meredith N et al. Resonance frequency analysis of implants subjected to immediate or early functional occlusal loading. Successful vs. failing implants. *Clin Oral Implants Res.* 2004; 15(4):428–434.

Gleiznys A, Skirbutis G, Harb A, Barzdziukaite I, Grinyte I. New approach towards mini dental implants and small-diameter implants: an option for long-term prostheses. *Stomatologija.* 2012; 14(2):39–45.

Goldstein BH, Bergersen L, Armstrong AK et al. Adverse events, radiation exposure, and reinterventions following transcatheter pulmonary valve replacement. *J Am Coll Cardiol.* 2020; 75(4):363–376.

Goswami MM. Comparison of crestal bone loss along two implant crest module designs. *Med J Armed Forces India.* 2009; 65(4):319–322.

Gupta S, Sabharwal R, Nazeer J et al. Platform switching technique and crestal bone loss around the dental implants: a systematic review. *Ann Afr Med.* 2019; 18(1):1–6.

Hägi TT, Enggist L, Michel D et al. Mechanical insertion properties of calcium-phosphate implant coatings. *Clin Oral Implants Res.* 2010; 21(11):1214–1222.

Hänggi MP, Hänggi DC, Schoolfield JD et al. Crestal bone changes around titanium implants. Part I: a retrospective radiographic evaluation in humans comparing two non-submerged implant designs with different machined collar lengths. *J Periodontol.* 2005; 76(5):791–802.

Hansson S. The implant neck: smooth or provided with retention elements. A biomechanical approach. *Clin Oral Implants Res.* 1999; 10(5):394–405.

Hermann F, Lerner H, Palti A. Factors influencing the preservation of the periimplant marginal bone. *Implant Dent.* 2007; 16(2):165–175.

Hermann JS, Schoolfield JD, Nummikoski PV et al. Crestal bone changes around titanium implants: a methodologic study comparing linear radiographic with histometric measurements. *Int J Oral Maxillofac Implants.* 2001; 16(4):475–485.

Hermann JS, Schoolfield JD, Schenk RK, Buser D, Cochran DL. Influence of the size of the microgap on crestal bone changes around titanium implants. A histometric evaluation of unloaded non-submerged implants in the canine mandible. *J Periodontol.* 2001; 72(10):1372–1383.

Hsu YT, Lin GH, Wang HL. Effects of platform-switching on peri-implant soft and hard tissue outcomes: a systematic review and meta-analysis. *Int J Oral Maxillofac Implants.* 2017; 32(1):e9–e24.

Ioannidis A, Gallucci GO, Jung RE et al. Titanium-zirconium narrow-diameter versus titanium regular-diameter implants for anterior and premolar single crowns: 3-year results of a randomized controlled clinical study. *J Clin Periodontol.* 2015; 42(11):1060–1070.

Jungner M, Lundqvist P, Lundgren S. Oxidized titanium implants (Nobel Biocare TiUnite) compared with turned titanium implants (Nobel Biocare mark III) with respect to implant failure in a group of consecutive patients treated with early functional loading and two-stage protocol. *Clin Oral Implants Res.* 2005; 16(3):308–312.

Junker R, Dimakis A, Thoneick M, Jansen JA. Effects of implant surface coatings and composition on bone integration: a systematic review. *Clin Oral Implants Res.* 2009; 20(Suppl 4):185–206.

Kohles SS, Clark MB, Brown CA, Kenealy JN. Direct assessment of profilometric roughness variability from typical implant surface types. *Int J Oral Maxillofac Implants.* 2004; 19(4):510–516.

Koller B, Att W, Strub JR. Survival rates of teeth, implants, and double crown-retained removable dental prostheses: a systematic literature review. *Int J Prosthodont.* 2011; 24(2):109–117.

Kong L, Hu K, Li D et al., Evaluation of the cylinder implant thread height and width: a 3-dimensional finite element analysis. *Int J Oral Maxillofac Implants.* 2008; 23(1):65–74.

Koodaryan R, Hafezeqoran A. Evaluation of implant collar surfaces for marginal bone loss: a systematic review and meta-analysis. *Biomed Res Int.* 2016; 2016:4987526.

Kullar AS, Miller CS. Are there contraindications for placing dental implants? *Dent Clin North Am.* 2019; 63(3):345–362.

Lavenus S, Louarn G, Layrolle P. Nanotechnology and dental implants. *Int J Biomater,* 2010; 2010:915327.

Lazzara RJ, Porter SS. Platform switching: a new concept in implant dentistry for controlling postrestorative crestal bone levels. *Int J Periodontics Restorative Dent.* 2006; 26(1):9–17.

Lazzara RJ, Testori T, Trisi P, Porter SS, Weinstein RL. A human histologic analysis of osseotite and machined surfaces using implants with 2 opposing surfaces. *Int J Periodontics Restorative Dent.* 1999; 19(2):117–129.

Lee JJ, Rouhfar L, Beirne OR. Survival of hydroxyapatite-coated implants: a meta-analytic review. *J Oral Maxillofac Surg.* 2000; 58(12):1372–1379; discussion 1379–1380.

Lee SY, Kim SJ, An HW et al. The effect of the thread depth on the mechanical properties of the dental implant. *J Adv Prosthodont.* 2015; 7(2):115–121.

Ma P, Liu H-C, Li D-H et al. [Influence of helix angle and density on primary stability of immediately loaded dental implants: three-dimensional finite element analysis]. *Zhonghua Kou Qiang Yi Xue Za Zhi.* 2007; 42(10):618–621.

Mendonça G, Mendonça DBS, Aragão FJL, Cooper LF. Advancing dental implant surface technology—from micron- to nanotopography. *Biomaterials.* 2008; 29(28):3822–3835.

Meng X, Kwon TY, Yang Y, Ong JL, Kim KH. Effects of applied voltages on hydroxyapatite coating of titanium by electrophoretic deposition. *J Biomed Mater Res B Appl Biomater.* 2006; 78(2):373–377.

Menini M, Bagnasco F, Calimodio I et al. Influence of implant thread morphology on primary stability: a prospective clinical study. *Biomed Res Int.* 2020; 2020: 69 74050.

Meredith N. A review of nondestructive test methods and their application to measure the stability and osseointegration of bone anchored endosseous implants. *Crit Rev Biomed Eng.* 1998; 26(4):275–291.

Minamikawa H, Ikeda T, Att W et al. Photofunctionalization increases the bioactivity and osteoconductivity of the titanium alloy Ti6Al4V. *J Biomed Mater Res A.* 2014; 102(10):3618–3630.

Misch CE. *Contemporary Implant Dentistry.* St. Louis, MO: Mosby; 1999.

Misch CE, Steignga J, Barboza E et al. Short dental implants in posterior partial edentulism: a multicenter retrospective 6-year case series study. *J Periodontol.* 2006; 77(8):1340–1347.

Morris HF, Ochi S, Crum P, Orenstein IH, Winkler S. AICRG, part I: a 6-year multicentered, multidisciplinary clinical study of a new and innovative implant design. *J Oral Implantol.* 2004; 30(3):125–133.

Morris HF, Ochi S, Spray JR, Olson JW. Periodontal-type measurements associated with hydroxyapatite-coated and non-HA-coated implants: uncovering to 36 months. *Ann Periodontol.* 2000; 5(1):56–67.

Nicholson W. Titanium alloys for dental implants: a review. *Prosthesis.* 2020; (2):17.

Norton MR. Marginal bone levels at single tooth implants with a conical fixture design. The influence of surface macro- and microstructure. *Clin Oral Implants Res.* 1998; 9(2):91–99.

Ogle OE. Implant surface material, design, and osseointegration. *Dent Clin North Am.* 2015; 59(2):505–520.

Ong JL, Chan DC. Hydroxyapatite and their use as coatings in dental implants: a review. *Crit Rev Biomed Eng.* 2000; 28(5–6):667–707.

Orsini E, Giavaresi G, Trirè A, Ottani V, Salgarello S. Dental implant thread pitch and its influence on the osseointegration process: an in vivo comparison study. *Int J Oral Maxillofac Implants.* 2012; 27(2):383–392.

Osman RB, Ma S, Duncan W et al. Fractured zirconia implants and related implant designs: scanning electron microscopy analysis. *Clin Oral Implants Res.* 2013; 24(5):592–597.

Osman RB, Swain MV, Atieh M, Ma S, Duncan W. Ceramic implants (Y-TZP): are they a viable alternative to titanium implants for the support of overdentures? A randomized clinical trial. *Clin Oral Implants Res.* 2014; 25(12):1366–1377.

Parekh RB, Shetty O, Tabassum R. Surface modifications for endosseous dental implants. *Int J Oral Implantol Clin Res.* 2012; 3(3):116–121.

Park K-H, Koak J-Y, Kim S-K, Han C-H, Heo S-J. The effect of ultraviolet-C irradiation via a bactericidal ultraviolet sterilizer on an anodized titanium implant: a study in rabbits. *Int J Oral Maxillofac Implants.* 2013; 28(1):57–66.

Puleo D, Nanci A. Understanding and controlling the bone–implant interface. *Biomaterials.* 1999; 20(23–24):2311–2321.

Pypen CM, Plenk H Jr, Ebel MF, Svagera R, Wernisch J. Characterization of microblasted and reactive ion etched surfaces on the commercially pure metals niobium, tantalum and titanium. *J Mater Sci Mater Med.* 1997; 8(12):781–784.

Quirynen M, Naert I, van Steenberghe D. Fixture design and overload influence marginal bone loss and fixture success in the Branemark system. *Clin Oral Implants Res.* 1992; 3(3):104–111.

Rokn A, Ghahroudi AR, Mesgarzadeh A, Miremadi AA, Yaghoobi S. Evaluation of stability changes in tapered and parallel wall implants: a human clinical trial. *J Dent (Tehran).* 2011; 8(4):186–200.

Romanos GE, Delgado-Ruiz RA, Sacks D, Calvo-Guirado JL. Influence of the implant diameter and bone quality on the primary stability of porous tantalum trabecular metal dental implants: an in vitro biomechanical study. *Clin Oral Implants Res.* 2018; 29(6):649–655.

Schroeder A. Gewebsreaktion auf ein Titan-Hohlzylinderimplantat mit Titan-Spritzschichtoberfläche. *Schweiz Monatsschr Zahnheilk.* 1976; 86:713.

Schwartz Z, Boyan B. Underlying mechanisms at the bone–biomaterial interface. *J Cell Biochemistry.* 1994; 56(3):340–347.

Schwarz F, Wieland M, Schwartz Z et al. Potential of chemically modified hydrophilic surface characteristics to support tissue integration of titanium dental implants. *J Biomed Mater Res B Appl Biomater.* 2009; 88(2):544–557.

Sennerby L, Meredith N. Implant stability measurements using resonance frequency analysis: biological and biomechanical aspects and clinical implications. *Periodontol* 2000. 2008; 47:51–66.

Shimada E, Pilliar RM, Deporter DA, Schroering R, Atenafu E. A pilot study to assess the performance of a partially threaded sintered porous-surfaced dental implant in the dog mandible. *Int J Oral Maxillofac Implants.* 2007; 22(6):948–954.

Simon Z, Watson PA. Biomimetic dental implants—new ways to enhance osseointegration. *J Can Dent Assoc.* 2002; 68(5):286–288.

Smeets R, Stadlinger B, Schwarz F et al. Impact of dental implant surface modifications on osseointegration. *Biomed Res Int.* 2016; 2016:6285620.

Stadlinger B, Lode AT, Eckelt U et al. Surface-conditioned dental implants: an animal study on bone formation. *J Clin Periodontol.* 2009; 36(10):882–891.

Steigenga JT, al-Shammari KF, Nociti FH, Misch CE, Wang HL. Dental implant design and its relationship to long-term implant success. *Implant Dent.* 2003; 12(4):306–317.

Sykaras N, Iacopino AM, Marker VA, Triplett RG, Woody RD. Implant materials, designs, and surface topographies: their effect on osseointegration. A literature review. *Int J Oral Maxillofac Implants.* 2000; 15(5):675–690.

Szmukler-Moncler S, Perrin D, Ahossi V, Magnin G, Bernard JP. Biological properties of acid etched titanium implants: effect of sandblasting on bone anchorage. *J Biomed Mater Res B Appl Biomater.* 2004; 68(2):149–159.

Szmukler-Moncler S, Salama H, Reingewirtz Y, Dubruille JH. Timing of loading and effect of micromotion on bone-dental implant interface: review of experimental literature. *J Biomed Mater Res.* 1998; 43(2):192–203.

Terheyden H, Lang NP, Bierbaum S, Stadlinger B. Osseointegration—communication of cells. *Clin Oral Implants Res.* 2012; 23(10):1127–1135.

Watzak G, Zechner W, Ulm C et al. Histologic and histomorphometric analysis of three types of dental implants following 18 months of occlusal loading: a preliminary study in baboons. *Clin Oral Implants Res.* 2005; 16(4):408–416.

Webster TJ, Ejiofor JU. Increased osteoblast adhesion on nanophase metals: Ti, Ti6Al4V, and CoCrMo. *Biomaterials.* 2004; 25(19):4731–4739.

Weinlaender M, Kenney EB, Lekovic V et al. Histomorphometry of bone apposition around three types of endosseous dental implants. *Int J Oral Maxillofac Implants.* 1992; 7(4):491–496.

Wennerberg A, Albrektsson T, Andersson B. Design and surface characteristics of 13 commercially available oral implant systems. *Int J Oral Maxillofac Implants.* 1993; 8(6):622–633.

Zhao G, Schwartz Z, Wieland M et al. High surface energy enhances cell response to titanium substrate microstructure. *J Biomed Mater Res A.* 2005; 74(1):49–58.

CHAPTER 29
Examination and treatment planning of the implant patient

Sejal R. Thacker

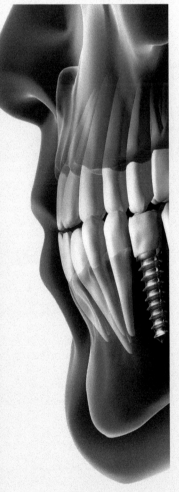

Contents

Essential Periodontics, First Edition. Edited by Steph Smith and Khalid Almas.
© 2022 John Wiley & Sons Ltd. Published 2022 by John Wiley & Sons Ltd.

Learning objectives

- Factors to consider in the general evaluation of the implant patient.
- How to clinically evaluate the implant patient.
- Anatomic landmarks of importance in the radiographic evaluation.
- Factors to consider regarding timing of placement of implants, the hard and soft tissues around implants, and the prosthetic considerations.

Introduction

Implant planning requires a multidisciplinary team-based approach. The initial assessment involves a preliminary screening of the patient for eligibility for an implant-supported prosthesis. This includes the patient's chief complaint, age, medical and medication history, past dental history, and behavioral patterns. This is followed by clinical extraoral and intraoral examination and radiographic evaluation, leading to a detailed diagnosis and treatment plan.

General evaluation of the patient

Age of the patient

Consideration should be given to patients seeking dental implants during the mixed dentition phase and to edentulous patients in the geriatric population. Implants inserted during the mixed dentition phase have low chances of being maintained in function, as osseointegrated implants remain stable in their position despite the growing surrounding bone, without any adaptation to remodeling (Oesterle et al. 1993). Typically, facial growth is complete by the age of 17 in females and 25 in males. Implants inserted during early adult life or the final period of puberty have a higher chance of longevity (Oesterle & Cronin 2000). Complications in the geriatric population are mainly related to systemic conditions and medications that could preclude surgical intervention and compliance, as well as compromise healing.

Behavioral pattern, chief complaint, and patient expectations

A patient's chief complaint and expectations can have a direct impact on treatment. Dysmorphophobia, unrealistic expectations, and other psychological disturbances are some behavioral contraindications to implant therapy. The patient's desires have to be in harmony with attainable outcomes projected by the clinician after assessment of the specific clinical situation (Lindhe et al. 2008). Furthermore, patient compliance and ability to follow postoperative instructions have to be assessed beforehand to avoid complications and dissatisfaction.

Systemic conditions and medications

Systemic diseases and medications such as bleeding disorders, malignancies, history of radiation therapy, uncontrolled diabetes, anticoagulant therapy, and antiresorptive medications are a few examples that may pose as relative contraindications to any surgical intervention. Patients with these conditions should be co-managed with consultation and clearance from their primary care physicians.

Osteoporosis results in decrease in bone mass and can result in bone fragility. Intraorally, an osteoporotic patient may present with poor bone quality. However, most reports have shown comparable survival rates of implants in these patients, especially with the advent of micro- and macro-modifications of the implant structure (Lindhe et al. 2008).

Poor glycemic control in uncontrolled diabetics results in slower wound healing and delay in implant stabilization (Oates et al. 2014). Marginally lower survival rates have been documented in diabetic patients. Increased HBA1C, age of onset, and the type of diabetes are some risk factors for higher morbidity in these patients (Fiorellini et al. 2000). Glycemic control, longer healing times, preoperative antibiotics, and coated implants are a few recommendations for successful management of these patients (Morris et al. 2000).

Surgical intervention in a minority of patients on antiresorptive and antiangiogenic medications, such as bisphosphonates and receptor activator of nuclear factor-kappa B (RANKL) inhibitors, can result in a condition called medication-related osteonecrosis of the jaw (MRONJ), which is defined as an unhealed site with bone exposure for more than 8 weeks. The prevalence of MRONJ in patients on oral bisphosphonates is as low as 0.004–0.21% and on intravenous medications is 0.017–6.7% (Ruggiero et al. 2014). A modified drug holiday of 2 months is recommended for patients on oral bisphosphonates for >2 years to reduce the risk of MRONJ, but the evidence behind this recommendation is extremely low (Ruggiero et al. 2014). Limited data exist on the effect of these medications on osseointegration, implant failure rates, or marginal bone loss (Chrcanovic et al. 2016). Due to significant uncertainty in this area, communication with the treating physician, risk–benefit assessment, and a thorough discussion with the patient should be considered (Lindhe et al. 2008).

Radiation therapy can result in oral soft tissue damage, non-healing ulcerations, and exposed bone, similar to MRONJ, called osteoradionecrosis (ORN), due to hypovascularity, hypocellularity, and hypoxia (Muller & Barter 2016). ORN occurs in 3–35% of patients undergoing radiation therapy (Marx & Johnson 1987). Evidence shows that radiotherapy can significantly affect successful dental implant healing and almost double the implant failure rates (Granström 2005; Muller & Barter 2016).

See also Chapter 31 for other systemic conditions and implant patients.

Habits

A threefold increase in implant failure rates in smokers has been shown, along with higher odds for postoperative infections and pronounced peri-implant bone loss (Chrcanovic et al. 2015; Vandeweghe & De Bruyn 2011). Smoking cessation and counseling, preoperative antibiotics, along with the use of coated implants have been suggested in smokers to reduce these risks (Bain 1996; Lambert et al. 2000).

Evidence for the correlation of bruxism and implant failure is lacking, but prosthetic complications such as fracture of prosthesis, screw loosening, and fractures seem to be a frequent occurrence in these patients (Lindhe et al. 2008).

Dental history

Present or past history of periodontal disease, patient compliance, and maintenance regimens are important to evaluate, since a history of periodontal disease can increase the odds ratio for having peri-implantitis by 3.7–4.1 (Ferreira et al. 2006; Kotsovilis et al. 2006). All periodontal therapy, caries control, extraction of hopeless teeth, restorations, patient motivation, oral hygiene, and maintenance should be assessed and accomplished prior to implant therapy.

Clinical evaluation

Extraoral evaluation

Any gross facial asymmetry in the form of swellings or lesions should be noted, evaluated, and managed. Extent of mouth opening will help determine access during surgical and prosthetic intervention.

For anterior implant cases, additional assessments are important in providing a comprehensive treatment plan and an outcome that is not only functional but also esthetic. This includes:

- Symmetry in facial thirds, facial form, vertical dimension of occlusion, maxillomandibular relationship.
- Horizontal reference lines such as interpapillary line and vertical reference lines such as midline.
- Smile line – assessed on the amount of display of the maxillary anterior teeth and gingiva when patient smiles:
  - High smile line: entire length of maxillary anterior teeth is visible along with variable part of gingiva.
  - Moderate smile line: 75–100% of teeth is visible along with interproximal papillae.
  - Low smile line: no more than 75% of teeth is visible (Tjan et al. 1984) (see Figures 29.1 to 29.3).

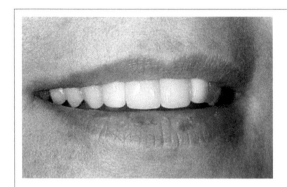

Figure 29.1 Low smile line.

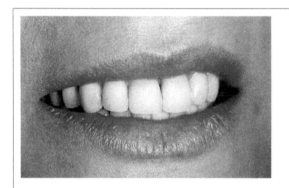

Figure 29.2 Average smile line.

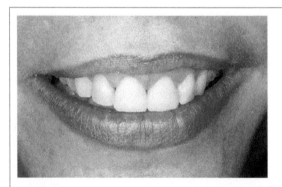

Figure 29.3 High smile line.

Intraoral evaluation

Oral cancer screening and general examination, to ascertain the absence of any intraoral pathology, should precede evaluation of the dentition (Lindhe et al. 2008). Dental evaluation and management of the following pathologies should be accomplished, if deemed necessary, using a team-based approach:

- Extraction of hopeless teeth.
- Caries excavation, endodontic treatment, and restorations.
- Management of periodontal disease and assessment of periodontal stability, oral hygiene, and compliance.
- Orthodontic management of malocclusion and misalignment of teeth.

Once dental and occlusal stability is achieved, the site planned for implant restoration should be evaluated from a surgical (hard and soft tissue adequacy) and prosthetic (interarch and interdental distance) standpoint.

Evaluation of hard tissue

An edentulous site planned for an implant prosthesis should be evaluated for hard tissue adequacy in mesio-distal, bucco-lingual, and apico-coronal dimensions.

- *Mesio-distal dimension*: This space is usually confined by the roots of the adjacent teeth in a partially edentulous patient. A space of at least 1.5 mm between the implant and the roots of the adjacent teeth is necessary to prevent damage to the existing roots (Esposito et al. 1993). In the esthetic zone, 3–4 mm of distance between the implant and the adjacent root is recommended for creation of a harmonious emergence profile and soft tissue fill in papillary areas (Gastaldo et al. 2004). When two adjacent implants are placed, an inter-implant distance of >3 mm is critical to maintain crestal bone levels (Tarnow et al. 2000). Assessment of the mesio-distal distance helps in the selection of implant diameter and design, and may also necessitate orthodontic intervention to create the necessary space between the roots.
- *Bucco-lingual dimension*: The adequacy of bone in the bucco-lingual dimension will determine implant selection and the need for bone grafting. Though bone volume in this dimension can be gauged clinically, for definitive assessment a three-dimensional cone beam scan is recommended. A buccal wall thickness of 2 mm facial to the implant is necessary to prevent bone loss and help with long-term stability (Merheb et al. 2014).
- *Apico-coronal dimension*: The vertical bone height available for implant placement can be restricted by anatomic structures such as the nasal floor, maxillary sinus, mental foramen, and inferior alveolar nerve. Radiographic assessment using either a two-dimensional or three-dimensional radiograph will be required to determine length of implant, need for sinus augmentation, and vertical ridge augmentation. A distance of at least 2 mm from vital structures such as the mental foramen and the inferior alveolar nerve canal is paramount to prevent damage and sensory dysfunction (Greenstein & Tarnow 2006).

Evaluation of soft tissue

Gingival thickness is an important factor to assess, not only for esthetic stability in anterior teeth, but also for maintenance of tissue closure when bone grafts are planned in posterior sextants of the mouth. A thick gingival phenotype is defined as tissue that is >1 mm versus a thin gingival phenotype being <1 mm in thickness (Kan et al. 2010). Keratinized tissue width from the free gingival margin to the mucogingival junction should also be assessed. Lack of keratinized tissue width and vestibular depth can pose difficulty in hygiene maintenance and result in higher gingivitis recordings around implant restorations and greater crestal bone loss (Oh et al. 2017). Based on these assessments, gingival grafting to thicken the tissue or to increase vestibular depth and keratinized tissue width may be planned either before, during, or after implant placement.

Prosthetic space

The interarch distance is sometimes restricted due to supra-eruption of opposing teeth and malocclusion. The space required is largely determined by the planned prosthesis, especially in completely edentulous patients, but an average distance of 7 mm from the implant platform to the opposing occlusal surface is necessary for implant-supported crown restorations in partially edentulous patients. The mesio-distal, bucco-lingual, and apico-coronal implant space and positioning influence the prosthetic outcome and longevity.

Radiographic evaluation

Periapical radiographs are suitable for implant treatment planning when performed according to the paralleling technique. A full mouth series will help ascertain overall dental stability of the remaining dentition and help evaluate the mesio-distal distance and apico-coronal height of bone.

A panoramic radiograph, though having significant magnification and distortion, can serve as a good screening tool to rule out any bone pathologies. It also helps evaluate proximity to anatomic structures such as the nasal floor, maxillary sinus, mental foramen, and inferior alveolar nerve.

With the advent of low-radiation three-dimensional cone beam computed tomography (CBCT), implant planning has become efficient and predictable. A CBCT scan provides cross-sectional images of the jaw and is highly accurate. A CBCT scan should be utilized when the edentulous site presents with narrow bucco-lingual thickness, proximity to vital structures, when a sinus graft is anticipated, and with immediate or esthetic implant cases.

Anatomic considerations for implant surgery

A proficient knowledge of oral anatomy is needed to provide effective implant dentistry and to avoid surgical complications (Greenstein et al. 2008).

Maxillary arch

- *Nasopalatine foramen and nerve*: The nasopalatine foramen (incisive canal) is about 4.6–7.4 mm wide and is housed in the midline on the maxillary palatal surface. The canal transmits the anterior branches of the descending palatine vessels and the nasopalatine nerves (Greenstein et al. 2008; Mraiwa et al. 2004). A large canal may pose a challenge with respect to bone availability for future implant surgery. In these case scenarios, the contents of the canal can be enucleated and grafted or displaced to facilitate implant placement (Artzi et al. 2000; Greenstein et al. 2008; Rosenquist 1994).

■ *Greater palatine foramen and nerve*: The greater palatine foramen contains the artery and the nerve, and is located approximately halfway between the osseous crest and the median raphe opposite the third or second molar in the palate. One may encounter this during soft tissue harvesting from the palate or during flap elevation, especially when the maxillary posterior edentulous ridge is atrophic and has lost height. Determination of the location and preparedness with local hemostatic agents to control bleeding are necessary when working in this sextant of the mouth (Greenstein et al. 2008).

■ *Maxillary sinus*: The maxillary sinus is the largest of the paranasal sinuses and is frequently encountered when restoring the edentulous posterior maxilla. The sinus ostium is located in the middle meatus, about 25–35 mm above the antral floor. It tends to increase in size over life and with extraction of maxillary posterior teeth (Chanavaz 1990). This pneumatization of the sinus can limit the height of bone available for implant placement. The classification proposed by Jensen (1999), shown in Table 29.1, can be used as a guide for placing implants in proximity to the maxillary sinus. Advances in implant design and the evolution in armamentarium have made it possible to successfully place short implants or do minimally invasive internal sinus grafts with simultaneous implant placement, even in class III cases with 4–6 mm of residual bone (see Figures 29.4–29.7).

When a lateral sinus augmentation is planned, a CBCT scan analysis is prudent to rule out sinus pathologies, make necessary Ear, Nose, and Throat (ENT) referrals, and evaluate the anatomy for sinus septa, surgical access, and ostium patency.

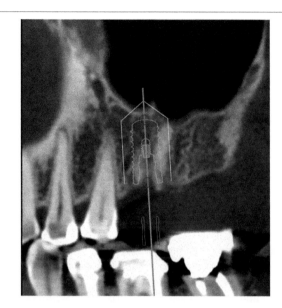

Figure 29.4 Class I: >10 mm remnant bone.

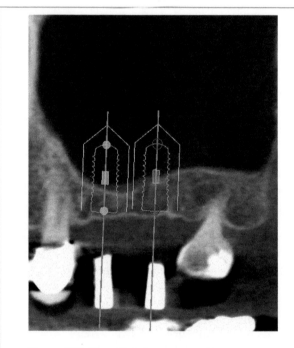

Figure 29.5 Class III: 4–6 mm remnant bone.

Table 29.1 Implant placement in proximity to maxillary sinus.

Class	Residual bone height	Suggested surgical technique
Class I	>10 mm	Direct implant placement
Class II	7–9 mm	Short implants Internal or lateral sinus elevation with simultaneous implant placement
Class III	4–6 mm	Lateral sinus elevation with simultaneous or staged implant placement
Class IV	1–3 mm	Lateral sinus elevation with staged implant placement
Class V		Removed or absent sinus

Source: Adapted from Jensen 1999.

Mandibular arch

■ *Inferior alveolar nerve (IAN) and canal*: The inferior alveolar canal in the posterior mandibular sextant houses the IAN, which traverses from the lingual to the buccal, and often in the first molar site is located midway between the buccal and lingual cortices (Greenstein et al. 2008; Gustinna Wadu et al. 1997). On average the canal is located 3.5–5.4 mm from the apices of the mandibular molars (Greenstein et al. 2008; Littner et al. 1986). In a mandibular edentulous

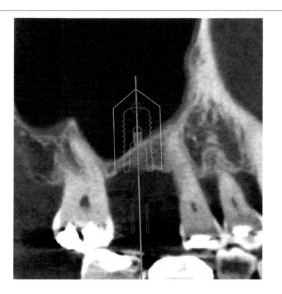

Figure 29.6 Class IV: 1–3 mm remnant bone.

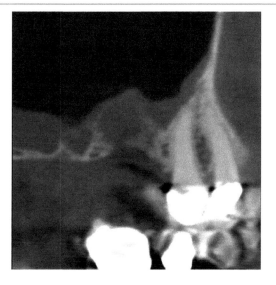

Figure 29.7 Scan showing Schneiderian membrane thickening and oro–antral communication.

ridge with vertical atrophy, the distance from the crest to the canal will be reduced. A panoramic radiograph or a CBCT scan is recommended for precise measurements for planning of implant length and the need for vertical augmentation (see Figure 29.8).

- *Mental foramen, anterior loop, and mental nerve*: The IAN branches into the mental and incisal nerve in the premolar region. The horizontal position of the mental foramen can vary, but is usually located between the first and second mandibular premolars (Greenstein & Tarnow 2006; Greenstein et al. 2008). Vertically the foramen may be situated coronal to the apex (38.6%), at the apex (15.4%), and apical to the apex (46%) (Fishel et al. 1976). In an edentulous site, due to loss of vertical height, this position may be altered bringing the foramen closer to the crestal portion. Caution and consideration to the foramen location should be exercised when placing immediate implants in the premolar site (Greenstein et al. 2008). It has been suggested to leave a 2 mm zone of safety between the implant and the coronal aspect of the nerve (Greenstein & Tarnow 2006). The anterior loop of the mental foramen refers to the IAN when it courses inferiorly and anteriorly to the foramen and loops back to emerge from the foramen (Greenstein et al. 2008). The anterior extent of this loop determines the antero-posterior positioning of interforaminal implants placed in a completely edentulous resorbed mandible planned for a full arch implant-supported prosthesis. A huge variability of 0–7.5 mm may exist with respect to the extent of this anterior loop (Greenstein & Tarnow 2006). Diagnostic scans and direct visualization with surgical exposure of the mental foramen have been recommended to avoid sensory nerve damage (Greenstein & Tarnow 2006) (see Figure 29.9).
- *Lingual nerve*: The lingual nerve is a branch of the mandibular nerve and it provides sensory innervation to the mucous membrane of the anterior two-thirds of the tongue and to the lingual tissues (Greenstein et al. 2008). The lingual nerve is located 3 mm apical to the osseous crest and 2 mm horizontally from the lingual cortical plate. However, in 15–20% of cases the nerve is situated at or above the bone crest, lingual to the mandibular third molars.

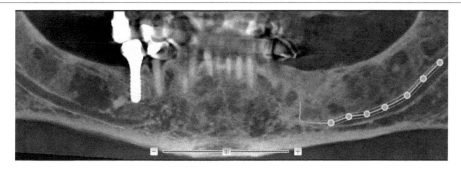

Figure 29.8 Inferior alveolar nerve traced on the right side in a cone beam computed tomography scan (in green).

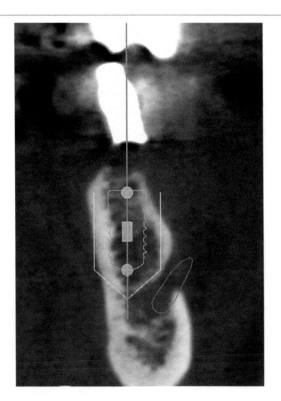

Figure 29.9 Locating the mental foramen for implant planning in mandibular premolars.

sions in these areas is recommended to avoid nerve injury (Greenstein et al. 2008).

- *Lingual concavity*: In the posterior mandible, a lingual undercut is a common finding and could result in perforation of the lingual plate during osteotomy, leading to damage of vital structures. Scan analysis studies have shown that the mean depth of this undercut can be 2.4 mm, being located about 11.7 mm from the cementoenamel junction of the second premolar (Chan et al. 2011).

Implant planning

Timing of implant surgery

Implants can be placed at different time points following extraction of a tooth. Multiple factors such as bone volume in all three dimensions, hard and soft tissue morphotype, and the surgeon's experience are involved in the decision-making process of timing of implant placement. The timing of implant placement in extraction sites, along with their advantages and disadvantages, are listed in Table 29.2.

Hard and soft tissue grafting around implants

Depending on the bone available at the implant site, adjunctive bone grafting may be required to provide adequate bone support for stability and longevity of the implant. This determination is based on clinical and radiographic examination of the site planned for implant surgery. Adequate soft tissue thickness and keratinized tissue width are important for the health of the implant and can help prevent recession and provide access for hygiene maintenance. Adjunctive procedures may need to be planned to increase bone and soft tissue volume around implants.

Additionally, 22% of the time the nerve may contact the lingual cortical plate (Behnia et al. 2000; Greenstein et al. 2008). The vertical distance of the nerve is about 9.6, 13, and 14.8 mm from the second molar, first molar, and second premolar sites, respectively (Chan et al. 2010). Gentle full-thickness flap elevation with no vertical inci-

Table 29.2 Timing of implant placement.

Classification	Timing	Advantages	Disadvantages
Type I	Implant placement immediately following extraction	Reduced surgical visits Reduced time Optimal availability of existing bone	Morphology may complicate optimal implant placement Adjunctive procedures may be required Technique-sensitive procedure
Type II	Implant placement after complete soft tissue coverage of the socket – 4–8 weeks	Increased soft tissue volume facilitates soft tissue adaptation Resolution of local pathology, if there was any during extraction	Site morphology may complicate implant surgery Varying degrees of socket wall resorption Adjunctive procedures may be required Increased treatment time
Type III	Substantial bone fill of the socket – typically 12–16 weeks	Substantial bone and soft tissue available	
Type IV	Healed site >16 weeks	Healed site with mature soft tissue available	Large variations in bone volume Increased treatment time

Source: Adapted from Hämmerle et al. 2004.

Prosthetic loading protocols

Implants can be loaded either immediately, early, or in a delayed manner. Immediate loading is when the implant is in function within 1 week of placement, early is between 1 and 2 months, while delayed is when it is put into function 2 months or more after placement (Esposito et al. 2013). The loading protocol is mainly determined by the ability to obtain primary stability of the implant. Other factors that influence this decision are the experience of the restorative dentist, the opposing dentition, and the need for adjunctive grafting of the implant.

REFERENCES

Artzi Z, Nemcovsky CE, Bitlitum I, Segal P. Displacement of the incisive foramen in conjunction with implant placement in the anterior maxilla without jeopardizing vitality of nasopalatine nerve and vessels: a novel surgical approach. *Clin Oral Implants Res.* 2000; 11(5):505–510.

Bain CA. Smoking and implant failure—benefits of a smoking cessation protocol. *Int J Oral Maxillofac Implants.* 1996; 11(6):756–759.

Behnia H, Kheradvar A, Shahrokhi M. An anatomic study of the lingual nerve. *J Oral Maxillofac Surg.* 2000; 58(6):649–651.

Chan HL, Brooks SL, Fu JH et al. Cross-sectional analysis of the mandibular lingual concavity using cone beam computed tomography. *Clin Oral Implants Res.* 2011; 22(2):201–206.

Chan H L, Leong DJM, Fu J-H et al. The significance of the lingual nerve during periodontal/implant surgery. *J Periodontol.* 2010; 81(3):372–377.

Chanavaz M. Maxillary sinus: anatomy, physiology, surgery, and bone grafting related to implantology—eleven years of surgical experience (1979–1990). *J Oral Implantol.* 1990; 16(3):199–209.

Chrcanovic BR, Albrektsson T, Wennerberg A. Smoking and dental implants: a systematic review and meta-analysis. *J Dent.* 2015; 43(5):487–498.

Chrcanovic BR, Albrektsson T, Wennerberg A. Bisphosphonates and dental implants: a meta-analysis. *Quintessence Int.* 2016; 47(4):329–342.

Esposito M, Ekestubbe A, Gröndahl K. Radiological evaluation of marginal bone loss at tooth surfaces facing single Brånemark implants. *Clin Oral Implants Res.* 1993; 4(3):151–157.

Esposito M, Grusovin MG, Maghaireh H, Worthington HV. Interventions for replacing missing teeth: different times for loading dental implants. *Cochrane Database Syst Rev.* 2013; 3:CD003878. doi: 10.1002/14651858.CD003878.pub5.

Ferreira SD, Silva GLM, Cortelli JR, Costa JE, Costa FO. Prevalence and risk variables for peri-implant disease in Brazilian subjects. *J Clin Periodontol.* 2006; 33(12):929–935.

Fiorellini JP, Chen PK, Nevins M, Nevins ML. A retrospective study of dental implants in diabetic patients. *Int J Periodontics Restorative Dent.* 2000; 20:366–373.

Fishel D, Buchner A, Hershkowith A, Kaffe I. Roentgenologic study of the mental foramen. *Oral Surg Oral Med Oral Pathol.* 1976; 41(5):682–686.

Gastaldo JF, Cury PR, Sendyk WR. Effect of the vertical and horizontal distances between adjacent implants and between a tooth and an implant on the incidence of interproximal papilla. *J Periodontol.* 2004; 75(9):1242–1246.

Granström G. Osseointegration in irradiated cancer patients: an analysis with respect to implant failures. *J Oral Maxillofac Surg.* 2005; 63(5):579–585.

Greenstein G, Cavallaro J, Tarnow D. Practical application of anatomy for the dental implant surgeon. *J Periodontol.* 2008; 79(10):1833–1846.

Greenstein G, Tarnow D. The mental foramen and nerve: clinical and anatomical factors related to dental implant placement: a literature review. *J Periodontol.* 2006; 77(12):1933–1944.

Gustinna Wadu S, Penhall B, Townsend GC. Morphological variability of the human inferior alveolar nerve. *Clin Anat.* 1997; 10(2):82–87.

Hämmerle CHF, Chen ST, Wilson TG. Consensus statements and recommended clinical procedures regarding the placement of implants in extraction sockets. *Int J Oral Maxillofac Implants.* 2004; 19:Suppl:26–28.

Jensen OT (ed.), *The Sinus Bone Graft.* Chicago, IL: Quintessence; 1999.

Kan JYK, Morimoto T, Rungcharassaeng K, Roe P, Smith DH. Gingival biotype assessment in the esthetic zone: visual versus direct measurement. *Int J Periodontics Restorative Dent.* 2010; 30(3):237–243.

Kotsovilis S, Karoussis IK, Fourmousis I. A comprehensive and critical review of dental implant placement in diabetic animals and patients. *Clin Oral Implants Res.* 2006; 17(5):587–599.

Lambert PM, Morris HF, Ochi S. The influence of smoking on 3-year clinical success of osseointegrated dental implants. *Ann Periodontol.* 2000; 5(1):79–89.

Lindhe J, Lang NP, Karring T. (eds), *Clinical Periodontology and Implant Dentistry.* Oxford: Blackwell Munksgaard; 2008.

Littner MM, Kaffe I, Tamse A, Dicapua P. Relationship between the apices of the lower molars and mandibular canal—a radiographic study. *Oral Surg Oral Med Oral Pathol.* 1986; 62(5):595–602.

Marx RE, Johnson RP. Studies in the radiobiology of osteoradionecrosis and their clinical significance. *Oral Surg Oral Med Oral Pathol.* 1987; 64(4):379–390.

Merheb J, Quirynen M, Teughels W. Critical buccal bone dimensions along implants. *Periodontol 2000.* 2014; 66(1):97–105.

Morris HF, Ochi S, Winkler S. Implant survival in patients with type 2 diabetes: placement to 36 months. *Ann Periodontol.* 2000; 5(1):157–165.

Mraiwa N, Jacobs R, Van Cleynenbreugel J et al. The nasopalatine canal revisited using 2D and 3D CT imaging. *Dentomaxillofacial Radiol.* 2004; 33(6):396–402.

Muller F, Barter S. ITI treatment guide. In: D Wismeiker, S Chen, D Buser (eds), *Implant Therapy in Geriatric Patients.* Chicago, IL: Quintessence; 2016: 88–89.

Oates TW, Galloway P, Alexander P et al. The effects of elevated hemoglobin A1c in patients with type 2 diabetes mellitus on dental implants: survival and stability at one year. *J Am Dent Assoc.* 2014; 145(12):1218–1226.

Oesterle LJ, Cronin RJ. Adult growth, aging, and the single-tooth implant. *Int J Oral Maxillofac Implants.* 15(2):252–260.

Oesterle LJ, Cronin RJ, Ranly DM. Maxillary implants and the growing patient. *Implant Dent.* 1993; 8(4):377–387. doi: 10.1097/00008505-199405000-00014.

Oh S-L, Masri RM, Williams DA, Ji C, Romberg E. Free gingival grafts for implants exhibiting lack of keratinized mucosa: a prospective controlled randomized clinical study. *J Clin Periodontol.* 2017; 44(2):195–203.

Rosenquist B. Implant placement in combination with nerve transpositioning: experiences with the first 100 cases. *Int J Oral Maxillofac Implants.* 1994; 9:522–531.

Ruggiero SL, Dodson TB, Fantasia J et al. American association of oral and maxillofacial surgeons position paper on medication-related osteonecrosis of the jaw – 2014 update. *J Oral Maxillofac Surg.* 2014; 72(10):1938–1956.

Tarnow DP, Cho SC, Wallace SS. The effect of inter-implant distance on the height of inter-implant bone crest. *J Periodontol.* 2000; 71(4):546–549.

Tjan AHL, Miller GD, The JG. Some esthetic factors in a smile. *J Prosthet Dent.* 1984; 51(1):24–28.

Vandeweghe S, De Bruyn H. The effect of smoking on early bone remodeling on surface modified Southern Implants®. *Clin Implant Dent Relat Res.* 2011; 13(3):206–214.

CHAPTER 30

Risk factors for implant therapy

Steph Smith

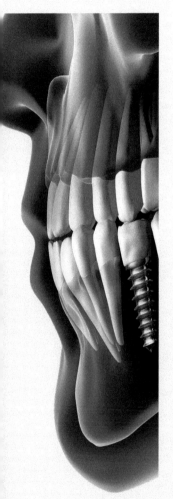

Contents

Learning objectives

- Anatomic risk factors in both mandible and maxilla associated with the placement of implants.
- Soft tissue–related factors that will influence esthetic results, and complications that can occur during implant placement.
- Presence of the biofilm around implants as related to the development of peri-implant mucositis and peri-implantitis.
- Various tobacco products influencing implant success.
- Influence of restorative design in both the supragingival and subgingival restorative zones on the development and diagnosis of peri-implant diseases.
- Influence of physiological occlusion and occlusal overload during application of axial, non-axial, and transverse occlusal forces.
- Aspects of patient compliance regarding implant planning and long-term success.

Essential Periodontics, First Edition. Edited by Steph Smith and Khalid Almas.
© 2022 John Wiley & Sons Ltd. Published 2022 by John Wiley & Sons Ltd.

Introduction

The incidence of dental implant success with regard to survival of implants and prostheses is potentially influenced by several factors (Alsaadi et al. 2008; Martin et al. 2009). These factors can be divided into local and systemic risk factors, influencing the early or late phase of implant therapy. A risk factor is a characteristic that is statistically associated with an increased risk of morbidity or mortality, but is not necessarily causally related to implant failure. More specifically, a local risk factor can pose a risk to successful osseointegration and restoration of a dental implant at the level of the implant site and surrounding teeth. Verified risk factors can be beneficial for treatment planning, establishing treatment protocols, and potentially improving clinical outcomes (Martin et al. 2009). Although the list of potential risk factors for implant therapy may be a comprehensive one, this chapter presents some important aspects of certain local risk factors, as well as patient compliance. Regarding systemic risk factors for implant therapy, see Chapter 31.

Anatomic factors

Knowledge of anatomic structures of the oral cavity that are relevant to implant placement is important so as to prevent bleeding and hematoma formation, which can lead to serious life-threatening complications (Box 30.1). It is also imperative to avoid nerve injuries to prevent varying degrees of sensory loss and pain (Ramanauskaite et al. 2019).

Soft tissue–related parameters

Commonly accepted criteria for the assessment of implant success are implant survival rates, continuous prosthesis stability, radiographic bone loss, and absence of infection in the peri-implant soft tissues. However, the focus has shifted from implant survival to include the creation of life-like implant restorations with natural-looking peri-implant soft tissues, thus underscoring the effect of esthetic outcomes and patient satisfaction (Chackartchi et al. 2019). Besides osseointegration, the quantity and quality of the bone surrounding an implant also influence the shape and contour of the overlying soft tissue, this being imperative for the esthetic outcome of treatment (Koutouzis 2019). Therefore, in implant-related treatment planning, various factors should be considered for the prevention of soft tissue complications (Chackartchi et al. 2019).

- An adequate width of keratinized attached mucosa around dental implants may lead to better soft and hard tissue stability, less plaque accumulation, less soft tissue recession, and a lower incidence of peri-implant mucositis (Bouri et al. 2008; Roccuzzo et al. 2016).
- In contrast to attached gingiva, peri-implant mucosa appears to have less capacity for an inflammatory response against external irritations, such as plaque accumulation, and tissue breakdown may progress faster at dental implants than at teeth (Zigdon & Machtei 2008).
- Long-term stability of pink esthetics around dental implant prostheses has been strongly correlated with a thick peri-implant soft tissue phenotype (Fu et al. 2011).

Box 30.1   Anatomic factors as contributing risk factors

Mandible
- The mandibular canal has a diameter of 2.1–5.0 mm (de Oliveira-Santos et al. 2012), is mostly located in the lower half of the mandible, and commonly follows the lingual cortical plate in 70% of cases (Kim et al. 2009).
- The distance from the mandibular canal to the buccal cortical margin of the mandible is about 4.9 ± 1.3 mm (range 1.3–7.8 mm) and tends to decrease with age (Levine et al. 2007).
- The vertical distance from the mandibular canal to the alveolar crest may vary considerably within and between partially and fully edentulous patients (Ramanauskaite et al. 2019).
- Mandibular canal bifurcations and related accessory foramina may be seen in 41.2–65% of patients (Shen et al. 2014).
- An anterior loop of the inferior alveolar nerve may be detected in 22–90% of patients, specifically in male subjects, and ranges in length between 0.4 and 6 mm. Accordingly, a safety distance of 3–6 mm is recommended for implant placement anterior to the

mental foramen (Ramanauskaite et al. 2019; Uchida et al. 2007).
- The mental foramen is usually located between, and apical to, the apices of the premolars in 46–62% of cases (Mraiwa et al. 2003).
- The incisive canal may feature poor corticalization and, when presenting with a large diameter, there may be associated pain and bleeding, thus preventing implant placement (Romanos & Greenstein 2009).
- The lingual foramina and their associated intraosseous canals are very common and are mainly located superior to the mental spine and in the premolar areas. These canals can be associated with branches from either the sublingual or submental vessels, or with anastomoses between both (Rosano et al. 2009).
- The prevalence of a lingual concavity (sublingual fossa) in the edentulous mandible (i.e. the second premolar and first molar region) can be up to 68%. The mean depth of the concavity can be 2.4 mm, being located about 11.7 mm from the cementoenamel junction of the second premolar (Chan et al. 2011).

- Proper assessment of the configuration of lingual concavities is crucial to avoid perforation of the lingual cortical plate during implant placement procedures. In some cases, there may be resultant damage to the lingual nerve or formation of a complex hematoma due to damage to the adjacent sublingual and/or submental arteries (Parnia et al. 2010).

Maxilla

- The diameter of the incisive foramen measures 4.45–4.6 mm and further enlarges after tooth loss, thus occupying larger parts of the atrophic anterior maxilla, and may emerge from the alveolar crest, thus potentially complicating implant placement (Mardinger et al. 2008).
- The maxillary sinus has a pyramidal shape and may extend anteriorly to the canine and premolar areas and posteriorly to the maxillary tuberosity, with its deepest extension in the first molar region. Due to continuous pneumatization, the sinus expands with age and after tooth loss (Sharan & Madjar 2008; van den Bergh et al. 2000).
- Bone dehiscences may be observed in the anterolateral wall of the sinus, leading to perforation of the Schneiderian membrane during flap elevation. Furthermore, if residual crestal bone is thin (<1.5 mm), this may compromise effective graft regeneration (Taschieri et al. 2015).

- During sinus floor elevation procedures, it is mandatory to ensure undisturbed ventilation of the maxillary sinus via the ostium naturale. Obturation of the ostium during sinus floor elevation (e.g. by dislocated bone fillers) may disturb the physiological ventilation and result in maxillary sinusitis (Hunter et al. 2009).
- Perforation of the Schneiderian membrane is a frequent complication during sinus floor elevation procedures, the risk of perforation increasing in the presence of septation of the maxillary sinus, especially in the premolar region of the atrophic edentulous maxilla (Krennmair et al. 1999).
- The incidence of septa varies from 16% to 58%, with an average of about 30%, and may be located in the anterior, middle, and posterior portions of the maxillary sinus, thereby interfering with the shape of the antrostomy (Kim et al. 2006).
- The posterior lateral nasal artery, the posterior superior alveolar artery, and the inferior orbital artery are the major branches of the maxillary artery that provide blood supply to the bony walls and membrane of the sinus. These arteries may be connected and form intraosseous and extraosseous anastomoses (Rosano et al. 2011).
- From a radiographic point of view, the intraosseous anastomoses may only be evident in approximately 50% of patients (Mardinger et al. 2007). Any injuries to these arteries can result in major bleeding (Rosano et al. 2011).

- Because of alveolar bone remodeling after tooth extraction, bone will not always be available in the correct buccolingual position, resulting in an unplanned dehiscence or thin bone at the buccal aspect of the implant (Araujo & Lindhe 2005). An absent or thin buccal bone will lead to soft tissue complications during healing (Bengazi et al. 2014).
- The distance between the implant surface and the outer contour of the buccal alveolar bony crest influences the degree of resorption of the buccal bone plate, thereby influencing the long-term stability of the underlining soft tissues (Bengazi et al. 2014; Chackartchi et al. 2019).
- Implants placed more buccally within the bucco-lingual bone envelope experience greater recession than implants placed lingually (Chen et al. 2009).
- Preservation of the width of the interproximal bone in the mesio-distal dimension is crucial for the preservation of the interdental papillae, so as to not result in soft tissue compromise (Song et al. 2017).
- Implant angulation may also pose a risk for tissue stability, leading to recession of the facial mucosal margin. This risk is increased through the combination of immediate implant placement and flapless surgeries, including a thin tissue biotype, a facial malposition of the implant, and a thin or

damaged facial bone wall at extraction (De Rouck et al. 2008; Lang et al. 2012).
- Failure to maintain flap closure in simultaneous implant installation and guided bone regeneration can lead to severe bone and soft tissue dehiscence, compromising esthetics and the long-term stability of implants (Ronda & Stacchi 2011). Flap tension is more crucial for complete wound stability than flap thickness (Burkhardt & Lang 2010).
- Various soft tissue augmentation procedures around dental implants represent a substantial part of ensuring long-term functional and esthetic stability (Chackartchi et al. 2019) (see also Chapter 17).

Dental biofilm

The success of dental implants extends beyond the lack of mobility, but also encompasses the maintenance of peri-implant health despite the constant microbial challenge in the oral environment (Papaspyridakos et al. 2012). Dental implants are placed in an oral microbial environment of commensal bacteria and potentially pathogenic microorganisms, whereby the initiation of peri-implant disease results from a bacterial challenge together with an excessive host response (Heitz-Mayfield & Lang 2010; Mombelli & Lang 1994).

- Initial bacterial colonization of dental implants happens quickly in the oral cavity for both dentate and fully edentulous patients (Quirynen & Van Assche 2011; Quirynen et al, 2006).
- Edentulous patients do not have a lower risk of developing peri-implantitis, as periodontal pathogens can reside in the buccal cheek cells of edentulous patients (Cortelli et al. 2008; Fernandes et al. 2010).
- The periodontal and peri-implant microbiomes are less similar than previously thought and may represent unique niches in the oral cavity (Dabdoub et al. 2013), indicating the complexity that includes not only titanium surfaces and the oral microbiome, but also the periodontal status of the patient (Daubert & Weinstein 2019).
- While preexisting species may colonize an implant rapidly, the microbial load has been shown to be higher at tooth sites compared to the peri-implant niche (Daubert & Weinstein 2019).
- Emerging evidence of the interplay between the titanium surface and the peri-implant biofilm indicates that bacterial adhesion on titanium is affected by surface roughness, free energy, chemistry, and titanium purity (Han et al. 2016; Pettersson et al. 2016; Safioti et al. 2017).
- Biofilm formation on implants may thus be dissimilar to teeth because of the above chemical and physical surface properties of the implant on which the biofilm is established (Lang et al. 2011).
- Biofilm at healthy implants and at sites of peri-implant disease are generally described as being similar to that associated with healthy teeth and chronic periodontitis, respectively (Charalampakis et al. 2012; Quirynen & Van Assche 2011).
- Marked differences have been reported in the composition of subgingival biofilm between healthy implants and implants with peri-implantitis (da Silva et al. 2014), including the peri-implantitis microbiome being occasionally linked to a different microbiome (Charalampakis et al. 2012; Quirynen & Van Assche 2011).
- The subgingival peri-implant biofilm has been described as one of the main etiological factors for the initiation and maintenance of peri-implant diseases and subsequent alveolar bone loss (Costa et al. 2012).
- Peri-implant soft tissues have been shown to develop a stronger inflammatory response to experimental plaque accumulation than gingival tissues (Salvi et al. 2012).
- There is however no clear consensus for a specific bacterial complex and/or a keystone microorganism that initiates peri-implant bone loss (Daubert & Weinstein 2019; Pérez-Chaparro et al. 2016).
- Microbial communities of peri-implant mucositis have been described to be intermediate in nature between those of healthy implants and implants with peri-implantitis, and periodontal pathogens may play a role in shifting from health to disease at implant sites (Zheng et al. 2015).
- Oral bacteria are capable of affecting titanium electroconductive properties, leading to spontaneous generation of electricity and corrosion of titanium implants (Pozjitkov et al. 2015; Sridhar et al. 2015).
- An eightfold increase in titanium corrosion products has been described in the plaque around implants with peri-implantitis compared to healthy ones (Safioti et al. 2017).
- Furthermore, titanium dissolution products may act as a modifier of the peri-implant microbiome structure (Daubert et al. 2018).
- For further detailed discussion on the peri-implant microbiome, see Chapter 35.1.

Tobacco products

A significant risk factor for peri-implant diseases is the habitual use of tobacco products (Keenan & Veitz-Keenan 2016). Tobacco smoke contains over 4000 potential toxins, of which nicotine is considered one of the most hazardous and addictive (with dopaminergic properties) (Javed et al. 2019). The oral cavities of tobacco smokers and users of smokeless tobacco products are exposed to high concentrations of nicotine, whereby the nicotine concentration can be up to 300 times higher in gingival crevicular fluid than in serum (Benowitz & Jacob 1984).

- High concentrations of nicotine adversely affect the proliferation of human gingival fibroblasts and their adhesion to root surfaces, thereby compromising gingival clinical attachment levels (Gonzalez et al. 1996).
- Nicotine enhances the growth and proliferation of osteoclasts that increase alveolar bone loss (Wu et al. 2013).
- Nicotine impairs the function of polymorphonuclear leucocytes (PMNs) and causes hypercoagulation of blood as a result of increased platelet activation and raised fibrinogen levels (Hom et al. 2016).
- Animal studies have shown decreased bone volume around implants and decreased bone-to-implant contact when exposed to nicotine (Soares et al. 2010; Yamano et al. 2010).
- Peri-implant marginal bone loss is statistically significantly higher in cigarette smokers than in ex-smokers and non-smokers (Levin et al. 2008). This may be due to increased production of interleukin (IL)-6 and tumor necrosis factor (TNF)-α by osteoblasts (Rosa et al. 2008).
- Nicotine and chemicals associated with waterpipe smoking can possibly induce a state of oxidative stress in peri-implant gingiva and alveolar bone, thereby increasing the likelihood of inflammatory peri-implant disease development (Javed et al. 2019).
- The prevalence of moderate and severe periodontitis is significantly higher in cigar and pipe smokers than in non-smokers, including an increase in the number of sites with clinical attachment loss of ≥5 mm, probing depth of ≥3 mm, and gingival recession (Albandar et al. 2000).

- Electronic cigarette smoking may negatively influence dental implant therapy outcomes in a manner similar to conventional smoking by enhancing oxidative stress in periodontal and peri-implant tissues and augmenting alveolar bone loss (Javed et al. 2019).
- Nicotine is an integral component in smokeless tobacco products, and it is hypothesized that peri-implant inflammatory parameters are worse in smokeless tobacco product users, especially around implants located in the buccal vestibule in which the smokeless tobacco product is placed (Javed et al. 2019).

Associated Risks with Restorative Design

Within the context of identifying the presence of peri-implant disease, two distinct and interrelated restorative zones have been proposed: (i) the supragingival restorative zone, which is represented by the portion of the prosthesis that emerges from the gingival sulcus, and extends from the gingival margin to the interproximal contact point, so as to establish the facial and lingual/palatal restorative contours; and (ii) the subgingival restorative zone, which contains the gingival sulcus, the tissue–abutment–restoration interface, and the abutment–implant interface (Dixon & London 2019).

Supragingival restorative zone

An imperative prosthetic goal is long-term implant health. This entails a subtle, vertical emergence pattern that is amenable to probing and hygiene instrumentation that most closely resembles the natural tooth emergence contours. Steps should thus be taken to minimize inflammatory states within the peri-implant tissue by placing the abutment–implant platform interface as far as possible above the bony crest for hygiene facilitation and maintenance procedures, but also vertically deep enough for emergence profile and esthetics. The correct implant prosthetic/restorative design will also allow for the early diagnosis and treatment of either peri-implant mucositis or peri-implantitis (Dixon & London 2019).

- Over-contouring of the restoration, which includes excessive heights of contour, extreme convex/concave profiles, or obstructing the gingival sulcus by means of a ridge lap/ partial ridge lap restoration or by means of restorative materials, will deflect/obstruct a periodontal probe entering into the gingival sulcus (Dixon & London 2019).
- Implants with over-contoured restorations may negatively impact proper oral hygiene by limiting accessibility to cleaning, especially when debriding deep bony defects around implants with peri-implantitis, which can lead to further disease progression (Serino & Ström 2009).
- Restorations with an emergence angle >30° in bone-level implants has been found to be a significant risk indicator for peri-implantitis (Katafuchi et al. 2018; Yi et al. 2020).
- A retrospective study has found that, during the first year after the development of peri-implantitis, implants with restoration emergence angles of >30° had around 1.74 mm more peri-implant bone loss than when restoration emergence angles were ≤30° (Majzoub et al. 2021).
- Implant position, if relatively off-center (mesial or distal) within the edentulous area, will also have a major impact on restorative contours to achieve interproximal contact. As the contact position shifts toward the middle or gingival positions, difficulties in both assessments of the gingival sulcus and oral hygiene measures increase (Dixon & London 2019).
- Implant width selection is another important consideration regarding the establishment of a proper emergence profile and thus the potential consequences for inflammation. Utilizing a wider implant platform under a wider tooth results in a more vertically directed emergence profile, easier and more direct probing, and easier hygiene procedures to maintain implant health (Dixon & London 2019).
- Implant platform switching can also result in a narrower start to the restorative emergence, which can result in an over-contoured profile, thus negating any benefit of preserving a small amount of bone initially (Dixon & London 2019).
- However, in cases where the implant diameter is close to the diameter of the natural tooth being replaced, then platform switching may be beneficial if the provisional and final restorative contours remain maintainable regarding oral hygiene and gingival health assessment (Dixon & London 2019).
- During surgery, vertical positioning of the implant platform will affect the restorative contour in creating an esthetic and hygienic emergence profile angle. Too shallow a placement will result in an acute angle of restorative material (horizontal contours) emanating from the implant abutment, and an implant placed slightly deeper (vertically) will create a more obtuse restorative angle, thereby allowing for less obstructed hygiene access (Dixon & London 2019).
- This implies that implant platforms of 4 mm may need to be placed vertically deeper relative to a 6 mm platform implant if one is to achieve the same profile dimensions. Thus, the 3 mm down rule may be too generalized to achieve proper vertical positioning (Dixon & London 2019).

Subgingival restorative zone

Crestal bone loss during the first year of function coincides with the time period when most treatment manipulations occur (Koutouzis 2019). A risk factor involved with initial bone remodeling around implants is related to implant placement procedures, namely osteotomy preparation and implant placement, as well as abutment connection procedures, coupled with the avascular nature of the implant and component systems, whereby approximately 86% of the total mean bone loss may occur before the final prosthesis placement (Cochran et al. 2009). Within minutes after implant placement, early bacterial colonization of implant surfaces and peri-implant tissues can occur (Fürst et al. 2007). Subsequent to this, manipulations will most likely occur, e.g. among others second-stage surgery for implant exposure, healing abutment connections/disconnections, and the fabrication of implant-supported provisional restorations (Koutouzis 2019). When a transmucosal prosthetic abutment is connected to a dental implant, a micro-gap is established between the components. Microorganisms may colonize the implant–abutment interface micro-gap and establish a bacterial reservoir, resulting in an area of inflamed soft tissue facing the implant–abutment junction (Callan et al. 2005; Quirynen & Van Steenberghe 1993).

- In general, the micro-gap space at the implant–abutment interface is approximately 10 μm; the mean diameter of bacteria, however, is smaller, <2.0 μm (Callan et al. 2005).
- in vitro studies have shown that complete prevention of bacterial penetration through the implant–abutment interface is difficult to achieve (Koutouzis 2019), and that the implant–abutment interface can therefore favour bacterial colonization, resulting in inflammation of peri-implant mucosa and peri-implantitis (Piattelli et al. 2001).
- However, implant–abutment interface contamination alone may not necessarily result in peri-mucositis or peri-implantitis (Callan et al. 2005; Rimondini et al. 2001).
- Implants with internal conical connections exhibit reduced risk for bacterial penetration into the implant–abutment interface under non-loaded and loaded experimental conditions, compared with implants with external and internal clearance-fit connections (Koutouzis et al. 2014; Tripodi et al. 2012).
- Some studies have also demonstrated differences in the risk of bacterial penetration to the implant–abutment interface among different internal conical connections (Jansen et al. 1997).
- Bacterial endotoxin penetration has also been shown in all specimens of implants with internal conical connections (Koutouzis 2019).
- in vivo studies are in agreement with in vitro study findings that elimination of bacterial colonization of the internal aspect of the implant has not been demonstrated (Koutouzis 2019).
- Implants with an external clearance-fit connection exhibit heavy contamination of the internal aspects of the implants.
- Implants with internal conical connection have lower counts of bacteria than external and internal clearance-fit connections.
- Trends for differences in the bacterial profiles for internal conical and internal clearance-fit connections have been shown in longitudinal studies (Koutouzis 2019).
- Animal studies have shown that positioning the implant–abutment interface at or below the bone-level crest results in greater bone loss than when positioning the interface above the level of the bone crest (Hermann et al. 2000).
- In addition, it has been demonstrated that mobility between the implant and abutment might be more important than the size of the micro-gap between those two components (Hermann et al. 2001).

- There is limited clinical evidence analyzing the relationship between internal contamination of implants through the implant–abutment interface, associated crestal bone loss, and peri-implant diseases, and the comparison of different types of implant–abutment connections (Koutouzis 2019).
- However, an association of bacterial penetration into the implant–abutment interface with crestal bone loss at the early stages of implant treatment may exist (Koutouzis 2019).
- Implant platform switching has been suggested as a method to help reduce initial marginal bone loss after implant placement, whereby the implant–abutment interface is moved inward, and thus farther away from bone. Implant platform switching may thus reduce the vertical component of the supracrestal tissue attachment (biological width) and create a greater horizontal distance to harbor the inflammatory cell infiltrate, thereby reducing initial bone remodeling (Dixon & London 2019). Furthermore, the narrowing of the abutment might distribute the biomechanical stress toward the central axis of the implant (Maeda et al. 2007), and also enable the placement of dental implants closer to adjacent teeth/implants (Baffone et al. 2012; Rodriguez-Ciurana et al. 2009).
- Other studies have however indicated that vertical mismatching (implant–abutment height) may have a greater influence on peri-implant bone preservation than does horizontal mismatching (Galindo-Moreno et al. 2016). A multivariate analysis study has shown significantly greater bone loss around implants with shorter versus longer abutments (Vervaeke et al. 2014a), and a study over a 2-year period showed significantly greater marginal bone loss around implants with abutments having vertical heights of <2 mm, 2 mm or 3 mm than around implants with abutments of ≥4 mm (Vervaeke et al. 2014b).
- When comparing titanium abutments to zirconia abutments, a statistically significant greater increase in mucosal inflammation, as depicted by bleeding on probing values, for titanium abutments has been observed in a systematic review and meta-analysis study (Sanz-Martín et al. 2018). This has been ascribed to the possibility of the surface properties of zirconia abutments showing less plaque retention, and hence inducing a lesser degree of inflammation (Nakamura et al. 2010).
- In contrast to that study, when zirconia and titanium implant abutments were compared in a 3-month split-mouth clinical trial, no differences in soft tissue health and bacterial composition were reported (van Brakel et al. 2012).
- Studies on the impact of surface roughness of abutments on soft tissue attachment have shown contradictory results. A study has demonstrated that soft tissue adhesion is not significantly influenced by material roughness on turned and acid-etched titanium abutments (Abrahamsson et al. 2002), and, on the contrary, moderately rough surfaces have been shown to be beneficial for soft tissue integration (Schwarz

et al. 2013). However, more studies are needed to be able to draw robust conclusions (Sanz-Martín et al. 2018).

- Zirconia implant surfaces show a difference in biofilm formation in comparison with titanium implant surfaces; however, the clinical appearance of peri-implantitis around titanium and ceramic implants may show some similarities (Cionca et al. 2017; Fretwurst et al. 2021). A pilot study assessing the histological classification of inflamed peri-implant soft tissue around ceramic implants in comparison with titanium implants demonstrated a similar histological appearance in the soft tissue of peri-implantitis lesions around ceramic and titanium implants (Fretwurst et al. 2021). Nevertheless, the study demonstrated interindividual distinctions regarding the immunohistological cellular composition on the patient level, irrespective of the implant material being used. It was suggested that the immune response, which is associated with patient-specific parameters rather than only the implant material used, is thus responsible for the interindividual distinctions regarding cell-type frequency. These patient-specific parameters were suggested to include implant biofilm/oral microbiome composition, different implant surface characteristics, different anatomic features like bone quality and soft tissue condition, different and/or combined etiology pathways, and individual genetic and epigenetic immunological conditions (Fretwurst 2021).

- The quality of soft tissue attachment may also play a role in the degree of inflammation. in vitro assessment of zirconia has been shown to promote a higher degree of fibroblast proliferation when compared to titanium (Nothdurft et al. 2015); however, these findings could not be translated to differential histological outcomes in experimental studies (Welander et al. 2008).

Occlusal forces

Dental/implant occlusion is complex, entailing multidirectional occlusal forces whereby axial, non-axial, and transversal force vectors occur simultaneously (Koyano & Esaki 2015). Occlusal forces (physiological and occlusal overload) are dissipated through the occlusal surfaces, prosthetic structure, implant–abutment connection, retention screw, implant body, implant–bone interface, and finally within the surrounding supporting bone (Delgado-Ruiz 2009; Glantz & Nilner 1998). Occlusal overload occurs when the occlusal load exerted through function or parafunction exceeds the resistance of the prosthesis, implant components, implant, and osseointegrated interface, thereby affecting the weakest part of the system, producing structural and/or biological failures (Klinge & Meyle 2012; Laney 2017). At the biological level, occlusal overload is produced when the amount of force overextends the adaptation capabilities of the host site (Menini et al. 2013).

- The magnitude of occlusal forces can range between 25 and 1000 N, with anterior teeth transmitting lower forces than posterior teeth, with the second molars exerting the maximum levels of force. Males generate higher biting forces when compared with females (Delgado-Ruiz et al. 2019).

- The number and location of teeth and implants, their inclinations within the dental arch, the kind of restoration, the bone quality, as well as the duration, distribution, direction, and magnitude of forces, will also influence the resultant occlusal forces (Michalakis et al. 2012; Sagat et al. 2010).

- The implant–bone interface does not possess an absorption shock mechanism able to reduce the impact of occlusal loading, thus all the forces will be absorbed by the interface (Michalakis et al. 2012).

- These forces produce a mechanical stimulus that has been recognized as crucial for the maintenance of osseointegration, or for its breakdown (Duyck et al. 2004).

- Ideal occlusal forces may produce the release of cytokines and hormones that alter the bone strength through changes in the bone mineral content, bone mass, and bone remodeling rates, characterized by increased bone-to-implant contacts and enhanced osseointegration (Fu et al. 2012; Joos et al. 2006).

- When axial loading is predominant, compressive stresses are transmitted to the implant apex, thereby generating a minimal component of stresses at the cortical bone. Non-axial and transverse loads produce a combination of compressive and tensile stresses within the cortical bone, and in the transition between the cortical and cancellous bone. The trabecular bone microstructure disperses the stress and strain, and functions as a load buffer through the trabecular network and the basal bone (Liao et al. 2016; O'Mahony et al. 2000).

- Occlusal forces transferred to the implant–bone interface will influence bone remodeling by modulating bone formation and resorption. This process of bone homeostasis is achieved by the process of mechano-transduction (Robling 2012). Mechano-transduction is the process of load transformation into biological and biochemical reactions (Ingber 2006).

- Occlusal forces are sensed by the bone and, by means of the mechanism of mechano-transduction, the loaded implant forms a dynamic complex in which forces, materials, interfaces, bone tissue, and cells (osteoblasts, osteocytes, osteoclasts, and mesenchymal stem cells) interact in an orchestrated manner, to achieve and maintain osseointegration, the stability of the implant, and the maintenance of bone homeostasis through the remodeling process (Delgado-Ruiz et al. 2019; Klein-Nulend et al. 2012).

- Thus, when an implant is osseointegrated and in function, and more bone–implant contact is achieved, then more efficient load transfer is reached. However, with overloading of the bone primarily due to improper occlusion (dominant lateral loads), as well as prosthesis and/or implant design, then loss of osseointegration may occur as well as an increase in bone loss (Korabi et al. 2017).

- When transverse occlusal forces are applied on an implant, bending of the implant components occurs and only a reduced portion of the supporting bone is involved in counteracting the load, leading to higher stress levels in particular portions of the implant–bone interface (Glantz & Nilner 1998).

- In that instance, a retrospective study has indicated that the length of the internal screw can influence the progression of marginal bone loss in the presence of peri-implantitis. With the application of transverse occlusal forces, the higher stress levels in particular portions of the implant–bone interface can be due to the transition of internal forces from the apical end of the internal screw to the supporting bone on the external side of the implant body, thereby leading to a faster progression of peri-implant bone loss in the presence of peri-implantitis (Majzoub et al. 2021). It was further indicated that this process will progress until the marginal bone level reaches the same level as the apical end of the internal screw, whereby the progression of peri-implant bone loss would then probably slow down (Majzoub et al. 2021).

- This same study, however, reiterated that occlusion is not a risk factor for peri-implantitis development, but raises a question about the possible influence of occlusion on peri-implant bone loss and even peri-implantitis progression (Majzoub et al. 2021).

Patient compliance

Patient compliance is one of the key factors for success in implant therapy. Patients thus need to be active partners in the prevention and, if needed, the treatment and management of peri-implant diseases (Cortellini et al. 2019).

- Proper oral hygiene measurements are crucial in patients rehabilitated with dental implants.

- It is imperative that the clinician creates optimal conditions (surgical and prosthetic considerations) for patients to perform adequate oral self-care and to help them improve their skills (Serino & Ström 2009).

- Elderly patients often have impaired manual skills and reduced visual capacity, and therefore have to be reinstructed in self-performed oral hygiene procedures (Dunne 2000).

- A lack of compliance has been shown to increase the risk of problems in peri-implant tissue (Cortellini et al. 2019).

- A significant correlation between increased probing pocket depth and lower compliance has been described (Frisch et al. 2014), and patient compliance has been shown to have a significant impact on peri-implant bone loss (Vervaeke et al. 2015).

- The prevalence of peri-implantitis has been reported to be greater in individuals with insufficient oral hygiene and in those who do not attend dental appointments (Charyeva et al. 2012).

- Compliance has been shown to be significantly lower for smoker patients (Lagervall & Jansson 2013), and smoking habits, as well as poor compliance, have been shown to be significantly associated with the prevalence of peri-implantitis (Rinke et al. 2011).

- Geographic distance has been found to be the most significant factor influencing non-compliance, followed by tobacco smoking and diabetes. However, pre-existing experience in prophylaxis programs (such as for periodontal disease) and the number of implants placed in the same patient have been shown to positively affect patient compliance (Frisch et al. 2014).

- It is suggested that patient compliance can be ensured by improvements in patient communication and motivation at the end of active therapy. Supportive periodontal therapy should also be presented as an essential part of the procedure prior to commencement of implant therapy (Cortellini et al. 2019).

SUMMARY

Knowledge of local risk factors during the planning and establishment of treatment protocols for implant therapy can potentially improve clinical outcomes of osseointegration and the restoration of dental implants. Surgical placement of implants into the mandible and maxilla requires precision so as to avoid vascular and neurological complications, as well as to maintain the integrity of the soft tissues around functioning implants. The prevention of plaque biofilm accumulation by means of effective access is necessary for the diagnosis and long-term avoidance of peri-mucositis and peri-implantitis, the emphasis thus being on the structural design of both supra- and subgingival implant components. An understanding of the effects of occlusal forces during functioning of dental implants is imperative for the avoidance of structural and/or biological failures, as well as for the maintenance of osseointegration and bone homeostasis. The long-term success of implant therapy is furthermore dependent on patient compliance throughout their lifetime.

REFERENCES

Abrahamsson I, Zitzmann NU, Berglundh T et al. The mucosal attachment to titanium implants with different surface characteristics: an experimental study in dogs. *J Clin Periodontol.* 2002; 29:448–455.

Albandar JM, Streckfus CF, Adesanya MR, Winn DM. Cigar, pipe, and cigarette smoking as risk factors for periodontal disease and tooth loss. *J Periodontol.* 2000; 71(12):1874–1881.

Alsaadi G, Quirynen M, Komarek A, van Steenberghe D. Impact of local and systemic factors on the incidence of late oral implant loss. *Clin Oral Implants Res* 2008; 19:670–676.

Araujo MG, Lindhe J. Dimensional ridge alterations following tooth extraction. An experimental study in the dog. *J Clin Periodontol.* 2005; 32(2):212–218.

Baffone GM, Botticelli D, Canullo L et al. Effect of mismatching abutments on implants with wider platforms – an experimental study in dogs. *Clin Oral Implants Res.* 2012; 23:334–339.

Bengazi F, Botticelli D, Favero V et al. Influence of presence or absence of keratinized mucosa on the alveolar bony crest level as it relates to different buccal marginal bone thicknesses. An experimental study in dogs. *Clin Oral Implant Res.* 2014; 25(9):1065–1071.

Benowitz NL, Jacob P 3rd. Daily intake of nicotine during cigarette smoking. *Clin Pharmacol Ther.* 1984; 35(4):499–504.

Bouri A Jr, Bissada N, Al-Zahrani MS, Faddoul F, Nouneh I. Width of keratinized gingiva and the health status of the supporting tissues around dental implants. *Int J Oral Maxillofac Implants.* 2008; 23(2):323–326.

Burkhardt R, Lang NP. Role of flap tension in primary wound closure of mucoperiosteal flaps: a prospective cohort study. *Clin Oral Implant Res.* 2010; 21(1):50–54.

Callan DP, Cobb CM, Williams KB. DNA probe identification of bacteria colonizing internal surfaces of the implant-abutment interface: a preliminary study. *J Periodontol.* 2005;76(1):115–120.

Chackartchi T, Romanos GE, Sculean A. Soft tissue-related complications and management around dental implants. *Periodontol 2000.* 2019; 81:124–138.

Chan HL, Brooks SL, Fu JH et al. Cross-sectional analysis of the mandibular lingual concavity using cone beam computed tomography. *Clin Oral Implants Res.* 2011; 22(2):201–206.

Charalampakis G, Leonhardt Å, Rabe P, Dahlén G. Clinical and microbiological characteristics of peri-implantitis cases: a retrospective multicentre study. *Clin Oral Implants Res.* 2012; 23(9):1045–1054.

Charyeva O, Altynbekov K, Zhartybaev R, Sabdanaliev A. Longterm dental implant success and survival – clinical study after an observation period up to 6 years. *Swed Dent J.* 2012; 36(1):1–6.

Chen ST, Darby IB, Reynolds EC, Clement JG. Immediate implant placement post-extraction without flap elevation. *J Periodontol.* 2009; 80(1):163–172.

Cionca N, Hashim D, Mombelli A. Zirconia dental implants: where are we now, and where are we heading? *Periodontol 2000.* 2017; 73:241–258.

Cochran DL, Nummikoski PV, Schoolfield JD, Jones AA, Oates TW. A prospective multicenter 5-year radiographic evaluation of crestal bone levels over time in 596 dental implants placed in 192 patients. *J Periodontol.* 2009; 80(5):725–733.

Cortelli JR, Aquino DR, Cortelli SC et al. Detection of periodontal pathogens in oral mucous membranes of edentulous individuals. *J Periodontol.* 2008; 79(10):1962–1965.

Cortellini S, Favril C, De Nutte M, Teughels W, Quirynen M. Patient compliance as a risk factor for the outcome of implant treatment. *Periodontol 2000.* 2019; 81:209–225.

Costa FO, Takenaka-Martinez S, Cota LOM et al. Peri-implant disease in subjects with and without preventive maintenance: a 5-year follow-up. *J Clin Periodontol.* 2012; 39(2):173–181.

da Silva ES, Feres M, Figueiredo LC et al. Microbiological diversity of peri-implantitis biofilm by Sanger sequencing. *Clin Oral Implants Res.* 2014; 25(10):1192–1199.

Dabdoub SM, Tsigarida AA, Kumar PS. Patient-specific analysis of periodontal and peri-implant microbiomes. *J Dent Res.* 2013; 92(12 Suppl):168S–175S.

Daubert D, Pozhitkov A, McLean J, Kotsakis G. Titanium as a modifier of the peri-implant microbiome structure. *Clin Implant Dent Relat Res.* 2018; 20(6):945–953.

Daubert DM, Weinstein BF. Biofilm as a risk factor in implant treatment. *Periodontol 2000.* 2019; 81:29–40.

de Oliveira-Santos C, Souza PH, de Azambuja Berti-Couto S et al. Assessment of variations of the mandibular canal through cone beam computed tomography. *Clin Oral Investig.* 2012; 6(2):387–393.

De Rouck T, Collys K, Cosyn J. Immediate single-tooth implants in the anterior maxilla: a 1-year case cohort study on hard and soft tissue response. *J Clin Periodontol.* 2008; 35(7):649–657.

Delgado-Ruiz RA, Calvo-Guirado JL, Romanos GE. Effects of occlusal forces on the peri-implant-bone interface stability. *Periodontol 2000.* 2019; 81:179–193.

Dixon DR, London RM. Restorative design and associated risks for peri-implant diseases. *Periodontol 2000.* 2019; 81:167–178.

Dunne JT. Prosthodontics for the elderly: diagnosis and treatment. *Spec Care Dentist.* 2000; 20(1):35–36.

Duyck J, De Cooman M, Puers R et al. A repeated sampling bone chamber methodology for the evaluation of tissue differentiation and bone adaptation around titanium implants under controlled mechanical conditions. *J Biomech.* 2004; 37:1819–1822.

Fernandes CB, Aquino DR, Franco GCN et al. Do elderly edentulous patients with a history of periodontitis harbor periodontal pathogens? *Clin Oral Implant Res.* 2010; 21(6):618–623.

Fretwurst T, Müller J, Larsson L et al. Immunohistological composition of peri-implantitis affected tissue around ceramic implants—a pilot study. *J Periodontol.* 2021; 92:571–579.

Frisch E, Ziebolz D, Vach K, Ratka-Krüger P. Supportive post-implant therapy: patient compliance rates and impacting factors: 3-year follow-up. *J Clin Periodontol.* 2014; 41(10):1007–1014.

Fu J, Hsu Y, Wang H. Identifying occlusal overload and how to deal with it to avoid marginal bone loss around implants. *Eur J Oral Implantol.* 2012; 5S:S91–S103.

Fu JH, Lee A, Wang HL. Influence of tissue biotype on implant esthetics. *Int J Oral Maxillofac Implants.* 2011; 26(3):499–508.

Fürst M, Salvi G, Lang NP, Persson R. Bacterial colonization immediately after installation of oral titanium implants. *Clin Oral Implants Res.* 2007; 18(4):501–508.

Galindo-Moreno P, León-Cano A, Monje A et al. Abutment height influences the effect of platform switching on peri-implant marginal bone loss. *Clin Oral Implants Res.* 2016; 27:167–173.

Glantz P, Nilner K. Biomechanical aspects of prosthetic implant-borne reconstructions. *Periodontol 2000.* 1998; 17:119–124.

Gonzalez YM, De Nardin A, Grossi SG et al. Serum cotinine levels, smoking, and periodontal attachment loss. *J Dent Res.* 1996; 75(2):796–802.

Han AF, Tsoi JKH, Rodrigues FP, Leprince JG, Palin WM. Bacterial adhesion mechanisms on dental implant surfaces and the influencing factors. *Int J Adhes Adhes.* 2016; 69:58–71.

Heitz-Mayfield LJ, Lang NP. Comparative biology of chronic and aggressive periodontitis vs. peri-implantitis. *Periodontol 2000.* 2010; 53:167–181.

Hermann JS, Buser D, Schenk RK, Cochran DL. Crestal bone changes around titanium implants. A histometric evaluation of unloaded non-submerged and submerged implants in the canine mandible. *J Periodontol.* 2000; 71(9):1412–1424.

Hermann JS, Schoolfield JD, Schenk RK, Buser D, Cochran DL. Influence of the size of the microgap on crestal bone changes around titanium implants. A histometric evaluation of unloaded non-submerged implants in the canine mandible. *J Periodontol.* 2001; 72(10):1372–1383.

Hom S, Chen L, Wang T et al. Platelet activation, adhesion, inflammation, and aggregation potential are altered in the presence of electronic cigarette extracts of variable nicotine concentrations. *Platelets.* 2016; 27(7):694–702.

Hunter WLT, Bradrick JP, Houser SM, Patel JB, Sawady J. Maxillary sinusitis resulting from ostium plugging by dislodged bone graft: case report. *J Oral Maxillofac Surg.* 2009; 67(7):1495–1498.

Ingber D. Cellular mechano-transduction: putting all the pieces together again. *FASEB J.* 2006; 20:811–827.

Jansen VK, Conrads G, Richter EJ. Microbial leakage and marginal fit of the implant-abutment interface. *Int J Oral Maxillofac Implants.* 1997; 12(4):527–540.

Javed F, Rahman I, Romanos GE. Tobacco-product usage as a risk factor for dental implants. *Periodontol 2000.* 2019; 81:48–56.

Joos U, Wiesmann H, Szuwart T, Meyer U. Mineralization at the interface of implants. *Int J Oral Maxillofac Surg.* 2006; 35:783–790.

Katafuchi M, Weinstein BF, Leroux BG, Chen YW, Daubert DM. Restoration contour is a risk indicator for peri-implantitis: a cross-sectional radiographic analysis. *J Clin Periodontol.* 2018; 45:225–232.

Keenan JR, Veitz-Keenan A. The impact of smoking on failure rates, postoperative infection and marginal bone loss of dental implants. *Evid Based Dent.* 2016; 17(1):4–5.

Kim MJ, Jung UW, Kim CS et al. Maxillary sinus septa: prevalence, height, location, and morphology. A reformatted computed tomography scan analysis. *J Periodontol.* 2006; 77:903–908.

Kim ST, Hu KS, Song WC et al. Location of the mandibular canal and the topography of its neurovascular structures. *J Craniofac Surg.* 2009; 20(3):936–939.

Klein-Nulend J, Bacabac R, Bakker A. Mechanical loading and how it affects bone cells: the role of the osteocyte cytoskeleton in maintaining our skeleton. *Eur Cell Mater.* 2012; 24:278–291.

Klinge B, Meyle J. EAO Consensus Report: peri-implant tissue destruction. The Third EAO Consensus Conference 2012. *Clin Oral Impl Res.* 2012; 23:108–110.

Korabi R, Shemtov-Yona K, Dorogoy A, Rittel D. The failure envelope concept applied to the bone-dental implant system. *Sci Rep.* 2017; 7:2051.

Koutouzis T, Mesia R, Calderon N, Wong F, Wallet S. The effect of dynamic loading on bacterial colonization of the dental implant fixture-abutment interface: an in vitro study. *J Oral Implantol.* 2014; 40(4):432–437.

Koutouzis T. Implant-abutment connection as contributing factor to peri-implant diseases. *Periodontol 2000.* 2019; 81:152–166.

Koyano K, Esaki D. Occlusion on oral implants: current clinical guidelines. *J Oral Rehabil.* 2015; 42:153–161.

Krennmair G, Ulm CW, Lugmayr H, Solar P. The incidence, location, and height of maxillary sinus septa in the edentulous and dentate maxilla. *J Oral Maxillofac Surg.* 1999; 57(6):667–671.

Lagervall M, Jansson LE. Treatment outcome in patients with peri-implantitis in a periodontal clinic: a retrospective study. *J Periodontol.* 2013; 84(10):1365–1373.

Laney WR. Glossary of oral and maxillofacial implants. *Int J Oral Maxillofac Implants.* 2017; 32:111.

Lang NP, Berglundh T, Working Group 4 of Seventh European Workshop on Periodontology. Periimplant diseases: where are we now? Consensus of the Seventh European Workshop on Periodontology. *J Clin Periodontol.* 2011; 38(11):178–181.

Lang NP, Pun L, Lau KY, Li KY, Wong MC. A systematic review on survival and success rates of implants placed immediately into fresh extraction sockets after at least 1 year. *Clin Oral Implant Res.* 2012; 23(Suppl 5):39–66.

Levin L, Hertzberg R, Har-Nes S, Schwartz-Arad D. Long-term marginal bone loss around single dental implants affected by current and past smoking habits. *Implant Dent.* 2008; 17(4):422–429.

Levine MH, Goddard AL, Dodson TB. Inferior alveolar nerve canal position: a clinical and radiographic study. *J Oral Maxillofac Surg.* 2007; 65(3):470–474.

Liao S, Zhu X, Xie J, Sohodeb V, Ding X. Influence of trabecular bone on peri-implant stress and strain based on micro-CT finite element modeling of beagle dog. *Biomed Res Int.* 2016; 2016: 3926941. doi: 10.1155/2016/3926941.

Maeda Y, Miura J, Taki I, Sogo M. Biomechanical analysis on platform switching: is there any biomechanical rationale? *Clin Oral Implants Res.* 2007; 18:581–584.

Majzoub J, Chen Z, Saleh I, Askar H, Wang HL. Influence of restorative design on the progression of peri-implant bone loss: a retrospective study. *J Periodontol.* 2021; 92(5):536–546.

Mardinger O, Abba M, Hirshberg A, Schwartz-Arad D. Prevalence, diameter and course of the maxillary intraosseous vascular canal with relation to sinus augmentation procedure: a radiographic study. *Int J Oral Maxillofac Surg.* 2007; 3:735–738.

Mardinger O, Namani-Sadan N, Chaushu G, Schwartz-Arad D. Morphologic changes of the nasopalatine canal related to dental implantation: a radiologic study in different degrees of absorbed maxillae. *J Periodontol.* 2008; 79(9):1659–1662.

Martin W, Lewis E, Nicol A. Local risk factors for implant therapy. *Int J Oral Maxillofac Implants.* 2009; 24(Suppl):28–38.

Menini M, Conserva E, Tealdo T et al. Shock absorption capacity of restorative materials for dental implant prostheses: an in vitro study. *Int J Prosthodont.* 2013; 26:549–556.

Michalakis K, Calvani P, Hirayama H. Biomechanical considerations on tooth-implant supported fixed partial dentures. *J Dent Biomech.* 2012; 3: 1758736012462025. doi: 10.1177/1758736012462025.

Mombelli A, Lang NP. Microbial aspects of implant dentistry. *Periodontol 2000.* 1994; 4:74–80.

Mraiwa N, Jacobs R, van Steenberghe D, Quirynen M. Clinical assessment and surgical implications of anatomic challenges in the anterior mandible. *Clin Implant Dent Relat Res.* 2003; 5(4):219–225.

Nakamura K, Kanno T, Milleding P, Ortengren U. Zirconia as a dental implant abutment material: a systematic review. *Int J Prosthodont.* 2010; 23:299–309.

Nothdurft FP, Fontana D, Ruppenthal S et al. Differential behavior of fibroblasts and epithelial cells on structured implant abutment materials: a comparison of materials and surface topographies. *Clin Implant Dent Relat Res.* 2015; 17:1237–1249.

O'Mahony A, Bowles Q, Woolswy G, Robinson S, Spencer P. Stress distribution in the single-unit osseointegrated dental implant: finite element analyses of axial and off-axial loading. *Implant Dent.* 2000; 9:207–218.

Papaspyridakos P, Chen CJ, Singh M, Weber HP, Gallucci GO. Success criteria in implant dentistry: a systematic review. *J Dent Res.* 2012; 91(3):242–248.

Parnia F, Fard EM, Mahboub F, Hafezeqoran A, Gavgani FE. Tomographic volume evaluation of submandibular fossa in patients requiring dental implants. *Oral Surg Oral Med Oral Pathol Oral Radiol Endod.* 2010; 109(1):e32–e36.

Pérez-Chaparro PJ, Duarte PM, Shibli JA et al. The current weight of evidence of the microbiologic profile associated with peri-implantitis: a systematic review. *J Periodontol.* 2016; 87(11):1295–1304.

Pettersson M, Kelk P, Belibasakis GN et al. Titanium ions form particles that activate and execute interleukin-1beta release from lipopolysaccharide-primed macrophages. *J Periodontal Res.* 2016; 52(1):21–32.

Piattelli A, Scarano A, Paolantonio M et al. Fluids and microbial penetration in the internal part of cement-retained versus screw-retained implant-abutment connections. *J Periodontol.* 2001; 72(9):1146–1150.

Pozhitkov AE, Daubert D, Brochwicz Donimirski A et al. Interruption of electrical conductivity of titanium dental implants suggests a path towards elimination of corrosion. *PLoS ONE.* 2015; 10(10):e0140393.

Quirynen M, Van Assche N. Microbial changes after full-mouth tooth extraction, followed by 2-stage implant placement. *J Clin Periodontol.* 2011; 38(6):581–589.

Quirynen M, van Steenberghe D. Bacterial colonization of the internal part of two-stage implants. An in vivo study. *Clin Oral Implants Res.* 1993; 4(3):158–161.

Quirynen M, Vogels R, Peeters W et al. Dynamics of initial subgingival colonization of "pristine" peri-implant pockets. *Clin Oral Implants Res.* 2006; 7(1):25–37.

Ramanauskaite A, Becker J, Sader R, Schwarz F. Anatomic factors as contributing risk factors in implant therapy. *Periodontol 2000.* 2019; 81:64–75.

Rimondini L, Marin C, Brunella F, Fini M. Internal contamination of a 2-component implant system after occlusal loading and provisionally luted reconstruction with or without a washer device. *J Periodontol.* 2001; 72(12):1652–1657.

Rinke S, Ohl S, Ziebolz D, Lange K, Eickholz P. Prevalence of periimplant disease in partially edentulous patients: a practice-based cross-sectional study. *Clin Oral Implants Res.* 2011; 22(8):826–833.

Robling A. The interaction of biological factors with mechanical signals in bone adaptation: recent developments. *Curr Osteoporos Rep.* 2012; 10:126–131.

Roccuzzo M, Grasso G, Dalmasso P. Keratinized mucosa around implants in partially edentulous posterior mandible: 10-year results of a prospective comparative study. *Clin Oral Implant Res.* 2016; 27(4):491–496.

Rodriguez-Ciurana X, Vela-Nebot X, Segala-Torres M et al. The effect of interimplant distance on the height of the interimplant bone crest when using platform-switched implants. *Int J Periodontics Restorative Dent.* 2009; 29:141–151.

Romanos GE, Greenstein G. The incisive canal. Considerations during implant placement: case report and literature review. *Int J Oral Maxillofac Implants.* 2009; 24(4):740–745.

Ronda M, Stacchi C. Management of a coronally advanced lingual flap in regenerative osseous surgery: a case series introducing a novel technique. *Int J Periodontics Restorative Dent.* 2011; 31(5):505–513.

Rosa GM, Lucas GQ, Lucas ON. Cigarette smoking and alveolar bone in young adults: a study using digitized radiographs. *J Periodontol.* 2008; 79(2):232–244.

Rosano G, Taschieri S, Gaudy JF, Testori T, Del Fabbro M. Anatomic assessment of the anterior mandible and relative hemorrhage risk in implant dentistry: a cadaveric study. *Clin Oral Implants Res.* 2009; 20(8):791–795.

Rosano G, Taschieri S, Gaudy JF, Weinstein T, Del Fabbro M. Maxillary sinus vascular anatomy and its relation to sinus lift surgery. *Clin Oral Implants Res.* 2011; 22(7):711–715.

Safioti LM, Kotsakis GA, Pozhitkov AE, Chung WO, Daubert DM. Increased levels of dissolved titanium are associated with peri-implantitis – a case-control study. *J Periodontol.* 2017; 88(5):436–442.

Sagat G, Yalcin S, Gultekin B, Mijiritsky E. Influence of arch shape and implant position on stress distribution around implants supporting fixed full-arch prosthesis in edentulous maxilla. *Implant Dent.* 2010; 19:498–508.

Salvi GE, Aglietta M, Eick S et al. Reversibility of experimental peri-implant mucositis compared with experimental gingivitis in humans. *Clin Oral Implants Res.* 2012; 23(2):182–190.

Sanz-Martín I, Sanz-Sánchez I, Carrillo de Albornoz A, Figuero E, *Sanz M. Effects of modified abutment characteristics on peri-implant soft tissue health: a systematic review and meta-analysis. Clin Oral Implants Res.* 2018; 29:118–129.

Schwarz F, Mihatovic I, Becker J et al. Histological evaluation of different abutments in the posterior maxilla and mandible: an experimental study in humans. *J Clin Periodontol.* 2013; 40:807–815.

Serino G, Ström C. Peri-implantitis in partially edentulous patients: association with inadequate plaque control. *Clin Oral Implants Res.* 2009; 20:169–174.

Sharan A, Madjar D. Maxillary sinus pneumatization following extractions: a radiographic study. *Int J Oral Maxillofac Implants.* 2008; 23(1):48–56.

Shen EC, Fu E, Fu MM, Peng M. Configuration and corticalization of the mandibular bifid canal in a Taiwanese adult population: a computed tomography study. *Int J Oral Maxillofac Implants.* 2014; 29(4):893–897.

Soares EV, Favaro WJ, Cagnon VH, Bertran CA, Camilli JA. Effects of alcohol and nicotine on the mechanical resistance of bone and bone neoformation around hydroxyapatite implants. *J Bone Miner Metab.* 2010; 28(1):101–107.

Song JW, Leesungbok R, Park SJ et al. Analysis of crown size and morphology, and gingival shape in the maxillary anterior dentition in Korean young adults. *J Adv Prosthodont.* 2017; 9(4):315–320.

Sridhar S, Wilson TG, Palmer KL et al. in vitro investigation of the effect of oral bacteria in the surface oxidation of dental implants. *Clin Implant Dent Relat Res.* 2015; 17(Suppl 2):e562–e575.

Taschieri S, Testori T, Corbella S et al. Platelet-rich plasma and deproteinized bovine bone matrix in maxillary sinus lift surgery: a split-mouth histomorphometric evaluation. *Implant Dent.* 2015; 24:592–597.

Tripodi D, Vantaggiato G, Scarano A et al. An in vitro investigation concerning the bacterial leakage at implants with internal hexagon and Morse taper implant-abutment connections. *Implant Dent.* 2012; 21(4):335–339.

Uchida Y, Yamashita Y, Goto M, Hanihara T. Measurement of anterior loop length for the mandibular canal and diameter of the mandibular incisive canal to avoid nerve damage when installing endosseous implants in the interforaminal region. *J Oral Maxillofac Surg.* 2007; 65(9):1772–1779.

van Brakel R, Meijer GJ, Verhoeven JW et al. Soft tissue response to zirconia and titanium implant abutments: an in vivo within-subject comparison. *J Clin Periodontol.* 2012; 39:995–1001.

van den Bergh JP, ten Bruggenkate CM, Disch FJ, Tuinzing DB. Anatomical aspects of sinus floor elevations. *Clin Oral Implants Res.* 2000; 11(3):256–265.

Vervaeke S, Collaert B, Cosyn J, De Bruyn H. A 9-year prospective case series using multivariate analyses to identify predictors of early and late peri-implant bone loss. *Clin Implant Dent Relat Res.* 2014a; 18(1):30–39.

Vervaeke S, Collaert B, Cosyn J, Deschepper E, De Bruyn H. A multifactorial analysis to identify predictors of implant failure and peri-implant bone loss. *Clin Implant Dent Relat Res.* 2015; 17(S1):e298–e307.

Vervaeke S, Dierens M, Besseler J, De Bruyn H. The influence of initial soft tissue thickness on peri-implant bone remodeling. *Clin Implant Dent Relat Res.* 2014b; 16:238–247.

Welander M, Abrahamsson I, Berglundh T. The mucosal barrier at implant abutments of different materials. *Clin Oral Implants Res.* 2008; 19:635–641.

Wu LZ, Duan DM, Liu YF et al. Nicotine favors osteoclastogenesis in human periodontal ligament cells co-cultured with CD4(+) T cells by upregulating IL-1beta. *Int J Mol Med.* 2013; 31(4):938–942.

Yamano S, Berley JA, Kuo WP et al. Effects of nicotine on gene expression and osseointegration in rats. *Clin Oral Implants Res.* 2010; 21(12):1353–1359.

Yi Y, Koo KT, Schwarz F, Ben Amara H, Heo SJ. Association of prosthetic features and peri-implantitis: a cross-sectional study. *J Clin Periodontol.* 2020; 47:392–403.

Zheng H, Xu L, Wang Z et al. Subgingival microbiome in patients with healthy and ailing dental implants. *Sci Rep.* 2015; 5:10948. doi: 10.1038/srep 10948.

Zigdon H, Machtei EE. The dimensions of keratinized mucosa around implants affect clinical and immunological parameters. *Clin Oral Implant Res.* 2008; 19(4):387–392.

CHAPTER 31

Dental implants and patients with systemic conditions

Fawad Javed

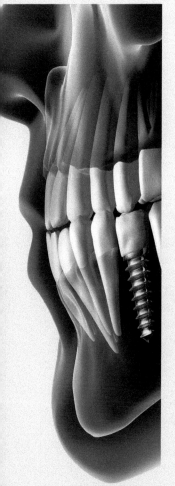

Contents

Learning objectives

- Various systemic diseases that can influence the success and/or survival of dental implants.
- Factors that may contribute toward the long-term success and survival of dental implants in medically challenged individuals.

Essential Periodontics, First Edition. Edited by Steph Smith and Khalid Almas.
© 2022 John Wiley & Sons Ltd. Published 2022 by John Wiley & Sons Ltd.

Introduction

Dental implants can osseointegrate and remain functionally and aesthetically stable over long durations, which includes high success and survival rates in systemically healthy individuals. Dental implant therapy has, however, also been reported to be successful among medically challenged patients, such as those with diabetes mellitus and AIDS. This chapter presents an evidence-based approach with the identification of original research studies that have assessed the success and/or survival of dental implants in patients with various systemic diseases.

Success and/or survival of dental implants in patients with various systemic diseases

Diabetes mellitus

- Poorly controlled diabetes mellitus (DM) jeopardizes periodontal health and is also a significant risk factor for dental implant failure (Javed & Romanos 2009; Javed et al. 2007; Oates et al. 2009).
- Diabetics have a 3–4-fold higher risk of peri-implantitis compared with normoglycemics (Naujokat et al. 2016).
- Chronic hyperglycemia increases the formation and accumulation of glucose-mediated advanced-glycation end-products (AGEs) in the periodontal and systemic tissues in patients with poorly controlled DM (Holla et al. 2001; Murillo et al. 2008).
- Animal studies have shown wound healing to be compromised with the potential of ulcer formation. This includes a reduction in re-epithelialization, as well as in insulin-like growth factor-1 and transforming growth factor-beta levels (Velander et al. 2008).
- Impaired wound healing is furthermore associated with increased expression of polymorphonuclear leucocytes (PMNs), reduced angiogenesis, reduction in the number of fibroblasts, reduced collagen deposition, and an increased expression of proinflammatory cytokines (Brizeno et al. 2016).
- Endothelial cells take up glucose passively in an insulin-independent manner, causing tissue damage (Ebersole et al. 2008).
- Chronic hyperglycemia is associated with alterations in host resistance, which includes defective migration of PMNs, impairment in phagocytosis, and an exaggerated inflammatory response to microbial products (Soory 2002).
- This is manifested in increased levels of inflammation associated with hyperglycemia, increased generation of reactive oxygen species and AGEs, a greater inflammatory response to bacterial challenge, and the possibility of a more pathogenic oral microbiota (Graves et al. 2020).
- Experimental studies furthermore have shown chronic hyperglycemia to interfere with osseointegration of implants by deferring expression of fibronectin and integrin alpha-5 beta-1 (Liu et al. 2015).

- AGEs have been shown to inhibit osseointegration and to compromise the biomechanical properties at the bone–implant interface (Quintero et al. 2010).
- Persistent hyperglycemia plays a role in abnormal differentiation of osteoclasts, thereby making bone tissue more susceptible to resorption (Catalfamo et al. 2013).
- This may explain the increased prevalence of peri-implant diseases (peri-implant mucositis and peri-implantitis) in patients with poorly controlled DM compared to non-diabetic controls (Ferreira et al. 2006; Gomez-Moreno et al. 2015).
- Clinical studies have indicated that chronic hyperglycemia is associated with peri-implant soft tissue inflammation, crestal bone loss, and implant failure (Javed & Romanos 2019). However, other studies have shown that patients with poorly controlled type 2 diabetes (HbA1c levels of 8% to 12%) can demonstrate high implant survival rates (96.6%) (Eskow & Oates 2017).
- Patients with well-controlled DM have been reported to have implants that remain functionally stable, in contrast to patients with poor metabolic control (Casap et al. 2008; de Molon et al. 2013; Kwon et al. 2005; Lee et al. 2013; Maguer et al. 2015; Tawil et al. 2008).
- Strict glycemic control can reduce microvascular complications in DM (Rocha et al. 2001). Maintenance of serum glycemic levels can improve the function of osteoblasts, and the progression of periodontal bone loss is markedly reduced in subjects with well-controlled DM compared to poorly controlled DM subjects (Taylor et al. 1998).
- Serum and gingival crevicular fluid (GCF) concentrations of proinflammatory cytokines are also significantly reduced in well-controlled DM patients compared to poorly controlled DM patients (Iwamoto et al. 2001; Javed et al. 2014).
- Maintenance of a healthy periodontal environment is essential for successful dental implant treatment (Mealey & Oates 2006), as higher scores for plaque index, bleeding on probing, and periodontal probing depths have been reported in DM patients compared to non-diabetic controls (Javed et al. 2007, 2009).
- Inflammatory reactions in the peri-implant tissues have been associated with the presence of dental plaque around implants, whereby inflammation may increase insulin resistance in a way similar to obesity, thereby also aggravating glycemic control (Maximo et al. 2009; Mealey & Oates 2006).
- Periodontal therapy has been shown to improve glycemic control in hyperglycemic patients, therefore control and treatment of periodontal infections are an important part of the overall management of DM patients, consequently playing an important role in successful implant therapy (Javed et al. 2014).
- Controversy exists over the use of antimicrobial agents in healthy candidates for dental implant therapy (Javed et al. 2013). However, the use of antimicrobial agents in DM reduces the risk of surgical wound infection and may

improve implant survival rates by 10.5%, compared to a rate of 4.5% in healthy candidates for implants (Laskin et al. 2000; Morris et al. 2000).

- A twice-daily use of an antiseptic mouthwash, such as chlorhexidine, has been suggested for the maintenance of dental implants, as effective reduction of viable *Porphyromonas gingivalis* infection and peri-implant mucositis has been shown (Ciancio et al. 1995; Leyes Borrajo et al. 2002).
- In conclusion, dental implants can osseointegrate and remain functionally stable in patients with DM provided glycemic levels are maintained. The role of routine dental hygiene maintenance therefore remains imperative.

Cardiovascular diseases

- A limited number of studies have assessed the influence of cardiovascular diseases (CVD) on osseointegration of dental implants (Khadivi et al. 1999).
- Studies have shown that patients with controlled CVD are not at an increased risk of failure of osseointegration (Khadivi et al. 1999; van Steenberghe et al. 2002).
- Patients with CVD, including hypertension and ischemic heart diseases, have been shown to be not statistically associated with an increased incidence of early implant failures (Alsaadi et al. 2007, 2008b).
- It has also been reported that oral rehabilitation with dental implants among patients with or without CVD is a valid treatment (Neves et al. 2018; Nobre et al. 2016).
- In conclusion, it seems that dental implants can osseointegrate and remain functionally stable in patients with CVD; however, further long-term follow-up studies are needed.

Hepatic disorders

- Aspartate aminotransferase (AST) is an enzyme mainly found in the liver, and plays an essential role in the metabolism of amino acids. When the liver is diseased, elevated levels of AST are released into the bloodstream. In this regard, AST level assessment is commonly performed for the diagnosis of hepatic disorders (Miura et al. 2017; Pokorska-Spiewak et al. 2016).
- Salivary AST levels are significantly higher in patients with chronic periodontitis (CP). However, mechanical debridement of plaque and calculus results in a statistically significant decrease in salivary AST levels in patients with CP (Kudva et al. 2014).
- Similarly, increased AST activity in peri-implant sulcular fluid has been associated with peri-implant bleeding on probing and bone loss (Paolantonio et al. 2000; Ruhling et al. 1999).
- No studies have assessed the influence of hepatic disorders on the success and survival of dental implants.
- However, since AST blood levels are significantly higher in patients with hepatic disorders, and increased AST activity has been associated with periodontal and peri-implant

diseases (Kudva et al. 2014), it is hypothesized that implant therapy outcomes may be compromised in patients with hepatic disorders.

HIV/AIDS

- Case reports and case series studies have reported that dental implants can remain functionally stable in HIV-positive patients with stable disease, provided that appropriate infection control protocols are adopted (Achong et al. 2006; Baron et al. 2004; Gay-Escoda et al. 2016; Gherlone et al. 2016a, b; Kolhatkar et al. 2011; May et al. 2016; Oliveira et al. 2011; Romanos et al. 2014; Stevenson et al. 2007; Strietzel et al. 2006; Vidal et al. 2017).
- There is however insufficient evidence to determine whether in the long term, dental implants can remain functionally stable in HIV-positive and AIDS patients. Hence, further studies are needed.

Crohn's disease

- Crohn's disease (CD) is an idiopathic chronic inflammatory disorder of the gastrointestinal tract, which may also affect the oral cavity (Scheper & Brand 2002).
- The prevalence rates of oral manifestations in adult patients with CD vary between 5% and 20% (Orosz & Sonkodi 2004), and may present as gingivitis, dental caries (Rikardsson et al. 2009), or ulcerative lesions involving the lips, tongue, buccal mucosa, and posterior pharynx (Estrin & Hughes 1985).
- In addition, clinical scores for periodontitis (bleeding on probing, probing pocket depth, clinical attachment loss) have been reported to be higher in patients with CD than in controls (Vavricka et al. 2013).
- Studies have shown that CD can be significantly associated with early implant failure (Alsaadi et al. 2007, 2008a, b; van Steenberghe et al. 2002; Vavricka et al. 2013), and on the contrary be associated with functionally and esthetically stable implants (Peron et al. 2017). Further long-term studies are therefore needed.

Psychological, autism spectrum, and eating disorders

- A limited number of studies have assessed the success and survival of dental implants in patients with psychological/psychiatric disorders (Addy et al. 2006; Ekfeldt et al. 2001; Griess et al. 1998; Kromminga et al. 1991; Kubo & Kimura 2004).
- Some studies have concluded that psychiatric disorders, including schizophrenia and Parkinson's disease, are not contraindicated for dental implant therapy (Addy et al. 2006; Griess et al. 1998; Kubo & Kimura 2004).
- In contrast, other studies have concluded that dental implant therapy outcomes are compromised among patients

with psychological disorders, including personal grief and depression, which have been found to be significant risk factors associated with dental implant failure (Ekfeldt et al. 2001; Kromminga et al. 1991).

- Patients with psychological/psychiatric disorders are more susceptible to periodontal disease, as poor oral hygiene status, bruxism, the repeated insertion of fingers in the mouth, and behavioral issues are common in such patients (Nayak et al. 2016; Stein et al. 2007).

- Periodontal inflammatory parameters (including bleeding on probing, probing depth, and dental calculus index) are poorer among patients with psychiatric disorders, such as schizophrenia and mood disorders (Nayak et al. 2016). Such factors may complicate dental implant therapy and jeopardize the long-term success and survival of dental implants.

- A compromised oral health status has been reported in adult patients with autism spectrum disorder (ASD) (Blomqvist et al. 2015).

- Patients with ASD can present with (i) ongoing social problems such as resistance to communication and interaction with others; (ii) repetitive behaviors and limited interests or activities; or (iii) symptoms that impair an individual's ability to function in various areas of life (Scott et al. 2017).

- A statistically significant association has been reported between ASD and the prevalence of dental caries due to a reduced salivary flow rate (Blomqvist et al. 2015). Other oral manifestations may include bruxism, self-perpetrated oral lesions, and dental malocclusions (most commonly anterior open bite) (Orellana et al. 2012).

- No studies have assessed the success and survival of dental implants in adults with ASD. Hence, further studies are needed.

- Eating disorders (EDs), such as anorexia nervosa and bulimia nervosa, are abnormal eating habits, involving either insufficient or excessive food consumption. These may jeopardize an individual's physical and/or mental health status (Bell et al. 2017; Fischer et al. 2014; Tortorella et al. 2014).

- There is insufficient evidence to determine whether dental implants can remain functionally stable in patients with EDs, and thus further studies are needed.

Conclusion

Systemic diseases are not a contraindication to dental implant therapy. Routine oral hygiene maintenance and a stabilized systemic health can contribute toward the long-term success and survival of dental implants in medically challenged individuals.

REFERENCES

Achong RM, Shetty K, Arribas A, Block MS. Implants in HIV-positive patients: 3 case reports. *J Oral Maxillofac Surg.* 2006; 64:1199–1203.

Addy L, Korszun A, Jagger RG. Dental implant treatment for patients with psychiatric disorders. *Eur J Prosthodont Restor Dent.* 2006; 14:90–92.

Alsaadi G, Quirynen M, Komarek A, van Steenberghe D. Impact of local and systemic factors on the incidence of oral implant failures, up to abutment connection. *J Clin Periodontol.* 2007; 34:610–617.

Alsaadi G, Quirynen M, Komarek A, van Steenberghe D. Impact of local and systemic factors on the incidence of late oral implant loss. *Clin Oral Implants Res.* 2008a; 19:670–676.

Alsaadi G, Quirynen M, Michiles K, Teughels W, Komarek A, van Steenberghe D. Impact of local and systemic factors on the incidence of failures up to abutment connection with modified surface oral implants. *J Clin Periodontol.* 2008b; 35:51–57.

Baron M, Gritsch F, Hansy AM, Haas R. Implants in an HIV-positive patient: a case report. *Int J Oral Maxillofac Implants.* 2004; 19:425–430.

Bell C, Waller G, Shafran R, Delgadillo J. Is there an optimal length of psychological treatment for eating disorder pathology? *Int J Eat Disord.* 2017; 50(6):687–692.

Blomqvist M, Bejerot S, Dahllof G. A cross-sectional study on oral health and dental care in intellectually able adults with autism spectrum disorder. *BMC Oral Health.* 2015; 15:81. doi: 10.1186/s12903-015-0065-z.

Brizeno LA, Assreuy AM, Alves AP et al. Delayed healing of oral mucosa in a diabetic rat model: implication of TNF-alpha, IL-1beta and FGF-2. *Life Sci.* 2016; 155:36–47.

Casap N, Nimri S, Ziv E, Sela J, Samuni Y. Type 2 diabetes has minimal effect on osseointegration of titanium implants in psammomys obesus. *Clin Oral Implants Res.* 2008; 19:458–464.

Catalfamo DL, Britten TM, Storch DL et al. Hyperglycemia induced and intrinsic alterations in type 2 diabetes-derived osteoclast function. *Oral Dis.* 2013; 19(3):303–312.

Ciancio SG, Lauciello F, Shibly O, Vitello M, Mather M. The effect of an antiseptic mouthrinse on implant maintenance: plaque and peri-implant gingival tissues. *J Periodontol.* 1995; 66:962–965.

de Molon RS, Morais-Camilo JA, Verzola MH et al. Impact of diabetes mellitus and metabolic control on bone healing around osseointegrated implants: removal torque and histomorphometric analysis in rats. *Clin Oral Implants Res.* 2013; 24:831–837.

Ebersole JL, Holt SC, Hansard R, Novak MJ. Microbiologic and immunologic characteristics of periodontal disease in Hispanic Americans with type 2 diabetes. *J Periodontol.* 2008; 79:637–646.

Ekfeldt A, Christiansson U, Eriksson T et al. A retrospective analysis of factors associated with multiple implant failures in maxillae. *Clin Oral Implants Res.* 2001; 12:462–467.

Eskow CC, Oates TW. Dental implant survival and complication rate over 2 years for individuals with poorly controlled type 2 diabetes mellitus. *Clin Implant Dent Relat Res.* 2017; 19(3):423–431.

Estrin HM, Hughes RW Jr. Oral manifestations in Crohn's disease: report of a case. *Am J Gastroenterol.* 1985; 80:352–354.

Ferreira SD, Silva GL, Cortelli JR, Costa JE, Costa FO. Prevalence and risk variables for peri-implant disease in Brazilian subjects. *J Clin Periodontol.* 2006; 33:929–935.

Fischer S, Meyer AH, Dremmel D, Schlup B, Munsch S. Short-term cognitive-behavioral therapy for binge eating disorder: long-term efficacy and predictors of long-term treatment success. *Behav Res Ther.* 2014; 58C:36–42.

Gay-Escoda C, Perez-Alvarez D, Camps-Font O, Figueiredo R. Long-term outcomes of oral rehabilitation with dental implants in HIV-positive patients: a retrospective case series. *Med Oral Patol Oral Cir Bucal.* 2016; 21:e385–e391.

Gherlone EF, Cappare P, Tecco S et al. A prospective longitudinal study on implant prosthetic rehabilitation in controlled HIV-positive patients with 1-year follow-up: the role of CD4+ level, smoking habits, and oral hygiene. *Clin Implant Dent Relat Res.* 2016a; 18:955–964.

Gherlone EF, Cappare P, Tecco S et al. Implant prosthetic rehabilitation in controlled HIV-positive patients: a prospective longitudinal study with 1-year follow-up. *Clin Implant Dent Relat Res.* 2016b; 18:725–734.

Gomez-Moreno G, Aguilar-Salvatierra A, Rubio Roldan J et al. Peri-implant evaluation in type 2 diabetes mellitus patients: a 3-year study. *Clin Oral Implants Res.* 2015; 26(9):1031–1035.

Graves DT, Ding Z, Yang Y. The impact of diabetes on periodontal diseases. *Periodontol 2000.* 2020; 82:214–224.

Griess M, Reilmann B, Chanavaz M. The multi-modal prosthetic treatment of mentally handicapped patients—necessity and challenge. *Eur J Prosthodont Restor Dent.* 1998; 6:115–120.

Holla LI, Kankova K, Fassmann A et al. Distribution of the receptor for advanced glycation end products gene polymorphisms in patients with chronic periodontitis: a preliminary study. *J Periodontol.* 2001; 72:1742–1746.

Iwamoto Y, Nishimura F, Nakagawa M et al. The effect of antimicrobial periodontal treatment on circulating tumor necrosis factor-alpha and glycated hemoglobin level in patients with type 2 diabetes. *J Periodontol.* 2001; 72:774–778.

Javed F, Ahmed HB, Mehmood A, Bain C, Romanos GE. Effect of nonsurgical periodontal therapy (with or without oral doxycycline delivery) on glycemic status and clinical periodontal parameters in patients with prediabetes: a short-term longitudinal randomized case-control study. *Clin Oral Investig.* 2014; 18(8):1963–1968.

Javed F, Al-Daghri NM, Wang HL, Wang CY, Al-Hezaimi K. Short-term effects of non-surgical periodontal treatment on the gingival crevicular fluid cytokine profiles in sites with induced periodontal defects: a study on dogs with and without streptozotocin-induced diabetes. *J Periodontol.* 2014; 85(11):1589–1593.

Javed F, Alghamdi AS, Ahmed A et al. Clinical efficacy of antibiotics in the treatment of peri-implantitis. *Int Dent J.* 2013; 63:169–176.

Javed F, Klingspor L, Sundin U et al. Periodontal conditions, oral candida albicans and salivary proteins in type 2 diabetic subjects with emphasis on gender. *BMC Oral Health.* 2009; 9:12.

Javed F, Nasstrom K, Benchimol D et al. Comparison of periodontal and socioeconomic status between subjects with type 2 diabetes mellitus and non-diabetic controls. *J Periodontol.* 2007; 78:2112–2119.

Javed F, Romanos GE. Chronic hyperglycemia as a risk factor in implant therapy. *Periodontol 2000.* 2019; 81:57–63.

Javed F, Romanos GE. Impact of diabetes mellitus and glycemic control on the osseointegration of dental implants: a systematic literature review. *J Periodontol.* 2009; 80:1719–1730.

Khadivi V, Anderson J, Zarb GA. Cardiovascular disease and treatment outcomes with osseointegration surgery. *J Prosthet Dent.* 1999; 81:533–536.

Kolhatkar S, Khalid S, Rolecki A, Bhola M, Winkler JR. Immediate dental implant placement in HIV-positive patients receiving highly active antiretroviral therapy: a report of two cases and a review of the literature of implants placed in HIV-positive individuals. *J Periodontol.* 2011; 82:505–511.

Kromminga R, Habel G, Muller-Fahlbusch H. [Failure of dental implants following psychosomatic disturbances in the stomatognathic system—a clinical-catamnestic study]. *Dtsch Stomatol.* 1991; 41:233–236.

Kubo K, Kimura K. Implant surgery for a patient with Parkinson's disease controlled by intravenous midazolam: a case report. *Int J Oral Maxillofac Implants.* 2004; 19:288–290.

Kudva P, Saini N, Kudva H, Saini V. To estimate salivary aspartate aminotransferase levels in chronic gingivitis and chronic periodontitis patients prior to and following non-surgical periodontal therapy: a clinico-biochemical study. *J Indian Soc Periodontol.* 2014; 18:53–58.

Kwon PT, Rahman SS, Kim DM et al. Maintenance of osseointegration utilizing insulin therapy in a diabetic rat model. *J Periodontol.* 2005; 76:621–626.

Laskin DM, Dent CD, Morris HF, Ochi S, Olson JW. The influence of preoperative antibiotics on success of endosseous implants at 36 months. *Ann Periodontol.* 2000; 5:166–174.

Lee SB, Retzepi M, Petrie A et al. The effect of diabetes on bone formation following application of the GBR principle with the use of titanium domes. *Clin Oral Implants Res.* 2013; 24:28–35.

Leyes Borrajo JL, Garcia VL, Lopez CG et al. Efficacy of chlorhexidine mouthrinses with and without alcohol: a clinical study. *J Periodontol.* 2002; 73:317–321.

Liu Z, Zhou W, Tangl S et al. Potential mechanism for osseointegration of dental implants in Zucker diabetic fatty rats. *Br J Oral Maxillofac Surg.* 2015; 53(8):748–753.

Mager DR, Iniguez IR, Gilmour S, Yap J. The effect of a low fructose and low glycemic index/load (fragile) dietary intervention on indices of liver function, cardiometabolic risk factors, and body composition in children and adolescents with nonalcoholic fatty liver disease. *J Parenter Enteral Nutr.* 2015; 39(1):73–84.

Maximo MB, de Mendonca AC, Renata Santos V et al. Short-term clinical and microbiological evaluations of peri-implant diseases before and after mechanical anti-infective therapies. *Clin Oral Implants Res.* 2009; 20:99–108.

May MC, Andrews PN, Daher S, Reebye UN. Prospective cohort study of dental implant success rate in patients with AIDS. *Int J Implant Dent.* 2016; 2:20. doi: 10.1186/s40729-016-0053-3.

Mealey BL, Oates TW. Diabetes mellitus and periodontal diseases. *J Periodontol.* 2006; 77:1289–1303.

Miura Y, Kanda T, Yasui S et al. Hepatitis A virus genotype IA-infected patient with marked elevation of aspartate aminotransferase levels. *Clin J Gastroenterol.* 2017; 10:52–56.

Morris HF, Ochi S, Winkler S. Implant survival in patients with type 2 diabetes: placement to 36 months. *Ann Periodontol.* 2000; 5:157–165.

Murillo J, Wang Y, Xu X et al. Advanced glycation of type I collagen and fibronectin modifies periodontal cell behavior. *J Periodontol.* 2008; 79:2190–2199.

Naujokat H, Kunzendorf B, Wiltfang J. Dental implants and diabetes mellitus—a systematic review. *Int J Implant Dent.* 2016; 2(1):5.

Nayak SU, Singh R, Kota KP. Periodontal health among non-hospitalized chronic psychiatric patients in Mangaluru City-India. *J Clin Diagn Res.* 2016; 10:Zc40–Zc43.

Neves J, de Araujo Nobre M, Oliveira P, Martins Dos Santos J, Malo P. Risk factors for implant failure and peri-implant pathology in systemic compromised patients. *J Prosthodont.* 2018; 27(5):409–415.

Nobre M de A, Malo P, Goncalves Y, Sabas A, Salvado F. Outcome of dental implants in diabetic patients with and without cardiovascular disease: a 5-year post-loading retrospective study. *Eur J Oral Implantol.* 2016; 9:87–95.

Oates TW, Dowell S, Robinson M, McMahan CA. Glycemic control and implant stabilization in type 2 diabetes mellitus. *J Dent Res.* 2009; 88:367–371.

Oliveira MA, Gallottini M, Pallos D et al. The success of endosseous implants in human immunodeficiency virus-positive patients receiving antiretroviral therapy: a pilot study. *J Am Dent Assoc.* 2011; 142:1010–1016.

Orellana LM, Silvestre FJ, Martinez-Sanchis S, Martinez-Mihi V, Bautista D. Oral manifestations in a group of adults with autism spectrum disorder. *Med Oral Patol Oral Cir Bucal.* 2012; 17:e415–e419.

Orosz M, Sonkodi I. Oral manifestations in Crohn's disease and dental management. *Fogorv Sz.* 2004; 97:113–117.

Paolantonio M, Di Placido G, Tumini V et al. Aspartate aminotransferase activity in crevicular fluid from dental implants. *J Periodontol.* 2000; 71:1151–1157.

Peron C, Javed F, Romanos GE. Immediate loading of tantalum-based implants in fresh extraction sockets in patient with Sjogren syndrome: a case report and literature review. *Implant Dent.* 2017; 26:634–638.

Pokorska-Spiewak M, Kowalik-Mikolajewska B, Aniszewska M et al. Predictors of liver disease severity in children with chronic hepatitis B. *Adv Clin Exp Med.* 2016; 25:681–688.

Quintero DG, Winger JN, Khashaba R, Borke JL. Advanced glycation end products and rat dental implant osseointegration. *J Oral Implantol.* 2010; 36(2):97–103.

Rikardsson S, Jonsson J, Hultin M, Gustafsson A, Johannsen A. Perceived oral health in patients with Crohn's disease. *Oral Health Prev Dent.* 2009; 7:277–282.

Rocha M, Nava LE, Vazquez de la Torre C et al. Clinical and radiological improvement of periodontal disease in patients with type 2 diabetes mellitus treated with alendronate: a randomized, placebo-controlled trial. J *Periodontol.* 2001; 72:204–209.

Romanos GE, Goldin E, Marotta L, Froum S, Tarnow DP. Immediate loading with fixed implant-supported restorations in an edentulous patient with an HIV infection: a case report. *Implant Dent.* 2014; 23:8–12.

Ruhling A, Jepsen S, Kocher T, Plagmann HC. Longitudinal evaluation of aspartate aminotransferase in the crevicular fluid of implants with bone loss and signs of progressive disease. *Int J Oral Maxillofac Implants.* 1999; 14:428–435.

Scheper HJ, Brand HS. Oral aspects of Crohn's disease. *Int Dent J.* 2002; 52:163–172.

Scott M, Jacob A, Hendrie D et al. Employers' perception of the costs and the benefits of hiring individuals with autism spectrum disorder in open employment in Australia. *PLoS ONE.* 2017; 12:e0177607.

Soory M. Hormone mediation of immune responses in the progression of diabetes, rheumatoid arthritis and periodontal diseases. *Curr Drug Targets Immune Endocr Metabol Disord.* 2002; 2:13–25.

Stein PS, Desrosiers M, Donegan SJ, Yepes JF, Kryscio RJ. Tooth loss, dementia and neuropathology in the NUN study. *J Am Dent Assoc.* 2007; 138:1314–1322.

Stevenson GC, Riano PC, Moretti AJ et al. Short-term success of osseointegrated dental implants in HIV-positive individuals: a prospective study. *J Contemp Dent Pract.* 2007; 8:1–10.

Strietzel FP, Rothe S, Reichart PA, Schmidt-Westhausen AM. Implant-prosthetic treatment in HIV-infected patients receiving highly active antiretroviral therapy: report of cases. *Int J Oral Maxillofac Implants.* 2006; 21:951–956.

Tawil G, Younan R, Azar P, Sleilati G. Conventional and advanced implant treatment in the type II diabetic patient:

surgical protocol and long-term clinical results. *Int J Oral Maxillofac Implants.* 2008; 23(4):744–752.

Taylor GW, Burt BA, Becker MP, Genco RJ, Shlossman M. Glycemic control and alveolar bone loss progression in type 2 diabetes. *Ann Periodontol.* 1998; 3:30–39.

Tortorella A, Brambilla F, Fabrazzo M et al. Central and peripheral peptides regulating eating behaviour and energy homeostasis in anorexia nervosa and bulimia nervosa: a literature review. *Eur Eat Disord Rev.* 2014; 22(5):307–320.

van Steenberghe D, Jacobs R, Desnyder M, Maffei G, Quirynen M. The relative impact of local and endogenous patient-related factors on implant failure up to the abutment stage. *Clin Oral Implants Res.* 2002; 13:617–622.

Vavricka SR, Manser CN, Hediger S et al. Periodontitis and gingivitis in inflammatory bowel disease: a case-control study. *Inflamm Bowel Dis.* 2013; 19: 2768–2777.

Velander P, Theopold C, Hirsch T et al. Impaired wound healing in an acute diabetic pig model and the effects of local hyperglycemia. *Wound Repair Regen.* 2008; 16(2):288–293.

Vidal F, Vidal R, Bochnia J, de Souza RC, Goncalves LS. Dental implants and bone augmentation in HIV-infected patients under HAART: case report and review of the literature. *Spec Care Dentist.* 2017; 37:150–155.

CHAPTER 32

Clinical considerations for implant-restorative procedures

Ahmad Kutkut

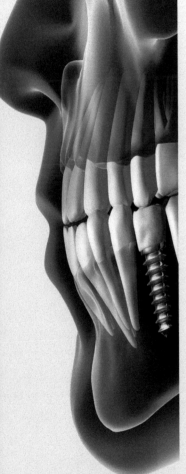

Contents

Learning objectives

- Considerations to be given for a non-restorable tooth requiring extraction and implant placement, including immediate implant placement, socket classification, and pre-surgical considerations.

- Considerations of occlusion, positioning of implants, factors influencing implant esthetics, number of teeth to be replaced, bone availability.

- Considerations regarding papilla preservation, emergence profile, space needed for single and multiple implant placement.

- Considerations for site development and soft tissue management and clinical follow-up of cases.

Essential Periodontics, First Edition. Edited by Steph Smith and Khalid Almas.
© 2022 John Wiley & Sons Ltd. Published 2022 by John Wiley & Sons Ltd.

Non-restorable tooth requiring extraction and implant placement

Cookot classification based on vascular supply

See Elian et al. (2007) and Chu et al. (2015b).

Type I *(Figure 32.1)*

- Soft tissue present.
- Intact buccal plate.

Type II *(Figure 32.2)*

- Soft tissue present
- No buccal plate.

Type III *(Figure 32.3)*

- No soft tissue.
- No buccal plate.

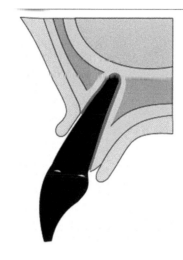

Figure 32.3 Type III socket.

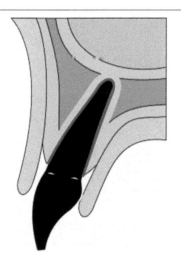

Figure 32.1 Type I socket.

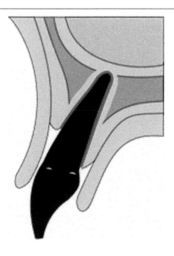

Figure 32.2 Type II socket.

Factors to consider

- Blood supply.
- Graft material.
- Membrane.

Recommendations to preserve the blood supply

- Avoid flap reflection during tooth extraction.
- Avoid creating a subperiosteal pocket during membrane insertion.
- Avoid advancement of the flap for primary closure (Elian et al. 2009; Greenstein et al. 2008).

Suggested type I socket treatment

- High scalloped, thin soft tissue, and thin bone:
  - Atraumatic extraction.
  - Graft material placement.
  - Membrane coverage.
  - Implant placement after healing.
- Low scalloped, thick soft tissue and bone:
  - Atraumatic extraction.
  - Immediate implant placement (Chu et al. 2015b; Elian et al. 2007, 2009; Greenstein et al. 2008).

Suggested type II socket treatment

- Atraumatic extraction.
- Graft material placement.
- Do not elevate a buccal flap or create a pocket (maintain buccal side blood supply).
- Membrane placement into the socket inside the defect on buccal bone area.
- Cover the socket orifice.
- Palatal single interrupted suture.
- No attempt to advance flap for primary closure (Chu et al. 2015b; Elian et al. 2007, 2009; Greenstein et al. 2008).

Suggested type III socket treatment

- Same as type II.
- Maintain soft tissue volume.
- Guided bone regeneration procedure (GBR) (Chu et al. 2015b; Elian et al. 2007, 2009; Greenstein et al. 2008).

Example of current atraumatic extraction socket preservation technique

Different techniques are reported in the literature; however, there is no evidence to support the superiority of one technique over another (Tan-Chu et al. 2014) (Figures 32.4–32.7).

Immediate implant placement in type I socket

Immediate implants *should not* routinely be placed during phase I treatment. Socket preservation with an interim partial denture (if needed) until phase I treatment is complete is the presumption. The surgeon should consider immediate implant

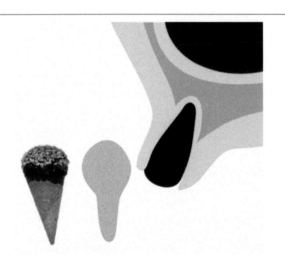

Figure 32.4 Atraumatic extraction.

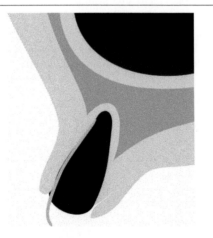

Figure 32.5 Membrane adaptation inside the socket.

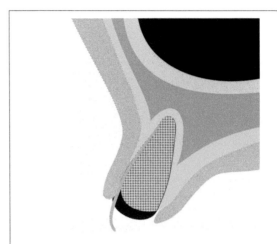

Figure 32.6 Socket preservation graft.

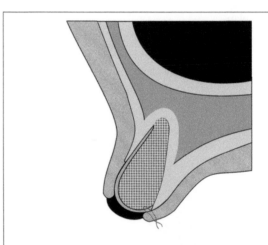

Figure 32.7 Sutures to stabilize membrane.

placement more to the lingual/palatal bone, with the long access of the implant aligned with the cingulum/central fossa of the proposed crown (Chu et al. 2012, 2014, 2015a, 2018; Sarnachiaro et al. 2016; Tarnow & Chu 2011; Tarnow et al. 2014) (Figures 32.8 and 32.9).

Pre-surgical needs

- Treatment site periapical X-rays.
- Panoramic radiograph, if needed.
- Cone beam computed tomography (CBCT).
- Mounted diagnostic casts.
- Diagnostic wax-up.
- Periodontal examination and charting.
- Surgical/radiographic guide.

Pre-surgical planning

- Age, sex, medical and dental history.
- Patient expectations.

- Smile line.
- Gingival biotype.
- Neighboring tooth position, shape, shade.
- Number of missing teeth.
- Implant size selection and papilla preservation.
- Provisionalization: removable or fixed.

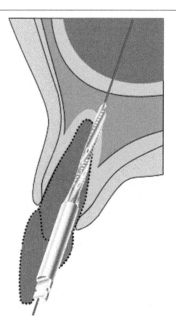

Figure 32.8 Osteotomy preparation using Lindemann Bur.

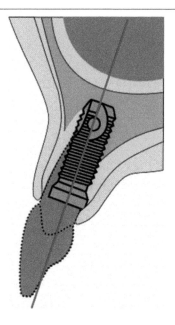

Figure 32.9 Osteotomy prepared to the palatal wall for immediate implant placement.

Pre-operative evaluation (Table 32.1)

Smile line (esthetic zone)

- High smile line: "gummy smile," showing buccal gingiva, "high esthetic demands."
- Moderate smile line: showing 75–100% of the tooth, only papilla.
- Low smile line: showing under 75% of the tooth and small papilla (Manjula et al. 2015).

Occlusion (bruxism)

Occlusal guard protection required in bruxers.

Implant occlusion considerations [14]

- Occlusal contact of the single-tooth implant crown should be lighter in casual intercuspation and equal to the natural teeth in firm closure. Some clinicians will reduce the size of contact in an attempt to compensate for the lack of periodontal ligament around the implant. If the implant prosthesis is taken out of occlusion, the risk is supra-eruption of the opposing natural dentition.
- The implant crown should avoid opposing contact in *all* excursive movements, if possible. This is especially true for posterior teeth.
- For molars, some clinicians suggest making the occlusal surface smaller buccolingually to prevent eccentric contact from decreasing the lever arm on the restorative complex (Koyano & Esaki 2015).

Factors affecting implant loading

- Cuspal inclination –> 30% torque ↑ per 10° increase in cuspal inclination.
- Implant inclination –> 5% torque ↑ per 10° change in implant inclination.
- Horizontal Implant offset –> 15% torque ↑ for every 1 mm of offset.
- Apical Implant offset –> 5% torque ↑ for every 1 mm of apical offset.

It is recommended to reduce cuspal inclination to reduce restorative complications (Sadid-Zadeh et al. 2015; Weinberg & Kruger 1995).

Periodontal phenotype (thin vs. thick)

- A flat periodontium is usually thick.
- A scalloped periodontium is usually thin (Bittner et al. 2019).

Bone sounding/bone mapping: cone beam computed tomography scan

See Hämmerly and Tarnow (2018) and Kutkut et al. (2013, 2015, 2016).

- *Three-dimensional implant positioning*: mesio-distal (M-D), bucco-lingual (B-L), and apico-coronal – implant should be

Table 32.1 Esthetic risk analysis for implant dentistry.

Esthetic risk factor	Low risk	Moderate risk	High risk
Medical status	Healthy	Under control with medication	Medically compromised
Smoking habit	Non-smoker	Smoker (<10 cigs/day)	Heavy smoker (>10 cigs/day)
Patient's esthetic expectations	Low	Medium	High
Lip line	Low	Medium	High
Gingival biotype	Flat, thick	Medium scalloped	High scalloped, thin
Shape of tooth crowns	Square	Rectangular	Triangular
Infection at implant site	None	Chronic	Acute
Bone level at adjacent teeth	<5 mm to contact point	5.5–6.5 mm to contact point	>7 mm to contact point
Restorative status of neighboring teeth	No restorations	Minor restorations	Major restorations
Width of edentulous span	1 tooth (>7 mm)	1 tooth (<7 mm)	2 teeth or more
Soft tissue anatomy	Intact soft tissue	Minor recession	Soft tissue defects
Bone anatomy of alveolar crest	No bone defect	Horizontal or vertical bone defect	Horizontal and vertical bone defect

Source: Adapted from International Team for Implantology esthetic risk assessment, www.iti.org.

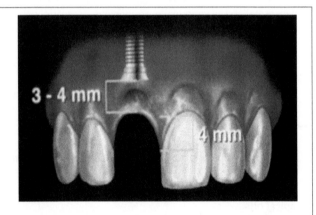

Figure 32.10 Implant platform positioned 3–4 mm subgingivally for optimal emergence profile formation.

centered mesio-distally to minimize leverage, and it should be as perpendicular as possible to the occlusal surface.

- *Apico-incisal positioning*: 3–4 mm if a bone-level implant is placed, depending on the room for emergence profile, and 1–2 mm if a tissue-level implant placed, depending on the esthetic demand (Figure 32.10).
- *Mesio-distal positioning*: 1.5–2 mm between natural tooth and implant and minimum 3 mm between implant and implant (Figure 32.11).
- *Labio-palatal positioning*: Recommended to place the implant minimum 1 mm, ideally 2 mm from the buccal bone. For cement-retained restorations, the implant should be in the center of the long axis of the implant crown. For screw-retained restorations (not common), the implant should be placed slightly palatal to the long axis of the crown (Figures 32.12 and 32.13).

Diagnostic assessment of a hopeless tooth

See Al-Sabbagh and Kutkut (2015) and Kutkut et al. (2012a, b).

Positive factors for favorable implant esthetics
- Tooth position/free gingival margin (FGM): more coronal.
- Gingival form: flat/not scalloped.
- Gingival biotype: thick.
- Tooth shape: square.
- Position of the osseous crest: high.

Negative factors for favorable implant esthetics
- Tooth position/FGM: receded.
- Gingival form: high scalloped.
- Biotype: thin.
- Tooth shape: triangular.
- Position of the osseous crest: apical.

Number of missing dentition

- Single implant:
  - High degree of predictability.
- Multiple adjacent implants:
  - Resorption of the ridge occurs after the loss of multiple teeth.

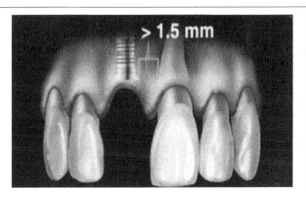
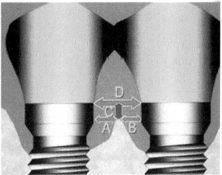

Figure 32.11 The minimum distance between an implant and a tooth is 1.5 mm, and between two implants is 3 mm.

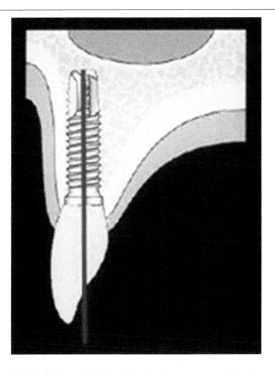

Figure 32.12 Labio-palatal positioning for a screw-retained crown.

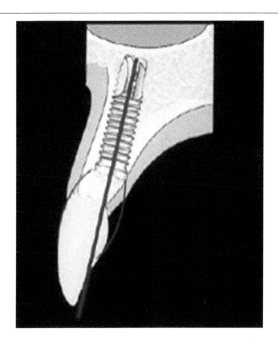

Figure 32.13 Labio-palatal positioning for a cement-retained crown.

- Difficulty in re-establishing a naturally appearing inter-implant papilla between two adjacent implants.
- Reducing the number of implants will help improve the esthetic outcome (Figure 32.14).

Bone availability and implant size

Implant size and type are to be determined based on the diagnostic wax-up of the edentulous site. If the optimal treatment site is unacceptable because there is not adequate bone available, GBR/grafting techniques will be employed, with the subsequent delayed placement of the implant. CBCT scan may be required as a diagnostic tool before the surgical treatment visit. Each student should become familiar with the basic treatment planning procedures for Straumann implants.

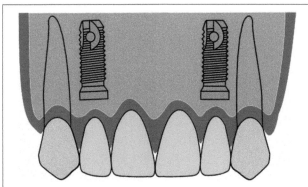

Figure 32.14 Reducing the number of implants will help improve the esthetic outcome. Given the example of four missing anterior teeth, considering two implants at the lateral incisor positions provides a better esthetic outcome by supporting a four-unit bridge with ovate pontics, instead of replacing the teeth with four implants individually.

Alveolar ridge defect classification

- Class I: Bucco-lingual loss of tissue with normal ridge height.
- Class II: Apico-coronal loss of tissue with normal ridge width.
- Class III: Combination bucco-lingual, apico-coronal loss of tissue resulting in loss of normal height and width (Greenstein & Tarnow 2006; Seibert 1983) (Figure 32.15).

CBCT imaging is becoming increasingly common for implant treatment planning. Analysis of the image using available software makes measuring heights and widths accurate and fairly easy.

In those cases where a CBCT is unavailable, the use of an X-ray template with X-ray reference spheres is recommended:

- The selected implant positions are marked on the study cast. The X-ray reference spheres are fixed at the marked points, and the vacuum-formed template is then made with the spheres.
- The subsequently taken X-ray shows the vertical bone availability and mucosal thickness from which the corresponding implant length and type can be derived, taking into account the enlargement factor.
- The X-ray reference sphere has a diameter of 5 mm. The image of the sphere on the X-ray provides the reference value for the magnification scale.

Interdental papillae preservation

If the distance from bone level on the adjacent tooth to the contact point is <5 mm it leads to 100% papilla regeneration (Figures 32.16 and 32.17) (Choquet et al. 2001; Elian et al. 2011; Esposito et al. 1993; Greenstein & Tarnow 2014; Grunder 2000; Tarnow et al. 1992).

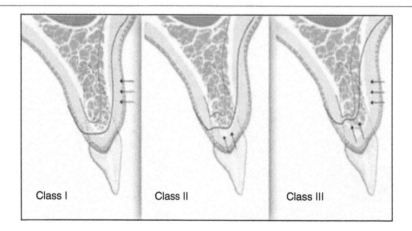

Figure 32.15 Seibert classification of alveolar ridge defects. Source: Adapted from Seibert 1983.

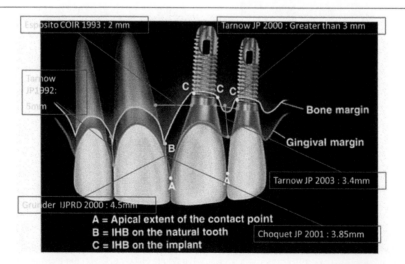

Figure 32.16 The ideal distance between an implant and a tooth is 2 mm, and the minimum distance between two implants is 3 mm. To maintain the papilla between restored implants, the distance between the interproximal bone and the contact area is less than 5 mm.

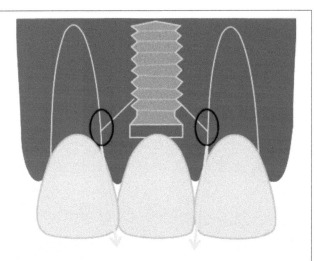

Figure 32.17 For the presence of a papilla, the bone level on the tooth side is the determining factor, not that on the implant side.

For the presence of a papilla, the bone level on the tooth side is the determining factor, not that on the implant side.

Emergence profile

The emergence profile is the contour of a restoration, such as a crown on a dental implant abutment, as it relates to the adjacent tissues (Kutkut et al. 2013, 2015) (Figures 32.18 and 32.19).

Space needed for placement – single missing tooth replacement *(Greenstein et al. 2019)*

The Straumann® dental implant system comprises four implant lines (Figure 32.20):

- Straumann *Standard* has a smooth neck section of 2.8 mm and is suitable for single-stage procedures, when the implant is not covered with soft tissues during the healing phase (transgingival healing).
- Straumann *Standard Plus* has a shorter smooth neck section of 1.8 mm, which allows for submerged healing as well as transgingival healing. It is useful in the anterior region and case of the thin periosteal flap.
- Straumann *Tapered Effect* is a combination of the two shapes, designed to mimic a tooth's alveolus.
- Straumann *Bone Level* is a CrossFit implant-abutment connection that is self-guiding and has simple positioning. It is used mainly in the anterior esthetic zone.

Depending upon the implant type, these four implants are available with the following specifications:

- Lengths from 6 to 16 mm (in 2 mm increments).
- Endosteal diameters of 3.3 mm, 4.1 mm, and 4.8 mm.
- Shoulder diameters:
  - 3.5 mm (narrow neck – NN).
  - 4.8 mm (regular neck – RN).
  - 6.5 mm (wide neck – WN).

Space requirements

Mesio-distal width

The shoulder diameter of the implant and the gap width (the available space between teeth) are vital dimensions for the restorative dentist (Table 32.2). Here is the sequence:

- As a first step, the distance between two teeth can be determined by measuring the width of the gap. Depending on the tooth shape, the gap width at the level of the proximal contact areas is about 1 mm (2 × 0.5 mm) *less* than the distance at bone level.
- The minimum gap width for the various implant types can be derived accordingly. For instance: mm (shoulder width) + (2 × 1 mm) ≥6.8 mm minimum gap width.

Bucco-lingual width
See Figure 32.20.

Vertical space

Prior to surgery, the restorative dentist will determine the available vertical space for a prosthetic clinical crown by measuring from the crest of the residual alveolar bone to the opposing dentition. This may be done either intraorally or on the mounted diagnostic casts (soft tissue thickness is estimated: maxillary ~2 mm; mandibular ~1 mm). If the actual

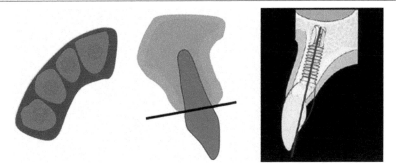

Figure 32.18 Ideally, the implant should be positioned lingually and 3–4 mm subgingivally.

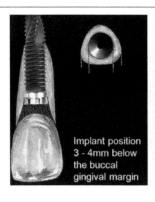
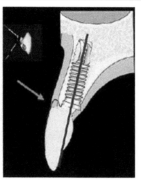

Implant position 3 - 4mm below the buccal gingival margin

Figure 32.19 If the implant is not apical enough, a ridge lap shape design is required.

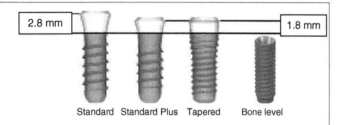

2.8 mm   1.8 mm

Standard   Standard Plus   Tapered   Bone level

Figure 32.20 Straumann dental implant system.

Table 32.2 Shoulder diameter of implant and gap width.

	Narrow neck	Regular neck	Wide neck
Implant shoulder	3.5 mm	4.8 mm	6.5 mm
Space on either side to adjacent tooth	1.0–1.5 mm	1.0–1.5 mm	1.0–1.5 mm
Minimum gap width	5.5 mm (6 mm is better)	6.8 mm (7 mm is standard)	8.5 mm (9 mm is better)

thickness is greater, the clinician will have more vertical space than anticipated. The minimum requirements are outlined in Table 32.3.

Maxillary premolar considerations

- Often, a buccal concavity in the bone exists due to tooth loss. If implants are placed palatally, the restoration is cantilevered buccally. Thus, a lever arm may be created, increasing the undesirable force on the components.
- Often, significant bone is lost in the vertical direction. If implants are placed in this situation, a longer tooth (occlusogingivally) may result (when viewed from the buccal). This tooth will not be in harmony with the height of the adjacent teeth.

Table 32.3 Vertical space requirements.

Solid abutment	PFM with metal occlusal Minimum space recommended	PFM with porcelain occlusal Minimum space recommended
4.0 mm RN abutment (yellow)	5.5 mm	6.0 mm
5.5 mm RN abutment (gray)	7.0 mm	7.5 mm
7.0 mm RN abutment (blue)	8.5 mm	9.0 mm
4.0 mm WN abutment (green)	5.5 mm	6.0 mm
5.5 mm WN abutment (brown)	7.0 mm	7.5 mm

PFM, porcelain fused to metal crown; RN, regular neck; WN, wide neck.

- Site preparation usually prevents these problems. Site preparation generally involves augmentation with bone only or with bone and soft tissue. Proper site preparation allows for optimal implant placement for the surgeon and better function and esthetics for the restoring dentist.

Mandibular premolar considerations

- Again, there may be a buccal concavity in the bone.
- The limiting factor for placement of an implant for a mandibular premolar may be the position of the mental nerve, foramen, and loop.
- There is often inadequate vertical height of bone superior to the nerve to allow for implant placement.

Single molar considerations

Before implant placement, the clinician will measure the mesio-distal space to be restored. If there has been a mesial drift of the second molar, the occlusal load on the implant restoration may be lessened due to the decreased mesio-distal space. The restoration may be only the size of a premolar, but a more predictable restoration is the result. Adequate vertical space is required.

The bucco-lingual width of the bone needed is >6.0 mm. This allows placement of a 4.1 mm wide implant with 1 mm of bone on each side. The bucco-lingual width of 7.0 mm allows placement of the 4.8 mm diameter implant.

- *Limitations*:
  - For a single missing maxillary molar, the most common limiting factor is the vertical bone height below the maxillary sinus and the opposing occlusion.

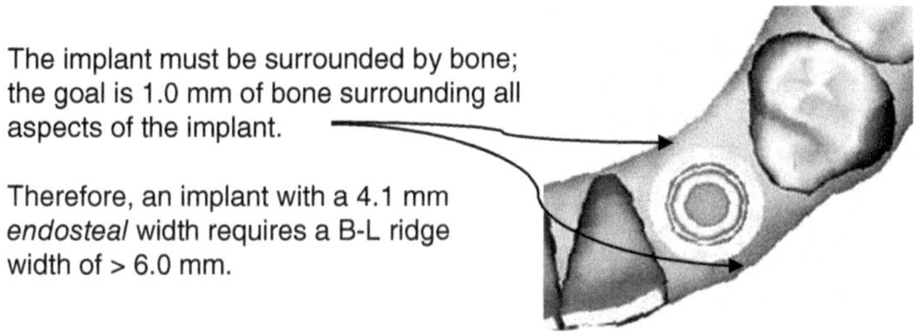

The implant must be surrounded by bone; the goal is 1.0 mm of bone surrounding all aspects of the implant.

Therefore, an implant with a 4.1 mm *endosteal* width requires a B-L ridge width of > 6.0 mm.

Figure 32.21 Bucco-lingual width. B, buccal; L, lingual.

- For a single missing mandibular molar, the most common limiting factor is the bone height above the inferior alveolar nerve and opposing occlusion.
- *Position*:
  - Center the implant mesio-distally to direct the force on the implant along the long axis.
  - If the implant is positioned to the mesial or distal, a cantilever is created, which tends to loosen or stress the screw joint.
- *Fabrication of the restoration*:
  - Narrowing the occlusal surface bucco-lingually will reduce the occlusal load on the restoration.
  - Reducing the cusp inclines of the restoration has been suggested to reduce the occlusal load in the horizontal direction.
  - Ideally, in mediotrusion, laterotrusion, and protrusion, the molar single-tooth replacement should be out of occlusion to guard against overloading. This is most important for patients with parafunctional habits and less than ideal anterior guidance.

Multiple missing teeth replacement

Bucco-lingual placement

The ideal placement is in the bucco-lingual center of the occlusal surface. This places the force primarily in the long axis and decreases the cantilever effect buccally or lingually, and thus reduces the bending moment. Implants placed to the lingual create a lever arm or cantilever to the buccal, which amplifies the load on the components.

In general, splinted implants have a mechanical advantage at the implant level.

Ideally, implants should be loaded along the long axis. Implants placed at an angle and prosthetically restored have an increase in shear force on the components. The clinician should be conservative in the design of the implant prosthesis on angled implants.

Vertical space

The minimum vertical space needed from the superior aspect of the implant to the opposing occlusion depends on the abutment selected.

Before implant placement, the clinician should analyze the vertical space and the plane of occlusion. If inadequate space is available, there are several options to gain additional space:

- Enameloplasty or occlusal adjustment of the opposing dentition.
- Restoration of the opposing dentition and "normalizing" of the plane of occlusion.
- Orthodontics.
- Segmental osteotomy plus orthodontics.

Distance between implants

The distance between implants, center to center, must be 7 mm (with 3.5 or 4.1 mm implants). This leaves 3 mm of vital bone between the implant surface or 1.5 mm of the bone surrounding each implant.

If a wider implant is utilized, this distance must be increased. When a 5 mm implant is used, the distance should be 8 mm center to center.

Determining the number of implants to be utilized

Measure the mesio-distal width of the edentulous space between the proximal tooth surfaces. Some clinicians use the following formula for RN implant shoulders (4.8 mm):

$$\frac{(x - 1\ mm)}{7} = \#\ of\ implants,$$ where x = the mesio-distal width

If x $\geq$22 mm, 3 implants are possible.
If x $\geq$15 mm, but <22 mm, 2 implants are possible.
If x <15 mm, 1 implant is possible.

If the team considers a mixture of RN and WN implant shoulders, this formula does not work as well. Refer to the Straumann product literature.

Ridge width

The clinician should confirm (through radiographs, CBCT, sounding, or other means) a 6.0 mm width ridge for the 3.5 mm or 4.1 mm and 7.0 mm for the 4.8 mm implant. This allows 1 mm of vital bone on the facial and lingual surface of the implant. See Figure 32.21.

Spaces required between implants based on tooth site and implant diameter are summarized in Figure 32.22.

Site development

Esthetic implant restorations depend on adequate bone volume and appropriate soft tissue quantity and quality (Elian

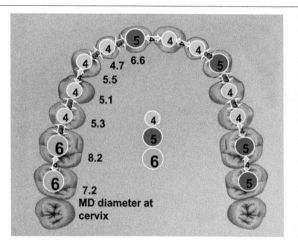
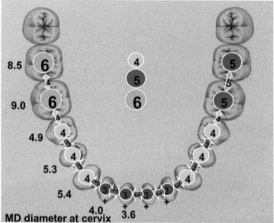

Figure 32.22 Summary of the spaces between implants based on tooth site and implant diameter.

et al. 2008; Gotta et al. 2008; Kutkut et al. 2011, 2012a, b; Ogihara & Tarnow 2015; Urbani et al. 1998; Wallace et al. 2012). Site development techniques include:

- *Extraction socket graft (ridge) preservation*: Immediate placement of a grafting material in the extraction socket following a tooth extraction to preserve the bone and soft tissue contour by avoiding bone resorption with a resultant ridge defect.
- *Guided bone/tissue regeneration (GBR/GTR)*: Any procedure designed to enlarge or increase the dimension of the existing deformed bone/soft tissue using a barrier membrane.
- *Maxillary sinus augmentation*: Augmentation of the antral floor with bone graft and/or bone substitutes to accommodate dental implant insertion.
- *Block grafts*: Onlay block of bone harvested intraorally (from ramus or anterior mandible) or extraorally (from the iliac crest).
- *Distraction osteogenesis (DO)*: Formation of new soft tissue and bone between vascular bone surfaces created by an osteotomy and separated by gradual and controlled distraction.
- *Forced eruption/orthodontic movement*: Formation of new soft tissue and bone by slow orthodontic extrusion of the non-restorable tooth.

Soft tissue management

Implants can achieve successful osseointegration. However, a clinically successful dental implant is one that not only achieves osseointegration, but also has a healthy soft tissue environment that helps to recreate a natural-looking restoration, and this may also reduce the potential risk of peri-implantitis (Berglundh et al. 2018).

The problems involved in soft tissue management include:

- Soft tissue recession.
- Loss of papilla.
- Peri-implantitis.

Its goals are to:

- Increase keratinized tissue.

- Increase the volume of soft tissue.
- Preserve the papilla.

Appropriate times for soft tissue surgery are:

- Before implant placement.
- During stage 1 surgery.
- During stage 2 surgery.
- After restoration.

Soft tissue management techniques include:

- Incision and flap design:
  - Papillae-saving incision flap.
  - H-design flap.
  - Apically positioned flap (APF).
- Grafting procedures:
  - Connective tissue graft (CTG).
  - Free gingival graft (FGG).
  - Allogenic graft (AG).
- Combined techniques: incision/flap design and grafting.

Follow-up

Clinical follow-up for completed implant cases should be performed every six months. Clinical examination to evaluate peri-implant soft and hard tissues along with the probing depth and occlusal evaluation is required. Radiographic assessment with peri-apical (PA), bitewing (BW), and/or panoramic (PAN) X-rays required as needed (in case of a deep pocket, tissue loss, or infection related to implant site). Regular radiographic assessment should be performed not less than three years after implant placement, PA or PAN may be advised for healthy implant sites every three years.

See also the following appendices:

- Appendix 4. Indications for Cone Beam CT in Implant Dentistry.
- Appendix 5. Imaging Modalities for Clinical Situations and Their Specific Indications.
- Appendix 6. Radiographic Selection Criteria for Dental Implants.

REFERENCES

Al-Sabbagh M, Kutkut A. Immediate implant placement: surgical techniques for prevention and management of complications. *Dent Clin North Am.* 2015; 59:73–95.

Berglundh T, Armitage G, Araujo MG et al. Peri-implant diseases and conditions: consensus report of workgroup 4 of the 2017 World Workshop on the Classification of Periodontal and Peri-Implant Diseases and Conditions. *J Periodontol.* 2018; 89:S313–S318.

Bittner N, Schulze-Späte U, Silva C et al. Changes of the alveolar ridge dimension and gingival recession associated with implant position and tissue phenotype with immediate implant placement: a randomised controlled clinical trial. *Int J Oral Implantol.* 2019; 12:469–480.

Choquet V, Hermans M, Adriaenssens P et al. Clinical and radiographic evaluation of the papilla level adjacent to single-tooth dental implants. A retrospective study in the maxillary anterior region. *J Periodontol.* 2001; 72:1364–1371.

Chu SJ, Hochman MN, Tan-Chu JH, Mieleszko AJ, Tarnow DP. A novel prosthetic device and method for guided tissue preservation of immediate postextraction socket implants. *Int J Periodontics Restorative Dent.* 2014; 34:9–17.

Chu SJ, Saito H, Salama MA et al. Flapless postextraction socket implant placement, part 3: the effects of bone grafting and provisional restoration on soft tissue color change – a retrospective pilot study. *Int J Periodontics Restorative Dent.* 2018; 38:509–516.

Chu SJ, Salama MA, Garber DA, et al. Flapless postextraction socket implant placement, part 2: the effects of bone grafting and provisional restoration on peri-implant soft tissue height and thickness – a retrospective study. *Int J Periodontics Restorative Dent.* 2015a; 35:803–809.

Chu SJ, Salama MA, Salama H et al. The dual-zone therapeutic concept of managing immediate implant placement and provisional restoration in anterior extraction sockets. *Compend Contin Educ Dent.* 2012; 33:524–532.

Chu SJ, Sarnachiaro GO, Hochman MN, Tarnow DP. Subclassification and clinical management of extraction sockets with labial dentoalveolar dehiscence defects. *Compend Contin Educ Dent.* 2015b; 36:516–522.

Elian N, Cho SC, Froum S, Smith RB, Tarnow DP. A simplified socket classification and repair technique. *Pract Proced Aesthet Dent.* 2007; 19:99–104.

Elian N, Ehrlich B, Jalbout Z, Cho SC, Froum S, Tarnow D. A restoratively driven ridge categorization, as determined by incorporating ideal restorative positions on radiographic templates utilizing computed tomography scan analysis. *Clin Implant Dent Relat Res.* 2009; 11:272–278.

Elian N, Jalbout Z, Ehrlich B et al. A two-stage full-arch ridge expansion technique: review of the literature and clinical guidelines. *Implant Dent.* 2008; 17:16–23.

Elian N, Bloom M, Dard M et al. Effect of interimplant distance (2 and 3 mm) on the height of interimplant bone crest: a histomorphometric evaluation. *J Periodontol.* 2011; 82:1749–1756.

Esposito M, Ekestubbe A, Gröndahl K. Radiological evaluation of marginal bone loss at tooth surfaces facing single Brånemark implants. *Clin Oral Implants Res.* 1993; 4:151–157.

Gotta S, Sarnachiaro GO, Tarnow DP. Distraction osteogenesis and orthodontic therapy in the treatment of malpositioned osseointegrated implants: a case report. *Pract Proced Aesthet Dent.* 2008; 20:401–405.

Greenstein G, Cavallaro J, Romanos G, Tarnow D. Clinical recommendations for avoiding and managing surgical complications associated with implant dentistry: a review. *J Periodontol.* 2008; 79:1317–1329.

Greenstein G, Cavallaro J, Tarnow D. Dental implantology: numbers clinicians need to know. *Compend Contin Educ Dent.* 2019; 40:e1–e26.

Greenstein G, Tarnow D. The mental foramen and nerve: clinical and anatomical factors related to dental implant placement: a literature review. *J Periodontol.* 2006; 77:1933–1943.

Greenstein G, Tarnow D. Using papillae-sparing incisions in the esthetic zone to restore form and function. *Compend Contin Educ Dent.* 2014; 35:315–322.

Grundei U. Stability of the mucosal topography around single-tooth implants and adjacent teeth: 1-year results. *Int J Periodontics Restorative Dent.* 2000; 20:11–17.

Hämmerle CHF, Tarnow D. The etiology of hard- and soft-tissue deficiencies at dental implants: a narrative review. *J Periodontol.* 2018; 89:S291–S303.

Koyano K, Esaki D. Occlusion on oral implants: current clinical guidelines. *J Oral Rehabil.* 2015; 42:153–161.

Kutkut A, Abu-Hammad O, Frazer R. A simplified technique for implant-abutment level impression after soft tissue adaptation around provisional restoration. *Dent J (Basel).* 2016; 4(2):E14.

Kutkut A, Abu-Hammad O, Mitchell R. Esthetic considerations for reconstructing implant emergence profile using titanium and zirconia custom implant abutments: fifty case series report. *J Oral Implantol.* 2015; 41:554–561.

Kutkut A, Andreana S, Kim HL, Monaco E Jr. Extraction socket preservation graft before implant placement with calcium sulfate hemihydrate and platelet-rich plasma: a clinical and histomorphometric study in humans. *J Periodontol.* 2012a; 83:401–409.

Kutkut A, Andreana S, Monaco E Jr. Clinical and radiographic evaluation of single-tooth dental implants placed in grafted extraction sites: a one-year report. *J Int Acad Periodontol.* 2013; 15:113–124.

Kutkut A, Andreana S, Monaco E. Esthetic consideration for alveolar socket preservation prior to implant placement: description of a technique and 80-case series report. *Gen Dent.* 2012b;60:e398–e403.

Kutkut AM, Andreana S, Kim HL, Monaco E. Clinical recommendation for treatment planning of sinus augmentation procedures by using presurgical CAT scan images: a preliminary report. *Implant Dent.* 2011; 20:413–417.

Manjula WS, Sukumar MR, Kishorekumar S, Gnanashanmugam K, Mahalakshmi K. Smile: a review. *J Pharm Bioallied Sci.* 2015; 7:S271–S275.

Ogihara S, Tarnow DP. Efficacy of forced eruption/enamel matrix derivative with freeze-dried bone allograft or with demineralized freeze-dried bone allograft in infrabony defects: a randomized trial. *Quintessence Int.* 2015; 46:481–490.

Sadid-Zadeh R, Kutkut A, Kim H. Prosthetic failure in implant dentistry. *Dent Clin North Am.* 2015; 59:195–214.

Sarnachiaro GO, Chu SJ, Sarnachiaro E, Gotta SL, Tarnow DP. Immediate implant placement into extraction sockets with labial plate dehiscence defects: a clinical case series. *Clin Implant Dent Relat Res.* 2016; 18:821–829.

Seibert JS. Reconstruction of deformed, partially edentulous ridges, using full thickness onlay grafts. Part I. Technique and wound healing. *Compend Contin Educ Dent.* 1983; 4:437–453.

Tan-Chu JH, Tuminelli FJ, Kurtz KS, Tarnow DP. Analysis of buccolingual dimensional changes of the extraction socket using the "ice cream cone" flapless grafting technique. *Int J Periodontics Restorative Dent.* 2014; 34:399–403.

Tarnow DP, Chu SJ, Salama MA et al. Flapless postextraction socket implant placement in the esthetic zone: part 1. The effect of bone grafting and/or provisional restoration on facial-palatal ridge dimensional change – a retrospective cohort study. *Int J Periodontics Restorative Dent.* 2014; 34:323–331.

Tarnow DP, Chu SJ. Human histologic verification of osseointegration of an immediate implant placed into a fresh extraction socket with excessive gap distance without primary flap closure, graft, or membrane: a case report. *Int J Periodontics Restorative Dent.* 2011; 31(5):515–521.

Tarnow DP, Magner AW, Fletcher P. The effect of the distance from the contact point to the crest of bone on the presence or absence of the interproximal dental papilla. *J Periodontol.* 1992; 63(12):995–996.

Urbani G, Lombardo G, Santi E, Tarnow D. Localized ridge augmentation with chin grafts and resorbable pins: case reports. *Int J Periodontics Restorative Dent.* 1998; 18:363–375.

Wallace SS, Tarnow DP, Froum SJ et al. Maxillary sinus elevation by lateral window approach: evolution of technology and technique. *J Evid Based Dent Pract.* 2012; 12:161–171.

Weinberg LA, Kruger B. A comparison of implant/prosthesis loading with four clinical variables. *Int J Prosthodont.* 1995; 8:421–433.

CHAPTER 33
Implant surgical procedures

Steph Smith, Khalid Almas, Nehal Almehmadi and Mohanad Al-Sabbagh

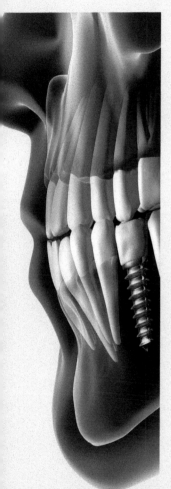

Contents

Essential Periodontics, First Edition. Edited by Steph Smith and Khalid Almas.
© 2022 John Wiley & Sons Ltd. Published 2022 by John Wiley & Sons Ltd.

Learning objectives

■ The fundamentals of placement of implants in the context of the needs and demands of patients, as well as the clinical considerations for implant-restorative procedures, the risk factors for implant therapy, and patients with systemic conditions.

■ Principles of implant surgery and different surgical protocols.

■ The basic concepts entailing the surgical placement of implants.

■ Understanding the fundamental principles, including the advantages and disadvantages involved in the timing of implant placement.

■ Knowledge of available advanced surgical implant procedures.

■ Aspects of postoperative care of patients undergoing implant surgery.

■ Factors determining success of surgical outcomes of implant placement.

■ Awareness of survival rates of implants placed in different time frames relative to tooth extraction.

Introduction

Implants offer a predictable solution for tooth replacement with high clinical success and survival rates. Implants with various designs are successfully placed in edentulous ridges, fresh extraction sockets, sites with ridge defects, and regenerated bony areas (Pjetursson et al. 2004).

Ideal conditions must be established for successful bone and soft tissue integration with implants. Therefore, aspects must be evaluated such as the overall objective of the treatment, the location of the proposed implant site(s) within the oral cavity (esthetic versus non-esthetic zone), the anatomy of the bone and soft tissue at the site(s), and the adaptive changes of the alveolar process following tooth loss/extraction (Hämmerle et al. 2015). Additionally, treatment must also satisfy patient demands regarding esthetic outcome. In such cases, the overall surgical and prosthetic treatment protocols become more demanding, as factors other than osseointegration and soft tissue integration may play an important role in the final esthetic outcome (Hämmerle et al. 2015). Thorough examination and treatment planning of implant patients are essential to achieve the desired outcome of the treatment (see Chapter 29). Implant-restorative procedures (see Chapter 32), risk factors for implant therapy (see Chapter 30), and patients'

systemic conditions (see Chapter 31) are among the factors that could influence implant success and, therefore, should be carefully assessed.

Basic principles of implant surgery

■ Implants must be placed in healthy, viable bone with good primary stability in order to achieve osseointegration (Hämmerle et al. 2015).

■ The best results are achieved when the bone-to-implant (BIC) contact is intimate at the time of implant placement. Anatomic features of bone quality of the recipient site influence the BIC interface. Cortical bone offers a much greater surface area for BIC than cancellous bone. Areas exhibiting thin layers of cortical bone and large marrow spaces of cancellous bone, such as the posterior maxilla, have lower success rates than areas of dense bone (Jaffin & Berman 1991).

■ An atraumatic technique is fundamental to avoid damage to bone. This includes the sequential incremental preparation of the implant bed for a precise fit of the implant (Lindhe & Lang 2015; Newman et al. 2019). Drilling of the bone without adequate cooling generates excessive heat, which injures bone and increases the risk of implant failure (Klokkevold 2019; Watanabe et al. 1992).

Timing of implant placement

In clinical practice, the decision to place an implant following tooth extraction is determined by specific soft and hard tissue characteristics of the healing socket (Hämmerle et al. 2004). In optimal cases, the decision can be made to place the implant(s) immediately after tooth extraction. However, a period of alveolar soft and hard tissue healing (weeks or months) should be allowed prior to implant placement in complicated cases. The decision regarding the timing of implant placement should be based on the knowledge of the structural/adaptive changes of the socket following tooth extraction (Hämmerle et al. 2015).

Adaptive changes occurring during socket healing

Hard tissue changes

A variety of factors may influence bone dimensional changes following tooth extraction. These factors may include the patient's systemic health and habits (e.g. smoking), local conditions such as the number and proximity of extracted teeth, presence of infection, the condition of the socket before and after tooth extraction, tissue phenotype, socket location in dental arches, the implementation of socket preservation procedures, and the type of interim prosthesis used (Chen et al. 2004). Bone formation within the center of the socket occurs simultaneously with loss of alveolar ridge height and width from the periphery. Most dimensional changes occur within the first three months following tooth extraction. Ridge dimensional loss occurs as a result of the destruction of the bundle bone–periodontal ligament (BB–PDL) complex following tooth extraction, and thus leads to resorption of the buccal ridge contour (Chen et al. 2004; Gluckman & Du Toit 2015).

Resorption of the alveolar ridge is more pronounced on the buccal aspect and may result in as much as 56% loss of the residual ridge dimensions (Araújo & Lindhe 2005). Alveolar ridge height reduction of 3–4 mm, or approximately half of the initial socket height, has been reported after 6 months of healing (Lekovic et al. 1997, 1998). Greater apico-coronal changes take place at multiple adjacent extraction sites than at a single extraction site (Lam 1960; Schropp et al. 2003b). Horizontal socket width reduction of 4–5 mm, or approximately two-thirds of the original socket width, has been shown after 6 months of healing (Lekovic et al. 1997, 1998). Approximately 5–7 mm of external horizontal bucco-lingual ridge reduction, representing about half of the initial ridge width, has been shown over a 6- to 12-month period of healing; most of these dimensional changes occur during the first 4 months of healing (Johnson 1963, 1969).

Thickness of the facial bone at the time of implant placement is also an important factor (Chen et al. 2007). Extraction sockets with thin facial bone may lose more vertical height and show less bone fill than sites with thicker bone. Residual bony defects following immediate implant placement may heal with either complete bone fill or residual crater-like defects, and a vertical loss of crestal bone height of 0.3–0.9 mm at re-entry can occur when the initial thickness of the facial bone is between 0.7 and 0.9 mm. In contrast, sites may heal with a dehiscence defect when the facial bone has an initial thickness of 0.5 mm and may show a vertical crestal bone loss of 2.1 mm at re-entry (Chen et al. 2007).

Pathological or traumatic processes may damage one or more of the bony walls of the socket, thereby altering the rate and pattern of bone resorption. It is likely that fibrous tissue may occupy part of the socket, thus preventing normal healing and osseous regeneration, which may lead to the formation of dehiscence defects (Chen et al. 2004; Nemcovsky et al. 2000; Schropp et al. 2003b). The location of the implant in relation to the socket is a critical determinant of the outcome of regenerative treatment at dehisced sites. Implants should be placed well within the confines of the socket to take advantage of the healing potential of the socket (Chen et al. 2004).

In summary, studies have shown that implant placement immediately after tooth extraction does not alter the pattern of the physiological phenomenon of bone resorption after dental extraction (Lanza et al. 2015). In general, the external socket walls of the alveolus undergo resorption, while the center of the socket is filled with cancellous bone, and the overall volume of the site becomes markedly reduced. In particular, the buccal wall of the edentulous site diminishes not only in the bucco-lingual/palatal direction, but also in the apico-coronal dimension (Hämmerle et al. 2015; Schropp et al. 2003b).

Soft tissue changes

During the first week after extraction, cell proliferation within the mucosa results in an increase of connective tissue volume (Hämmerle et al. 2015). Although complete epithelialization of the socket is established by the fifth week of healing, organization and maturation of the collagen in the underlying lamina propria take longer time to occur. Matrix synthesis begins at 7 days and peaks at 3 weeks; this is followed by a continuous process of maturation until complete tensile strength is restored several months later (Chen et al. 2004). The soft tissue wound eventually becomes epithelialized and a keratinized mucosa covers the extraction site. The contour of the mucosa subsequently adapts to follow the changes that occur in the external profile of the hard tissue of the alveolar process (Hämmerle et al. 2015).

Lack of tensile strength in the mucosa of healing extraction sockets may result in wound dehiscence. Dehiscence rates of 5–24% have been reported at delayed implant sites treated with both resorbable and non-resorbable membranes, despite the presence of adequate tissue volume to achieve primary closure (Chen et al. 2004). The volumetric change of the alveolar ridge is the net result of bone and connective tissue loss. Also, healing does not necessarily follow rigid time frames, and may vary according to site and patient factors. Furthermore, no ideal time point can be specified where there is maximum socket bone fill and soft tissue maturation (Hämmerle et al. 2015). Figure 33.1 depicts the changes in the soft and hard tissues following tooth extraction over time.

Classification of type 1–4 implant placements

Based on the morphological, dimensional, and histological changes of soft and hard tissue after tooth extraction (Figure 33.1), a classification has been developed representing four different time points for implant placement. The classification was proposed at the Third International Team for Implantology (ITI) Consensus Conference (Hämmerle et al. 2004). Table 33.1 depicts the classification of type 1–4 implant placements, together with the advantages and disadvantages of each type (Chen & Buser 2009; Hämmerle et al. 2015).

Clinical approach to type 1–4 implant placement (Hämmerle et al. 2004)

Patient assessment

All patients planned for post-extraction implant placement should meet the same general screening criteria as regular implant patients, regardless of the timing of implant placement (see also Chapter 29).

Antibiotics

There are inconclusive studies regarding antibiotic use in conjunction with implant therapy. There is general agreement that the use of antibiotics is advantageous when augmentation procedures are performed. In most studies reviewed, broad-spectrum systemic antibiotics have been used in conjunction with implant placement types 1, 2, and 3.

Tooth extraction

An atraumatic extraction technique should be utilized to limit trauma to hard and soft tissues. The sectioning of multirooted teeth is advised. All granulation tissue should be removed and the socket thoroughly irrigated.

Site evaluation

Site evaluation is critical to determine the appropriate treatment modality, and should include the following factors:

- Overall patient treatment plan.
- Esthetic expectations of the patient.
- Soft tissue quality, quantity, and morphology.
- Bone quality, quantity, and morphology.
- Presence of pathology.
- Condition of adjacent teeth and supporting structures (see also Chapters 29 and 32).

Primary implant stability

Implants should not be placed at the time of tooth extraction if the residual ridge morphology precludes attainment of primary stability of an appropriately sized implant in an ideal restorative position.

Periodontal tissue phenotype

- Patients with a thin, scalloped phenotype, even those with an intact buccal plate, are at high risk of buccal plate resorption and marginal tissue recession. Therefore, esthetic risk assessment should be considered for such patients. Concomitant augmentation procedures at the time of type 1 implant placement should be considered.

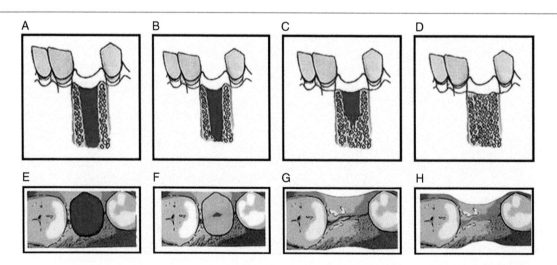

Figure 33.1 Hard and soft tissue changes following tooth extraction. (A, E) Axial and occlusal view of the socket immediately after extraction. (B, F) 4–8 weeks after extraction. (C, G) 12–16 weeks after extraction. (D, H) More than 16 weeks after extraction.

Table 33.1 Classification of type 1–4 implant placements.

Classification	Definition	Advantages	Disadvantages
Type 1	Implant placement as part of the same surgical procedure and immediately following tooth extraction	Reduced number of surgical procedures Reduced overall treatment time Optimal availability of existing bone	Site morphology may complicate optimal placement and anchorage Thin tissue phenotype may compromise optimal outcome Potential lack of keratinized mucosa for flap adaptation Adjunctive surgical procedures may be required Technique-sensitive procedure
Type 2	Complete soft tissue coverage of the socket (typically 4–8 weeks)	Increased soft tissue area and volume facilitate soft tissue flap management Allows resolution of local pathology to be assessed	Site morphology may complicate optimal placement and anchorage Increased treatment time Varying amounts of resorption of the socket walls Adjunctive surgical procedures may be required Technique-sensitive procedure
Type 3	Substantial clinical and/or radiographic bone fill of the socket (typically 12–16 weeks)	Substantial bone fill of the socket facilitates implant placement Mature soft tissues facilitate flap management	Increased treatment time Adjunctive surgical procedures may be required Varying amounts of resorption of the socket walls
Type 4	Healed site (typically >16 weeks).	Clinically healed ridge Mature soft tissues facilitate flap management	Increased treatment time Adjunctive surgical procedures may be required Large variation in available bone volume

Source: Adapted from Hämmerle et al. 2015.

- Patients with a thick, less scalloped phenotype with an intact buccal plate may not need concomitant augmentation procedures at the time of type 1 implant placement. Thick periodontal phenotypes have lower risk of buccal plate resorption compared to thin phenotypes. The need for augmentation procedures is of importance for thick phenotype sites if buccal plate integrity is lost.
- If buccal plate integrity is compromised, a condition that might negatively impact the predictability of treatment outcomes of immediate implant placement (type 1), it is not recommended to place implants immediately after extraction. Rather, ridge augmentation procedures should be performed, and either type 2, 3, or 4 implant placements should be utilized.
- When the jumping distance in type 1 implants (the horizontal defect dimension between the implant and the internal socket wall) is greater than 2 mm, concomitant bone grafting needs to be performed (Figure 33.2).
- In general, type 2 implants are preferred to type 1 implants when advanced or complete soft tissue healing is desired to improve flap handling and primary closure in case of concomitant augmentation procedures. Type 3 and 4 implant placements are the treatment of choice when hard tissue healing is desired (Hämmerle et al. 2004).

- Adjunctive hard and/or soft tissue augmentation procedures may be indicated in any of the above situations to optimize esthetic treatment outcomes.

Implant placement

The three-dimensional positioning of dental implants should be prosthetically driven. Implants should be placed with reference to the three dimensions dictated by the position of the final restoration and not by the availability of bone. The ideal implant position entails the surgical placement into the alveolus according to apico-coronal, mesio-distal, and bucco-lingual parameters, as well as the implant angulation relative to the final prosthetic restoration and gingival margins (Figure 33.3) (Newman et al. 2019). Proper planning of the correct three-dimensional implant position is established traditionally using a diagnostic wax-up of the proposed prosthesis and radiographic imaging with radiopaque markers to indicate the desired tooth position(s) relative to the available bone. Digital wax-up and implant planning software has been extensively used in recent years to serve the same purpose. Accurate planning will prevent incorrect bodily placement, potential esthetic complications, or violation of neighboring anatomy such as encroaching on adjacent tooth roots (see also Chapter 32).

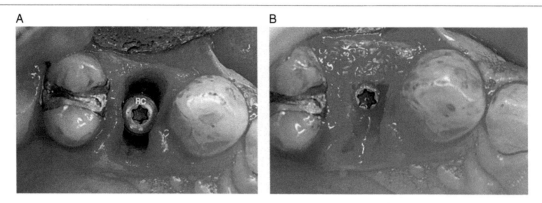

Figure 33.2 Clinical photograph of the jumping distance around type 1 implant placed immediately after extraction of maxillary right first premolar. (A) Buccal and lingual horizontal jumping distance around the implant. (B) The jumping distance was filled with bone graft particulates.

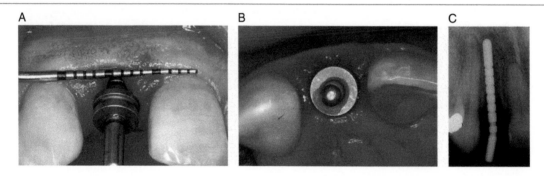

Figure 33.3 Placement of prosthetically driven implant in the correct three-dimensional position. (A) Depth gauge is inserted to check the apico-coronal dimension of the osteotomy. (B) Bucco-lingual, mesio-distal, and angulation of the osteotomy are verified. (C) Periapical radiograph using a paralleling pin verifying relation of the prepared implant site to neighboring vital structures.

The implant surgical procedure

Flap design, incisions, and elevation

The location and objective of the planned surgery will dictate the incision/flap design for implant surgery. The most common flap design is the envelope flap with crestal incision (Figure 33.4). This involves an incision that runs along the crest of the alveolar ridge and bisects the existing zone of keratinized mucosa. Remote incisions and layered suturing techniques can be utilized when extensive bone augmentation is planned to minimize the incidence of bone graft exposure. However, closure of crestal incisions is easier to manage and typically results in less bleeding and edema, and faster healing (Scharf & Tarnow 1993).

Following the crestal incision, buccal and lingual/palatal full-thickness flaps are reflected to or slightly beyond the level of the mucogingival junction, exposing the alveolar ridge of the implant surgical sites. At this step, the bone at the implant site should be thoroughly debrided of all soft tissue tags or

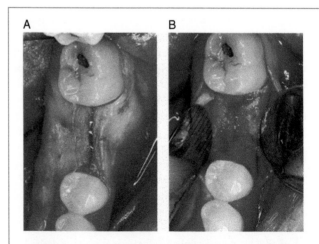

Figure 33.4 Flap design, incisions, and elevation. (A) Crestal incision was made to dissect the soft tissue and the periosteum. (B) Elevation of mucoperiosteal envelope flap on both buccal and lingual sides to expose the alveolar bone.

granulation tissue. In the case of one-stage surgical approach selection, a crestal incision bisecting the existing keratinized tissue is utilized. Vertical releasing incisions may be needed at one or both ends of the flap to facilitate access to the bone or osteotomy site. Full-thickness flaps are elevated facially and lingually (Newman et al. 2019).

Bone evaluation at implant site

"Knife-edge" alveolar ridges could be flattened with a large round bur to provide a wider, leveled surface for implant site preparation, given that sufficient alveolar bone height exists to allow for acceptable distance from vital structures (e.g. inferior alveolar nerve). However, if the vertical height of the alveolar bone is limited (e.g. <10 mm), the knife-edge alveolar bone crest should be preserved. Bone augmentation procedures can be then used to increase the ridge width while preserving alveolar bone height (Newman et al. 2019).

Preparation of the implant osteotomy site

A series of drills are used to prepare the osteotomy site precisely and incrementally. A surgical guide should preferably be used throughout the surgical procedure to ensure proper implant positioning. Copious irrigation and gentle surgical techniques are imperative while using the sequential twist drills to avoid bone overheating and necrosis. Combination of long and short drills, with or without extensions, may be necessary in some patients who present with limited access for instrumentation. Implant site preparation for the one-stage approach is identical in principle to the two-stage implant surgical approach. The primary difference is that the coronal aspect of the implant (tissue level) or the healing abutment (bone level) is placed approximately 2–3 mm above the bone crest and the soft tissues are approximated around the implant neck/implant abutment (Newman et al. 2019).

Table 33.2 depicts various drills and drilling sequence for preparation of the osteotomy site.

Implant placement

Implants are either inserted with a handpiece rotating at slow speeds (e.g. 25 rpm) or manually using a wrench. Insertion of the implant must follow the path of the osteotomy site. When multiple implants are placed, guide pins are inserted in other osteotomy sites to serve as a visual guide for implant path of insertion (Figure 33.5) (Newman et al. 2019).

Flap closure and suturing

Most threaded endosseous implants can be placed using either a one-stage or a two-stage protocol.

One-stage protocol

- The implant or the abutment emerges through the mucoperiosteum/gingival tissue at the time of implant placement (Klokkevold 2019).

- Tissue-level implants are specifically designed with a polished collar that is positioned approximately 2–3 mm above the crest of bone, extending through the gingival tissues at the time of placement. The flap is adapted around the implant collar (Figure 33.6).
- A bone-level implant platform is placed at the level of the bone crest and thus requires a healing abutment to be attached to the implant at the time of placement if a one-stage protocol is considered. The flap is adapted around the healing abutment.
- The keratinized edges of the flap are sutured with either resorbable or non-resorbable sutures using a single interrupted suturing technique.
- Scalloping the soft tissue around the implant collar/abutment could provide better flap adaptation. Scalloping could be considered only when keratinized tissue is abundant.
- A one-stage surgical approach simplifies the procedure because a second-stage exposure surgery is not needed (Klokkevold 2019).

Two-stage protocol

- The implant platform and cover screw are completely covered by the mucoperiosteal flap.
- Tension-free primary closure of the flap over the implant is essential (Figure 33.7).
- Flap tension is eliminated with a superficial horizontal incision that runs on the fibrous, non-elastic periosteum (periosteal releasing incision) at the apical end of the flap.
- Flap primary closure can be achieved using a number of suturing techniques, the best of which is a combination of alternating horizontal mattress and interrupted sutures. Horizontal mattress sutures evert the wound edges and approximate the inner, connective tissue surfaces of the flap to facilitate closure and wound healing. Interrupted sutures help to bring the wound edges together while counterbalancing the eversion caused by horizontal mattress sutures.
- In cases where primary closure is difficult to achieve, e.g. type 1 implant placement, a resorbable collagen membrane can be used and the flap is allowed to heal by secondary intension (Figure 33.8).
- The application of resorbable suture materials simplifies patient management as it does not require removal at the postoperative visit. However, when moderate to severe postoperative swelling is anticipated, a non-resorbable suture material is recommended to counteract flap tension caused by swelling and to maintain longer primary closure. Nonetheless, non-resorbable sutures will require removal at a postoperative visit (Newman et al. 2019).
- Implants are allowed to heal for an average of three months, without loading or micromovement, to allow for osseointegration to occur.
- The implant must be surgically exposed following the healing period.
- In the second-stage (exposure) surgery, the implant is uncovered and a healing abutment is connected to allow

Table 33.2 Drilling sequence for implant bed preparation.

1

Needle bur

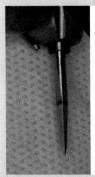 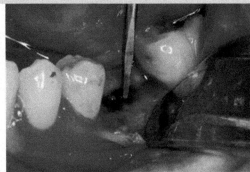

Round bur

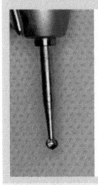 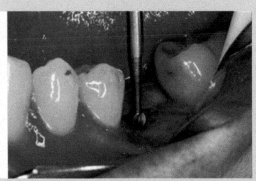

Needle bur is to make the initial penetration into bone for the implant site preparation. Initial marks are checked for their appropriate buccal-lingual and mesial-distal location, as well as the positions relative to each other, in case of multiple adjacent implants, and adjacent teeth. Each marked site is then prepared to a depth of 1–2 mm with the round bur, breaking through the cortical bone and creating a starting point for the 2 mm twist drill. Initial marks for adjacent implants should be separated by at least 7 mm (center to center) for 4 mm standard-diameter implants. This will ensure that implants are positioned approximately 3 mm between one another, and that sufficient interimplant bone and soft tissue is present for optimum health and to facilitate oral hygiene procedures. More space will be needed for wide-diameter implants.

2

1st twist drill

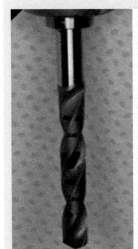 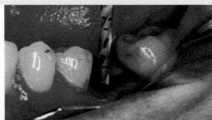

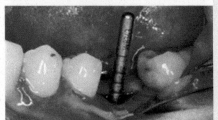

A 1st twist drill, marked to indicate drilling depth corresponding to the implant height, is then used to establish the depth and angulation of the osteotomy. The drilling speed is set between 600 to 1200 rpm. Copious irrigation (external or internal irrigation) is important to prevent overheating and necrosis of alveolar bone. Clinicians should pump the drill (up and down) intermittently and avoid using a constant "pushing" of the drill in the apical direction, to facilitate irrigation and clearance of bone debris from the cutting surfaces of the drill. If multiple osteotomies are prepared, a guide pin should be placed in the prepared osteotomy sites while drilling for the next to check alignment, parallelism, and proper prosthetic spacing throughout the preparation process. The relationship to neighboring vital structures (e.g. nerve and tooth roots) can be determined by taking a periapical radiograph with a guide pin or radiographic marker in the osteotomy site. The 1st twist drill is used to establish the final depth of the osteotomy corresponding to the length of each planned implant. During this stage, the clinician should evaluate bone quality (density) to assess the need for modification of the drilling sequence.

Table 33.2 (Continued)

Radiographic verification

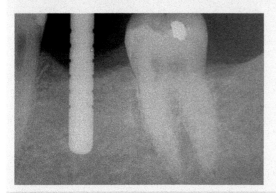

| 3 | A pilot drill with a non-cutting "guide" at the apical end and a cutting (wider) midsection is used to enlarge the osteotomy site at the coronal end, thus facilitating the insertion of the subsequent drills in the sequence. |
| Pilot drill | |

| 4 | The osteotomy is prepared using a set of sequential twist drills with increasing diameter until reaching the required preparation width for the planned implant. The twist drill is used to widen the entire depth of the osteotomy from the previous diameter to the final diameter of the planned osteotomy. Implant stability is dependent on the final preparation of the osteotomy. The diameter of the final drill may be slightly increased or decreased to enhance implant stability, depending on bone density. It is of extreme importance that the final drilling is accomplished with a steady hand, without wobbling or changing direction, so that the site is not overprepared. |
| Sequential twist drills | |

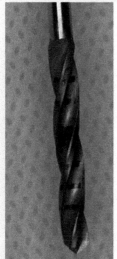
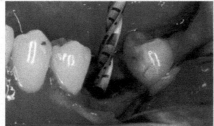
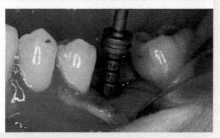
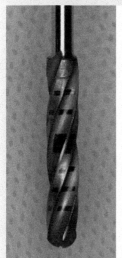
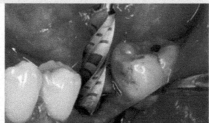
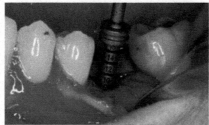

Table 33.2 (Continued)

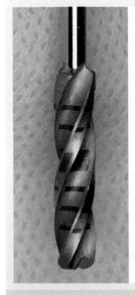

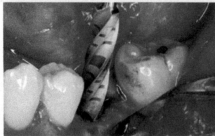

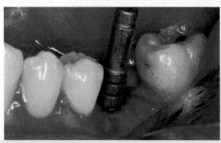

5 Countersink drill 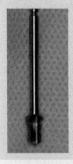	Countersink drilling is used to shape or flare the crestal aspect of the osteotomy site when the cover screw is placed at or slightly below the crestal bone. This will allow the coronal flare of the implant head and cover screw to fit within the osteotomy site.
6 Bone tap 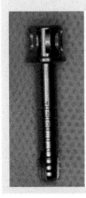 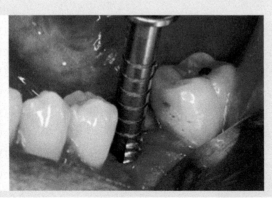	Bone tapping refers to the creation of threads in the osteotomy site before implant placement. Tapping facilitates implant insertion and to reduce the risk of implant binding when implants are placed in dense bone, or when longer self-tapping implants are placed into moderately dense bone. Bone tapping and implant insertion are both established at a very slow speed, i.e. 20–40 rpm.

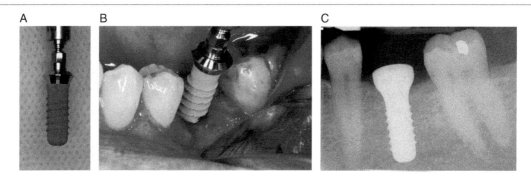

Figure 33.5 Implant placement. (A) Clinical picture showing the implant attached to the implant carrier ready to be inserted. (B) Motor-driven placement of the implant into the osteotomy. (C) Radiographic verification of implant complete seating and crestal bone level immediately following implant placement.

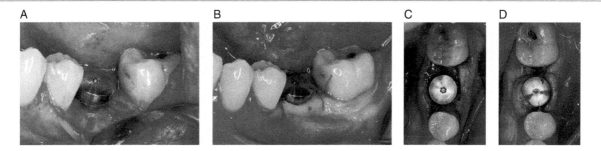

Figure 33.6 Clinical photograph of one-stage (transmucosal) implant healing. (A) Buccal view of a tissue-level implant and healing abutment at the time of implant placement in the left mandibular first molar site. (B) Buccal view of the same implant after suturing of the full-thickness flap around the healing abutment. (C, D) Occlusal view of the same implant before and after flap closure.

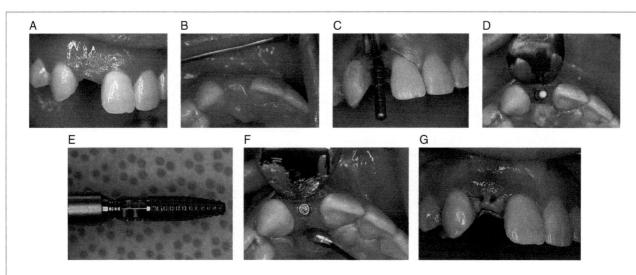

Figure 33.7 Two-stage implant placement. (A) Buccal view of edentulous ridge at the site of missing right maxillary lateral incisor. (B) Occlusal view of the same edentulous site. (C, D) After initial drilling, the apico-coronal, bucco-lingual, mesio-distal, and angulation of the osteotomy are verified. (E) Clinical photograph of the tapered implant. (F) Occlusal view of the implant in place with the closure screw. (G) The implant was completely submerged under the mucoperiosteal flap and primary closure was achieved using resorbable internal horizontal mattress sutures.

A

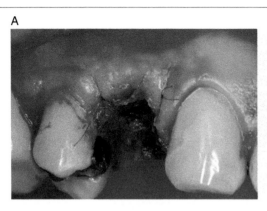

B

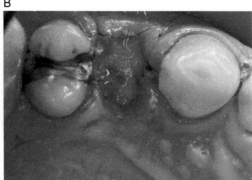

Figure 33.8 Clinical photograph of secondary intension closure of two-stage implant procedure. (A) Buccal view of the sutured flap and the collagen membrane covering the occlusal aspect. (B) Occlusal view showing clearly the exposed collagen membrane.

emergence of the abutment through the soft tissues. Once healing has occurred, the restorative dentist proceeds with the prosthodontic aspects of the implant therapy (impressions and fabrication of prosthesis) (Klokkevold 2019).

- The two-stage, submerged approach is advantageous for certain situations, such as when simultaneous bone or connective tissue augmentation procedures are performed (Klokkevold 2019), or when less than optimum implant primary stability was achieved.

Postoperative care of surgical implant patients (Klokkevold 2019)

- Simple implant surgery does not require a postoperative course of antibiotic therapy in healthy patients. However, antibiotic coverage (e.g. one week of either amoxicillin, 500 mg three times a day [TID], or clindamycin, 150 mg four times a day [QID], in cases of penicillin allergy) could be prescribed if surgery is extensive, biological grafting materials are used, or patients are medically compromised. This antibiotic dose and frequency serves as an example. Choice of the type and dosage of antibiotic should be based on the patient's medical history and must be adjusted according to their age and systemic health conditions.
- Postoperative swelling is common after flap surgery, especially if the periosteal releasing incision is used. As a preventive measure, patients are instructed to apply cold packs for the first 24–48 hours.
- 0.012% chlorhexidine gluconate oral rinse is beneficial in facilitating plaque control, especially immediately after surgery when oral hygiene is typically compromised.
- Adequate pain medication should be prescribed (e.g. ibuprofen, 600–800 mg TID).
- Patients should be instructed to maintain a relatively soft diet after surgery for 7–10 days, and gradually to return to a normal diet as healing progresses.

- Patients should refrain from tobacco or alcohol use during the healing after surgery.
- Patients have to be reminded of the need for good oral hygiene around the implant and adjacent teeth.
- Patients should be instructed to avoid brushing the surgical area if repositioned flaps or soft tissue grafts were used.
- Implant-supported immediate provisional restorations should be checked and adjusted (out of occlusion) to minimize trauma to the implant in the critical early period of osseointegration.
- Provisional removable prostheses should be adjusted and relieved to avoid direct pressure or movement of soft tissue at the surgical area, which could delay the healing process.
- Regular monitoring of soft tissue healing is advisable, and constant relief and soft relining of provisional prostheses would minimize postoperative complications.
- Patients should be advised to avoid chewing in the area of the implant.
- Prosthetic appliances should not be used if direct chewing forces are transmitted to the implant, particularly in the early healing period.
- Depending on healing and maturation of soft tissues, impressions for final prostheses fabrication can begin about 2–6 weeks after implant exposure surgery.

Second-stage exposure surgery (Newman et al. 2019)

Second-stage exposure surgery is necessary when using a two-stage "submerged" surgical protocol. Uncovering the implant can be accomplished with different incision designs, depending on the amount of keratinized tissue available at the implant site. Soft tissues may be thinned, repositioned, or augmented at the second-stage surgery to increase the zone of keratinized tissue or to improve soft tissue thickness surrounding the implant (Newman et al. 2019). Second-stage implant exposure modalities are described in this section.

A 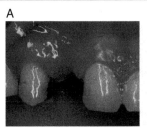 B 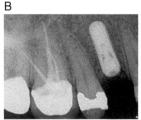 C 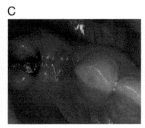 D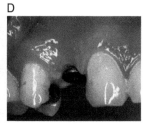

Figure 33.9 Clinical photograph of second-stage (implant exposure) surgery. (A) Buccal view of the completely healed soft tissue at the implant site. Adequate amount of keratinized mucosa is present at the implant site. (B) Periapical radiograph was taken to confirm the integration of the implant. (C) Circular tissue punch was used to expose the implant after 3 months of healing time. (D) Implant was exposed, and the cover screw replaced with a healing abutment of sufficient height to allow for soft tissue healing and adaptation around the healing abutment. Sutures are not needed when the tissue punch implant exposure modality is utilized.

Simple circular "punch"

In areas with a sufficient zone of keratinized tissue, the gingiva covering the head of the implant can be exposed with a circular or "punch" incision (Figure 33.9). The punched-out soft tissue will leave the implant head exposed. The cover screw is then removed from the implant and an appropriate size healing abutment/provisional prosthesis is screwed to the implant to sculpt the soft tissue. A sufficient period of time is then allowed for soft tissue adaptation (3–4 weeks) before an impression is taken to fabricate the implant-supported prosthesis.

Crestal incision–full-thickness flap reflection

As an alternative to the punch technique, a mid-crestal incision through the keratinized tissue and full-thickness flap reflection can be used to expose implants. This technique is utilized when the amount of keratinized tissue is inadequate, where an excision of soft tissue (as in the punch technique) will result in less than 2 mm of keratinized tissue around the implant. Another indication for this technique is when a connective tissue graft is planned at the time of second-stage surgery.

Partial-thickness repositioned flap

An insufficient zone of keratinized tissue at the implant site can be corrected using a partial-thickness repositioned flap technique at the time of second-stage surgery. The objective of this approach is to expose the implant while increasing the width of keratinized tissue at the same time. The initial incision is made within the zone of keratinized tissue. If the initial amount of keratinized tissue is less than 2 mm, the flap may be started at the labial edge of the keratinized tissue, allowing that zone to remain on the lingual aspect of the implant. Vertical releasing incisions are placed on both mesial and distal ends of the flap. A partial-thickness flap is then raised, leaving a firm periosteum attached to the underlying bone (thus without exposing the alveolar bone). The flap, containing a narrow band of keratinized tissue, is repositioned apical to the facial side of the

emerging head of the implant and sutured to the periosteum. A free gingival graft may then be harvested from the palate and sutured to the periosteum coronal to the sutured edge of the partial-thickness flap on the facial surface of the implants to increase the zone of keratinized tissue. Thereafter, the excess tissue coronal to the cover screw is excised, and the cover screw is removed. The head of the implant is thoroughly cleaned of any soft or hard tissue overgrowth, and the healing abutments or standard abutments are placed on the implant. Figure 33.10 depicts the sequence of the entire procedure of type 4 implant placement.

Advanced surgical implant procedures

As part of a team approach, awareness of the general availability and scope of advanced surgical implant procedures is necessary, so as to enable the practitioner to recommend them as part of comprehensive dental care. Table 33.3 depicts various advanced surgical implant placement procedures, together with the indications for each.

Postoperative complications of surgical implant placement

Implant surgical procedures are not without complications and risks (Newman et al. 2019). As part of the overall planning and surgical placement of implants, clinicians should be able to anticipate any potential surgical complications that may occur. Table 33.4 depicts such complications.

Post-treatment evaluation and maintenance of implants

An important component of successful treatment includes the periodic post-treatment examination of implants, implant-supported prostheses, and the condition of the surrounding peri-implant tissues. Peri-implant mucositis or peri-implantitis might go unnoticed by the patient, but could be detected early during implant maintenance visits. Peri-implant complications

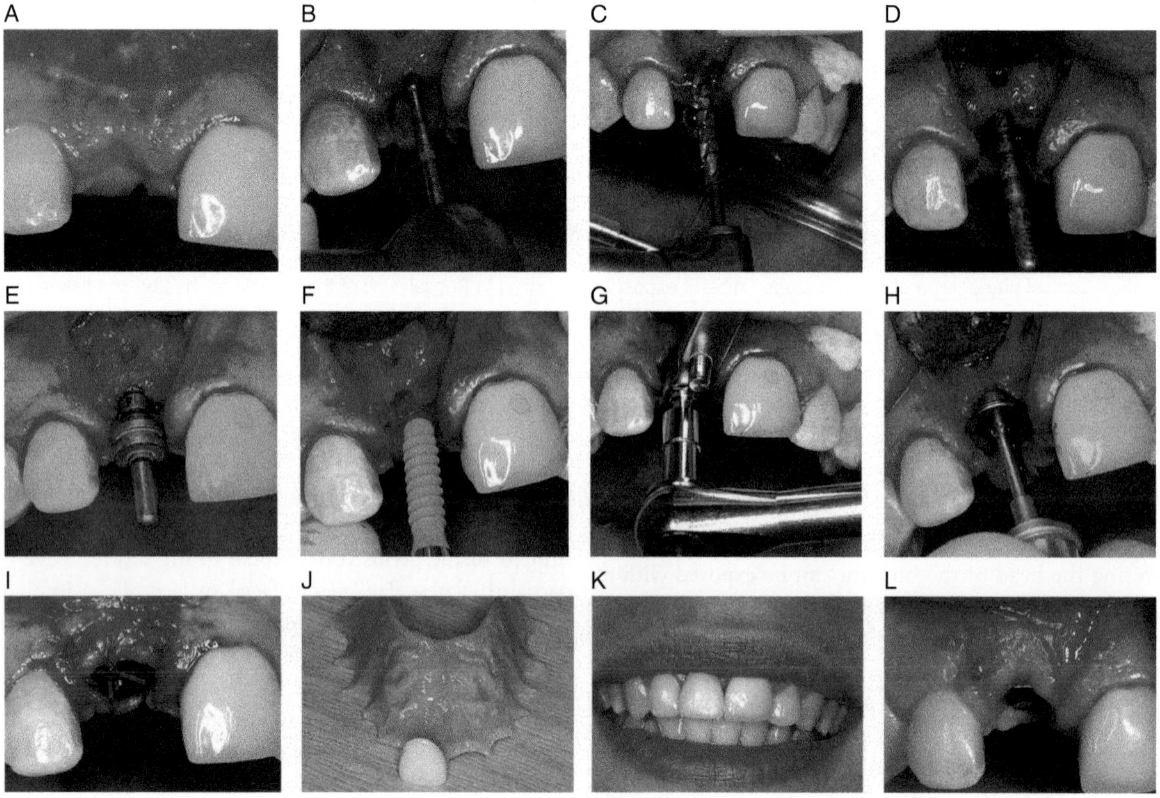

Figure 33.10 Implant placement procedure. (A) Preoperative view of missing tooth #8. (B) Incision was made and full-thickness flap was raised, then initial drilling was made with a round bur to penetrate the cortical bone. (C) Osteotomy preparation with a 2 mm twist drill. (D) A 2 mm guide pin used to check alignment, parallelism, and proper prosthetic spacing. (E) A depth gauge corresponds to the final osteotomy preparation size used to verify final implant depth, position, and angulation. (F, G) Manual implant placement using a wrench. (H) One-stage healing abutment tightened with a screwdriver. (I) Flap re-opposed and sutured to allow transmucosal healing. (J) Provisional tooth replacement during healing. (K) Patient smile with the provisional tooth replacement in place. (L) Soft tissue healing around the healing abutment.

can often be treated if discovered early. Radiographic monitoring is essential to detect marginal or peri-implant bone changes. The reader is referred to Appendix 4. For long-term follow-up and maintenance of implants, see Chapter 36.

Factors determining success of surgical outcomes of type 1–4 implant placement

The focus on treatment goals has shifted from merely implant survival to treatment success. Treatment success includes optimal esthetic outcomes, healthy peri-implant tissues, restoration of function, and long-term maintenance (Annibali et al. 2012). Factors other than timing of implant placement may affect the outcomes of implant placement procedures (Lang et al. 2012). These factors include but are not limited to the following:

- *History of disease*: Subjects with a history of periodontitis might be at greater risk for peri-implant infections and show decreased survival rates (Renvert & Persson 2009).

Significantly greater peri-implant marginal bone loss has been shown in periodontitis-susceptible subjects than in non-susceptible subjects (De Boever et al. 2009). Few studies have compared implants placed in extraction sockets for non-periodontally related reasons and for mixed periodontal and non-periodontal reasons. Although comparable implant survival rates were reported between the two groups, the non-periodontal group survival rate has been slightly higher (Annibali et al. 2012; Polizzi et al. 2000).

- *Primary stability and bone quality*: Secondary to the dimensions of the extraction socket, the relative proportion of the load-bearing lamellar bone versus cancellous bone in a given implant site determines primary stability. The mandible is composed of a larger proportion of lamellar bone than in the maxilla. Therefore, it is speculated that implant survival rates will be more favorable in the mandible. Although not statistically significant, studies have shown an estimated annual failure rate of 0.73% in the maxilla compared to an annual failure rate of 0.50% in the mandible (Annibali et al. 2012).

Table 33.3 Advanced surgical implant procedures.

Socket preservation	Prevention of alveolar ridge deficiency after tooth extraction. Facilitates bone formation by osteoconduction, osteoinduction, or osteogenesis. Socket preservation is performed using a combination of bone graft materials, such as alloplasts, xenografts, allografts or autografts, in conjunction with resorbable or non-resorbable membranes. Socket preservation could be performed using membrane alone without bone grafting.
Guided bone regeneration (GBR)	To reconstruct lost alveolar bone in horizontal or vertical dimensions so that implants can be placed in the correct position. GBR could be performed with either particulate bone grafts or monocortical block graft, together with barrier membranes.
Simultaneous implant placement with GBR or sinus elevation	Implant placement simultaneously with either sinus elevation or bone augmentation procedures is considered an advanced procedure that requires adequate clinical skills and experience. Implants could be placed only if sufficient native bone exist to stabilize the implant in the desired location.
Ridge splitting	The division of a narrow alveolar ridge into two plates to effectively widen the bone while simultaneously placing the implant.
Vertical bone augmentation	Indicated for the reconstruction of severely atrophic edentulous ridges. Includes using bone graft filler materials and titanium-reinforced membranes.
Maxillary sinus elevation and bone augmentation (lateral window approach)	Indicated when vertical alveolar bone height in the posterior maxilla is less than 5 mm.
Closed sinus lift technique (trans-crestal approach)	The elevation of the sinus membrane through a vertical osteotomy within the implant site and the placement of a particulate graft to increase bone volume. Osteotomes are used to elevate push the particulate graft and consequently elevate the sinus membrane.
Distraction osteogenesis	Increase alveolar bone height using native autogenous bone and intraoral devices activated periodically by the patient.
Inferior alveolar nerve (IAN) lateralization	Allows the placement of implants in the posterior mandible where the residual bone height above the IAN is less than adequate.
Partial extraction therapy (PET) (Gluckman et al. 2016b, 2017)	Maintain bucco-lingual/palatal ridge dimension, prevent horizontal ridge collapse, and preserve the alveolar ridge contour for pontic sites. PET can be performed prior to, or simultaneously with, implant placement. PET includes root submergence (Salama et al. 2007), socket shield (Hürzeler et al. 2010), pontic shield (Gluckman et al. 2016a), and proximal socket shield (Kan & Rungcharassaeng 2013) techniques.
Growth factors in bone augmentation	Induction of bone formation using bone morphogenetic proteins (BMP), platelet-rich plasma (PRP), or platelet-rich fibrin (PRF).
Soft tissue augmentation procedures	Improve the quality and quantity of the peri-implant soft tissues. The procedure is done using either autogenous connective tissue grafts, allogenic grafts, or xenogeneic collagen.

Source: Adapted from Newman et al. 2019.

- *Initial bone-to-implant contact (BIC):* The basic prerequisites for successful bone healing in immediate and delayed implant sites are the same as for implants placed in healed alveolar ridges. A space (jumping distance) often exists between the surface of the implant and the socket walls that needs to be filled with bone to achieve an optimal outcome. Bone healing is dependent on stabilization of the initially formed coagulum occupying the jumping distance. The distance from the bone to the implant and the surface characteristics of the implant are thus critical factors for

stabilization of the coagulum (Akimoto et al. 1999; Botticelli et al. 2003). Clot stabilization and bone formation may be adversely affected by lack of intact bony walls. In such situations, techniques utilizing barrier membranes and/or membrane-supporting materials have been shown to be effective in regenerating bone and allowing osseointegration of the placed implants (Akimoto et al. 1999; Gher et al. 1994).

Studies have shown that peri-implant defects with gaps of less than 2 mm following type 1 and 2 implant placement

Table 33.4 Postoperative complications.

Infection	Failure to attain primary stability
Hemorrhage and hematoma	Early implant failure and loss
Pain	Membrane exposures
Swelling and bruising	Neurosensory disturbances (neuropathies)
Suture granuloma	Devitalization of adjacent teeth
Wound dehiscence	Jaw fractures
Implant malposition	Sinusitis
Bone harvesting and grafting failures	Maxillary sinus complications
Perforation of mucosa after grafting	Displacement of implants into maxillary sinuses

may heal with spontaneous bone regeneration, defect resolution, and osseointegration (Chen & Buser 2009). Other studies showed that when implants were placed with a horizontal defect of 2 mm or less, spontaneous bone healing and osseointegration can take place provided implants have a rough surface (Schwartz-Arad & Chaushu 1998; Wilson et al. 1998, 2003).

Horizontal defects greater than 2 mm have shown less predictable bone fill and reduced spontaneous bone regeneration (Chen & Buser 2009; Wilson et al. 1998). However, it may be possible to achieve predictable bone fill in such situations by using collagen barrier membranes over implants with a sand-blasted and acid-etched surface (Wilson et al. 2003). A combination of a barrier membrane and bone graft has been shown to enhance the percentage of BIC in large horizontal defects in animal models (Stentz et al. 1997).

- *Bone augmentation procedures*: Clinical studies investigating bone augmentation procedures in combination with immediate (type 1) and early (type 2) implant placement have shown statistically and clinically significant bone fill and defect resolution of peri-implant horizontal defects (Chen & Buser 2009; Chen et al. 2005, 2007). Furthermore, bone augmentation in conjunction with type 1 placement reduces horizontal resorption of the facial bone. Interestingly enough, bone augmentation procedures do not appear to influence vertical resorption of the facial bone (Chen & Buser 2009). Schropp et al. (2003a) have shown greater bone fill at sites with intact bone walls compared to sites with dehiscence defects. Extraction sites that present with damage to the facial bone and undergo augmentation procedures with type 1 or 2 implant placement show greater resorption of the facial bone, thus having significant implications for esthetic outcomes (Schropp et al. 2003a). This is backed up by the high incidence of facial gingival recession reported by Kan et al. (2007), where type 1 implants were placed with simultaneous bone augmentation using deproteinized bovine bone mineral (DBBM) and a collagen membrane in sockets with facial bone defects.

In general, augmentation procedures are more successful with immediate (type 1), early (type 2), and delayed (type 3) implant placement than with late placement (type 4). Regenerative outcomes are better with type 2 placement compared to type 1 placement in the presence of bony dehiscence defects. This could be explained by the presence of adequate soft tissue characteristics in type 2 placement. However, with intact bone walls, type 1 and 2 placements achieve similar results with respect to bone fill of the peri-implant horizontal defect (Chen & Buser 2009).

- *Location and dimension of the implant site*: It has been speculated that there is a decreased amount of implant surface in direct contact with the adjacent bony walls in multirooted tooth sites, thereby negatively affecting optimal primary stability. However, differences in survival rates between implants placed in anterior single-rooted and posterior multirooted sockets have been shown to be negligible. Survival rates of 89–100% (median 99.5%) for implants placed into multiroot extraction sites have been shown to be similar for implants placed in single-root extraction sites (Cafiero et al. 2008; Chen & Buser 2009). This can be attributed to the surgical protocol, which includes minimal insertion torque and engagement of bone apical to the socket, as well as utilization of different-diameter implants that match various socket dimensions (Lang et al. 2012).

- *Wound dehiscence and membrane exposure*: Delaying implant placement for several weeks after tooth extraction allows time for bone regeneration to occur at the base and periphery of the socket, thereby avoiding the need for augmentation procedures (Nir-Hadar et al. 1998). However, the concomitant resorption of buccal bone may increase the need for augmentation bucco-lingually. Although no conclusions can be drawn from the available data regarding the optimal bone augmentation technique (Chen et al. 2004), wound dehiscence and early exposure of non-resorbable barrier membrane may lead to reduced quality and volume of bone regeneration in peri-implant defects (Augthun et al. 1995; Gher et al. 1994; van Steenberghe et al. 2000). Wound dehiscence is the most common postoperative complication with immediate implant placement, when either collagen or e-PTFE membranes are used in conjunction with submerged healing (Chen & Buser 2009). Resorbable membranes, however, appear to be effective and are associated with lower rates of wound dehiscence and membrane exposure than non-resorbable membranes (Chen et al. 2004). Also, studies have shown lower incidences of wound dehiscence and membrane exposure with delayed implant placement, irrespective of the type of membrane used (Nemcovsky & Artzi 2002; Zitzmann et al. 1997).

- *Soft tissue adaptation and esthetics*: There are no controlled studies available evaluating the esthetic treatment outcomes in type 1, 2, and 3 procedures (Hämmerle et al. 2004). Timing of implant placement following tooth removal is critical, and the decision on the type of implant placement should be based on whether the biological aspects of the implant site are adequate or there is a need to take advantage of a period of healing. Delayed implant placement offers advantages such as resolution of infection at the site, as well as an increase in the volume of soft tissue for flap adaptation and acceptable soft tissue esthetics (Chen et al. 2004). However, this advantage is offset by resorption of bone and loss of ridge dimensions. A delay of 3 months or more after tooth extraction in the anterior maxilla may result in such an advanced stage of bone resorption that only narrow-diameter implants can be used (de Wijs et al. 1995). Thus, 4–8 weeks appears to be the optimal period to defer implant placement to allow adequate soft tissue healing to take place without undue loss of bone volume (Chen et al. 2004). Adjunctive techniques to mobilize flaps and to augment soft tissue volume for wound closure at immediate implant sites may be beneficial in achieving acceptable esthetic results (Chen & Dahlin 1996; Goldstein et al. 2002; Nemcovsky et al. 2000).

- *Recession*: Midfacial mucosal recession, even when bone augmentation is performed, is a common complication with type 1 placement, and occurs soon after immediate restoration of implants. Implants placed without flap elevation are at increased risk of recession. The frequency of recession with type 1 placement has been reported in a high proportion of sites, ranging from 8.7% to 45.2% (median 39%), with recession of 1 mm or more ranging from 8% to 40.5% (median 21.4%) of sites (Chen & Buser 2009). Recession of the midfacial mucosa ranging from 0.5 to 0.9 mm (median 0.75 mm) has been reported with type 1 implant placement (Cornelini et al, 2005; Evans & Chen 2008). Furthermore, sites with thin tissue phenotype have shown a higher frequency of recession of >1 mm than sites with thick tissue phenotype when type 1 implants were placed (Chen et al. 2007). Another significant risk factor for mucosal recession is damage to the facial bony wall encountered at the time of type 1 implant placement. The risk of recession can also increase with the presence of an existing dehiscence of the facial bone (Kan et al. 2007).

- Early placement (type 2) may also be associated with recession (mean recession of 0.6–0.7 mm) (Chen & Buser 2009). However, early placement with soft tissue healing (type 2) is associated with a relatively low incidence of recession when implant placement is combined with guided bone regeneration (GBR) procedures using DBBM (Chen & Buser 2009). There is also evidence that early placement with partial bone healing (type 3) is associated with a lower frequency of recession compared to type 1 placement (Chen & Buser 2009). In studies with an average observation period of 3 years, about 20% of patients who have undergone immediate implant placement and delayed restorations had suboptimal esthetic outcomes due to buccal soft tissue recession. Further studies are needed to determine the influence of gingival phenotypes and the bucco-lingual implant position on buccal soft tissue levels (Lang et al. 2012). Also, novel techniques, including non-submerged immediate implant placement and flapless procedures, need further evaluation with respect to esthetic outcomes (Rocci et al, 2003; Schwartz-Arad & Chaushu 1998).

- *Periapical pathology*: The data for survival of implants in sites with apical pathology are contradictory (Chen & Buser 2009). In a controlled study, the survival rate was shown to be lower for type 1 compared to type 3 implant placement (Lindeboom et al. 2006). Another controlled clinical study including type 1 implant placement in 17 tooth sites with apical pathology was compared to 17 tooth sites without apical pathology. After 12 months, the survival rates for both groups were 100% (Siegenthaler et al. 2007).

- *Loading protocols*: The data on survival rates of immediately loaded implants placed in post-extraction sites are unclear. A wider range of survival rates of 65–100% (median 91%) has been reported for type 1 implants, indicative of less survival predictability, compared to 94–100% (median 95%) for type 4 implants placed in a similar clinical situation (Chen & Buser 2009). When implants are placed in extraction sockets of teeth with chronic periodontitis, a much lower survival rate has been reported for type 1 placement (65%) compared to type 4 placement (94%) (Horwitz et al. 2007). A study conducted on immediately loaded and conventionally loaded implants has reported implant survival rates of 98.2% and 98.5%, respectively, after a 2-year observation period. However, the immediately inserted restorations were free of contacts in centric occlusion and during excursive movements, thereby limiting micromovements of implants (Lang et al. 2012).

- *Antibiotics*: There is paucity of studies evaluating survival outcomes with or without systemic antibiotic therapy (Gluckman & Du Toit 2015). However, the implant annual failure rate in patients who received only preoperative prophylactic dosages of antibiotic was statistically higher than in patients treated with a postoperative course of antibiotic. This indicates that antibiotic coverage for implant patients might be of clinical importance (Lang et al. 2012).

Survival rates for type 1–4 implant placements

Due to the heterogeneity of studies with respect to implant surfaces, loading protocols, and relatively short-term observation periods for the majority of studies, data should be cautiously interpreted. However, it appears that survival rates for immediate implant placement are high, with the majority of studies reporting survival rates of over 95% (Chen & Buser 2009).

- *Type 1 implant placement*: Type 1 implant placement is a successful and predictable clinical method (Covani et al. 2004; Lang et al. 1994). Short-term studies with mean observation periods of 1–3 years have indicated survival rates ranging from 65% to 100% (median 99%). Studies with follow-up periods of 3–5 years have shown survival rates to range from 90% to 100% (median 95.5%). A recent systematic review showed that implants placed immediately in fresh extraction sockets yielded a low annual failure rate of 0.82% (95% confidence interval [CI]: 0.48–1.39%) translating to a 2-year survival rate of 98.4% (Lang et al. 2012).

- *Type 2 implant placement*: Short-term studies of 1–3 years have shown survival rates ranging from 91% to 100% (Chen & Buser 2009).

- *Type 3 implant placement*: Few studies have reported data on early implant placement with partial bone healing. Chen and Buser (2009) reported a survival rate ranging between 96% and 100%.

- *Type 1 versus type 2 implant placement*: Short-term retrospective studies and prospective cohort studies with a 5-year follow-up period have reported survival rates for type 1 implant placement ranging from 90% to 99% (median 90%) and from 90% to 100% (median 94%) for type 1 and 2 implant placements, respectively (Perry & Lenchewski 2004; Polizzi et al. 2000; Watzek et al. 1995). However, increased failure rates were noted in patients with a history of periodontitis (Evian et al. 2004; Polizzi et al. 2000).

- *Type 1 versus type 3 implant placement*: One study compared the outcome of type 1 and 3 implant placements in 50 patients with a single tooth site and radiographic evidence of chronic apical periodontitis. Using a submerged healing protocol, implants were followed up for 12 months. The study reported that the survival rates of implants were 92% and 100% for type 1 and 3 implants, respectively (Lindeboom et al. 2006).

- *Type 1 versus type 4 implant placement*: Two clinical studies have reported similar success and survival rates for type 1 and 4 implants (Lam 1960; Lekovic et al. 1998). Retrospective and prospective clinical studies showed survival rates of type 1 implants ranging from 90% to 100% (median 99%), compared to from 60% to 100% (median 94%) for type 4 implants (Degidi et al. 2006, 2007). However, with immediate loading, type 1 implants may have lower survival rates than implants placed into healed sites (Chen & Buser 2009).

Summary

Implant therapy is currently the first line of treatment to replace missing teeth. Satisfactory results can be obtained by correct three-dimensional implant placement, together with management of the peri-implant tissues. Careful diagnosis, treatment planning and execution, including the use of diagnostic imaging, surgical guides, meticulous surgical techniques, and adherence to evidence-based principles, are central to avoid surgical complications and to achieve predictable results. Thorough understanding of anatomy, biology, wound healing, and osseointegration principles are of paramount importance to facilitate decision making on the timing of implant placement. The fundamental protocols of implant placement presented in this chapter apply to all implant systems. Knowledge of advanced implant surgical procedures guides clinicians to manage complex implant placement in the most time- and cost-effective manner.

Even though osseointegration of dental implants and subsequent restoration are milestones in patient management, they should not be the endpoint of treatment. Placement of implant patients on a long-term maintenance program is momentous for avoidance, early detection, and treatment of implant-related complications. Maintenance should include long-term stability of volume, health, and esthetics of the supporting tissues. Training, knowledge, and the level of clinical expertise have a significant impact on the outcome of implant treatment (Chappuis et al. 2013; Lanza et al. 2015; Newman et al. 2019).

Future recommendations

Analysis of implant success rates is complex because the outcome is multifactorial. The assessment of clinical performance based only on implant survival rate is insufficient, as that ignores peri-implant soft and hard tissue conditions, esthetic outcomes, and patient-related outcome measurements (Graziani et al. 2019). There is a need to develop standards for long-term assessment of implant success and complications, especially in the esthetic zone. Thus, better evaluation of outcomes allows for generation of evidence-based guidelines for clinicians. Future research is also necessary to better understand the influence of potential prognostic factors like tissue phenotype, dimensions of the socket, and defect morphology on the regenerative capacity of an implant site (Graziani et al. 2019). Digital biomedical imaging techniques may further assist in assessment of regenerative outcomes and identification of the most suitable biomaterials for the preservation and maintenance of the facial bone wall dimensions. Well-designed and -conducted randomized clinical trials are needed to elucidate the long-term success and cost-effectiveness of early implant placement protocols (Graziani et al. 2019).

REFERENCES

Akimoto K, Becker W, Donath K, Becker BE, Sanchez R. Formation of bone around titanium implants placed into zero wall defects: pilot project using reinforced e-PTFE membrane and autogenous bone grafts. *Clin Implant Dent Relat Res.* 1999; 12:98–104.

Annibali S, Bignozzi I, La Monaca G, Cristalli MP. Usefulness of the aesthetic result as a success criterion for implant therapy: a review. *Clin Implant Dent Relat Res.* 2012; 14(1):3–40.

Araújo MG, Lindhe J. Dimensional ridge alterations following tooth extraction. An experimental study in the dog. *J Clin Periodontol.* 2005; 32:212–218.

Augthun M, Yildirim M, Spiekermann H, Biesterfeld S. Healing of bone defects in combination with immediate implants using the membrane technique. *Int J Oral Maxillofac Implants.* 1995; 10:421–428.

Botticelli D, Berglundh T, Buser D, Lindhe J. The jumping distance revisited: an experimental study in the dog. *Clin Oral Implants Res.* 2003; 141:35–42.

Cafiero C, Annibali S, Gherlone E et al. Immediate transmucosal implant placement in molar extraction sites: a 12-month prospective multicenter cohort study. *Clin Oral Implants Res.* 2008; 19:476–482.

Chappuis V, Buser R, Brägger U et al. Long-term outcomes of dental implants with a titanium plasma sprayed surface: a 20-year prospective case series study in partially edentulous patients. *Clin Implant Dent Relat Res.* 2013; 15(6):780–790.

Chen ST, Buser D. Clinical and esthetic outcomes of implants placed in post extraction sites. *Int J Oral Maxillofac Implants.* 2009; 24(Suppl):186–217.

Chen ST, Dahlin C. Connective tissue grafting for primary closure of extraction sockets treated with an osteopromotive membrane technique: surgical technique and clinical results. *Int J Periodontics Restorative Dent.* 1996; 164:348–355.

Chen ST, Darby IB, Adams GG, Reynolds EC. A prospective clinical study of bone augmentation techniques at immediate implants. *Clin Oral Implants Res.* 2005; 16:176–184.

Chen ST, Darby IB, Reynolds EC. A prospective clinical study of non-submerged immediate implants: clinical outcomes and esthetic results. *Clin Oral Implants Res.* 2007; 18:552–562.

Chen ST, Wilson TG Jr, Hämmerle CHF. Immediate or early placement of implants following tooth extraction: review of biologic basis, clinical procedures, and outcomes. *Int J Oral Maxillofac Implants.* 2004;19(Suppl):12–25.

Cornelini R, Cangini F, Covani U, Wilson TG Jr. Immediate restoration of implants placed into fresh extraction sockets for single-tooth replacement: a prospective clinical study. *Int J Periodontics Restorative Dent.* 2005; 25:439–447.

Covani U, Crespi R, Cornelini R, Barone A. Immediate implants supporting single crown restoration: a 4-year prospective study. *J Periodontol.* 2004; 75:982–988.

De Boever AL, Quirynen M, Coucke W, Theuniers G, De Boever JA. Clinical and radiographic study of implant treatment outcome in periodontally susceptible and non-susceptible patients: a prospective long-term study. *Clin Oral Implants Res.* 2009; 20:1341–1350.

de Wijs FLJA, Cune MS, de Putter C. Delayed implants in the anterior maxilla with the IMZ-implant system. *J Oral Rehabil.* 1995; 22:319–326.

Degidi M, Piattelli A, Carinci F. Immediate loaded dental implants: comparison between fixtures inserted in postextractive and healed bone sites. *J Craniofac Surg.* 2007; 18:965–971.

Degidi M, Piattelli A, Gehrke P, Felice P, Carinci F. Five-year outcome of 111 immediate nonfunctional single restorations. *J Oral Implantol.* 2006; 32:277–285.

Evans CJD, Chen ST. Esthetic outcomes of immediate implant placements. *Clin Oral Implants Res.* 2008; 19:73–80.

Evian CI, Emling R, Rosenberg ES et al. Retrospective analysis of implant survival and the influence of periodontal disease and immediate placement on long-term results. *Int J Oral Maxillofac Implants.* 2004; 19:393–398.

Gher ME, Quintero G, Assad D, Monaco E, Richardson AC. Bone grafting and guided bone regeneration for immediate dental implants in humans. *J Periodontol.* 1994; 65:881–991.

Gluckman H, Du Toit J. The management of recession midfacial to immediately placed implants in the aesthetic zone. *International Dentistry African Ed.* 2015; 5:6–15.

Gluckman H, Du Toit J, Salama M. The pontic shield: partial extraction therapy for ridge preservation and pontic site development. *Int J Periodontics Restorative Dent.* 2016a: 36;417–423.

Gluckman H, Salama M, Du Toit J. Partial extraction therapies (PET). Part 1: maintaining alveolar ridge contour at pontic and immediate implant sites. *Int J Periodontics Restorative Dent.* 2016b; 36:681–687.

Gluckman H, Salama M, Du Toit J. Partial extraction therapies (PET). Part 2: procedures and technical aspects. *Int J Periodontics Restorative Dent.* 2017; 37:377–385.

Goldstein M, Boyan BD, Schwartz Z. The palatal advanced flap: a pedicle flap for primary coverage of immediately placed implants. *Clin Oral Implants Res.* 2002; 13(6):644–650.

Graziani F, Chappuis V, Molina A et al. Effectiveness and clinical performance of early implant placement for the replacement of single teeth in anterior areas: a systematic review. *J Clin Periodontol.* 2019; 46(Suppl. 21):242–256.

Hämmerle CHF, Chen ST, Wilson TG Jr. Consensus statements and recommended clinical procedures regarding the placement of implants in extraction sockets. *Int J Oral Maxillofac Implants.* 2004; 19(Suppl):26–28.

Hämmerle CHF, Araújo M, Lindhe J. Timing of implant placement. In: J Lindhe & NP Lang (eds), *Clinical Periodontology and Implant Dentistry.* Oxford: Wiley-Blackwell; 2015: 1073–1088.

Horwitz J, Zuabi O, Peled M, Machtei EE. Immediate and delayed restoration of dental implants in periodontally susceptible patients: 1-year results. *Int J Oral Maxillofac Implants*. 2007; 22:423–429.

Hürzeler MB, Zuhr O, Schupbach P et al. The socket-shield technique: a proof-of-principle report. *J Clin Periodontol*. 2010; 37:855–862.

Jaffin RA, Berman CL. The excessive loss of Brånemark fixtures in type IV bone: a 5-year analysis. *J Periodontol*. 1991; 62:2–4.

Johnson K. A study of the dimensional changes occurring in the maxilla after tooth extraction. Part 1: normal healing. *Aust Dent J*. 1963; 8:428–434.

Johnson K. A study of the dimensional changes occurring in the maxilla following tooth extraction. *Aust Dent J*. 1969; 14:241–244.

Kan JY, Rungcharassaeng K. Proximal socket shield for interimplant papilla preservation in the esthetic zone. *Int J Periodontics Restorative Dent*. 2013; 33:e24–e31.

Kan JYK, Rungcharassaeng K, Sclar A, Lozada JL. Effects of the facial osseous defect morphology on gingival dynamics after immediate tooth replacement and guided bone regeneration: 1-year results. *J Oral Maxillofac Surg*. 2007; 65(suppl 1):13–19.

Klokkevold PR. Basic implant surgical procedures. In: MG Newman, HH Takei, PR Klokkevold et al. (eds), *Newman and Carranza's Clinical Periodontology*. St. Louis, MO: Elsevier Saunders; 2019: 4247–4276.

Lam RV. Contour changes of the alveolar processes following extraction. *J Prosthet Dent*. 1960; 10:25–32.

Lang NP, Bragger U, Hämmerle CH, Sutter F. Immediate transmucosal implants using the principle of guided tissue regeneration. I. Rationale, clinical procedures and 30-month results. *Clin Oral Implants Res*. 1994; 5:154–163.

Lang NP, Lui P, Lau KY, Li KY, Wong MCM. A systematic review on survival and success rates of implants placed immediately into fresh extraction sockets after at least 1 year. *Clin Oral Impl Res*. 2012; 23(Suppl 5):39–66.

Lanza A, Scognamiglio F, Femiano F, Lanza M. Immediate, early, and conventional implant placement in a patient with history of periodontitis. *Case report. Case Rep Dent*. 2015; 2015:217895.

Lekovic V, Camargo PM, Klokkevold PR et al. Preservation of alveolar bone in extraction sockets using bioabsorbable membranes. *J Periodontol*. 1998; 69(9):1044–1049.

Lekovic V, Kenney EB, Weinlaender M et al. A bone regenerative approach to alveolar ridge maintenance following tooth extraction. Report of 10 cases. *J Periodontol*. 1997; 686:563–570.

Lindeboom JA, Tjiook Y, Kroon FH. Immediate placement of implants in periapical infected sites: a prospective randomized study in 50 patients. *Oral Surg Oral Med Oral Pathol Oral Radiol Endod*. 2006; 101:705–710.

Lindhe J, Lang NP (eds) *Clinical Periodontology and Implant Dentistry*. Oxford: Wiley-Blackwell; 2015.

Nemcovsky CE, Artzi Z. Comparative study of buccal dehiscence defects in immediate, delayed, and late maxillary implant placement with collagen membranes: clinical healing between placement and second-stage surgery. *J Periodontol*. 2002; 73(7):754–761.

Nemcovsky CE, Artzi Z, Moses O. Rotated palatal flap in immediate implant procedures. Clinical evaluation of 26 consecutive cases. *Clin Oral Implants Res*. 2000; 11:83–90.

Newman MG, Takei HH, Klokkevold PR et al. *Newman and Carranza's Clinical Periodontology*. St. Louis, MO: Elsevier Saunders; 2019.

Nir-Hadar O, Palmer M, Soskolne WA. Delayed immediate implants: alveolar bone changes during the healing period. *Clin Oral Implants Res*. 1998; 9:26–33.

Perry J, Lenchewski E. Clinical performance and 5-year retrospective evaluation of Frialit-2 implants. *Int J Oral Maxillofac Implants*. 2004; 19:887–891.

Pjetursson BE, Tan K, Lang NP et al. A systematic review of the survival and complication rates of fixed partial dentures (FPDS) after an observation period of at least 5 years. *Clin Oral Implants Res*. 2004; 15(6):625–642.

Polizzi G, Grunder U, Goene R et al. Immediate and delayed implant placement into extraction sockets: a 5-year report. *Clin Implant Dent Relat Res*. 2000; 2:93–99.

Renvert S, Persson GR. Periodontitis as a potential risk factor for peri-implantitis. *J Clin Periodontol*. 2009; 36(Suppl 10):9–14.

Rocci A, Martignoni M, Gottlow J. Immediate loading in the maxilla using flapless surgery, implants placed in predetermined positions, and prefabricated provisional restorations: a retrospective 3-year clinical study. *Clin Implant Dent Relat Res*. 2003; 5(suppl 1):29–35.

Salama M, Ishikawa T, Salama H, Funato A, Garber D. Advantages of the root submergence technique for pontic site development in esthetic implant therapy. *Int J Periodontics Restorative Dent*. 2007; 27:521–527.

Scharf DR, Tarnow DP. The effect of crestal versus mucobuccal incisions on the success rate of implant osseointegration. *Int J Oral Maxillofac Implants*. 1993; 8:187–190.

Schropp L, Kostopoulos L, Wenzel A. Bone healing following immediate versus delayed placement of titanium implants into extraction sockets: a prospective clinical study. *Int J Oral Maxillofac Implants*. 2003a; 182:189–199.

Schropp L, Wenzel A, Kostopoulos L, Karring T. Bone healing and soft tissue contour changes following single-tooth extraction: a clinical and radiographic 12-month prospective study. *Int J Periodontics Restorative Dent*. 2003b; 23:313–323.

Schwartz-Arad D, Chaushu G. Immediate implant placement: a procedure without incisions. *J Periodontol*. 1998; 697:743–750.

Siegenthaler DW, Jung RE, Holderegger C, Roos M, Hämmerle CH. Replacement of teeth exhibiting periapical pathology by immediate implants. A prospective, controlled clinical trial. *Clin Oral Implants Res*. 2007; 18:727–737.

Stentz WC, Mealey BL, Gunsolley JC, Waldrop TC. Effects of guided bone regeneration around commercially pure titanium and hydroxyapatite-coated dental implants. *II. Histologic analysis. J Periodontol.* 1997; 68(10):933–949.

van Steenberghe D, Callens A, Geers L, Jacobs R. The clinical use of deproteinized bovine bone mineral on bone regeneration in conjunction with immediate implant installation. *Clin Oral Implants Res.* 2000; 11:210–216.

Watanabe F, Tawada Y, Komatsu S et al. Heat distribution in bone during preparation of implant sites: heat analysis by real-time thermography. *Int J Oral Maxillofac Implants.* 1992; 7:212–219.

Watzek G, Haider R, Mensdorff-Pouilly N, Haas R. Immediate and delayed implantation for complete restoration of the jaw following extraction of all residual teeth: a retrospective study comparing different types of serial immediate implantation. *Int J Oral Maxillofac Implants.* 1995; 10:561–567.

Wilson TG Jr, Carnio J, Schenk R, Cochran D. Immediate implants covered with connective tissue membranes: human biopsies. *J Periodontol* 2003; 743:402–409.

Wilson TG Jr, Schenk R, Buser D, Cochran D. Implants placed in immediate extraction sites: a report of histologic and histometric analyses of human biopsies. *Int J Oral Maxillofac Implants.* 1998; 133:333–341.

Zitzmann NU, Naef R, Schärer P. Resorbable versus nonresorbable membranes in combination with Bio-Oss for guided bone regeneration. *Int J Oral Maxillofac Implants.* 1997; 12:844–852.

CHAPTER 34
Peri-implant diseases and conditions

Steph Smith

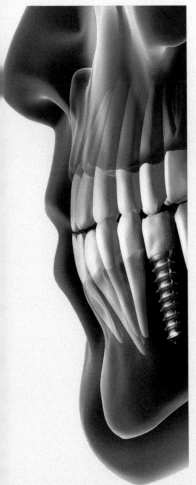

Contents

Learning objectives

- Histological features of peri-implant tissues in health.
- Development and risk indicators of peri-implant mucositis.
- Overview of features of peri-implantitis.
- Case definitions and diagnostic criteria for peri-implant health, peri-implant mucositis and peri-implantitis.
- Factors associated with and/or causing soft and hard tissue deficiencies of dental implants.

Essential Periodontics, First Edition. Edited by Steph Smith and Khalid Almas.
© 2022 John Wiley & Sons Ltd. Published 2022 by John Wiley & Sons Ltd.

Introduction

The tissues occurring around osseointegrated dental implants are referred to as peri-implant tissues, being divided into soft and hard tissue compartments. The soft tissue compartment is denoted peri-implant mucosa, and is formed during the wound-healing process following implant/abutment placement. The hard tissue compartment forms a contact relationship to the implant surface, thereby securing implant stability (Albrektsson & Sennerby 1991; Berglundh et al. 2007). The peri-implant mucosa protects the underlying bone, while the bone supports the implant (Araujo & Lindhe 2018).

Peri-implant health

Peri-implant mucosa

Following implant placement, usually 6–8 weeks afterward, a mature peri-implant mucosal adhesion to the implant surface is established comprising a core of connective tissue covered by either non-keratinized or often orthokeratinized squamous epithelium (Araujo & Lindhe 2018). Keratinized mucosa may be present at many implant sites, extending from the margin of the peri-implant mucosa to the lining oral mucosa. It consists of a fibrous connective tissue lamina propria, including fibroblasts and equal amounts of type I and III collagen. The thickness of the facial keratinized mucosa can be greater at implants than at teeth (2.0 mm vs. 1.1 mm, respectively) (Chang et al. 1999; DeAngelo et al. 2007). Controversy exists as to the need for a minimum amount of keratinized mucosa to maintain peri-implant tissue health (Brito et al. 2014; Wennström & Derks 2012). Studies have failed to associate the lack of a minimum amount of keratinized mucosa with mucosal inflammation (Kim et al. 2009; Schrott et al. 2009), while other studies have suggested plaque build-up and marginal inflammation to be more frequent at implant sites with <2 mm of keratinized mucosa (Bouri et al. 2008; Boynueğri et al. 2013).

When measured from the mucosal margin to the peri-implant bone crest, the peri-implant mucosa is 3–4 mm in height. The portion of the peri-implant mucosa facing the implant (abutment) is designated as the peri-implant supracrestal tissue attachment (old term: biological width) (Kao et al. 2020). The coronal portion of the supracrestal tissue attachment consists of a thin, non-keratinized barrier epithelium (similar to the junctional epithelium of the gingiva), with a basal lamina and hemidesmosomes facing the implant or abutment surface (Listgarten et al. 1991), and a non-keratinized peri-implant sulcular epithelium (Kao et al. 2020). In total, this portion is usually about 2 mm long (Araujo & Lindhe 2018). The apical segment of the supracrestal tissue attachment is designated as the zone of connective tissue adhesion, which appears to be in direct contact with the implant surface (Araujo & Lindhe 2018) (Figure 34.1).

The connective tissue adhesion zone is comprised of collagen fibers and matrix elements (85%), comparatively few fibroblasts (3%), and vascular units (5%). In the connective tissue immediately lateral to the barrier and sulcular epithelium is a delicate plexus of vascular structures, similar to the dentogingival vascular plexus (Berglundh et al. 1994). The connective tissue adhesion zone appears to harbor only limited amounts of vascular structures. The connective tissue adhesion zone furthermore includes two distinct layers: an inner layer, about 40 μm wide, harboring large numbers of fibroblasts (32% of volume) that appear to be in intimate contact with the surface of the implant; and an outer layer, about 160 μm wide, dominated by collagen fibers (83%), smaller numbers of fibroblasts (11%), and larger volumes of vascular structures (3%) (Moon et al. 1999). At implants placed into masticatory mucosa, the main collagen fiber bundles are anchored in the crestal bone and extend in a marginal direction parallel to the surface of the metal device. It is assumed that circular fibers may also be present in this type of peri-implant mucosa (Araujo & Lindhe 2018; Kao et al. 2020) (Figure 34.1).

An inflammatory cell infiltrate in the connective tissue adjacent to the epithelial barrier represents the host's defense against the bacterial challenge. The barrier epithelium and the presence of scattered inflammatory cells constitute the soft tissue seal separating the healthy peri-implant attachment from the oral cavity (Heitz-Mayfield & Salvi 2018; Tonetti et al. 1995). The absence of Sharpey's fibers and cementum around dental implants constitutes a weak coronal seal, thereby rendering implants more susceptible to pathogenic challenges and tissue inflammation (Kao et al. 2020).

The soft tissue cuff around implants has been suggested to show less resistance to probing than the gingiva at adjacent tooth sites. This property may lead to mechanically induced bleeding on probing on dental implants that are clinically healthy (Abrahamsson & Soldini 2006). In general, the

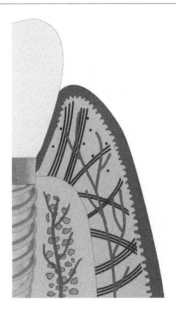

Figure 34.1 Peri-implant health. Courtesy of Dr. Abdulqader Alhammadi.

probing depth associated with peri-implant health should be ≤5.0 mm (Araujo & Lindhe 2018). Peri-implant tissue health can also exist following treatment of peri-implantitis with variable levels of bone support (Renvert et al. 2018).

Bone tissue around implants

Modeling of the bone occurs following implant installation and loading, whereby some crestal bone height may be lost during this healing phase (Berglundh & Stavropoulos 2012; Hermann et al. 1997). This crestal bone reduction apparently varies between implant brands and seems to be related to the design of the implant system used (implant–abutment interface) (Berglundh & Stavropoulos 2012; Ekelund et al. 2003; Hermann et al. 1997). After this initial period, osseointegration takes place and about 75% of implants experience no additional bone loss (Araujo & Lindhe 2018). Most implant sites that exhibit crestal bone loss of >1 mm appear to be associated with soft tissue inflammation, or with an apparent absence thereof (Derks et al. 2015). For a detailed description of implant surfaces and osseointegration, see Chapter 28.

Peri-implant mucositis

Peri-implant mucositis is an inflammatory lesion of the mucosa surrounding an endosseous implant without loss of supporting peri-implant bone (Heitz-Mayfield & Salvi 2018; Zitzmann & Berglundh 2008).

The clinical sign of inflammation is bleeding on probing, and may additionally include signs of erythema, swelling, and suppuration (Heitz-Mayfield & Salvi 2018).

Pathognomonic features of peri-implant mucositis

Peri-implant mucositis develops from healthy peri-implant mucosa following accumulation of bacterial biofilms around osseointegrated dental implants. A cause-and-effect relationship between bacterial biofilms around titanium dental implants and the development of an inflammatory response (i.e. experimental peri-implant mucositis) has been demonstrated in humans (Meyer et al. 2017; Salvi et al. 2012). When comparing biopsies from gingiva at teeth and biopsies from peri-implant mucosa, the size of the inflammatory cell infiltrate and number of immune cell populations were found not to be significantly different (Zitzmann et al. 2001). Biofilm-induced peri-implant mucositis has also been shown to be a reversible disease (Meyer et al. 2017), although it may take longer than 3 weeks for complete clinical resolution thereof (Heitz-Mayfield & Salvi 2018). Peri-implant mucositis may be present for extensive periods of time without progression to peri-implantitis; however, sites with peri-implant mucositis should be considered at increased risk for the development of peri-implantitis (Costa et al. 2012; Heitz-Mayfield & Salvi 2018).

Studies have shown that, even though the plaque index may be significantly higher at tooth sites as compared to implant sites, a higher proportion of bleeding sites can be found in the peri-implant mucosa. Furthermore, even with a comparable bacterial challenge at implant and tooth sites, a significantly higher increase of gingival inflammation may be observed at implant sites (Meyer et al. 2017; Salvi et al. 2012).

Risk indicators/factors for peri-implant mucositis

General risk indicators that have been identified for peri-implant mucositis are cigarette smoking, radiation therapy, and diabetes mellitus (Gómez-Moreno et al. 2015; Karbach et al. 2009). Major local risk indicators are a significant dose-dependent association between plaque scores and peri-implant mucositis; the compliance/lack of compliance with supportive implant therapy; implants with submucosal restoration margins; and excess cement (Heitz-Mayfield & Salvi 2018). Evidence for the presence or a minimum width of keratinized peri-implant mucosa is controversial (Heitz-Mayfield & Salvi 2018). A lack of or inadequate width of less than 2 mm at implant sites has been shown to be associated with higher rates of peri-implant mucositis (Lin et al. 2013).

Peri-implantitis

Peri-implantitis is a pathological condition occurring in tissues around dental implants, characterized by inflammation in the peri-implant mucosa and progressive loss of supporting bone (Schwarz et al. 2018).

2017 World Workshop evidence-based overview on peri-implantitis

A narrative review by Schwarz et al. (2018) provides an evidence-based overview on peri-implantitis as determined by the 2017 World Workshop on the Classification of Periodontal and Peri-Implant Diseases and Conditions. The following conclusions were reached:

- The histopathological and clinical conditions leading to the conversion from peri-implant mucositis to peri-implantitis are not completely understood.
- The onset of peri-implantitis may occur early during follow-up and the disease progresses in a non-linear and accelerating pattern.
- Peri-implantitis sites exhibit clinical signs of inflammation and increased probing depths compared to baseline measurements.
- At the histological level, compared to periodontitis sites, peri-implantitis sites often have larger inflammatory lesions.
- Surgical entry at peri-implantitis sites often reveals a circumferential pattern of bone loss.
- There is strong evidence that there is an increased risk of developing peri-implantitis in patients who have a history of chronic periodontitis, poor plaque control skills, and no regular maintenance care after implant therapy. Data identifying "smoking" and "diabetes" as potential risk factors/indicators for peri-implantitis are inconclusive.

- There is some limited evidence linking peri-implantitis to other factors such as post-restorative presence of submucosal cement, lack of peri-implant keratinized mucosa, and positioning of implants that makes it difficult to perform oral hygiene and maintenance.
- There is currently no evidence that occlusal overload constitutes a risk factor/indicator for the onset or progression of peri-implantitis.
- Available evidence does not allow for an evaluation of the role of titanium or metal particles in the pathogenesis of peri-implant diseases.
- Evidence suggests that progressive crestal bone loss around implants in the absence of clinical signs of soft tissue inflammation is a rare event.

For a more detailed description of the diagnosis and treatment of peri-implantitis, see Chapter 35.

Clinical case definitions for peri-implant health, peri-implant mucositis, and peri-implantitis

To enable the clinician to assign a proper diagnosis and treatment plan in cases where disease is present, a state of peri-implant health must be differentiated from clearly defined conditions of peri-implant mucositis and peri-implantitis (Renvert et al. 2018). In the absence of a standard therapeutic protocol for the management of peri-implant diseases, there remains a need to establish applicable clinical guidelines for the diagnosis of peri-implant mucositis and peri-implantitis (Mattheos et al. 2012; Renvert et al. 2018). The clinical diagnostic guidelines for the case definitions of peri-implant health, peri-implant mucositis, and peri-implantitis are depicted in Table 34.1.

Peri-implant soft and hard tissue deficiencies

Tissue deficiencies at implant sites are common clinical findings (de Souza Nunes et al. 2013). Their presence may lead to an increase in marginal bone loss, soft tissue inflammation, and soft tissue recession (Hämmerle & Tarnow 2018). Hard tissue defects at implant sites encompass intra-alveolar defects, dehiscence, fenestration, horizontal ridge defects, and vertical ridge defects (Benic & Hammerle 2014). Soft tissue defects include volume and quality deficiencies, i.e. lack of keratinized tissue (Thoma et al. 2014). The factors associated with and/or causing soft and hard tissue deficiencies of dental implants are depicted in Table 34.2. For a more detailed description of these factors, the reader is referred to Hämmerle and Tarnow (2018).

Table 34.1 Case definitions for peri-implant health, peri-implant mucositis, and peri-implantitis.

Case definition	Diagnostic criteria
Peri-implant health	• Visual inspection demonstrating the absence of peri-implant signs of inflammation: pink as opposed to red, no swelling as opposed to swollen tissues, firm as opposed to soft tissue consistency • Lack of profuse (line or drop) bleeding on probing • Probing pocket depths could differ depending on the height of the soft tissue at the implant location. An increase in probing depth over time, however, conflicts with peri-implant health • Absence of further bone loss following initial healing, which should not be ≥ 2 mm
Peri-implant mucositis	• Visual inspection demonstrating the presence of peri-implant signs of inflammation: red as opposed to pink, swollen tissues as opposed to no swelling, soft as opposed to firm tissue consistency • Presence of profuse (line or drop) bleeding and/or suppuration on probing • Increase in probing depths compared to baseline • Absence of bone loss beyond crestal bone-level changes resulting from initial remodeling
Peri-implantitis	• Evidence of visual inflammatory changes in the peri-implant soft tissues combined with bleeding on probing and/or suppuration • Increasing probing pocket depths compared to measurements obtained at placement of the supra-structure • Progressive bone loss in relation to the radiographic bone-level assessment at 1 year following delivery of the implant-supported prosthetics reconstruction • In the absence of initial radiographs and probing depths, radiographic evidence of bone level ≥ 3 mm and/or probing depths ≥ 6 mm in conjunction with profuse bleeding represents peri-implantitis

Source: Adapted from Renvert et al. 2018.

Table 34.2 Factors affecting hard and soft tissue deficiencies at dental implants.

Hard tissue deficiencies prior to implant placement	These deficiencies encompass situations where the available amount of bone does not allow placing of a standard implant fully embedded in the local host bone	Tooth loss, trauma from tooth extraction, periodontitis, endodontic infections, longitudinal root fractures, general trauma, bone height in posterior maxilla, systemic diseases
Hard tissue deficiencies after implant placement	These deficiencies may be associated with healthy situations and those associated with diseases and malfunctions	Defects in healthy situations, malpositioning of implants, peri-implantitis, mechanical overload, soft tissue thickness, systemic diseases
Soft tissue deficiencies prior to implant placement	These deficiencies encompass the available amount of soft tissue not easily allowing coverage of bone volume augmentation; tension-free primary coverage of implant placement site; tension-free adaptation of keratinized soft tissue flap around neck of placed implant	Tooth loss, periodontal disease, systemic diseases
Soft tissue deficiencies after implant placement		Lack of buccal bone, papilla height, keratinized tissue, migration of teeth, life-long skeletal changes

Source: Adapted from Hämmerle & Tarnow 2018.

REFERENCES

Abrahamsson I, Soldini C. Probe penetration in periodontal and peri-implant tissues. An experimental study in the beagle dog. *Clin Oral Implants Res.* 2006; 17:601–605.

Albrektsson T, Sennerby L. State of the art in oral implants. *J Clin Periodontol.* 1991; 18:474–481.

Araujo MG, Lindhe J. Peri-implant health. *J Clin Periodontol.* 2018; 45(Suppl 20):S230–S236.

Benic GI, Hammerle CH. Horizontal bone augmentation by means of guided bone regeneration. *Periodontol 2000.* 2014; 66:13–40.

Berglundh T, Abrahamsson I, Welander M, Lang NP, Lindhe J. Morphogenesis of the peri-implant mucosa: an experimental study in dogs. *Clin Oral Implants Res.* 2007; 18:1–8.

Berglundh T, Lindhe J, Jonsson K, Ericsson I. The topography of the vascular systems in the periodontal and peri-implant tissues in the dog. *J Clin Periodontol.* 1994; 21:189–193.

Berglundh T, Stavropoulos A. Preclinical in vivo research in implant dentistry. Consensus of the eighth European workshop on periodontology. *J Clin Periodontol.* 2012; 39(Suppl. 1):1–5.

Bouri A, Bissada N, Al-Zahrani MS, Faddoul F, Nouneh I. Width of keratinized gingiva and the health status of the supporting tissues around dental implants. *Int J Oral Maxillofac Implants.* 2008; 23:323–326.

Boynueğri D, Nemli SK, Kasko YA. Significance of keratinized mucosa around dental implants: a prospective comparative study. *Clin Oral Implants Res.* 2013; 24:928–933.

Brito C, Tenenbaum HC, Wong BKC, Schmitt C, Nogueira-Filho G. Is keratinized mucosa indispensable to maintain peri-implant health? A systematic review of the literature. *J Biomed Mater Res B Appl Biomater.* 2014; 102:643–650.

Chang M, Wennström JL, Odman P, Andersson B. Implant supported single-tooth replacements compared to contralateral natural teeth. Crown and soft tissue dimensions. *Clin Oral Implants Res.* 1999; 10:185–194.

Costa FO, Takenaka-Martinez S, Cota LOO et al. Peri-implant disease in subjects with and without preventive maintenance: a 5-year follow-up. *J Clin Periodontol.* 2012; 39:173–181.

de Souza Nunes LS, Bornstein MM, Sendi P, Buser D. Anatomical characteristics and dimensions of edentulous sites in the posterior maxillae of patients referred for implant therapy. *Int J Periodontics Restorative Dent.* 2013; 33:337–345.

DeAngelo SJ, Kumar PS, Beck FM, Tatakis DN, Leblebicioglu B. Early soft tissue healing around one-stage dental implants: clinical and microbiologic parameters. *J Periodontol.* 2007; 78:1878–1886.

Derks J, Håkansson J, Wennström JL et al. Effectiveness of implant therapy analyzed in a Swedish population: early and late implant loss. *J Dent Res.* 2015; 94:44S–51S.

Ekelund J-A, Lindquist LW, Carlsson GE, Jemt T. Implant treatment in the edentulous mandible: a prospective study on Brånemark system implants over more than 20 years. *Int J Prosthodont.* 2003; 16:602–608.

Gómez-Moreno G, Aguilar-Salvatierra A, Rubio Roldán J et al. Peri-implant evaluation in type 2 diabetes mellitus patients: a 3-year study. *Clin Oral Implants Res.* 2015; 26:1031–1035.

Hämmerle CHF, Tarnow D. The etiology of hard- and soft-tissue deficiencies at dental implants: a narrative review. *J Clin Periodontol.* 2018; 45(Suppl 20):S267–S277.

Heitz-Mayfield LJA, Salvi GE. Peri-implant mucositis. *J Clin Periodontol.* 2018; 45 (Suppl 20):S237–S245.

Hermann JS, Cochran DL, Nummikoski PV, Buser D. Crestal bone changes around titanium implants. A radiographic evaluation of unloaded non-submerged and submerged implants in the canine mandible. *J Periodontol.* 1997; 68:1117–1130.

Kao RT, Curtis DA, Kim DM et al. American Academy of Periodontology best evidence consensus statement on modifying periodontal phenotype in preparation for orthodontic and restorative treatment. *J Periodontol.* 2020; 91:289–298.

Karbach J, Callaway A, Kwon Y-DD, d'Hoedt B, Al-Nawas B. Comparison of five parameters as risk factors for peri-mucositis. *Int J Oral Maxillofac Implants.* 2009; 24:491–496.

Kim B-S, Kim Y-K, Yun P-Y et al. Evaluation of peri-implant tissue response according to the presence of keratinized mucosa. *Oral Surg Oral Med Oral Pathol Oral Radiol Endod.* 2009; 107:e24–e28.

Lin G-HH, Chan H-LL, Wang H-LL. The significance of keratinized mucosa on implant health: a systematic review. *J Periodontol.* 2013; 84:1755–1767.

Listgarten MA, Lang NP, Schroeder HE, Schroeder A. Periodontal tissues and their counterparts around endosseous implants. *Oral Implants Res.* 1991; 2:1–19.

Mattheos N, Collier S, Walmsley AD. Specialists' management decisions and attitudes towards mucositis and peri-implantitis. *Br Dent J.* 2012; 212:E1.

Meyer S, Giannopoulou C, Courvoisier D et al. Experimental mucositis and experimental gingivitis in persons aged 70 or over. Clinical and biological responses. *Clin Oral Implants Res.* 2017; 28(8):1005–1012.

Moon IS, Berglundh T, Abrahamsson I, Linder E, Lindhe J. The barrier between the keratinized mucosa and the dental implant. An experimental study in the dog. *J Clin Periodontol.* 1999; 26:658–663.

Renvert S, Persson GR, Pirih FQ, Camargo PM. Peri-implant health, peri-implant mucositis, and peri-implantitis: case definitions and diagnostic considerations. *J Clin Periodontol.* 2018; 45(Suppl 20):S278–S285.

Salvi GE, Aglietta M, Eick S et al. Reversibility of experimental peri-implant mucositis compared with experimental gingivitis in humans. *Clin Oral Implants Res.* 2012; 23:182–190.

Schrott AR, Jimenez M, Hwang J-W, Fiorellini J, Weber H-P. Five-year evaluation of the influence of keratinized mucosa on peri-implant soft-tissue health and stability around implants supporting full-arch mandibular fixed prostheses. *Clin Oral Implants Res.* 2009; 20:1170–1177.

Schwarz F, Derks J, Monje A, Wang H-L. Peri-implantitis. *J Clin Periodontol.* 2018;45(Suppl 20):S246–S266.

Thoma DS, Buranawat B, Hammerle CH, Held U, Jung RE. Efficacy of soft tissue augmentation around dental implants and in partially edentulous areas: a systematic review. *J Clin Periodontol.* 2014; 41(Suppl. 15):S77–91.

Tonetti MS, Imboden M, Gerber L, Lang NP. Compartmentalization of inflammatory cell phenotypes in normal gingiva and peri-implant keratinized mucosa. *J Clin Periodontol.* 1995; 22:735–742.

Wennström JL, Derks J. Is there a need for keratinized mucosa around implants to maintain health and tissue stability? *Clin Oral Implants Res.* 2012; 23(Suppl 6):136–146.

Zitzmann NU, Berglundh T. Definition and prevalence of peri-implant diseases. *J Clin Periodontol.* 2008; 35:286–291.

Zitzmann NU, Berglundh T, Marinello CP, Lindhe J. Experimental peri-implant mucositis in man. *J Clin Periodontol.* 2001; 28:517–523.

CHAPTER 35
Peri-implantitis

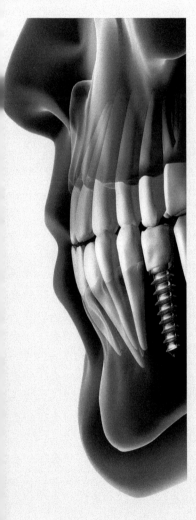

Contents

Essential Periodontics, First Edition. Edited by Steph Smith and Khalid Almas.
© 2022 John Wiley & Sons Ltd. Published 2022 by John Wiley & Sons Ltd.

35.1 THE PERI-IMPLANT MICROBIOME

Steph Smith

Contents

Learning objectives

- Considerations for differences between periodontitis and peri-implant associated microbiomes.
- Various mechanisms involved in initial peri-implant biofilm formation.
- Effects of implant surface topography on biofilm formation.
- Effects of bio-tribocorrosion on implant surfaces, biofilm formation, tissue responses, and allergies/hypersensitivity.
- Bacterial composition on healthy and diseased implant surfaces.
- Modifications of implant surfaces for the prevention of bacterial surface contamination.

Introduction

Peri-implantitis is a biofilm-related, immune-mediated chronic inflammation that affects implant sites and is characterized by loss of implant supporting bone (Kinane et al. 2017). It has been suggested that approximately one-third of all patients and one-fifth of all implants will experience peri-implantitis. Epidemiological observations hrefreave identified the primary risk factors to be ill-fitting or ill-designed fixed and cement-retained restorations, as well as a history of periodontitis (Kordbacheh Changi et al. 2019). Smoking is also an important risk factor, particularly in combination with poor oral hygiene (Kumar 2019). Furthermore, the most common complications related to implants initiate at the implant–bone interface (Figuero et al. 2014).

Implant surfaces are engineered to integrate with bone. This integration is facilitated by adhesion of proteins to the implant surface. However, this protein deposition generates an ideal surface for bacterial colonization and biofilm formation (Hickok et al. 2018). Similar to biofilm formation on natural teeth, bacterial colonization of implant surfaces is rapid and reflective of the native microbiota, occurring within 30 minutes after the implantation procedure and throughout the life cycle of an implant (Belibasakis & Manoil 2021; Furst et al. 2007; Hickok et al. 2018). After implant insertion, during the next 2 weeks, bacterial colonization leads to the establishment of an organized biofilm community in the peri-implant niche, whereby bacterial communities reach a symbiotic equilibrium with the host that is compatible with peri-implant health (Belibasakis & Manoil 2021). Modifications in the microenvironment that promote biofilm growth and also favor the initiation of tissue inflammation cause dysbiotic shifts in the peri-implant microbiota, leading to biofilm-induced peri-implantitis (Belibasakis & Manoil 2021). Peri-implantitis can lead to inefficient osseointegration due to contamination during insertion (early failure) or of already osseointegrated implants (late failure), or lead to compromised bone regeneration/re-osseointegration during the surgical reconstructive phase of treatment (Belibasakis & Manoil 2021).

Both periodontal and peri-implant inflammation are associated respectively with the presence of periodontal or peri-implant biofilms. It has been assumed that these seemingly identical inflammatory phenotypes that are related to bacterial biofilms share similar clinical phenotypes, including signs of soft tissue inflammation, increased depth/bleeding on probing of the gingival pocket area, and destruction of the supporting bones (Esposito et al. 2012; Meffert 1996). Also, both periodontal and peri-implant inflammation share similar pathogenetic mechanisms, which include the histological appearance of associated leukocytic infiltration and intense pro-inflammatory signaling (Kotsakis & Olmedo 2021; Koutouzis et al. 2013; Meffert 1996). Nonetheless, there are fundamental histological and immunophysiological differences between natural teeth and dental implants that render implants more susceptible to endogenous oral infections (Belibasakis 2014; Belibasakis et al. 2015). Furthermore, there is also a difference between bone loss associated with periodontitis and that found in peri-implantitis (Kotsakis & Olmedo 2021). The progression of inflammatory destructive disease around implants, which includes the rate of progression, has been described to be rampant, as substantial bone destruction can be seen clinically as early as 6 months following implant placement (Konstantinidis et al. 2015). Natural teeth are supported in the alveolus via the periodontal ligament (PDL), whereas osseointegrated implants are directly anchored to bone. The resulting lack of PDL limits the blood supply to supraperiosteal vessels, thereby restricting the amount of nutrients and immune cells needed to tackle the early stages of bacterial infection. Also, fibers of the supracrestal connective tissues are positioned circumferentially around implants, not perpendicularly as into natural teeth. These factors therefore reduce the physical barrier against bacterial invasion into the submucosa and thus places peri-implant tissues in an "open wound" conformation (Belibasakis & Manoil 2021).

The primary etiology for bone loss is considered to be specific anaerobic pathogens during biofilm accumulation (Haraguchi et al. 2020). Consequently, treatment protocols for peri-implantitis have been modeled according to those used for periodontitis (Meffert 1996). However, peri-implantitis treatments have been shown to yield only short-term benefits, with some interventions showing a disease recurrence rate of up to 100% at 1 year post treatment (Esposito et al. 2012). Furthermore, resistance to antibiotic regimens that are normally efficacious against periodontitis has been shown in peri-implant microbiotas. A study targeting putative periodontal pathogens in patients with peri-implantitis, utilizing tetracycline or amoxicillin plus metronidazole, reported that 42% of implants had either failed clinically and were lost, or continued to lose peri-implant bone (Leonhardt et al. 2003). A 6-month follow-up study that included the administration of azithromycin as an adjunct to non-surgical debridement to patients with peri-implant mucositis showed no difference in probing depth measurements or bacterial composition between those who did or did not receive adjunctive antibiotics (Hallstrom et al. 2012).

These unsuccessful adaptations of periodontitis treatment strategies for peri-implantitis have thus revealed the need to distinguish peri-implantitis pathogens from the ones associated with periodontitis (Kotsakis & Olmedo 2021). It has therefore been suggested that differences between the disease phenotypes of periodontitis and peri-implants may be ascribed to dissimilarities between the periodontal microbiome and a distinct peri-implant microbiome, this being fundamentally due to different microbiome–biomaterial interactions during biofilm formation (Kostakis & Olmedo 2021).

Peri-implant biofilm formation

Surface energy, topography, wettability, and electrochemical charges of all substrata affect bacterial adhesion and succession during biofilm formation (Busscher et al. 2010; Song et al. 2015). Distinct biofilm structures will thus result from chemically different substrata dictating initial bacterial colonization and subsequent bacterial accumulation (Song et al. 2015). Another fundamental risk factor for the development of peri-implantitis is the abiotic implant surface, which may alter the microbiota as the pathogenic biofilm develops (Lima et al. 2008; Sanchez et al. 2014). Physicochemical and electrochemical characteristics of these different substrata will therefore define each ecological niche, thereby affecting bacterial adhesion with which early colonizers have to contend, leading to further enrichment for selected taxa (Busscher et al. 2010; Song et al. 2015). For example, the wettability properties and adsorption kinetics of intentionally microrough and hydrophilic implant surfaces are different from those of dentin, which affects the organization of pellicle components (Aroonsang et al. 2014; Hannig & Hannig 2009). Despite the existence of a core microbiome that includes early colonizers with strong adhesion properties (e.g. *Streptococcus* spp.) and bridging organisms that support complex biofilms (e.g. *Fusobacterium* spp.), the end result is a microbial community that is distinctly shaped by a specific substratum (Kotsakis & Olmedo 2012). The effects of micro- and nanoscale implant surface topography on bacterial attachment are determined by various mechanisms, namely physicochemical forces, cell membrane deformation, chemical gradients at the solid–liquid interface, hydrodynamics, surface wettability and air entrapment, topography-induced cell ordering and segregation, and conditioning films (Cheng et al. 2019). The various factors mediating peri-implant biofilm formation are shown in Figure 35.1.1.

The titanium surface and initial bacterial colonization

When titanium (Ti) is exposed to fluid medium or air, it quickly develops a layer of titanium dioxide, forming a boundary at the interface between the biological medium and the metal structure. It produces passivation of the metal, thus determining the degree of biocompatibility and the biological response to the implant (Kotsakis & Olmedo 2012). Differences between implant- and tooth-bound biofilms appear as early as bacterial adhesion commences. The electrostatic forces and ionic bonding that drive initial bacterial adhesion are fundamentally different for titanium dioxide compared with mineralized organic hydroxyapatite (Yeo et al. 2012). The adsorption of macromolecules (i.e. proteins) to the implant surface, forming the conditioning film, is governed by the interplay of various physicochemical factors. Upon adsorption, proteins may undergo conformational changes at the liquid–solid interface, which may lower the total free energy of the system; and the extent of unfolding of these proteins is dependent on the hydrophobicity of the solid surface, which, after conditioning, makes the surface energy less predictable (Cheng et al. 2019). This conditioning film will then affect bacterial attachment, as the macromolecules adhered to the implant surface can significantly modify its physicochemical and topographical properties. This includes both surface smoothening and surface-roughening effects (Bakker et al. 2004). Consequently, this can lead to unpredictable deviations from the anticipated outcome of bacteria–surface interactions. However, various studies have reported contradictory results on the effects of this conditioning film on bacterial attachment, which include both inhibitory and opposite effects (Garrido et al. 2013; Hwang et al. 2013).

Immediately after exposure to the oral environment, *Streptococcus* spp. employ their molecular surface milieu, including adhesins, to colonize implant surfaces. However, the distinct microenvironment created by metal implant surfaces and their local dissolution products appears to dictate a very different ecological succession, compared with dental mineralized organic hydroxyapatite. On hydroxyapatite, adhesion of *Streptococcus* spp. is typically succeeded by *Actinomyces naeslundii*, while on titanium substrates there are significantly lower

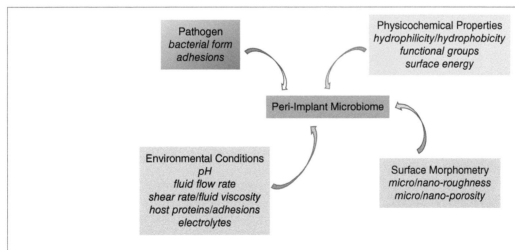

Figure 35.1.1 Factors mediating peri-implant biofilm formation. Source: Adapted from Narayana & Srihari 2019.

numbers of *A. naeslundii*, and coaggregation with *Veillonella* spp. is observed in early biofilms (Bermejo et al. 2019; Yu et al. 2019).

Effects of surface topography on biofilm formation

Surface topography shapes the near surface microenvironment, and therefore plays a central role in controlling bacteria–surface interactions, and thus the outcome of bacterial attachment. Bacterial attachment to a surface involves stages of locating, approaching, and sensing the proximity of the surface. Bacterial cells take in physicochemical or biological signals from their immediate surroundings within each stage and respond accordingly by employing a variety of mechanisms to colonize terrains with diverse surface topographies. This furthermore involves the regulation of gene expression by bacteria responding to the above signals (Cheng et al. 2019).

Bacterial mobility near surfaces can be influenced by the scale of the surface topographies, and consequently influence the spatial organization of biofilms (Chang et al. 2018). Surface topography of a scale comparable with microbial cell dimensions (about 1–2 μm) has been recognized as a crucial and positive contributing factor to bacteria–surface interaction and bacterial attachment (Friedlander et al. 2013; Hsu et al. 2013). By contrast, when the dimensions of surface topography are much larger than those of microbial cells, the attachment behavior seems to be independent of the size of surface features (Scheuerman et al. 1998). Micrometric-scale topography, which is comparable to that of bacterial cells, impacts attachment via hydrodynamics, topography-induced cell ordering, and air entrapment. Nanometric topography impacts attachment via alteration of chemical gradients, physicochemical force fields, and cell membrane deformation. Multiple anti-attachment mechanisms are also involved at the same time, with different ranges of action. Some of these mechanisms may be turned "on" at a certain scale, while others may be turned "off" (Cheng et al. 2019).

Scientific reports describing the effects of topography on bacterial attachment have often led to contradictory conclusions, as topographical effects may be further compounded by other physicochemical factors, e.g. surface chemistry (Cheng et al. 2019). The physical topography and chemistry of implant surfaces determine the wettability of a surface (Genzer & Efimenko 2006). Surface wetting is a very important factor in bacterial attachment. Surface wetting is also affected by surface hydrophobicity/hydrophilicity of implant surfaces. In general, hydrophobic interactions are favoured between relatively hydrophobic bacteria and apolar surfaces, while hydrophilic bacteria prefer to adhere to hydrophilic surfaces (Hori & Matsumoto 2010). *Porphyromonas gingivalis* has been shown to exhibit hydrophobic activity (Naito et al. 1993), and therefore are less adherent to hydrophilic surfaces (Almaguer-Flores et al.

2012). Similarly, *Aggregatibacter actinomycetemcomitans* and *Fusobacterium nucleatum* also have shown reduced levels on hydrophilic surfaces in culture mediums (Almaguer-Flores et al. 2012).

As previously discussed, the presence of a conditioning film often leads to changes in surface chemistry and surface topography (Cheng et al. 2019). Surface topographies with nanometric height and/or depth are susceptible to complete masking of the topography by conditioning films, as the dimensions of adsorbed macromolecules, such as proteins, are also in the nanometer range (Anselme et al. 2010). Surface topography features in the micrometric range are more resistant to such masking effects (Cheng et al. 2019).

Bacteria can employ a variety of mechanisms to colonize diverse surface topographies and, as previously mentioned, are able to actively sense and respond to surface topography, which in turn affects attachment. Certain species, e.g. *Staphylococcus epidermidis*, produce surface-associated adhesins that facilitate cell–cell cohesion, allowing early colonizers to provide a foothold for subsequent colonizers. Further cell–cell interactions occurring between bacteria from different species lead to the development of symbiotic microbial biofilm communities (Rickard et al. 2003). Bacterial appendages have also been shown to interact directly with various surface topographies (Friedlander et al. 2013). Flagellated bacterial cells can explore recessed topography that may be inaccessible to cell bodies, by using their flagellar filaments. Such filaments are able to form networks that bridge large interfeature spacings like a "hammock," resulting in improved attachment of additional cells (Cheng et al. 2019).

Surface roughness has been found to have a significant impact on biofilm formation. The surface roughness at micrometer level can increase the surface area and hence increase the bacterial colonization (Pita et al. 2015). Various in vitro studies have been performed to assess biofilm formation on dental implants with different surface microtopography, which included moderate-roughness surfaces being compared to minimal-roughness surfaces. The results of these studies showed that multispecies biofilms grew in both implant surfaces, without significant structural or qualitative differences; however, quantitatively a higher biomass volume and higher numbers of total bacteria were found on moderate-roughness surface implants. Furthermore, these studies also demonstrated significantly higher concentrations of pathogenic bacteria, namely *F. nucleatum* and *A. actinomycetemcomitans* in moderate-roughness surfaces when compared to minimal-roughness surface implants, within a similar biofilm structure (Bermejo et al. 2019; Bevilacqua et al. 2018; Drago et al. 2016).

In summary, in vitro studies have indicated that wettability, chemical composition, surface energy, hydrophobicity, and surface roughness affect the bacterial adhesion to surfaces of implant components (Cheng et al. 2019).

Bio-tribocorrosion and the peri-implant microbiome

Bio-tribocorrosion of implant surfaces

It is well established that the titanium dioxide layer covering the implant surface makes it highly resistant to corrosion. However, studies have described the presence of particles of implants in peri-implant tissues, strongly suggesting that a corrosive process has occurred on the titanium implant (Kim et al. 2019; Martini et al. 2003). Titanium corrosion is of the electrochemical type and is produced in wet environments, in the presence of water or other electrolytic fluids. The most common type of corrosion is galvanic, in which a breakage or displacement is produced in the titanium oxide surface layer. The breakdown of the titanium passive film leads to a localized corrosion failure such as intergranular attack, pitting, or corrosion fatigue. Corrosion can furthermore lead to numerous corrosive species such as hydrogen ions, sulfur compounds, oxygen-free radicals, and chlorine ions, which can trigger alterations to the implant surface and peri-implant tissues (Comino-Garayoa et al. 2020).

Released titanium particles can come from the titanium coating layer or from the titanium implant itself (Kim et al. 2019). Ions/particles can be released as a result of friction against the bone upon implant placement (Franchi et al. 2004); or due to wear caused by micromovements between contacting surfaces at implant connections (Cruz et al. 2011); as well as micromovements at the implant–bone tissue interface (Mathew et al. 2009). Wear can also be generated by debridement of implants at maintenance visits (Suarez-Lopez Del Amo et al. 2018). An in vitro study has shown that ultrasonic scaling around implants can lead to the release of titanium microparticles (Eger et al. 2017). Corrosion (i.e. electrochemical processes interacting with body fluids) can be combined with these wear mechanisms (Jacobs et al. 1998; Olmedo et al. 2003). The release of ions/particles can also be caused by the corrosive effect of therapeutic bleaching agents, a low pH, or high concentrations of fluoride, lactic acid, and hydrogen peroxide (Kim et al. 2019; Peñarrieta Juanito et al. 2015; Souza et al. 2015a). It is thus suggested that wear and corrosion in the contacting surfaces of implant fixtures and implant abutments can cause the failure of dental implant systems (Kim et al. 2019).

The human body, and specifically the oral cavity, represents a challenging condition for any biomaterial due to mechanical, chemical, biochemical, and microbiological degradation processes (Apaza-Bedoya et al. 2017). Various authors have suggested that long-standing accumulation of an oral microbial biofilm on implant surfaces combined with mechanical strain may cause titanium implant surfaces to deteriorate (Mombelli et al. 2018; Souza et al. 2010). According to a statement published by the European Association for Osseointegration (EAO) Consensus Conference 2018 (Schliephake et al. 2018), a number of in vitro studies have reported that the acidity of the oral environment caused by bacterial biofilm metabolism and/or inflammatory processes can provoke titanium particle release in a process known as biocorrosion. Tribocorrosion is defined as a tribosystem that incorporates three interrelated components: tribology (friction, wear, and lubrication), corrosion (material and environmental factors), and biochemistry (interactions between cells and protein) (Souza et al. 2015b). Furthermore, in the oral environment, the synergism of biocorrosion, metabolic, immunological, biochemical, and microbiological processes, mechanical wear, environmental factors, and contact with chemical agents will lead in some cases to material degradation in a process called bio-tribocorrosion (Dini et al. 2020; Mombelli et al. 2018).

On the whole, due to bacteria and inflammatory reaction products causing higher corrosion of titanium, the surface roughness of titanium can increase, favoring microbial attachment, and thus further influence the bio-tribocorrosion of titanium material (Dini et al. 2020). However, proof of a unidirectional sequence of causative events does not exist. It has been suggested that higher concentrations of titanium in peri-implantitis lesions could be the consequence of the presence of biofilms and inflammation, rather than being the trigger for disease (Mombelli et al. 2018).

Titanium particles/ions and peri-implant microbiome composition

The presence of metallic particles, or their interaction or synergistic effect with periodontal pathogens, may be associated with the possible onset of peri-implantitis (Kotsakis & Olmedo 2012). An in situ study has shown that titanium products, especially titanium ions, have the potential to change the microbiological composition of in situ biofilms formed on titanium surfaces (Souza et al. 2020). In this study, when biofilms were exposed to titanium products, the particles were used as a substrate for bacterial adhesion and coaggregation, favouring biofilm growth. Although titanium particles did not profoundly change the biofilm composition, the levels of *Streptococcus anginosus*, *Prevotella nigrescens*, *Capnocytophaga sputigena*, and *Actinomyces israelli* were statistically elevated. However, biofilms exposed to titanium ions showed a dose-dependent increase in the microbial load of 16 bacterial species, which included several known periodontal/peri-implant pathogens, such as *Tannarella forsythia*, *Treponema socranskii*, *Eubacterium nodatum*, *P. nigrescens*, and *Campilobacter* spp. The combination of titanium particles + ions showed an increase in the growth of 10 bacterial species. It was thus concluded in the study that titanium ions can cause a biofilm dysbiosis that includes a progressive increase in the proportions of periodontal pathogens, leading to peri-implantitis, and furthermore that a synergistic effect can be expected between the concentration of titanium products and biofilm virulence, since titanium products can increase anaerobic bacterial levels, and biofilm formation can enhance implant biocorrosion and degradation (Schliephake et al. 2018; Souza et al. 2020). It has thus been suggested that titanium creates a unique niche in the oral cavity, causing changes in microbiome structure (Daubert et al. 2018).

Another study also showed a strong role of titanium particles in shaping the peri-implant microbiome, whereby higher titanium concentrations in plaque were found to be associated with peri-implantitis, with a less diverse microbiota, and included the enrichment for *Veillonella* spp. (Daubert et al. 2018). *Veillonella* spp. have potent lipopolysaccharides that activate rapid bone loss, they are resistant to penicillins and metals (titanium), they can coaggregate on titanium substrates with streptococci, and their biofilms have high antibiotic resistance (Daubert et al. 2018; Kotsakis & Olmedo 2012). Titanium dissolution products in peri-implantitis, via enrichment for selected oral taxa, may thus play a role as a modifier of peri-implant microbiota, thereby causing a shift of the peri-implant microbiome toward dysbiosis and peri-implant inflammation (Daubert et al. 2018; Domingo et al. 2019). Furthermore, due to differences in microbiome structures that are dependent on the presence of titanium, it has been hypothesized that different phenotypes of peri-implantitis may exist, which may have distinct etiologies (Daubert et al. 2018).

The mechanisms by which titanium particles and ions increase bacterial growth are still unknown. It has been suggested that the different charges between titanium and bacterial cell walls may induce ionic bonding coaggregation, as bacterial cell membranes are composed of negatively charged lipids, and the titanium dioxide layer on titanium implants is positively charged (Koch & Manzhos 2017; Pöyry & Vattulainen 2016). Furthermore, the dose-dependent direct effect of titanium ions' high oxygen vacancies, which reduces oxygen availability in the biofilm microenvironment, may favour the shift of the microbial community toward a specific anaerobic bacterial species (Wen et al. 2018).

Oral bacterial taxa may also have the potential to disrupt the biocompatible titanium dioxide surface layer (Rakic et al. 2016). For example, *Streptococcus mutans* has been shown to be capable of affecting titanium electro-conductive properties, which can lead to spontaneous generation of an electrical potential with an increase in the corrosion current, causing an accelerated titanium dissolution from titanium implants (Daubert et al. 2018; Fukushima et al. 2014; Pozhitkov et al. 2015; Sridhar et al. 2015).

Titanium particles/ions and tissue interactions

Studies of peri-implantitis as a multifactorial entity have established a strong association between titanium dissolution particles and the prevalence of peri-implantitis (Fretwurst et al. 2018; Safioti et al. 2017; Rodrigues et al. 2013). Titanium dissolution particles in increased concentrations have been observed under inflammatory conditions as compared to relative clinical health, thereby suggesting their role in peri-implant inflammation (Kotsakis et al. 2021). Titanium dissolution particles have also been observed in peri-implant plaque (Safioti et al. 2017). A study has indicated that biofilm presence alone is adequate to increase titanium dissolution particles by nearly fourfold in untreated versus sterile titanium surfaces (Kotsakis et al. 2021). By implication, this represents a distinct biomaterial-related factor that may be involved in the initiation of and/or progression of peri-implant inflammatory bone loss (Kotsakis et al. 2021). The host immune response has furthermore been shown to vary along with the amount of titanium dissolution products (Daubert et al. 2019). This highlights the complex dynamics that define the peri-implant milieu, which includes biomaterial surfaces, oral biofilms, and host immunity (Daubert et al. 2018; Safioti et al. 2017). Concentrations of titanium ions between 100 and 300 ppm have been discovered in peri-implant tissues (Goutam et al. 2014). Furthermore, titanium particles in the range of 1–10 um diameter have been shown to be most biologically reactive compared to larger particle sizes (Eger et al. 2017). Titanium particles from corrosion processes may accumulate in the gingival sulcus and diffuse into the adjacent tissues, causing blue-gray pigmentation of the gingiva and root dentin. Titanium needle-like deposits have been described to be present in the extracellular matrix around fibroblasts and macrophages (Suarez-Lopez Del Amo et al. 2018; Venclikova et al. 2007). Released titanium ions and micro- or nanoparticles diffusing into the surrounding implant tissues may also potentiate an inflammatory response (Apaza-Bedoya et al. 2017). Titanium may act as the priming agent of the inflammatory immune response, whereby the microbial component is deemed necessary for instigating inflammation (Belibasakis & Menoil 2021). Titanium particles can activate leukocytes leading to the secretion of superoxide anions, which cause damage to peri-implant tissue cells (Kotsakis et al. 2021). M1 macrophages, neutrophils, and T lymphocytes activated by titanium can secrete metallic proteinases and pro-inflammatory cytokines, such as tumor necrosis factor (TNF)-α, interleukin (IL)-1α, IL-1β, IL-6, IL-10, and prostaglandin (PGE2), which can promote bone resorption (Eger et al. 2017; Fretwurst et al. 2016; Kumazawa et al. 2002; Noronha Oliveira et al. 2018; Souza et al. 2015b).

Titanium ions may also inhibit osteoblast differentiation and alter the receptor activator for nuclear factor-kappa B ligand (RANKL)/osteoprotegerin ratio responsible for osteoclast differentiation. Titanium ions could thus have adverse effects on bone remodeling at the interface between implants and surrounding tissues (Albrektsson et al. 2018; Mine et al. 2010). The mechanical treatment of titanium implant surfaces with titanium brushes can lead to surface alterations and increased titanium dissolution from the surface, causing biologically adverse changes that may hinder the osteoconductivity of treated surfaces (Kotsakis et al. 2021). In addition, metal ions and particles can induce differentiation and maturation of osteoclasts, thereby increasing the function of peri-prosthetic osteolysis (Mine et al. 2010). Also, during inflammatory defense processes, osteoblasts are capable of internalizing and phagocytosing wear debris, which can modify basic osteoblastic cell mechanisms, leading to cell necrosis (Noronha Oliveira et al. 2018).

Titanium has been observed both inside and outside epithelial cells and macrophages (Olmedo et al. 2013). By means of cellular DNA damage, titanium wear particles can be toxic to epithelial cells, thereby affecting the integrity of the epithelial barrier. This can facilitate bacterial colonization and infection, thereby increasing inflammatory reactions (Noronha Oliveira et al. 2018).

Titanium allergies/hypersensitivity

Although the causes of implant failures have been widely studied (i.e. infection, impaired healing, and overload) (Esposito et al. 1999), some implant failures remain unexplained (Sicilia et al. 2008). These failures include spontaneous rapid exfoliation of the implant (Deas et al. 2002), or the successive failure of implants in the same patient, known as the "cluster phenomenon," this being in the absence of any infection or overload risk factors (Chuang et al. 2005; Goutam et al. 2014). This has led to the question of whether there may be a systemic determinant of failure that has not been identified or understood. One of the causes of implant failure can be attributed to allergic reactions to titanium (Lim et al. 2012).

Many patients can suffer from multiple allergies, including metal allergy, which is possibly genetically based (Ruiz & Maestro 2008). Individuals with previous reactions to metals or jewelry may have a greater risk of developing hypersensitivity reactions to metal implants (Hallab et al. 2001). The risk of titanium toxicity has been found to be significantly low (Ruiz & Maestro 2008), and contact sensitization to titanium in the oral cavity is not very common (Fabian et al. 2008; Kim et al. 2019). From an immunological point of view, the oral mucosa has a lower reactivity than skin, as the mucosa-associated lymphoid tissue contains a lesser number of Langerhans cells compared to skin-associated lymphoid tissue (Sicilia et al. 2008). In order to cause tissue microscopic reactions, the oral mucosa must be exposed to allergen concentrations 5–12 times greater than the skin. Furthermore, contact between the metal and the host is hampered, due to the implant–host contact surface being limited, and due to surface stabilization and corrosion resistance being formed by the titanium dioxide layer on implant surfaces. Furthermore, bone also has low reactivity, and the implant and prosthetic structures in the oral cavity are coated with a layer of salivary glycoprotein, which acts as a protective barrier (Goutam et al. 2014; Sicilia et al. 2008).

Titanium ions (haptens), due to their high affinity to proteins, can combine with endogenous proteins to form protein–metal complexes, which may become immunogenic, thereby triggering hypersensitivity reactions (Campbell et al. 2014).

These complex molecules are captured by Langerhans cells, which may lead to type I, III, or IV hypersensitivity immune responses in the orofacial regions (Chaturvedi 2013; Hallab et al. 2001; Olmedo et al. 2012). Hypersensitivity reactions are initiated by sensitized lymphocytes that release proteolytic enzymes in response to antigen, causing a resultant inflammatory response (Campbell et al. 2014). A common type of allergy found in the oral cavity is type IV, whereby the clinical appearance associated with the allergy can start from a few days to several years from contact with allergens. Histologically, sensitivity to titanium is characterized locally by abundant M1 macrophages and T lymphocytes (CD4 and CD8 cells) and the absence of B lymphocytes, indicating type IV hypersensitivity (Chaturvedi 2013; Hunt et al. 1994; Mine et al. 2010). Leukopenia has also been observed in patients with adverse skin reactions to titanium-based implants in the head and neck region (Holgers et al. 1992). It is however also important to take cognizance of the fact that there are two different typologies of titanium implants, i.e. pure titanium and alloy dental implants (e.g. titanium, vanadium, and aluminum; Stenport & Johansson 2008), which are dissimilar in the rate of corrosion, and this dissimilarity influences the antigenicity of released metals in surrounding tissue (Pigatto et al. 2009). Titanium per se also contains impurities that can trigger allergic reactions. These include traces of aluminum, beryllium, cadmium, iron, manganese, molybdenum, nickel, chromium, palladium, or vanadium (Comino-Garayoa et al. 2020). It has been hypothesized that some of these trace elements, rather than titanium, may be responsible for triggering hypersensitivity reactions (Harloff et al. 2010; Javed et al. 2013).

Signs or symptoms associated with allergy that have been reported after implant placement may not always be uniform (Campbell et al. 2014). Patients may present with subjective complaints affecting the oral mucosa, including burning mouth and painful mucositis of peri-implant tissues, and more objective conditions, including rash, urticaria, pruritus, exfoliative cheilitis, swelling in the orofacial region, oral or facial erythema, eczematous lesions of the cheeks, hyperplastic lesions of the peri-implant mucosa, necrosis, and bone loss (Campbell et al. 2014; Lim et al. 2012; Mitchell et al. 1990). Systemic disease can also occur due to titanium, with numerous reports showing an association between titanium and "yellow nail syndrome," including titanium being judged to be a pathogen of the syndrome (Ataya et al. 2015; Dos Santos 2016; Kim et al. 2019). Yellow nail syndrome is characterized by a change in the nails, which includes growing slowly, thicker, and yellowish in color (Berglund & Carlmark 2011). Other related signs and symptoms include lymphedema, inflammation in the maxillary sinus, postnasal drip and cough-associated sinusitis, recurrent pleural effusion, bronchial obstruction, and intermittent coughing with bronchial asthma accompanied by sputum and bronchiectasis (Berglund & Carlmark 2011). Pleural effusion has been reported to have a high protein content associated with a reduction in systemic albumin (D'Alessandro et al. 2001).

Allergies and hypersensitivity reactions related to titanium release in oral tissues are unlikely to play a major role in the epidemiology of peri-implant diseases (Souza et al. 2010). However, due to the risk for titanium, alternative implant materials are under investigation. These include zirconia and polyether ether ketone (PEEK) dental implants (Kim et al. 2019; Pieralli et al. 2017; Sagomonyants et al. 2008).

Bacterial composition on implant surfaces

Identification of biofilm composition

Bacteria colonize the peri-implant crevice soon after implant placement to establish polymicrobial communities (Quirynen et al. 2006). Various techniques have been utilized to study the peri-implant microbiota; these techniques may include, among others, the culture technique, the DNA–DNA checkerboard hybridization technique, and gene polymerase chain reaction (PCR) and 16S rRNA gene pyrosequencing (Martellacci et al. 2019). However, there is controversy among researchers about whether the composition of biofilms in peri-implantitis is really different from the composition of biofilms in periodontitis-affected sites, or even from the microflora around healthy dental implants (Faveri et al. 2015; Lafaurie et al. 2017; Sousa et al. 2017). A systematic review and meta-analysis study has indicated, however, that comparing the results from studies that utilize different microbiological techniques may also be problematic (Sahrmann et al. 2020). Furthermore, the onset and progression of peri-implantitis may not merely be dependent on the composition of the related biofilms, but might also depend on risk factors, such as smoking, and diseases affecting general health, such as diabetes mellitus (Kumar et al. 2012). Other more difficult factors to assess are psychic stress and nutrition, which are known to substantially influence the course of inflammatory diseases, and are furthermore also likely to influence peri-implant health (Baumgart & Sandborn 2012; Singh et al. 2017). Nonetheless, there seems to be general consensus that peri-implant and periodontal sites behave as distinct ecosystems that differently shape the quantitative and qualitative composition of their residing microbiota, with limited influence from nearby niches (Belibasakis & Manoil 2021). Genome-wide metatranscriptome analysis (RNA-seq) and function-based assignment studies of messenger RNA (mRNA) sequences, especially focusing on putative virulence genes, have furthermore described peri-implantitis and periodontitis to be associated with similar virulence factors, whereas distinct virulence profiles have been found between healthy periodontal sites and peri-implantitis sites, the latter being characterized by significant complex associations between some species, which have not been observed in periodontitis (Duran-Pinedo et al. 2014; Shiba et al. 2016).

The periodontal/peri-implant microbiome

Contemporary culture-free methods for identifying microbes have shown distinct dissimilarities between the periodontal microbiome and the peri-implant microbiome. 16S RNA sequencing studies used to analyze adjacent peri-implant and periodontal microbiomes in states of health and disease have found that 85% of individuals shared less than 8% of abundant species between teeth and implants (Dabdoub et al. 2013). Other studies have demonstrated peri-implant communities to also have less diversity than periodontal microbial communities (Kumar et al. 2012; Payne et al. 2017; Tamura et al. 2013). In patients with a controlled periodontal status, who have a history of chronic periodontitis, a study described healthy periodontal sites as also exhibiting a more diverse microbiota, associated with increased abundance of the genera *Actinobacillus* and *Streptococcus* (Apatzidou et al. 2017).

The peri-implant/peri-implantitis microbiome

Studies have reported that the bacterial flora around implants are mostly composed of *Streptococci* (45–86%), *Actinomyces naeslundii*, *A. oris*, *A. meyeri*, *Neisseria* spp., and *Rothia* spp. (Elter et al. 2008; Quirynen et al. 2005). Other studies utilizing culture-based microbial identification methods as well as the DNA–DNA checkerboard hybridization technique (Persson & Renvert 2014) have shown that sometimes known periodontal pathogens can be identified in peri-implantitis patients, even in the absence of obvious signs of inflammation. These may include *F. nucleatum*, *Prevotella intermedia*, *P. gingivalis*, *A. actinomycetemcomitans*, and *Filifactor alocis* (Casado et al. 2011; Leonhardt et al. 1999; Persson & Renvert 2014). Other species such as *Actinomyces*, *Neisseria*, and *Rothia* spp. have also been more frequently found in supragingival peri-implant biofilms (Martellacci et al. 2019).

In peri-implantitis sites, periodontal pathogens associated with such diseased sites have been found to include *P. gingivalis*, *Treponema denticola*, *Tannerella forsythia*, *A. actinomycetemcomitans*, *P. intermedia*, *P. nigrescens*, *F. nucleatum*, *Bacteroides forsythes*, *Peptostreptococcus micros*, and *Campylobacter* (Hultin et al. 2002; Leonhardt et al. 1999; Shibli et al. 2008). *Staphylococcus* spp., enterics, and *Candida* spp. may also contribute to peri-implant infections (Leonhardt et al. 1999; Slots & Rams 1991).

When comparing plaque samples from healthy implant sites to those of peri-implantitis sites, a study showed that peri-implantitis sites harbored statistically significantly more diverse bacterial communities than healthy sites, with microbial communities of peri-implantitis sites having the most phylogenetic diversity, and those of healthy implant sites having the least phylogenetic diversity (Zheng et al. 2015). Other studies have also detected fewer species in healthy implant sites compared to peri-implantitis sites (Maximo et al. 2009; Shibli et al. 2008). Studies supporting these findings of a higher microbial diversity in peri-implantitis sites than in healthy implant sites have specifically reported on the prevalence of *Bacteroidetes* spp., *Actinomyces* spp., *Peptococcus* spp., *Campylobacter* spp., *Streptococcus* spp., and *Butyrivibrio* spp. (Dabdoub et al. 2013; Sanz-Martin et al. 2017). *Prevotella* spp. and *Porphyromonas* spp. have also been found to be most discriminative of peri-implantitis (Apatzidou et al. 2017). Contrary to these findings, a study utilizing 16S gene pyrosequencing revealed that the microbial profile of healthy implants was significantly more diverse than that of peri-implantitis sites (Kumar et al. 2012). However, another study evaluating the prevalence of individual species using DNA–DNA hybridization methods found no difference in microbial diversity between peri-implantitis sites and healthy sites (Renvert et al. 2007).

The peri-implant mucositis microbiome

A core microbiome has been described to exist in healthy implant, peri-implant mucositis, and peri-implantitis sites, which includes *Streptococcus, Leptotrichia, Actinomyces, Capnocytophaga, Prevotella, Fusobacterium, Neisseria, Rothia,* and TM7 (Saccharibacteria) (Zheng et al. 2015). Periodontal pathogens such as *Porphyromonas gingivalis, T. forsythia, P. intermedia,* and *Capnocytophaga ochracea* have furthermore been observed to be clustered together in peri-implant mucositis sites, suggesting that periodontal pathogens may play important roles in the pathogenesis of peri-implant diseases. The microbial communities of peri-implant mucositis sites have been described to be intermediate in nature between those of healthy implants and peri-implantitis sites, and thus from a microbial viewpoint peri-implant mucositis may appear to be a transitional phase on the course to peri-implantitis (Zheng et al. 2015). Peri-implant mucositis has furthermore also been found to be associated with greater bacterial diversity than healthy implant sites, but to have a lower diversity than peri-implantitis sites (Zheng et al. 2015). However, it has also been stressed that it cannot presently be concluded that peri-implant mucositis will definitely progress to peri-implantitis (Zheng et al. 2015).

A study using 16S rRNA gene sequence analysis investigated the microbiome at peri-implant mucositis sites with and without clinical signs of suppuration (Wang et al. 2020). Sites with suppuration demonstrated a more disordered microbiome structure than sites without suppuration, with lower microbial richness and more distinct pathogenic microbiota. Specifically, this included the genera of *Fusobacterium* and *Tannerella* (Wang et al. 2020). These genera are also strongly associated with peri-implantitis (Jakobi et al. 2015; Kroger et al. 2018; Zheng et al. 2015), and the suggestion has thus been made that suppuration is possibly a sign of active progression of inflammation, and that peri-implant mucositis sites with suppuration are more prone to progress into peri-implantitis (Wang et al. 2020). The higher pathogenicity and disordered community associated with suppuration in peri-implant mucositis sites could thus be an indication of increased risk of aggravating destruction, as other studies have demonstrated a threefold increased susceptibility of bone loss in peri-implantitis sites showing the clinical presence of suppuration (Fransson et al. 2008; Roos-Jansaker et al. 2006; Wang et al. 2020).

Implant surface modifications for antibacterial applications

The ideal implant surface modification should enhance the interaction between the implant's surface and its surrounding bone, which will facilitate osseointegration while minimizing bacterial colonization to reduce the risk of biofilm formation (Kligman et al. 2021). Therefore, there should be a fine balance between antimicrobial activity and the desired osteoconductive properties (Hickok et al. 2018). This balance is difficult to achieve, as greater surface roughness promotes firmer bone fixation, but is however also directly proportional to bacterial retention, which may promote biofilm formation in the long run (Berglundh et al. 2007). Presently, a diversity of implant surface modifications, including different physical, chemical, and biological techniques, have been applied to a broad range of materials, such as titanium, zirconia, and PEEK, to achieve these goals (Kligman et al. 2021). Conceptually, the ideal implant should prevent mature biofilm formation; display a non-selective effect on bacterial, fungal, and viral pathogens; and prevent antibiotic resistance, in the mid- or long-term follow-up (Chouirfaa et al. 2019). However, once a mature biofilm has developed on any implant surface, bacterial eradication becomes very difficult despite the use of antibiotic therapy and repeated surgical irrigation and debridement. Factors contributing to bacterial eradication include an exopolysaccharide matrix that inhibits the penetration of antibiotics, scarce vascularization, and a high implant surface. Also, small colony variants or persister cells, through mutations of metabolic genes, can show reduced antibiotic sensitivity. These factors will therefore necessitate the performance of hardware removal whenever simple irrigation and debridement procedures are ineffective in curing infections related to implanted devices. The emergence of resistant bacterial strains (persisters) presents additional issues whenever antibiotics are administered (Chouirfaa et al. 2019). Conditions are ideal within polymicrobial biofilms for the acquisition of plasmids that carry antibiotic resistance genes. Persisters are bacteria that are recalcitrant to the effects of high antibiotic levels. These persisters are usually in an inactive state until antibiotic concentrations wane. They then emerge from quiescence, whereby they regain their proliferative phenotype. In this manner, persisters can repopulate a depleted region or initiate biofilm formation (Hickok et al. 2018). It has also been suggested that the numbers of persisters are significantly higher in the biofilm state than in planktonic cultures (Lewis 2012). Resistant bacteria, whether planktonic or localized to biofilms, are thus difficult to eradicate at antibiotic levels that are non-toxic (Hickok et al. 2018). Long-term clinical success is dependent upon the antimicrobial properties of implanted materials. To date, no surface treatment guarantees rapid and complete biofilm destruction or prevents infection recurrence (Chouirfaa et al. 2019).

Various methods have been devised to create/engineer implants with surfaces that minimize bacterial colonization and biofilm formation. The aim is to create surfaces that resist bacterial adherence and/or promote bacterial killing (Chouirfaa et al. 2019). The challenge, however, is to generate surfaces that fulfill these criteria while remaining biocompatible and that also promote osseointegration (Hickok et al. 2018; Kligman et al. 2021). Three classes of antimicrobial surfaces have been created: (i) structured surfaces, often with nanoscale topography, which decrease bacterial adhesion to retard establishment of infection; (ii) surfaces that actively elute antimicrobials to avert bacterial adhesion and promote killing; and (iii) surfaces containing permanently bonded agents that generate antimicrobial surfaces that prevent long-term bacterial adhesion (Hickok et al. 2018). Some of the various types and features of titanium implant antimicrobial surfaces are depicted in what follows.

Structured surfaces

Physical modifications can be categorized at the macro, micro, and nano levels (Kligman et al. 2021). These include engineered metal topographies and molecular structures, as well as nanoparticle- and nanotube-modified surfaces (Hickok et al. 2018). Topographical modifications include alterations in charge, hydrophobicity, roughness, and porosity (Hasan & Chatterjee 2015). Micro-level modifications include machining, grit blasting, and sand-blasting combined with acid etching. Nano-level modifications include laser ablation and nanocomposites (Kligman et al. 2021). Various nanoparticles, such as titanium dioxide (TiO_2), silver (Ag), hydroxyapatite (HA), pectins, cubic zirconia, ultra-nanocrystalline diamond, and carbon nanotubes, can be added to titanium using both physical and chemical techniques (Cheng et al. 2019; Kligman et al. 2021). Other methods include chemical and biological modifications, heat treatment, anodic oxidation/anodization, discrete crystalline deposition, fluoride treatment, and exposure to UV light (photofunctionalization) (Hickok et al. 2018; Kligman et al. 2021; Rodriguez y Baena et al. 2012).

Increased surface roughness for better osteogenic potential is however associated with higher risks of biofilm formation, as more stabilized microbe–substrate linkage is established by increasing the surface area for bacterial attachment and protecting bacteria from fluid shear forces (Achinas et al. 2019; Subramani et al. 2009). Thread structure has an impact on biofilm formation, as biofilm microcolonies can be mostly deposited on the lateral surfaces and peaks of the implant threads, with little deposits on the area between threads (Bermejo et al. 2019). Although physicochemical properties, such as roughness and wettability, can be dramatically changed at the micro level, these features can make a significant impact on biofilm formation as they have a similar topographical size to the colonizing microorganisms (Kligman et al. 2021). When comparing machined and acid-etched only surfaces, sand-blasted, large-grit, acid-etched (SLA) modification has been shown to induce the most severe colonization in vitro (Schmidlin et al. 2013). Nanoscale topographies have been found to decrease bacterial adhesion and limit the establishment of infection (Hickok et al. 2018). An in vitro study has suggested that laser-ablated titanium shows significantly lower biofilm formation than machined and grit-blasted implants, as well as human enamel surfaces (Ionescu et al. 2018). Coating silver nanoparticles on titanium surfaces has shown statistically significant antibacterial features against *Staphylococcus aureus*, assisting in preventing peri-implantitis (Lampe et al. 2019).

Chemical modifications bringing about increased hydrophilicity discourage hydrophobic interactions, and create repulsion between hydrophobic bacteria and the implant surface, thus preventing their adhesion and activity (Yuan et al. 2017). Studies have shown that both superhydrophobic and superhydrophilic surfaces could reduce bacterial adhesion and inhibit biofilm formation (Mi & Jiang 2014; Zhang & Levänena 2013), and therefore have potential applications to improve the antifouling properties of dental implants (Kligman et al. 2021).

Discrete crystalline deposition (DCD) is a sol-gel process that includes a double acid-etched surface that is modified with calcium phosphate particles of 20–100 nm (Bonfante et al. 2013). Compared to machined and acid-etched implant surfaces, DCD-modified surfaces have shown a significant reduction in bacterial attachment (Rodriguez y Baena et al. 2012). Adhesion of *A. actinomycetemcomitans*, *S. mutans*, and *S. sanguis* has been shown to be significantly reduced on DCD-modified surfaces in comparison with acid-etched surfaces, this being attributed to the decrease in surface roughness of this material (Rodriguez y Baena et al. 2012).

Electrochemical deposition of fluoridated HA may also have antibacterial effects against specifically *S. aureus* and *P. gingivalis* (Kulkarni Aranya et al. 2017). However, long-term stability and clinical outcomes of HA-coated implants, which include bacterial microleakage and peri-implant tissue complications, are still uncertain, causing existing controversy (Ong & Chan 2017).

Photofunctionalization has been shown to have antibacterial effects of prohibiting biofilm formation (Karthik et al. 2013). Anodized heat-treated titanium followed by ultraviolet light treatment has also exhibited a reduction in the attachment of *S. mutans*, *S. salivarius*, and *S. sanguis* (Del Curto et al. 2005).

Elution systems

Antibiotic elution systems inhibit bacterial growth and prevent bacterial adhesion to the implant surface and adjacent tissues (Jepsen & Jepsen 2016). Supratherapeutic levels of antibiotics are only achieved within the first week, with lower, continued elution (exponential decline) for some time afterward (Bormann et al. 2014; Humphrey et al. 1998). Depending on the antibiotic and the local environment, including tissue fluid volume, pH, and circulation, initial quantities can be toxic to already compromised bone (Antoci et al. 2007a). With high antibiotic concentrations, a small percentage of bacteria will convert to a persister phenotype. Continued elution of antibiotics to subtherapeutic levels may enhance selection of bacteria exhibiting a survival/growth advantage, thereby fostering enrichment/emergence of antibiotic-resistant bacteria (Lewis 2012). Despite this, these systems are used quite successfully to treat implant-associated infections (Da Rocha et al. 2015). Elution methods developed to treat peri-implantitis include use of (i) antiseptics such as chlorhexidine digluconate; (ii) minocycline spheres and tetracycline periodontal fibers; and (iii) metals such as silver and copper (Humphrey et al. 1998). Study results are however inconclusive concerning the best local, chemical approach, and there is no clarity as to whether they offer an advantage over systemic antibiotic therapy and mechanical debridement (Javed et al. 2013). Chemotherapeutic agents such as chlorhexidine can be adsorbed by titanium surfaces with protracted cytotoxic effects, thereby adversely compromising cellular reattachment to implant surfaces (Kotsakis et al. 2016; Kozlovsky et al. 2006; Parlar et al. 2009). Silver-eluting dental implants are being developed (Matsubara et al. 2015). The antimicrobial effects of silver are attributed to the production of Ag+ ions, which are toxic to bacterial cells, and toxicity may be related to the affinity of silver for bacterial cell membranes (Brennan et al. 2015). Silver elution/dissolution can occur over long time periods, where its antimicrobial activity may be enhanced by surface area and shape (Kumari et al. 2017). There are however toxicity concerns with silver. This toxicity includes mitochondrial respiratory chain interruptions, interactions with sulfur-containing proteins, altered membrane permeability, and reactive oxygen species production (McShan et al. 2014).

Permanent antimicrobial surfaces

This system depends on tethering or cross-linking an antimicrobial molecule to the surface of the implant so that bacteria are killed upon adherence. These surfaces rely on the ability of the antimicrobial agent to retain its activity, even when covalently bonded to a surface (Jose et al. 2005; Lawson et al. 2010). Tethered antimicrobial compounds include various chitosans and amines (Actis et al. 2013), antimicrobial peptides (de la Fuente-Nunez et al. 2016), and antibiotics (Hickok & Shapiro 2012). Using a number of different linkages, antibiotics can be attached to titanium, titanium alloy, cobalt chromium molybdenum alloys, and stainless steel. It is important that antibiotics like vancomycin and members of the tetracycline family, including the glycylcyclines, reversibly bind to target groups within the bacterium, thus enabling antibiotic-coated implant surfaces to be repeatedly challenged with bacteria, so as to retain their biocidal activity (Kotsakis et al. 2016). Surfaces bearing the antibiotic gentamicin, an aminoglycoside, show high biocidal activity; however, when bacterially rechallenged, the antibiotic wanes and loses activity, presumably due to irreversibly binding to the bacterial ribosome (Kotsakis et al. 2016). Biodegradable hydrogels can also be used to bind to metal surfaces, whereby their chemistry can be controlled to display and/or release antimicrobial agents (de la Fuente-Nunez et al. 2016). Proteins derived from saliva or blood might however mask antimicrobial activity associated with these surfaces (Antoci et al. 2007b). This can further be confounded by the role of pH, electrolyte composition, and flow conditions (Darrene & Cecile 2016). Questions do however also remain concerning antimicrobial resistance when permanent antibiotic surfaces are used. If resistant bacteria are cultured in the presence of the surface, it is possible that they could populate the implant (Hickok et al. 2018).

Future considerations

It should be kept in mind that in vitro biofilm formation on surfaces cannot be transferred to clinical settings. However, advances in understanding and controlling bacteria–surface interactions via surface topography can provide promising solutions to biofilm control in many areas that directly affect human oral and systemic health (Cheng et al. 2019). However, the absolute lack of studies comparing metagenomic, culturomic, 16S gene pyrosequencing gene analyses and other techniques for identifying peri-implant microbiota necessitates an analytic and systematic approach, so as to give greater specific weight to scientific knowledge (Quirynen et al. 2006).

Further research is warranted on functional and virulence differences between strains of the same bacterial species, expressed as altered transcriptional profiles, and may thus provide a more finite understanding of peri-implant ecological pathways leading to the functional pathogenicity of the specialized peri-implant bacterial community. More importantly, though, efforts should be invested in deciphering the ecological triggers of functional pathogenicity that might prove to be more beneficial in building improved strategies for risk assessment, prevention, diagnosis, or supportive therapy when required. This would ultimately prove to be beneficial for the long-term retention of dental implants (Belibasakis & Manoil 2021).

Further understanding of the interplay between the periodontal microbial community and titanium particles may provide insight into the prevention of peri-implant disease (Daubert et al. 2018). Despite recent scientific advances, there is no consensus on the complete effects of titanium degradation products. Little is known regarding the possible cytotoxicity in human cells related to the amount, size, and chemical composition of titanium wear debris. Moreover, the long-term biological effect of bio-tribocorrosion in the survival of dental implants and prostheses is still unknown. Further studies are required to clarify the role of titanium degradation products in the mechanisms of cytotoxicity and genotoxicity in peri-implant tissues (Dini et al. 2020).

Investigations focused on a proper combination of implant site osteotomy, implant material, and various implant surface modification strategies can potentially improve implant success rates, especially in patients who have poor bone quality in implant sites (Kligman et al. 2021). The quest for a cheap and scalable engineered implantable surface that can promote cell adhesion, guarantee biocompatibility, and ensure over a 99.9% non-selective biocidal effect remains a major challenge. Multiple barriers have yet to be overcome, due to most studies reporting strictly in vitro results. Furthermore, to this date, no study has assessed the interaction with animal or human immune cells. in vivo studies are scarce that correspond to the actual application of studied biomaterials (Chouirfaa et al. 2019). The antibacterial effects of antibiotic-coated surfaces appear to be promising; however, there is considerable variability in the test conditions employed, and therefore it is difficult to compare between trials. Investigations using animal models that recapitulate disease phenotypes thus become even more important for guiding future strategies for developing anti-infective biomaterials (Hickok et al. 2018; Narayana & Srihari 2019). If permanent surfaces showing sustained in vitro efficacy can withstand the mechanical, chemical, and immunological assaults associated with an infected implant, then it may be possible to significantly reduce the implant failures and associated bone loss that accompany peri-implantitis (Hickok et al. 2018). Nanosurface modeling on bulk materials has been extensively described. It entails the engineering of uncoated surfaces producing physical surface characteristics that will promote cell adhesion and repel bacteria, thereby facilitating biocompatibility or tissue integration. This is now becoming a mature technology that is currently available to clinicians (Chouirfaa et al. 2019).

Most studies recommending interventions for implant surface cleaning have been developed based on simple antibacterial assays, without specific attention to titanium surface properties and dissolution (Kotsakis et al. 2021). The goal of future peri-implantitis research should thus include prospective longitudinal clinical studies assessing titanium dissolution in vivo, thereby enabling the identification of peri-implantitis treatments that will effectively remove biofilms while maintaining the electrochemical properties of titanium, so as to avoid accelerated titanium dissolution in peri-implant tissues.

This will allow the regrowth of osteoblastic cells on the treated surface, which is a proxy for clinical re-osseointegration, thus maintaining the biocompatibility of titanium implants (Kotsakis et al. 2021).

Titanium can accumulate in the body through various pathways, with implant erosion being an additional pathway (Skocaj et al. 2011). Although titanium causes fewer hypersensitive reactions than other metals, it does not mean that allergy symptoms related to titanium do not exist (Kim et al. 2019). The role of titanium as a potential allergen is under-investigated (Goutam et al. 2014). It seems possible that the incidence of allergic reaction to titanium implants may be under-reported due to dentists not being aware of, or not considering, titanium allergy to be a possible etiological factor for implant failure (Campbell et al. 2014; Pigatto et al. 2009; Siddiqi et al. 2011). Many patients suffer from multiple allergies (Forte et al. 2008), and those with a history of allergy to metals or jewelry have a greater risk of developing a hypersensitivity reaction to a metal implant (Friedlander et al. 2013). The prevalence of these cases is also likely to increase (Goutam et al. 2014). Patients with yellow nail syndrome with titanium implants further demonstrate the possibility of systemic disease due to titanium implants. More studies are therefore needed to determine the relationship between titanium and yellow nail syndrome and the pathogenesis thereof (Kim et al. 2019). Any history or suspicion of a titanium allergy should be considered prior to dental implant placement, which includes carrying out metal allergy assessments and making use of a worldwide standardized patch test for titanium (Hosoki et al. 2016; Pigatto & Guzzi 2007; Pigatto et al. 2009).

From a clinical point of view, implant surfaces, with various topographical anatomy, need daily meticulous oral hygiene. If this condition is met, then the choice of implant surface characteristics may be salient to the long-term health of any implant placed. However, if the biofilm is allowed to grow uncontrolled, the influences of different titanium surfaces become irrelevant (Schmidlin et al. 2013).

REFERENCES

Achinas S, Charalampogiannis N, Euverink G-J. A brief recap of microbial adhesion and biofilms. *Appl Sci.* 2019; 9:2801.

Actis L, Gaviria L, Guda T, Ong JL. Antimicrobial surfaces for craniofacial implants: state of the art. *J Korean Assoc Oral Maxillofac Surg.* 2013; 39(2):43–54.

Albrektsson T, Chrcanovic B, Mölne J, Wennerberg A. Foreign body reactions, marginal bone loss and allergies in relation to titanium implants. *Eur J Oral Implant.* 2018; 11:S37–S46.

Almaguer-Flores A, Olivares-Navarrete R, Wieland M et al. Influence of topography and hydrophilicity on initial oral biofilm formation on microstructured titanium surfaces in vitro. *Clin Oral Implant Res.* 2012; 23:301–307.

Anselme K, Davidson P, Popa AM et al. The interaction of cells and bacteria with surfaces structured at the nanometre scale. *Acta Biomater.* 2010; 6:3824–3846.

Antoci V Jr, Adams CS, Hickok NJ, Shapiro IM, Parvizi J. Antibiotics for local delivery systems cause skeletal cell toxicity in vitro. *Clin Orthop Relat Res.* 2007a; 462:200–206.

Antoci V Jr, King SB, Jose B et al. Vancomycin covalently bonded to titanium alloy prevents bacterial colonization. *J Orthop Res.* 2007b; 25(7):858–866.

Apatzidou D, Lappin DF, Hamilton G et al. Microbiome of peri-implantitis affected and healthy dental sites in patients with a history of chronic periodontitis. *Arch Oral Biol.* 2017; 83:145–152.

Apaza-Bedoya K, Tarce M, Benfatti CAM et al. Synergistic interactions between corrosion and wear at titanium-based dental implant connections: a scoping review. *J Periodontal Res.* 2017; 52:946–954.

Aroonsang W, Sotres J, El-Schich Z, Arnebrant T, Lindh L. Influence of substratum hydrophobicity on salivary pellicles: organization or composition? *Biofouling.* 2014; 30(9):1123–1132.

Ataya A, Kline KP, Cope J, Alnuaimat H. Titanium exposure and yellow nail syndrome. *Respir Med Case Rep.* 2015; 16:146–147.

Bakker DP, Busscher HJ, van Zanten J et al. Multiple linear regression analysis of bacterial deposition to polyurethane coatings after conditioning film formation in the marine environment. *Microbiology.* 2004; 150:1779–1784.

Baumgart DC, Sandborn WJ. Crohn's disease. *Lancet.* 2012; 380:1590–1605.

Belibasakis GN. Microbiological and immuno-pathological aspects of peri-implant diseases. *Arch Oral Biol.* 2014; 59(1):66–72.

Belibasakis GN, Manoil D. Microbial community-driven etiopathogenesis of peri-implantitis. *J Dent Res.* 2021; 100(1):21–28.

Belibasakis GN, Charalampakis G, Bostanci N, Stadlinger B. Periimplant infections of oral biofilm etiology. *Adv Exp Med Biol.* 2015; 830:69–84.

Berglund F, Carlmark B. Titanium, sinusitis, and the yellow nail syndrome. *Biol Trace Elem Res.* 2011; 143:1–7.

Berglundh T, Gotfredsen K, Zitzmann NU, Lang NP, Lindhe J. Spontaneous progression of ligature induced periimplantitis at implants with different surface roughness: an experimental study in dogs. *Clin Oral Implant Res.* 2007; 18:655–661.

Bermejo P, Sanchez MC, Llama-Palacios A et al. Biofilm formation on dental implants with different surface micro-topography: an in vitro study. *Clin Oral Implants Res.* 2019; 30(8):725–734.

Bevilacqua L, Milan A, Del Lupo V, Maglione M, Dolzani L. Biofilms developed on dental implant titanium surfaces with different roughness: comparison between in vitro and in vivo studies. *Curr Microbiol.* 2018; 75(6):766–772.

Bonfante E, Granato R, Marin C et al. Biomechanical testing of microblasted, acid-etched/microblasted, anodized, and discrete crystalline deposition surfaces: an experimental study in beagle dogs. *Int J Oral Maxillofac Implant.* 2013; 28:136–142.

Bormann N, Schwabe P, Smith MD, Wildemann B. Analysis of parameters influencing the release of antibiotics mixed with bone grafting material using a reliable mixing procedure. *Bone.* 2014; 59:162–172.

Brennan SA, Ni Fhoghlu C, Devitt BM et al. Silver nanoparticles and their orthopaedic applications. *Bone Joint J.* 2015; 97B(5):582–589.

Busscher HJ, Rinastiti M, Siswomihardjo W, van der Mei HC. Biofilm formation on dental restorative and implant materials. *J Dent Res.* 2010; 89(7):657–665.

Campbell S, Crean St J, Ahmed W. Titanium allergy: fact or fiction? *Faculty Dent J.* 2014; 5(1):18–25.

Casado PL, Otazu IB, Balduino A et al. Identification of periodontal pathogens in healthy periimplant sites. *Implant Dent.* 2011; 20:226–235.

Chang YR, Weeks ER, Ducker WA. Surface topography hinders bacterial surface motility. *ACS Appl Mater Interfaces.* 2018; 10:9225–9234.

Chaturvedi TP. Allergy related to dental implant and its clinical significance. *Clin Cosmet Investig Dent.* 2013; 5:57–61.

Cheng Y, Feng G and Moraru CI. Micro- and nanotopography sensitive bacterial attachment mechanisms: a review. *Front Microbiol.* 2019; 10:191.

Chouirfaa H, Bouloussa H, Migonneya V, Falentin-Daudré C. Review of titanium surface modification techniques and coatings for antibacterial applications. *Acta Biomaterialia.* 2019; 83:37–54.

Chuang S, Cai T, Douglass C, Wei L, Dodson T. Frailty approach for the analysis of clustered failure time observation in dental research. *J Dent Res.* 2005; 84:54–58.

Comino-Garayoa R, Brinkmann J C-B, Peláez J et al. Allergies to titanium dental implants: what do we really know about them? *A scoping review. Biology.* 2020; 9:404.

Cruz HMV, Souza JCM, Henriques M, Rocha LA. Tribocorrosion and bio-tribocorrosion in the oral environment: the case of dental implants. *Biomed Tribol.* 2011; 1(1):3–33.

D'Alessandro A, Muzi G, Monaco A et al. Yellow nail syndrome: does protein leakage play a role? *Eur Respir J.* 2001; 17:149–152.

Da Rocha HA, Silva CF, Santiago FL et al. Local drug delivery systems in the treatment of periodontitis: a literature review. *J Int Acad Periodontol.* 2015; 17(3):82–90.

Dabdoub SM, Tsigarida AA, Kumar PS. Patient-specific analysis of periodontal and peri-implant microbiomes. *J Dent Res.* 2013; 92(12 Suppl):168S–S175.

Darrene LN, Cecile B. Experimental models of oral biofilms developed on inert substrates: a review of the literature. *Biomed Res Int.* 2016; 2016: 74 61047.

Daubert D, Pozhitkov A, McLean J, Kotsakis G. Titanium as a modifier of the peri-implant microbiome structure. *Clin Implant Dent Relat Res.* 2018; 20(6):945–953.

Daubert DM, Pozhitkov AE, Safioti LM, Kotsakis GA. Association of global DNA methylation to titanium and periimplantitis: a case-control study. *JDR Clin Trans Res.* 2019; 4:284–291.

de la Fuente-Nunez C, Cardoso MH, de Souza Candido E, Franco OL, Hancock RE. Synthetic antibiofilm peptides. *Biochim Biophys Acta.* 2016; 1858(5):1061–1069.

Deas DE, Mikotowicz JJ, Mackey SA, Moritz AJ. Implant failure with spontaneous rapid exfoliation: case reports. *Implant Dent.* 2002; 11:235–242.

Del Curto B, Brunella MF, Giordano C et al. Decreased bacterial adhesion to surface-treated titanium. *Int J Artif Organs.* 2005; 28:718–730.

Dini C, Costa RC, Sukotjo C et al. Progression of bio-tribocorrosion in implant dentistry. *Front Mech Eng.* 2020; 6:1.

Domingo MG, Ferrari L, Aguas S et al. Oral exfoliative cytology and corrosion of metal piercings. *Tissue implications. Clin Oral Investig.* 2019; 23(4):1895–1904.

Dos Santos VM. Titanium pigment and yellow nail syndrome. *Skin Appendage Disord.* 2016; 1:197.

Drago L, Bortolin M, De Vecchi E et al. Antibiofilm activity of sandblasted and laser-modified titanium against microorganisms isolated from peri-implantitis lesions. *J Chemother.* 2016; 28(5):383–389.

Duran-Pinedo AE, Chen T, Teles R et al. 2014. Community-wide transcriptome of the oral microbiome in subjects with and without periodontitis. *ISME J.* 8(8):1659–1672.

Eger M, Sterer N, Liron T, Kohavi D, Gabet Y. Scaling of titanium implants entrains inflammation-induced osteolysis. *Sci Rep.* 2017; 7:39612.

Elter C, Heuer W, Demling A et al. Supra- and subgingival biofilm formation on implant abutments with different surface characteristics. *Int J Oral Maxillofac Implant.* 2008; 23:327–334.

Esposito M, Grusovin MG, Worthington HV. Interventions for replacing missing teeth: treatment of peri-implantitis. *Cochrane Database Syst Rev.* 2012; 1:CD004970. doi: 10.1002/14651858.CD004970.pub5.

Esposito M, Hirsch J, Lekholm U, Thomsen P. Differential diagnosis and treatment strategies for biologic complications and failing oral implants: a review of the literature. *Int J Oral Maxillofac Implants.* 1999; 14:473–490.

Fabian E, Landsiedel R, Ma-Hock L et al. Tissue distribution and toxicity of intravenously administered titanium dioxide nanoparticles in rats. *Arch Toxicol.* 2008; 82:151–157.

Faveri M, Figueiredo LC, Shibli JA, Pérez-Chaparro PJ, Feres M. Microbiological diversity of peri-implantitis biofilms. *Adv Exp Med Biol.* 2015; 830:85–96.

Figuero E, Graziani F, Sanz I, Herrera D, Sanz M. Management of peri-implant mucositis and peri-implantitis. *Periodontol 2000.* 2014; 66:255–273.

Forte G, Petrucci F, Bocca B. Metal allergens of growing significance: epidemiology, immunotoxicology, strategies for testing and prevention. *Inflamm Allergy.* 2008; 7:1–18.

Franchi M, Bacchelli B, Martini D et al. Early detachment of titanium particles from various different surfaces of endosseous dental implants. *Biomaterials.* 2004; 25(12):2239–2246.

Fransson C, Wennstrom J, Berglundh T. Clinical characteristics at implants with a history of progressive bone loss. *Clin Oral Implants Res.* 2008; 19:142–147.

Fretwurst T, Buzanich G, Nahles S et al. Metal elements in tissue with dental peri-implantitis: a pilot study. *Clin Oral Implants Res.* 2016; 27:1178–1186.

Fretwurst T, Nelson K, Tarnow DP, Wang HL, Giannobile WV. Is metal particle release associated with peri-implant bone destruction? *An emerging concept. J Dent Res.* 2018; 97:259–265.

Friedlander RS, Vlamakis H, Kim P et al. Bacterial flagella explore microscale hummocks and hollows to increase adhesion. *Proc Natl Acad Sci U.S.A.* 2013; 110:1–6.

Fukushima A, Mayanagi G, Nakajo K, Sasaki K, Takahashi N. Microbiologically induced corrosive properties of the titanium surface. *J Dent Res.* 2014; 93: 525–529.

Furst MM, Salvi GE, Lang NP, Persson GR. Bacterial colonization immediately after installation on oral titanium implants. *Clin Oral Implant Res.* 2007; 18:501–508.

Garrido KD, Palacios RJS, Le C, Kang S. Impact of conditioning film on the initial adhesion of *E. coli* on polysulfone ultrafiltration membrane. *J Ind Eng Chem.* 2013; 20:1438–1443.

Genzer J, Efimenko K. Recent developments in superhydrophobic surfaces and their relevance to marine fouling: a review. *Biofouling.* 2006; 22:339–360.

Goutam M, Giriyapura C, Mishra SK, Gupta S. Titanium allergy: a literature review. *Indian J Dermatol.* 2014; 59:630.

Hallab N, Merritt K, Jacobs J. Metal sensitivity in patients with orthopaedic implants. *J Bone Joint Surg Am.* 2001; 83:428–436.

Hallstrom H, Persson GR, Lindgren S, Olofsson M, Renvert S. Systemic antibiotics and debridement of peri-implant mucositis. A randomized clinical trial. *J Clin Periodontol.* 2012; 39(6):574–581.

Hannig C, Hannig M. The oral cavity—a key system to understand substratum-dependent bioadhesion on solid surfaces in man. *Clin Oral Investig.* 2009; 13(2):123–139.

Haraguchi T, Ayukawa Y, Shibata Y et al. Effect of calcium chloride hydrothermal treatment of titanium on protein, cellular, and bacterial adhesion properties. *J Clin Med.* 2020: 9:2627.

Harloff T, Hönle W, Holzwarth U et al. Titanium allergy or not? "Impurity" of titanium implant materials. *Health.* 2010; 2:306–331.

Hasan J, Chatterjee K. Recent advances in engineering topography mediated antibacterial surfaces. *Nanoscale.* 2015; 7(38):15568–15575.

Hickok NJ, Shapiro IM. Immobilized antibiotics to prevent orthopaedic implant infections. *Adv Drug Deliv Rev.* 2012; 64(12):1165–1176.

Hickok NJ, Shapiro IM, Chen AF. The impact of incorporating antimicrobials into implant surfaces. *J Dent Res.* 2018; 97(1):14–22.

Holgers KM, Roupe G, Tjellstrom A, Bjursten LM. Clinical, immunological and bacteriological evaluation of adverse reactions to skin-penetrating titanium implants in the head and neck region. *Contact Dermatitis.* 1992; 27:1–7.

Hori K, Matsumoto S. Bacterial adhesion: from mechanism to control. *Biochem Eng J.* 2010; 48:424–434.

Hosoki M, Nishigawa K, Miyamoto Y, Ohe G, Matsuka Y. Allergic contact dermatitis caused by titanium screws and dental implants. *J Prosthodont Res.* 2016; 60:213–219.

Hsu L, Fang J, Borca-Tasciuc D, Worobo R, Moraru CI. The effect of micro- and nanoscale topography on the adhesion of bacterial cells to solid surfaces. *Appl Environ Microbiol.* 2013; 79:2703–2712.

Hultin M. Gustafsson A, Hallström H et al. Microbiological findings and host response in patients with peri-implantitis. *Clin Oral Implants Res.* 2002; 13:349–358.

Humphrey JS, Mehta S, Seaber AV, Vail TP. Pharmacokinetics of a degradable drug delivery system in bone. *Clin Orthop Rel Res.* 1998; 349:218 224.

Hunt J, Williams D, Ungersbock A, Perrin S. The effect of titanium debris on soft tissue response. *J Mater Sci Mater Med.* 1994; 5:381–383.

Hwang G, Liang J, Kang S, Tong M, Liu Y. The role of conditioning film formation in *Pseudomonas aeruginosa* PAO1 adhesion to inert surfaces in aquatic environments. *Biochem Eng J.* 2013; 76:90–98.

Ionescu AC, Brambilla E, Azzola F et al. Laser microtextured titanium implant surfaces reduce in vitro and in situ oral biofilm formation. *PLoS One.* 2018; 13:e0202262.

Jacobs JJ, Gilbert JL, Urban RM. Corrosion of metal orthopaedic implants. *J Bone Joint Surg Am.* 1998; 80(2):268–282.

Jakobi ML, Stumpp SN, Stiesch M, Eberhard J, Heuer W. The peri-implant and periodontal microbiota in patients with and without clinical signs of inflammation. *Dent J (Basel).* 2015; 3:24–42.

Javed F, Al-Hezaimi K, Almas K, Romanos GE. Is titanium sensitivity associated with allergic reactions in patients with dental implants? A systematic review. *Clin Implant Dent Relat Res.* 2013; 15:47–52.

Javed F, Alghamdi AS, Ahmed A et al. Clinical efficacy of antibiotics in the treatment of peri-implantitis. *Int Dent J.* 2013; 63(4):169–176.

Jepsen K, Jepsen S. Antibiotics/antimicrobials: systemic and local administration in the therapy of mild to moderately advanced periodontitis. *Periodontol 2000.* 2016; 71(1):82–112.

Jose B, Antoci V Jr, Zeiger AR, Wickstrom E, Hickok NJ. Vancomycin covalently bonded to titanium beads kills *Staphylococcus aureus. Chem Biol.* 2005; 12(9):1041–1048.

Karthik K, Sivaraj S, Thangaswamy V. Evaluation of implant success: a review of past and present concepts. *J Pharm Bioallied Sci.* 2013; 5:S117–S119.

Kim KT, Eo MY, Nguyen TTH, Kim SM. General review of titanium toxicity. *Int J Implant Dent.* 2019; 5:10.

Kinane DF, Stathopoulou PG, Papapanou PN. *Periodontal diseases. Nat Rev Dis Primers.* 2017; 3:17038.

Kligman S, Ren Z, Chung C-H et al. The impact of dental implant surface modifications on osseointegration and biofilm formation. *J Clin Med.* 2021; 10:1641.

Koch D, Manzhos S. On the charge state of titanium in titanium dioxide. *J Phys Chem Lett.* 2017; 8:1593–1598.

Konstantinidis IK, Kotsakis GA, Gerdes S, Walter MH. Cross-sectional study on the prevalence and risk indicators of peri-implant diseases. *Eur J Oral Implantol.* 2015; 8(1):75–88.

Kordbacheh Changi K, Finkelstein J, Papapanou PN. Peri-implantitis prevalence, incidence rate, and risk factors: a study of electronic health records at a U.S. dental school. *Clin Oral Implants Res.* 2019; 30(4):306–314.

Kotsakis GA, Black R, Kum J et al. Effect of implant cleaning on titanium particle dissolution and cytocompatibility. *J Periodontol.* 2021; 92:580–591.

Kotsakis GA, Lan C, Barbosa J et al. Antimicrobial agents used in the treatment of peri-implantitis alter the physicochemistry and cytocompatibility of titanium surfaces. *J Periodontol.* 2016; 87:809–819.

Kotsakis GA, Olmedo DG. Periimplantitis is not periodontitis: scientific discoveries shed light on microbiome-biomaterial interactions that may determine disease phenotype. *Periodontol 2000.* 2021; 86(1):231–240. doi: 10.1111/prd.12372.

Koutouzis T, Catania D, Neiva K, Wallet SM. Innate immune receptor expression in peri-implant tissues of patients with different susceptibility to periodontal diseases. *J Periodontol.* 2013; 84(2):221–229.

Kozlovsky A, Artzi Z, Moses O, Kamin-Belsky N, Greenstein RB. Interaction of chlorhexidine with smooth and rough types of titanium surfaces. *J Periodontol.* 2006; 77:1194–1200.

Kroger A, Hulsmann C, Fickl S et al. The severity of human peri-implantitis lesions correlates with the level of submucosal microbial dysbiosis. *J Clin Periodontol.* 2018; 45:1498–1509.

Kulkarni Aranya A, Pushalkar S, Zhao M et al. Antibacterial and bioactive coatings on titanium implant surfaces. *J Biomed Mater Res A.* 2017; 105:2218–2227.

Kumar PS. Systemic risk factors for the development of periimplant diseases. *Implant Dent.* 2019; 28:115–119.

Kumar PS, Mason MR, Brooker MR, O'Brien K. Pyrosequencing reveals unique microbial signatures associated with healthy and failing dental implants. *J Clin Periodontol.* 2012; 39(5):425–433.

Kumari M, Pandey S, Giri VP et al. Tailoring shape and size of biogenic silver nanoparticles to enhance antimicrobial efficacy against MDR bacteria. *Microb Pathog.* 2017; 105:346–355.

Kumazawa R, Watari F, Takashi N et al. Effects of Ti ions and particles on neutrophil function and morphology. *Biomaterials.* 2002; 23:3757–3764.

Lafaurie GI, Sabogal MA, Castillo DM, Rincón MV, Chambrone L. Microbiome and microbial biofilm profiles of peri-implantitis: a systematic review. *J Periodontol.* 2017; 88:1066–1089.

Lampe I, Beke D, Biri S et al. Investigation of silver nanoparticles on titanium surface created by ion implantation technology. *Int J Nanomed.* 2019; 14:4709–4721.

Lawson MC, Hoth KC, Deforest CA, Bowman CN, Anseth KS. Inhibition of *Staphylococcus epidermidis* biofilms using polymerizable vancomycin derivatives. *Clin Orthop Relat Res.* 2010; 468(8):2081–2091.

Leonhardt A, Dahlen G, Renvert S. Five-year clinical, microbiological, and radiological outcome following treatment of peri-implantitis in man. *J Periodontol.* 2003; 74(10):1415–1422.

Leonhardt Å, Renvert S, Dahlén G. Microbial findings at failing implants. *Clin Oral Implants Res.* 1999; 10(5):339–345.

Lewis K. Persister cells: molecular mechanisms related to antibiotic tolerance. *Handb Exp Pharmacol.* 2012; 211:121–133.

Lim HP, Lee KM, Koh YI, Park SW. Allergic contact stomatitis caused by a titanium nitride-coated implant abutment: a clinical report. *J Prosthet Dent.* 2012; 108:209–213.

Lima EM, Koo H, Vacca Smith AM, Rosalen PL, Del Bel Cury AA. Adsorption of salivary and serum proteins, and bacterial adherence on titanium and zirconia ceramic surfaces. *Clin Oral Implant Res.* 2008: 19:780–785.

Martellacci L, Quaranta G, Patini R et al. A literature review of metagenomics and culturomics of the peri-implant microbiome: current evidence and future perspectives. *Materials* 2019; 12:3010.

Martini D, Fini M, Franchi M et al. Detachment of titanium and fluorohydroxyapatite particles in unloaded endosseous implants. *Biomaterials.* 2003; 24:1309–1316.

Mathew MT, Pai P, Pourzal R, Fischer A, Wimmer M. Significance of Tribocorrosion in biomedical applications: overview and current status. *Adv Tribol.* 2009; 2009: 250986.

Matsubara VH, Igai F, Tamaki R et al. Use of silver nanoparticles reduces internal contamination of external hexagon implants by *Candida albicans. Braz Dent J.* 2015; 26(5):458–462.

Maximo MB, de Mendonça AC, Renata Santos V et al. Short-term clinical and microbiological evaluations of peri-implant diseases before and after mechanical anti-infective therapies. *Clin Oral Implants Res.* 2009; 20:99–108.

McShan D, Ray PC, Yu H. Molecular toxicity mechanism of nanosilver. *J Food Drug Anal.* 2014; 22(1):116–127.

Meffert RM. Periodontitis vs. peri-implantitis: the same disease? The same treatment? *Crit Rev Oral Biol Med.* 1996; 7(3):278–291.

Mi L, Jiang S. Integrated antimicrobial and nonfouling zwitterionic polymers. *Angew Chem Int Ed Engl.* 2014; 53:1746–1754.

Mine Y, Makihira S, Nikawa H et al. Impact of titanium ions on osteoblast-, osteoclast- and gingival epithelial-like cells. *J Prosthodont Res.* 2010; 54:1–6.

Mitchell DL, Synnott SA, Van Dercreek JA. Tissue reaction involving an intraoral skin graft and CP titanium abutments: a clinical report. *Int J Oral Maxillofac Implants.* 1990; 5:79–84.

Mombelli A, Hashim D, Cionca N. What is the impact of titanium particles and biocorrosion on implant survival and complications? A critical review. *Clin Oral Implants Res.* 2018; 29(Suppl 18):37–53.

Naito Y, Tohda H, Okuda K, Takazoe I. Adherence and hydrophobicity of invasive and noninvasive strains of *Porphyromonas gingivalis. Oral MicroBiol Immunol.* 1993; 8:195–202.

Narayana PSVVS, Srihari PSVV. Biofilm resistant surfaces and coatings on implants: a review. *Mater Today: Proc.* 2019; 18(7):4847–4853.

Noronha Oliveira M, Schunemann WVH, Mathew MT et al. Can degradation products released from dental implants affect peri-implant tissues? *J Periodontal Res.* 2018; 53:1–11.

Olmedo D, Fernandez MM, Guglielmotti MB, Cabrini RL. Macrophages related to dental implant failure. *Implant Dent.* 2003; 12(1):75–80.

Olmedo DG, Nalli G, Verdú S, Paparella ML, Cabrini RL. Exfoliative cytology and titanium dental implants: a pilot study. *J Periodontol.* 2013; 84:78–83.

Olmedo DG, Paparella ML, Spielberg M et al. Oral mucosa tissue response to titanium cover screws. *J Periodontol.* 2012; 83:973–980.

Ong JL, Chan DCN. A review of hydroxyapatite and its use as a coating in dental implants. *Crit Rev Biomed Eng.* 2017; 45:411–451.

Parlar A, Bosshardt DD, Cetiner D et al. Effects of decontamination and implant surface characteristics on re-osseointegration following treatment of peri-implantitis. *Clin Oral Implants Res.* 2009; 20:391–399.

Payne JB, Johnson PG, Kok CR et al. Subgingival microbiome colonization and cytokine production during early dental implant healing. *mSphere.* 2017; 2(6):e00527–17.

Peñarrieta Juanito GM, Morsch C, Benfatti C et al. Effect of fluoride and bleaching agents on the degradation of titanium: literature review. *Dentistry.* 2015; 2015:5. doi: 10.4172/2161-1122.1000273.

Persson GR, Renvert S. Cluster of bacteria associated with peri-implantitis. *Clin Implant Dent Relat Res.* 2014; 16:783–793.

Pieralli S, Kohal RJ, Jung RE, Vach K, Spies BC. Clinical outcomes of zirconia dental implants: a systematic review. *J Dent Res.* 2017; 96:38–46.

Pigatto PD, Guzzi G. The link between patch testing and dental material. *Contact Derm.* 2007; 56:301–302.

Pigatto PD, Guzzi G, Brambilla L, Sforza C. Titanium allergy associated with dental implant failure. *Clin Oral Implants Res.* 2009; 20(8):857. doi: 10.1111/j.1600-0501.2009.01749.x.

Pita PPC, Rodrigues JA, Ota-Tsuzuki C et al. Oral streptococci biofilm formation on different implant surface topographies. *BioMed Res Int.* 2015; 2015:159625.

Pöyry S, Vattulainen I. Role of charged lipids in membrane structures—insight given by simulations. *Biochim Biophys Acta.* 2016; 1858:2322–2333.

Pozhitkov AE, Daubert DM, Brochwicz DA et al. Interruption of electrical conductivity of titanium dental implants suggests a path towards elimination of corrosion. *PLoS One.* 2015; 10:e0140393.

Quirynen M, Vogels R, Pauwels M et al. Initial subgingival colonization of "pristine" pockets. *J Dent Res.* 2005; 84:340–344.

Quirynen, M, Vogels R, Peeters W et al. Dynamics of initial subgingival colonization of "pristine" peri-implant pockets. *Clin Oral Implants Res.* 2006; 17:25–37.

Rakic M, Grusovin MG, Canullo L. The microbiologic proile associated with peri-implantitis in humans: a systematic review. *Int J Oral Maxillofac Implants.* 2016; 31:359–368.

Renvert S, Roos-Jansaker AM, Lindahl C, Renvert H, Rutger Persson G. Infection at titanium implants with or without a clinical diagnosis of inflammation. *Clin Oral Implants Res.* 2007; 18:509–516.

Rickard AH, Gilbert P, High NJ, Kolenbrander PE, Handley PS. Bacterial coaggregation: an integral process in the development of multi-species biofilms. *Trends Microbiol.* 2003; 11:94–100.

Rodrigues D, Valderrama P, Wilson T et al. Titanium corrosion mechanisms in the oral environment: a retrieval study. *Materials.* 2013; 6:5258–5274.

Rodriguez Y Baena R, Arciola CR, Selan L et al. Evaluation of bacterial adhesion on machined titanium, Osseotite(R) and Nanotite(R) discs. *Int J Artif Organs.* 2012; 35:754–761.

Roos-Jansaker AM, Renvert H, Lindahl C, Renvert S. Nine- to fourteen-year follow-up of implant treatment. Part III: factors associated with peri-implant lesions. *J Clin Periodontol.* 2006; 33:296–301.

Ruiz E, Maestro A. Titanium allergy in dental implant patients: a clinical study on 1500 consecutive patients. *Clin Oral Impl Res.* 2008; 19:823–835.

Safioti LM, Kotsakis GA, Pozhitkov AE, Chung WO, Daubert DM. Increased levels of dissolved titanium are associated with peri-implantitis—a cross-sectional study. *J Periodontol.* 2017; 88:436–442.

Sagomonyants KB, Jarman-Smith ML, Devine JN, Aronow MS, Gronowicz GA. The in vitro response of human osteoblasts to polyetherether ketone (PEEK) substrates compared to commercially pure titanium. *Biomaterials.* 2008; 29:1563–1572.

Sahrmann P, Gilli F, Wiedemeier DB et al. The microbiome of peri-implantitis: a systematic review and meta-analysis. *Microorganisms.* 2020; 8:661.

Sanchez MC, Llama-Palacios A, Fernandez E et al. An in vitro biofilm model associated to dental implants: structural and quantitative analysis of in vitro biofilm formation on different dental implant surfaces. *Dent Mater.* 2014; 30:1161–1171.

Sanz-Martin I, Doolittle-Hall J, Teles RP, Patel M, Teles FRF. Exploring the microbiome of healthy and diseased peri-implant sites using Illumina sequencing. *J Clin Periodontol.* 2017; 44:1274–1284.

Scheuerman TR, Camper AK, Hamilton MA. Effects of substratum topography on bacterial adhesion. *J Colloid Interface Sci.* 1998; 208:23–33.

Schliephake H, Sicilia A, Al-Nawas B et al. Drugs and diseases: summary and consensus statements of group 1. The 5th EAO Consensus Conference 2018. *Clin Oral Implant Res.* 2018; 29:93–99.

Schmidlin PR, Müller P, Attin T et al. Polyspecies biofilm formation on implant surfaces with different surface characteristics. *J Appl Oral Sci.* 2013; 21(1): 48–55.

Shiba T, Watanabe T, Kachi H et al. Distinct interacting core taxa in co-occurrence networks enable discrimination of polymicrobial oral diseases with similar symptoms. *Sci Rep.* 2016; 6:30997.

Shibli JA, Melo L, Ferrari DS et al. Composition of supra- and subgingival biofilm of subjects with healthy and diseased implants. *Clin Oral Implants Res.* 2008; 19:975–982.

Sicilia A, Cuesta S, Coma G et al. Titanium allergy in dental implant patients: a clinical study on 1500 consecutive patients. *Clin Oral Impl Res.* 2008; 19:823–835.

Siddiqi A, Payne AGT, De Silva RK, Duncan WJ. Titanium allergy: could it affect dental implant integration? *Clin Oral Impl Res.* 2011; 22:673–680.

Singh RK, Chang HW, Yan D, Lee KM, Liao W. Influence of diet on the gut microbiome and implications for human health. *J Transl Med.* 2017; 15:73.

Skocaj M, Filipic M, Petkovic J, Novak S. Titanium dioxide in our everyday life; is it safe? *Radiol Oncol.* 2011; 45:227–247.

Slots J, Rams TE. New views on periodontal microbiota in special patient categories. *J Clin Periodontol.* 1991; 18(6):411–420.

Song F, Koo H, Ren D. Effects of material properties on bacterial adhesion and biofilm formation. *J Dent Res.* 2015; 94(8):1027–1034.

Sousa V, Nibali L, Spratt D, Dopico J, Donos N. Peri-implant and periodontal microbiome diversity in aggressive periodontitis patients: a pilot study. *Clin Oral Implants Res.* 2017; 28:558–570.

Souza JC, Barbosa SL, Ariza EA et al. How do titanium and Ti6Al4V corrode in fluoridated medium as found in the oral cavity? An in vitro study. *Mater Sci Eng C Mater Biol Appl.* 2015a; 47:384–393.

Souza JC, Henriques M, Oliveira R et al. Do oral biofilms influence the wear and corrosion behavior of titanium? *Biofouling.* 2010; 26(4):471–478.

Souza JCM, Henriques M, Teughels W et al. Wear and corrosion interactions on titanium in oral environment: literature review. *J Bio Tribo Corros.* 2015b; 1:13.

Souza JGS, Costa Oliveira BE, Bertolini M et al. Titanium particles and ions favor dysbiosis in oral biofilms. *J Periodontal Res.* 2020; 55:258–266.

Sridhar S, Wilson TG, Palmer KL et al. in vitro investigation of the effect of oral bacteria in the surface oxidation of dental implants. *Clin Implant Dent Relat Res.* 2015; 17(Suppl 2):e562–e575.

Stenport VF, Johansson CB. Evaluations of bone tissue integration to pure and alloyed titanium implants. *Clin Implant Dent Relat Res.* 2008; 10:191–199.

Suarez-Lopez Del Amo F, Garaicoa-Pazmino C, Fretwurst T, Castilho RM, Squarize CH. Dental implants-associated release of titanium particles: a systematic review. *Clin Oral Implants Res.* 2018; 29(11):1085–1100.

Subramani K, Jung RE, Molenberg A, Hammerle CH. Biofilm on dental implants: a review of the literature. *Int J Oral Maxillofac Implant.* 2009; 24:616–626.

Tamura N, Ochi M, Miyakawa H, Nakazawa F. Analysis of bacterial flora associated with peri-implantitis using obligate anaerobic culture technique and 16S rDNA gene sequence. *Int J Oral Maxillofac Implants.* 2013; 28(6):1521–1529.

Venclikova Z, Benada O, Bartova J, Joska L, Mrklas L. Metallic pigmentation of human teeth and gingiva: morphological and immunological aspects. *Dent Mater J.* 2007; 26:96–104.

Wang Q, Lu H, Zhang L et al. Peri-implant mucositis sites with suppuration have higher microbial risk than sites without suppuration. *J Periodontol.* 2020; 91:1284–1294.

Wen B, Hao Q, Yin WJ et al. Electronic structure and photo absorption of Ti(3+) ions in reduced anatase and rutile TiO(2). *Phys Chem Chem Phys.* 2018; 20:17658–17665.

Yeo IS, Kim HY, Lim KS, Han JS. Implant surface factors and bacterial adhesion: a review of the literature. *Int J Artif Organs.* 2012; 35(10):762–772.

Yu XL, Chan Y, Zhuang L et al. Intra-oral single-site comparisons of periodontal and peri-implant microbiota in health and disease. *Clin Oral Implants Res.* 2019; 30(8):760–776.

Yuan Y, Hays MP, Hardwidge PR, Kim J. Surface characteristics influencing bacterial adhesion to polymeric substrates. *RSC Adv.* 2017; 7:14254–14261.

Zhang XWL, Levänena E. Superhydrophobic surfaces for the reduction of bacterial adhesion. *RSC Adv.* 2013; 3:12003–12020.

Zheng H, Xu L, Wang Z et al. Subgingival microbiome in patients with healthy and ailing dental implants. *Sci Rep.* 2015; 5:10948.

35.2   DIAGNOSIS AND TREATMENT OF PERI-IMPLANTITIS

Pierluigi Balice

Contents

Learning objectives

- Definition and prevalence of peri-implantitis.
- How to diagnose peri-implantitis.
- The etiology and pathogenesis of peri-implantitis.
- Treatment modalities in the management of peri-implantitis.
- Prevention of peri-implantitis.

Introduction

More than five million implants are placed annually in the United States, with a predicted annual growth rate of 12–15% (Misch 2015). A major challenge in the field of implant dentistry is the prevention and effective management of the biological complications of peri-implant diseases. Peri-implantitis is considered the most challenging biological complication, and if untreated may lead to implant loss (Berglundh et al. 2019).

Prevalence of peri-implantitis

Controversy exists regarding the threshold of bone loss to determine peri-implantitis (Tomasi & Derks 2012). Due to inconsistent consensus on the definition, reporting methods, and study characteristics, the prevalence of peri-implant disease varies significantly in studies. Hence, it is challenging to outline the exact prevalence of peri-implantitis. Recent meta-analysis data have reported the prevalence of peri-implantitis to be 18.5% at patient level and 12.8% at implant level (Rakic et al. 2018). These values were based on the Sanz and Chapple (2012) criteria defining peri-implantitis as the presence of bone loss >2 mm, positive bleeding on probing, and probing depth >5 mm.

Diagnosis of peri-implantitis

Peri-implantitis is a plaque-associated pathological condition occurring in tissues around dental implants, characterized by inflammation in the peri-implant mucosa and subsequent progressive loss of supporting bone. Peri-implantitis sites exhibit clinical signs of inflammation, bleeding on probing and/or suppuration, increased probing depths and/or recession of the mucosal margin, in addition to radiographic bone loss compared to previous examinations. Such bone loss, in the absence of treatment, seems to progress in a non-linear and accelerating pattern.

The diagnosis of peri-implantitis should include visual inspection, probing with a periodontal probe and digital palpation. Probing of peri-implant tissues is necessary to assess the presence of bleeding on probing and to monitor probing depth changes, including mucosal margin migration. This assessment may alert the clinician to the need for therapeutic intervention. Usage of a light probing force is considered a safe and important component of a complete oral examination. However, it is not possible to define a range of probing depths compatible with health, especially in light of the variety of implant designs and their interface with the soft tissues (Derks et al. 2016). Concerns about the accuracy of probing around implants as a result of the design of the supragingival implant components and the position of the implants have led the dental community to recommend a more flexible plastic probe for examination of the peri-implant pockets (Renvert & Polyzois 2015).

It is recommended that the clinician obtain baseline radiographic and probing measurements following the completion of the implant-supported prosthesis. An additional radiograph after a one-year loading period should be taken to establish a bone-level reference following physiological remodeling. If the patient presents for the first time with an implant-supported prosthesis, the clinician should try to obtain clinical records including previous radiographs in order to assess changes in bone levels.

The diagnosis of peri-implantitis requires:
- Presence of bleeding and/or suppuration on gentle probing.
- Increased probing depth compared to previous examinations.
- Marginal bone level changes of ≥2 mm after one year of loading.

In the absence of previous examination data, the diagnosis of peri-implantitis can be based on the combination of:
- Presence of bleeding and/or suppuration on gentle probing.
- Probing depths of ≥6 mm.
- Bone levels ≥3 mm apical of the most coronal portion of the intraosseous part of the implant (Berglundh et al. 2019).

Etiology of peri-implantitis

Biofilm growth on the implant surface is considered the main etiological factor associated with the development of peri-implant mucositis and peri-implantitis (Singh 2011). The build-up of a plaque biofilm on an implant follows the same sequence of bacterial colonization as that on teeth (Kilian et al. 2016); however, no specific or unique bacteria or proinflammatory cytokines have been identified. A systematic review revealed that significantly more patients developed peri-implantitis who had a prior history of periodontitis-associated tooth loss (Schou et al. 2006). There is strong evidence that there is an increased risk of developing peri-implantitis in patients who have a history of severe periodontitis, including an absence of regular maintenance care after implant therapy (Caton et al. 2018). Periodontitis should thus be treated before placement of dental implants, and regular maintenance care must be emphasized in patients with a history of periodontitis, so as to avoid the initiation of peri-implant disease.

Data identifying smoking and diabetes as potential risk indicators for peri-implantitis are still inconclusive. Implants that have been placed under less than ideal circumstances are often encountered in day-to-day practice. As a result, there may be an increased prevalence of peri-implantitis associated with these situations and, therefore, the etiology of peri-implantitis could be contributing to iatrogenic factors. There is some limited evidence linking peri-implantitis to the presence of post-restorative submucosal cement, as well as positioning of implants that does not facilitate oral hygiene and maintenance.

The role of peri-implant keratinized mucosa, occlusal overload, titanium particles release, bone compression necrosis, overheating, micromotion, and biocorrosion as risk indicators for peri-implantitis remains to be determined (Caton et al. 2018). However, lack of keratinized mucosa in patients with inadequate oral hygiene could be regarded as a predisposing factor for peri-implant diseases, since it is associated with more recession, less vestibular depth, and more plaque accumulation. This, in turn, may be predisposing to inflammation and therefore peri-implantitis (Monje et al. 2019). Recent meta-analysis has shown that an adequate amount of keratinized mucosa around implants favors peri-implant health and gingival indices (Caton et al. 2018). A growing body of evidence shows advantages in patient comfort and ease of plaque removal (Thoma et al. 2018).

Current evidence indicates that peri-implant mucositis is the precursor of peri-implantitis, this being similar to gingivitis being the precursor of periodontitis. Furthermore, there is evidence to suggest that peri-implant mucositis, like gingivitis, is reversible when effectively treated with indicated therapeutic regimens (Lang et al. 2011).

Management of peri-implantitis

While the non-surgical treatment of peri-implant mucositis is effective, the treatment of peri-implantitis is a highly controversial topic in implant dentistry, representing complex scenarios for clinicians. The severity and extensiveness of the lesion are crucial factors for successful and maintainable outcomes (Schou et al. 2006). Currently, there is not a single treatment protocol that is the preferred approach for treating peri-implantitis (Khoshkam et al. 2016). This presents a challenge for clinicians to make evidence-based decisions regarding choice of treatment, and warrants further studies to support the efficacy of available treatment protocols. A variety of conservative and surgical therapies have been introduced for the treatment of peri-implantitis; however, these studies show high heterogeneity, particularly regarding defect morphology, surgical protocols, patient factors, and selection of biomaterials (Daugela et al. 2016). Surgical approaches are commonly more appropriate and suitable in cases of extended severity of the disease. Nevertheless, non-surgical therapy should always be performed before any surgical intervention. Ideally, the treatment of peri-implantitis should entail the removal of the offending etiology in conjunction with the regeneration of supporting bone around the implant.

Various management strategies suggested for the treatment of peri-implantitis are as follows.

Mechanical therapy

- In conditions of inflammation of peri-implant tissues, mechanical therapy, with or without adjunctive use of antiseptic rinses, is usually the treatment of choice.
- Elimination of biofilm from the implant surface can be challenging. Most modern implants have a moderately rough surface structure. This surface facilitates osseointegration and increases the bone–implant contact area.

- On the other hand, it can complicate the management of infections, as the increased surface area and surface roughness may facilitate microbial colonization and enhance biofilm formation (Teughels et al. 2006).
- Instruments, such as titanium scalers, regular sonic and ultrasonic scalers with plastic tips, or piezoelectric scalers with carbon or plastic tips, can be used around dental implants and seem to be safe with regard to subgingival biofilm disruption and causing reduced damage to implant surfaces.
- The combination of professional irrigation of the sulci with chlorhexidine and professional administration of local delivery antimicrobials can be performed as an adjunct to mechanical therapy.
- Air-abrasive methods have been used to debride implant surfaces. They employ a small, thin, disposable plastic nozzle in order to gain access into the peri-implant pocket. The biofilm is removed by irrigation with a water/glycine powder mix. This treatment has been recognized as safe (Renvert & Polyzois 2015).

Decontamination/detoxification

- Decontamination is a large challenge for clinicians. Currently, there is no specific decontamination protocol that has been shown to be superior to others.
- Decontamination with laser therapy does not appear to be more advantageous than other surface decontamination methods (Mailoa et al. 2014).
- Rotating titanium brushes seem to be an effective instrument for mechanical cleansing (Louropoulou et al. 2014).
- Among the proposed methods to detoxify the implant surfaces, chlorhexidine gluconate, EDTA, and tetracycline hydrochloride are the most frequently used approaches. Simple saline irrigation can be also used in some cases, but only for cleaning the defect after debridement, not for detoxification (Renvert & Polyzois 2015).
- Once detoxification is accomplished, studies show that re-osseointegration is possible in both animal and human models, yet the degree of the bone-to-implant contact (BIC) is unpredictable (Fletcher et al. 2017; Renvert et al. 2009; Wohlfahrt et al. 2011).

Regeneration

- Clinicians are often presented with the decision of whether to attempt to save the implant using a regenerative procedure.
- Regenerative procedures utilizing bone-replacement grafts with or without barrier membranes have been proposed (see Figures 35.2.1–35.2.8).
- However, due to the variety of surgical techniques, decontamination methods, grafting materials, and barrier membranes available, it is challenging to draw conclusions regarding the effectiveness of each method (Esposito et al. 2012).

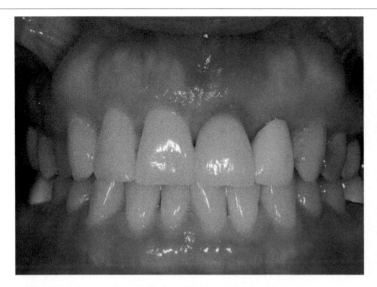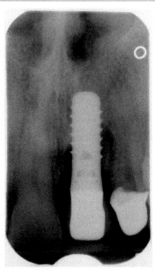

Figure 35.2.1 A 55-year-old Caucasian female (left) with no history of systemic disease or smoking showed peri-implantitis of the left maxillary incisor (#9). Intra-oral examination revealed slight erythema around the peri-implant soft tissues and buccal plate resorption on palpation. Bleeding and suppuration were induced on probing and buccal probing depths ranged from 3 to 8 mm. The implant #9, placed 8 years prior, was identified as a Straumann 4.8 × 12 mm Soft Tissue Level, regular neck (RN), SLA Active with a cement retained crown on a RN solid abutment, with a machined collar 1.8 mm in height. A peri-apical X-ray was taken (right) that revealed bone loss around the implant, with two threads exposed on the mesial side and three threads on the distal side.

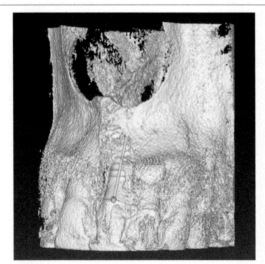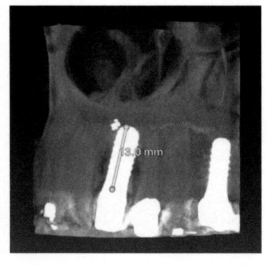

Figure 35.2.2 On the cone beam computed tomography scan, a buccal lesion of 11.2 mm (13 mm minus 1.8 mm of the machined Straumann STL implant collar height) was noted along with a 5 mm long tooth fragment located on the disto-labial aspect of the implant, which may have been the iatrogenic cause of the peri-implantitis. The reasons why a regenerative procedure was preferred over explantation by both the clinician and patient were first, considering the size of the implant (4.8 × 12 mm), explantation would have posed a more challenging rehabilitation process with a difficult restoration of the bone ridge anatomy and soft tissues. In addition, the contained anatomy of the bony defect and the thick gingival phenotype of the patient would facilitate the outcome of a possible graft. The patient's esthetic demand and her preference for a less invasive and time-consuming treatment also played a role. The patient was informed about the possible collapse of the mesial papilla of the adjacent lateral maxillary incisor (#10) after the regenerative treatment due to flap incision and a possible need for a new crown for #10, with a lower marginal preparation to overcome the exposed margin. She accepted the option of a new crown for #10, especially in light of a color mismatch with the adjacent teeth.

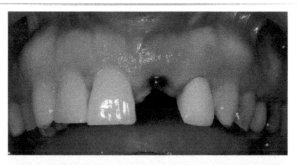

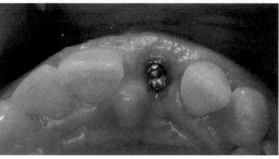

Figure 35.2.3 The cemented crown was removed from #9 and a cover screw applied. A non-surgical therapy was performed, consisting of intrasulcular irrigation with chlorhexidine 0.12% and ultrasonic debridement with plastic tips to decrease the level of inflammation prior to surgery. An essix retainer was delivered to the patient at the end of the appointment.

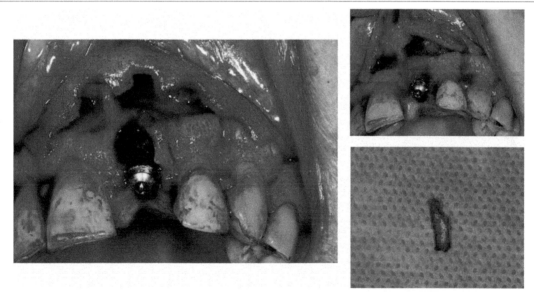

Figure 35.2.4 Two weeks later, the surgery was performed (left). A full-thickness flap was raised buccally and palatally. A bony defect was observed on the buccal (five to six threads exposed) and palatal aspects (two threads exposed), along with a tooth fragment on the disto-labial aspect of the implant (right).

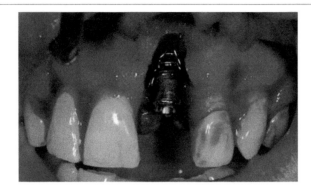

Figure 35.2.5 Thorough debridement of the implant surface was performed with titanium hand scalers and a rotary titanium brush comprising titanium alloy bristles (TiBrush™, Straumann®, Basel, Switzerland). The implant surface was decontaminated with abundant irrigations with saline solution and chlorhexidine gluconate 0.12%, and 0.6 mL of 24% EDTA surface gel conditioner (Emdogain PrefGel®, Straumann) was applied for 120 seconds on the implant surface.

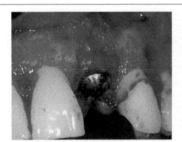
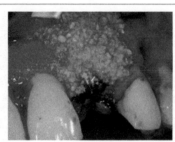
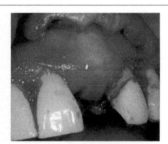

Autogenous Graft   Xenograft   Resorbable Membrane
and Tacks

Figure 35.2.6 Autogenous bone was obtained from the exostosis with a bone scraper, mixed with gentamicin sulfate 80 mg/2 mL and used to fill the defect (left). The existing graft was bulked with 0.5 g bovine-derived xenograft (Geistlich Bio-Oss®, Wolhusen, Switzerland; small granules 0.25–1 mm) mixed with enamel matrix derivative (Emdogain®, Straumann) to enhance the viscosity and stabilization of the graft (centre). A resorbable bilayer collagen membrane (Geistlich Bio-Gide®, 13 x 25 mm) was trimmed following the ridge anatomy, applied, and then stabilized with two tacks (TRUtacks, ACE Surgical Supply Co., Brockton, MA, USA) on the buccal plate (right). Primary closure was achieved. Amoxicillin 500 mg, ibuprofen 600 mg, and hydrocodone bitrate and acetaminophen 5 mg/300 mg were prescribed to the patient. A new essix retainer was delivered for esthetics, avoiding pressure on the surgical wound. The patient was dismissed and did not report significant postoperative discomfort.

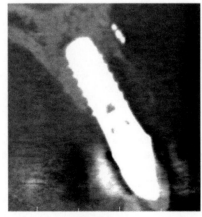
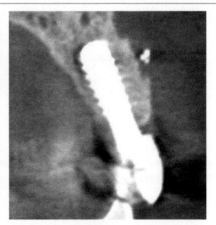

Preoperative   Postoperative at 9 months

Figure 35.2.7 A new cone beam computed tomography (CBCT) scan was performed 9 months from the procedure (right). The comparison between pre- (left) and postoperative CBCT showed a vertical bone-level gain of 11.2 mm buccally, 2.3 mm palatally, and a 2.5 mm thick buccal plate. Calibrated measurements comparing pre- and postoperative CBCT scans were performed with ImageJ software (National Institute of Health, NIH), knowing the 1.25 mm thread pitch of the 4.8 mm wide Straumann implant.

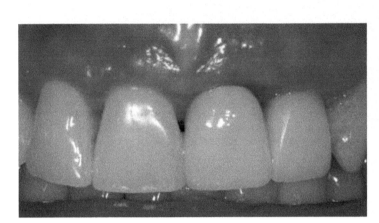
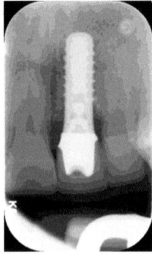

Figure 35.2.8 The final restoration for #9 and crown on #10 were delivered (left). At 36 months follow-up a peri-apical X-ray was taken, showing preserved marginal bone levels. Probing depths were within normal limits, ranging from 2 to 3 mm, and no alteration of marginal soft tissues was noted. The patient was happy with the result (right) and declined any additional soft tissue augmentation to improve esthetics.

Resection and implantoplasty

- Resective procedures consist of eliminating the bony defect via ostectomy and/or osteoplasty of the surrounding bone.
- It is usually associated with open flap debridement, apical flap positioning, and implantoplasty, which includes the mechanical removal of the implant threads in order to smooth the contaminated rough surface (see Figures 35.2.9–35.2.12).
- Recent studies show implantoplasty not to be associated with any remarkable mechanical or biological complication (Stavropoulos et al. 2019).

Explantation

- An alternative treatment is the explantation of the implant, which may result in morbidity, additional time, and expenses in order to restore the explanted site for placement of a new implant (see Figures 35.2.13–35.2.17).
- Additionally, studies have not indicated specific indications for explantation, unless the implant is clinically mobile (Froum et al. 2012).
- Currently, no guidelines are available to treat a complex case of peri-implantitis, including no clear indications and cut-off for implant explantation, making the clinical approach empirical as well as surgeon preference oriented (Esposito et al. 2012).

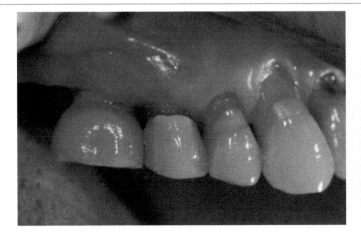
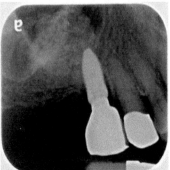

Figure 35.2.9 The patient presented with peri-implantitis on implant #3 (left). Probing depths ranged from 5 mm to 9 mm. Due to financial constraints and the extent of treatment involving implant explantation, ridge preservation via bone grafting, and new implant placement, the treatment of choice was represented by a resective procedure. The peri-apical X-ray showed a mesio-distal bony defect around the implant previously placed after sinus grafting (right).

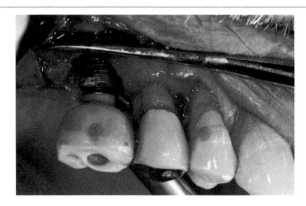

Figure 35.2.10 Full-thickness flap showing peri-implant bony defect and surface contamination.

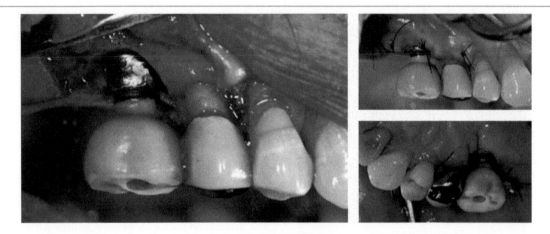

Figure 35.2.11 Implantoplasty with round diamond finishing burs and Arkansas stone burs was performed along with surface decontamination (via glycine powder air polishing, copious chlorhexidine gluconate 0.12% and saline solution rinses) and osteoplasty (left). The flaps were sutured with vertical mattress and simple interrupted sutures (right).

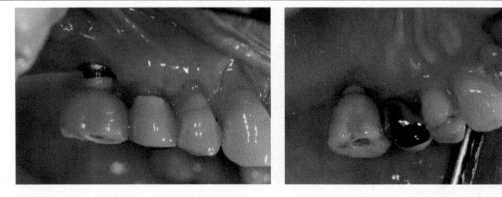

Figure 35.2.12 Follow-up at more than 6 weeks showing healing with recessions along with decrease in probing depths (ranging from 3 to 4 mm).

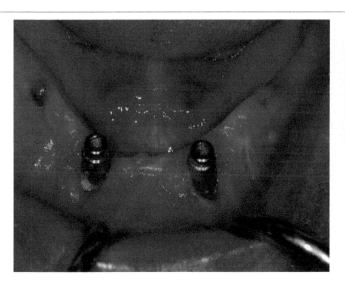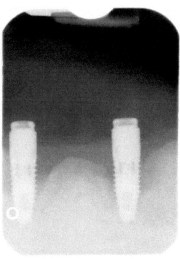

Figure 35.2.13 A 74-year-old patient with no contributory medical history presented peri-implantitis on implant #23 and #26, with probing depths ranging from 5 to 10 mm. Implants lacked marginal keratinized tissue and had been presumably placed too buccal over the alveolar ridge (left). Peri-apical X-ray shows severe bone loss (right).

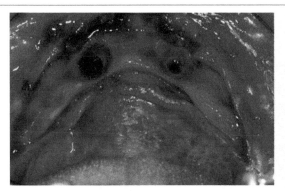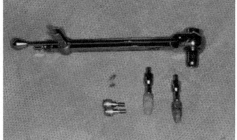

Figure 35.2.14 Implants explanted with reverse torque device.

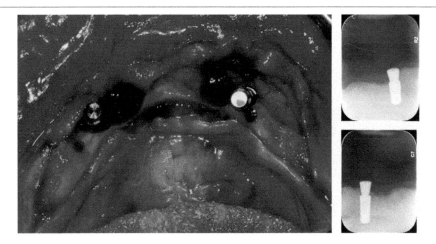

Figure 35.2.15 New implants were placed (left) and alveolar defects were grafted with Xenograft (Geistlich BioOss) using collagen resorbable membranes (Geistlich Bio-Gide) (right). Peri-apical X-rays show placement of new implants (bottom).

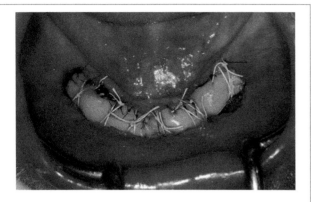

Figure 35.2.16 Implants were submerged to prepare the sites for a second-stage approach consisting of bilateral free gingival grafts, secured with simple interrupted monofilament nylon sutures and cross-mattress PTFE sutures.

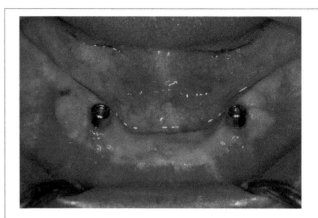

Figure 35.2.17 Follow-up results at more than 6 weeks after placement of free gingival grafts.

Soft tissue augmentation

See Figures 35.2.18–35.2.22.

Maintenance therapy

- Since peri-implant mucositis precedes peri-implantitis and is evidently reversible, the initial stage of the disease is the best time to diagnose peri-implantitis and to reverse it before it becomes an unpredictable issue (Lang & Berglundh 2011).

- Prevention of the disease is therefore the best form of treatment and should be a high priority in everyday clinical practice to minimize the occurrence and the severity of the problem (Tonetti et al. 2015).
- It has been demonstrated that peri-implant health can be maintained throughout implant maintenance therapy.
- Thus, following implant placement, patients should be closely monitored with regular recalls to evaluate periodontal and implant health, including compliance with oral hygiene (Lin et al. 2019; Salvi & Zitzmann 2014).

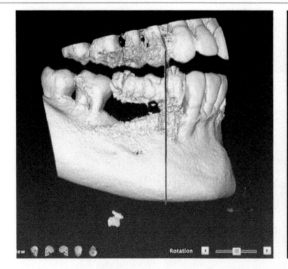
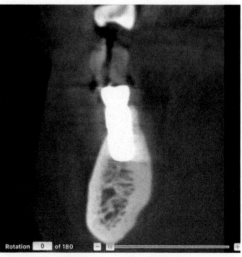

Figure 35.2.18 The patient presented with stable buccal marginal bone loss, with no signs of inflammation and therefore no peri-implantitis on implant #28. Marginal dehiscence was probably due to iatrogenic factors. The patient had previously lost implant #30.

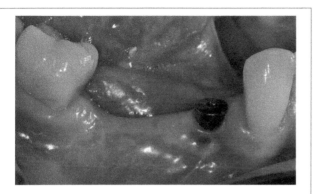

Figure 35.2.19 Peri-implant soft tissues looked thin, showing a fenestration and lack of keratinized tissue. In order to avoid implant explantation, ridge reconstruction, and new implant placement, the treatment of choice was soft tissue augmentation.

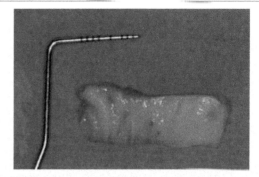

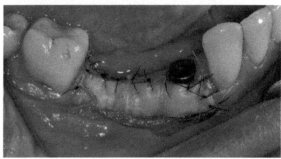

Figure 35.2.21 Free gingival graft applied (top) and secured with interrupted and cross-mattress sutures (bottom).

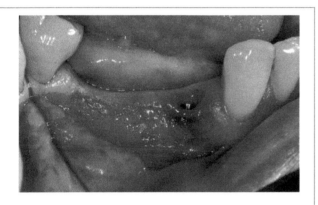

Figure 35.2.20 Partial-thickness flap was performed to create an even recipient bed for a free gingival graft.

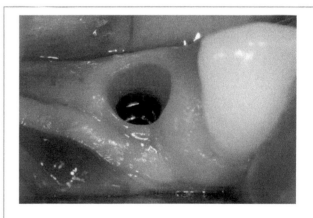

Figure 35.2.22 Follow-up at more than 6 weeks with clear thickening of peri-implant soft tissues to preserve long-term stability in combination with a recall regimen.

REFERENCES

Berglundh T, Jepsen S, Stadlinger B, Terheyden H. Peri-implantitis and its prevention. *Clin Oral Implants Res.* 2019; 30(2):150–155.

Caton JG, Armitage G, Berglund T et al. A new classification scheme for periodontal and peri-implant diseases and conditions – introduction and key changes from the 1999 classification. *J Periodontol.* 2018; 89:(Suppl 1):S1–S8.

Daugela P, Cicciù M, Saulacic N. Surgical regenerative treatments for peri-implantitis: meta-analysis of recent findings in a systematic literature review. *J Oral Maxillofac Res.* 2016; 7(3):e15. doi: 10.5037/jomr.2016.7315.

Derks J, Schaller D, Hakansson J et al. Peri-implantitis—onset and pattern of progression. *J Clin Periodontol.* 2016; 43:383–388.

Esposito M, Grusovin MG, Worthington HV. Treatment of peri-implantitis: what interventions are elective? A Cochrane systematic review. *Eur J Oral Implantol.* 2012; 5(suppl):s21–s41.

Fletcher P, Deluiz D, Tinoco EMB et al. Human histologic evidence of re-osseointegration around an implant affected with peri-implantitis following decontamination with sterile saline and antiseptics: a case history report. *Int J Periodontics Restorative Dent.* 2017; 37(4):499–508.

Froum SJ, Froum SH, Rosen PS. Successful management of peri-implantitis with a regenerative approach: a consecutive series of 51 treated implants with 3- to 7.5-year follow-up. *Int J Periodontics Restorative Dent.* 2012; 32:11–20.

Khoshkam V, Suárez-López Del Amo F, Monje A et al. Long-term radiographic and clinical outcomes of regenerative approach for treating peri-implantitis: a systematic review and meta-analysis. *Int J Oral Maxillofac Implants.* 2016; 31(6):1303–1310.

Kilian M, Chapple IL, Hannig M et al. The oral microbiome – an update for oral healthcare professionals. *Br Dent J.* 2016; 221(10):657–666.

Lang NP, Berglundh T. Periimplant diseases: where are we now? Consensus of the Seventh European Workshop on Periodontology. *J Clin Periodontol.* 2011; 38 (Suppl 11):178–181.

Lin CY, Chen Z, Pan WL, Wang HL. The effect of supportive care in preventing peri-implant diseases and implant loss: a systematic review and meta-analysis. *Clin Oral Implants Res.* 2019; 30(8):714–724.

Louropoulou A, Slot DE, Van der Weijden F. The effects of mechanical instruments on contaminated titanium dental implant surfaces: a systematic review. *Clin Oral Implants Res.* 2014; 25(10):1149–1160.

Mailoa J, Lin GH, Chan HL, MacEachern M, Wang HL. Clinical outcomes of using lasers for peri-implantitis surface detoxification: a systematic review and meta-analysis. *J Periodontol.* 2014; 85(9):1194–1202.

Misch CE. Rationale for dental implants. In: *CE Misch, Dental Implant Prosthetics.* St. Louis, MO: Elsevier Mosby; 2015: 11.

Monje A, Insua A, Wang HL. Understanding peri-implantitis as a plaque-associated and site-specific entity: on the local predisposing factors. *J Clin Med.* 2019; 8(2):279. doi: 10.3390/jcm8020279.

Rakic M, Galindo-Moreno P, Monje A. How frequent does peri-implantitis occur? A systematic review and meta-analysis. *Clin Oral Investig.* 2018; 22(4):1805–1816.

Renvert S, Polyzois I, Maguire R. Re-osseointegration on previously contaminated surfaces: a systematic review. *Clin Oral Implants Res.* 2009; 20(suppl 4):216–227.

Renvert S, Polyzois IN. Clinical approaches to treat peri-implant mucositis and peri-implantitis. *Periodontol 2000.* 2015; 68(1):369–404.

Salvi GE, Zitzmann NU. The effects of anti-infective preventive measures on the occurrence of biologic implant complications and implant loss: a systematic review. *Int J Oral Maxillofac Implants.* 2014; 29(suppl):292–307.

Sanz M, Chapple IL, Working Group 4 of the VIII European Workshop on Peri-odontology. Clinical research on peri-implant diseases: consensus report of Working Group 4. *J Clin Periodontol.* 2012; 39 (Suppl 12):202–206.

Schou S, Holmstrup P, Worthington HV et al. Outcome of implant therapy in patients with previous tooth loss due to periodontitis. *Clin Oral Implants Res.* 2006; 17:104–213.

Singh P. Understanding peri-implantitis: a strategic review. *J Oral Implantol.* 2011; 37:622–626.

Stavropoulos A, Bertl K, Eren S, Gotfredsen K. Mechanical and biological complications after implantoplasty—a systematic review. *Clin Oral Implants Res.* 2019; 30(9):833–848.

Teughels W, Van Assche N, Sliepen I, Quirynen M. Effect of material characteristics and or surface topography on bio-film development. *Clin Oral Implants Res.* 2006; 17(Suppl 2):68–81.

Thoma DS, Naenni N, Figuero E et al. Effects of soft tissue augmentation procedures on peri-implant health or disease: a systematic review and meta-analysis. *Clin Oral Implants Res.* 2018; 29:(Suppl 15):32–49.

Tomasi C, Derks J. Clinical research of peri-implant diseases – quality of reporting, case definitions and methods to study incidence, prevalence and risk factors of peri-implant diseases. *J Clin Periodontol.* 2012; 39(Suppl. 12):207–223.

Tonetti MS, Chapple IL, Jepsen S, Sanz M. Primary and secondary prevention of periodontal and peri-implant diseases: introduction to, and objectives of the 11th European Workshop on Periodontology consensus conference. *J Clin Periodontol.* 2015; 42(Suppl 16):S1–S4.

Wohlfahrt JC, Aass AM, Ronold HJ, Lyngstadaas SP. Micro CT and human histological analysis of a peri-implant osseous defect grafted with porous titanium granules: a case report. *Int J Oral Maxillofac Implants.* 2011; 26(1):e9–e14.

CHAPTER 36
Maintenance of implants

Khalid Almas and Avinash S. Bidra

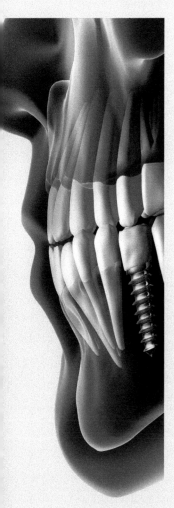

Contents

Learning objectives

- The need for implant maintenance.
- The assessment of risk for implant failures.
- Determination of frequency of recall maintenance.
- Mechanical and chemical methods of implant maintenance.
- Occlusal aspects of implant maintenance.
- Common complications encountered during maintenance therapy.

Essential Periodontics, First Edition. Edited by Steph Smith and Khalid Almas.
© 2022 John Wiley & Sons Ltd. Published 2022 by John Wiley & Sons Ltd.

Introduction

Osseointegration is considered as the most important factor in maintaining implant stability, whereas the role of soft tissue healing and maintenance around implants has been somewhat neglected (Albrektsson et al. 2012, 2013, 2014; Schwarz et al. 2012). More recently, evidence has demonstrated that the long-term survival of osseointegrated implants is also partly dependent on the transmucosal healing and stability around the implant collar, termed "peri-implant mucosa" (Lindhe et al. 2008). This attachment of the soft tissue to the coronal portion of an implant acts to provide a protective seal that prevents the development of bacterial invasion and future inflammation (Berglundh et al. 1991; Kawahara et al. 1998). Thus, the soft tissue seal is necessary for stable osseointegration and long-term survival of implants (Koka 1998; Koutouzis et al. 2016; Romanos et al. 2016).

One of the key findings relating to peri-implant mucosa is the direction of gingival fibers compared with the natural tooth. This key difference explains the increased ability of bacteria to penetrate the epithelial layer and subsequent connective tissue, thus increasing the breakdown of soft tissues around implants (Ikeda et al. 2002). Therefore, if patient compliance is not fully obtained and proper oral hygiene is not maintained, inflammatory changes in the soft tissues surrounding dental implants will develop (Pontoriero et al. 1994). This inflammatory process in the peri-implant mucosa begins with reddening and swelling, and once bleeding on probing is initiated, the condition is then termed peri-implant mucositis. If this condition is left untreated, it may lead to progressive and irreversible destruction of the implant-surrounding tissues, including the loss of alveolar bone, ultimately leading to implant failure (Heitz-Mayfield 2008). Thus, the structural and biological events that take place during osseointegration and soft tissue attachment are important components of implant survival and maintenance.

Lifelong implant maintenance

The survival of implants in suitably selected patients is generally very high. However, implants do fail and can be lost for a variety of reasons. Scientific evidence suggests that the longevity of implants may not be superior to that of a diseased but well-restored natural dentition. A key factor for long-term implant survival is the quality of periodontal and implant maintenance. Recent surveys have shown that there appears to be contradictory advice on how best to monitor and maintain dental implants in function. Peri-implant disease is increasingly being shown to be common, with an incidence rate ranging from 5% to 56% (ADA 2012).

Dental implant complications can be divided into two types:

- *Early complications*: Early implant failures usually arise from failure of initial integration occurring during the biological healing phase. Poor surgical technique, inability to achieve primary fixation, inadvertent implant loading during the integration phase, infection, and systemic conditions such as uncontrolled diabetes are some of the factors that could cause early implant loss.
- *Late complications*: Late complications are caused by one or both of the following two fundamental reasons:
  - *Biological failures*: caused by plaque-induced peri-implant disease. If untreated, the progressive crestal bone loss results in implant mobility.
  - *Mechanical failures*: caused by unfavorable loading conditions due to poor restorative design or failure to control occlusal interferences. Typically, mechanical failures are manifested by screw or abutment loosening or porcelain fractures. Implant fractures have also been reported, but these tend to occur in reduced-diameter implants.

Early failures are difficult to predict, measure, or prevent. Late failures, on the other hand, can be identified and treated successfully if they are intercepted in the early stages of the disease process. In this respect, any clinician who accepts an implant patient for maintenance assumes significant responsibilities and duty of care for monitoring dental implants and the health of the peri-implant soft tissues. This requires a systematic recall program of monitoring and maintenance.

Risk assessment

Periodontal risk assessment

Several periodontal risk assessment tools have been developed and validated to varying extents (Heitz-Mayfield 2005; Lang et al. 2015). At the 11th European Workshop on Periodontology (Tonetti et al. 2015), five risk assessment tools were addressed in a systematic review (Lang et al. 2015). Of the five, one risk assessment tool, the Periodontal Risk Assessment (PRA; Lang & Tonetti 2003), was highlighted as having been validated in nine international studies. These studies indicated that patients at high risk for periodontal reinfection and progression of disease after active periodontal treatment could be identified by using the six criteria of the PRA (www.perio-tools.com/PRA).

Implant disease risk assessment

As the etiology and pathogenesis of peri-implant diseases have received increasing attention, a similar risk assessment tool for the prediction of the development of peri-implantitis has been developed. While a risk assessment predominantly evaluates the subject risk, it may also address the implant site. The Implant Disease Risk Assessment (IDRA; Heitz-Mayfield et al. 2020) is used with the purpose of minimizing the chance of developing peri-implant tissue breakdown. As for the PRA, there is not one single factor that can be attributed to the development of peri-implant disease. However, eight parameters have been identified (Table 36.1). By understanding the key factors associated with the development of peri-implant diseases, the clinician may then selectively address such factors to improve the outcomes of implant therapy. The IDRA may be

Table 36.1 Parameters for Implant Disease Risk Assessment (IDRA).

History of periodontitis	History of periodontitis (yes/no).
BOP%	Percentage of implant and tooth sites with positive bleeding on probing (BOP).
PD ≥5 mm	Number of sites with pocket depth (PD) ≥5 mm at implants and teeth.
BL/age	Periodontal bone loss (BL) in relation to the patient's age. Bone loss is estimated from a periapical or bitewing radiograph at the most severely affected tooth. In periapical radiographs, the % alveolar bone loss is compared with the distance 1 mm apical from the cementoenamel junction to the root apex. In bitewing radiographs, the % alveolar bone loss is calculated with 10% per 1 mm.
Perio susceptibility	The patient's susceptibility to periodontitis. Staging and grading according to the 2017 World Workshop on Classification of Periodontal Diseases (Tonetti et al. 2018).
SPT	Supportive periodontal therapy (SPT) – compliant with SPT, recall interval ≤5 months, recall interval 6 months, casual attender, no supportive therapy.
RM–bone	Distance from the restorative margin (RM) of the implant prosthesis to the marginal bone crest (soft tissue level [STL] implant >1.5 mm, <1.5 mm). This is determined from a radiograph.
Prosthesis	Assessment of factors related to the implant-supported prosthesis – cleansable, poor fit with supramucosal margins, poor fit with submucosal margins, excess cement, not cleansable.

Table 36.2 Implant Disease Risk Assessment (IDRA).

Parameter	Low L	Moderate M	High H	Your patient's values	Your patient's risk L, M, H
History of periodontitis	No	–	Yes		
BOP%	9	25	>49		
PD ≥5 mm	2	6	≥10		
BL/age	0.5	1.0	1.5		
Periodontal susceptibility	1A	3A/B	4C		
SPT	Compliant	6 months	No		
RM–bone	STL	>1.5 mm	<1.5 mm		
Prosthesis	Cleansable	Poor fit Supramucosal	Not cleansable		

BL, bone level; BoP, bleeding on probing; PD, pocket depth; Prosthesis: fixed, removable, removable fixed; RM–bone, restoration margin–marginal bone crest; SPT, supportive periodontal therapy; STL, soft tissue level.

used to evaluate risk for both edentulous and partially dentate patients. However, with edentulous patients, there may be some limitations (Heitz-Mayfield et al. 2020).

The eight parameters have been combined in an octagon that visualizes the risk for disease development (see Appendix 7). A comprehensive evaluation using this functional diagram will provide an individual total risk profile and determine the need for measures targeting risk reduction. Each vector represents one risk parameter with an area of relative risk.

Based on these criteria, a table has been developed for the individual patient's use on initial and follow-up appointments or recall maintenance visits. For long-term monitoring, the risk assessment and modification and frequency of recall maintenance can be easily tailored from this table (see Table 36.2).

- *Low risk (L)*: A low IDRA risk patient has all parameters in the low-risk categories or at the most 1 of the 8 parameters in the moderate-risk category (1 M). Recall 2 times/year.
- *Moderate risk (M)*: A moderate IDRA risk patient has at least 2 of the 8 parameters in the moderate-risk category but at most 1 of the 8 parameters in the high-risk category (2 M + 1 H). A moderate IDRA patient may also have 1 of the 8 parameters in the high-risk category with all other parameters in the low-risk categories (1H + All others L). Recall 3 times/year.
- *High risk (H)*: A high IDRA risk patient has at least 2 of the 8 parameters in the high-risk category (2H). Recall 4 times/year for the first year.

Note: Recall frequency will be adjusted after the reduced/modified risk from the second year follow-up.

Implant maintenance protocols

Various implant maintenance protocols are in practice (Tarawali 2015). Generally, it is recommended that patients treated with implant-supported restorations are seen at least on an annual basis, but in some cases they will all require routine hygienist treatment at 3-, 4-, or 6-monthly intervals, according to individual requirements (Palmer & Pleasance 2006). This is also in line with the UK National Institute for Health and Care Excellence (NICE) guidelines (2004).

The following assessments should be made at review appointments:
- Peri-implant soft tissue health and oral hygiene.
- Marginal bone levels (radiographs at appropriate intervals).
- Conditions of prosthetic replacement and occlusion.
- Hygiene maintenance requirements.

At every check-up appointment, the dental clinician should assess the following:
- Soft tissue assessment.
- Assessment of plaque and calculus.
- Probing – bleeding, depth, suppuration.
- Occlusal assessment.
- Mobility.
- Radiographic assessment.
- Integrity of restoration: for overdentures – check bars, balls, locator attachments, and the respective inserts that are housed in the dentures.

Various controversies do however exist regarding the evaluation of the implant–tissue interface. Review studies have indicated that periodontal indices do not seem to be reliable indicators for appropriate diagnosis and treatment needs around dental implants, and furthermore that they do not provide better information than visual inspection and detection of mucosa redness (Coli & Sennerby 2019). Probing around dental implants is more uncomfortable for the patient compared to probing around teeth. Probing around implants could potentially create a trauma in the peri-implant scar tissue that could become difficult to manage. All the information gathered from probing (bleeding on probing [BOP], periodontal pocket depth [PPD], clinical attachment loss [CAL]) needs to be associated with the radiographic assessment of crestal bone levels to establish a definitive diagnosis so as to avoid overtreatment. Therefore, it appears to be more logical to avoid any risks of disturbing the peri-implant tissues with probing and to proceed with a clinical examination that includes:
- A visual inspection of the peri-implant tissues for the assessment of oral hygiene and the detection of potential redness and swelling.
- Palpation of the peri-implant tissues for assessment of the potential presence of swelling, bleeding, and suppuration.
- Radiography for the assessment of crestal bone levels for comparison with previous radiographs to evaluate potential progressive bone loss, even if there is a need for more scientific evidence of the true value of the first two clinical testing modes (Coli & Sennerby 2019).

Cumulative Interceptive Supportive Therapy

Based on the parameters collected at follow-up visits, the Cumulative Interceptive Supportive Therapy (CIST) protocol has been suggested (Lang et al. 2004). This protocol includes four treatment modalities for different peri-implant tissue conditions, such as mechanical debridement, antiseptic treatment, antibiotic treatment, and regenerative or resective surgery. Although this is an interesting protocol, to date no study has evaluated the effect of this therapy on the incidence of peri-implant diseases. The CIST protocol is presented in Table 36.3.

This protocol supposes that probing depths range from 2 to 4 mm under peri-implant healthy tissue conditions. However, it should be noted that probing depth around implants may be related to implant position. Factors that may influence probing depth include but are not restricted to implant position related to the bone crest (epi- or subcrestal), the width of peri-implant tissues, and the type of implant/abutment connection. In some cases, increased probing depths may not imply peri-implant disease. For this reason, it is very important to establish the baseline bone level when the prosthesis is installed (Rösing et al. 2019).

Clinical practice guidelines for recall and maintenance

The American College of Prosthodontists in collaboration with the American Dental Association, the Academy of General Dentistry, and the American Dental Hygiene Association developed clinical practice guidelines (CPGs) for recall and maintenance (professional and at-home) of patients with dental implants (Bidra et al. 2016) (Table 36.4). These baseline

Table 36.3 Cumulative Interceptive Supportive Therapy protocol.

Peri-implant tissue condition	Treatment modality
a. Pocket depth (PD) <3 mm, no plaque or bleeding on probing (BOP)	No therapy
b. PD <3 mm with plaque and/or BOP	Mechanical cleaning, polishing, oral hygiene instructions
c. PD 4–5 mm without radiographic bone loss	Mechanical cleaning, polishing, oral hygiene instructions plus local anti-infective therapy (e.g. chlorhexidine) for 3–4 weeks
d. PD >5 mm with <2 mm radiographic bone loss	Mechanical cleaning, polishing, microbiological test, local and systemic anti-infective therapy
e. PD >5 mm with >2 mm radiographic bone loss	Resective or regenerative surgery

Table 36.4 Professional and at-home maintenance of implants.

Professional maintenance

	Biological	Mechanical
Implant-borne removable restorations (partial and overdentures)	– Extra-oral and intra-oral health and dental examination – Oral hygiene instructions and interventions – Oral topical chlorhexidine gluconate – Glycine powder air-polishing system	– Examination of intra- and extra-oral prosthetic components – Adjustment, repair, replacement, or remake of components that could compromise function
Implant-borne fixed restorations (single crowns, partial fixed and complete arch)	– Extra-oral and intra-oral health and dental examination – Oral hygiene instructions and interventions – Oral topical chlorhexidine gluconate – Glycine powder air-polishing system	– Examination of the prosthesis, prosthetic components – Reassess prosthesis contours – Adjustment, repair, replacement, or remake of components that could compromise function – Using new prosthetic screws

At-home maintenance

Implant-borne removable restorations (partial and overdentures)	– Education regarding brushing existing natural teeth, restorations, and intra-oral implant components twice daily, the usage of dental floss, water flossers, air flossers, interdental cleaners, soft and electric toothbrushes – Usage of professional recommended denture-cleaning agent – Removal of restoration while sleeping and storing in a prescribed cleaning solution	
Implant-borne fixed restorations (single crowns, partial fixed and complete arch)	– Education regarding brushing existing natural teeth, restorations, and intra-oral implant components twice daily, the usage of dental floss, water flossers, air flossers, interdental cleaners, soft and electric toothbrushes – Usage of toothpaste containing 0.3% triclosan – Supplemental short-term use of chlorhexidine gluconate if indicated – Usage of prescribed occlusal devices during sleep, advice about cleaning before and after use with a soft brush and prescribed cleaning agent, methods for storage	

guidelines intend to improve patient care protocols, but are not intended to be a standard of care. The outlined CPGs should be supplemented with professional judgment and consideration of the unique needs of each patient.

Frequency of patient recall

In order to maintain peri-implant health, patients should receive individualized, regular supportive care so as to assure the longevity and success of dental implants. The management of systemic and local risk factors, including biofilm control, smoking, diabetes, and peri-implant inflammation, is paramount to prevent peri-implantitis and peri-implant mucositis. Besides these factors, a previous history of periodontitis and the complexity of the rehabilitation should be taken into consideration to establish the maintenance protocol and its frequency. Furthermore, replacing compromised teeth with dental implants does not guarantee a long-term functional dentition, since underlying genetics, microbiology, functional demands, and behavioral habits associated with oral diseases do not necessarily change with the placement of dental implants (Rösing et al. 2019). Also, patients with complex implant-borne restorations require a lifelong professional recall regimen

to provide biological and mechanical maintenance. Therefore, based upon age, ability to perform oral self-care. the biological or mechanical complications of remaining natural teeth, as well as those of tooth-borne restorations and implant-borne restorations (fixed or removable), patients should be advised to obtain a dental professional examination visit at various recall visits, depending upon the clinical situation and tailored to the individual patient (Bidra et al. 2016).

The risk classification and recall maintenance have been standardized, based on evidence as presented in Table 36.2 and Appendix 7. Low risk has been assigned every six months, moderate risk every four months, and high-risk patients every three months for recall. Emergency mechanical or biological situations can be dealt with at any time apart from the risk classification.

Professional and at-home maintenance

After the recall maintenance schedule has been decided upon, then both professional and at-home maintenance has to be performed for patients with fixed and removable implant-borne restorations. This includes both biological and mechanical aspects of maintenance (see Table 36.4 and Figures 36.1–36.4).

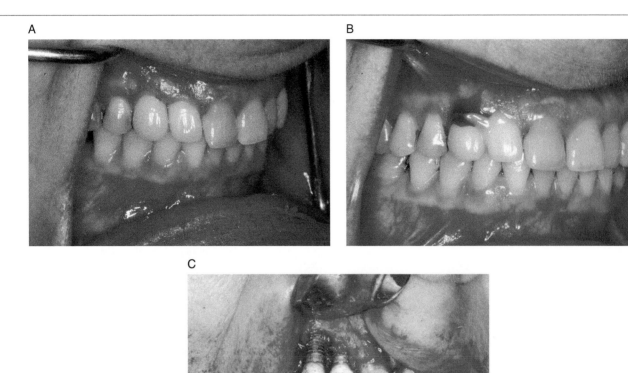

Figure 36.1 (A) Patient with dental implants at maxillary canine and lateral incisors restored 10 years ago. This patient had not returned to the dentist for regular professional maintenance and had poor compliance. (B) Severe bleeding was noticed on probing, indicating inflammation. Purulence was also noted on clinical palpation, indicating peri-implantitis. (C) After elevation of the mucoperiosteal flap, severe loss of bone was noticed. Both implants were eventually removed due to severe destruction of bone and poor prognosis.

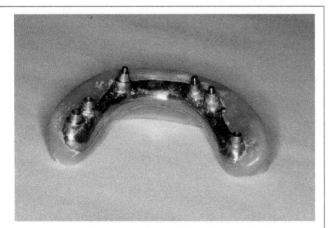

Figure 36.2 Poor oral hygiene in a patient with a metal resin complete arch fixed implant-supported prosthesis (CAFIP) that was exacerbated by a poorly contoured prosthesis. Notice the labial flange that impedes access to oral hygiene. Such flanges should be removed and the prosthetic contours should be corrected.

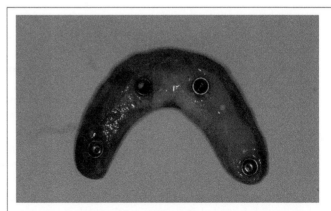

Figure 36.3 Poor oral hygiene underneath a complete arch fixed implant-supported prosthesis (CAFIP) despite proper contours of the tissue surface. This was due to poor patient compliance and absence of oral hygiene instruction.

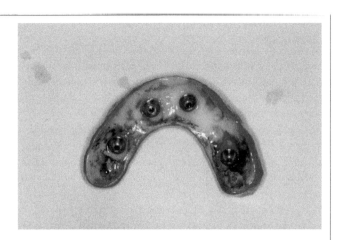

Figure 36.4 Poor oral hygiene in a patient with a monolithic zirconia complete arch fixed implant-supported prosthesis (CAFIP) that was exacerbated by a poorly contoured prosthesis. Irrespective of the type of material, poor oral hygiene can compromise the success of treatment.

Tooth versus implants

The biophysiological differences between a natural tooth and endosseous dental implants are well known. From the available evidence, it can be speculated that osseointegrated implants without periodontal receptors would be more susceptible to occlusal overloading, because the load-sharing ability, adaptation to occlusal forces, and mechanoreception are significantly reduced in dental implants (Kim et al. 2005). However, the potential biomechanical characteristics derived from the differences remain controversial (Carr & Laney 1987; Cho &

Chee 1992; Glantz & Nilner 1998; Lundgren & Laurell 1994; Rangert et al. 1991; Schulte 1995; Sekine 1967). The differences between teeth and dental implants are summarized in Table 36.5.

Implant occlusal maintenance

It is important to replicate or approximate the patient's natural occlusal scheme for proper functioning of the prosthesis as well as patient comfort. Care should be taken to distribute the occlusal load evenly onto the implants to minimize biomechanical complications. Owing to lack of the periodontal ligament, osseointegrated implants, unlike natural teeth, react biomechanically in a different manner from occlusal forces. It is therefore believed that dental implants may be prone to occlusal overloading, resulting in late failure of the implant/implant prosthesis. Overloading factors that may have a negative influence on implant longevity include:

- Large distal cantilevers.
- Parafunctional habits.
- Unfavorable occlusal design.
- Improper selection of implant geometry (e.g. narrow-diameter implants, short implants).

Masticatory forces developed by a patient restored with implant-supported restorations are equivalent to those of a natural dentition (Carr & Lancy 1987). There are studies supporting the finding that implants are more susceptible to occlusal overloading than natural teeth (Mericske-Stern et al. 1992). Hence, it is important to control implant occlusion within physiological limits and thus to provide optimal implant load to ensure long-term implant success. The occlusion should be evaluated and

Table 36.5 Comparison between tooth and implant.

Variables	Tooth	Implant
Connection	Periodontal ligament (PDL)	Osseointegration, functional ankylosis
Proprioception	Periodontal mechanoreceptors	Osseoperception
Tactile sensitivity	High	Low
Axial mobility	25–100 μm	3–5 μm
Movement phases	Two phases Primary: non-linear and complex Secondary: linear and elastic	One phase Linear and elastic
Movement patterns	Primary: immediate movement Secondary: gradual movement	Gradual movement
Fulcrum to lateral force	Apical third of root	Crestal bone
Load bearing characteristics	Shock absorption function Stress distribution	Stress concentration at crestal bone
Signs of overloading	PDL thickening, mobility, wear facets, fremitus, pain	Screw loosening or fracture, abutment or prosthesis fracture, bone loss, implant fracture

Source: Adapted from Kim et al. 2005.

organized so that there is anterior guidance and disclusion of posterior teeth on lateral excursion. Ideally, there should be no contact of posterior teeth on both working and non-working sides. If the canine is compromised, partial group function or premolar guidance is acceptable. Initial occlusal contact should occur on the natural dentition. The centric occlusal contact should be adjusted with light occlusal contact on the implants (Javraj & Chee 2006). Due to continued lifelong growth of human jaws (Thilander 2009), natural teeth can be expected to move and migrate at various levels, and this can result in opening of proximal contacts between adjacent natural teeth and implant-supported restorations. Therefore, at every professional recall and maintenance visit, proximal contacts should be evaluated for the long-term success and survival of both the implant-supported prostheses and the adjacent natural teeth.

Implant complications during maintenance therapy

There is still a substantial lack of well-performed longitudinal reports on implant-supported restorations over an observation period of 10 or more years (Lang & Zitzmann 2012). Some studies have shown technical complications to occur in about 20% of all implants, comparable with 31.1% in another study over a 16-year period (Simonis et al. 2010). The most common complication over a 10-year follow-up period was abutment/screw loosening, which occurred in 5.3% of all implants. Chipping has also been observed in 4.0% of all implant-supported restorations, which is comparable with chipping of the veneering material of fixed dental prosthesis (4.1%), which was shown in a review over 5 and 10 years (Thoma et al. 2017) (see Figures 36.5–36.9).

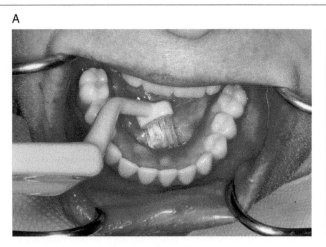
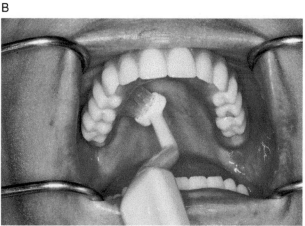

Figure 36.5 (A) Patients should be instructed to brush underneath the tissue surface twice daily using an angled soft brush ("TePe brush") dipped in an antimicrobial rinse, such as 0.12% chlorhexidine gluconate. (B) Palatal access to tissue surfaces of maxillary prosthesis is often challenging for patients, but can be resolved by the use of an angled soft brush.

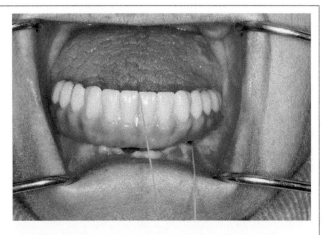

Figure 36.6 Using floss designed for bridges (such as "Super floss") is an excellent option for patients whose manual dexterity allows such oral hygiene aids.

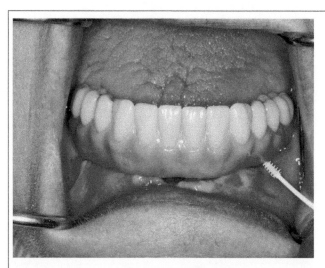

Figure 36.7 Use of rubber tips underneath the tissue surface is another alternative. Patients should be encouraged to try a variety of oral hygiene aids until they find those that they are most comfortable with.

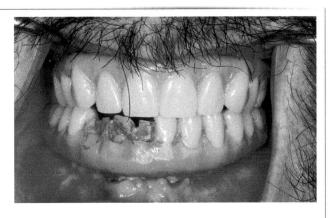

Figure 36.8 Fracture of acrylic resin and denture teeth is the most common mechanical complication noticed in complete arch fixed implant-supported prosthesis (CAFIP). Contemporary methods to mitigate this complication include use of monolithic materials such as zirconia.

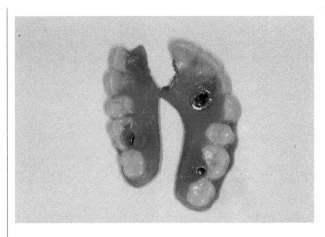

Figure 36.9 Fracture of the entire metal resin prosthesis including the metal bar can occur as a mechanical complication, especially in bruxism patients.

SUMMARY

Various in-office and home care, chemical and mechanical methods are available for the long-term maintenance of dental implants. The dental provider has a role in guiding implant stability following osseointegration; however, proper maintenance of the peri-implant soft tissue health is largely in the control of the patient's own oral hygiene regimen. Patient self-management includes mechanical methods and chemical ways to control biofilm formation and subsequent plaque/calculus accumulation. Implant disease risk assessment should be followed to customize recall maintenance frequency for individual patients (Heitz-Mayfield et al. 2020). Emphasis should also be placed on home care, compliance, and regular recall visits for a predictable outcome of implant therapy in motivated patients. It must be emphasized that currently there is not an evidence-based, implant-specific concept of occlusion. Future studies are recommended to clarify the relationship between occlusion and implant success (Kim et al. 2005). Furthermore, there is always room for reconsideration of existing protocols or guidelines in the advent of emerging evidence. Clinicians should therefore keep themselves updated regarding developments in biological and mechanical complications so as to improve or modify their clinical preventive, curative, and recall maintenance protocols.

REFERENCES

Association of Dental Implantology (ADI). A dentist's guide to implantology. ADI; 2012. https://www.adi.org.uk/resources/guidelines_and_papers.aspx.

Albrektsson T, Buser D, Sennerby L. Crestal bone loss and oral implants. *Clin Implant Dent Relat Res.* 2012; 14(6):783–791.

Albrektsson T, Buser D, Sennerby L. On crestal/marginal bone loss around dental implants. *Int J Periodontics Restorative Dent.* 2013; 33(1):9–11.

Albrektsson T, Dahlin C, Jemt T et al. Is marginal bone loss around oral implants the result of a provoked foreign body reaction? *Clin Implant Dent Relat Res.* 2014; 16(2):155–165.

Berglundh T, Lindhe J, Ericsson I et al. The soft tissue barrier at implants and teeth. *Clin Oral Implants Res.* 1991; 2:81–90.

Bidra AS, Daubert DM, Garcia LT et al. Clinical practice guidelines for recall and maintenance of patients with tooth-borne and implant-borne dental restorations. *J Am Dent Assoc.* 2016; 147(1):67–74.

Carr AB, Laney WR. Maximum occlusal force levels in patients with osseointegrated oral implant prosthesis and patients with complete dentures. *Int J Oral Maxillofac Implants.* 1987; 2:101–108.

Cho GC, Chee WWL. Apparent intrusion of natural teeth under an implant-supported prosthesis: a clinical report. *J Prosthet Dent.* 1992; 68:3–5.

Coli P, Sennerby L. Is peri-implant probing causing over-diagnosis and over-treatment of dental implants? *J Clin Med.* 2019; 8:1123–1135.

Glantz PO, Nilner K. Biomechanical aspects of prosthetic implant-borne reconstructions. *Periodontol 2000.* 1998; 17:119–124.

Heitz-Mayfield, LJ. Disease progression: identification of high-risk groups and individuals for periodontitis. *J Clin Periodontol.* 2005; 32(Suppl 6):196–209.

Heitz-Mayfield LJ. Diagnosis and management of periimplant diseases. *Aust Dent J.* 2008; 53(Suppl 1):S43–S48.

Heitz-Mayfield LJA, Fritz Heitz F, Lang NP. Implant Disease Risk Assessment (IDRA) – a tool for preventing peri-implant disease. *Clin Oral Implants Res.* 2020; 31(4):397–403.

Ikeda H, Shiraiwa M, Yamaza T et al. Difference in penetration of horseradish peroxidase tracer as a foreign substance into the peri-implant or junctional epithelium of rat gingivae. *Clin Oral Implants Res.* 2002; 13:243–251.

Javraj S, Chee W. Treatment planning of implants in the posterior quadrants. *Br Dent J.* 2006; 201:13–23.

Kawahara H, Kawahara D, Hashimoto K, Takashima Y, Ong JL. Morphologic studies on the biologic seal of titanium dental implants. Report I. in vitro study on the epithelialization mechanism around the dental implant. *Int J Oral Maxillofac Implants.* 1998; 13(4):457–464.

Kim Y, Oh TJ, Misch CE, Wang HL. Occlusal considerations in implant therapy: clinical guidelines with biomechanical rationale. *Clin Oral Implants Res.* 2005; 16(1):26–35.

Koka S. The implant-mucosal interface and its role in the long-term success of endosseous oral implants: a review of the literature. *Int J Prosthodont.* 1998; 11:421–432.

Koutouzis T, Gadalla H, Lundgren T. Bacterial colonization of the Implant-Abutment Interface (IAI) of dental implants with a sloped marginal design: an in-vitro study. *Clin Implant Dent Relat Res.* 2016; 18(1):161–167.

Lang NP, Berglundh T, Heitz-Mayfield LJ et al. Consensus statements and recommended clinical procedures regarding implant survival and complications. *Int J Oral Maxillofac Implants.* 2004; 19(Suppl):150–154.

Lang NP, Suvan JE, Tonetti MS. Risk factor assessment tools for the prevention of periodontitis progression a systematic review. *J Clin Periodontol.* 2015; 42(Suppl 16):S59–S70.

Lang NP, Tonetti MS. Periodontal risk assessment (PRA) for patients in supportive periodontal therapy (SPT). *Oral Health Prev Dent.* 2003; 1(1):7–16.

Lang NP, Zitzmann NU. Clinical research in implant dentistry: evaluation of implant supported restorations, aesthetic and patient-reported outcomes. *J Clin Periodontol.* 2012; 39(Suppl 12):133–138.

Lindhe J, Lang NP, Karring T. *Clinical Periodontology and Implant Dentistry*. Oxford: Wiley-Blackwell; 2008.

Lundgren D, Laurell L. Biomechanical aspects of fixed bridgework supported by natural teeth and endosseous implants. *Periodontol 2000.* 1994; 4:23–40.

Mericske-Stern R, Geering AH, Burgin WB, Graf H. Three-dimensional force measurements on mandibular implants supporting overdentures. *Int J Oral Maxillofac Implants.* 1992; 7:185–194.

National Institute for Health and Care Excellence. NICE CG19. Dental checks: intervals between oral health reviews. NICE; 2004. https://www.nice.org.uk/guidance/cg19.

Palmer RM, Pleasance C. Maintenance of osseointegrated implant prostheses. *Dent Update.* 2006; 33:84–92.

Pontoriero R, Tonelli MP, Carnevale G et al. Experimentally induced peri-implant mucositis. A clinical study in humans. *Clin Oral Implants Res.* 1994; 5:254–259.

Rangert B, Gunne J, Sullivan DY. Mechanical aspects of a Brånemark implant connected to a natural tooth: an in vitro study. *Int J Oral Maxillofac Implants.* 1991; 6:177–186.

Romanos GE, Biltucci MT, Kokaras A, Paster BJ. Bacterial composition at the implant-abutment connection under loading in vivo. *Clin Implant Dent Relat Res.* 2016; 18(1):138–145.

Rösing CK, FiorinI T, Haas AN et al. The impact of maintenance on peri-implant health. *Braz Oral Res.* 2019; 33(suppl 1):0074.

Schulte W. Implants and the periodontium. *Int Dent J.* 1995; 45:16–26.

Schwarz F, Iglhaut G, Becker J. Quality assessment of reporting of animal studies on pathogenesis and treatment of peri-implant mucositis and peri-implantitis. A systematic review using the ARRIVE guidelines. *J Clin Periodontol.* 2012; 39(Suppl 12):63–72.

Sekine M. Problems of occlusion from the standpoint of prosthetic dentistry, with reference to the significance of balanced occlusion in the denture and biological considerations on the abutment teeth in relation to occlusion pressure in the partial denture. *Shikwa Gakuho.* 1967; 7:859–867.

Simonis P, Dufour T, Tenenbaum H. Long-term implant survival and success: a 10-16-year follow-up of non-submerged dental implants. *Clin Oral Implants Res.* 2010; 21(7):772–777.

Tarawali K. Maintenance and monitoring of dental implants in general dental practice. *Dent Update.* 2015; 42:513–518.

Thilander B. Dentoalveolar development in subjects with normal occlusion. A longitudinal study between the ages of 5 and 31 years. *Eur J Orthod.* 2009; 31(2):109–120.

Thoma DS, Sailer I, Ioannidis A et al. A systematic review of the survival and complication rates of resin-bonded fixed dental prostheses after a mean observation period of at least 5 years. *Clin Oral Implants Res.* 2017; 28(11):1421–1432.

Tonetti MS, Chapple IL, Jepsen S, Sanz M. Primary, and secondary prevention of periodontal and peri-implant diseases: introduction to, and objectives of the 11th European Workshop on Periodontology consensus conference. *J Clin Periodontol.* 2015; 42(Suppl 16):S1–S4.

Tonetti MS, Greenwell H, Kornman KS. Staging and grading of periodontitis: framework and proposal of a new classification and case definition. *J Periodontol.* 2018; 89(Suppl 1):S159–S172.

CHAPTER 37

Future advances and research in periodontics

Yasir Dilshad Siddiqui

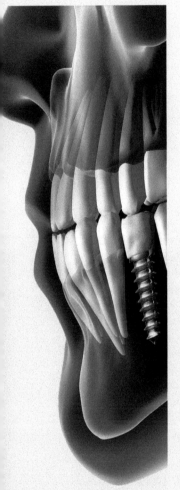

Contents

Essential Periodontics, First Edition. Edited by Steph Smith and Khalid Almas.
© 2022 John Wiley & Sons Ltd. Published 2022 by John Wiley & Sons Ltd.

Introduction

The field of periodontics is a central focus of research and advancement because of its bi-directional relationship with other branches of dentistry, as well as systemic conditions. Various research areas are currently under investigation. In this chapter, some current developments and their expected future advancements are mentioned that can aid in reshaping periodontal therapy in the future.

Inflammation and dysbiosis in periodontitis

The temporal relationship between oral dysbiosis and periodontal inflammation remains elusive. The evidence for a dysbiosis being associated with the overgrowth of putative periodontal pathogens preceding destructive inflammation is weak and inconclusive (Yost et al. 2015). Furthermore, control of excess inflammation reverses the pathogenic shift of the microbiome, leading to a paradigm shift of periodontitis from being an infectious disease to an inflammatory disease (Lee et al. 2016). This distinction changes the treatment paradigm from trying to control the composition of the commensal flora to the control of inflammation (Van Dyke 2008). Researchers will thus be focusing on the identification of new molecules that are not antibacterial in nature, but are aimed to control the excess inflammation that could reverse the non-specific microbial composition. This could manifest in the form of new mimetic drugs for the control of inflammatory diseases, without the side-effect profile that plagues the current anti-inflammatory pharmacopoeia. Furthermore, investigation of cross-talks between subgingival microorganisms with the host response will refine our understanding of inflammation-mediated dysbiosis in periodontitis.

Proresolving lipid mediators and periodontal disease

Resolution of inflammation is an active biochemical and metabolic process, not merely a passive termination of inflammation, and is mediated by specialized proresolving lipid mediators (SPMs) (Serhan & Chiang 2013; Serhan et al. 2008). These SPMs include lipoxins, resolvins, protectins, and maresins. At the site of injury, SPMs stereo-selectively reduce excessive polymorphonuclear neutrophil (PMN) trafficking, cytokine production, and bacterial burden (local and systemic), while increasing peritoneal mononuclear cells, macrophage phagocytosis, and intracellular generation of phagosomal reactive oxygen species for microbial killing (Spite et al. 2009). Furthermore, SPMs promote resolution by preventing the generation of activated Th1 and Th17 cells and enhance the differentiation of regulatory T cells, which is typically altered during chronic inflammatory and autoimmune diseases (Chiurchiu et al. 2016). In future, research will advance to involve more in vivo and human trials, so that these exogenous SPMs can be used in the form of medications for periodontal disease. Furthermore, it will open avenues to study the impact of these molecules on proinflammatory mediators, and on hyperactive immune cells responsible for the progression of disease.

Periodontal regeneration

Various products and techniques have been explored to achieve periodontal regeneration, and these have generally involved various membranes, and the implantation of bone substitutes into periodontal defects. Yet, despite efforts to improve periodontal regeneration, each of these procedures remains technique sensitive and is clinically unpredictable. Thus, new approaches are needed to regain loss of periodontal tissues. This could be made possible by a complete understanding of the events and mechanisms of inflammation in the development of periodontitis, and identifying the molecules that affect resident stem cells that can drive the shift from a destructive phase to a regenerative phase.

Nexus between inflammatory resolution and periodontal regeneration

Neutrophils and macrophages play a key role during inflammation and are responsible for phagocytosing bacteria and removing tissue debris. Uncontrolled inflammation leads to chronic disease that is due to defective resolution of initial proinflammatory responses that are deemed to impact stem cell behavior (Kizil et al. 2015). Knowledge about the interactions of neutrophils and stem cells is presently rather limited. It has been suggested that the interaction between dental mesenchymal stem cells (MSCs) and the immune system is reciprocal, because the immunomodulatory activity of MSCs is strongly regulated by immune cells producing leukotrienes, prostaglandins, cytokines, and chemokines (Andrukhov et al. 2019). MSCs produce and respond to lipoxins and resolvins, and regulate PMN functions related to inflammation resolution and bacterial killing (Cianci et al. 2016). Besides promoting resolution of inflammation, they reverse tissue destruction caused by excessive PMN influx, and consequently may facilitate stem cell activation, presumably alveolar bone stem/progenitor cells and periodontal ligament stem/progenitor cells, and induce calcification (Cianci et al. 2016). Thus, in the future, research will be designed to understand the mechanism and cross-talk between immune and stem cells. However, recent data suggest that specialized lipid mediators are key molecules that drive a shift from proinflammation to proresolution, but there are insufficient data that elucidate the mechanism of SPM interactions on regeneration and differentiation of stem cells. It is likely that in future researchers would work on products that have dual actions, i.e. inflammatory resolution, stem cell regeneration, and tissue-specific differentiation.

Therapeutics of stem cells in periodontal regeneration

Periodontal ligament stem cells (PDLSCs) are considered to be a subpopulation of the MSCs, with a resemblance to pericytes present in the perivascular space of the periodontal ligament (Zhu & Liang 2015). Successful periodontal regeneration has been noted after transplantation of PDLSCs in surgically created bone defects in rats (Iwasaki et al. 2019). A future challenge would be to develop suitable delivery devices that can successfully deliver cells to sites of interest. Furthermore, the development of biocompatible scaffolds will be crucial in the next phase of this technology (Bartold et al. 2006). This is also an active area of research involving the development of biodegradable materials, smart materials, and three-dimensional bioprinting (Rasperini et al. 2015); however, considerable work needs to be done before such modalities become a reliable and effective approach to treatment. In future, this will involve large-scale collaborative efforts between bioengineers, nanotechnologists, cell biologists, and molecular biologists. Furthermore, it will focus on combining cell-based therapies and the controlled delivery of regulatory molecules using tissue-engineering techniques. As the field advances, other significant issues will include biosafety and sound manufacturing principles, as well as controlling the cost of such technologies.

Guided tissue regeneration

Recent advances in guided tissue regeneration (GTR) barrier membranes have focused on the optimization of degradation and mechanical properties, and the incorporation of new functions into GTR membranes. Membranes have been prepared from composites that combine different biomaterials, such as natural and synthetic polymers, thereby integrating bioactive molecules (Wang et al. 2016). GTR membranes have also been utilized to serve as carriers for drug delivery so as to enhance tissue regeneration (Caballé-Serano et al. 2019), as the loading of antibacterial drugs inhibits local infection and inflammation, thereby facilitating periodontal ligament tissue formation (Sam & Pillai 2014). Furthermore, multilayered GTR membranes with different functions in each layer have also been developed to enhance periodontal tissue regeneration (Rad et al. 2017). However, the outcomes of GTR treatment are unpredictable in several types of periodontal defects. Besides membrane stability, future research may focus on the combination of GTR membranes with other approaches, such as SPM-based molecules and inorganic nano-composites. These efforts may provide better regenerative outcomes.

Extracorporeal shock wave therapy

Extracorporeal shock wave therapy (ESWT) has been widely used in medical practice for the management of urolithiasis, cholelithiasis, and in various orthopedic and musculoskeletal disorders. Its efficacy to stimulate osteoblasts, fibroblasts, induce neovascularization, and increase expression of bone morphogenic proteins has been well documented (Prabhuji et al. 2014). In ESWT shock waves of a certain energy are used to cause a sudden and transient pressure disturbance in targeted tissues. Loss of alveolar bone is a common consequence of periodontal disease. The documented evidence on the use of ESWT in periodontics, however, is very limited. Studies report that ESWT has a potential for rapid periodontal healing and bone regeneration, and has anti-inflammatory properties (Prabhuji et al. 2014). Furthermore, its impact on the periodontal microflora, various immune cells, and periodontal ligament stem cells could be studied in the future.

Proteomics, genomics, and nanotechnology

Proteomics is the study of proteomes and their functions. A quantitative proteomic analysis of saliva from severe periodontitis subjects has revealed an altered abundance in 15 proteins (Haigh et al. 2010). These alterations in proteins have the potential to act as biomarkers for detecting and monitoring periodontal disease, as well as serving as targets for disease intervention (Haigh et al. 2010; Singh & Sarkar 2019).

Nutrigenomics includes the study of epigenetic variations (like histone modifications, DNA methylation, and chromatin remodeling) in genes regulating nutrients, which can cause an increase in the probability of micronutrient diseases like obesity and type 2 diabetes mellitus that impact periodontal health (Chawla et al. 2018).

Infectogenomics deals with the influence of host genetic variability on microbial colonization and governs the outcome of infection by various pathogens (Kellam & Weiss 2006). Mutations in genes expressing pattern recognition receptors can induce an altered host response to microbial invasion (Chawla et al. 2018; Kaur et al. 2018). Polymorphisms in the interleukin (IL)-1 gene have also been extensively implicated in the pathogenesis of chronic periodontitis (Karimbux et al. 2012). In future, the field of periodontal infectogenomics may determine different pathogenic pathways in different forms of periodontitis, and possibly assist in early prevention and management of disease. Further research is needed to evaluate the ability of different genotypes to predict disease initiation and to evaluate the effectiveness of genotyping in making diagnostic or treatment intervention strategies.

With the advent of nanotechnology, controlled drug release can be achieved in combination with nanomaterials in the form of nanotubes, hollow spheres, and core shell structures. Triclosan-loaded nanoparticles have been tested through an emulsification-diffusion process and have shown a positive response (Pinon-Segundo et al. 2005). Scaffold systems have also been constructed at a nanoscale for periodontal tissue regeneration procedures. In future, nanotechnology could directly manipulate periodontal tissues. More research is still ongoing to improve existing nanomaterials.

Probiotics

Applications of probiotics (e.g. lactobacillus acidophilus) are encouraging, as they reduce the pH of the oral cavity, and retain antioxidant properties that reduce the formation of plaque and calculus. Dendritic cells up-regulate the expression of Th1 and Th2 cells after being stimulated by probiotics. Probiotics enhance immunity by means of binding to Toll-like receptors (Chatterjee et al. 2011). The research on the effect of probiotics on periodontics is still in a preliminary stage, however. More long-term studies are required to evaluate their effectiveness.

Periodontal vaccine

A promising avenue for research has opened after realization of the prospective application of a periodontal vaccine. Hence, inventing new prevention methods is compelling. Periodontal vaccination can be active, passive, or genetic (Kudyar et al. 2011). It has been proposed that *Porphyromonas gingivalis* heat shock protein could potentially be developed as a vaccine to inhibit periodontal disease induced by multiple pathogenic bacteria (Lee et al. 2006). In the future, more basic and clinical research will be conducted on making an efficient vaccine against periodontitis.

Micro-dentistry

Micro-dentistry can be defined as the practice of minimally invasive dentistry with the help of advanced tools or optical devices that aid in the operative field. The benefits thereof may be lower stress levels, effective control of the operatory field, less fatigue, improved ergonomics, and more efficiency. Micro-dentistry in the context of periodontology includes a periodontal endoscope (the Perio-Scope) that utilizes fiber-optic technology for illumination, magnification, and video-recording for visualizing subgingival tissues (Ganesh et al. 2015). This allows for instrumentation in the most efficient way, including thorough debridement. Similarly, endoscopic capillaroscopy systems have been developed for the imaging of periodontal pocket and gingival crevice microvasculature, and in the future may prove to be an effective diagnostic aid (Townsend & D'Aiuto 2010).

Biophotonics

The term biophotonics denotes the interaction of biology and photons. Photodynamic therapy (PDT) is one such application where it is used an as adjunct to scaling and root planing. The three elements of photodynamic therapy are oxygen, a photosensitizer, and light. The triplet-state photosensitizer, which forms after excitation of a photosensitizer with light, can react with biomolecules in two ways, type I and type II (Kumar et al. 2015). In type I, it reacts through direct electron/hydrogen transfer, and in type II through formation of singlet oxygen. Photodynamic antimicrobial chemotherapy (PACT) has been observed to show efficacy against bacteria (including drug-resistant strains), yeasts, and parasites (Wainwright 1998). Future research will be conducted to analyze its impact on the diagnosis of periodontal disease and treatment.

Artificial intelligence

Software is being developed that combines more precise cone beam computed tomography (CBCT) scans with machine learning to detect even the slightest anomalies based on several previous scans and to provide an appropriate treatment plan. This can include the automatic selection of optimal implant sites and angulations for a given patient. In periodontics, two visuohaptic systems named Periosim and Periodontal Simulator (University of Illinois at Chicago, USA) have been produced that simulate three dental instruments, i.e. an explorer, a periodontal probe, and a scaler. They are used to train students in different aspects of periodontology (Mallikarjun et al. 2014). Artificial intelligence continues to evolve, with the expectation being that commercially available and reliable detection tools will be able to detect bone loss and changes in bone density, as well as assisting in the diagnosis and treatment planning of periodontal disease (Mallikarjun et al. 2014).

SUMMARY OF FUTURE RESEARCH GOAL

- Better understanding of the shift from gingivitis to periodontitis in the context of inflammation and dysbiosis.
- Further understanding of SPMs using animal data and clinical trials to formulate precise therapies to achieve active resolution of periodontal inflammation.
- Clarifying whether dysbiosis is a cause or a consequence of periodontal disease.
- Identification of molecular mechanisms by which periodontal bacteria inhibit antimicrobial or killing mechanisms without suppressing overall inflammation.

- Genome-wide studies to identify transcriptome sequencing and epigenomes of host cells in periodontal health and disease.
- Clarifying the mode of progression of periodontitis, whether it is linear or comprises episodes of active and quiescent periods.
- Application of increasing knowledge regarding the development of individually tailored therapeutic modalities.
- Development of an efficient vaccine against periodontitis.
- Application of stem cell-based therapeutics in clinical reality.

REFERENCES

Andrukhov CB, Blufstein A, Rausch-Fan X. Immunomodulatory properties of dental tissue-derived mesenchymal stem cells: implication in disease and tissue regeneration. *World J Stem Cells.* 2019; 11(9):604.

Bartold PM, Xiao Y, Lyngstaadas SP, Paine ML, Snead ML. Principles and applications of cell delivery systems for periodontal regeneration. *Periodontol 2000.* 2006; 41:123–135.

Caballé-Serrano J, Abdeslam-Mohamed Y, Munar-Frau A et al. Adsorption and release kinetics of growth factors on barrier membranes for guided tissue/bone regeneration: a systematic review. *Arch Oral Biol.* 2019; 100:57–68.

Chatterjee A, Bhattacharya H, Kandwal A. Probiotics in periodontal health and disease. *J Indian Soc Periodontol.* 2011; 15(1):23–28.

Chawla K, Bhardwaj S, Garg V. A capsulate on nutrigenomics in periodontitis. *EJPMR.* 2018; 206–223.

Chiurchiu V, Leuti A, Dalli J et al. Proresolving lipid mediators resolvin D1, resolvin D2, and maresin 1 are critical in modulating T cell responses. *Sci Transl Med.* 2016; 8:353ra111.

Cianci E, Recchiuti A, Trubiani O et al. Human periodontal stem cells release specialized proresolving mediators and carry immunomodulatory and prohealing properties regulated by lipoxins. *Stem Cells Transl Med.* 2016; 5:20–32.

Ganesh PR, Karthikeyan R, Malathi K. Perio-scopy: a new paradigm in periodontal therapy. *Int J Dent Med Res.* 2015; 1:168–171.

Haigh BJ, Stewart KW, Whelan JRK et al. Alterations in the salivary proteome associated with periodontitis. *J Clin Periodontol.* 2010; 37(3):241–247.

Iwasaki K, Akazawa K, Nagata M et al. The fate of transplanted periodontal ligament stem cells in surgically created periodontal defects in rats. *Int J Mol Sci.* 2019; 20(1):192.

Karimbux NY, Saraiya VM, Elangovan S et al. Interleukin-1 gene polymorphisms and chronic periodontitis in adult whites: a systematic review and meta-analysis. *J Periodontol.* 2012; 83(11):1407–1419.

Kaur G, Grover V, Bhaskar N, Kaur RK, Jain A. Periodontal infectogenomics. *Inflamm Regen.* 2018; 38:8.

Kellam P, Weiss RA. Infectogenomics: insights from the host genome into infectious diseases. *Cell.* 2006; 24;124(4):695–697.

Kizil C, Kyritsis N, Brand M. Effects of inflammation on stem cells: together they strive? *EMBO Reports.* 2015; 16(4):416–426.

Kudyar N, Dani N, Mahale S. Periodontal vaccine: a dream or reality. *J Indian Soc Periodontol.* 2011; 15(2):115–120.

Kumar V, Sinha J, Verma N et al. Scope of photodynamic therapy in periodontics. *Indian J Dent Res.* 2015; 26(4):439–442.

Lee CT, Teles R, Kantarci A et al. Resolvin E1 reverses experimental periodontitis and dysbiosis. *J Immunol.* 2016; 197(7):2796–2806.

Lee JY, Yi NN, Kim US et al. *Porphyromonas gingivalis* heat shock protein vaccine reduces the alveolar bone loss induced by multiple periodontopathogenic bacteria. *J Periodontal Res.* 2006; 41:10–14.

Mallikarjun SA, Tiwari S, Sathyanarayana S, Devi PR. Haptics in periodontics. *J Indian Soc Periodontol.* 2014; 18(1):112–113.

Pinon-Segundo E, Ganem-Quintanar A, Alonso-Perez V, Quintanar-Guerrero D. Preparation and characterization of triclosan nanoparticles for periodontal treatment. *Int J Pharm.* 2005; 294(1–2):217–232.

Prabhuji MLV, Khaleelahmed S, Vasudevalu S, Vinodhini K. Extracorporeal shock wave therapy in periodontics: a new paradigm. *J Indian Soc Periodontol.* 2014; 18(3):412–415.

Rad MM, Khorasani SN, Ghasemi-Mobarakeh L et al. Fabrication and characterization of two-layered nanofibrous membrane for guided bone and tissue regeneration application, *Mater Sci Eng C Mater Biol Appl.* 2017; 80:75–87.

Rasperini G, Pilipchuk SP, Flanagan CL et al. 3D-printed bioresorbable scaffold for periodontal repair. *J Dent Res.* 2015; 94(Suppl 9):S153–S157.

Sam G, Pillai BR. Evolution of barrier membranes in periodontal regeneration. Are the third-generation membranes really here? *JCDR.* 2014; 8:ZE14–ZE17.

Serhan CN, Chiang N. Resolution phase lipid mediators of inflammation: agonists of resolution. *Curr Opin Pharmacol.* 2013; 13(4):632–640.

Serhan CN, Chiang N, Van Dyke TE. Resolving inflammation: dual anti-inflammatory and pro-resolution lipid mediators. *Nat Rev Immunol.* 2008; 8(5):349–361.

Singh DDK, Sarkar S. Recent advancement in periodontics. *Int J Sci Nat.* 2019; 10(1):1–10.

Spite M, Norling LV, Summers L et al. Resolvin D2 is a potent regulator of leukocytes and controls microbial sepsis. *Nature.* 2009; 461:1287–1291.

Townsend D, D'Aiuto F. Periodontal capillary imaging in vivo by endoscopic capillaroscopy. *J Med Biol Eng.* 2010; 30:119–123.

Van Dyke TE. The management of inflammation in periodontal disease. *J Periodontol.* 2008; 79:1601–1608.

Wainwright M. Photodynamic antimicrobial chemotherapy (PACT). *J Antimicrob Chemother.* 1998; 42(1):13–28.

Wang J, Wang L, Zhouet Z et al. Biodegradable polymer membranes applied in guided bone/tissue regeneration: a review. *Polymers.* 2016; 8:4.

Yost S, Duran-Pinedo AE, Teles R, Krishnan K, Frias-Lopez J. Functional signatures of oral dysbiosis during periodontitis progression revealed by microbial metatranscriptome analysis. *Genome Med.* 2015; 7(1):27.

Zhu W, Liang M. Periodontal ligament stem cells: current status, concerns, and future prospects. *Stem Cells Int.* 2015; 972313. doi: 10.1155/2015/972313.

Appendix 1: Periodontal chart

PERIODONTAL CHART

Date [ ]

Patient Last Name [ ]   First Name [ ]   Date Of Birth [ ]

☐ **Initial Exam**   ☐ **Reevaluation**   Clinician [ ]

	18	17	16	15	14	13	12	11		21	22	23	24	25	26	27	28
Mobility	0	0	0	0	0	0	0	0		0	0	0	0	0	0	0	0
Implant																	
Furcation																	
Bleeding on Probing																	
Plaque																	
Gingival Margin	0 0 0	0 0 0	0 0 0	0 0 0	0 0 0	0 0 0	0 0 0	0 0 0		0 0 0	0 0 0	0 0 0	0 0 0	0 0 0	0 0 0	0 0 0	0 0 0
Probing Depth	0 0 0	0 0 0	0 0 0	0 0 0	0 0 0	0 0 0	0 0 0	0 0 0		0 0 0	0 0 0	0 0 0	0 0 0	0 0 0	0 0 0	0 0 0	0 0 0

Buccal

Lingual

	18	17	16	15	14	13	12	11		21	22	23	24	25	26	27	28
Gingival Margin	0 0 0	0 0 0	0 0 0	0 0 0	0 0 0	0 0 0	0 0 0	0 0 0		0 0 0	0 0 0	0 0 0	0 0 0	0 0 0	0 0 0	0 0 0	0 0 0
Probing Depth	0 0 0	0 0 0	0 0 0	0 0 0	0 0 0	0 0 0	0 0 0	0 0 0		0 0 0	0 0 0	0 0 0	0 0 0	0 0 0	0 0 0	0 0 0	0 0 0
Plaque																	
Bleeding on Probing																	
Furcation	I	I	I		I							I		I	I	I	
Note																	

Essential Periodontics, First Edition. Edited by Steph Smith and Khalid Almas.
© 2022 John Wiley & Sons Ltd. Published 2022 by John Wiley & Sons Ltd.

	Mean Probing Depth =	0 mm	Mean Attachment Level =	0 mm	0% Plaque	0% Bleeding on Probing

Note														
Furcation														
Bleeding on Probing														
Plaque														
Gingival Margin	0 0 0	0 0 0	0 0 0	0 0 0	0 0 0	0 0 0	0 0 0	0 0 0	0 0 0	0 0 0	0 0 0	0 0 0	0 0 0	0 0 0
Probing Depth	0 0 0	0 0 0	0 0 0	0 0 0	0 0 0	0 0 0	0 0 0	0 0 0	0 0 0	0 0 0	0 0 0	0 0 0	0 0 0	0 0 0

Lingual

Buccal

Gingival Margin	0 0 0	0 0 0	0 0 0	0 0 0	0 0 0	0 0 0	0 0 0	0 0 0	0 0 0	0 0 0	0 0 0	0 0 0	0 0 0	0 0 0
Probing Depth	0 0 0	0 0 0	0 0 0	0 0 0	0 0 0	0 0 0	0 0 0	0 0 0	0 0 0	0 0 0	0 0 0	0 0 0	0 0 0	0 0 0
Plaque														
Bleeding on Probing														
Furcation														
Implant														
Mobility	0	0	0	0	0	0	0	0	0	0	0	0	0	0
	48	47	46	45	44	43	42	41	31	32	33	34	35	36	37	38

www.periodontalchart-online.com

Copyright © 2010 by Department of Periodontology, University of Bern, Switzerland

Source: Periodontal Chart. © 2010 by www.perio-tools.com.

Appendix 2: Periodontal indices

A variety of index systems have been developed for the scoring of specific parameters that reflect the periodontal status of a given individual. Some of these index systems have been designed to exclusively examine patients in a dental practice set-up, while others have been developed for use in epidemiological research. At the time these systems were introduced, the various scores reflected the knowledge of the etiology and pathogenesis of periodontal diseases, as well as concepts related to contemporary therapeutic approaches and strategies (Papapanou & Lindhe 2015). With the development of the new periodontal disease classification system, there is a need to redefine or develop new indices in accordance with this new classification. This appendix gives a brief description of a limited number of indices that are currently being used.

Contents

Essential Periodontics, First Edition. Edited by Steph Smith and Khalid Almas.
© 2022 John Wiley & Sons Ltd. Published 2022 by John Wiley & Sons Ltd.

Assessment of chronic inflammatory periodontal disease

Community Periodontal Index of Treatment Needs

The Community Periodontal Index of Treatment Needs (CPITN) was originally designed to assess chronic inflammatory periodontal disease in epidemiological surveys (Ainamo et al. 1982), which is intended to provide data as a basis for estimating the overall population needs in terms of treatment categories, and in the clinical care situation the procedure offers a simple screening method for determining the level of intervention required (Cutress et al. 1987). A substantial amount of data generated by the use of CPITN has been accumulated in the World Health Organization Global Oral Data Bank (Miyazaki et al. 1991a, b). The CPITN is however not meant to describe the prevalence, extent, or severity of periodontal disease (Papapanou & Lindhe 2015).

The CPITN is primarily a screening procedure that requires clinical assessment for the presence or absence of periodontal pockets, calculus, and gingival bleeding. Use of a special CPITN periodontal probe (or its equivalent) is recommended (Cutress et al. 1987). For epidemiological purposes in adult populations, 10 specified index teeth are examined; for persons under 20 years of age, only 6 index teeth are specified. In dental practice all teeth are examined and only the most severe measure in the sextant is chosen to represent the sextant (Cutress et al. 1987; Papapanou & Lindhe 2015). The treatment need (TN) scores range from 0 to 4 and are based on the most severe periodontal condition code in the entire dentition (Papapanou & Lindhe 2015) (Table A2.1).

Basic Periodontal Examination

The Basic Periodontal Examination (BPE) was developed from the CPITN. It is a fast and simple general practice system to screen for the presence or absence of periodontal diseases.

It should *not* be used for the full assessment of patients with periodontal diseases or for the monitoring of patients who have been treated for periodontal diseases.

It is a hierarchical scoring system, which means that the higher the score, the greater the level of disease (Briggs 2015). The BPE scores are as follows:

0 = Health, pockets less than 3.5 mm
1 = Pockets less than 3.5 mm, bleeding on probing
2 = Pockets less than 3.5 mm, calculus or another plaque retentive factor is present
3 = Pocket depth between 3.5 and 5.5 mm
4 = Pocket deeper than 5.5 mm
* = Furcation involvement.

If a * is recorded, both the number and the * should be recorded for that sextant, for example 4* would indicate that there is at least one tooth with pocketing deeper than 5.5 mm in the sextant and at least one tooth with a furcation involvement.

Table A2.1 Treatment need scores.

Periodontal condition	Code	Treatment need (TN)
No pockets, calculus, or overhangs of fillings, and no bleeding on probing	0	No treatment needed (TN0)
No pockets, calculus, or overhangs of fillings, but gingival bleeding on probing	1	Need for improving oral hygiene (TN1)
Dental calculus and plaque-retaining factors are identified subgingivally	2	Need for scaling, removal of overhangs, and improved oral hygiene (TN2)
Teeth with 4–5 mm deep pockets	3	Need for scaling and improved oral hygiene (TN3)
Pathological pockets >6 mm	4	Need for scaling and improved oral hygiene and complex periodontal treatment (TN4)

Assessment of plaque

Plaque is assessed by determining a plaque score. Various indices used are as follows:

Plaque Index

The Plaque Index (Silness & Löe 1964) has possible scores of 0, 1, 2, or 3:
Score 0 – Absence of plaque deposits.
Score 1 – A film of plaque adhering to the free gingival margin and adjacent area of the tooth. The plaque may only be recognized by running a probe across the tooth surface.
Score 2 – Moderate accumulations of soft deposits within the gingival pocket, on the gingival margin, and/or adjacent tooth surface, which can be seen by the naked eye.
Score 3 – Abundance of soft matter within the gingival pocket and/or on the gingival margin and adjacent tooth surface.

Simplified Plaque Index

Ainamo and Bay (1975) introduced a simplified version of the Plaque Index. This is probably one of the most commonly used and reliable methods of assessing plaque. In the Simplified Plaque Index, there are two scores, 0 or 1:
Score 0 – No plaque detected.
Score 1 – Visible plaque detected.

Quigley Hein Index

This plaque index (as modified by Turesky et al. 1970) assigns a score of 0–5 to each buccal/labial and lingual/palatal non-restored surface of all the teeth except third molars, as follows:

0 – No plaque.

1 – Separate flecks of plaque at the cervical margin of the tooth.

2 – A thin continuous band of plaque up to 1 mm at the cervical margin of the tooth.

3 – A band of plaque wider than 1 mm but covering less than one-third of the crown of the tooth.

4 – Plaque covering at least one-third but less than two-thirds of the crown of the tooth.

5 – Plaque covering two-thirds or more of the crown of the tooth.

A score for the entire mouth is determined by dividing the total score by the number of surfaces (a maximum of 2 × 2 × 14 = 56 surfaces) examined.

Plaque Control Record

The Plaque Control Record (O'Leary et al. 1972) was developed to give a simple method of recording the presence of plaque on individual tooth surfaces. These surfaces are mesial, distal, buccal and lingual. A suitable plaque-disclosing solution, such as Bismarck brown, double tone, or a proprietary brand, is painted on all exposed tooth surfaces. After the patient has rinsed, the operator, using the tip of a probe, examines each stained surface for soft accumulations at the dentogingival junction. When found, deposits are recorded as present. The surfaces that do not have soft accumulations at the dentogingival junction are not recorded. After all teeth are examined and scored, the index is calculated by dividing the number of plaque-containing surfaces by the total number of available surfaces. It is expressed as a percentage.

Gingival indices

Gingival Index

This has a score of 0, 1, 2, or 3 (Löe & Silness 1962):

0 – Normal gingiva.

1 – Mild inflammation: slight change in color, slight edema, no bleeding on probing.

2 – Moderate inflammation: redness, edema, glazing and bleeding on probing.

3 – Severe inflammation: marked redness, edema and ulceration. Tendency to spontaneous bleeding.

Simplified Gingival Index

Ainamo and Bay (1975) developed the Simplified Gingival Index. It has two scores, 0 or 1:

Score 0 – No bleeding from the gingival margin detected after a periodontal probe is briefly run along the gingival margin.

Score 1 – Bleeding from the gingival margin detected after a periodontal probe is briefly run along the gingival margin.

Sulcus Bleeding Index

Mühlemann & Son (1971) introduced the Sulcus Bleeding Index (SBI), which is defined as follows:

Score 0 – gingiva of normal texture and color, no bleeding.

Score 1 – gingiva apparently normal, bleeding on probing.

Score 2 – bleeding on probing, change in color, no edema.

Score 3 – bleeding on probing, change in color, slight edema.

Score 4 – either (a) bleeding on probing, change in color, obvious edema; or (b) bleeding on probing, obvious edema.

Score 5 – bleeding on probing and spontaneous bleeding, change in color, marked edema.

Assessment of calculus

A number of systems for assessing calculus have been proposed. The main disadvantage of many of them is the difficulty in interpretation of the criteria set down. A simple visual assessment should be made of the presence or absence of both supragingival and subgingival calculus (Briggs 2015).

Assessment of tooth mobility

Most systems for assessing tooth mobility have developed criteria to define mild, moderate, or severe tooth mobility. The most commonly used index system to record tooth mobility is that devised by Miller (1950) (see Chapter 12).

Assessment of furcation involvement

According to the glossary of terms of the American Academy of Periodontology, a furcation involvement exists when periodontal disease has caused resorption of bone into the bi- or trifurcation area of a multirooted tooth (Glickman 1972; Hamp et al. 1975; Lindhe & Nyman 1975; Tarnow & Fletcher 1985). Currently, the proposed classifications are based on the extension of the defect and the degree of horizontal/vertical attachment loss (see Chapter 11).

Classification of cervical enamel projection

Masters and Hoskins (1964) suggested a classification system that was based on the extent of cervical enamel projecting into the furcation area:

Grade I – Enamel projection extends from cementoenamel junction of tooth toward furcation entrance.

Grade II – Enamel projection approaches entrance to furcation. It does not enter furcation, and therefore no horizontal component is present.

Grade III – Enamel projection extends horizontally into furcation.

REFERENCES

Ainamo J, Barmes D, Beagrie G et al. Development of the World Health Organization (WHO) Community Periodontal Index of Treatment Needs (CPITN). *Int Dent J.* 1982; 32:281–291.

Ainamo J, Bay I. Problems and proposals for recording gingivitis and plaque. *Int Dent J.* 1975; 25:229–235.

Briggs, L. Assessment and monitoring of a periodontal patient. In: K Eaton, P Ower (eds), *Practical Periodontics*. St. Louis, MO: Elsevier; 2015: 93–110.

Cutress TW, Ainamo J, Sardo-Infirri J. The community periodontal index of treatment needs (CPITN) procedure for population groups and individuals. *Int Dent J.* 1987; 37(4):222–233.

Glickman I. *Clinical Periodontology: Prevention, Diagnosis, and Treatment of Periodontal Disease in the Practice of General Dentistry*. Philadelphia, PA: Elsevier Saunders; 1972.

Hamp SE, Nyman S, Lindhe J. Periodontal treatment of multirooted teeth. Results after 5 years. *J Clin Periodontol.* 1975; 2:126–135.

Lindhe J, Nyman S. The effect of plaque control and surgical pocket elimination on the establishment and maintenance of periodontal health. A longitudinal study of periodontal therapy in cases of advanced disease. *J Clin Periodontol.* 1975; 2:67–79.

Löe H, Silness J. Periodontal disease in pregnancy. *Prevalence and severity. Acta Odontol Scand.* 1963; 21:533–551.

Masters DH, Hoskins SW. Projection of cervical enamel into molar furcations. *J Periodontol.* 1964; 35:49–53.

Miller SC. *Textbook of Periodontia*. Philadelphia, PA: Blackiston; 1950.

Miyazaki H, Pilot T, Leclercq MH, Barmes DE. Profiles of periodontal conditions in adolescents measured by CPITN. *Int Dent J.* 1991a; 41:61–73.

Miyazaki H, Pilot T, Leclercq MH, Barmes DE. Profiles of periodontal conditions in adults measured by CPITN. *Int Dent J* 1991b; 41:74–80.

Mühlemann HR, Son S. Gingival sulcus bleeding—a leading symptom in initial gingivitis. *Helv Odontol Acta.* 1971; 15(2):107–113.

O'Leary TJ, Drake RB, Naylor JE. The plaque control record. *J Periodontol.* 1972; 43:38.

Papapanou PN, Lindhe J. Epidemiology of periodontal diseases. In: NP Lang, J Lindhe (eds), *Clinical Periodontology and Implant Dentistry*. Oxford: Wiley-Blackwell; 2015: 125–166.

Silness J, Löe H. Periodontal disease in pregnancy. II. Correlation between oral hygiene and periodontal condition. *Acta Odontol Scand.* 1964; 22:121–135.

Tarnow D, Fletcher P. Classification of the vertical component of furcation involvement. *J Periodontol.* 1985; 55:283–284.

Turesky S, Gilmore ND, Glickman I. Reduced plaque formation by the chloromethyl analogue of vitamin C. *J Periodontol.* 1970; 41:41–43.

Appendix 3: Smoking cessation

Substance abuse affects more than one-sixth of the world's population. More importantly, the nature of the abuse and the type of addictive substance available to individuals are increasing exponentially. Evidence strongly supports the efficacy of professionally delivered cessation counseling. Dentists, dental therapists, and dental hygienists are ideally placed to deliver these messages, and to spearhead efforts to provide behavioral and pharmacological support for cessation (Kumar 2020).

The most popular counseling algorithms are the *five As* (Ask, Advise, Assess, Assist, Arrange), the *three As* (Ask, Advise, Act), and the *ABC* (Ask, Brief Advice, Cessation Support). The five and three As intervention strategies are based on the stages of change philosophy (2008 PHS Guideline Update Panel 2008), and the ABC framework was developed out of recogni-tion that even the most unmotivated patients might be willing to change their behavior in response to the right trigger. Therefore, the ABC framework recommends that all smokers should be advised to stop regardless of their stage of change (Aveyard et al. 2012).

Smoking Cessation: 5 As

ASK patients if they use tobacco.
ADVISE patients to quit in a manner that is clear, strong, and personalized.
ASSESS readiness to quit using tobacco.
ASSIST them to quit by offering brief suggestions.
ARRANGE follow-up to prevent relapse.

REFERENCES

2008 PHS Guideline Update Panel, Liaisons, and Staff. Treating tobacco use and dependence: 2008 update U.S. Public Health Service Clinical Practice Guideline executive summary. *Respir Care.* 2008; 53(9):1217–1222.

Aveyard P, Begh R, Parsons A, West R. Brief opportunistic smoking cessation interventions: a systematic review and meta-analysis to compare advice to quit and offer of assistance. *Addiction.* 2012; 107(6):1066–1073.

Kumar PS. Interventions to prevent periodontal disease in tobacco-, alcohol-, and drug-dependent individuals. *Periodontol 2000.* 2020; 84:84–101.

Essential Periodontics, First Edition. Edited by Steph Smith and Khalid Almas.
© 2022 John Wiley & Sons Ltd. Published 2022 by John Wiley & Sons Ltd.

Appendix 4: Indications for cone beam computed tomography in implant dentistry

CBCT is always indicated	
When a site development procedure is planned	Examples: • Sinus lift • Block grafting • Ramus or symphysis grafting • The impacted tooth in the area of interest • Pathology in the area of interest
CBCT is indicated for preoperative evaluation in	
Anterior maxillary region: teeth area # 6–11	• Limited alveolar bone height; less than 10 mm from the nasal floor (to be able to place at least 8 mm implant) • Anatomic limitations: severe labial concavity width: less than 6 mm bucco-lingually • CAD/CAM guided surgery is planned
Posterior maxillary region: premolars and molars area	• Limited alveolar bone height; less than 5 mm from sinus floor (to decide for implant placement simultaneously with vertical sinus lift procedure) • CAD/CAM guided surgery is planned
Anterior mandibular region: teeth area # 22–27	• Knife-edge ridge and alveoloplasty are planned • Limited alveolar bone height; less than 8 mm from mental foramen and/or anterior loops (to be able to place implant) with a 2 mm safety zone around the anatomic structures • Anatomic limitations: lingual undercut, genial tubercles, and incisive canals • CAD/CAM guided surgery is planned
Posterior mandibular region: premolars and molars area	• Limited alveolar bone height; less than 8 mm from Inferior alveolar nerve canal, mental foramen, and anterior loop (to be able to place implant) with 2 mm safety zone around the anatomic structures • Anatomic limitations: any clinically visible lingual undercut, including sublingual fossa • CAD/CAM guided surgery is planned
CBCT is indicated for postoperative evaluation	
	• Altered sensation • Infection (sinusitis) • Post-augmentation assessment

CAD/CAM, computer-aided design/computer-aided manufacturing; CBCT, cone beam computed tomography. Source: Adapted from Bornstein et al. 2014; Tyndall et al. 2012.

REFERENCES

Bornstein MM, Scarfe WC, Vaughn VM, Jacobs R. Cone beam computed tomography in implant dentistry: a systematic review focusing on guidelines, indications, and radiation dose risks. *Int J Oral Maxillofac Implants.* 2014; 29:55–77.

Tyndall DA, Price JB, Tetradis S,et al.; American Academy of Oral and Maxillofacial Radiology. Position statement of the American Academy of Oral and Maxillofacial Radiology on selection criteria for the use of radiology in dental implantology with emphasis on cone beam computed tomography. *Oral Surg Oral Med Oral Pathol Oral Radiol.* 2012; 113:817–826.

Essential Periodontics, First Edition. Edited by Steph Smith and Khalid Almas.
© 2022 John Wiley & Sons Ltd. Published 2022 by John Wiley & Sons Ltd.

Appendix 5: Imaging modalities for clinical situations and their specific indications

Imaging modality	Clinical situation	Specific indication(s)
Panoramic and periapical radiography	Initial examination	
Cone beam computed tomography Radiographic guide	Preoperative evaluation: • Clinical doubt of alveolar bone height, width, and/or shape • Bone density • Anterior esthetic zone • Specific anatomic sites	Specific anatomic sites: • Anterior maxilla (nasal floor, incisive fossa) • Posterior maxilla (maxillary sinus, posterior superior alveolar canal) • Anterior mandible (lingual foramen, genial tubercles, incisive canal) • Posterior mandible (inferior alveolar nerve canal, mental foramen, anterior loop, lingual undercut, retromolar foramen) • Zygomatic region (orbital floor, infraorbital foramen, zygomatic bone)
	• Site development	• Sinus lift • Block or particulate bone grafting • Ramus or symphysis grafting • Pathology/impaction in the area of interest • Before traumatic injury
	• Computer-assisted treatment planning	• Follow manufacturer recommendations
Periapical and bitewing radiography Panoramic radiography in extensive implant therapy	• Postoperative integration	• Marginal peri-implant bone height • Bone–implant interface • Post-augmentation assessment • Implant mobility
Cone beam computed tomography	• Postoperative complications	• Altered sensation • Infection (sinusitis)

Source: Adapted from Bornstein et al. 2014; Tyndall et al. 2012.

REFERENCES

Bornstein MM, Scarfe WC, Vaughn VM, Jacobs R. Cone beam computed tomography in implant dentistry: a systematic review focusing on guidelines, indications, and radiation dose risks. *Int J Oral Maxillofac Implants.* 2014; 29:55–77.

Tyndall DA, Price JB, Tetradis S et al.; American Academy of Oral and Maxillofacial Radiology. Position statement of the American Academy of Oral and Maxillofacial Radiology on selection criteria for the use of radiology in dental implantology with emphasis on cone beam computed tomography. *Oral Surg Oral Med Oral Pathol Oral Radiol.* 2012; 113:817–826.

Essential Periodontics, First Edition. Edited by Steph Smith and Khalid Almas.
© 2022 John Wiley & Sons Ltd. Published 2022 by John Wiley & Sons Ltd.

Appendix 6: Radiographic selection criteria for dental implants

Treatment planning	• Panoramic film: imaging modality of choice • Periapical radiographs: anterior region or to supplement the information from the panoramic film • Lateral cephalometric: orthosystem and some cases of mandibular overdenture • Cone beam computed tomography (CBCT): as needed
Day of surgery	• During surgery: periapical radiographs are the imaging modality of choice • Immediately after surgery: panoramic radiographs are the modality of choice, except for the maxillary anterior region where the periapical film may be adequate
Healing assessment	• Periapical radiographs are the modality of choice • Panoramic films if periapical are inadequate
Complications	• A periapical radiograph is the modality of choice. • Panoramic radiographs if the sinus lift procedure was performed • CBCT must be taken when there is a neurosensory change and/or when radiographic images do not provide adequate information
Day of crown cementation	• A periapical radiograph is the modality of choice for an anterior implant • A bitewing radiograph is the modality of choice for a posterior implant
Maintenance	• Periapical radiographs are appropriate for monitoring the implant during maintenance visits • The implant should be followed radiographically at six months and one year of the first year after the surgical placement of the dental implant

Source: Adapted from Bornstein et al. 2014; Tyndall et al. 2012.

REFERENCES

Bornstein MM, Scarfe WC, Vaughn VM, Jacobs R. Cone beam computed tomography in implant dentistry: a systematic review focusing on guidelines, indications, and radiation dose risks. *Int J Oral Maxillofac Implants.* 2014; 29:55–77.

Tyndall DA, Price JB, Tetradis S et al.; American Academy of Oral and Maxillofacial Radiology. Position statement of the American Academy of Oral and Maxillofacial Radiology on selection criteria for the use of radiology in dental implantology with emphasis on cone beam computed tomography. *Oral Surg Oral Med Oral Pathol Oral Radiol.* 2012; 113:817–826.

Essential Periodontics, First Edition. Edited by Steph Smith and Khalid Almas.
© 2022 John Wiley & Sons Ltd. Published 2022 by John Wiley & Sons Ltd.

Appendix 7: Implant Disease Risk Assessment (IDRA) functional diagram

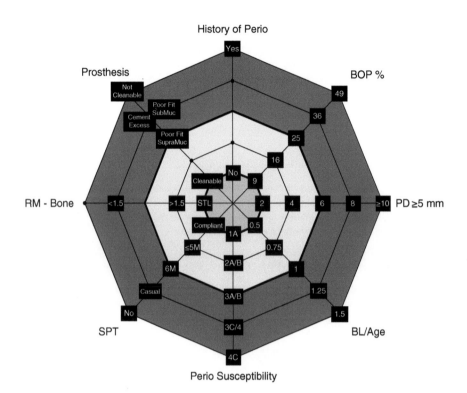

When factors are evaluated together

- *Low risk* is represented by the area within the center of the octagon (green shading).
- *Moderate risk* is represented by the area of the octagon between the first and second rings in bold (yellow shading).
- *High risk* is represented by the area outside the second bold ring of the octagon (red shading).

Essential Periodontics, First Edition. Edited by Steph Smith and Khalid Almas.
© 2022 John Wiley & Sons Ltd. Published 2022 by John Wiley & Sons Ltd.

Appendix 8: Periodontal and implant journals, societies, and useful websites

Recommended journals in periodontics

Chirurgie Buccale
Clinical Advances in Periodontics
Contemporary Clinical Dentistry
International Journal of Periodontics and Restorative Dentistry
Journal of Adhesive Dentistry
Journal of Clinical Periodontology
Journal of Indian Society of Periodontology
Journal of International Academy of Periodontology
Journal of Korean Academy of Periodontology
Journal of Oral Medicine and Oral Surgery
Journal of Oral Pathology and Medicine
Journal of Periodontal and Implant Science
Journal of Periodontal Research
Medecine Buccale
Periodontology 2000
The Journal of Periodontology

Recommended journals in implant dentistry

Clinical Implant Dentistry and Related Research
Clinical Oral Implants Research
International Journal of Implant Dentistry
Journal of Dental Implants
Journal of Periodontal & Implant Science
The International Journal of Oral & Maxillofacial Implants
The Journal of Oral Implantology

Periodontal and implant societies

American Academy of Periodontology (AAP), www.perio.org
British Society of Periodontology (BSP), www.bsperio.org.uk
European Federation of Periodontology (EFP), www.efp.org
Indian Society of Periodontology (ISP), https://ispperio.com
International Academy of Periodontology (IAP), www.perioiap.org
Japanese Society of Periodontology (JSP), www.perio.jp
Korean Academy of Periodontology (KAP), www.kperio.org
Saudi Society of Periodontology (SSP), https://saudiperio.org

Useful websites

AB Dental USA, www.ab-dentusa.com
A. Titan Instruments, Inc, www.atitan.com
Accurate Manufacturing, Inc, www.accurategelpacks.com
ACE Surgical Supply Company, www.acesurgical.com
ACTEON North America, www.acteonusa.com
AD Surgical, www.ad-surgical.com
Adin Implants, www.adin-implants.com
Aegis Communications LLC, www.aegiscomm.com
Almitech Inc., www.almitechimplants.com
AlphaDent, www.alphadent.com
Alpine Pharmaceuticals, www.alpinepharm.com
American Dental Society of Anesthesiology, www.adsahome.org
Anatomage, www.anatomage.com
Aseptico, Inc, www.aseptico.com
Astra Tech Inc., https://www.dentsplysirona.com/en/explore/implantology.html
Atec Dental GmbH, www.atec-dental.de
B & H Photo Video Digital Cameras, www.bhphotovideo.com
Benco Dental Company, www.benco.com
Beutlich Pharmaceuticals, LLC
Bicon Dental Implants, www.bicon.com
Bident International, www.bidcnt.com
Bien-Air Dental, www.bienair.com
BioHorizons, www.biohorizons.com
BIOLASE, www.biolase.com
Biomet 3i, www.zimmerbiometdental.com
Bioplant Inc.– E-dental.com, www.e-dental.com
BQ Ergonomics LLC, www.BQE-USA.com
Brasseler USA, www.brasselerusa.com
BTI of North America, www.bti-implant.com
Cain, Watters & Associates, PLLC, www.cainwatters.com
Camlog Biotechnologies, www.camlog.com
CareCredit, www.carecredit.com
Carestream Dental, www.carestreamdental.com
CeraRoot zirconia dental implants, www.ceraroot.com
Colgate, www.colgateprofessional.com
Community Tissue Service– Maxxeus, www.maxxeus.com
Consult Pro, www.consult-pro.com
Crescent Products, www.crescentproducts.com
Crest Oral-B, www.dentalcare.com
Curasan, Inc, www.curasaninc.com
DCIDS Tissue Bank, www.dcids.org
DecisionBase, Inc, www.decisionbase.com
Dental– Collagen Matrix, http://collagenmatrix.com
Dental Tribune, www.dentaltribune.com
Dentalfone, www.dentalfone.com
DentalVibe, www.dentalvibe.com

Essential Periodontics, First Edition. Edited by Steph Smith and Khalid Almas.
© 2022 John Wiley & Sons Ltd. Published 2022 by John Wiley & Sons Ltd.

Dentatus USA Ltd, www.dentatus.com

Dentis USA, https://dentisusa.com

Dentium USA, www.dentiumUSA.com

DENTSPLY Professional Division, www.dentsplysirona.com

Dentsply Sirona USA, www.dentsplysirona.com

Designs for Vision, Inc, www.designsforvision.com

DEXIS Digital X-Ray, https://www.kavo.com/en-us/dexis

3D Diagnostix, Inc, www.3ddx.com

Digital Education Solutions dental practice, https://education.avadent.com

Doctor.com, www.doctor.com

Dowell Dental Products, Inc, www.dowelldentalproducts.com

Dr. Fuji/Acigi Relaxation, www.fujichair.com

DSN Software, Inc, www.perioexec.com

Dyna Dental Engineering, www.dynadental.com

Elsevier, Inc., www.elsevier.com

Enova Illumination, www.goenova.com

Enovative Technologies, https://www.pinterest.com/enovativetech

Euro Dental Implant/euroteknica USA, www.Euroteknica.com

Exactech, Inc, www.exac.com

Froncare Inc, www.froncare.com

Geistlich Biomaterials, www.geistlich-na.com

Gendex/NOMAD/SOREDEX/Instrumentarium, www.kavo.com

GIDE Institute, www.gidedental.com

Global Surgical Corporation, www.globalsurgical.com

Glustitch, Inc, www.glustitch.com

Guided Surgery Solutions LLC, www.guidedsurgerysolutions.com

Gumchucks at Oralwise, Inc, www.gumchucks.com

Hamilton Capital Management, www.hamiltoncapital.com

Handpiece Solutions, Inc, www.handpiecesolutions.com

G. Hartzell & Son– Dental Evolution, www.dentalevolution.com

Harvest Technologies Corp., https://www.terumobct.com/biologics

http://www.somnotec.net/portfolio-items/harvest-prp-cellular-therapy

Hawaiian Moon, www.aloecream.biz

HealthFirst, www.healthfirstcorp.com

Henry Schein Dental, www.henryschein.com

Hi Tec Implants, www.dentalimplanttech.com

Hiossen, Inc, www.hiossen.com

HUBERMED, INC, www.hubermed.com

Hu-Friedy Manufacturing Company, LLC, www.hufriedygroup.com

i-CAT Imaging Sciences, https://www.kavo.com/en-us/i-cat

IDEA Interdisciplinary Dental, Education Academy www.ideausa.net

ids/Megagen USA, Inc, www.megagen.us

Impladent, Ltd, www.impladentltd.com

Implant dentistry– Dentsply Sirona, www.dentsplysirona.com

Implant Direct LLC, www.implantdirect.com

Implants Diffusion International, www.idisystem.fr

Institute for Advanced Laser Dentistry, www.theiald.com

Intra-Lock International, www.intra-lock.com

J. Morita USA, Inc, www.morita.com

Keystone Dental, Inc, www.keystonedental.com

Kilgore International, Inc, https://kilgoreinternational.com

Surgical instruments– KLS Martin, www.klsmartin.com

Laschal Surgical Instruments, Inc, www.laschaldental.com

Lasers4Dentistry Products, Fotona, https://www.dentalproductshopper.com/new-products

LED Dental, Inc, www.velscope.com

Lester A. Dine, Inc, www.dinecorp.com

Lexi Comp Publishing, https://www.wolterskluwer.com/en/know/drug-decision-support-solutions

LightScalpel, www.LightScalpel.com

Look/Surgical Specialties, www.angiotech.com

LumaDent, Inc, www.LumaDent.com

Mectron Dental, https://dental.mectron.com

Medical Protective, www.medpro.com

Medtronic, www.medtronic.com

Microsurgery Instruments, Inc, www.microsurgeryusa.com

Millennium Dental Technologies, www.LANAP.com

Miltex, An Integra Company, www.integralife.com/integramiltex

MIS Implants Technologies, Inc, www.misimplants.com

Neodent USA, Inc, https://www.straumann.com/neodent/us/en/dental-professionals.html

Neoss, www.neoss.com

Nobel Biocare, www.nobelbiocare.com

NSK Dental, LLC, www.nskdental.us

OCO Biomedical, www.ocobiomedical.com

Officite, www.officite.com

OMNIA, LLC, www.omniaspa.us

Oral IceBerg, LLC, www.ceraroot.com

Oraltronics Dental Implant Technology GmbH– CompanyList.org, https://companylist.org

OraPharma, Inc, www.orapharma.com

Orascoptic, www.orascoptic.com

Osada, Inc, www.osadausa.com

Osseous Technologies of America, www.henryschein.com

Osstell, Inc., www.osstell.com

OsteoCare implant System Limited, www.osteocare.uk.com

Osteogenics Biomedical, www.osteogenics.com

Osteohealth, www.dentalproductshopper.com

Osteo-Ti, www.osteo-ti.com

Otto Trading Inc, www.irestmassager.com

Pallisades Dental, www.palisadesdental-llc.com

Panda Perio, www.pandaperio.com

Patient Marketing Specialist, www.patientmarketingspecialists.com

PBHS Web Site Design & Marketing, www.pbhs.com

PDT, Inc, www.pdtdental.com

PeriOptix, Inc, https://www.denmat.com/loupe-configurator

PeriOptix Loupes and Headlights– DenMat, www.denmat.com

Perioscopy, Inc/Danville Materials LLC, https://
dentistchannel.online/dental-directory/
perioscopy-incorporated-danville-materials-llc

Phase II Dental, https://phasetwodental.com

Philips Sonicare and Zoom Whitening, www.
philipsoralhealthcare.com

PhotoMed, www.photomed.net

Piezosurgery, Inc, www.piezosurgery.us

Pinhole Academy, https://pinholesurgicaltechnique.com

Planmeca USA, Inc, www.planmecausa.com

PREAT Corporation, www.prcat.com

Progressive Dental Marketing, www.
progressivedentalmarketing.com

ProphyMagic, https://www.medidenta.com/product-category/
hygiene

ProSites, www.prosites.com

Quality Aspirators/Q-Optics, www.q-optics.com

Quintessence Publishing Company, Inc, www.quintpub.com

Reputation, www.reputation.com

RGP Dental, Inc, www.rgpergo.com

Rx Honing (Sharpening) Machine, www.rxhoning.com

Sabra Dental: Dental Supplies and Surgical Tools, www.
sabradent.com

Salvin Dental Specialties, Inc, www.salvin.com

Schumacher Dental Instruments, www.karlschumacher.com

Snap On Optics, www.snaponoptics.com

Snoasis Medical, www.snoasismedical.com

Solutionreach, www.solutionreach.com

Southern Anesthesia + Surgical, Inc, www.southernanesthesia.
com

Steiner Bio, www.steinerbio.com

STMD Corporation, www.stmdmedical.com

Straumann, www.straumannusa.com

Sunstar Americas, Inc, www.gumbrand.com

SurgiTel/General Scientific Corp, www.surgitel.com

TePe Oral Health Care, Inc, www.tepeusa.com

Thommen Medical USA, www.thommenmedical.com

Treloar & Heisel, Inc, www.treloaronline.com

TRI Dental Implants, https://tri-implants.swiss

Trinon Titanium GmbH Q-Implant, www.Trinon.com

UltraLight Optics, https://ultralightoptics.com

Unicare Biomedical, Inc, www.unicarebiomedical.com

USHIO America, Inc, www.ushio.com

Vatech America, www.vatechamerica.com

W&H IMPEX, Inc, www.wh.com/na

WaterPik, Inc, www.waterpik.com

Wiley, www.wiley.com

Wiley-Blackwell, www.wiley.com/wiley-blackwell

Xemax Surgical Products, Inc, www.xemax.com

Yodle, https://enspireforenterprise.com

Young's Dental, www.youngsdental.com

Zest Dental Solutions, www.zestdent.com

Zimmer Dental, www.zimmerbiometdental.com

Zoll-Dental, www.zolldental.com

Index

N.B. Pages in *italics* refer to figures, pages in **bold** refer to tables.